Connections© ©for Health

Fourth Edition
Connections for Health

Kathleen D. Mullen
University of North Carolina at Greensboro

Robert J. McDermott
University of South Florida

Robert S. Gold
University of Maryland

Philip A. Belcastro
Borough of Manhattan Community College

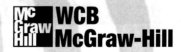

WCB McGraw-Hill

Boston, Massachusetts   Burr Ridge, Illinios   Dubuque, Iowa
Madison, Wisconsin   New York, New York   San Francisco, California   St. Louis, Missouri

WCB/McGraw-Hill

A Division of The McGraw·Hill Companies

Book Team

Publisher *Bevan O'Callaghan*
Managing Editor *Ed Bartell*
Developmental Editor *Megan Rundel*
Production Editor *Patricia A. Schissel*
Proofreading Coordinator *Carrie Barker*
Designer *Lu Ann Schrandt*
Art Editor *Miriam Hoffman*
Photo Editor *Laura Fuller*
Permissions Coordinator *LouAnn Wilson*
Visuals/Design Developmental Consultant *Rachel Imsland*
Production Manager *Beth Kundert*
Production/Costing Manager *Sherry Padden*
Production/Imaging and Media Develoment Manager *Linda Meehan Avenarius*
Marketing Manager *Pamela S. Cooper*
Copywriter *Sandy Hyde*

Basal Text *10/12 Goudy*
Display Type *Journal*
Typesetting System *Macintosh*™
  Quark XPress™
Paper Stock *50# Mirror Matte*

Vice President of Production and New Media Development *Vickie Putman*
Vice President of Sales and Marketing *Bob McLaughlin*
Vice President of Business Development *Russ Domeyer*
Director of Marketing *John Finn*

The credits section for this book begins on page 671 and is considered an
extension of the copyright page.

Front cover image: Cheryl Maeder/FPG International Corp.
Back cover image and interior design: Corel Professional Photos; LetraSet: Phototone

Proofread by Francine Buda Banwarth

Library of Congress Catalog Card Number: 95–78142

ISBN 0–697–21565–1

Printed in the United States of America

10 9 8 7 6 5 4 3

To those who
seek to live life
to the fullest,
exploring the
connections
along the way.

BRIEF Contents

Contents

Chapter 11

Chapter 12

Chapter 13

UNIT IV MINIMIZING NEGATIVE HEALTH-RELATED BEHAVIORS 455

Chapter 14

Chapter 15

Chapter 19

Preface

For years, personal health textbooks have been based on the theme of disease prevention. Such textbooks have focused almost entirely upon what an individual can do to 1) prevent diseases from occurring, 2) detect diseases at their earliest stage, and 3) recover from diseases as optimally as possible. While disease prevention is an undeniably important component of a comprehensive personal health course, it does not address another very important concern—*wellness*.

Wellness, with its emphasis on the importance of quality of life issues, is theoretically very different from disease prevention. Wellness does not focus on avoiding disease, but rather on functioning optimally and adapting creatively on a daily basis in order to enhance your life both now and in the future. We have found the concept of wellness to be of particular interest to young adults, who often have great difficulty focusing on preventing a disease from occurring twenty or thirty years down the road. Choosing to focus attention on how diet and exercise, for instance, can enhance the enjoyment and quality of life, often provides an important motivational element that encourages people to actually try to incorporate wellness activities and attitudes into their lifestyles.

Research into the components of wellness has pointed out that the present focus on the individual and on self-responsibility accounts for only one-half of the wellness concept. As individuals, we do not live in a vacuum. Rather, we must function and adapt within a social and cultural context. Therefore, an examination of social supports and barriers to a wellness lifestyle is essential, as is fostering an awareness of our roles and responsibilities toward the larger community.

Connections for Health was written as a comprehensive personal health textbook—one that incorporates and integrates the themes of both wellness and disease prevention. We believe that, as a wellness text, each edition of *Connections for Health* has advanced a new focus for the study of personal health—one that emphasizes the importance of quality as well as quantity of life.

Connections for Health has also been designed to assist students in achieving high-level wellness through active participation and critical thinking. We are gratified by the positive responses we received from the first three editions of *Connections*, and we trust that the fourth edition will be even more effective in helping instructors and students facilitate their quest for wellness.

Explore personal health issues further with the following educational materials:

- NEW! **HealthQuest,** an interactive CD-ROM, includes activities and assessments that give instant feedback and help students learn about wellness in a rich multimedia environment. *HealthQuest* provides you with an opportunity to interact with the *Connections for Health* material by assessing your current health status and predicting future outcomes of risky behaviors as well as the predicted benefits of risk-reduction efforts. Additionally, you can personalize your interaction with *HealthQuest* to investigate your specific circumstances, receiving guidance on a variety of health-related behavior changes you may be considering or undertaking. A glossary that provides audio pronunciation of terms, and interactive knowledge quizzes are also included.
- NEW! **Explorations in Health and Human Behavior.** This exciting CD-ROM gives you the opportunity to investigate ten vital health-related topics as they should be explored—with movement, color, sound, and interaction.
- A **Student Workbook** to accompany *Connections for Health* contains self-assessment activities, a review of important concepts, questions to help you apply information from the text, as well as reading and activities for further study.

Additionally, a wellness contract and nutrient analysis tables are found in appendices. The workbook supplements *Connections for Health* and can be used during classroom instruction and as a study guide for exam preparation.

- Updated twice a year, **The AIDS Booklet** by Frank D. Cox conveys the latest information on AIDS.

- **Taking Sides: Clashing Views on Controversial Issues on Health and Society** offers supplemental previously published essays from conflicting viewpoints on a variety of topics including health care, mind-body issues, substance use and abuse, sexuality, nutrition, exercise, and environmental and consumer health.

- **Annual Editions: Health** contains an assortment of previously published, contemporary articles on many topics including health, stress, sexuality, disease, drugs, and consumer health.

All of these materials are designed to help you get the most out of your personal health course. The more information you have, the better educated you'll be in order to make the best decisions about your lifestyle and personal health.

Acknowledgments

There are many people who contributed support and guidance to this text. First, we would like to thank the members of the Brown & Benchmark editorial and production teams for both the current and past editions. Their understanding, advice, and careful attention to detail are sincerely appreciated. We would especially like to recognize the contributions of our fourth edition editors: Ed Bartell, Editor; Megan Rundel, Developmental Editor; and Pat Schissel, Production Editor.

Several colleagues provided valuable assistance in preparing first-edition drafts of chapters within their areas of expertise. These include Dr. Gerald Costello (medical care consumerism), Dr. Richard Detert (stress management), and Dr. David Duncan (mental wellness and psychoactive drug use). We greatly appreciate their contributions to *Connections for Health*. Additionally, a special word of thanks goes to Ms. Keri Gross, co-author of the instructor's manual and test item file, and to Ms. Deborah Horne,

co-author of the student workbook that accompanies this text. We would also like to thank our reviewers, both past and present, whose feedback was important to the development and writing of this text.

Kathleen Akpom
Youngstown State University

Carolyn M. Allred
Central Piedmont Community College

Elizabeth H. Barrington
San Diego Mesa College

John A. Bavaro
Slippery Rock University

Shelia C. Harbet
California State University–Northridge

George Jacobson
Salem State College

Herb Jones
Ball State University

Seth C. Kalichman
Medical College of Wisconsin

Rebecca Rutt Leas
Clarion University of Pennsylvania

Pat Lefler
Lexington Community College

Wendy Loren
Lane Community College

Sharon McNeely
Northeastern Illinois University

Carolyn K. Mikanowicz
Youngstown State University

Susan Mitchell
University of Central Florida

J. Dirk Nelson
Missouri Southern State College

Richard Riggs
University of Kentucky

Dell Smith
Mendocino College

Patrick Kidd Tow
Old Dominion University

Parris R. Watts
University of Missouri

Finally, we would like to offer special thanks to our families and friends, who offered understanding and support when writing deadlines took precedence over personal time. These individuals are companions in our explorations of wellness and add an important dimension to both our personal and professional endeavors.

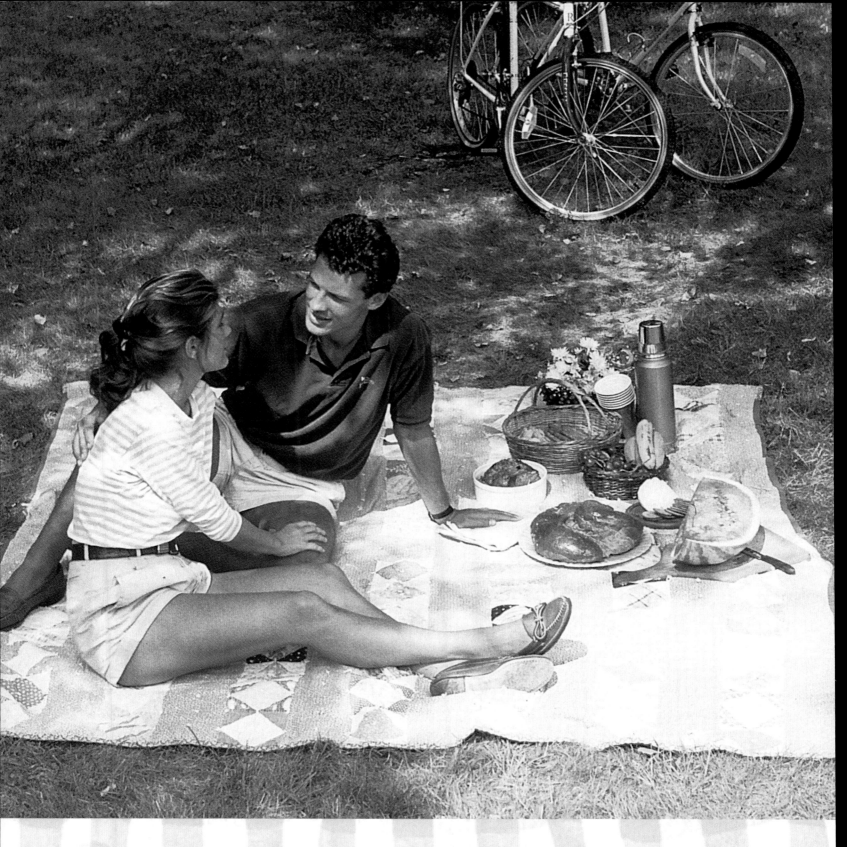

Baselines of Health and Well-Being

Health has traditionally been defined as the freedom from disease. Well-being, though, involves much more than that. In Unit I we will introduce a fresh approach to personal health called "wellness."

Wellness is a self-designed and dynamic style of living. It aims at optimal functioning and creative adapting both personally and in our interactions with others and the environment. Wellness involves a capacity to live life to the fullest.

An important key to wellness lies in self-responsibility and self-initiative. Unless you take an active role in your own well-being and recognize your capacity to set and achieve personal goals, high-level wellness is inconceivable. Chapters 1 through 5 will help you establish those goals by exploring the basics of personal well-being and by offering practical guidelines on how to implement a wellness lifestyle. We will consider how mental wellness and a positive approach to life's stressors can improve your well-being. We will also discuss how nutrition, weight control, and physical fitness contribute to helping you live your life to the fullest.

Wellness: A Quality of Living

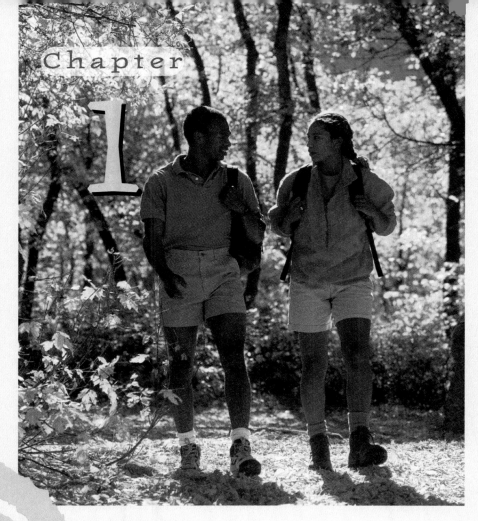

Chapter 1

Student Learning Objectives

Upon completion of this chapter, you should be able to:

1. define and give an example of the three levels of disease prevention;

2. list and briefly describe the four major components of health as defined by the "environment of health" model;

3. define the term lifestyle factor, and cite five examples;

4. explain why understanding the risk factors for various types of injury or disease is useful when making health- and safety-related decisions;

5. explain the differences between the "state" of health and the "process" of wellness as viewed by Halbert Dunn;

6. list and explain the three criteria advanced by Dunn that affect an individual's level of wellness;

7. differentiate between the wellness elements of adaptation and functioning;

8. discuss the concept of "rights" and "responsibilities" with respect to personal health as alluded to by John Knowles;

9. list the five health habits that significantly affect health and life expectancy, according to the research of Berkman, Breslow, and Wingard;

10. explain the three major goals of the Surgeon General's report *Healthy People 2000*;

11. analyze why poverty is an important risk factor for many types of disease and injury;

12. give two examples each of factors that predispose, enable, and reinforce a risky behavior such as cigarette smoking;

13. explain why the results from *one* scientific study do not, in and of themselves, *prove* something;

14. discuss how predisposing, enabling, and reinforcing factors combine to influence health behaviors and affect decision making;

15. assess your current level of positive health-related behaviors;

16. analyze the impact social norms have made on the development of health-related lifestyle factors;

17. assess the current social and cultural norms that exist within your inner circle of friends and family, and in your community;

18. list and explain the six stages of change as delineated by Prochaska, Norcross, and DiClemente.

Wellness is a term that has gained widespread popularity in recent years. Community wellness programs are springing up around the country; local bookstores are stocking up on wellness literature. Wellness centers and wellness programs are now found on many college campuses, as well as in businesses where you may work both during and after college. People in general are becoming more aware of and interested in their own health and wellness: witness the unprecedented number of fitness and health-food enthusiasts alone.

What is this "wellness movement," and what can it mean for you? Is wellness different from health? This chapter will introduce you to the concepts of health and wellness and the role they can play in your life.

Descriptions of Health

Traditionally, health has been viewed as freedom from disease. If you had no signs or symptoms of illness, you were well. In 1947 the World Health Organization (WHO) defined health in broader terms: "Health is a state of complete physical, mental, and social well-being, and not merely the absence of disease and infirmity."[1] While this definition started health professionals and the general public thinking of health as a state of well-being, the process has been slow. Many of us still tend to believe the false notion that if we are not sick we must be healthy. Personal health care is viewed by many solely in terms of the yearly physical. We have standard employee benefit packages of "disease insurance" and "sick days." We measure our nation's health status by **morbidity** (disease) and **mortality** (death) rates. In general, we are part of a "disease-care," not a "health-care," system.

One of the major indicators of health in our current disease-care system is **infant mortality,** or the number of deaths within the first year of life per 1,000 live births. Overall, infant mortality in the U.S. is decreasing (see figure 1.1). However, minority groups in the U.S. are still disproportionately affected by infant mortality. African-Americans, Native Americans, and Puerto Ricans all have infant mortality rates significantly higher than the U.S. average.[2] Additionally, compared to other developed countries, the U.S. ranks about 24th in infant deaths.[3] Many people cite this high level of infant mortality in the U.S. as evidence that the health of U.S. citizens is not what it should be.

Looking past the first year of life, other causes of death become important factors in measuring health. As illustrated in figure 1.2, for all age groups combined the top five causes of death in the U.S. are heart disease, cancer (malignant neoplasms), stroke (cerebrovascular diseases), chronic obstructive lung disease (i.e., emphysema and chronic bronchitis), and unintentional injury (sometimes referred to as accidents). These five causes of death accounted for over 71 percent of the 2,169,518 U.S. deaths in 1993.[4] Looking more specifically at young people, the leading causes of death change. Unintentional injury, homicide and legal intervention, and suicide lead the list for people fifteen to twenty-four years of age (see figure 1.3).

Deaths alone, however, are not an adequate measure of the health status of a country. Recently, health scientists have begun to calculate the **years of potential life lost (YPLL)** for a variety of causes of death. This measure considers the age at which deaths occur; thus, unintentional and intentional injuries, which often take the lives of very young people, carry a very high cost to society in terms of the loss of human potential and productivity. For instance, it is estimated that injuries to persons under the age of forty take more than 2 million potential years of life from U.S. citizens each year.[5]

An important goal of the present health-care system involves the prevention of death and disability and years of productive life lost due to disease or injury. **Disease prevention** activities, as they are called, can be grouped into three distinct categories. **Primary prevention** involves activities that prevent a disease from ever occurring. For example, cutting down on the amount of saturated fats in your diet or not smoking cigarettes both constitute activities that are believed to decrease the risk of developing coronary artery disease. **Secondary prevention** involves those activities that detect a disease condition early so that the duration and severity of the disease can be shortened. Women who have regular Pap smears are

Years of potential life lost (YPLL): the difference between a person's life expectancy and that person's age at death. This is used as one measure of the consequences of early death for society.

Disease prevention: activities undertaken to decrease the likelihood of the occurrence of a disease or injury, to detect disease as early as possible, or to rehabilitate people when disease or injury occurs. Such activities all seek to prevent death and disability from disease and injury.

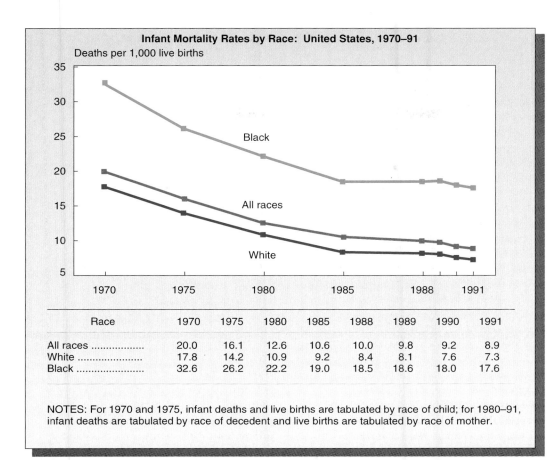

Infant Mortality Rates by Race: United States, 1970–91

Deaths per 1,000 live births

Race	1970	1975	1980	1985	1988	1989	1990	1991
All races	20.0	16.1	12.6	10.6	10.0	9.8	9.2	8.9
White	17.8	14.2	10.9	9.2	8.4	8.1	7.6	7.3
Black	32.6	26.2	22.2	19.0	18.5	18.6	18.0	17.6

NOTES: For 1970 and 1975, infant deaths and live births are tabulated by race of child; for 1980–91, infant deaths are tabulated by race of decedent and live births are tabulated by race of mother.

Figure 1.1: What Do You Think?

1. What variables may have contributed to the decreasing infant mortality rates illustrated above?
2. In 1991, infant mortality rates for Blacks were 2.4 times higher than for Whites in the U.S. Compare the 1991 Black infant mortality rate with the 1970 White infant mortality rate. Why do you think Black infants are at a greater risk for death than White infants in the U.S.?

Source: Data from Centers for Disease Control and Prevention, National Center for Health Statistics, National Vital Statistics System.

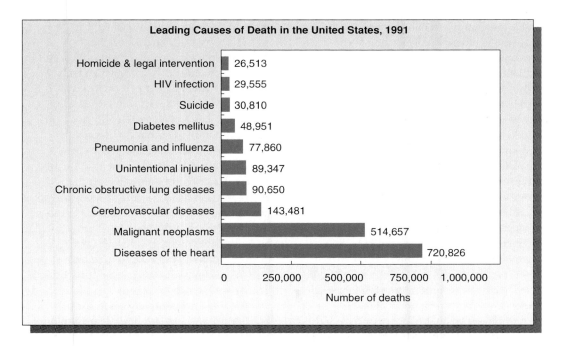

Leading Causes of Death in the United States, 1991

Cause	Number of deaths
Homicide & legal intervention	26,513
HIV infection	29,555
Suicide	30,810
Diabetes mellitus	48,951
Pneumonia and influenza	77,860
Unintentional injuries	89,347
Chronic obstructive lung diseases	90,650
Cerebrovascular diseases	143,481
Malignant neoplasms	514,657
Diseases of the heart	720,826

Number of deaths

Figure 1.2: What Do You Think?

1. There were 2,169,518 deaths from all causes in the U.S. in 1991. What percent of those deaths were caused by chronic disease (heart disease, cancer, cerebrovascular disease, chronic lung disease, and diabetes)?
2. What percent of the 1991 deaths were caused by injury (unintentional and intentional)?
3. For how many of the ten leading causes of death have we identified lifestyle-related risk factors? List the known risk factors.

Source: Data from National Center for Health Statistics in *Health, United States, 1993*. Hyattsville, MD: Public Health Service, 1994.

1. How do the leading causes of death for people 15 to 24 years of age compare with the overall leading causes of death in the U.S.? (Refer to figure 1.2.)
2. How do the number of deaths in the U.S. from various causes for all ages (figure 1.2) compare with the number of deaths from various causes for people age 15 to 24?

Source: Data from National Center for Health Statistics in *Health, United States, 1993.* Hyattsville, MD: Public Health Service, 1994.

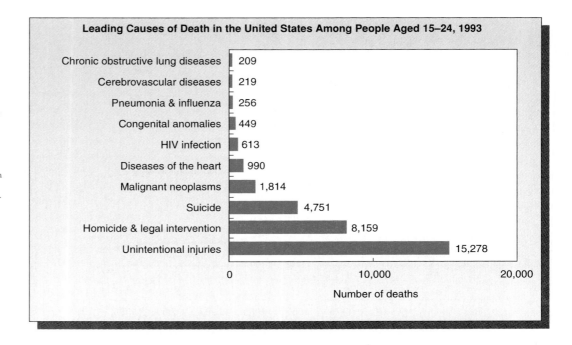

Leading Causes of Death in the United States Among People Aged 15–24, 1993

Cause	Number of deaths
Chronic obstructive lung diseases	209
Cerebrovascular diseases	219
Pneumonia & influenza	256
Congenital anomalies	449
HIV infection	613
Diseases of the heart	990
Malignant neoplasms	1,814
Suicide	4,751
Homicide & legal intervention	8,159
Unintentional injuries	15,278

Number of deaths

Risk factors: variables that, when present, increase the probability that disease or injury will occur in the future.

Down's syndrome: a congenital disease caused by the presence of an extra number-21 chromosome, resulting in mental deficiency and a variety of physical defects.

Sickle-cell anemia: a hereditary disease that affects primarily people of African descent. Defective hemoglobin causes the red blood cells to become sickle shaped, resulting in anemia and often severe complications such as kidney or heart failure.

practicing a measure of secondary prevention—screening for the early detection of cervical cancer. Finally, some prevention activities are characterized as **tertiary prevention.** These activities are used to rehabilitate someone from a particular disease. A person who has had a heart attack and joins a cardiac rehabilitation exercise program would be involved in tertiary prevention. The goal is to help the individual achieve the highest level of functioning possible following a disease or health problem. Disease prevention efforts are extremely important to both individuals and society and should receive more attention and funding.

Disease prevention efforts hinge on our understanding of the factors that are known to be associated with disease and injury. Health planners have developed a model that suggests that health (often defined as the absence of disease) is determined by four main elements: environment, behavior, heredity, and health-care services (see figure 1.4). Most disease and injury **risk factors** fit under one of the elements of this "environment of health" model.

In this model of health the environment is conceptualized in a very broad sense, beginning with the fetal environment. Is a fetus exposed to drugs or chemicals via the mother's circulatory system? Does a fetus receive adequate nutrition? From this beginning environment we expand outward to include our physical surroundings (the air we breathe, the water we drink), our social interactions with significant others and people in general, our level of education, and the type of job we have. All these environmental factors have been shown to have an effect on our level of health.

Heredity is another important determinant of our health. Certain diseases or health problems, such as **Down's syndrome, sickle-cell anemia,** and certain types of alcoholism, are believed to have genetic causes. This is one area of health risk over which the individual has little control.

Health-care services is the third determinant in the environment of health model. This determinant refers to the availability and accessibility of medical-care personnel, technology, and facilities. It is hypothesized that those people with available and accessible medical care will have a greater probability of overcoming major health problems and staying healthy through primary prevention programs.

Last, but certainly not least, is the behavior of individuals. This determinant of health is often referred to as lifestyle factors. The foods you choose to consume, whether or not you use or abuse drugs, your exercise habits, and how you control the stress in your life are all examples of behaviors known to influence health.

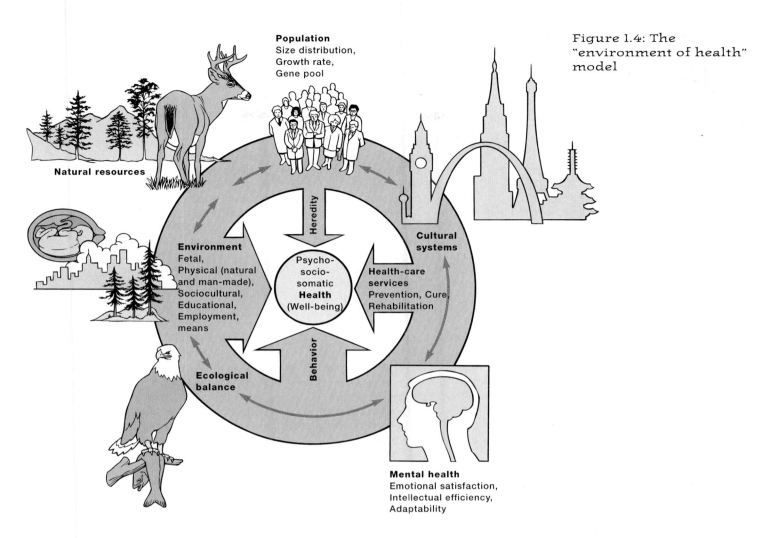

Henrick Blum, a health planner who devised the environment of health model, designed the model so that the width of the arrows of each determinant indicates his view of the importance each element plays in health promotion and disease prevention. Other health planners, however, make the assumption that all four determinants have an equal impact on health.[6] The elements in the circle surrounding the arrows are factors believed to influence the determinants of health. These include population, culture, mental health, ecological balance, and natural resources.

Health researchers at the Centers for Disease Control and Prevention, using an environmental model of health, have estimated the role of each determinant in the leading causes of death in the U.S.[7] On the average, 43 percent of the leading causes of death in the U.S. are thought to be related to **lifestyle factors.** When environmental factors are added to this, it appears that U.S. citizens have some measure of control over approximately 43 to 62 percent of the current leading causes of death. Disease prevention programs aim at these known behavioral and environmental risk factors.

Throughout this textbook you will find scientific information about a large number of potential health problems. Additionally, you will read about specific actions that you could take to decrease your risk of death and disability. It will be up to you to decide which of these behaviors you will adopt and which you might simply ignore. To make informed choices, however, you need to understand what it means when you learn that certain behaviors or characteristics are risk factors, while other behaviors may decrease your risk.

When we talk about risk, we are speaking in terms of probabilities—not guarantees. If you do not smoke cigarettes, for instance, you will decrease your chances of developing lung cancer dramatically. Research studies indicate

Lifestyle factors: individual practices that are part of an established pattern of long-term behavior. Lifestyle factors may be habits or cultural practices, and often affect health status and wellness levels. Examples include food consumption patterns, exercise habits, drug use and abuse, stress management techniques, and the like.

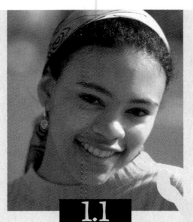

Activity for Wellness

Low Risk, High Risk: Taking Control of Your Health

How would you answer the following questions?

1. You are about to plan a 1,000-mile journey, and you aren't pressed for time. Rank the following means of transportation from the safest (#1) to the riskiest (#4):
   ___ bus ___ train ___ plane
   ___ passenger car

2. What would you say kills more Americans annually?
   a. heart disease
   b. cancer
   c. automobile accidents

3. You're a healthy 45-year-old man, slightly overweight. Your father and his brother both died in their fifties of heart disease. Your mother, now 65, has had Type II diabetes for several years. Are you likely to get one of these ailments?
   a. yes
   b. no

4. Winston Churchill, not to mention your Aunt Harriet, drank brandy, smoked habitually, and was overweight. Both lived into their eighties and died peacefully in their sleep. Does that prove there's something health experts don't know?
   a. yes
   b. no

5. You're 50, female, and a smoker. Your last checkup showed that both your blood pressure and blood cholesterol level were somewhat higher than they should be. You know this means that you risk a heart attack or stroke, but you read an article that said that even 50-year-old male smokers with high blood pressure and elevated cholesterol have only a 13 percent chance of getting sick within six years. So you're looking on the bright side: you've got an 87% chance of staying healthy for the next six years. Is this a constructive attitude?
   a. yes
   b. no

Answers

Questions 1 and 2: Figuring the Odds

Of these questions, only the first two have fairly straight-forward answers. You're safest in a bus, and in greatest danger in an automobile. (More than 10 people die per billion automobile and taxi miles; but it takes more than 2 billion bus miles to produce a fatality. Trains and planes are 10 times safer than cars, but only about half as safe as buses.) But whether they travel or stay at home, more people in the U.S. die from heart disease each year than from anything else. The purpose of the questions above however—all of which will be discussed in the course of this article—is not so much to produce correct answers as to invite you to figure your odds.

Efforts to identify health risks—and reduce them, if possible—are as old as medicine itself. Hippocrates advised his fellow physicians to "consider the seasons of the year and what effects each of them produces" and to take note of what people drank and ate and how they lived. Scientists today are still looking for the determinants of health, albeit with a little more sophistication and scientific knowledge. Epidemiology (literally, the study of epidemics) is the attempt to identify the factors that cause diseases and injuries to determine what the probabilities are that they *will* cause them, and to determine how to decrease or eliminate the identified risk. This is often referred to as risk hazard appraisal, which is of growing importance in medical science, especially in the effort to prevent disease and promote health. Once the risk factors are known, the next job is to make changes in the environment (for example, to persuade manufacturers to install seat belts of a certain design) and to persuade people to change their behavior (for example, convince them to fasten the belt).

When we speak of risk, like a horseplayer at the race track, we're simply quoting odds. No one can honestly assure you that doing one thing will kill you, while refraining from doing it will keep you safe. For example, on the average, 1 out of 10 smokers gets lung cancer, but only a rare nonsmoker gets it. If you are an average smoker, your chances of getting lung cancer at any time of life are 24 times higher than those for nonsmokers, and the risk increases as the amount of smoking increases.

that at least 80 percent of lung cancer victims smoked cigarettes. Still, we cannot guarantee that if you do not smoke cigarettes you will not get lung cancer, or that if you do smoke you will definitely get lung cancer. What we can tell you is that in a group of 100 lung cancer victims, research has shown that about 80 of them will have been cigarette smokers. We also know that smoking increases a person's chances of developing lung cancer; the average smoker is 24 times more likely to develop lung cancer as compared to someone who never smoked.

Risk is a group concept that is used by individuals as guidance in making decisions. Imagine that you have been told by your physician that you need to have surgery and that your chances of survival are 50 percent. Would you want to have that surgery? What if the chance of survival were 95 percent?

Thus you're asked to draw your own conclusions. In the science of risk assessment, there's no such thing as absolute safety, but you can choose to widen or narrow your safety margins. And though scientists may assess the risks, how you manage your life is up to you. It's often hard to evaluate what the experts say, and the press seldom makes your task simpler. The headline "Alcohol shown to cause breast cancer" will attract more readers than "Study suggests alcohol intake slightly increases breast cancer risk for some women." It is always easier to oversimplify than to tell people how complicated things really are.

Questions 3 and 4: Heredity Is Not Destiny

If your father died young of a heart attack, you have a good chance of following in his footsteps. Knowing your inherited liabilities, though, gives you an excellent opportunity to alter them. The genetic odds may be lowered significantly if you are not overweight, keep your blood pressure under control, and maintain a low blood cholesterol level. If your mother has diabetes, that's an indication that weight control and exercise are crucially important for you.

For many of us, familial tendencies constitute an emotional trap. People whose parents or grandparents died at comparatively young ages of heart disease or cancer, or some other disease with a genetic component, usually realize that this heritage works against them and may falsely conclude that taking care of their own health is irrelevant. On the other hand, if all your relatives were as indestructible as Winston Churchill or the hypothetical Aunt Harriet, you may have an equally false sense of invulnerability.

Researchers may one day unravel the genetic code and come closer to accurately predicting your chances of getting a disorder such as heart disease or hypertension. But today only a few diseases are known to have purely genetic causes, for example, hemophilia, in which a blood-clotting factor is absent; sickle-cell anemia, a blood disorder that occurs most commonly among people of African descent; cystic fibrosis; and certain forms of kidney disease.

In many ailments that show signs of running in families, such as cancer, heart disease, or diabetes, heredity is only one factor in the mix. Your biological and cultural heritage and your environment interact, and it's the interaction that counts. Your diet or exercise habits or your environment may foster, or foil, the tendencies you were born with.

Question 5: Heart Attack Roulette

A 50-year-old smoker, male or female, with elevated blood cholesterol and blood pressure is seriously courting cardiovascular disease. You may have only a 13 percent chance of developing it, since neither you nor your doctor has any way of predicting whether you'll fall into the lucky 87 percent who do not develop heart disease or the unlucky 13 percent who do. If these sound like favorable odds, you may decide not to make any changes in your habits. However, a more realistic way to consider the odds is as follows. If your risk factors were low (that is, you didn't smoke and your blood pressure and blood cholesterol levels were low), your chances of having a heart attack between age 40 and 64 would be only 6 percent. However, if you continue to smoke and do nothing about your other risk factors, your chance of having a heart attack during these years is 40 percent. This is a very big difference. Giving up cigarettes, controlling your blood pressure, and lowering your blood cholesterol level would significantly widen your safety margin. Obviously, that's the constructive action to take.

Another example of this kind of reasoning can be seen in the relationship between oral contraceptives and heart attacks. High-dose oral contraceptives increase the risk of heart attack by a factor of 4.7. This sounds like a very large increase. However, if you're a 20- to 24-year-old woman, your heart attack risk is less than 1 in 500,000. Thus a fivefold increase represents only about 5 in 500,000 (or 1 in 100,000). This means that if all 8.5 million women in the U.S. in this age group were to take oral contraceptives, 80 of them (instead of the expected 17) would have heart attacks. This would produce many fewer deaths than might result from unwanted pregnancies in the same age group. And even this small risk has been markedly reduced by the new low-dose estrogen contraceptives.

Risk in Perspective

So be cautious in interpreting articles that talk about doubling or tripling your risk of getting a specific disease. To make sense of a twofold or threefold increase in risk, first you have to know how likely you are to get the disease anyway. For example, if your chances of developing a certain illness are 1 in 100,000, a doubled risk brings you up to 2 in 100,000 (or 1 in 50,000). Those are still pretty low odds. However, if 1 out of 10 people develops this illness and you do something that doubles your risk, your chances are now 1 in 5. That's a very significant increase.

Reprinted by permission from the *University of California at Berkeley Wellness Letter,* © Health Letter Associates, 1988.

What does it mean to have a 95 percent chance of survival? Simply, in a group of 100 patients who have had that type of surgery, 95 of them lived through the surgery. But remember, five of them also died. Can your surgeon guarantee that you will be one of the 95 who live? Of course that is impossible, but the *odds* of survival would be in your favor with a procedure that had a 95 percent survival rate. Your actual risk, however, is either 100 or 0 percent—you will live or you will die. For any given individual we cannot predict the outcome in advance. This is true of all the risk factors we will discuss in this text book. How much risk are you willing to take with your health and your life? That may be one of the most important decisions you make in life. Activity for Wellness 1.1 will help you learn to weigh scientific evidence as a part of health decision making.

Although disease prevention is a necessary component of an improved health-care system, it continues to place a major emphasis on disease and leads us to rely on the medical-care system as our primary means to health. Is there more to well-being than health as it is currently depicted? Advocates of a new concept—wellness—believe so.

The Wellness Concept

Wellness has been described as a process involving a zest for living,[8] a self-designed style of living that allows you to live your life to the fullest.[9] Because the wellness concept has recently become popular, many believe it to be a phenomenon of a 1980s health consciousness. Actually, the concept of high-level wellness was first proposed by Halbert Dunn during the 1950s. Dunn was a well-known physician and statistician who served from 1935 to 1960 as Chief of the National Office of Vital Statistics. Dunn's idea of high-level wellness was based on the World Health Organization's definition of health.[10] Dunn saw WHO's definition of health as a positive statement of well-being with implications for the existence of multiple levels of wellness. Dunn was careful to point out, however, that the "state" of health was different from the "process" of wellness. He saw health as a relatively passive state of homeostasis or balance; he viewed wellness as a dynamic concept or a process of continuously moving toward one's potential for optimal functioning.

Dunn believed that a person's level of wellness was dependent on three criteria: (1) direction and progress, (2) the total individual, and (3) how the individual functions.[11] The first criterion—direction and progress—implies that wellness is not a static state but rather a movement toward ever-higher potentials of functioning (see figure 1.5). You cannot attain a "state" of wellness and then stop. If you are not moving forward and upward toward high-level wellness, then you must be moving backward, away from your wellness potential. Wellness is active and requires individual initiative.

Dunn's second criterion for wellness maintains that we must be concerned with the total person, including the physical, mental (intellectual), emotional (feeling), social, and spiritual dimensions. Robert Russell, a professor of health education at Southern Illinois

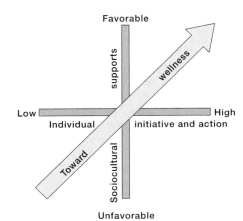

Figure 1.5: Direction and progress toward wellness.
Wellness involves both personal initiative and action and the availability of social support networks. Improvements in both dimensions will be necessary for achieving higher levels of wellness.

University, has developed a model that unites this total-person concept with Dunn's third criterion of functioning[12] (see figure 1.6).

Russell's model depicts an individual surrounded by the five dimensions of the total person. In Russell's view, the spiritual dimension unites all other dimensions—mental, physical, emotional, and social. Spiritual well-being may be, but is not necessarily, of a religious nature. It is also considered to encompass your philosophy of life, your values, or what gives meaning and purpose to your life. Individuals in their many-faceted dimensions, function daily in the environment that surrounds them. Functioning implies skills or activities of daily living (lifestyle) that impact on the five dimensions. These daily activities include lifestyle choices such as what we eat, how and when we exercise, the ways we choose to relax and cope with stress, how we communicate with other people, the types and quantity of products we consume, and how we treat the environment.

Adaptation is an essential element of wellness. Daily life brings sudden, unexpected opportunities or challenges that call for adaptation. Our world is changing at an increasingly rapid pace, and such change requires creative and frequent adaptation. The number of complete value changes

Wellness: a process of optimal functioning and creative adapting that involves the total person (physical, mental, emotional, social, and spiritual dimensions) and strives for an ever-increasing quality of life.

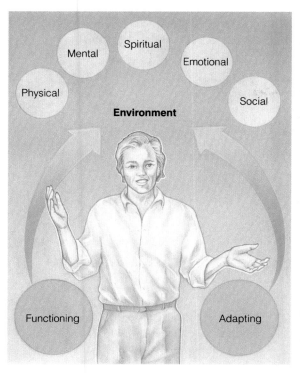

Figure 1.6: A model of well-being.
A well person is one who, within a given
environment, is constantly moving toward
wellness in all dimensions of being both during
daily functioning and during times of challenge,
when adaptation is necessary.

Source: From Dr. Robert Russell, Southern Illinois University at
Carbondale, Department of Health Education, Carbondale, IL.

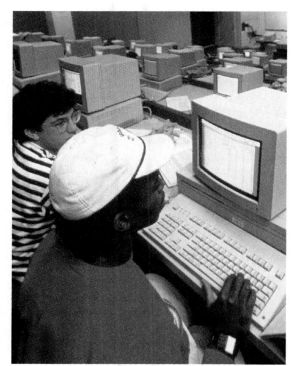

Figure 1.7: What Do You Think?

1. New technologies trigger rapid changes in society
   as a whole. How has changing technology affected
   your life?

taking place in the world during a typical life
span has increased steadily.[13] In the past, the
values of one generation had meaning and
application for the next. There was little
change in the world from generation to
generation. If you were raised on a farm,
chances were you would be a farmer, and the
skills and values you attained during your
formative years would be relevant to your
survival and well-being. With the industrial
revolution the pace of world change
increased; a person could have a complete
change of world values within a single life
span. Today, with the advent of the
technological revolution, the pace continues
to increase. How many changes will we have
to make during this life span? How many
changes will our children be expected to
make? How can we be well with such constant
change and adaptation required of us?

In 1970, Alvin Toffler documented the
problems inherent in rapid change and
labeled the syndrome "future shock."[14] Such
rapid change continues (see figure 1.7). Ten
years before Toffler's work, however, Halbert
Dunn spoke to the same concern:[15]

> In today's world . . . the spurts of
> change are becoming a turbulent,
> racing torrent. There seem to be no
> quiet pools in this flood of change
> which permit one to slow down and
> rest for a bit, to become accustomed to
> an altered situation before facing the
> next disturbance. Can we, as
> individuals and families, attain and
> maintain wellness while riding the
> crest of a social millrace? This is the
> problem that we must face up to,
> because we cannot slow down the
> social changes now in process.

Dunn believed that wellness and change
could coexist. This would require that we be
willing to face inconsistencies in our thinking
and reexamine our beliefs and practices in
light of contradictions that come to our

attention as a result of changes in our world. Knowing how and when to question is an essential wellness skill we must cultivate in ourselves and others. Such adaptation requires creative coping and greater energy output. When it is successful, adaptation returns us to a balanced level of functioning.

A well person then is one who, within a given environment, is constantly moving toward wellness in all dimensions of being (physical, mental, emotional, social, and spiritual), both during daily functions and during times of challenge when adaptation is necessary. Wellness is not based on a concern for disease and its prevention but rather on optimal functioning and creative adapting.

Wellness is not simply a concept to be applied at an individual level. Dunn believed that wellness could be expanded to include the family, the community, and eventually the world.[16] Just as the ripples on a pond expand outward when a stone is thrown in, so does individual wellness expand and ripple outward to affect the family, the community, and the world. It is easier to seek high-level wellness for yourself if you are a member of a well family, community, and world.

Using the work of Halbert Dunn and other current wellness articles and books as a starting point, a panel of health professionals recently undertook the task of developing a contemporary model of wellness.[17] Over the course of a year the panel reviewed a variety of suggested components of wellness and rated them as to their usefulness in describing the most important elements of a wellness program. This model of wellness points out that while individual initiative is an important dimension of wellness, it is not *the* key to wellness. Equally important is a sense of community. Being able to cooperate with others in reaching goals, being aware of your role and responsibility within your community, relating thoughtfully to your environment (including the people in it), having a wellness mentor to help you with your wellness efforts (or being a mentor for someone else), and building reinforcements into your wellness lifestyle (including providing rewards to others for seeking wellness) are all important elements of a wellness program.

Self-Responsibility for Health and Wellness

Americans have, in recent years, grown increasingly vocal about their "rights." Articles and books on such topics as the "right to health care" and the "right to health" abound. But what of a balance between rights and responsibilities? In 1975 John Knowles, physician and president of the Rockefeller Foundation, convened a group of physicians, philosophers, social scientists, and medical administrators to study health as a means for influencing the quality of life in the U.S. The proceedings of this meeting, "Doing Better and Feeling Worse: Health in the United States," contained strong statements regarding health as a right and a responsibility. His words still ring true today.[18]

> The cost of sloth, gluttony, alcoholic intemperance, reckless driving, sexual frenzy, and smoking is now a national, and not an individual, responsibility. This is justified as individual freedom— but one man's freedom in health is another man's shackle in taxes and insurance premiums. I believe the idea of a "right" to health should be replaced by the idea of an individual moral obligation to preserve one's own health—a public duty if you will. The individual then has the "right" to expect help with information, accessible services of good quality, and minimal financial barriers.

A prime example of individual involvement in achieving a state of health was demonstrated by Lisa Berkman, Lester Breslow, and Deborah Wingard.[19] Their research findings indicate that a number of simple health habits significantly affect health and life expectancy. These health habits include (1) regular moderate exercise during leisure time (such as long walks, bicycling, swimming, gardening), (2) no cigarette smoking, (3) no alcohol or only moderate use, (4) moderate weight, and (5) seven or eight hours sleep a night. This study followed nearly 7,000 adults, aged thirty to sixty-nine, for nine years. Men in the study who practiced two or less of these health-related behaviors had almost three times the risk of dying during the nine year follow-up as those men who practiced four of five of the health-related behaviors. For women, the

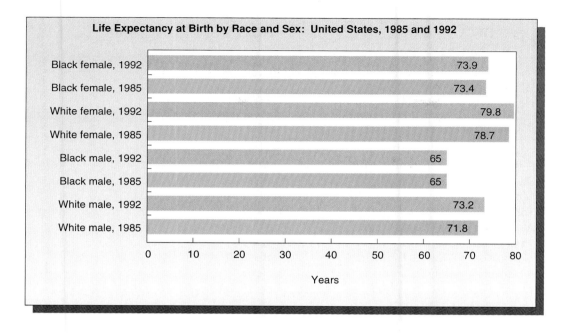

Life Expectancy at Birth by Race and Sex: United States, 1985 and 1992

	Years
Black female, 1992	73.9
Black female, 1985	73.4
White female, 1992	79.8
White female, 1985	78.7
Black male, 1992	65
Black male, 1985	65
White male, 1992	73.2
White male, 1985	71.8

Figure 1.8: What Do You Think?

1. What trends in life expectancy at birth have occurred for females in the U.S. between 1985 and 1992 as compared with males? What might account for the differences?
2. How do life expectancy rates at birth for Whites compare with those for Blacks in the U.S.? What might account for the differences?

Source: Data from National Center for Health Statistics.

risk of dying was 3.2 times higher for those practicing two or fewer of the health-related behaviors.

Self-responsibility, or an active sense of accountability for your own well-being, is also an important factor in achieving a high level of wellness. The first step in becoming responsible for your personal level of wellness is to recognize that you make choices that impact on your total being—physically, mentally, emotionally, socially, and spiritually. This realization should result in a freeing experience. If you are experiencing high-level wellness through your daily lifestyle choices you have good reason to celebrate. Just as important, however, is that if you find yourself falling somewhat short of your wellness potential, you have the power, the right, and the responsibility to choose differently. While health educators, physicians, hospitals, YMCA/YWCAs, and the like can provide valuable knowledge and assistance in carrying out your wellness plan, the initiative and action must come from you. As Halbert Dunn once commented, "We cannot take high-level wellness like a pill out of a bottle. It will come only to those who work at following its precepts."[20]

Healthy People 2000

In 1991 the U.S. Surgeon General's Office issued a report entitled *Healthy People 2000*, which delineated health promotion and disease prevention goals and objectives for the nation, to be accomplished by the year 2000. *Healthy People 2000* cites three main goals for improving the nation's health.[21] The first and central goal is to increase the span of healthy life for people in the U.S. This goal involves increasing the number of years a person can expect to live, as well as enhancing the quality of life during those years. According to *Healthy People 2000*, "healthy life means a vital, creative, and productive citizenry contributing to thriving communities and a thriving Nation."

In 1991, the average life expectancy at birth in the U.S. was 75.5 years.[22] This means that a child born in 1991 could expect to live to the age of 75.5. As you can see in figure 1.8, however, life expectancy at birth varies by race and sex. In general, Blacks have a significantly shorter life expectancy at birth in the U.S. than Whites. Additionally, between 1985 and 1991 the gap between life expectancy at birth of Whites and Blacks widened, from six to seven years.

The National Center for Health Statistics has cited several reasons for the decline in life expectancy for Black people including a slowing of improvement in infant mortality rates, the high homicide rate for Black men, and the increase in deaths from AIDS, especially among young Black women.[23]

The disparity in life expectancy between White and Black people is only one example of many health problems disproportionately affecting minorities in the U.S. The second goal of *Healthy People 2000* is to reduce the health disparities

Healthy People 2000	Connections for Health
Priority Areas	Chapters

Health Promotion: Strategies related to individual lifestyle—personal choices made in a social context—that can have a powerful influence over one's health prospects.

Physical Activity & Fitness	Chapters 5 and 18
Nutrition	Chapters 3 and 4
Tobacco	Chapter 15
Alcohol and Other Drugs	Chapters 14 and 16
Family Planning	Chapter 8
Mental Health & Mental Disorders	Chapter 2
Violent and Abusive Behavior	Chapter 9

Health Protection: Strategies related to environmental or regulatory measures that confer protection on large population groups.

Unintentional Injuries	Chapters 9 and 18
Occupational Safety & Health	Chapters 2 and 9
Environmental Health	Chapter 19
Food and Drug Safety	Chapters 3 and 14
Oral Health	Chapter 3

Preventive Services: Counseling, screening, immunization, or drug interventions for individuals in clinical settings.

Maternal and Infant Health	Chapter 7
Heart Disease and Stroke	Chapter 10
Cancer	Chapter 11
Diabetes and Chronic Disabling Conditions	Chapters 10 and 18
HIV Infection	Chapter 12
Sexually Transmitted Diseases	Chapter 12
Immunization and Infectious Diseases	Chapter 12
Clinical Preventive Services	Chapters 17 and 18

Source: Data from *Healthy People 2000 National Promotion and Disease Prevention,* Department of Health and Human Services, Washington, D.C.

among persons living in the U.S. A variety of groups are targeted in this report as being disproportionately affected by certain health problems. These target groups may be a certain age group, members of a racial or ethnic group, people with low income (see A Social Perspective 1.1), or people with disabilities. As you read further in this text, you will notice that *Healthy People 2000* objectives for health promotion, health protection, and preventive services are highlighted in the appropriate chapters (see table 1.1).

The final goal of *Healthy People 2000* is to have preventive services available to all people in the U.S. Prevention services such as prenatal care, childhood immunizations, blood pressure and blood cholesterol

screening, and screenings for the early detection of cancer are just a few of the prevention services that should be available to all people.

Personal and Social Influences

Our individual habits and behavior choices, as well as the social environment in which we make such choices, have a significant influence on our level of wellness at any point in time. An understanding of what influences us to behave in certain ways, and not in others, can provide a valuable perspective upon which to build a personal wellness program.

People with Low Income

Nearly one of every eight persons in the U.S. lives in a family with an income below the federal poverty level. Nearly a quarter of children younger than six are members of such families.* Low income itself (or low socioeconomic status) is a shorthand label that encompasses family groups with individuals who have poorly paid jobs or are unemployed, families living in substandard housing, and families more likely to have only a single parent in residence. Health disparities between poor people and those with higher incomes are almost universal for all dimensions of health.

For virtually all of the chronic diseases that lead the nation's list of killers, low income is a special risk factor. For example, the risk of death from heart disease is more than 25 percent higher for low-income people than for the overall population.† The incidence of cancer increases as family income decreases, and survival rates are lower for low-income cancer patients. The association of cancer and low income varies by cancer site; lung, esophageal, oral, stomach, cervical, and prostate cancers are more frequent among the poor, while breast and colorectal cancers are not.‡, § Infectious diseases, like HIV infection and tuberculosis, are also often found disproportionately among the poor.

Similar vulnerability for low-income people is found with some causes of traumatic injury and death. These individuals, more than those with higher incomes, are the victims of violent crime. Poverty appears to be a major predisposing factor associated with a higher risk for murder of acquaintances and family members, as well as robbery-motivated killings of strangers. Injuries and deaths among children from fires, drowning, and suffocation are strongly related to low socioeconomic status.*

No single indicator of health status makes the connection between poverty and poor health more clear than does infant mortality. Poor pregnancy outcomes including prematurity, low birth weight, birth defects, and infant death are linked to low income, low educational level, low occupational status, and other indicators of social and economic disadvantage.∞

Just as poor health is more likely among persons of low income, so are some, but not all, of the major risk factors for poor health. Higher-than-average rates of obesity and high blood pressure, which are major risks for heart disease and stroke, have been linked directly with low-income status.# Tobacco use, which has declined dramatically in the past two decades for the population as a whole, has remained virtually constant since 1966 for those who completed less than 12 years of schooling. Smoking levels among blue-collar workers are about 20 percent higher than among others.**

For the coming decade, perhaps no challenge is more compelling than that of equity. The disparities experienced by people who are born and live their lives at the lowest income levels define the dimensions of that challenge. The relationships between poverty and health are complex and cannot be reduced to a simple one-to-one relationship between dollars available and level of health. Low income may, in fact, be a product of poor health, just as poor health may be caused by environmental exposures, material deficiencies, and lack of access to health services that adequate income might correct or improve. While, from a public health perspective, the leverage available to effect improvements is limited largely to the availability and the quality of health services, improvements in education, job training, and other social services are necessary to erase the health effects of current income disparities.

Source: Data from *Healthy People 2000 National Health Promotion and Disease Prevention,* Department of Health and Human Services, Washington, D.C., 1991.

References: *National Center for Children in Poverty. *A Statistical Profile of Our Poorest Young Citizens.* New York: National Center for Children in Poverty, 1990.
†National Heart, Lung, and Blood Institute; National Cholesterol Education Program. *Report of the Expert Panel on*

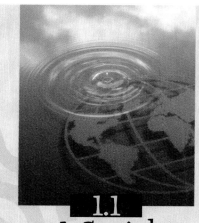

1.1
A Social Perspective

Population Strategies for Blood Cholesterol Reduction. Washington, D.C.: U.S. Department of Health and Human Services, 1990.
‡Amler, R. W. and Dull, H. B., *Closing the Gap: The Burden of Unnecessary Illness.* New York: Oxford University Press, 1987.
§U.S. Department of Health and Human Services. *Report of the Secretary's Task Force on Black and Minority Health.* Washington, D.C.: U.S. Department of Health and Human Services, 1985.
∞Institute of Medicine. *Preventing Low Birthweight.* Washington, D.C.: National Academy Press, 1985.
#Public Health Service. *The Surgeon General's Report on Nutrition and Health.* Washington, D.C.: U.S. Department of Health and Human Services, 1988.
**Office on Smoking and Health. Unpublished data from the 1987 National Health Interview Study.

What Do You Think?

1. Referring to the environmental model of health illustrated in figure 1.4, how do you think poverty interplays with the four determinants of health?
2. For each of these dimensions of health, what intervention strategies might improve levels of health and well-being for those of low socioeconomic status in the U.S.? Do you think your suggestions are feasible? Explain.

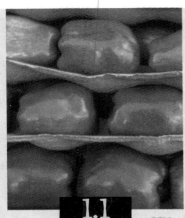

1.1
Of Special Interest

"A recent study proves . . ."

You pick up the newspaper or turn on the television and you're greeted by major news in the health field. A study in the latest issue of the *Extraordinarily Prestigious Journal* shows a definite link between caffeine and heart disease. Men who drink five cups of coffee daily have more heart attacks than other people. You're a heavy coffee drinker. Does this mean you're a goner? Does a study always *prove* something? What is a study, anyway?

Almost anything can be called a study or be so designated by the press. Major journals in the medical field attempt to limit unproven or overstated claims by carefully reviewing what's submitted to them. However, a phenomenal amount of research is published each year: an average of 240,000 biomedical articles in English alone are indexed each year by the National Library of Medicine. If every study "proved" something, there would be no questions left unanswered. A dose of skepticism is always in order, even when the study comes from an important institution and appears in a respected journal.

In fact in 1986 a leading journal published a study from Johns Hopkins showing that heavy coffee drinkers had two to three times the risk of heart disease—a study conducted over many years and using many subjects. From reports in the media, it sounded like proof positive, unless you actually had a copy of the study and read it all the way to the end. The authors didn't ask participants about important risk factors such as their diet (did they habitually eat a lot of fat and cholesterol?), smoking habits, and exercise levels. It wasn't clear, therefore, whether the coffee was at fault, or the diet, or other factors altogether. "A need for further investigation" was the final word—though this hasn't kept writers and reporters from citing this study as proof of the dangers of caffeine.

It is helpful to keep the following pointers in mind:

A single study cannot prove anything. Scientific findings should be duplicated by others for validity, and even then there's an element of uncertainty.

No matter how enthusiastically a finding is hailed in the press, see what the experts are saying next week and next month.

Be wary of any study cited in advertising or in another context where the motive is to sell you something.

What Do You Think?

1. What is your major source of health information? Television? Newspapers? Magazines? Friends? How carefully do you analyze the health information presented?
2. Who should be responsible for the accuracy of health reports presented by mass media representatives? What is the consumer's role in interpreting health news stories?

Predisposing factors: knowledge, attitudes, beliefs, values, and confidence levels that serve as either motivators or barriers to practicing health-related behaviors.

Enabling factors: skills and resources that help one implement a health promotion plan.

Reinforcing factors: feedback that either rewards or punishes certain behaviors, thus enhancing or diminishing the likelihood that a health-related behavior will be continued.

Health and Wellness Behavior

A great deal of research has been conducted in the area of health behavior in an attempt to discover why we do what we do concerning our health and wellness. This body of research makes one point quite clear. Human behavior is a complex and not easily understood phenomenon.

One contemporary theory of health behavior suggests three major determinants: **predisposing, enabling,** and **reinforcing factors.**[24]

Predisposing Factors

All individuals accumulate a number of health beliefs, attitudes, and values during their life spans, along with a wide variety of health knowledge. Together, these personal preferences and motivations toward health and wellness accumulate and interact to help shape our health and wellness behaviors. Some of the health knowledge, beliefs, and habits we pick up along the way come from accurate and reliable sources and tend to serve us well. Others, however, are picked up through advertisements, articles in popular magazines, conversations with well-meaning relatives and friends, and the like. These beliefs, many of which may have no scientific basis, often become intertwined with our more reliable health beliefs and values.

Knowledge. An accurate and reliable health knowledge base is a sound foundation on which to build a wellness lifestyle (see Of Special Interest 1.1). Most of us, however, can think of numerous personal instances where our health behavior was in direct conflict with our knowledge. How many of us, for instance, continue to drive our automobiles without fastening our seat belts or even after consuming too many alcoholic drinks? Knowledge must be combined with other motivating factors if we are to move toward high-level wellness.

Pleasure and Pain. Pleasure and pain can be viewed as flip sides of the same coin. Both are strong human motivators. Basically, people tend to seek pleasurable sensations and to avoid painful ones. Sometimes, however, pleasure is delayed and comes to us at some expense of pain. To understand this pleasure/pain dichotomy better let's analyze three bicyclers, Mike, Greg, and Dacia, all of whom meet three mornings a week to exercise together.

Mike took up the sport of long-distance cycling after his doctor prescribed it in order to help increase his work capacity, which was slowly decreasing as a result of heart disease. Bicycling is not an especially thrilling experience for Mike; however, because of his bicycling, he has increased the amount of activity he can do before having signs of chest pain. The consequences of his bicycling—being able to play with his children, keep up with his friends and colleagues on the tennis courts, and so forth—bring Mike his greatest pleasurable motivation.

Greg has always been athletically inclined; he played football and track in both high school and college. Greg enjoys the pleasure of pushing his physical self to the limits of his endurance. He finds that long-distance cycling is one means to the pleasurable state of knowing he has done his best. The pleasure of the moment is an essential motivator for Greg.

Dacia was a jogger throughout her college years and had enjoyed the challenge, but after a while she became bored and decided to try long-distance cycling as an alternative. Dacia has found that she enjoys the pleasurable company of Greg and Mike and is constantly amazed by the beauty of nature on these early morning jaunts. In addition to the pleasures of the moment, Dacia finds that her bicycling pleasures carry over into all dimensions of her life. She feels mentally and emotionally refreshed on the days she cycles and enjoys her work, family, and friends more. Dacia's motivation appears to be spread throughout her lifestyle. All three bicyclers are moving in a positive

direction toward creative ada[...] optimal functioning within their environment and circumstances.

Fulfillment of Needs. Another strong motivator of our health and wellness behavior is the fulfillment of needs. Maslow has developed a model that depicts our basic human needs as a triangular hierarchy, placing basic survival needs at the base (see figure 1.9).[25] As our physical and psychological survival needs are met we move upward in the triangle to safety, love, esteem, and finally self-actualization needs. Maslow's theory is based on the belief that we must satisfy lower-level needs before we can attempt the higher levels. Ultimately, a healthy person will be motivated by a need for self-actualization, or a striving to become everything one is capable of becoming. Self-esteem and love/belongingness needs are also strong wellness motivators. Most of our daily lifestyle activities are tied into how we see ourselves and how we view others' perceptions of us.

Although we are often motivated by the desire to fulfill our various needs, these actions are not always healthy or socially acceptable. We have a very basic need for food, which we satisfy by eating. If we choose to satisfy this need with potato chips and soft drinks much of the time, however, we will not be meeting our nutritional needs adequately. We must combine our motivations with a reliable knowledge base.

The Created Need. Our industrial society, based on principles of mass production and consumption, has produced a new category of human need. We must contend with the "created need" daily. Advertising executives are masters of the "created need." People in the U.S. have become convinced that they need everything from electric toothbrushes to automatic garage-door openers. Every time we open a magazine, turn on the television, or walk down the street, we are bombarded with messages trying to convince us of another "need" to add to our list. A sound knowledge base does not seem adequate in helping us to avoid such unnecessary, and often harmful, creation of needs. We must be consciously aware of our environment and begin to question ourselves about our personal values, beliefs, attitudes, and knowledge regarding these "created needs" and their possible impact on our levels of well-being.

Figure 1.9: Maslow's hierarchy of human needs

Source: Data (for diagram) based on Hierarchy of Needs, in "A Theory of Human Motivation," in *Motivation and Personality*, 2nd edition by Abraham H. Maslow, 1970.

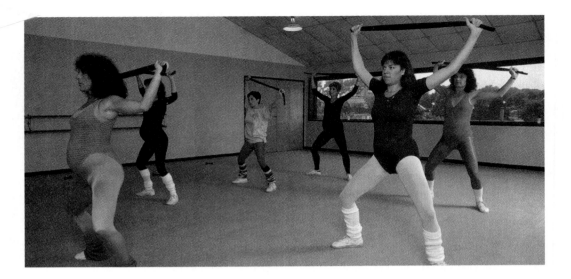

Figure 1.10: What do You think? Support is growing

1. America accessible wellness resources, such as this exercise class for pregnant women. What wellness resources are you aware of on your campus and in your hometown? Do you make use of these resources?

Enabling and Reinforcing Factors

Once we have the personal initiative to attempt a wellness lifestyle, implementation and maintenance become the important focus. Skills and resources are the enabling factors that help us implement our wellness plan. Joe, a college sophomore, has noticed that he is under a good deal of stress lately, and he believes that relaxation would be helpful. Joe has tried to relax on his own but it doesn't seem to be helping. In order to "relax," he needs to learn the skills involved in deep muscle relaxation. While reading the local paper Joe discovers that there are several stress-management classes offered on campus that teach such skills and allow time and facilities for practice. He decides to sign up for one of the free evening workshops to enhance his wellness lifestyle.

The availability and accessibility of wellness resources is an important concern. Factors such as cost, distance, transportation, hours open for use, and so forth must all be considered. Many options for wellness are impractical because the recreation center's swimming pool closes too early, the wellness center's cooking class is all the way across town, or we cannot afford to take three hours a week to attend the relaxation training class. Social support in the U.S. for readily available and easily accessible wellness resources is growing slowly (see figure 1.10). In the meantime, we must learn to be more flexible and creative in our personal lifestyle efforts.

Once we have the necessary skills and resources we are back, once again, to the motivation issue—how do we maintain our initiative? Reinforcing factors are especially important during this phase. We do not live in a vacuum. Others react, both positively and negatively, to our various behaviors. Some of the more common sources of feedback and reinforcement include our family, peers, instructors, employers, and physicians. At different points in our life the reinforcement and support of certain individuals will carry more weight than others. For instance, children are significantly influenced by the beliefs and behaviors of their parents, siblings, and peers. As we become adults, relationships with a spouse or "significant other" become more important influences on our health behavior.

Let's check in on Joe's stress-management efforts and see how he has been reinforced. Joe is really excited by the new skills he has learned in his stress-management workshop. These skills give him a new sense of mastery over his life. Through the evening workshop he has also met several new friends who have interests similar to his own. These new friends offer each other positive support and feedback. In addition to their daily relaxation sessions, they decide to try jogging a mile several times a week, both for the social outlet and the reduction of stress.

Joe needs his new support group, however, because his roommates are not equally accepting of his new activities. They do not understand why Joe wants to take a good twenty minutes to relax when he could be partying with them. Joe will undoubtedly have setbacks in his stress-management program. Having some friends who support his desire to improve in managing stress, however, will increase his chances for success.

As we have seen, predisposing, enabling, and reinforcing factors work together in a

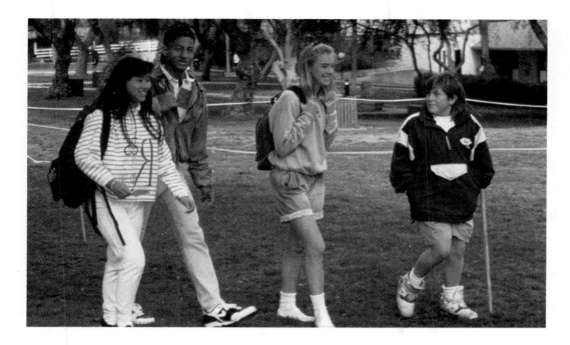

Figure 1.11: What Do You Think?

1. A strong social support network can encourage and complement your wellness lifestyle. Do you have a group of friends that you can talk with easily, and who support your efforts to improve your well-being? Do you take actions to support family and friends in their attempts to improve their health?

cyclical manner to influence our wellness lifestyles. As we interact with others and the environment we receive feedback that cycles into our health and wellness decision-making process. How healthy is your lifestyle? Activity for Wellness 1.2 will help you assess your current lifestyle in terms of those health-related behaviors that are believed to promote health and prevent disease.

Social Norms

Your lifestyle is not completely a result of individual behavior, as many would have you believe. Rather, lifestyles are a combination of personal behavior modified and influenced by a lifelong process of socialization. Socialization is carried on by the institutions with which we interact, such as families, churches, schools, unions, businesses, and clubs. Robert Allen, author of the book *Lifegain,* believes that we live in an antihealth and antiwellness culture: one that actually encourages us to be "overweight, underexercised, improperly nourished, tense, accident prone, and unfit."[26] We are encouraged in these antiwellness lifestyles through the social norms exhibited by our culture. **Social norms** are the behaviors expected, exhibited, and rewarded by a given culture. Our Western culture seems to set up barriers to wellness at every turn. Many people, for stance, would enjoy a nutritious snack on their daily work breaks. When they go to the refreshment area, however, they find the snack machines loaded with candy bars, potato chips, and cookies—no fresh fruit or other nutritious alternative is readily available.

Allen suggests that a combination of self-responsibility and building supportive environments is one way to circumvent the antiwellness social norms bombarding us daily. You are responsible for assessing social traps that may impede your wellness planning. You must choose which social norms you will maintain and which you wish to change. When you choose to change, include in your planning the creation of a social support network that expects and encourages you to move toward higher levels of wellness (see figure 1.11). Join a group that exercises together. Share your wellness plan with a friend or two. Ask your friends for emotional support or other forms of assistance that would be helpful. Encourage your family and friends to join in your wellness program. And provide strokes and encouragement for those around you who may also be seeking high-level wellness (see Activity for Wellness 1.3).

Wellness: Where Do You Start?

Wellness, that process of optimal functioning and creative adapting, does not just happen. You must supply the initiative and action for the journey toward high-level wellness. But what is the best way to go about making the changes in your life that will help you to achieve greater levels of well-being?

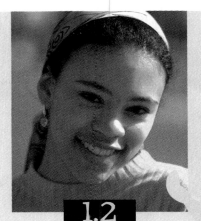

1.2
Activity for Wellness

Health-Style: A Self-Test

All of us want good health. But many of us do not know how to be as healthy as possible. Health experts now describe *lifestyle* as one of the most important factors affecting health. In fact, it is estimated that as many as seven of the ten leading causes of death could be reduced through commonsense changes in lifestyle. That's what this brief test, developed by the Public Health Service, is all about. Its purpose is simply to tell you how well you are doing to stay healthy. The behaviors covered in the test are recommended for most people. Some of them may not apply to persons with certain chronic diseases or handicaps, or to pregnant women. Such persons may require special instructions from their physicians.

Key:
A = Almost always
S = Sometimes
N = Almost never

Cigarette Smoking

If you never smoke, enter a score of 10 for this section and go the next section on *Alcohol and Drugs*.

	A	S	N
1. I avoid smoking cigarettes.	2	1	0
2. I smoke only low-tar and low-nicotine cigarettes *or* I smoke a pipe or cigars.	2	1	0

Smoking score: _____

Alcohol and Drugs

	A	S	N
1. I avoid drinking alcoholic beverages *or* I drink no more than one or two drinks a day.	4	1	0
2. I avoid using alcohol or other drugs (especially illegal drugs) as a way of handling stressful situations or the problems in my life.	2	1	0
3. I am careful not to drink alcohol when taking certain medicines (for example, medicine for sleeping, pain, colds, and allergies), or when pregnant.	2	1	0
4. I read and follow the label directions when using prescribed and over-the-counter drugs.	2	1	0

Alcohol and drugs score: _____

Eating Habits

	A	S	N
1. I eat a variety of foods each day, such as fruits and vegetables, whole-grain breads and cereals, lean meats, dairy products, dry peas and beans, and nuts and seeds.	4	1	0

	A	S	N
2. I limit the amount of fat, saturated fat, and cholesterol I eat (including fat on meats, eggs, butter, cream, shortenings, and organ meats such as liver).	2	1	0
3. I limit the amount of salt I eat by cooking with only small amounts, not adding salt at the table, and avoiding salty snacks.	2	1	0
4. I avoid eating too much sugar (especially frequent snacks of sticky candy or soft drinks).	2	1	0

Eating habits score: _____

Exercise/Fitness

	A	S	N
1. I maintain a desired weight, avoiding overweight and underweight.	3	1	0
2. I do vigorous exercises for fifteen to thirty minutes at least three times a week (examples include running, swimming, brisk walking).	3	1	0
3. I do exercises that enhance my muscle tone for fifteen to thirty minutes at least three times a week (examples include yoga and calisthenics).	2	1	0
4. I use part of my leisure time participating in individual, family, or team activities that increase my level of fitness (such as gardening, bowling, golf, and baseball).	2	1	0

Exercise/fitness score: _____

Stages of Change

Most of us realize that changing our health-related behaviors, like losing weight or quitting smoking, is often a lengthy and challenging process. Sometimes we seem to have more success changing than at other times. In order to help people be more effective in their behavior-change attempts, psychologists James Prochaska, John Norcross, and Carlo DiClemente decided to study individuals who had successfully changed health-related behaviors on their own. Prochaska and his colleagues wanted to find out which behavior-change techniques successful changers found to be the most helpful. Yet what these researchers

Stress Control

	A	S	N
1. I have a job or do other work that I enjoy.	2	1	0
2. I find it easy to relax and express my feelings freely.	2	1	0
3. I recognize early, and prepare for, events or situations likely to be stressful for me.	2	1	0
4. I have close friends, relatives, or others whom I can talk to about personal matters and call on for help when needed.	2	1	0
5. I participate in group activities (such as church and community organizations) or hobbies that I enjoy.	2	1	0

Stress control score: _____

Safety

	A	S	N
1. I wear a seat belt while riding in a car.	2	1	0
2. I avoid driving while under the influence of alcohol and other drugs.	2	1	0
3. I obey traffic rules and the speed limit when driving.	2	1	0
4. I am careful when using potentially harmful products or substances (such as household cleaners, poisons, and electrical devices).	2	1	0
5. I avoid smoking in bed.	2	1	0

Safety score: _____

What Your Scores Mean to You

Scores of 9 and 10

Excellent! Your answers show that you are aware of the importance of this area to your health. More important, you are putting your knowledge to work for you by practicing good health habits. As long as you continue to do so, this area should not pose a serious health risk. It's likely that you are setting an example for your family and friends to follow. Since you got a very high test score on this part of the test, you may want to consider other areas where your scores indicate room for improvement.

Scores of 6 to 8

Your health practices in this area are good, but there is room for improvement. Look again at the items you answered with a "Sometimes" or "Almost never." What changes can you make to improve your score? Even a small change can often help you achieve better health.

Scores of 3 to 5

Your health risks are showing! Would you like more information about the risks you are facing and about why it is important for you to change these behaviors? Perhaps you need help in deciding how to successfully make the changes you desire. In either case, help is available.

Scores of 0 to 2

Obviously, you were concerned enough about your health to take the test, but your answers show that you may be taking serious and unnecessary risks with your health. Perhaps you are not aware of the risks and what to do about them. You can easily get the information and help you need to improve, if you wish. The next step is up to you.

Where Do You Go from Here?

Start by asking yourself a few frank questions: *Am I really doing all I can to be as healthy as possible? What steps can I take to feel better? Am I willing to begin now?* If you scored low in one or more sections of the test, decide what changes you want to make for improvement. You might pick that aspect of your lifestyle where you feel you have the best chance for success and tackle that one first. Once you have improved your score there, go on to other areas.

If you already have tried to change your health habits (to stop smoking or exercise regularly, for example), don't be discouraged if you haven't yet succeeded. The difficulty you have encountered may be due to influences you've never really thought about—such as advertising—or to a lack of support and encouragement. Understanding these influences is an important step toward changing the way they affect you.

There's Help Available

In addition to personal actions you can take on your own, there are community programs and groups (such as the YMCA or the local chapter of the American Heart Association) that can assist you and your family to make the changes you want to make. If you want to know more about these groups or about health risks, contact your local health department. There's a lot you can do to stay healthy or to improve your health—and there are organizations that can help you. Start a new HEALTH STYLE today!

Source: Data from *Health-Style: A Self-Test.* Office of Disease Prevention and Health Promotion, Department of Health and Human Services, Washington, D.C., 1980.

---

discovered during their years of studying behavior change is that individuals progressed through very distinct *stages of change* on their way to improved well-being.[27] These stages include precontemplation, contemplation, preparation, action, maintenance, and in some instances termination. Prochaska and his colleagues also noted that certain behavior-change techniques worked better in some stages of change than in others.

Gaining an appreciation of the stages of change and the techniques that are most useful during each stage should help you make health-related behavior changes more successfully. In order to better understand the stages of change,

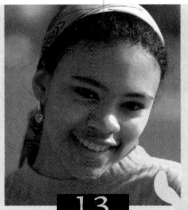

1.3
Activity for Wellness

Cultural Norm Assessment

How supportive is your social/cultural environment? What cultural norms may be either enhancing or acting as barriers to your personal quest for wellness? Read the following lists of norms that enhance wellness and norms that are barriers to wellness. Place a check in the boxes following each item if they are true of your close friends and family, or of your local community in general.

Norms That Enhance Wellness

On the average, do your family and close friends, or local community, as a group, believe in and act upon the following recommended health-related behaviors?

	Family and close friends	Local community
1. Routinely look for enjoyment and pleasure in everyday events?	❑	❑
2. Strive for a balance between work, play, and rest?	❑	❑
3. Regularly use stress-management techniques such as relaxation, time management, humor, and exercise?	❑	❑
4. Ask for help in times of trouble, both at home and at work?	❑	❑
5. Express feelings openly, honestly, and lovingly?	❑	❑
6. Eat a nutritious low-fat diet that follows the food pyramid's daily recommendations, such as 1–2 servings of fish, poulty, meat, nuts, and eggs; 4–6 servings of vegetables and beans; 2–4 servings of fruit?	❑	❑
7. Read food labels to help select nutritious foods?	❑	❑
8. Strive to balance the amount of calories eaten with an appropriate amount of exercise, not just in youth but throughout life?	❑	❑
9. Exercise the recommended 30 minutes daily?	❑	❑
10. View exercise as "play" rather than work?	❑	❑
11. Seek to have loving, intimate relationships in life that offer care and support in both good times and bad?	❑	❑
12. Handle conflict constructively and nonviolently?	❑	❑
13. Keep firearms and ammunition locked up separately, or not own firearms at all?	❑	❑
14. Wear seat belts whenever driving or riding in an automobile, truck, or van?	❑	❑
15. Wear helmets when roller blading, or riding a bicycle or motorcycle?	❑	❑
16. Drink alcohol rarely or not at all?	❑	❑

Norms That Are Barriers to Wellness

On the average, do your family and close friends, or local community, as a group, believe in or act upon the following health risk-related attitudes and behaviors?

	Family and close friends	Local community
1. Look at life with the attitude that one's cup is half empty rather than half full, or see stressors as problems rather than opportunities?	❑	❑
2. Focus the most time and attention on work, often at the expense of time and attention for family and close friends?	❑	❑
3. Regularly use alcohol, cigarettes, and other drugs as a way to cope with the stressors of everyday life?	❑	❑
4. View the world as "us" versus "them," such as Republicans versus Democrats, Black-Americans versus White-Americans, old people versus young people, or big business versus environmentalists?	❑	❑
5. Keep feelings bottled up inside?		
6. Skip breakfast, or have a doughnut or sausage biscuit and coffee on the run?	❑	❑
7. Regularly eat high-fat desserts such as ice cream, cake, or cookies?	❑	❑
8. View overeating at meals as a "pleasure" or "treat?"	❑	❑
9. Believe that becoming overweight is a natural part of aging?	❑	❑
10. Regularly watch sports on television, but rarely participate in exercise?	❑	❑
11. Try to solve problems by yelling at or hitting other people?	❑	❑
12. Drive a motor vehicle after drinking too much alcohol or taking other psychoactive drugs?	❑	❑
13. Believe that being a good party host means keeping everyone's glass filled with an alcoholic beverage?	❑	❑
14. View being able to drink large amounts of alcohol as an accomplishment?	❑	❑
15. Drive motor vehicles at speeds over the posted limit?	❑	❑
16. View aging as an unfortunate consequence of life?	❑	❑

Review your assessment of cultural norms. Do you have more supports or barriers for a life of high-level wellness? How can you make the most of your supports and minimize your barriers? What role could you play in improving cultural supports in your intimate support groups (family and friends) and in your local community?

Source: From Judd Allen and Robert F. Allen, "From Short-term Compliance to Long-term Freedom: Culture-based Health Promotion by Health Professionals," *American Journal of Health Promotion,* Vol. 1, No. 2 Health Promotion, Birmingham, MI.

let's follow Gina, a college freshman, through the various stages as she attempts to improve her level of wellness by stopping smoking.

Precontemplation

People at the precontemplation stage of change "usually have no intention of changing their behavior, and typically deny having a problem. Although their families, friends, neighbors, doctors, or coworkers can see the problem quite clearly, the typical precontemplator can't."[28]

This description aptly describes Gina during her high school years. Gina had her first cigarette at the age of fourteen. She began smoking because her friends did, and it seemed like the thing to do. Her parents were unhappy that she smoked and gave her pamphlets about the dangers of smoking; Gina wouldn't read them. She didn't want to believe that smoking cigarettes could really hurt her.

Then Gina went to college. Because of the hazards of environmental tobacco smoke, most buildings on campus had been designated as nonsmoking areas. This made smoking more inconvenient. Gina's roommate Elizabeth smoked when they started their freshman year, but decided to quit smoking one month into the fall semester. Elizabeth wanted Gina to quit too, and offered to help her. Finally, Gina studied the effects of cigarette smoking in her personal health course. When she read about pregnancy and the effects of smoking on a fetus, that really hit home. Gina wants to have a family of her own when she graduates from college and she would never want to knowingly do something that would harm an unborn child. All of these factors combined to influence Gina to *consider* trying to quit smoking cigarettes. During the fall semester, Gina had moved from the stage of precontemplation to contemplation.

Contemplation

"In the contemplation stage, people acknowledge that they have a problem and begin to think seriously about solving it. Contemplators struggle to understand their problem, to see its causes, and to wonder about possible solutions. Many contemplators have indefinite plans to take action within the next six months or so."[29]

Gina had realized that she should seriously consider stopping smoking. But she didn't know how to proceed. Gina decided to take her roommate up on her offer to help. Elizabeth had attended a stop smoking class when she quit smoking, and one activity that really helped her was to keep a diary for several days, tracking each cigarette she smoked, when she smoked it, and why. Gina followed Elizabeth's advice and kept a smoking diary for a week. She learned a great deal about her smoking habit. Additionally, Gina tried to imagine herself as a nonsmoker, focusing on the benefits she would receive. After thinking about quitting for several months, and with Elizabeth's help, Gina was ready to move to the next stage of change—preparation.

Preparation

"Most people in the preparation stage are planning to take action within the very next month, and are making the final adjustments before they begin to change their behavior."[30]

Gina had definitely decided to quit smoking and, like many smokers, was determined to do it without taking a class. However, she did read the materials that Elizabeth received in her stop smoking class. Elizabeth's stop smoking booklet recommended that Gina set a specific date to quit and announce that date to her family and friends, asking for their support. Additionally, Gina decided to cut back on the number of cigarettes she smoked each day in preparation for her quit day. She also read about techniques that would help her cope once she did stop smoking, and then wrote her plan in the form of a contract (see figure 1.12) that both she and Elizabeth signed. Gina's quit date was approaching fast. She was now ready to take action.

Action

"Action is the most obviously busy period, and the one that requires the greatest commitment of time and energy. Changes made during the action stage are more visible to others than those made during other stages, and therefore receive the greatest recognition."[31]

Gina quit smoking at the beginning of her spring break. She chose this time because she would be back home with her parents, who would support her efforts to quit. Gina knew the first week would be especially difficult. Additionally, by beginning her action stage away from school, she would be away from the normal environmental cues to smoke, like having a cigarette and a cup of coffee with friends after her 8:00 A.M. class. Gina began to chew sugarless gum in place of smoking, and also used techniques such as relaxation

Area for Improvement: *Smoking Cessation*

Goal: *To become a former smoker*

Current status: *Score of 9 (indicating addiction) on the Fagerstrom Nicotine Tolerance Scale (see Student Workbook); Currently smoke 1 1/2 packs of cigarettes each day.*

Resources:
(1) American Lung Association. "21 Days to Freedom" (smoking cessation program).
(2) Centers for Disease Control. (1990) "Out of the Ashes: Choosing a Method to Quit Smoking." [Washington, D.C.: U.S. Government Printing Office.]
(3) James O. Prochaska, John C. Norcross, and Carlo C. DiClemente. (1994) Changing for Good. (New York: William Morrow and Company, Inc.).

Objectives:
(1) I will smoke 0 cigarettes.
(2) I will swim 3 times a week as a way to control stress and avoid smoking cues.
(3) I will practice relaxation techniques to help manage the stress of quitting smoking.
(4) I will substitute chewing gum for cigarettes when I get an urge to smoke.

Scheduling:
(1) I will not smoke any cigarettes after March 6.
(2) On Mondays and Wednesdays I will swim at the student recreation center after my 8:00am class, rather than going for coffee and cigarettes with Pilar and Sam.
(3) On Saturday morning I will swim at the student recreation center with my roommate at 10:00 am.
(4) I will practice deep muscle relaxation as soon as I get up each morning, for 15 minutes.
(5) I will purchase a six pack of chewing gum on Saturdays, and carry a pack in my purse at all times.

Reinforcing and enabling factors:
(1) My roommate quit smoking three months ago and has agreed to swim with me and provide support when I need it.
(2) The student recreation center on campus is open at convenient hours for my swims.
(3) My family will support my quit effort; I will spend the first week of my quit program with them.

Barriers:
(1) My good friends Pilar and Sam are smokers and smoke in my presence.
(2) Final exams are approaching soon and I used to cope with the stress of exams by smoking.

I will begin this action on *March 6.*

Gina Smith	*Elizabeth Jones*
My signature	**My supporter's signature**

Note: A blank copy of this wellness contract is included in the *Connections for Health: Student Workbook.*

Figure 1.12
Personal wellness contract

strategies and cognitive coping techniques to help her control both her stress and urges to smoke. (Chapter 2 describes these stress-management techniques in detail.)

Gina had some rough days, but with her friends and family supporting her efforts Gina remained a former smoker for six months. At that point in the change process, maintaining her status as a nonsmoker was Gina's biggest concern.

Maintenance

"It is during maintenance that you must work to consolidate the gains you attained during the action and other stages, and struggle to prevent lapses and relapse. Change never ends with action. . . . Maintenance . . . is a critically important continuation that can last from as little as six months to as long as a lifetime."[32]

Gina is now beginning her sophomore year in the maintenance stage. She had relied heavily on the nonsmoking environment and social support her family had given her all summer. But now Gina will be faced with situations that, in the past, were her cues to light up a cigarette. How Gina responds to these temptations will determine whether her change will be successful.

Gina will need to take some proactive steps, such as avoiding situations which would be too great a temptation. For instance, Gina has decided to forego the trip to the coffee shop after class with her friends who still smoke. Instead, she plans to go to the student recreation center and swim; swimming is a new and enjoyable hobby Gina began as a technique to help her stop smoking.

In all likelihood, Gina may find herself in the situation where she has, once again, smoked a cigarette or two. If she learns to view this as a temporary *lapse* in her nonsmoking lifestyle she will be more likely to maintain her status as a former smoker. But, if she views this lapse as a catastrophe where all her hard work is lost, she is likely to *relapse* and return to her smoking lifestyle. This would take Gina back to the precontemplation or contemplation stages of change. Having support persons you can confide in about lapses, such as Gina's roommate and family who will provide positive strokes for returning to her nonsmoking lifestyle, has been shown to prevent relapse.[33]

Termination

"The termination stage is the ultimate goal for all changers. Here, your former addiction or problem will no longer present any temptation or threat; your behavior will never return, and you will have complete confidence that you can cope without fear of relapse."[34]

We are uncertain whether Gina will ever reach the stage of termination in terms of her addiction to cigarettes. Some people do appear to reach this point and claim that they have no temptation to smoke, even in the presence of others who are smoking. Yet, many former smokers report urges to smoke ten or more years after they smoke that last cigarette. This pattern is true for many other health-related behavior changes as well. We all know people, for instance, who started to exercise regularly and, after maintaining that change for a year or more, relapsed to their former sedentary ways. Still, many health researchers believe that our new understanding of the stages of change, and especially the maintenance stage, may help more people reach a stage of termination.

Achieving Higher Levels of Wellness

As you begin your formal study of personal health this semester, begin to think about how you could enhance your current level of well-being. What areas of your life need special attention for cultivating better functioning, adaptation, and growth? Activity for Wellness 1.2, "Health-Style: A Self-Test" will help you identify health-related behaviors that you may want to begin to change.

Once you have identified a behavior that you want to enhance, you need to determine what stage of change you are in regarding that behavior. Activity for Wellness 1.4 will help you assess the stages of change for any behavior you are interested in changing. Additionally, in each chapter throughout this textbook, you will find tables that provide you with tips for behavior change for each of the stages of change.

One of the best general tips we can offer for achieving higher levels of wellness is to start slowly. You have spent a number of years building your current lifestyle. To increase the chance that changes you make will be permanent, choose to focus on one change at a time. Don't attempt to completely overhaul your life all at once. As you read this textbook and study about health, take the time to explore the options and opportunities available to you. Take the time to develop a sound lifestyle of high-level wellness.

Assessing Your Stage of Change

Directions: Once you have a fairly clear idea of what action you need to take, respond [yes or no] to the following four simple statements to assess the stage of change you are in for a particular problem behavior.

Yes No

___ ___ 1. I solved my problem more than six months ago.

___ ___ 2. I have taken action on my problem within the past six months.

___ ___ 3. I am intending to take action in the next month.

___ ___ 4. I am intending to take action in the next six months.

Scoring: If you answered no to all statements, you are in the *precontemplation stage*. *Contemplators* will have answered yes to statement 4 and no to all the others. Those in the *preparation stage* will have answered yes to statements 3 and 4 and no to the others.

If you answered yes to statement 2 and no to statement 1, you are in the *action stage*. You've reached the *maintenance stage* when you can answer yes truthfully to statement 1.

From James O. Prochaska et al., *Changing for Good: The Revolutionary Program that Explains the Six Stages of Change and Teaches You How to Free Yourself from Bad Habits*, 1994, William Morrow and Company.

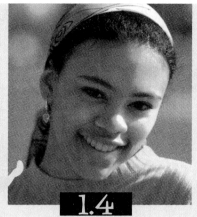

1.4

Activity for Wellness

Summary

1. Current health promotion efforts typically focus on prevention of death and disability and years of potential life lost due to injury and disease. These activities are known as disease prevention.

2. There are three major types of disease prevention activities: primary, secondary, and tertiary prevention.

3. Traditionally, health has been viewed as freedom from disease. One model of health suggests that there are four major determinates of health status: lifestyle, environment, heredity, and health-care services. Most risk factors for disease and injury fall into one of these categories.

4. Disease prevention activities attempt to decrease your risk by modifying risk factors. Changing risk factors, however, does not provide any guarantees; rather, it decreases the odds that you will experience a particular disease or injury.

5. Although disease prevention is a necessary component of an improved health-care system, it does not adequately address quality of life issues.

6. Wellness is an active process that focuses on moving toward optimal functioning and creative adapting. Wellness is a self-designed style of living that allows people to live life to the fullest. Both individual initiative and community interaction are necessary components of wellness.

7. According to Halbert Dunn, the father of the wellness concept, three criteria are essential for the wellness process. Moving toward both individual action and improved social supports is important. Also, we must consider our complete selves, including our emotional, mental, social, and spiritual aspects in addition to our physical being. Lastly, how we function on a daily basis and how we adapt to unusual events impacts on our level of well-being.

8. Self-responsibility is an important element of both health and wellness. One study of self-responsibility for lifestyle factors has indicated that people who practiced four or five common good health habits had a significantly decreased risk of dying than individuals who practiced two or fewer of these good health habits.

9. The Surgeon General's Office has issued a report entitled *Healthy People 2000*, which delineates the leading causes of death, disability, and years of potential life lost in the U.S. This report then suggests strategies to be accomplished by the year 2000 to improve the health and well-being of the nation.

10. Low income is an important risk factor for almost every chronic disease and injury that are leading causes of death in the United States. Living in poverty may result in poor health due to environmental exposure to hazardous conditions, lack of adequate material goods such as food and shelter, and inadequate access to health- and medical-care services.

11. Human behavior is a complex phenomenon. One behavior model suggests that there are three major determinants of health behavior—predisposing, enabling, and reinforcing factors. These factors work together in a cyclical manner to influence our wellness lifestyles.

12. The news media often reports the sensational finding of a new research study. When you interpret study results presented to you by the media, it is important to remember that one study cannot *prove* anything. Rather, it takes many studies done by different researchers to show a pattern of similar results. With such

a pattern of evidence we can place more trust in the answers provided by the body of research.

13. Another important key to health and wellness is a social support network. U.S. society is presently constructed with many barriers to health and wellness. Creating a social support group is an important motivator and reinforcer in our attempt to live a wellness lifestyle.

14. Psychologists have identified six distinct stages of change that individuals progress through when attempting to change health-related behaviors. These include precontemplation, contemplation, preparation, action, maintenance, and sometimes termination.

15. If you are trying to improve any specific health-related behavior, it is helpful to assess the stage of change you are at. Different strategies and behavior-change techniques are recommended for the various stages of change.

Recommended Readings

Pelletier, Kenneth R. (1994) *Sound Mind, Sound Body: A New Model for Lifelong Health*. (New York: Simon & Schuster).

This well-written book details the results of Dr. Pelletier's five-year research project that focused on fifty-one prominent people who have achieved high levels of well-being. Dr. Pelletier's work sheds new light on the characteristics that people of sound mind and body have in common, leaving us a road map to follow on our own quests for high-level wellness.

Prochaska, James O., John C. Norcross, and Carlo C. DiClemente. (1994) *Changing for Good: The Revolutionary Program that Explains the Six Stages of Change and Teaches You How to Free Yourself from Bad Habits*. (New York: William Morrow and Company, Inc.).

Prochaska, Norcross, and DiClemente propose a model of behavior change based upon years of research into the processes followed by individuals who successfully changed health-related behaviors. These psychologists outline six stages of change and the techniques that work best at each

stage. They also offer advice for changing specific behaviors such as smoking and alcohol abuse.

U.C. Berkeley Wellness Letter.

This highly regarded monthly newsletter carries articles on a variety of health topics. It provides up-to-date information in an easy to read, yet accurate style. Subscription information is available by writing: Wellness Letter, Subscription Department, P.O. Box 420148, Palm Coast, Florida 32142.

References

1. World Health Organization. (1947) "Constitution of the World Health Organization," *Chronicle of the World Health Organization*. 1: 29–43.

2. National Center for Health Statistics. (1994) *Health, United States, 1993*. (Hyattsville, Maryland: Public Health Service), 80.

3. *Health United States 1993*, 88.

4. *Health United States 1993*, 97.

5. Department of Health and Human Services. (1991) *Healthy People 2000: National Health Promotion and Disease Prevention Objectives*. (Washington D.C.: U.S. Government Printing Office), 64.

6. Dever, G. E. Alan. (1991) *Community Health Analysis: Global Awareness at the Local Level*. 2d ed. (Gaithersburg, Md: Aspen Publishers).

7. Green, Lawrence W. and Judith M. Ottoson. (1994) *Community Health* (St. Louis: Mosby).

8. Dunn, Halbert L. (1961) *High-Level Wellness* (Arlington, Va.: R. W. Beatty), 4.

9. Ardell, Donald B. (1982) *Fourteen Days to a Wellness Lifestyle* (Mill Valley, Calif.: Whatever Publishing).

10. Dunn, *High-Level Wellness*, 4.

11. Dunn, Halbert L. (1962) "High-level wellness in the world of today." *Journal of the American Osteopathic Association*. 61: 9.

12. Russell, Robert. Unpublished paper (Carbondale, Ill.: Southern Illinois University, Health Education Department).

13. Dunn, "High-level wellness in the world of today."

14. Toffler, Alvin. (1970) *Future Shock* (New York: Bantam Books).

15. Dunn, "High-level wellness in the world of today."

16. Dunn, *High-Level Wellness*.

17. Mullen, Kathleen D. and Robert S. Gold. (1988) "Wellness construct delineation: A Delphi study." *Health Education Research* 3(4):353–66.

18. Knowles, John. (1977) "Doing better and feeling worse: Health in the United States." *Daedalus*, Winter: 59.

19. Berkman, L. F. & L. Breslow. (1983) *Health and Ways of Living: The Alameda County Study*. (New York: Oxford University Press).

20. Dunn, "High-level wellness in the world of today."

21. *Healthy People 2000*, p. 43.

22. *Health, United States, 1993*.

23. "Life expectancy drops among black Americans." (1990) *Nutrition Week* XX (47):3.

24. Green, Lawrence, and Marshall W. Kreuter. (1991) *Health Promotion Planning: An Education and Environmental Approach* 2nd ed. (Mountain View, Calif.: Mayfield Publishing Company).

25. Maslow, Abraham. (1968) *Toward a Psychology of Being*, 2d ed. (New York: Van Nostrand).

26. Allen, Robert. (1981) *Lifegain* (New York: Appleton-Century-Crofts).

27. Prochaska, James O., John C. Norcross, and Carlo C. DiClemente. (1994) *Changing for Good: The Revolutionary Program That Explains the Six Stages of Change and Teaches You How to Free Yourself from Bad Habits*. (New York: William Morrow and Company, Inc.).

28. Prochaska et al., *Changing for Good*, p. 40.

29. Prochaska et al., *Changing for Good*, p. 41–42.

30. Prochaska et al., *Changing for Good*, p. 43.

31. Prochaska et al., *Changing for Good*, p. 44.

32. Prochaska et al., *Changing for Good*, p. 45.

33. Prochaska et al., *Changing for Good*, p. 250.

34. Prochaska et al., *Changing for Good*, p. 46.

Mental Well-Being and Stress: Coping Positively

Chapter 2

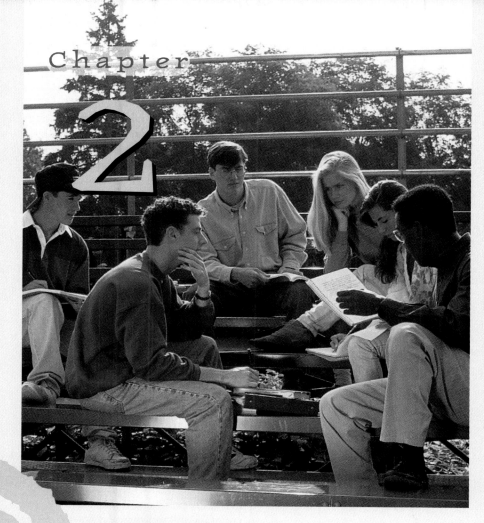

Student Learning Objectives

Upon completion of this chapter, you should be able to:

1. list and briefly describe at least five characteristics of a mentally well person;
2. list and discuss five characteristics of Roger's "fully functioning person";
3. list and briefly describe at least eight characteristics of Maslow's "self-actualized person";
4. compare and contrast Maslow's self-actualized person" with Pelletier's characteristics of "a healthy balance of mind, body, and environment";
5. compare the signs and symptoms of mild depression to those of severe or clinical depression;
6. list at least five self-help strategies that could be used to relieve mild depression;
7. compare and contrast the treatments for mild depression with the treatments for severe depression;
8. define the terms *stress* and *stressor*;
9. explain how individual perception of stressors can affect the stress response;
10. define eustress and distress, and give several examples of each;
11. describe the seven strengths of resilient people;
12. describe the physiological reactions that occur during the stress response;
13. analyze how both positive and negative "marker events" have affected your mental well-being;
14. define and compare social engineering and personality engineering strategies for coping with and managing the stress response;
15. define the "relaxation response";
16. describe at least two relaxation techniques that can lead to the "relaxation response";
17. discuss at least three methods of promoting mental wellness through enhancing personal awareness;
18. discuss at least three methods of promoting mental wellness through enhancing personal experience;
19. analyze social and cultural factors that tend to block our attempts to achieve mental wellness.

Self-concept, self-responsibility, competence, and realism are among the keys to wellness. Mental wellness may, in fact, be the heart of wellness in general. One recent study found that experts on wellness considered the mental and emotional aspects of health to be among the most important elements of wellness.[1]

One of the most promising strategies for promoting mental wellness involves the challenges of managing stress for personal growth. The college years are known to be a stressful time for most students. In a recent study, college students identified the most important stressors in their lives.[2] Finding the time to do course work, especially if working while attending college, was cited by most students as one of their major stressors. Other stressors noted by these college students included financial concerns, worry over what they would do following graduation from college, and problems with interpersonal relationships. Commuter students felt the added pressure of traffic and parking problems, as well as the stress of meeting home and school responsibilities.

In this chapter we will focus on the concept of mental wellness and how to achieve it in our daily lives through improving self-concept and competence, expanding awareness and experience, and learning to effectively manage life's stressors. We begin this chapter with a description of our goal—mental wellness.

An Attempt at Synthesis: What Mental Wellness Is

A review and synthesis of the literature reveals ten characteristics of mental wellness that seem to be constant. The concept of mental wellness continues to evolve, but these important elements stand out.

1. The mentally well are *real*. Mentally well people respond in a genuine, spontaneous way to events. The mentally well say what they mean and feel no need to censor their words or actions to get approval or to make an impression. They are unself-consciously themselves in the here and now. This quality of being real is sometimes called authenticity.

2. The mentally well are *realistic*. Realism means knowing the difference between what is and what ought to be; between what we can change and what we cannot change. The realistic person is capable of modifying beliefs in light of new evidence. The mentally well person possesses what Saint Francis prayed for— the strength to accept the things that cannot be changed, the courage to change those that can be, and the wisdom to know the difference.

3. The mentally well are *able to satisfy their needs*. Mentally well people recognize their own needs and do what they must to satisfy them. They are not hung up at a low level of their need hierarchy, wasting energy on needs that do not promote personal growth. They are competent—that is, they know how to satisfy their needs. They are not helpless, nor do they pretend to be.

4. The mentally well are *free and responsible*. Mentally well people are autonomous. They feel that they are in control of their own lives. They are inner-directed, accepting responsibility for their own actions or feelings.

5. The mentally well are *open to experience*. Mentally well individuals experience both their internal and external realities accurately and fully. They welcome new experiences and often seek them out but are not compulsive thrill seekers. Even experiences that brought pain, grief, or other unpleasantness are seen by the mentally well person as having potential for personal growth; the unpleasantness can often be defused by humor.

6. The mentally well are *capable of intimate relationships*. In many ways this is an extension of an openness to experience. The healthy person is open to the risks and the satisfactions of both physical and emotional intimacy. The ability to give and receive love is basic to healthy human development. Equally basic is the ability to trust in another and to be open in sharing one's feelings. Physical intimacy with romantic partners is a natural and fully enjoyed extension of emotional intimacy for the mentally well person.

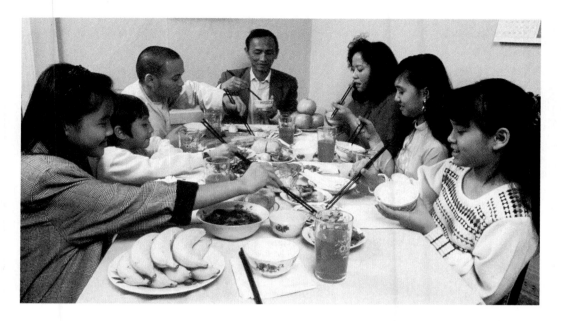

Figure 2.1: What Do You Think?

1. Why would enjoyment of ordinary daily activities, such as sharing a meal with your family, be a sign of mental wellness?
2. What ordinary daily activities do you routinely enjoy?

7. The mentally well are *tolerant and accepting of others*. Mental wellness is not compatible with racism, sexism, or ageism. A healthy person judges people on their individual merits and does not expect them to fit within a narrow limit of belief and behavior. A mentally well person is able to like a person while rejecting some part of that person's behavior.

8. The mentally well are *capable of reacting in a wide variety of ways*. In a mentally well person, the ability to lead is balanced by the ability to follow; the ability to judge, by the ability to empathize; the ability to act, by the ability to yield.

9. The mentally well are *capable of joie de vivre*. Enjoying life is a major characteristic of mental wellness (see figure 2.1). The healthy person enjoys the major elements of life—family, community, and job. These elements do not have to be perfect; the mentally well enjoy the pleasures of ordinary life (see Activity for Wellness 2.1).

10. The mentally well are *self-accepting*. Probably the most crucial characteristic of the mentally well personality is a positive self-concept. A deep and confident sense of liking oneself and feeling worthwhile is one of the most universally recognized characteristics of mental wellness. Most of these characteristics of mental wellness are predicated on accepting and liking oneself and all are facilitated by a positive self-concept.

What Mental Wellness Is Not

Marie Jahoda argued that we cannot define mental wellness or "positive mental health" in terms of normality, nor of absence of symptoms, nor of happiness.[3] Normality, she points out, is a statistical concept—not an ideal. **Normal** is whatever state is shared by most of the people in a population at a given time. As H. G. Wells pointed out, in the land of the blind the sighted man may be thought insane with his "ravings" about "seeing" things.

We also cannot define mental wellness on the basis of a lack of symptoms alone. Unhealthy people may not show any symptoms. In mental health as in physical health, wellness is more than the mere absence of symptoms of illness. We cannot expect the mentally healthy individual to be happy all the time. Everyone has emotional ups and downs. And we all must at times face experiences to which happiness would be an abnormal response.

Moreover, mental wellness cannot be defined in terms of "adjustment," "functioning," or "never having needed help." The problem with adjustment as a criterion is much the same as with normality. Joining the SS and murdering Jews, for instance, was a

Normal: in a mental-health context, the state of mind and behavior shared by most people at a particular point in time.

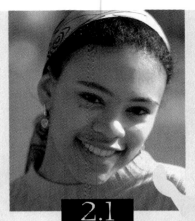

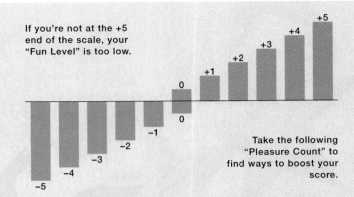

If you're not at the +5 end of the scale, your "Fun Level" is too low.

+5
+4
+3
+2
+1
0
0
−1
−2
−3
−4
−5

Take the following "Pleasure Count" to find ways to boost your score.

2.1

Activity for Wellness

What's Your "Fun Level"?

Having fun is good for your health. If you find that surprising, you probably could benefit from the following "pleasure assessment" profile.

Step 1. Just for the fun of it, place yourself on the Fun and Pleasure Scale above. Zero (0) is neutral; you don't think much about fun, one way or the other. Plus 5 means that your life is filled with pleasant activities. Minus 5 means that you never have fun, that you get no pleasure out of life.

Step 2. List your top ten favorite activities, and the number of times you have done them this week:

Activity   Times Done

1. _____
2. _____
3. _____
4. _____
5. _____
6. _____
7. _____
8. _____
9. _____
10. _____

What is the total number of times you've had fun this week?

If your weekly "fun count" was less than ten, you're not doing pleasurable things as often as you should. Make time for at least one of these activities every day. If anyone asks why you're having so much fun, explain it's for your health!

Warning: Serious, prolonged bouts of depression should be dealt with by a mental-health professional. Contact your mental-health agencies for assistance.

Source: Data from Dr. Arthur Ulene, Feeling Fine Productions, Inc., Los Angeles, CA.

---

very successful adjustment to society in Nazi Germany, but we would not point to it as an example of mental health. Those who refused to adjust to society in Nazi Germany were more likely to have been the mentally well members of that society.

Ability to function is no better a criterion. While mentally healthy people are able to function in all areas of their lives (family, work, play), the ability to function is not exclusive to healthy individuals. Even some individuals with a variety of mental illnesses may be able not only to function well but to excel in many roles.

Finally, we cannot define mental wellness in terms of never having needed help with an emotional problem. We would not say that someone who has never been treated by a physician is necessarily physically well. There are many people who have never had any kind of treatment but may be in need of such help.

Major Contributions to the Concept of Mental Wellness

Although the term *wellness* is of relatively recent origin, essentially the same concept has been explored under other names by a number of theorists. We will discuss the contributions of a few of the most prominent ones.

Rogers and the Fully Functioning Person

Psychologist Carl Rogers, originator of client-centered therapy and one of the founders of

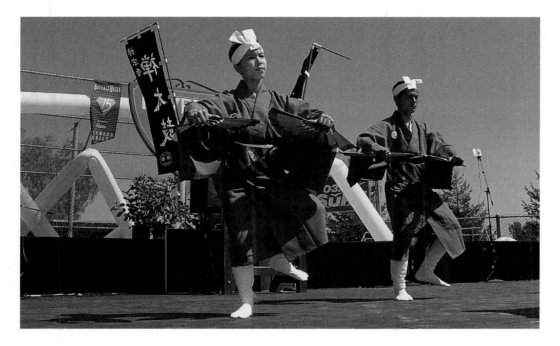

Figure 2.2: What Do You Think?

Figure 2.2: What Do You Think?

1. Do you regularly participate in a variety of cultural events that are different from your own culture?
2. How might this help you to be a "fully functioning person?"

the human-potential movement, has described what he termed the **fully functioning person.**[4] In Rogers' view most people do not function at their full potential. Most people only maintain life, whereas fully functioning people enhance life. According to Rogers the fully functioning person can be recognized by five characteristics.

1. The fully functioning person has *an openness to experience*, which is clearly the opposite of the defensiveness characteristic of the partially functioning majority. Every stimulus is freely attended to without distortion by any defense mechanism. New experiences are welcomed and sought out. Different perspectives are examined and accepted on their own merits. The fully functioning person can disagree with others without disliking them and can find friends on both sides of a conflict without feeling disloyal.

   This openness is internal as well as external. The fully functioning person is aware of his or her own feelings, needs, and weaknesses. These too are seen without defensiveness and are accepted for what they are. Whatever deficiencies the fully functioning person may have, he or she is aware of them and seeks to cope with them rather than deny them.

2. The fully functioning person *experiences life to its fullest every moment*, rather than

according to some fixed, preconceived script. Living in this way lends itself to the possibility of experiencing many new things (see figure 2.2).

   The fully functioning person is able to adapt to new situations. Instead of trying to impose some preconceived structure *on* experience, the fully functioning person finds structure *in* experience. A flowing, continuously changing reorganization of self and personality emerges from experience. This concept of existential living might be described as living flexibly, adaptably, and spontaneously.

3. **Organismic trusting** is Rogers' name for the third characteristic. By *trusting your own organism*, Rogers means a willingness to accept answers, decisions, and other feelings that come from within but without conscious process. It can be called intuition, gut reaction, or a hunch, but whatever you call it, the fully functioning person learns to trust and rely on the organism.

   The fully functioning person, who is open to all experience, brings to bear on any problem all the data from sensory impressions, memory, previous learning and internal visceral states without distortion by any defense mechanisms. With this data store to draw on, the fully functioning person often can arrive at

Fully functioning person: a concept offered by Carl Rogers, indicating that an individual is able to be open to new experiences, live life to its fullest, accept intuition as a legitimate source of information, make rational choices from alternatives, and engage in creative thought and activity.

Organismic trusting: a characteristic of Rogers' fully functioning person involving the ability to trust one's own judgments and intuitions.

correct decisions immediately and without conscious thought. Knowing that this decision is not merely projection or rationalization imposed on experience, the fully functioning person can trust these intuitions or gut reactions.

4. The fourth characteristic is **experimental freedom**—*the freedom to make choices between alternate courses of action.* Rogers' fully functioning person feels in control, acting and not just being acted upon. The fully functioning person adjusts to experience through a series of choices, not through a series of simple reactions.

   Like everyone else, the fully functioning person's ability to choose may be limited by prior experience, the environment, or bodily limitations. The fully functioning person feels in control and experiences an exhilarating sense of personal power in which all things seem possible. Openness to experience, existential living, and organismic trusting probably make the fully functioning person far freer from any conditioning or other constraints of the past than any other person can possibly be.

5. The fifth characteristic, which flows out of the four preceding characteristics, is **creativity.** Rogers does not confine his definition of creativity to artistic endeavors such as painting or composing music. Creativity refers more broadly to *the production of new and effective thoughts, actions, or things.* All of that external and internal experience, channeled by a person of flexibility, organismic trust, and decisiveness, could scarcely fail to produce something new and useful.

These five characteristics describe a fully functioning person who leads a life that "involves a wider range, a greater richness, than the constricted living in which most of us find ourselves."[5] But with that greater range, greater variety, and greater richness come challenge and uncertainty. The fully functioning person has given up the defenses to which most of us cling for fear of what we would surely face if we were open, flexible, and in control. As Rogers put it: "This process of living the full life is not, I am convinced, a life for the fainthearted. It involves the stretching and growing of becoming more and more of one's potentialities."[6]

Maslow and the Self-Actualized Person

Abraham Maslow is a major contributor to modern motivation theory, he is one of the founders of humanistic psychology, and he may come to be regarded as second only to Halbert Dunn in shaping the wellness movement. Maslow's contributions to the concept of mental wellness flowed out of his theory of human motivation.[7]

Other psychologists had described human needs as a conglomerate, with all needs present at once and competing for gratification. Maslow described a hierarchy of needs motivating human behavior. You will remember from chapter 1 that at the primary level are the physiological needs—for food, water, oxygen, protection from extreme temperature, and so on. Only when these needs have been met do the second level of needs become felt—the need for safety and security. Only when a basic level of safety and security has been achieved does the third level of need become felt—the need to feel loved and accepted. When this need is minimally satisfied it is succeeded by the fourth level—the need for self-esteem.

Finally, when all the more basic levels of needs, from the physiological through self-esteem, have been satisfied, the highest level of need emerges. This is the need for **self-actualization**—a drive to achieve your full potential, to be all that you can possibly be. It is the need to do that "stretching and growing" that Rogers also mentioned.

Not everyone, however, reaches this highest level of need. Poverty and deprivation keep many at the first and second levels of need, struggling to meet their basic physiological needs and to achieve some security that those needs will be met in the future. Others, also less economically fortunate, may never achieve self-esteem or a sense of being loved and accepted and thus remain trapped at those need levels. Still others may never overcome insecurity and fear learned early in life and may spend their entire lives desperately and compulsively building up wealth as a bulwark against their fears. Only a few people ever reach the level of the need for self-actualization.

Maslow set out to identify persons—both among his own acquaintances and among historical figures—who had lived rich, fulfilling lives and seemed to be motivated by

Self-actualization: a concept popularized by Abraham Maslow, the self-actualized person is one who is able to achieve his or her full potential. Self-actualization sits atop the pinnacle of a series of needs that begin with basic human physiological needs, the need for security, the need for love and acceptance, and the need for self-esteem.

the need for self-actualization. Maslow could not definitely identify anyone as being purely motivated by self-actualization, but he compiled a list of forty-eight persons he believed might be self-actualizers. Among those he listed were Albert Einstein, Abraham Lincoln, Eleanor Roosevelt, Franklin Roosevelt, and five-time presidential candidate Eugene V. Debs.

Both the listing and his descriptions of the individuals were inevitably subject to Maslow's own biases and preconceptions. Despite any such biases, Maslow seems to have made a sincere attempt at objectivity in developing his list. The similarities to the descriptions given by Rogers and other psychologists give further support to the validity of Maslow's conclusions. The sixteen common characteristics of self-actualizing individuals include the following.

1. Self-actualizers *perceive reality accurately* and without distortion, even when reality is unpleasant or painful. This is clearly similar to the openness described by Rogers.

2. Self-actualizers show a *high level of self-acceptance and of acceptance of others* as they really are. Such self-acceptance is to be expected in a person whose need for self-esteem has been satisfied. It is also consistent with the other personality descriptions we have previously examined.

3. Self-actualizers *have loving intimate relationships* with one or several people. Although many of Maslow's subjects were unpopular people, they all had at least one loving intimate relationship. Again, this seems self-evident in persons who have already satisfied their needs for love and acceptance.

4. Self-actualizers *possess a high degree of autonomy or independence*. They judge for themselves what is right or wrong and stick by their judgments even if this makes them unpopular. They have the strength to stand alone when necessary. This does not mean that they are rebellious or loners but that they have the courage to stand up for what they believe.

5. Self-actualizers *show a natural, effortless, and highly individual spontaneity in thought and in emotion*. They respond in fresh and different ways to the events of the day

instead of becoming trapped in a limited repertoire of responses.

6. Self-actualizers *are task-oriented* rather than preoccupied with self. They are genuinely concerned with the tasks they perform and see them as more than a means to personal gratification. To them a job is not just a way to make money or achieve status—it is a meaningful and important activity in itself. They are likely to have a commitment to some larger cause or purpose toward which their work is directed.

7. Unlike so many people who are only comfortable with the familiar and who resist change, self-actualizers *are attracted to the new, the different, and the unexpected*.

8. Not only are they attracted by new experiences, self-actualizers *possess a continued freshness of appreciation* that enables them to approach familiar experiences from a fresh perspective. They see something new each day in the familiar. They avoid lumping experiences into categories and dismissing each new instance as merely one more instance of a familiar category. Instead, each time the familiar is reexperienced, it is seen as though it were the first time.

9. Self-actualizers *possess a sense of spirituality* that may or may not be religious in a formal sense. Maslow found that this spirituality is typically centered on a sense of unity with nature or with the universe and is shaped by one or more "peak experiences." This spiritual sense of oneness is related to a sense of belonging to all humankind. Peak experiences, sometimes called "mystical" or "oceanic" experiences, involve a sense of exhilaration and feelings that your boundaries as a person have suddenly dissolved and that you have become part of all nature. Such experiences are sometimes achieved through, or caused by, meditation, prayer, drugs, or stress. They may also occur spontaneously with no specific trigger phenomenon.

10. Related to these characteristics, self-actualizers *have a sense of belonging to all humankind*—Maslow uses the German word *gemeinschaftsgefuhl*, meaning brotherly feeling, to describe this feeling. For them the connectedness of humankind is a felt reality, not a

1. Self-actualized individuals feel great empathy for people in other cultures, such as the people affected by the war in Bosnia. How would such a concern for others around the world lead to an individual being able to achieve his or her full potential?

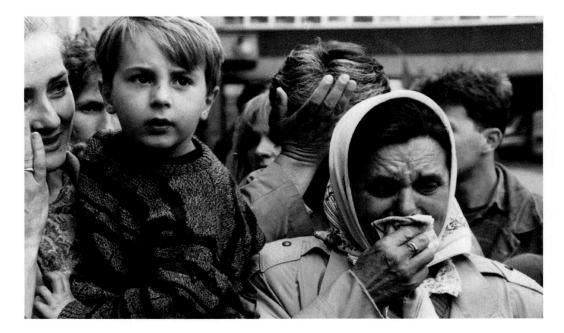

platitude. Their view of humankind does not divide into "us" versus "them"; they see everyone as a part of "us." Possessing this sense of belonging allows them to feel empathy for the situations of persons in other cultures with the same acuteness of empathy that they feel for their own family and close friends (see figure 2.3).

11. Self-actualizers have a tendency to *relate to others as unique individuals* rather than as types or group members. The self-actualizing person is essentially uninfluenced by prejudice or bias. This characteristic is logically related to traits 8 and 9.

12. Self-actualizers *have a firm sense of right and wrong*. Their ethical views usually are not wholly conventional, but they are consistently applied. Their behavior is guided by their own ethical principles, which they place above convention, peer pressure, or even the law.

13. Self-actualizers *exhibit a resistance to acculturation*. Although they usually seem outwardly to accept the norms of their society, privately they are casual and detached about them. They show a rather calm and good-humored rejection of the stupidities and imperfections of their culture. They are a part of their culture without being dominated or limited by it, seeming to select from their culture what they judge to be good about it and to reject what they find to be bad.

This may bring them into conflict with institutions of their culture. When it does, they are able to fight vigorously against social pressures that persons still struggling for acceptance or not yet confident of their self-esteem would be unable to resist.

14. Although self-actualizers enjoy being with people, they *are also able to tolerate and even enjoy solitude*. They seek solitude on occasion and use it for meditation or for periods of intense concentration.

15. Self-actualizers *are creative and inventive* in some areas of their lives. They are not necessarily artistically creative, but they have their own unique ways of doing and thinking rather than being followers of the usual. This is identical to Rogers' use of the concept of creativity.

16. Self-actualizers *possess a benign sense of humor*. They laugh at common human failings, pretensions, and foolishness rather than more hostile subjects.

Pelletier's Sound Mind, Sound Body Study

Many of the features of Maslow's theory of the self-actualized person have been recently confirmed by Kenneth Pelletier. Pelletier, an associate professor at the Stanford University School of Medicine, spent five years studying prominent people in the U.S. who had exhibited high levels of well-being.[8] He interviewed each of the fifty-one participants

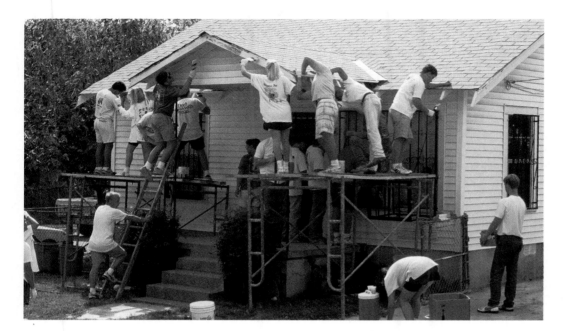

What Do You Think?

1. Many people volunteer to help the homeless. How does their service to others make them healthier?

for several hours, attempting to learn how they had approached life and why they thought they had developed "a healthy balance of mind, body, and environment."[9] Pelletier's *Sound Mind, Sound Body* study findings include the following.

1. The *Sound Mind, Sound Body* participants exhibited a strong sense of **self-efficacy** or a belief that they could overcome any challenges life offered. This belief was usually a result of having overcome a major childhood trauma, such as a death, divorce, or illness. These individuals had reacted to trauma in a constructive way, learning from the experience that they could and would control their own lives to a large extent.

2. The *Sound Mind, Sound Body* participants "demonstrated a healthy way of utilizing stress."[10] They seemed to have a positive attitude toward both themselves and the world around them. As the old saying goes, they viewed their cup as half full, rather than half empty. Stressors were perceived as growth opportunities.

3. The *Sound Mind, Sound Body* participants had a "deep and abiding sense of purpose . . . [with] service to others as the highest mission."[11] For many of these people, this sense of purpose was related to spiritual beliefs, much as Maslow described the spirituality of self-actualizers. Yet, the spirituality of the *Sound Mind, Sound Body* participants

was translated into active service to others, such as starting a program to feed the homeless.

4. The *Sound Mind, Sound Body* participants focused on the immediate here and now, rather than dwelling on the past or the future. They were more concerned with dealing constructively with current challenges they faced.

5. The *Sound Mind, Sound Body* participants demonstrated a "commitment to fully relating to others."[12] Like Maslow's self-actualizers, supportive relationships with immediate family members and one or two close friends were most important to a sense of mental well-being. The *Sound Mind, Sound Body* participants valued giving support as much as getting support.

6. The *Sound Mind, Sound Body* participants routinely practiced a variety of techniques that helped them to quiet their bodies and minds, such as meditation or relaxation.

7. Like Maslow's self-actualizers, the *Sound Mind, Sound Body* participants reported that they were directed more by inner beliefs and values rather than by social rules or mores.

Mental wellness, as described by Rogers, Maslow, Pelletier and others, is a goal worthy of pursuit. The road to mental well-being, however, is seldom an easy one. There are many potential roadblocks to challenge us on our way.

Self-efficacy: a person's sense of personal adequacy or competency; one's confidence in being able to attain goals through individual effort.

1. **Reduce the prevalence of mental disorders (exclusive of substance abuse) among adults living in the community to less than 10.7 percent.** (Baseline: One-month point prevalence of 12.6 percent in 1984.)

2. **Reduce to less than 35 percent the proportion of people aged 18 and older who experienced adverse health effects from stress within the past year.** (Update: 40.6 percent in 1990, down from 44.2 percent in 1985.) (Special Population Target: people with disabilities.)

3. **Increase to at least 45 percent the proportion of people with major depressive disorders who obtain treatment.** (Update: 36 percent in 1983, up from 31 percent in 1982.)

4. **Increase to at least 20 percent the proportion of people aged 18 and older who seek help in coping with personal and emotional problems.** (Update: 12.5 percent in 1990, up from 11.1 percent in 1985.) (Special Population Target: People with disabilities.)

5. **Decrease to no more than 5 percent the proportion of people aged 18 and older who report experiencing significant levels of stress who do not take steps to reduce or control their stress.** (Update: 28 percent in 1990 up from 24 percent in 1985.)

6. **Increase to at least 40 percent the proportion of worksites employing 50 or more people that provide programs to reduce employee stress.** (Update: 37 percent in 1992, up from 26.6 percent in 1985.)

Source: Data from *Healthy People 2000 National Health Promotion and Disease Prevention Objectives,* pp. 213–218, 1991; and from National Center for Health Statistics, *Healthy People 2000 Review, 1993, 1994.* U.S. Gov. Printing Office, Washington, D.C.

Mental Health Objectives for the Year 2000

In its *Healthy People 2000* report, the U.S. Department of Health and Human Services has set a number of mental health objectives to be accomplished by the year 2000. As you can see in table 2.1, depression and stress are two barriers to mental well-being highlighted by the *Healthy People 2000* objectives.

Since these objectives were first published, progress has been made in improving the mental health of people in the U.S. The prevalence of stress has dropped. In 1990, 40.6 percent of U.S. citizens reported experiencing adverse health effects from stress, down from 44.2 percent in 1987. The number of people seeking help for emotional problems has increased to 12.5 percent in 1990, compared with only 11.1 percent in 1987. Additionally, more worksites now offer stress-management programs for their employees (37 percent of worksites in 1992 compared with 26.6 percent in 1987). However, we have moved farther away from the year 2000 target regarding the proportion of people who report being stressed but who do not take steps to manage it. In 1990, 28 percent of people reported they were not taking such steps to manage their stress, up from 24 percent in 1987. The remainder of this chapter will explore both depression and stress as barriers to mental well-being. Strategies for coping with stress and depression will be highlighted.

Depression: Moving Away from Mental Wellness

We all have experienced days when we felt so "low" that not even winning the million-dollar lottery could have raised our spirits. Such negative emotion can occur from the loss of a close friendship or love relationship, being humiliated in front of peers, receiving a failing grade at school, losing the "big game," or facing another type of disappointment. These kinds of events are a normal part of the "human condition" and are to be expected. Writes John Langone:[13]

Indeed, those days when the corners of your mouth turn down may also be good for you in the long run, for they are part of the daily rhythm that gives life meaning, that raises it from the ordinary and makes living interesting. If we never knew what it was like to be depressed, then not only would we be considered abnormal but our lives would be one big snore, a soft existence so full of good things and good luck that we could never begin to understand the plight and anguish of others not so fortunate. Even the anxiety, that uneasiness of mind that so often accompanies depression, can be positive. It can loosen creative forces, give us drive and ambition. Anxiety, because it helps us respond to situations and get things done, is often found in the lives of our most successful and accomplished individuals.

Depression is a term widely used to represent a variety of conditions, from occasional episodes of mild sadness or discouragement to serious incapacitating mental illness that involves feelings of utter hopelessness and helplessness. Moreover, reactions to depression can range from a sense of being "down in the dumps" to suicide.

If it seems that conversations about depression and being "bummed out" are widespread among college students and other young adults, it is because depression *is* widespread. Depression is one of the most frequently experienced mental-health problems among college students. Depression is, in fact, so common that it is often referred to as the common cold of mental illness.

Although depression can occur anytime in the life cycle, it is least common in middle adulthood, a time of life when most people feel secure. During adolescence and young adulthood, however, and again in late adulthood, when lives are undergoing significant and stressful transitions, people may be more susceptible to episodes of recurrent or persistent depression.

Depression may be a response to a traumatic or stressful event such as the death of a loved one, the loss of a job, the breakup of an important relationship, a serious illness or physical disorder, a major disappointment, or another significant change in a person's living situation.[14] Some disruption as a result of any of these events is a natural expectation. Experiencing an overwhelming number of life changes might bring on distress in even the hardiest of individuals.

Depression may also be caused by a genetic predisposition. Research focusing on the incidence of depression in twins has provided valuable insights into the link between family history and an increased risk of depression. A 1992 study of female twins indicated that the risk of depression was 66 percent higher for an individual if their identical twin suffered from clinical depression. When fraternal twins, who are not genetically identical, were studied the risk of depression dropped to 27 percent for an individual whose fraternal twin had

experienced clinical depression.[15] The actual mechanism for this genetic predisposition is as yet unknown.

Depression might also be caused by low self-esteem.[16] People who do not think highly of themselves, who are critical of themselves and others, and who are pessimistic seem to be more prone to depression.

According to the National Institute of Mental Health, traumatic events from our childhood may predispose us to depression later in life.[17] In 1991 a study conducted by Stanford University researchers indicated that up to 35 percent of the difference in depression rates between men and women may be due to the sexual abuse of women when they were children.[18] This may explain, in part, the higher rates of depression in women.

Regardless of the cause of depression, the biochemical process is the same. Researchers believe that certain **neurotransmitters** in the brain become imbalanced, resulting in clinical depression.

Mild versus Severe Depression

Mild depressions that last longer than a few days most often are associated with a realistic perception of a negative event. You may feel down because you are grieving over a loss of something important to you. Coming to terms with the fact that a situation did not develop the way you hoped it would may include experiencing a period of mild depression (e.g., not getting a promotion, failing to attain a particular goal, or finding out your boyfriend or girlfriend just wants to be "friends"). If your sense of self-esteem is tied too closely to a job, a social position, the love of a person, or the attainment of a particular goal, the lost pride, bruised ego, and diminished self-efficacy when things do not work out may be painful. The duration of the depression is dependent on the length of time it takes you to realize that you are valuable to yourself and to other people, regardless of the thing that has been lost.

A "blue period" also is not an unusual occurrence following a time of great achievement or unusually high mental or physical productivity. Becoming "psyched" for a big exam, preparing for college graduation, getting married, returning from a summer vacation, gearing up for the holiday season, and many other essentially positive events may produce a letdown that is draining and causes symptoms of depression.

Depression: a state of altered mood ranging in severity and duration; in its mild form, it consists of sadness and discouragement, usually of brief duration. In more severe forms, called clinical depression, it consists of prolonged or recurrent mental incapacitation, possibly with thoughts of self-destruction or death.

Neurotransmitters: chemicals that transmit nerve impulses from one nerve cell to another. The neurotransmitters thought to be related to depression include serotonin, norepinephrine, and dopamine.

TABLE 2.2   *Self-Help Strategies to Relieve Mild Depression*

- If you feel sad, admit it. Acceptance enhances healing.
- Identify sources for your "blues," and if possible, change your surroundings in a way that may prevent similar reactions and feelings in the future.
- Tell people you are feeling depressed. It may be therapeutic. Do not cut yourself off from others. Talk especially to a friend or family member in whom you can confide.
- Take a brisk walk, or engage in some other form of exercise. It can be relaxing and improve your psychological outlook.
- Engage in some activity that you are good at—something that will promote a feeling of immediate success or accomplishment. Play a musical instrument, plant some flowers, rearrange the furniture, or paint the walls of a room.
- Do not vary from your normal routine. When things seem abnormal in your life, seek out the things you would normally do. The structure of doing this may minimize other stress and help you to maintain a sense of being in control.

- Pamper yourself just a little. Treat yourself to a special meal, a new item of clothing, or something else that you enjoy.
- Find some quiet time at the end of the day—after school or after work—to give yourself an opportunity to shift gears, refuel, and regain your strength.
- Minimize contact with other people who are depressed. Having someone unload his or her problems on you is unlikely to make you feel better about your own situation.
- Be realistic about your reaction to the situation that has brought on your low feeling. Ask yourself if you are exaggerating the significance of a particular event.
- Avoid any temptation to ease your depression by taking alcohol or other drugs. While these substances may bring about temporary relief, taking them may initiate a cycle that is difficult to break.

Source: From "Depression: Getting Down, Coming Up," 1982, Life Skills Education, Weymouth, MA.

The symptoms of mild depression usually are not difficult to recognize. They include a decreased ability to derive pleasure in the course of daily living, a loss of energy, and a feeling that even routine tasks are too much trouble to perform. Normal contacts with friends, sleep patterns, appetite, moods, and other things may be affected. Mild depression occurs in just about everyone occasionally and seldom requires intervention by a mental-health professional. People who recognize the existence of mild depression in themselves often can help themselves overcome these occasional "blues." Some suggestions for moving once again toward a higher level of mental wellness are identified in table 2.2. It is important to remember that recurrent symptoms may indicate the presence of a more serious form of depression, however, and should not be taken lightly (see Activity for Wellness 2.2).

According to the National Institute of Mental Health, 25 percent of all women and 12 1/2 percent of all men can expect a major depressive episode at least once in their lives.[19] While a precise diagnosis of severe clinical depression can be made only by a psychiatrist, it is unnatural for sadness, a lack of life satisfaction, and an inability to enjoy the company of friends and others to persist for more than about two weeks. Severe depression must be suspected under these circumstances, especially if accompanied by

any of the following additional warning signs: excessive use of alcohol and other drugs or increased dependence on these substances; behavioral changes such as crying, sleeplessness, and loss of appetite; suicidal statements or threats; and the belief that one's actions no longer can change the course of events, resulting in a sense of being helpless and out of control. While the passage of time can alleviate some of the symptoms of severe depression, symptoms may be recurrent, or even seasonal. Quite possibly, only professional intervention can adequately address the associated complications of serious depression.

Treatments for Depression

Clinical depression is the most treatable mental disorder. With therapy, 80 percent of depressed individuals will show marked improvement.[20] Yet, it is estimated that only 25 to 30 percent of people experiencing depression will seek professional help.[21]

There are several treatments currently used for individuals suffering clinical depression. These include drug therapy, counseling or "talk therapy," and electroconvulsive therapy. Each of these therapies has both strengths and potential side effects.

Drug Therapy

Drug therapy is widely used to treat depression. There are several types of drugs

The Center for Epidemiologic Studies Depression Scale

Depression is one of the most common mental-health problems of college students. The Center for Epidemiologic Studies of the National Institute of Mental Health has developed a short self-report scale designed to assess symptoms of depression in the general population. Lenore Sawyer Radloff has studied the reliability and validity of the instrument. This scale is shown below. It asks you to report the frequency with which each of twenty events was experienced during the previous week. On this scale, circle the number next to each item that best reflects how frequently you experienced that event in the past seven days.

To determine your "depression score," you are going to add each of the numbers you circled to get a sum. First, however, you must "reverse" the scale for items 4, 8, 12, and 16 so that 0 = 3, 1 = 2, 2 = 1, and 3 = 0. Notice that these four items reflect positive experiences rather than negative ones. Now add the twenty numbers together. Your score will be somewhere in the range of 0 to 60. If your total is 16 or greater, you may have experienced some depression in the past week. This scale should be used simply as an indicator of the degree of depression in your life. Only a competent mental-health professional can make a reliable clinical diagnosis of depression. Occasional symptoms of depression are normal experiences for college students. If you find yourself feeling this way often, though, by all means seek out the help of your college counseling center or health service. Even occasional bouts of depression are unpleasant and may lead to unfortunate consequences. A positive wellness decision is made when one seeks out resources that can assist in the recovery and maintenance of positive mental health.

2.2

Activity for Wellness

During the past week:

	Rarely or none of the time (less than 1 day)	Some or a little of the time (1–2 days)	Occasionally or a moderate amount of time (3–4 days)	Most or all of the time (5–7 days)
1. I was bothered by things that usually don't bother me.	0	1	2	3
2. I did not feel like eating; my appetite was poor.	0	1	2	3
3. I felt that I could not shake off the blues even with help from my family or friends.	0	1	2	3
4. I felt that I was just as good as other people.	0	1	2	3
5. I had trouble keeping my mind on what I was doing.	0	1	2	3
6. I felt depressed.	0	1	2	3
7. I felt that everything I did was an effort.	0	1	2	3
8. I felt hopeful about the future.	0	1	2	3
9. I thought my life had been a failure.	0	1	2	3
10. I felt fearful.	0	1	2	3
11. My sleep was restless.	0	1	2	3
12. I was happy.	0	1	2	3
13. I talked less than usual.	0	1	2	3
14. I felt lonely.	0	1	2	3
15. People were unfriendly.	0	1	2	3
16. I enjoyed life.	0	1	2	3
17. I had crying spells.	0	1	2	3
18. I felt sad.	0	1	2	3
19. I felt that people disliked me.	0	1	2	3
20. I could not get going.	0	1	2	3

currently prescribed by physicians, including MAO inhibiters, tricyclics, and the newer SSRI (Prozac, Paxil, and Zoloft) and SNRI antidepressant drugs. All of these drugs are believed to act on the neurotransmitters in the brain, correcting imbalances (see figure 2.4). An individual must take antidepressant drugs for four to six weeks before they will begin to feel the full effects of the medication. Side effects are common with many of the antidepressant medications and should be carefully monitored (see table 2.3).

Figure 2.4: How antidepressants work.

Depression is thought to be caused by a chemical imbalance in the brain. Chemicals known as neurotransmitters, particularly serotonin and norepinephrine, act as "messengers" transmitting signals from one nerve cell (neuron) to the next at the gap, or synapse, between cells. When a nerve cell sends neurotransmitters to another cell, some bind to the receptors on the next nerve cell, but others are reabsorbed by the sending cell in a process called reuptake.

Scientists think that the excessive reabsorption of neurotransmitters from the synapse creates a chemical imbalance that may lead to a depressive disorder. Prozac and other "selective serotonin reuptake inhibitors" (SSRIs) block the reuptake of serotonin, allowing it to remain in the synapse for a longer time. Other antidepressants block the reuptake of both serotonin and norepinephrine, as well as other neurotransmitters.

From *CQ Researcher*, August 19, 1994, Vol. 4 No. 31, p. 724. Reprinted by permission of Congressional Quarterly, Inc., Washington, D.C.

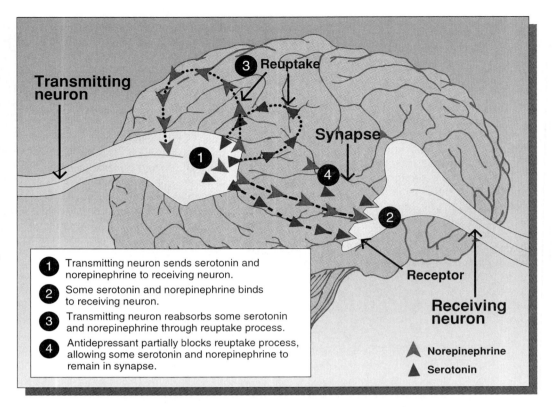

1. Transmitting neuron sends serotonin and norepinephrine to receiving neuron.
2. Some serotonin and norepinephrine binds to receiving neuron.
3. Transmitting neuron reabsorbs some serotonin and norepinephrine through reuptake process.
4. Antidepressant partially blocks reuptake process, allowing some serotonin and norepinephrine to remain in synapse.

▲ Norepinephrine
▲ Serotonin

Prozac, one of the new SSRI antidepressant drugs, has been the subject of great controversy since its introduction in 1988. Mental health professionals initially found Prozac to be an attractive drug for the treatment of depression because it has fewer and less severe effects and it is more difficult to take a lethal overdose with Prozac.[22] However, shortly after its introduction, psychiatrists and psychologists expressed concerns that Prozac was being over prescribed. Additionally, they noted that less than half of the prescriptions for Prozac are being written by psychiatrists, and that many patients are not receiving other appropriate therapies for depression along with the medication. Current research indicates that a patient will receive the best results when antidepressant drugs are combined with "talk therapy."[23] Other concerns about Prozac have been raised, including allegations that its use causes violent or suicidal behavior in some individuals. In October 1991, after reviewing the allegations and research on Prozac, the FDA's Psychopharmacological Drugs Advisory Committee ruled that the available data did not support a causal link between the use of Prozac and violent or suicidal behavior. The debate continues in the courts, however, as product liability suits against the manufacturer come forward.

Antidepressant drugs are only one of several important treatments currently available to people suffering from severe depression. As mentioned previously, counseling is an important tool in helping individuals cope with depression.

Talk Therapy

There are four major approaches to the use of talk therapy for the treatment of depression. These include psychoanalytic therapy, cognitive therapy, interpersonal therapy, and behavioral therapy.[24]

Psychoanalytic therapy originated with the work of Freud, and attempts to discover unconscious childhood conflicts that may be causing the patient's depression. Psychoanalysts believe that by remembering the childhood trauma, the depressed individual can better deal with it, thus gaining relief from his/her depression as well.

Cognitive therapy attempts to deal with issues of self-esteem and pessimism. The goal of cognitive therapy is to help depressed persons learn to think about themselves, others, and the world in more realistic and optimistic terms. This therapy is often used in patients with moderate levels of depression.

Interpersonal therapy seeks to establish more satisfying ties with significant others in

TABLE 2.3   *Antidepressants Available in the U.S.*

Type	Name	Effect	Side Effects
Tricyclics	Elavil (amitriptyline) Tofranil (imipramine) Norpramin (desipramine) and 29 other brand names (six other compounds)	Believed to increase levels of serotonin and/or norepinephrine, neurotransmitters associated with mood elevation.	Danger of overdose by suicidal patients. Serious side effects include irregular heartbeat, muscle tremors, nervousness, weight gain, sexual impairment.
MAO Inhibitors	Marplan (isocarboxazid) Nardil (phenelzine) Parnate (tranylcypromine)	Inhibits action of the enzyme monoamine oxidase (MAO), which breaks down serotonin, norepinephrine and dopamine.	Can be lethal if overdosed or taken with certain foods. Side effects include dizziness, difficult urination, blurred vision.
Bupropion	Wellbutrin	May inhibit reuptake of dopamine, a neurotransmitter.	Side effects include agitation, anxiety, irregular heartbeat, severe headache.
Selective Serotonin Reuptake Inhibitors (SSRI)	Prozac (fluoxetine) Paxil (paroxetine) Zoloft (setraline)	Enhances action of serotonin by increasing its concentration at the synapse between brain cells. Effective in about 60 percent of cases like earlier antidepressants.	Minimal overdose risk though some claim it prompts ideas of suicide. Fewer side effects than older drugs, including agitation, nausea, drowsiness.
Serotonin-Norepinephrine Reuptake Inhibitors (SNRI)	Effexor (venlafaxine)	Enhances action of both serotonin and norepinephrine.	Side effects similar to SSRIs. May help patients who don't respond to SSRIs.

From *CQ Researcher,* August 19, 1994, Vol. 4 No. 3, p. 732. Reprinted by permission of Congressional Quarterly, Inc., Washington, D.C.

a depressed person's life. This type of therapy is most useful when the depression was caused by a broken relationship, or possibly caused strain on important relationships. Often, significant others, such as family or friends, participate actively in the therapy sessions.

Behavior therapy attempts to address negative behavior patterns of a depressed individual. Learning to substitute more positive behaviors is the goal of this form of therapy.

Talk therapy is considered a very helpful tool in dealing with depression. However, talk therapy is usually a lengthy process. In some cases, a form of treatment with more immediate results is needed.

Electroconvulsive Therapy

Electroconvulsive therapy (ECT), also known as electroshock therapy, was first used to treat depression in the 1930s. With the advent of antidepressant drugs, this form of treatment lost favor. Recently, however, improvements in ECT techniques have increased the perceived value of this treatment for depression.[25] ECT consists of the application

of electrodes to the patient's head and the delivery of a brief dose of low-voltage electric shock. ECT usually requires six to twelve shock treatments. The most important side effect of this treatment appears to be the temporary loss of memory. According to the National Institute of Mental Health, most patients who agree to use ECT to treat depression are "successful doctors, lawyers, and businessmen who become depressed and want to get over it as soon as possible. They don't want to wait out the time it takes for a drug to work."[26]

The most important thing to remember about depression is that it is currently the most treatable mental disorder. It is very important to learn to recognize the signs and symptoms of depression, and then seek help if you or someone you know is depressed. Table 2.4 will help you locate appropriate help for dealing with depression.

Like depression, stress can be a barrier to mental wellness. However, as Kenneth Pelletier's *Sound Mind, Sound Body* study illustrated, learning to effectively cope with stress can enhance your chance of experiencing high-level wellness.

TABLE 2.4 — Resources for the Treatment of Depression

If you are seeking therapy, potential sources of referrals include teaching hospitals, university departments of psychology and social work, and local self-help groups. Increasingly, employee assistance programs are offering confidential counseling and referrals. Resources are voluminous, and your local library is a good place to start. You can also check the "Mental Health" section of the Yellow Pages.

Two Useful Sources

- *The Family Guide to Mental Health* (Prentice Hall, 1991), edited by Benjamin Wolman, offers brief descriptions in lay terms of a wide range of treatments and defines various disorders.
- The free pamphlet *A Consumer's Guide to Mental Health Services* is available from the Public Health Service, Alcohol, Drug Abuse, and Mental Health Administration, Rockville, MD 20857.

Professional Associations (partial listing)

- The American Psychiatric Association offers a series of pamphlets on mental disorders, substance abuse, and how to choose a psychiatrist. Single copies are free. Write to the APA Division of Public Affairs, 1400 K Street, NW, Washington, DC 20005.
- The American Psychological Association also publishes pamphlets on mental-health problems, as well as lists of psychological associations in your area. Send a self-addressed stamped envelope to 750 First Street, NE, Washington, DC 20002–4242.
- The National Association of Social Workers can refer you to a licensed practitioner in your area. Write to them at 750 First Street, NE, Washington, DC 20002; or call 202–408–8600.
- The American Association for Marriage and Family Therapy will send you a brochure and list of therapists in your area. Write to them at 1100 Seventeenth Street, NW, 10th floor, Washington, DC 20036; or call 800-374-2638.

Self-Help Groups

- The American Self-Help Clearinghouse can direct you to groups in your area. Write to 25 Pocono Road, St. Clares-Riverside Medical Center, Denville, NJ 07834; or call 201–625–7101.

Reprinted by permission from the *University of California at Berkeley Wellness Letter,* © Health Letter Associates, 1992.

Stress: A Mental Wellness Challenge

Dealing with stress in a productive manner is one of the biggest challenges we face in our search for mental wellness. Stress management may be more appropriately referred to as **life management.** Life management refers to everything that you do to adapt and remain functioning as a person. It includes the simple little things that come naturally and the more complex strategies that require constant effort. Managing your life more effectively does not call for the elimination of stress. Rather, life management directs us to channel stress, thus promoting stimulation, challenge, and growth experiences. Before we introduce you to a variety of life-management skills, it is helpful for you to have an understanding of the stress response.

The Meaning of Stress

Hans Selye, a pioneer researcher on stress, has described **stress** as the "nonspecific response of the body to any demand made upon it."[27] Although each demand is unique or specific, according to Selye, each event calls for adaptation by the body. It is this demand for readjustment that is referred to as nonspecific. Selye further states that, whether we consider a demand or situation to be pleasant or unpleasant, each demand requires us to readjust or adapt, thus creating the stress response.

This description of stress depicts three key points. First, stress is the "reaction" or mobilization of bodily resources in response to a stimulus. Second, there is mobilization of resources for adaptive or adjustment purposes. Third, the stimulus can be pleasant and desirable or unpleasant and undesirable.

Life management: everything a person does to adapt and attain optimal functioning. Life management involves channeling stress so that it leads to higher levels of wellness.

Stress: the body's response to a stimulus, either pleasant or unpleasant. The stress response consists of a mobilization of bodily resources for adaptation.

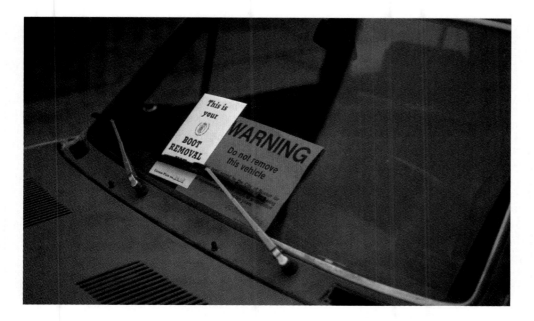

Figure 2.5: What Do You Think?

1. Stressors come in many forms. Would a boot placed on your car, making it impossible for you to drive until you paid a fine, be a stressor for you?
2. What other events in your life would you label stressors?

Stressors

The agent or stimulus that elicits the stress reaction is referred to as the **stressor.** Each day you encounter a variety of stressors with a range of intensity. Types of stressors include bioecological stressors, such as noise and jet lag; personality stressors, such as anxiety, frustration, and worry; and psychosocial stressors, such as a new girlfriend or boyfriend, a new job, and crowded conditions.[28] These categories are not exhaustive, but they do illustrate that in each of our lives there are numerous potential triggers for eliciting stress (see figure 2.5).

Intensity of Stressors

In addition to a variety of stressors, there is also a range in the strength of the response the stressor elicits. This is referred to as intensity and can be viewed as a continuum with **minor stressors** on the one end and **major stressors** on the other. Most of the stressors encountered daily are minor stressors, such as getting up late, running to class, and exhilaration over an unexpectedly high grade on a test. They are encountered and adapted to with varying degrees of regularity. More intense stressors, such as the death of a friend or family member, pregnancy or fathering a pregnancy, or transferring to another school, can be major stressors. It is a mistake, however, to assume that major stressors are harmful and minor stressors are not harmful. All stressors elicit the stress response to some degree and require that we adapt or cope.

Perception of Stressors

According to Hans Selye, it is not the stressor that is important, but "how you take it." One interpretation of "how you take it" is how you perceive the event and the meaning attached to it. This partially explains why people do not respond to the same stimulus with the same intensity or duration. What is a stressor for your friends, roommates, or family may not be a stressor for you. Each person's unique combination of personality, behavior patterns, life experiences, socialization experiences, and beliefs is involved. The kind and amount of stress, as well as how one copes with stress, are directly related to perception (see Of Special Interest 2.1).

Desirability: Eustress and Distress

Into every person's life some stress must fall; to be alive is to experience stress. It is our mind's and body's way of adapting. In this context, the only way you can be totally free of stress is to be dead. Selye coined the term **eustress** to designate desirable stress. Eustress is the stress that is experienced to maintain life, such as through cardiovascular regulation, digestion, and hormonal secretions. Desirable stress also includes life events in which the individual is taxed, challenged, and perceives a potential for personal growth. How one reacts to a stressor is a prime determinant of eustress (see figure 2.6). College athletes, for instance, commonly experience stress, both before and during their competition. Most athletes

Minor stressors: pleasant or unpleasant stimuli that one encounters and adapts to on a regular or daily basis.

Major stressors: pleasant or unpleasant stimuli that tend to evoke an intense stress response.

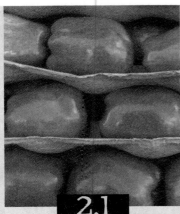

2.1
Of Special Interest

Resilience: The Seven Strengths

If you've lived through a troubled child-hood and come out on top, you can probably thank a handful of personal strengths that have allowed you to build a better life. Some of these are person-ality traits with which you were born; others you developed at an early age. Psychiatrist Steven Wolin and develop-mental psychologist Sybil Wolin identify seven such strengths, which they call resiliencies, in their book, *The Resilient Self*, based on their work with adult sur-vivors of adversity.

Insight: You ask tough questions of yourself and others and don't shy away from honest answers. As a child you became a careful observer and learned to rely on your own interpretations of events, not on what others told you. As an adult you've learned to see things as they are and refuse to blame yourself for your family's troubles.

Independence: You've learned to separate yourself both physically and emotionally from your family's problems. As a child, when things got tough at home, you escaped—to a friend's house, into school activities, into your books or hobbies. When you grew up you may have moved out of town and curtailed visits home. When you do visit, you've learned to avoid letting family members draw you into their unhappiness.

Relationships: You've developed close relationships to substitute for the ones you couldn't achieve with those who failed you. As a child you learned to keep an eye out for concerned adults and became skilled at recruiting their attention and affection. You've cultivated a close circle of friends as a substitute family and in choosing a mate may have picked one with the type of close-knit family you always wished you had.

Initiative: You believe you are master of your fate. Resilient children are often hardworking. They welcome challenges and develop clear and realistic goals. Resilient adults manage to build secure and happy homes for themselves and their children.

Creativity: You've learned to bring order out of confusion in a way that makes your life more pleasing. As a child at play in a rich imaginary world, you practiced overcoming the evil forces that threatened your happiness. As you grew, you learned to express your inner turmoil through writing, music, art, or dance.

Humor: You keep your pain in perspective by finding the lighter side of your troubles. Children from unhappy homes often use humor to defuse difficult situations. Resilient adults are often adept at finding the absurd amid the pathos of their troubled pasts.

Morality: Your painful childhood prompted you to develop a sense of compassion and concern for others. Resilient children early on develop a clear sense of right and wrong. Resilient adults often take risks to pursue what they think is right and find meaning in serving others.

It's important to acknowledge your inner strengths, the Wolins say, in order to develop a healthy dose of survivor's pride. That in turn will help you avoid the victim's trap—the mind-set that dwells on pain rather than accomplishment. "Get revenge by living well instead of squandering your energy by blaming and faultfinding," the Wolins suggest. "Break the cycle of your family's troubles and put the past in its place."

What Do You Think?

1. Do you know anyone personally who has had a difficult life, yet has managed to cope well and live a good life? Describe that person in terms of lifestyle and personality characteristics.
2. Does the person you described fit the Wolin's description of resiliency? If so, does that person seem to you to have a high level of wellness?

---

perceive this stress as eustress. Before the competition the stress response helps them "get up for the game." During competition, controlled and channeled stress helps bring out the athlete's best effort.

The flip side of eustress is **distress.** Generally, distress is taken to mean too much stress. But how much stress is too much? Broadly speaking, distress is experiencing too many stressors in a short time. It may also be too many stressors over the long haul, exceeding your ability to cope effectively and remain in control. Intense, prolonged, and unrelenting stress carries with it the potential to wear the mind and body down, affect system and organ functioning, and upset physical and psychological balance. How much is too much varies from person to person.

The Physiology of Stress

Stress is a response to a stimulus—a response involving interaction between the brain and subsequent reactions throughout varying

Distress: a state of physical or psychological imbalance resulting from exposure to intense, prolonged, or unrelenting stressors.

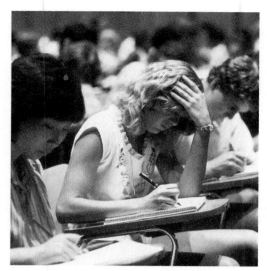

Figure 2.6: What Do You Think?

1. Exams can seem less of a stressor if you view them as an opportunity to learn or demonstrate what you know. How do you perceive exams? Does your perception of the stressfulness of exams relate to how well you prepared for them?

organs of the body. These complex reactions maintain the **homeostasis,** or balanced state, of the body. Homeostasis involves coordinated processes that keep the body from deviating so far from the norm that illness, disease, or death might result. The physiology of the stress response is essential for homeostasis.

The stress response occurs through two major pathways in the body: the **central nervous system** and the **endocrine system.** The manifestations each person recognizes when under stress include increased heart rate, increased breathing rate, increased perspiration, increased muscle tension, a dry mouth, and a general overall increase in body metabolism. Central nervous system stimulation and endocrine secretions are responsible for these manifestations.

The Nervous System Pathway

The central nervous system (CNS) consists of the brain and spinal cord. Brain function is divided into two parts: a voluntary system and an autonomic system. The **autonomic nervous system (ANS)** regulates bodily functions not normally controlled voluntarily, such as heart rate, breathing rate, and glandular secretions.

Nervous system involvement begins immediately when a stressor is encountered. As soon as a stressor is perceived, the outer layer of the brain transmits certain chemical messages to the **hypothalamus.** The hypothalamus is then responsible for stimulation of the autonomic nervous system. Since energy expenditure is required to meet a stressor, the ANS stimulates body metabolism, affecting various bodily functions (see figure 2.7). One of the major targets of the ANS stimulation are the **adrenal glands,** which, when stimulated, release the hormones **adrenalin** and **noradrenalin.** Adrenalin and noradrenalin are the action preparation hormones of the body and are often responsible for the remarkable feats accomplished during emergencies.

The demands most likely to trigger the ANS, with subsequent release of the action preparation hormones, are fear, severe pain, anger, and any situation that threatens physical harm.

The Endocrine System Pathway

Simultaneously with nervous system stimulation, the hypothalamus releases a hormone called **corticotropin releasing factor (CRF),** whose function is to activate the pituitary glands. The pituitary glands, when stimulated by CRF, secrete another hormone, called **adrenocorticotrophic hormone (ACTH),** into the general body circulation. Once in the bloodstream, the ACTH circulates to its target, the adrenal glands. The adrenal glands then secrete hormones into the bloodstream to assist in meeting the demands of stressors.

The **endocrine pathway hormones** increase body metabolism for greater energy, both during stress and during recovery from stress. Fat and protein substances are processed to form **glucose,** the energy provider. The body also retains extra sodium (salt), resulting in increased water retention. This, in turn, increases blood volume, blood pressure, and the amount of blood to be pumped by the heart with each beat. Effects from the endocrine pathway are presented in figure 2.7.

These two pathways of the stress response have evolved to provide humans with the ability to meet the demands of living; however, as the stress response became more refined during its evolutionary development, the demands of living changed drastically. New demands, rapid change, the breakdown of traditional ways of responding to life events, and countless other

Endocrine system: all glands that secrete hormones directly into the blood or body fluids. This system consists of the pituitary, thyroid, parathyroid, and adrenal glands, as well as the pancreas, ovaries, testes, pineal gland, and thymus gland.

Hypothalamus: a small portion of the brain that is involved in the regulation of a number of body functions including water metabolism, temperature regulation, appetite, thirst, blood-sugar level, growth, sleep, certain emotions such as anger, and cycles of the reproductive system. It is also the center of the autonomic nervous system.

Adrenal glands: endocrine glands located on the tops of the kidneys.

Endocrine pathway hormones: substances released directly into blood or body fluids from the endocrine system.

Glucose: a form of carbohydrate (simple sugar) that is the major energy-supplying molecule for the brain.

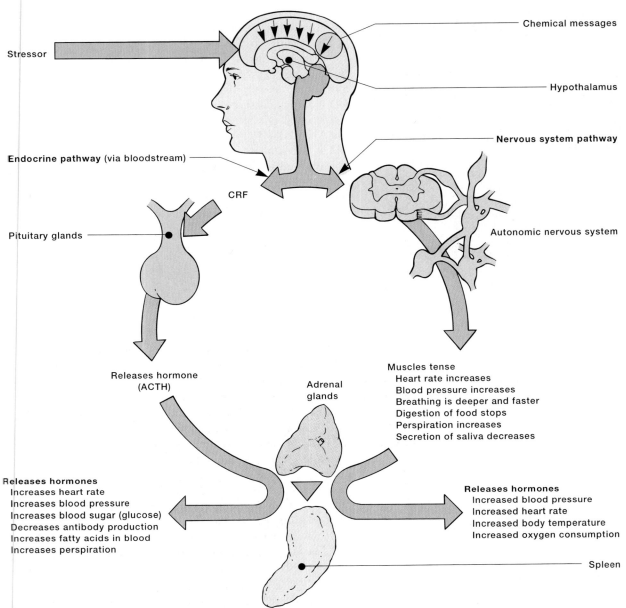

Figure 2.7: Stressors affect various bodily functions.

The following labels appear in the figure:

Stressor

Chemical messages

Hypothalamus

Nervous system pathway

Endocrine pathway (via bloodstream)

CRF

Pituitary glands

Autonomic nervous system

Releases hormone (ACTH)

Adrenal glands

Muscles tense
Heart rate increases
Blood pressure increases
Breathing is deeper and faster
Digestion of food stops
Perspiration increases
Secretion of saliva decreases

Releases hormones
Increases heart rate
Increases blood pressure
Increases blood sugar (glucose)
Decreases antibody production
Increases fatty acids in blood
Increases perspiration

Releases hormones
Increased blood pressure
Increased heart rate
Increased body temperature
Increased oxygen consumption

Spleen

Release of more RBCs
Blood clotting ability increases
More white blood cells produced

complexities of contemporary society have led to an assortment of stress-related problems and new challenges for its management.

The Problem and the Challenge of Stress

The stress response of our ancestors was a survival skill and prepared them to stalk game and protect themselves from human and animal intruders. When the stress response was elicited it was for life-threatening reasons. Physical activity usually followed the stress arousal. Excess energy was burned up and hormones broken down and disposed.

We are symbolic reactors today. Rather than confronting life-threatening stressors, life today centers around events that hold symbolic meaning. Should this symbolism be perceived to be threatening, the stress response is elicited. Today's norms do not readily allow appropriate release of the

TABLE 2.5 — Stress-Related Disorders Dubbed "Diseases of Adaptation"

- Coronary heart disease
- Hypertension
- Stroke
- Diabetes
- Cancer

- Colitis
- Peptic ulcer
- Gout
- Diarrhea, constipation

- Allergies
- Asthma
- Thyroid malfunction
- Headache

available energy. Rarely is physically attacking the source of stress acceptable, neither is fleeing from it. An upcoming test, a disagreement with a friend, the boredom of a job, or the lack of money to finance school are all examples of situations where both fighting and fleeing are unacceptable. Each of these stressors has some symbolic representation to the person experiencing them; none is life-threatening. These stressors may not bring about a complete stress reaction, but the result is significant physiological changes within the body.

Distress, or stress gone bad, can be described as encountering too many stressors within a short period of time, thus exceeding a person's ability to cope effectively. Should distress continue over time, body organs and systems can become fatigued. This wear and tear can result in illness or dysfunction. Many modern afflictions are conditions that result from a maladjustment of human beings to their physical and social environment. For this reason, the stress-related disorders have been dubbed "diseases of adaptation" (see table 2.5). This list does not include emotional and mental problems such as depression, suicide, and human abuse, which number in the millions and have also been linked to distressed individuals.

Most diseases have multiple causes, including factors such as heredity, personality, and ability to cope. It would be inappropriate to conclude that stress is *the* cause of diseases of adaptation, or that by effectively managing stress these problems will disappear. Human beings and disease causation are far too complex to reduce to a simplistic and narrow view. (A variety of diseases and their possible causes are discussed in more detail in chapters 10, 11, and 12.)

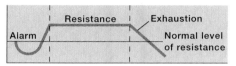

Figure 2.8: Stressors can cause greater susceptibility to disease and illness.

The General Adaptation Syndrome

One theory that attempts to explain the relationship between stress and disease was advanced by Selye. As early as 1936, Selye noticed in animal experiments a predictable way of responding to stress. Later, this became known as the **general adaptation syndrome (GAS).**[29] Its three stages—the alarm reaction, the stage of resistance, and the stage of exhaustion—describe the stress response and the adaptability of the body to stress.

When the human body experiences homeostasis, it is able to maintain a normal level of resistance to disease and can function at an optimal level. When exposed to stressors, however, the human body reacts in the manner illustrated in figure 2.8.

Alarm

First, during the **alarm stage,** the body awakens to the stressor. It is during the alarm phase that people experience the typical signs and symptoms of the stress response, such as muscle tension, a pounding heart, and butterflies in the stomach. The body gears up to deal with the stressor. During the alarm stage, general resistance to disease is decreased. Table 2.6 presents some of the more common signs and symptoms of the stress response. Take a moment to assess which of these symptoms you usually notice while experiencing stress.

TABLE 2.6 — Some of the More Common Signs and Symptoms of Stress

Emotional	Cardiorespiratory
Forgetfulness	Heart pounding
Nervousness	Cold, sweaty hands
Worrying	Headaches (throbbing pain)
Difficulty sleeping	Shortness of breath
	Rapid breathing

Muscular	Gastrointestinal
Shaky hands	Upset stomach
Back pain	Constipation
Tension headaches	Diarrhea
Stiff muscles	
Twitches	

Resistance

The second stage, **resistance,** is characterized by a rebound effect aimed at resisting the stressor. During this stage, the body attempts to adapt to the stressor and return to a balanced state of functioning. Successful adaptation leads to an increased level of resistance to disease and a disappearance of the alarm reaction. All people experience the first two stages of the GAS many times. Only under extreme conditions do most people enter the third stage—exhaustion.

Exhaustion

In the **stage of exhaustion** the body once again experiences the symptoms of the stress response. Exhaustion is the result of continued exposure to a stressor to which the body has already adjusted. Prolonged wear and tear of stressors can cause organs to become fatigued, leading to greater susceptibility to disease and illness. (In figure 2.8, note the line crossing below the normal level of resistance.)

Change and Adaptation

All change requires adjustment by the human body. Energy is used to adapt to new or novel circumstances. In contemporary society, change is inherent in the life cycle. Gail Sheehy, author of *Passages: Predictable Crises of Adult Life,* has written that throughout the life cycle there are predictable **marker events.**[30] Marker events are changes or events that are intense stressors when experienced. They are specific to developmental stages of

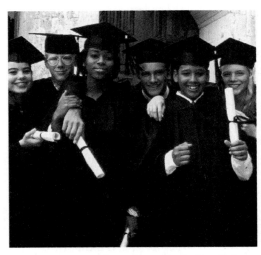

Figure 2.9: What Do You Think?

1. College graduation is the kind of marker event that can prove both exhilarating and stressful. What other marker events have you previously experienced that were both positive yet stressful?
2. Can you predict marker events you are likely to experience in the near future? How will you cope with them?

growth, as well as to social and cultural factors that influence them. Going to school for the first time is a marker event, as are graduating from high school, marriage, divorce, singlehood, having children, beginning a new career, and retirement. Marker events, as well as other less intense life events, can be either positive or negative. Graduation, marriage, and your first child are generally viewed as positive life changes (see figure 2.9). Each, however, requires adaptation specific to the event as well as prior to and after the event.

It has been discovered that the number, clustering, and intensity of major life changes experienced by a person in a short time can serve as a predictor of illness, injury, or psychological problems. The original instrument used to predict this relationship was the Social Readjustment Rating Scale (SRRS) developed by Thomas Holmes and Richard Rahe.[31] The SRRS has been researched with thousands of people from all walks of life. It lists forty-three life events that require significant adaptation or coping behavior. Theoretically, the more life changes per unit of time, the greater the physiological changes and use of body energy to resist stressors. The scoring mechanism of these forty-three events makes it possible to predict with some consistency the onset of an illness, injury, or depression.

Being a college student is a marker event. Many new life changes are occurring. A version of the SRRS for college students was developed to reflect more accurately life events of college students.[32] To see how recent events are affecting you, fill in the scale in Activity for Wellness 2.3.

Before reaching conclusions about predicting illness, two important facts about major life changes must be recognized. First, people vary in their ability to handle change. Some can adjust to major change with little distress, while others do not cope as well. The scale presented here only "predicts"; it is not absolute. Some students with a very high score will remain well; others with a very low score will become ill. Second, major life changes do not and need not produce distress. The adverse effects of change can be controlled. One obvious way to manage the stress of major life events involves planning. Using the Scores for Life-Change Events inventory as a self-assessment tool, watch for times in your life when you have a large score due to recent major life changes. At these times it makes sense to postpone or reschedule any major voluntary life changes. For instance, if you are just about to graduate from college, start a new job, and take out a loan for that much-needed car, it may be wise to delay another voluntary life change such as marriage. Planning can give you time to adapt to changes that have already occurred or changes over which you have little control before you undertake additional stressors.

Stimulation, challenge, and change are important ingredients for personal growth. They are also stressful. Stress can control us or we can learn to control it. Understanding more about yourself, life changes, and managing stress can equip you to deal with stress. Stress does not have to be delegated to a painful part of life to be endured. Illness, disease, and dysfunction are only one side of the stress issue. There is a more positive side of stress; stress can also be a challenge that leads to mental wellness.

Learning to control stress, not avoiding it, is the challenge. Controlling stress encourages us to view life in a positive manner regardless of our circumstances. Controlling stress is a challenge to become more sensitive to our physical selves in an artificial world. It is learning how to become more congruent, more real, and more alive. It is a challenge to make your life work better. There are no promises with this challenge. There are no guarantees that one will live longer. But those who accept the challenge to manage life's stress will tell you that it is a richer, fuller, healthier way to be alive. Developing your personal stress-management strategies and coping skills is one way to assume the challenge of enhancing mental wellness.

Promoting Mental Wellness through Stress Management

Managing stress is an ongoing process. It is learning more about who we are as human beings, why we act and react to the world around us as we do, and how to deal more effectively with life's insults and frustrations as well as its joys and pleasures. Some specific techniques are offered in this section. They are presented in light of the following principles.

1. Learning to manage life and stress requires an understanding of the stress response and appropriate management strategies to use when stress is out of control. Awareness is developed through conscious and regular assessment. It is consciously paying attention to the mental, physical, and social forces that impinge upon our lives. Awareness is learning to recognize and channel stress appropriately, thus reducing distress.

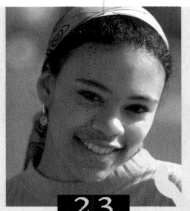

Activity for Wellness

Scores for Life-Change Events

To find your score on this scale, in Column A place the number of times during the last twelve months that you have experienced the event listed. Multiply the number under Column B by the number in Column A and place it in Column C. Remember to count *each* time you experienced the event. Finally, total Column C. If your score totals 1,435 or higher, you are in the "high" category for developing an illness. If your total is 347 or less, you fall into the "low" category. The "medium" score is 890.

Column A	Life-Change Event	Column B	Column C
_____	1. Entered college	50	_____
_____	2. Married	77	_____
_____	3. Trouble with your boss	38	_____
_____	4. Held a job while attending school	43	_____
_____	5. Experienced the death of a spouse	87	_____
_____	6. Major change in sleeping habits	34	_____
_____	7. Experienced the death of a close family member	77	_____
_____	8. Major change in eating habits	30	_____
_____	9. Change in or choice of major field of study	41	_____
_____	10. Revision of personal habits	45	_____
_____	11. Experienced the death of a close friend	68	_____
_____	12. Found guilty of minor violations of the law	22	_____
_____	13. Had an outstanding personal achievement	40	_____
_____	14. Experienced pregnancy, or fathered a pregnancy	68	_____
_____	15. Major change in health or behavior of family member	56	_____
_____	16. Had sexual difficulties	58	_____
_____	17. Had trouble with in-laws	42	_____
_____	18. Major change in number of family get-togethers	26	_____
_____	19. Major change in financial state	53	_____
_____	20. Gained a new family member	50	_____
_____	21. Change in residence or living conditions	42	_____
_____	22. Major conflict or change in values	50	_____
_____	23. Major change in church activities	36	_____
_____	24. Marital reconciliation with your mate	58	_____
_____	25. Fired from work	62	_____
_____	26. Were divorced	76	_____
_____	27. Changed to a different line of work	50	_____

2. Too much distress can lead to health problems, yet short-term distress forces us to turn our conscious attention to the source. We may discover a new insight, clarify a value, or modify a health habit that contributed to the distress. A wiser person emerges; personal growth has taken place. The principle is to benefit from distress by having it work for you rather than against you.

3. There is no single stress-management technique that will work for every person

Column A	Life-Change Event	Column B	Column C
_____	28. Major change in number of arguments with spouse	50	_____
_____	29. Major change in responsibilities at work	47	_____
_____	30. Had your spouse begin or cease work outside the home	41	_____
_____	31. Major change in working hours or conditions	42	_____
_____	32. Marital separation from mate	74	_____
_____	33. Major change in type and/or amount of recreation	37	_____
_____	34. Major change in use of drugs	52	_____
_____	35. Took on a mortgage or loan of less than $10,000	52	_____
_____	36. Major personal injury or illness	65	_____
_____	37. Major change in use of alcohol	46	_____
_____	38. Major change in social activities	43	_____
_____	39. Major change in amount of participation in school activities	38	_____
_____	40. Major change in amount of independence and responsibility	49	_____
_____	41. Took a trip or a vacation	33	_____
_____	42. Engaged to be married	54	_____
_____	43. Changed to a new school	50	_____
_____	44. Changed dating habits	41	_____
_____	45. Trouble with school administration	44	_____
_____	46. Broke or had broken a marital engagement or steady relationship	60	_____
_____	47. Major change in self-concept or self-awareness	57	_____
		Total	_____

Source: Data from M.T. Mark et al., "The Influence of Recent Life Experiences on the Health of College Freshmen," in *Journal of Psychosomatic Research*, vol. 19, p. 87, 1975.

or for the same person in different stress situations. The total-person approach to stress management is one that recognizes the multidimensionality of humans. The whole person is a dynamic interplay between the physical, mental, emotional, social, and spiritual dimensions. An exercise program alone is not sufficient to manage stress, nor is relaxation training, better time management, or improved communication. Each strategy serves a specific purpose, but if done to the exclusion of other strategies, and without consideration for the whole person, it may be less effective.

4. Given the magnitude of options to manage stress, how a person selects the most appropriate strategy at the right time is paramount. One approach is to match the coping technique to the situation at hand. Personal management or organizing skills are particularly effective for the times when life seems out of control, when the work to be done exceeds the available time, or when goals are unclear and values uncertain. Valuing, personal planning, commitment, time management, or pacing might be the skill of choice when organization is the issue.

5. Another approach is to match the coping technique to a person's individual strengths and preferences. Although capitalizing on strengths is often helpful, it can have its drawbacks as Donald Tubesing and Nancy Tubesing point out.

> A person who relies almost exclusively upon organizational skills . . . will probably handle certain job pressures (numerous demands, time pressures, tight deadlines, multiple responsibilities) very effectively. That same person may have difficulty responding appropriately to job or personal situations that evoke a grief reaction. The stress and pain of loss simply does not respond very well to getting better organized. In this situation the individual may want to focus on obtaining some personal support.[33]

The principle is to choose the most appropriate skill based on personal preference and the situation at hand.

6. Trying to learn and implement too many new strategies at one time may become a stressor. On the one hand, you may experience frustration from trying too hard, and on the other, too much change can result in stress. Change, growth, learning new strategies, and refining old ones all take time. Take time to gain insights about the underlying nature of your stressors. Explore a variety of skills to manage your reaction to those stressors. Experience each personal exploration to its fullest.

The primary purpose for developing coping and management skills is to reduce either the frequency or the intensity of the stress response. Daniel Girdano, George Everly, and Dorothy Dusek have presented a categorical scheme of strategies for controlling stress.[34] The scheme encompasses social engineering strategies, personality engineering strategies, and relaxation training. The categories presented here have been adapted to include medical treatment, as health-care providers are important in a comprehensive approach to managing stress.

Social engineering, personality engineering, and relaxation training involve a great number of skills that can be learned and employed by each person prior to the development of distress symptoms. These skills can be learned through self-direction or with the assistance of a professional.

Controlling and channeling stress for wellness includes employing strategies both prior to and during the stress response. Using life-management skills and techniques to prevent too much stress or to improve well-being on a regular basis helps prevent distress. Additionally, these same skills can be used as a part of a midsight approach to stress management. A midsight approach involves intervening in the stress cycle once you become aware that you are experiencing too much stress.

Although life-management strategies are presented here in four categories, it is difficult to separate them. Skills may overlap categories, and some could just as well be presented in a different category, depending upon one's intention for using the skill. For example, Brenda wants to help reduce the intensity of the stress response after taking an exam. She recognizes an increase in tension from a stressor and sets out to do a twenty-minute progressive muscle-relaxation exercise. For this purpose it is listed in the relaxation training category. Deb, however, practices relaxation daily to maintain well-being and for better sleep onset at night; for Deb, relaxation may serve as a social engineering strategy. How and why a skill is used determines its category. The four categories reflect various life-management strategies.

Social Engineering

One option for dealing with the stress response is to deal with the stressor itself. In this **social engineering** approach, stressors are

---

Social engineering strategies: stress management strategies based on the assumption that certain stressors cannot be changed and that managing the stress response calls for modifying one's position or response to such a stressor.

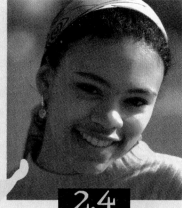

Social Engineering

Skill Development

1. *Identify stressors:* a conscious selection of events that cause stress.
2. *Analyze underlying cause:* determine if the stressor is the result of frustration, overload, deprivation, and so on.
3. *Rationally develop alternatives:* seek new ways of responding to stressors.
4. *List barriers to new ways of responding:* determine the obstacles that may prevent implementation of alternatives.
5. *Rank from most to least desirable:* choose the best alternative and formulate a new plan of action.
6. *Implement new plan:* test the plan in your daily schedule.
7. *Evaluate:* examine the effectiveness of the new plan as a stress-control strategy.
8. *Assess:* determine the need to modify the existing plan or adopt a new approach.

Exercise

Select a current stressor and use the above steps to change or modify your position in relation to the stressor.

2.4

Activity for Wellness

Stressor	Why	Alternatives	Barriers	Rank
Example:				
Rush-hour traffic	Slows me down and loud honking horns	1. leave earlier	may interfere with course schedule	1
		2. leave later		2
		3. try alternate route	takes longer to drive it	3

givens; for instance, you could be experiencing too many changes, frustration, overload, or any number or types of stressors. Once you have assessed the stressor, you may seek alternatives or you may modify your position rather than expend energy trying to change the stressor. In either case, your goal is to reduce how frequently you elicit the stress response.

A simple but effective way to reduce how frequently you elicit the stress response is to analyze your stressors on paper. As you list stressors, try to determine why these events are stressors for *you*. Next, list possible ways of alleviating each stressor. This is a brainstorming session so go for quantity in listing your ideas. Alongside each of the possibilities, identify any barriers to these new ways of responding to stressors. Finally, rank your possibilities from the most feasible to implement to the least feasible. For example, Hollis finds driving home from classes during rush hour very stressful. The slow pace and the honking car horns produce the stress response. Hollis decides that she could arrange her class schedule next semester so that she can either leave campus earlier or later in the day in order to avoid rush-hour traffic. Alternatively, she could look for a

route home that had less traffic at that time of the day. After weighing the barriers and benefits, Hollis decides that scheduling her classes earlier in the day and leaving campus earlier is her best alternative for avoiding the stress caused by rush-hour traffic.

By using this formal approach, you are getting at the source of the problem. The stressor remains the same; you have not changed it. What you have done is to use awareness and effective planning. Like most new approaches, however, it is important to do this in written form. It takes more time to write everything down, but you will quickly discover that in your analysis of stressors and in your brainstorming, there is more completeness and greater understanding of the process. Eventually, the process of alternative selection and ranking will become automatic. If what you chose does not turn out to be the best alternative for you, then you can select again from the many options you originally listed. Activity for Wellness 2.4 provides an opportunity to practice this strategy.

Personality Engineering

Personality includes values, attitudes, and behavior patterns, all of which help to define how one perceives and reacts to stressors.

Personality engineering strategies help to reduce stress by deliberately modifying some aspect of one's personality that has transformed a neutral life event into a psychosocial stressor. Personality engineering strategies also attempt to enhance one's self-concept.

Constructive self-talk is one technique that offers many positive stress-reduction benefits. We all talk to ourselves. Much of the time our self-talk is quite negative. We say things like, "Boy, was that ever a dumb thing to do!" or "I am such a weak person." This type of self-talk can be quite destructive, often keeping people in a state of stress. Self-talk, however, can also be used as a stress-control technique. People can learn to speak pleasantly to themselves, reinforcing the positive aspects of life. Statements such as "I did a good job on that" or "I will do better next time" help to enhance one's level of wellness.

One way to practice positive self-talk is to make affirmations. An **affirmation** is a verbal description of a desired condition stated as if it were present reality. It is something you repeat to yourself over and over again until you become convinced of its reality and your conviction then helps to make it become objectively true.

This approach was introduced by Emile Coué, a French physician, as part of his method of autosuggestion. Coué recommended repeating the phrase, "Every day, in every way, I'm getting better and better." It appears that repetition of this phrase or others like it can have an impact on self-concept and self-confidence.

Write your own affirmation and practice repeating it to yourself five times just before going to bed every night and the next morning when you get up. Think through your affirmation—"I am always on time" may not be as good as "I am easily on time"—and make it a simple statement of what you hope to achieve. Start with just one affirmation. Later, you may want to develop several.

There are a number of other ways you may want to try using affirmations.

a. Type or write your affirmation on a slip of paper and paste it to your mirror, your telephone, or anywhere you will see it often during the day.

b. Sing or chant your affirmation aloud while you are driving or some other time when you are alone—or maybe even if you are not alone.

c. Write your affirmation ten times in the first person—"I, Linden, feel relaxed and confident in front of a group." Then write it ten times in the second person—"You, Linden, feel relaxed and confident in front of a group." Then write it ten times in the third person—"Linden feels relaxed and confident in front of a group."

d. Tape-record yourself reciting your affirmation and listen to them while you are working, driving, or going to sleep.

e. Visualize the desired end result happening right now, with yourself in the picture enjoying it.

f. Draw or paint a picture of yourself living out your affirmation and put it up where you will see it often.

Some personality engineering skills are directed toward offsetting distress that results from the type A behavior pattern. The **type A personality** construct was first described by two cardiologists, Meyer Friedman and Ray Rosenman.[35] They noted common behavioral characteristics in a number of their patients who had manifested cardiovascular problems. Behaviors such as a chronic sense of time urgency (always in a hurry); being time conscious, deadline oriented, and impatient (hostility surfaces quickly when they are delayed); having a preoccupation with describing things in terms of numbers (quantitative rather than qualitative in orientation); being polyphasic (attempting to do or think about more than one task at a time); and being highly competitive are major descriptors of the type A personality. Persons not generally displaying these characteristics, and having seemingly less coronary disease, are referred to as **type B individuals.** Chapter 10 provides an in-depth discussion of type A behavior as a risk factor for coronary artery disease.

Planning, pacing, and commitment skills are the most useful personality engineering strategies for the type A person. The goal is not to change the personality of these individuals but to provide skills that can help them cope more effectively with stress. Thus, it is a person's perceptions of stressors that change, not the stressors themselves.

Like social engineering strategies, the goal of personality engineering is to reduce

Constructive self-talk: a personality engineering strategy that involves talking pleasantly to oneself, repeating statements that focus on positive aspects of one's life.

Type A personality: a personality type exhibited by a person who feels an urgency about time, is competitive, impatient, and is driven to complete tasks as quickly as possible.

Type B personality: a personality type exhibited by a person who is more easy going and less concerned with time pressures.

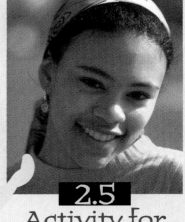

2.5
Activity for Wellness

Personality Engineering

Skill Development

1. *Valuing skills:* developing a philosophy of life, getting in touch with a core meaning to existence.
2. *Planning skills:* establishing goals and choosing to pursue certain goals over others via prioritizing.
3. *Commitment skills:* proactive assertiveness without feeling guilty for saying no, without violating someone else's rights or personhood.
4. *Pacing skills:* determining if one is a "racehorse" or a "turtle" and developing the ability to predict how much one can handle.
5. *Conversation skills:* developing friendships, self-disclosing, attending to nonverbal cues, pursuing details, facilitating questions, listening with empathy.
6. *Relabeling skills:* viewing problems as challenges, opportunities, or amusing vignettes can lead to a more positive outlook on life events, changing perceptions, attitudes, and behaviors.
7. *Whisper skills:* the art of positive self-talk via positive affirmations.
8. *Gentleness skills:* treating yourself kindly, giving yourself pats on the back, and energizing playfulness.

Exercise

Using these skills, modify or change an attitude, value, or behavior in regard to a large project that is due and for which you have had negative thoughts.

1. Identify a large overwhelming project that is due in several weeks

_____

_____

Example: Making a presentation in class next month.

2. Relabel: Make a positive statement about this project several times each day using words like "challenge" or "opportunity." My statement is

_____

_____

Example: This presentation is my opportunity to share what I have learned with my classmates.

3. Plan a steady course of action: use the "Swiss cheese" method of identifying what needs to be accomplished by breaking it down into smaller, more manageable units according to available time or work amount.

Example:

   a. Go to the library and research my topic.
   b. Read and synthesize the research I find.
   c. Write an outline for the presentation.
   d. Write out the text of the presentation based on my outline.
   e. Write and make copies of a summary handout for my classmates.
   f. Practice delivering my presentation in front of the mirror.
   g. Make an affirmation "I, Stephen, will feel relaxed and

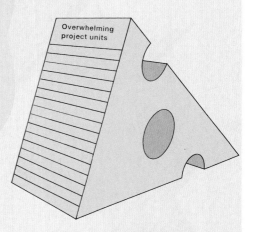

Overwhelming project units

confident when making my presentation."

4. Begin NOW—today—on one unit.
5. Pace: maintain a steady pace by doing something every day even if it is only for fifteen minutes.

---

the frequency with which the stress response is elicited. Activity for Wellness 2.5 illustrates a few personality engineering skills, and provides an opportunity to practice several of them.

Relaxation Training

The third category of life-management strategies encompasses various relaxation skills. The primary purpose of **relaxation training** is to induce systematically a physiological condition that is almost the opposite of the stress response. Table 2.7 compares the physiological response during stress and during relaxation.

There is a growing body of evidence that systematic relaxation training, when performed on a regular basis, is beneficial to health.[36] These benefits can be summarized by saying that relaxation:

1. is enjoyable;
2. can decrease symptoms of illness such as headache, nausea, and diarrhea;

T ABLE 2.7	**Relaxation Is Almost the Opposite of the Stress Response**

Stress	Relaxation
Increased body metabolism	Decreased body metabolism
Increased heart rate	Decreased heart rate
Increased blood pressure	Decreased blood pressure
Increased breathing rate	Decreased breathing rate
Increased oxygen consumption	Decreased oxygen consumption
Increased cardiac output	Decreased cardiac output
Increased muscular tension	Decreased muscular tension
Decreased blood-clotting time	Increased blood-clotting time
Increased blood flow to the major muscle groups involved in the fight-or-flight (including the arms and legs)	

From *Learn to Relax,* 1992, 2nd edition, page 21 by John D. Curtis. Reprinted by permission of Coulee Press, Lacrosse, WI.

3. can increase levels of physical activity;

4. can increase the ability to handle problems and increase overall efficiency and performance;

5. is helpful in the treatment of insomnia, depression, pain, drug abuse, fear and phobias, as well as backache;

6. can lower blood pressure; and

7. can increase resistance to stress, which may explain why some individuals do not overreact to stress as much as others.

While relaxation skills are easily learned, their benefits occur only if they are practiced regularly, preferably every day for a minimum of ten to twenty minutes (see figure 2.10). Researchers have found that people who report that they relax on such a regular basis:[37]

1. are less anxious;

2. feel in greater control of their lives; and

3. generally have a positive mental outlook.

There are many types of relaxation exercises that will, with daily use, lead to these benefits. Activity for Wellness 2.6 outlines a number of relaxation skills and provides more detailed instructions on one simple, but effective, relaxation technique.

In addition to deep muscle relaxation exercises, there are several other skills listed in this category. Brief relaxation, massage, mental diversion, and exercise provide

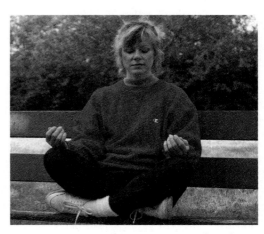

Figure 2.10: What Do You Think?

1. Relaxation skills like yoga, when practiced regularly, lead to important benefits. Do you currently practice a form of relaxation on a daily basis? If so, what benefits have you noticed?

2. If you do not currently practice a relaxation technique daily, how could you motivate yourself to make time for this in your daily routine?

additional relaxing strategies. These skills do not provide deep relaxation in the same way as other relaxation procedures, thus they do not necessarily provide all of the physical and psychological benefits discussed earlier. They do, however, help control mental and physical tension and can be a good adjunct to systematic relaxation training. Many experts, in fact, suggest that a relaxation exercise should follow twenty to thirty minutes of physical exercise (see figure 2.11). Together, they are a powerful combination for physical, mental, and spiritual restoration.

Relaxation Training

Skill Development

1. *Sensory awareness skills:* reeducating yourself to what is happening within your body (perceptions, functions, sensations) at a more conscious level.
2. *Progressive muscle relaxation:* development of "muscle sense" via alternately tensing and relaxing skeletal muscles of the forehead, face, and limbs in a progressive manner to induce physical and mental relaxation.
3. *Benson's relaxation response:* using mental repetition of a word devoid of special meaning (such as the word "one"), a passive attitude, a relaxed posture, and a quiet environment to induce relaxation.
4. *Meditation:* a variety of procedures used to evoke altered states of consciousness for the purposes of peace, enlightenment, or spiritual growth.
5. *Yoga:* assumption of certain postures and control of breathing to increase vital capacity, flexibility, balance, and relaxation.
6. *Biofeedback training:* use of instruments to provide auditory or visual feedback to help yourself learn how to make changes voluntarily in body processes such as muscle tension, heart rate, and blood pressure.
7. *Breathing rhythm skills:* using the breathing rhythm with associative sensations to evoke desired perceptions or physiological occurrences.
8. *Visualization exercises:* a group of exercises that employ conscious intentional imagery, making use of self-suggestions for psychological or physiological purposes.
9. *Brief relaxation exercises:* awareness exercises that aid in managing muscular tension or pace without the physiological benefits of total body relaxation.
10. *Mental diversion skills:* activities such as hiking, gardening, reading, fishing, exercising, and the like that divert attention from stressors and help maintain physical and mental balance.
11. *Massage:* kneading, pummeling, and stroking of muscle groups to increase metabolism, release substances back into circulation, improve lymph drainage, and evoke mental and physical relaxation.

Exercise: Benson's Relaxation Response

Follow the guidelines for Benson's relaxation response. Try the exercise once each day for the next four days for a minimum of ten minutes. Do not be concerned about doing it correctly. Read the exercise description several times until you are familiar with it. Then select an environment where there is minimal interruption and begin.

The four components presented by Benson are:

1. *A Quiet Environment.* While learning to elicit the response, you need a quiet, calm environment where you can be alone for the duration of the exercise. Interruptions or background noise can, in the beginning, change your focus and prevent relaxation. A bedroom seems to be the best place in the home. At work, a private office or a conference room may be adequate. You may want to invest in a "Do Not Disturb" sign to hang on the door. (Even the bathroom can serve as your quiet place, especially if it is the only room in which you can be sure you won't be disturbed.)
2. *A Mental Device.* A relaxation state may be difficult to elicit because your mind is so busy with thoughts about daily activities. Repetition of a single-syllable word, in time with your exhalations, helps you to focus away from thoughts that are distracting and perhaps stressful. The word should be repeated silently or in a low, soothing tone. Some people prefer to picture a word or an object, and some gaze at an object—a flower or a stone. Traditionally, many different words, or "mantras," have been used. Because of its simplicity, follow Benson's suggestion and use the word "one."

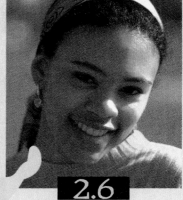

2.6
Activity for Wellness

3. *A Passive Attitude.* The opposite of stress and tension is relaxation. Unlike stress and tension, which can be generated within the body, relaxation cannot be forced to occur. Relaxation is a state that you can only allow to happen. Once you have learned the sequence of the technique, there is no need to be concerned about whether or not relaxation is happening. The harder you work at making it happen, the less likely you are to relax. If your focus on the mental device is interrupted by sounds or people, or if your thoughts wander, passively disregard them. Just return to focusing on your exhalations and your mental device.
4. *A Comfortable Position.* This method can be learned in any of the basic positions. Your body needs to be comfortable and well supported, so that muscle tension is reduced as much as possible. If you find yourself drifting into sleep from a lying position, use a sitting position. Remove or loosen any tight-fitting clothes.

From John D. Curtis and Richard A. Detert, *How to Relax: A Holistic Approach to Stress Management.* Copyright © 1981 by Mayfield Publishing Company, Mountain View, CA.

1. Physical exercise can be a positive
way of managing stress. What types
of physical exercise do you engage in
regularly? Do you use physical
activity as a stress-management
technique?

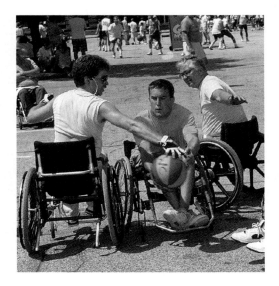

Medical Treatment

In contrast to the first three categories of life-management strategies where the individual is able to assume responsibility, the very nature of **medical treatment** means that some personal responsibility for controlling stress is given up. People normally seek out a medical specialist or health-care provider because of overt physical and mental symptoms or dysfunction. Often this results in a diagnosis and subsequent intervention efforts aimed at returning the person to a state of no discernible illness.

The health-care provider can prescribe medication for treating certain stress symptoms and diseases. In addition, the health-care provider has access to many of the same strategies of social engineering, personality engineering, and relaxation training. For example, a counselor is directly involved in facilitating individuals to examine their belief systems, attitudes, or behavior patterns that may be causing distress. A patient educator might monitor a fitness program to control high blood pressure.

The promise of stress is found in the challenge of its management. There are countless strategies to develop should you decide to accept this challenge.

Expanding Mental Wellness through Awareness and Experience

There is no easy path to wellness. In striving for mental wellness, we must try to practice the elements of mental wellness such as being real, being open to experience, and accepting others without prejudice. Those are not easy tasks, nor is there any single path to wellness. We must each find our own way to wellness.

Expand Your Awareness

Mental wellness incorporates an openness to experience and a joy in the large and the small things in life. It requires a level of awareness that is greater than that of most people. Here are a few activities that may help you to achieve an expanded awareness.

a. Think of some place you have been recently. Write down a detailed description of that place. Then go back and compare your description to the actual place. Try it again. You should get better.

b. Watch a sunrise or sunset without thinking about anything else. Take a walk in the country. Listen carefully to the sounds that are produced by different species of birds. Try to imagine the nature of the communication going on between them. Examine the shapes of the leaves of different kinds of trees. Observe the varied fragrances of wild flowers, and notice the variation in the insects that gather around them. Look at the evening sky. Imagine yourself going from star to star, not in a space vehicle, but just moving in the infinite openness of space. Such undivided attention is far from ordinary.

c. Put together an assortment of foods with contrasting tastes, textures, and temperatures—hot and cold; smooth, crisp, crumbly, and crunchy; sweet, sour, salty, and bitter; and so on. Then try them one after another. Contrast the tastes and try different combinations. Better still, wear a blindfold while a friend feeds bites of the different foods to you; this works best if you haven't seen the foods first.

d. Remember times that you enjoyed touching or being touched by someone (do not just think about sexual touching). Make a point of touching friends—a hug, a pat on the back, squeezing a hand, and so on. This may involve overcoming some anxieties and expanding your behavior options.

e. Exchange massages with a friend. Or massage your own head and neck or your feet. Focus on each of your senses.

f. Keep a private journal. Make a daily record of what you do, what you think, and what you feel. Review your diary or journal once each week at a regular time. Look for patterns in how you react and in how you feel. You may learn a lot about yourself in this way. As you try other activities for wellness, record them in your journal. Look to see what changes, if any, they have stimulated.

As you identify problem areas, set goals for behavior change. Then record the frequency of the goal behavior in your journal and record the consequences that follow the behavior. Changing the consequences is one of the best ways to change the behavior.

Expand Your Experience

It is important for you to be open to experiences and to be able to try new behavior options if you are to achieve mental wellness. The following activities may help you make a start at increasing your openness.

a. When you have choices to make, try brainstorming. Make a list of all the alternatives you can think of without weighing or evaluating any of them until you cannot think of any more alternatives. Then consider them all seriously.

b. For the next three weeks, make a point each week of doing something you never did before. Do not cheat—only significant new somethings count.

c. Do something (legal and not really dangerous) that you never had the nerve to do before. Enter a talent contest, learn to dance, perform a new activity, or do something else daring for you.

d. Explore another culture or lifestyle by living it for a while. You could do this at home or by traveling somewhere.

e. Live a day backwards. Start your day with supper and end it with breakfast. Relax, watch television during the morning; do your work in the evening. Try to think of other things you can reverse for one day. For many of you, this may be impractical but it can be a fascinating experience if you try it.

Personal and Social Influences on Mental Well-Being

Underlying all health attitudes and behaviors are a combination of cultural values, social pressures, and individual needs. The dynamic interaction of these factors can open a person to change and growth or serve as "barriers" to self-understanding and problem solving.

Personal, social, and cultural factors are not isolated from one another. The individual develops and matures as the result of socialization experiences, which are often the result of enculturation and ethnic patterns. We learn through these life experiences how to adjust, adapt, and cope in the world. Here is a sample of factors that impact on mental wellness.

An Inability to Perceive Stress

Odd as it may seem, some individuals do not recognize that they are overstressed. Pressure, tension, and stress symptoms have become a "way of life." This is the way they have been, are, and will continue. Without recognition of stress, there can be little motivation for control of it.

Defense Mechanisms

Defense mechanisms are our natural way to defend ourselves against stressors. For the most part they are unconscious ways of responding. They are learned and used in combination to protect ourselves against distress. Denial, intellectualization, and avoidance are three of the more important ways we use to defend ourselves against distress. When using **denial** as a coping tool we simply refuse to accept reality. This is especially common when coping with a loss such as a death or serious illnesses such as cancer. **Intellectualism** occurs when we transform our feelings into thoughts. This allows us to block unwanted feelings. **Avoidance** is also used to block unwanted emotions. For instance, you may know a fellow student who avoids going to class on the day a test is to be returned in order to avoid the feelings that might accompany a poor grade.

Defense mechanisms can be great pressure valves and serve as buffers to our ego and self-concept. Defense mechanisms can also serve as barriers to managing stress effectively. When overused they can hinder the development of new and exciting ways of

Avoidance: a defense mechanism whereby a person stays away from situations that are perceived to be distressful.

responding to stressful situations. They can keep people from expanding their repertoire of coping skills, thus blocking a more effective match between stressors and management strategies.

Poverty

As we have seen, Maslow's concept of a hierarchy of needs indicates that we cannot move to higher motivational levels until our more basic needs are met. A starving man only feels a need for food. Many people in the U.S. are living at the two lower levels of human needs. If they are not struggling to get enough to eat or to keep a roof over their heads, they are struggling to achieve some degree of security in order to continue to meet those needs in the future.

Stereotypes and Prejudices

A regrettably large part of our cultural learning includes stereotypes and prejudices. It is hard to grow up in our society without becoming influenced by some elements of racism, sexism, ageism, and the whole mass of stereotypes and prejudices that are a part of our culture. Prejudices render us intolerant and unable to accept the differentness of others; they also keep us from seeing things as they are. We cannot be realistic or open to experience in areas in which we are prejudiced and influenced by stereotypes.

In the words of Halbert Dunn:[38]

> The human brain is required to solve problems as they arise in daily life. The brain is so constructed that it will come up with correct solutions if it can. It does its work well to the degree that it has access to the information it needs for the solution of the problem in hand. But erroneous beliefs fixed in the mind, hate and prejudices, and the lack of essential information keep the brain from doing its job and, in the course of time, bring about mental and physical illness.

To whatever extent we accept that a stereotype applies to us and try to live up to it, we are abandoning our authenticity—our realness. By living in a stereotyped fashion we abandon our ability to react in a variety of ways and deny our freedom and responsibility. Our ability to meet our own needs may be vitally impaired by accepting a stereotype for ourselves.

The "Traditional" Nuclear Family

Many of us continue to believe that the typical, "normal" U.S. family is composed of mom and dad and the kids—the "traditional" nuclear family. In fact, such a family pattern is not truly traditional in our society. Prior to World War II, most families in the U.S. were extended families with several generations of adults and their children living together. Only on the frontiers were two-generation families common; the pioneers reared their children alone in their new home. As time passed and the pioneer families became established, they too became multigenerational, extended families. The increasing mobility of the postwar era broke up extended families and the nuclear family became the new norm.

The child raised in an extended family had an assortment of adults to look to for guidance, sympathy, support, and example. There were grandparents, aunts, uncles, and grown-up cousins as well as parents of other children. Such a diversity of role models offered a degree of protection against any bad examples. The normal development of children has always been threatened by disturbed, indifferent, or brutal parents, and in the nuclear family, the harmful influence is undiluted by equally close contact with other adults.

In addition to diluting the effect of bad role models, the extended family exposed children to an array of role models. A diversity of role models does not guarantee that a child will grow up to be tolerant of differences and capable of reacting in a variety of ways, but it does make such elements of mental wellness more likely to be learned.

Today, the nuclear family is once again a minority among U.S. families. Unfortunately, much of the shift away from the nuclear family is due to the growing number of single-parent families, predominantly female-headed. The barriers to wellness are thus heightened rather than diminished. Day care, Big Brother and Big Sister programs, and other arrangements can help give children broader exposure to adult models, but they are not adequate substitutes for family (see A Social Perspective 2.1).

The Pace of Life in the U.S.

U.S. society continues to be transformed at a rapid pace. In less than one hundred years we moved from a predominantly agricultural

Isolation of the Family

Mobility is a cultural trademark for U.S. success. It has reshaped our society several times over the past two centuries. The westward expansion culminated in California becoming our most populous state. Through continual waves of immigration it has also become the most culturally-diverse state. The migration of southern Blacks has fundamentally changed the character of northern cities. Much of the wealth, accumulated in upper and middle income majority groups in the industrial cities of the Northeast and Midwest, has been shifted to suburban areas and to other regions of the country.

The sum of these geographic and demographic changes has been to produce a society in which many families are more isolated from one another and from their extended family heritage than ever before. This does not apply evenly to all ethnic groups; indeed, it appears that certain groups have succeeded in preserving neighborhoods in some cities. Nonetheless, among families who do move, those with the financial means are able to compensate for the loss of neighborhood and extended family by purchasing the lost resources as commodities (i.e., day care, private education, self-controlling entertainment devices). Families in poverty find themselves caught in a fragmenting social process that breeds despair, hopelessness, poor health, undereducation, and violence. These urban areas have been largely abandoned by those who have the resources to move out. Society's general disregard for those (mostly Black and Hispanic) who are locked in urban poverty, dovetails with a fear of urban violence to further enforce a degree of isolation. This type of isolation is obviously much more debilitating than the type based on the mobility that characterizes the more affluent groups. What they have in common is a quality that jeopardizes children by distancing them from committed adults other than their parents and from the human resources these individuals bring to any encounter with a child.

What Do You Think?

1. What type of stressor would children from upper and middle income families experience when isolated from their extended families because of moving to another city or state? How could families and communities cope with these stressors to help their children attain higher levels of wellness?

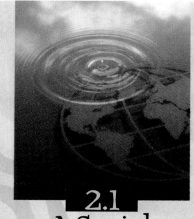

2.1
A Social Perspective

2. Why is the stress of poverty considered more debilitating for children than the stressors associated with mobility? What resources and assistance would help children in poverty attain higher levels of wellness? How could these resources and assistance be made readily available to families living in poverty?

Source: Data from Earls, Felton, and Mary Carlson. (1993) "Towards Sustainable Development for American Families" in *Daedalus 122* (1): 108–109, 1993.

---

society to an industrial society. The last four decades have led to another major shift—from the industrial era to the information era. In the information society, creating, processing, and distributing information "is" the job, not just a part of it. Computers are now the way to manage information. As Anthony Hordern points out, "In 1945 there were no microcircuits; no technology existed, there was no microelectronics industry. The pace of development in the next thirty-five years is analogous to having progressed from the Wright Brothers' first aeroplane (1903) to the space shuttle (1981) within a decade."[39] Rapid cultural changes have become the rule, not the exception. Change will continue to accelerate into the twenty-first century.

Acceleration in the external environment is translated into acceleration within the internal environment. The psychological and physical arousal characteristic of the stress response is increased to accommodate rapid change. For many, the increased arousal is used to embrace change. Change is viewed as contributing to a wider range of lifestyles, increased freedom, and greater diversity. The stress response can be directed for positive adapting and purposeful functioning.

Unfortunately, the acceleration is too much for many individuals. A state of anomie develops. **Anomie** is a state characterized by confusion, disorientation, and anxiety. A person is unable to adjust adequately or to engage in adjustment strategies.

Acceleration from within also tends to increase the pace of life. We are a people on the move; for many, good or bad days are measured by how much was accomplished. There is no time for stress management. It may be nice, but it is a low-priority item. For others, taking time to manage stress is perceived as being "lazy" or "wasting daylight hours." And for still others, taking time to manage stress signifies personal failure to keep up with others who do not appear to need recuperation. Individually, or collectively, getting caught in the mainstream of the rapid pace of life can divert attention away from managing the pace to surviving within it.

Career-Advancement Norms

For many people in the U.S., a large portion of each day is spent at the worksite. A stimulating occupation coupled with the perceived satisfaction of pay, autonomy, peer and supervisory interaction, and security can be a rewarding and fulfilling way to spend this part of the day. Job-related stress is reduced when people are made to feel a part of the organization and have input into it.

Generally, however, the advancement norms in this country are stress producers and serve as barriers to taking action to reduce stress. Financial incentives, promotion, and retention are used as "carrots" for increased productivity. Striving for these carrots is stressful. For many it means long workdays, weekends at the office, reduced personal and family time, work-related travel, and the like. The job becomes all-encompassing, and personal time is sacrificed in order to get the job done. Ulcers, hypertension, or headaches are used as a measure of "how hard one is working." Even when a certain measure of job success is reached, there are new stressors associated with maintaining it. Some become trapped by a desire to manage stress but are unwilling to simplify their lives or reduce their standard of living. Our society promotes the idea that who we are as persons is closely tied to our occupation and financial status. As long as these norms are prevalent, certain barriers will exist to taking steps to reduce stress. There will always be the fear by some that to admit a need to control stress is a sign of incompetence. Theirs is the fear that one is losing "drive" or "initiative"—qualities that are highly desirable in certain occupations. If perceived in this manner, promotion, salary, reputation, or even continued employment could be at stake. Some are not willing to risk these to manage stress more effectively. Yet learning to cope effectively with the stress of career-advancement norms, the pace of life in the U.S., family-related stressors, and other social and personal stressors can help you to achieve higher levels of well-being.

Improving Your Coping Skills

Managing stress effectively can seem like an overwhelming task. Yet learning to enhance your stress-management abilities may be one of the most important things you can do to enhance your level of wellness.

In chapter 1 the stages of behavior change were discussed in some detail. Look back at Activity for Wellness 1.4 and determine which stage of change you are in, in terms of enhancing your stress-management abilities. Then use the information in table 2.8 to help you focus your efforts on managing the stressors in your life.

Enjoying life and its many challenges is a goal worth seeking. Taking the time to invest in life-management skills while expanding your level of awareness and personal experience are important steps toward that goal.

Summary

1. A review of the literature indicates that mentally well people possess particular traits. The mentally well are real, realistic, able to satisfy their needs, free and responsible, open to experience, capable of intimate relationships, tolerant and accepting of others, capable of reacting in a variety of ways, capable of *joie de vivre*, and self-accepting.

2. Often the term *mental health* is confused with mental illness.

3. Mental health cannot be defined in terms of absence of symptoms or by ability to function.

4. A number of theorists have contributed to our concept of mental wellness including Rogers' fully functioning person, Maslow's self-actualized person, and Pelletier's Sound Mind, Sound Body study.

5. Depression and stress are potential roadblocks to achieving mental wellness.

6. Though depression is common on occasion to everyone, it can be severe and should never be taken lightly or ignored. Depressive symptoms that last longer than two weeks are an indication that professional help is needed.

7. Depression is a very treatable condition. For mild depression self-help strategies can be helpful. For severe or clinical depression, help from a medical professional is recommended. Treatment for severe depression most commonly includes a combination of drugs and talk therapy.

8. Stress is a state characterized by distinct physiological changes, such as an increased heart rate, increased breathing rate, increased perspiration, increased muscle tension, and a dry mouth.

Making changes in how you manage stressors is not an easy process. You will probably find that you go through a series of steps, like those listed below, each time you try to make healthy changes in your behavior. The following tips will help you as you progress through the stages of behavior change.*

Precontemplation → Contemplation

If you have never thought about making healthy changes in how you manage stressors or you do not intend to make any changes within the next six months you might want to consider:

- assessing how much stress you have in your life (Activity 2.3).
- assessing whether you are exhibiting any of the major signs and symptoms of stress (table 2.6).

Contemplation → Preparation

If you have been seriously considering making some changes in managing stressors, but have not yet attempted any changes, try to thoughtfully answer the following questions:

- How do I think or feel about taking time from my schedule to learn and regularly practice a relaxation technique, or exercise, or planning my time? Am I willing to change my lifestyle permanently to achieve a higher level of mental well-being through stress management?

Preparation → Action

If you are ready to make some definite plans for more effectively managing stressors during the next month, or if you have already made small changes in the past but were not able to maintain those changes as a permanent part of your lifestyle, consider the following actions:

- Make a resolution to yourself to begin a certain change in management of stressors; for instance, make a commitment to yourself to begin practicing relaxation every day.
- Set a specific date to begin your new behavior, for example "starting Monday I will relax in my room for fifteen minutes, every day."

Action → Maintenance

If you have recently started to make some healthy changes in how you manage stressors, the following tips will help you continue on this healthy path:

- Write a behavior change contract, such as found in chapter 1, and find a support person who will help you keep with your plan; have your support person sign your contract.
- Give yourself rewards *often* for meeting your goals and objectives; rewards should be things you really enjoy, but that you are willing to do without if you do not meet your goal.

Maintenance

You have made important changes in managing stressors that you have practiced for six months or longer; now you need to focus on maintaining your healthy choices every day:

- Keep a diary of how you feel each day before and after practicing your relaxation strategy.
- Teach a friend how to relax; offer each other support for regularly practicing relaxation.
- If you miss a day of relaxation, learn to view it as a temporary lapse in your routine; make your relaxation time a priority so that it becomes a permanent habit.

*Based on Prochaska, Norcross, and DiClemente's transtheoretical model. See Prochaska, J. O., Norcross, J. C., & DiClemente, C. C. (1994). *Changing for Good.* New York: William Morrow and Company, Inc.

9. Stressors are the stimuli that elicit the state of stress, also called the stress response.

10. Not all stressors elicit the same intensity of stress response. Some stressors may be very minor while others are quite devastating. Additionally, people perceive stressors differently—what may stimulate the stress response for you may not for a friend.

11. Selye has coined the term *eustress* to describe stress that is perceived as good, or leading to personal growth and fulfillment. Distress is stress that upsets your physical and psychological balance negatively, as a result of either too many stressors or a lack of effective coping skills.

12. Many people experience great trauma in their lives and yet still achieve high levels of mental wellness. Psychologists believe that these individuals often have the seven strengths of resilience: insight, independence, relationships, initiative, creativity, humor, and morality.

13. Physiologically, the stress response occurs through two major pathways of the body: the nervous system pathway and the endocrine pathway. Chemical nerve transmitters and hormones activate the body to deal physically with stress.

14. Throughout our lives there are predictable "marker events" that are likely to cause either distress or eustress. The Social Readjustment Rating Scale is an instrument that measures the number of specific marker events you have experienced in the past year. This scale then predicts one's risk of illness, injury, or psychological problems based on the number, clustering, and intensity of major life changes.

15. In today's society there are few options for physically coping with stressors; thus we are often unable to use the stress response as it was

originally intended. When fighting and running are not viable options, many people hold their stress inside and fail to cope effectively. Stress researchers believe this is one cause of the "diseases of adaptation."

16. Many options exist that can contribute to mental well-being including social engineering and personality engineering strategies, relaxation training, and expanding your awareness and experience base.

17. Social influences that may act as barriers to mental wellness abound. Poverty, stereotypes and prejudices, family relationships, the pace of U.S. life, and career advancement norms are all capable of decreasing our level of wellness.

18. Strategies to manage stress and treat depression are readily available. Making changes in your life to better manage stress is an investment in your current and future well-being.

Recommended Readings

Girdano, Daniel A., George S. Everly, Jr., and Dorothy E. Dusek. *Controlling Stress and Tension: A Holistic Approach*, 3d ed. Englewood Cliffs, N.J.: Prentice-Hall, 1990.

Girdano, Everly, and Dusek provide a well-written guide to assessing and managing stress. The book abounds with self-assessment exercises. For each type of assessment (psychosocial, bioecological, and personality), appropriate coping strategies are suggested.

Pelletier, Kenneth R. (1994) *Sound Mind, Sound Body: A New Model for Lifelong Health*. (New York: Simon & Schuster).

Pelletier's book presents the results of his five-year study of fifty-one prominent people in the U.S. who have successfully managed life's challenges and attained a high level of wellness. Additionally, this well-written text suggests important strategies each of us could use to enhance our own quests for wellness.

Peterson, Christopher, and Lisa M. Bossio. *Health and Optimism*. The Free Press. 1991.

Peterson and Bossio present evidence to document the notion that optimists enjoy better health.

Additionally, they present the major theories that address how psychological states translate into physical ones.

References

1. Mullen, Kathleen D., and Robert S. Gold. (1988) "Wellness construct delineation: A Delphi study." *Health Education Research* 3 (4): 353–66.

2. Hale, Janet F., Jerrold S. Greenberg, and Sheila A. Ramsey. (1990) "Assessment of college-student stress and stress-management needs: A pilot study." In James H. Humphrey, Ed. *Human Stress: Current Selected Research*, Vol. 4 (New York: AMS Press, Inc.), 77–88.

3. Jahoda, Marie. (1958) *Current Concepts of Positive Mental Health* (New York: Basic Books).

4. Rogers, Carl. (1961) *On Becoming a Person*. (Boston: Houghton Mifflin).

5. Rogers, *On Becoming a Person*, 195.

6. Rogers, *On Becoming a Person*, 196.

7. Maslow, Abraham. (1954) *Motivation and Personality*. (New York: Harper & Row); "Deficiency motivation and growth motivation," (1955) In ed. M. R. Jones. *Nebraska Symposium on Motivation* (Lincoln, Nebr.: Univ. of Nebraska Press); and *Toward a Psychology of Being*, (1968) 2d ed. (New York: Van Nostrand).

8. Pelletier, Kenneth R. (1994) *Sound Mind, Sound Body: A New Model for Lifelong Health* (New York: Simon & Schuster).

9. Pelletier, *Sound Mind, Sound Body*, 31.

10. Pelletier, *Sound Mind, Sound Body*, 106.

11. Pelletier, *Sound Mind, Sound Body*, 109, 121.

12. Pelletier, *Sound Mind, Sound Body*, 137.

13. Langone, John. (1986) *Dead End* (Boston: Little, Brown and Co.), 19–20.

14. "Defeating depression." (1993) *American Health* XII (10): 38–45, 86.

15. "Defeating depression," 43.

16. "Women and depression: Facing the illness." (1994) *Women's Health Matters* 4 (1): 1, 3.

17. "Women and depression," 3.

18. "Defeating depression," 43.

19. "Women and depression," 3.

20. "Depression." (1992) *CQ Researcher* 2 (37): 857–880.

21. "Depression," 857; "Women and depression," 3.

22. "Prozac controversy." (1994) *CQ Researcher* 4 (31): 721–744.

23. "Defeating depression," 44.

24. "Depression," 871.

25. "Depression," 865.

26. "Depression," 866.

27. Selye, Hans. (1976) *The Stress of Life* (New York: McGraw-Hill), 74.

28. Girdano, Daniel A., George S. Everly, Jr., and Dorothy E. Dusek. (1990) *Controlling Stress and Tension: A Holistic Approach*, 3d ed. (Englewood Cliffs, N.J.: Prentice-Hall).

29. Selye, Hans. (1974) *Stress Without Distress*. (New York: Signet, The New American Library), 27.

30. Sheehy, Gail. (1976) *Passages: Predictable Crises of Adult Life* (New York: E. P. Dutton and Co.), 20–21.

31. Holmes, Thomas H., and Richard Rahe. (1967) "The social readjustment rating scale," *Journal of Psychosomatic Research* 11: 213.

32. Mark, Martin B., Thomas F. Garrity, and Frank R. Bowers. (1975) "The influence of recent life experiences on the health of college freshmen," *Journal of Psychosomatic Research* 19: 87–98.

33. Tubesing, Donald, and Nancy Tubesing. (1981) "The treatment of choice: Selecting stress skills to suit the individual and the situation," Paper presented at The First National Burnout Conference, Philadelphia, Pa., 3 November, 1981.

34. Girdano et al., *Controlling Stress and Tension*, 158–66.

35. Friedman, Meyer, and Ray Rosenman. (1974) *Type A Behavior and Your Heart* (New York: Alfred A. Knopf).

36. Greenberg, Jerrold S. (1990) *Comprehensive Stress Management*, 3d ed. (Dubuque, Ia.: Wm. C. Brown Publishers).

37. Greenberg, *Comprehensive Stress Management*.

38. Dunn, Halbert. (1956) *Your World and Mine* (New York: Exposition Press), 91.

39. Hordern, Anthony. (1985) "The spectrum of stress," *Stress Medicine* 1: 17–25.

Nutrition: Eating for Health

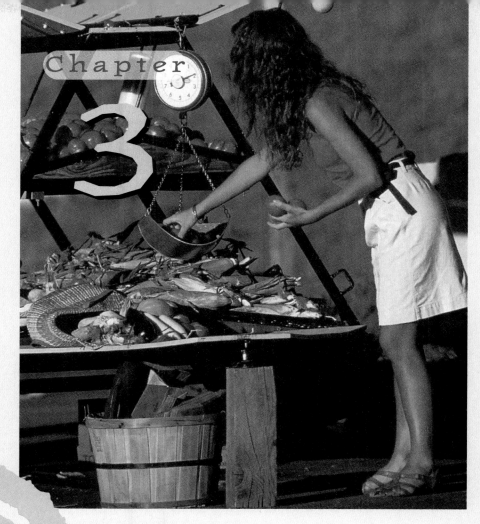

Chapter 3

Student Learning Objectives

Upon completion of this chapter, you should be able to:

1. describe the strengths and weaknesses of the typical U.S. diet;

2. list the National Research Council's dietary recommendations for people in the U.S., and describe at least three strategies for implementing each goal;

3. evaluate the strengths and weaknesses of your current dietary pattern;

4. describe how to read a food label, including how to interpret the percent daily value for your daily dietary needs;

5. identify the functions of fats, protein, and carbohydrates;

6. describe what is meant by the phrase "empty calories";

7. describe the benefits of consuming between 20 and 30 grams of fiber daily, and list five high-fiber foods;

8. discuss the link between diets high in saturated fats and coronary artery disease;

9. identify the possible influence of trans-fatty acids, HDL and LDL cholesterol on health and disease;

10. discuss the controversy surrounding interventions to lower the U.S. population's blood cholesterol level;

11. describe what a fat substitute is and identify possible health benefits of consuming them;

12. describe how to mix and match plant and low-fat animal sources of protein in your diet;

13. discuss the role of vitamins, minerals, and water in one's diet;

14. describe the current debate regarding the effectiveness of antioxidants in reducing the risk of various chronic diseases;

15. discuss the relationship between excess sodium in the diet and hypertension, osteoporosis, and stomach cancer;

16. describe the role calcium plays in the development, treatment, and prevention of osteoporosis;

17. compare and contrast your diet with the recommendations of the Center for Science in the Public Interest's Healthy Eating Pyramid;

18. describe how the four major types of food-borne infection occur, and list at least five ways to prevent such infection;

19. discuss the various special nutritional needs of athletes, vegetarians, pregnant women, and the elderly, as compared to general dietary recommendations for healthy adults;

20. analyze how variables such as cost, cultural influences, convenience, and taste may influence one's choice of foods;

21. describe the problem of hunger in the United States and identify at least ten potential solutions.

Nutrition is a topic of great interest to many people. Advertisers spend large sums of money to sell us the newest culinary delights. Bookstores across the country carry hundreds of different books that advise us on what and how much to eat. Community classes on healthy diets and cooking skills abound; stores selling "health foods" proliferate.

Nutrition may be of special interest or concern to college students. The college years are the first time many students choose or prepare their own meals. Many important nutritional questions arise. What are the best food selections in the campus cafeterias? Are fast foods and processed foods nutritious options? In order to make informed decisions regarding personal nutritional requirements, students need a sound background in the science of nutrition.

Knowing the basics of nutrition will help you decipher the many nutritional controversies prevalent today. Additionally, this chapter will help you consider the impact of personal and social influences on your food choices. A tasty yet nutritious diet can add great enjoyment to life and make a considerable contribution to higher levels of wellness.

The Typical U.S. Diet: A Status Report

Dietary patterns in the U.S. have changed dramatically over the past eighty years. In the early 1900s, people in the U.S. consumed much greater amounts of grains, fruits, and vegetables than now. In fact, 56 percent of the typical U.S. diet of the early 1900s came from carbohydrate sources. At the same time, people at the turn of the century consumed lesser amounts of fat, salt, and refined and processed sugars. Today, the typical diet consists of approximately 50 percent carbohydrates, 34 percent fat, and 16 percent protein.[1] These drastic changes in our diet have been unplanned and largely result from our affluent lifestyle.

Many respected scientists have suggested that there are major associations between the typical U.S. diet and many of the chronic and degenerative diseases prevalent today. In 1988, after much deliberation and review of expert testimony, the U.S. Department of Health and Human Services issued *The Surgeon General's Report on Nutrition and Health*.[2] This major report points out that the dietary habits of people in the U.S. represent a great threat to public health because they are linked to cardiovascular disease, cancer, hypertension, stroke, and diabetes. Other national health organizations, such as the American Heart Association and the National Cancer Institute, have recommended U.S. dietary guidelines to help improve the health of all through informed dietary selection. The National Research Council's dietary recommendations are presented in table 3.1. Additionally, recognizing the importance of a healthy diet for both disease prevention and wellness, the U.S. Public Health Service has issued many nutrition-related objectives for the nation. Table 3.2 presents an overview of some of the nutrition objectives for the year 2000. Since these objectives were published in 1991, progress has been made on one third of the nutrition objectives, including the objectives for reducing dietary fat intake, achieving informative nutrition labeling, and increasing the number of restaurant low-fat, low-calorie food choices. One objective, increasing the availability of low-fat and low-saturated fat processed foods, has already met the target set for the year 2000. Even with this success, however, we have moved away from our targets on other important nutritional objectives, such as the proportion of people in the U.S. who are overweight and the percent of overweight individuals who are engaged in weight loss efforts. Table 3.2 contains the updated information for a selection of the nutrition objectives.

These dietary guidelines have great potential for improving U.S. dietary patterns. They could intensify and expand the current nutritional consciousness. Although these guidelines and objectives may not be perfect, most people could benefit from closely examining their dietary habits and making the recommended dietary changes.

How does your diet rank nutritionally? You can assess the strengths and weaknesses of your diet by completing Activity for Wellness 3.1.

TABLE 3.1 — National Research Council Dietary Recommendations

1. Reduce total fat intake to 30 percent or less of calories. Reduce saturated fatty acid intake to less than 10 percent of calories and the intake of cholesterol to less than 300 mg daily.
2. Every day eat five or more servings of a combination of vegetables and fruits, especially green and yellow vegetables and citrus fruits. Also, increase starches and other complex carbohydrates by eating six or more daily servings of a combination of breads, cereals, and legumes.
3. Maintain protein intake at moderate levels.
4. Balance food intake and physical activity to maintain appropriate body weight.
5. Alcohol consumption is not recommended. For those who drink alcoholic beverages, limit consumption to the equivalent of 1 ounce of pure alcohol in a single day.
6. Limit total daily intake of salt to 6 grams or less.
7. Maintain adequate calcium intake.
8. Avoid taking dietary supplements in excess of the RDA in any one day.
9. Maintain an optimal intake of fluoride, particularly during the years of primary and secondary tooth formation and growth.

Reprinted with permission from *Diet and Health: Implications for Reducing Chronic Disease Risk.* Copyright © 1989 by the National Academy of Sciences. Courtesy of the National Academy Press, Washington, D.C.

The ABCs of Nutrition

We cannot live for long without food to fuel our bodies. Food supplies us with essential nutrients that provide the body with energy and the materials necessary for growth and maintenance of body tissues. Of the six major nutrients, three—carbohydrates, fats, and protein—actually contribute energy or **calories** to our diet. A calorie is a unit that measures the amount of energy we derive from a given food. Technically, a calorie is defined as the amount of heat needed to raise the temperature of a gram of water by 1 degree Celsius. The calorie used to measure the energy available in food is 1,000 times larger and is called a kilocalorie. It is common, however, to refer to a kilocalorie as simply a calorie. Although they do not contribute calories, the remaining three nutrients— vitamins, minerals, and water—are important aids in utilizing the energy received from carbohydrates, fats, and protein.

In order for our bodies to function at an optimal level, we need a balanced diet that supplies us with the appropriate amounts of each of the six essential nutrient groups. The Food and Nutrition Board of the National Research Council periodically reviews the current information on nutritional needs of healthy people in order to set recommended amounts of the various nutrients. These recommendations are known as the **RDA,** or Recommended Dietary Allowances. The RDAs are average amounts of nutrients that should be consumed *over time*, rather than minimal amounts to be consumed on any

given day. RDAs vary by sex and age and are intended to meet the needs of 98 percent of the healthy U.S. population.[3] The RDAs are especially useful to researchers and policy makers who focus on the nutritional status of the U.S. population. Appendix A contains the most recent RDA information.

One important step in improving your diet is to become knowledgeable about the six major nutrient groups and which foods contain adequate amounts of these nutrients. Learning how to read food labels will help you in identifying the foods that will contribute to a balanced and varied diet.

Food Labels

On December 9, 1992 the U.S. Food and Drug Administration (FDA) announced that, by May 1994, a new food label, titled "Nutrition Facts," would appear on packaged foods, meat and poultry, many fruits and vegetables, and raw fish. The new food label provides consumers with more useful information than food labels of the past.

How helpful are the Nutrition Facts labels? The story of Erin, a college freshman, will show you the value of Nutrition Facts. Erin decided to go to the local convenience store to get a treat. She was celebrating the fact that she got an A– on her first exam of the semester. Erin doesn't read food labels so she really doesn't know whether or not the treat she picked was a healthy one. She grabbed a bag of cheese crackers and ate the whole bag along with a soft drink. Figure 3.1 is the food label from Erin's cheese crackers. Let's analyze her snack.

Calorie: a unit of measure equal to a kilocalorie; a term used to express the energy value of food.

RDA: recommended dietary allowance, or the amount of various nutrients, recommended by the Food and Nutrition Board of the National Research Council, considered to be adequate for the maintenance of good nutrition in most healthy persons in the U.S.

1. **Reduce dietary fat intake to an average of 30 percent of calories or less and average saturated fat intake to less than 10 percent of calories among people aged 2 and older.** (Update: 34 percent of calories from total fat and 12 percent from saturated fat for people aged 20 through 74 in 1988–91, down from 35 percent total fat and 13 percent saturated fat in 1976–80.)

2. **Increase complex carbohydrate and fiber-containing foods in the diets of adults to 5 or more daily servings for vegetables (including legumes, such as beans and peas) and fruits, and to 6 or more daily servings for grain products.** (Baseline: 4 servings of vegetables and fruits in 1989–90 and 3 servings of grain products for women aged 19 through 50 in 1985.)

3. **Increase calcium intake so at least 50 percent of youth aged 12 through 24 and 50 percent of pregnant and lactating women consume 3 or more servings daily of foods rich in calcium, and at least 50 percent of people aged 25 and older consume 2 or more servings daily.** (Update: 7 percent of women and 14 percent of men aged 19 through 24 consumed 3 or more servings in 1989, unchanged from 1985–86; 16 percent of pregnant and lactating women consumed 3 or more servings in 1989, down from 24 percent in 1985–86; 16 percent of women and 23 percent aged 25 through 50 consumed 2 or more servings in 1989, up from 15 percent of women in 1985–86 and unchanged for men.) (Note: a serving is considered to be 1 cup of skim milk or its equivalent in calcium [302mg]).

4. **Decrease salt and sodium intake so at least 65 percent of home meal preparers prepare foods without adding salt, at least 80 percent of people avoid using salt at the table, and at least 40 percent of adults regularly purchase foods modified or lower in sodium.** (Baseline: 54 percent of women aged 19 through 50 who served as the main meal preparer did not use salt in food preparation, and 68 percent of women aged 19 through 50 did not use salt at the table in 1985; 20 percent of all people aged 18 and older regularly purchased foods with reduced salt and sodium content in 1988.)

5. **Reduce iron deficiency to less than 3 percent among children aged 1 through 4 and among women of childbearing age.** (Baseline: 9 percent for children aged 1 through 2, 4 percent for children aged 3 through 4, and 5 percent for women aged 20 through 44 in 1976–80.)

6. **Increase to at least 85 percent the proportion of people aged 18 and older who use food labels to make nutritious food selections.** (Update: 74 percent used labels to make food selections in 1991, a rate unchanged from the 1987 percent.)

7. **Achieve useful and informative nutrition labeling for virtually all processed foods and at least 40 percent of fresh meats, poultry, fish, fruits, vegetables, baked goods, and ready-to-eat carry-away foods.** (Update: 66 percent of sales of processed foods regulated by FDA had nutrition labeling in 1990, up from 60 percent in 1988; 77 percent of fresh produce and 75 percent of fresh seafood had nutrition labeling in 1993.)

8. **Increase to at least 5,000 brand items the availability of processed food products that are reduced in fat and saturated fat.** (Update: 5,618 items reduced in fat in 1993, up from 2,500 items in 1986.)

9. **Increase to at least 90 percent the proportion of restaurants and institutional food service operations that offer identifiable low-fat, low-calorie food choices, consistent with the *Dietary Guidelines for Americans.*** (Update: About 75 percent of fast food and family restaurant chains with 350 or more units had at least one low-fat, low-calorie item on their menu in 1990, up from 70 percent in 1989–90.)

10. **Reduce infections caused by key food-borne pathogens to incidences of no more than: 16 per 100,000 for Salmonella species** (Baseline: 18 per 100,000 in 1987; 14 per 100,000 in 1992); **25 per 100,000 for Campylobacter jejuni** (Baseline: 50 per 100,000 in 1987); **4 per 100,000 for Escherichia coli 0157:H7** (Baseline: 8 per 100,000 in 1987); **and 0.5 per 100,000 for Listeria monocytogenes** (Baseline: 0.7 per 100,000 in 1987).

11. **Reduce outbreaks of infections due to Salmonella enteridis to fewer than 25 outbreaks yearly.** (Update: 60 outbreaks in 1992, down from 77 outbreaks in 1989.)

12. **Increase to at least 75 percent the proportion of households in which principal food preparers routinely refrain from leaving perishable food out of the refrigerator for over two hours and wash cutting boards and utensils with soap after contact with raw meat and poultry.** (Baseline: For refrigeration of perishable foods, 70 percent; for washing cutting boards with soap, 66 percent; and for washing utensils with soap, 55 percent, in 1988.)

13. **Increase to at least 45 percent the proportion of people aged 35 through 44 who have never lost a permanent tooth due to dental caries or periodontal diseases.** (Baseline: 31 percent of employed adults had never lost a permanent tooth for any reason in 1985–86.)

Source: Data from *Healthy People 2000 National Health Promotion and Disease Prevention Objectives;* Healthy People 2000 Review 1993, Department of Health and Human Services, Washington, D.C., 1994.

The first thing to note as you look at the food label is the serving size. The FDA has now standardized serving sizes, attempting to set them in amounts that consumers would typically consume. Some serving sizes, however, have been set too large or small. For instance, the standard serving size for meat has been set at three ounces, a portion size smaller than what many people eat. In addition to serving size, the package label will indicate the number of servings per container. For instance, the food label in figure 3.1 tells us that there are two servings in this container. Erin ate the entire bag, or two servings. In order to interpret the rest of the nutrient information correctly, we will

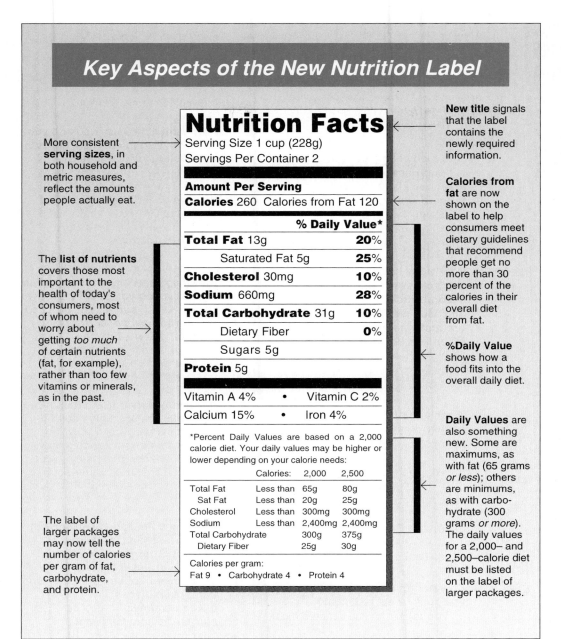

Key Aspects of the New Nutrition Label

More consistent serving sizes, in both household and metric measures, reflect the amounts people actually eat.

The **list of nutrients** covers those most important to the health of today's consumers, most of whom need to worry about getting *too much* of certain nutrients (fat, for example), rather than too few vitamins or minerals, as in the past.

The label of larger packages may now tell the number of calories per gram of fat, carbohydrate, and protein.

Nutrition Facts
Serving Size 1 cup (228g)
Servings Per Container 2

Amount Per Serving
Calories 260 Calories from Fat 120

	% Daily Value*
Total Fat 13g	**20**%
Saturated Fat 5g	**25**%
Cholesterol 30mg	**10**%
Sodium 660mg	**28**%
Total Carbohydrate 31g	**10**%
Dietary Fiber	**0**%
Sugars 5g	
Protein 5g	

Vitamin A 4%	•	Vitamin C 2%
Calcium 15%	•	Iron 4%

*Percent Daily Values are based on a 2,000 calorie diet. Your daily values may be higher or lower depending on your calorie needs:

	Calories:	2,000	2,500
Total Fat	Less than	65g	80g
Sat Fat	Less than	20g	25g
Cholesterol	Less than	300mg	300mg
Sodium	Less than	2,400mg	2,400mg
Total Carbohydrate		300g	375g
Dietary Fiber		25g	30g

Calories per gram:
Fat 9 • Carbohydrate 4 • Protein 4

New title signals that the label contains the newly required information.

Calories from fat are now shown on the label to help consumers meet dietary guidelines that recommend people get no more than 30 percent of the calories in their overall diet from fat.

%Daily Value shows how a food fits into the overall daily diet.

Daily Values are also something new. Some are maximums, as with fat (65 grams *or less*); others are minimums, as with carbohydrate (300 grams *or more*). The daily values for a 2,000– and 2,500–calorie diet must be listed on the label of larger packages.

Figure 3.1:
A number of consumer studies conducted by the FDA, as well as outside groups, enabled the FDA and the Food Safety and Inspection Service of the U.S. Department of Agriculture to agree on a new nutrition label. The new label is seen as offering the best opportunity to help consumers make informed food choices and to understand how a particular food fits into the total daily diet.

Source: From *FDA Consumer*, May 1993, pp. 22–27, U.S. Government Printing Office.

have to multiply the values given by two. For instance, Erin did not consume 260 total calories, 120 of which were from fat; rather she consumed double that, or 520 total calories, 240 of them from fat.

As you look further down the new label you will see information on the amounts of fat, cholesterol, sodium, carbohydrates, and protein in the food product. These nutrients are considered to be the most important for the health of consumers today. Looking at figure 3.1, we can see how much of these nutrients Erin consumed with her quick snack. The column to the right of the

amounts, titled % Daily Value, will help us interpret what these amounts really mean for Erin's overall diet.

The % Daily Value tells us how a food fits into our overall daily diet. It is calculated by comparing the amount of a given nutrient in a food with a new standard called the **Daily Reference Values (DRVs).** The DRVs are amounts of certain nutrients that a person should consume as part of a 2,000 calorie daily diet. A 2,000 calorie diet standard would be appropriate for most women, children, and men over age fifty. Younger men, teenage boys, and all very active people

Daily Reference Values (DRVs): the amount of fat, saturated fatty acids, cholesterol, total carbohydrates, fiber, sodium, potassium, and protein adults and children over four should consume daily for maintenance of good nutrition. These values are based on a 2,000 calorie diet, and are listed on the "Nutrition Facts" food label.

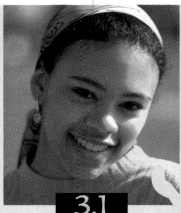

3.1

Activity for Wellness

How's Your Diet?

The forty questions below will help you focus on the key features of your diet. The (+) or (–) numbers under each set of answers instantly pat you on the back for good habits or alert you to problems you may not even realize you have.

The Grand Total rates your overall diet, on a scale from "Great" to "Arrgh!"

The quiz focuses on fat, saturated fat, cholesterol, sodium, sugar, fiber, and vitamins A and C. It doesn't attempt to cover everything in your diet. Also, it doesn't try to measure precisely how much of these key nutrients you eat.

What the quiz will do is give you a rough sketch of your current eating habits and, implicitly, suggest what you can do to improve them.

And don't despair over a less-than-perfect score. We didn't get a + 117 either.

Instructions

- Under each answer is a number with a + or – sign in front of it. Circle the number that is directly beneath the answer you choose. That's your score for the question. (If you use a pencil, you can erase your answers and give the quiz to someone else.)
- Circle only one number for each question, unless the instructions tell you to "average two or more scores if necessary."
- *How to average.* In answering question 18, for example, if you drink club soda (+3) and coffee (–1) on a typical day, add the two scores (which gives you +2) and then divide by 2. That gives you a score of +1 for the question. If averaging gives you a fraction, round it to the nearest whole number.

- If a question doesn't apply to you, skip it.
- Pay attention to serving sizes. For example, a serving of vegetables is 1/2 cup. If you usually eat one cup of vegetables at a time, count it as two servings.
- Add up all your + scores and your – scores.
- Subtract your – scores from your + scores. That's your GRAND TOTAL.

Quiz

1. **How many times per week do you eat unprocessed red meat (steak, roast beef, lamb or pork chops, burgers, etc.)?**
   (a) 0   (b) 1 or less (c) 2–3
   +3   +2   0
   (d) 4–5   (e) 6 or more
   –1   –3

2. **How many times per week do you eat processed meats (hot dogs, bacon, sausage, bologna, luncheon meats, etc.)?** *(OMIT products that contain one gram of fat or less per serving.)*
   (a) 0   (b) less than 1 (c) 1
   +3   +2   0
   (d) 2–3   (e) 4 or more
   –1   –3

3. **What kind of ground meat or poultry do you usually eat?**
   (a) regular or lean ground beef
                    –3
   (b) extra lean ground beef
                    –2
   (c) ground round   (d) ground turkey
          –1   +1
   (e) Healthy Choice
          +3
   (f) don't eat ground meat
          +3

4. **Do you trim the visible fat when you cook or eat red meat?**
   (a) yes (b) no (c) don't eat red meat
   +1   –3   0

5. **After cooking, how large is the serving of red meat you usually eat?** *(To convert from raw to cooked, reduce by 25 percent. For example, 4 oz. of raw meat shrinks to 3 oz. after cooking. There are 16 oz. in a pound.)*
   (a) 8 oz. or more (b) 6–7 oz. (c) 4–5 oz.
          –3   –2   –1
   (d) 3 oz. or less (e) don't eat red meat
          0   +3

6. **What type of bread, rolls, bagels, etc., do you usually eat?**
   (a) 100% whole wheat
          +3

   (b) whole wheat as 1st or 2nd ingredient
                    +2
   (c) rye, pumpernickel, or oatmeal
                    +1
   (d) white, French, or Italian
                    –1

7. **How many times per week do you eat deep-fried foods (fish, chicken, vegetables, potatoes, etc.)?**
   (a) 0 (b) 1–2 (c) 3–4 (d) 5 or more
   +3   0   –1   –3

8. **How many servings of nonfried vegetables do you usually eat per day?** *(One serving = 1/2 cup. INCLUDE potatoes.)*
   (a) 0 (b) 1 (c) 2 (d) 3 (e) 4 or more
   –3   0   +1   +2   +3

9. **How many servings of cruciferous vegetables do you usually eat per week?** *(ONLY count kale, broccoli, cauliflower, cabbage, Brussels sprouts, greens, bok choy, kohlrabi, turnip, and rutabaga. One serving = 1/2 cup.)*
   (a) 0 (b) 1–3 (c) 4–6 (d) 7 or more
   –3   +1   +2   +3

10. **How many servings of vitamin-A-rich fruits or vegetables do you usually eat per week?** *(ONLY count cantaloupe, apricots, or cooked carrots, pumpkin, sweet potatoes, spinach, winter squash, or greens. One serving = 1/2 cup.)*
    (a) 0 (b) 1–3 (c) 4–6 (d) 7 or more
    –3   +1   +2   +3

11. **How many times per week do you eat at a fast-food restaurant?** *(INCLUDE burgers, fried fish or chicken, croissant or biscuit sandwiches, topped potatoes, and other main dishes. OMIT plain baked potatoes, broiled skinned chicken, or low-fat salads.)*
    (a) 0 (b) less than 1 (c) 1 (d) 2
    +3   +1   0   –1
    (e) 3   (f) 4 or more
    –2   –3

12. **How many servings of grains do you eat per day?** *(One serving = 1 slice of bread, 1 large pancake, 1 cup cold cereal, or 1/2 cup cooked cereal, rice, pasta, bulger, wheat berries, kasha, or millet. OMIT heavily-sweetened cold cereals.)*
    (a) 0   (b) 1–3   (c) 4–5
    –3   0   +1
    (d) 6–8   (e) 9 or more
    +2   +3

13. **How many times per week do you eat fish or shellfish?** (*OMIT deep-fried items, tuna packed in oil, and mayonnaise-laden tuna salad—a little mayo is okay.*)

(a) 0   (b) 1   (c) 2
0   +1   +2

(d) 3 or more   (e) 0 (vegetarians)
+3   +3

14. **How many times per week do you eat cheese?** (*INCLUDE pizza, cheeseburgers, veal or eggplant parmigiana, cream cheese, etc. OMIT low-fat or fat-free cheeses.*)

(a) 0   (b) 1   (c) 2–3   (d) 4 or more
+3   +1   −1   −3

15. **How many servings of fresh fruit do you eat per day?**

(a) 0 (b) 1 (c) 2 (d) 3 (e) 4 or more
−3   0   +1   +2   +3

16. **Do you remove the skin before eating poultry?**

(a) yes   (b) no   (c) don't eat poultry
+3   −3   0

17. **What do you usually put on your bread or toast?** (*AVERAGE two or more scores if necessary.*)

(a) butter or cream cheese
−3

(b) margarine   (c) peanut butter
−2   −1

(d) diet margarine (e) jam or honey
−1   0

(f) 100% fruit butter   (g) nothing
+1   +3

18. **Which of these beverages do you drink on a typical day?** (*AVERAGE two or more scores if necessary.*)

(a) water or club soda   (b) fruit juice
+3   +1

(c) diet soda (d) coffee or tea
−1   −1

(e) soda, fruit "drink," or fruit "ade"
−3

19. **Which flavorings do you most frequently add to your foods?** (*AVERAGE two or more scores if necessary.*)

(a) garlic or lemon juice
+3

(b) herbs or spices   (c) olive oil
+3   −1

(d) salt or soy sauce   (e) margarine
−1   −2

(f) butter   (g) nothing
−3   +3

20. **What do you eat most frequently as a snack?** (*AVERAGE two or more scores if necessary.*)

(a) fruits or vegetables   (b) yogurt
+3   +2

(c) crackers (d) nuts
+1   −1

(e) cookies or fried chips (f) granola bar
−2   −2

(g) candy bar or pastry   (h) nothing
−3   0

21. **What is your most typical breakfast?** (*SUBTRACT an extra 3 points if you also eat bacon or sausage.*)

(a) croissant, danish, or doughnut
−3

(b) whole eggs (c) pancakes or waffles
−3   −2

(d) cereal or toast   (e) low-fat yogurt
+3   or cottage cheese
+3

(f) don't eat breakfast
0

22. **What do you usually eat for dessert?**

(a) pie, pastry, or cake (b) ice cream
−3   −3

(c) fat-free cookies or cakes
−1

(d) frozen yogurt or ice milk
0

(e) non-fat ice cream or sorbet
+1

(f) fruit   (g) don't eat dessert
+3   +3

23. **How many times per week do you eat beans, split peas, or lentils?**

(a) 0   (b) 1   (c) 2   (d) 3   (e) 4 or more
−3   0   +1   +2   +3

24. **What kind of milk do you drink?**

(a) whole (b) 2% fat (c) 1% low-fat
−3   −1   +2

(d) 1/2% or skim   (e) don't drink milk
+3   0

25. **Which items do you choose at a salad bar?** (*ADD two or more scores if necessary.*)

(a) nothing, lemon, (b) fat-free
    or vinegar   dressing
+3   +2

(c) low- or reduced-calorie dressing
+1

(d) regular dressing (e) croutons or
−1   bacon bits
−1

(f) cole slaw, pasta salad, or
    potato salad
−1

26. **What sandwich fillings do you eat most frequently?** (*AVERAGE two or more scores if necessary.*)

(a) regular luncheon meat
−3

(b) cheese   (c) roast beef
−2   −1

(d) peanut butter (e) low-fat luncheon
0   meat
+1

(f) tuna or chicken salad
+1

(g) fresh turkey breast or bean spread
+3

(h) don't eat sandwiches
0

27. **What do you usually spread on your sandwiches?** (*AVERAGE two or more scores if necessary.*)

(a) mayonnaise (b) light mayonnaise
−2   −1

(c) catsup, mustard, or fat-free
    mayonnaise
+1

(d) nothing
+2

28. **How many egg yolks do you eat per week?** (*ADD 1 yolk for every slice of quiche you eat.*)

(a) 2 or less (b) 3–4
+3   0

(c) 5–6   (d) 7 or more
−1   −3

29. **How many times per week do you eat canned or dried soups?** (*OMIT low-sodium, low-fat soups.*)

(a) 0 (b) 1–2 (c) 3–4 (d) 5 or more
+3   0   −2   −3

30. **How many servings of a rich source of calcium do you eat per day?** (*One serving = 2/3 cup milk or yogurt, 1 oz. cheese, 1 1/2 oz. sardines, 3 1/2 oz. canned salmon (with bones), 5 oz. tofu made with calcium sulfate, 1 cup greens or broccoli, or 200 mg of a calcium supplement.*)

(a) 0   (b) 1   (c) 2   (d) 3 or more
−3   +1   +2   +3

31. **What do you usually order on your pizza?** (*Vegetable toppings include green pepper, mushrooms, onions, and other vegetables. SUBTRACT 1 point from your score if you order extra cheese.*)

(a) no cheese with vegetables
+3   *Continued*

(b) cheese with vegetables
    +1

(c) cheese
    0

(d) cheese with meat toppings
    −3

(e) don't eat pizza
    +2

32. What kind of cookies do you usually eat?

(a) don't eat cookies
    +3

(b) fat-free cookies
    +2

(c) graham crackers or ginger snaps
    +1

(d) oatmeal
    −1

(e) sandwich cookies (like Oreos)
    −2

(f) chocolate coated, chocolate chip, or peanut butter
    −3

33. What kind of frozen dessert do you usually eat? (*SUBTRACT 1 point from your score for each topping you use—whipped cream, hot fudge, nuts, etc.*)

(a) gourmet ice cream
    −3

(b) regular ice cream
    −2

(c) frozen yogurt, ice milk
    0

(d) sorbet, sherbet, or ices
    +1

(e) non-fat frozen yogurt or fat-free ice cream
    +1

(f) don't eat frozen desserts
    +3

34. What kind of cake or pastry do you usually eat?

(a) cheesecake, pie, or any microwave cake
    −3

(b) cake with frosting
    −2

(c) cake without frosting
    −1

(d) unfrosted muffin, banana bread, or carrot cake
    0

(e) angel food or fat-free cake
    +1

(f) don't eat cakes or pastries
    +3

35. How many times per week does your dinner contain grains, vegetables, or beans, but little or no animal protein (meat, poultry, fish, eggs, milk, or cheese)?

(a) 0 (b) 1–2 (c) 3–4 (d) 5 or more
   −1   +1   +2   +3

36. Which of the following "salty" snacks do you typically eat? (*AVERAGE two or more scores if necessary.*)

(a) potato chips, corn chips, or pre-popped popcorn
    −3

(b) tortilla chips, reduced-fat potato chips, or microwave popcorn
    −2

(c) salted pretzels
    −1

(d) light microwave popcorn
    0

(e) unsalted pretzels
    +1

(f) fat-free tortilla or potato chips
    +2

(g) homemade air-popped popcorn
    +3

(h) don't eat salty snacks
    +3

37. What do you usually use to sauté vegetables or other foods? (*Vegetable oil includes safflower, corn, canola, sunflower, and soybean.*)

(a) butter or lard   (b) margarine
    −3   −2

(c) vegetable oil   (d) olive oil
    −1   +1

(e) broth   (f) water or cooking spray
    +2   +3

38. What kind of cereal do you usually eat?

(a) whole grain (like oatmeal or Shredded Wheat)
    +3

(b) low-fiber (like Cream of Wheat or Corn Flakes)
    0

(c) sugary low-fiber (like Frosted Flakes)
    −1

(d) regular granola
    −2

39. With what do you make tuna salad, pasta salad, chicken salad, etc.?

(a) mayonnaise (b) light mayonnaise
    −2   −1

(c) non-fat mayonnaise
    0

(d) low-fat yogurt (e) non-fat yogurt
    +2   +3

40. What do you typically put on your pasta? (*ADD one point if you also add sautéed vegetables. AVERAGE two or more scores if necessary.*)

(a) tomato sauce, with or without a little parmesan
    +3

(b) white clam sauce
    0

(c) meat sauce or meat balls
    −2

(d) Alfredo, pesto, or other creamy or oily sauce
    −3

Your Grand Total

+59 to +117 GREAT!
You're a nutrition superstar. Give yourself a big (nonbutter) pat on the back.

0 to +58   GOOD
You're doing just fine. Pin your Quiz to the nearest wall.

−1 to −58   FAIR
Hang in there. Continue to read this chapter for a little friendly help.

−59 to −116 ARRGH!
Empty your refrigerator and cupboard. It's time to start over. Read this chapter for suggestions on how to improve your diet.

Daily Reference Values (DRVs)*

Food Component	DRV
fat	65 grams (g)
saturated fatty acids	20 g
cholesterol	300 milligrams (mg)
total carbohydrate	300 g
fiber	25 g
sodium	2,400 mg
potassium	3,500 mg
protein**	50 g

*Based on 2,000 calories a day for adults and children over 4 only

**DRV for protein does not apply to certain populations; Reference Daily Intake (RDI) for protein has been established for these groups: children 1 to 4 years: 16 g; infants under 1 year: 14 g; pregnant women: 60 g; nursing mothers: 65 g.

Source: Data from *FDA Consumer*, May 1993.

need a greater number of calories daily.[4] Individuals who consume more or less than 2,000 calories daily will need to adjust the Daily Values accordingly. Table 3.3 presents the new DRVs. Additionally, the bottom of each food label provides the DRVs for both a 2,000 and a 2,500 calorie diet.

Looking again at figure 3.1 you will notice that when Erin ate her snack, she consumed 40 percent (with two servings) of the total fat she should eat in one day. Erin's snack was very high in fat, and even higher in saturated fat (50 percent of her Daily Value). Generally, if a food has 20 percent or more of your Daily Value you should consider it "high" in that nutrient. "Low" would be daily values of 5 percent or less.[5] You will notice that there is no Daily Value on the food label for sugars or protein. The FDA did not set a Daily Value for added sugar because previous nutrition policy recommendations have not set a standard for how much added sugar we should consume as part of a healthy diet. The Center for Science in the Public Interest (CSPI) recommends that consumers limit their added sugar intake to 50 grams a day.[6] Using this value, Erin's snack provided 10

grams of sugars or 20 percent (10÷50) of the CSPIs recommended sugar intake for the day.

Food manufacturers are not required to list a Daily Value for protein. However, they can voluntarily list a percent based on a DRV of 50 grams. This DRV applies to everyone except children one to four years, infants under one year, and pregnant or nursing mothers. Table 3.3 provides the protein DRV for these special populations. You will notice that Erin's snack provided her with 10 grams of protein, or 20 percent of a daily value based on 50 grams.

In reviewing the Daily Values for Erin, you can see that her snack choice was high in fat, saturated fat, cholesterol, sodium, carbohydrates, sugars, and protein. But what about vitamins and other minerals? As you can see in figure 3.1, information is provided for vitamins A and C, and for the minerals calcium and iron. This information is required on all food labels. Daily values for other essential vitamins and minerals may be provided voluntarily by manufacturers. The percent daily values for these vitamins and minerals are based on **Reference Daily Intakes (RDIs),** formerly known as the USRDA (see table 3.4). Looking at the "Nutrition Facts" for Erin's snack, we can easily see that it contained a good amount of calcium, but was low in Vitamins A and C, as well as iron.

In past years, food products have often made health claims that were misleading. Consider the case of the potato chip manufacturer that on the bag claimed the chips were "cholesterol free," implying that they contributed to a healthy diet that would reduce the risk of coronary heart disease. While the potato chips did not contain cholesterol (because they are a plant food), they did contain high levels of saturated fat that when consumed will elevate blood cholesterol levels, which is a risk factor for coronary artery disease. The new food labels have regulations to control such misleading labeling. Figure 3.2 presents the seven health claims that can now be put on food labels.

Learning more about each of the major nutrient groups—carbohydrates, fats, protein, vitamins, minerals, and water—will help you better understand the information you find on food labels. Additionally, it will clarify the role that a balanced diet plays in your overall level of well-being.

Reference Daily Intakes (RDIs): formerly known as the USRDA, the amount of certain vitamins and minerals that should be consumed daily by adults in the U.S. The current RDIs are identical to the USRDA established in 1968.

TABLE 3.4

Reference Daily Intakes (RDIs)*

Nutrient	Amount
vitamin A	5,000 International Units (IU)
vitamin C	60 milligrams (mg)
thiamin	1.5 mg
riboflavin	1.7 mg
niacin	20 mg
calcium	1.0 gram (g)
iron	18 mg
vitamin D	400 IU
vitamin E	30 IU
vitamin B$_6$	2.0 mg
folic acid	0.4 mg
vitamin B$_{12}$	6 micrograms (mcg)
phosphorus	1.0 g
iodine	150 mcg
magnesium	400 mg
zinc	15 mg
copper	2 mg
biotin	0.3 mg
pantothenic acid	10 mg

*Based on National Academy of Sciences' 1968 Recommended Dietary Allowances.

Source: Data from *FDA Consumer,* May 1993.

Carbohydrates

All **carbohydrates** consist of a combination of carbon, oxygen, and hydrogen atoms. Carbohydrates derive their name from the fact that their hydrogen and oxygen atoms are always in the same proportion as in water—H_2O. Thus the name carbo (carbon) hydrate (water).

The major function of carbohydrates is to provide energy for the body. Carbohydrates are the body's preferred form of energy. Over the years, carbohydrates have been mislabeled as the "fattening nutrient." This is a fallacy of great significance. Carbohydrates provide only four calories per gram, the same number of calories provided by a gram of protein and less than one-half the calories supplied by a gram of fat. In addition to their caloric value, carbohydrates can also be a rich source of vitamins, minerals, fiber, and water—all vital nutrients contributing significantly to health and levels of wellness.

Carbohydrates are typically divided into two categories: simple and complex. There are several major distinctions between these groups that merit a closer look.

Simple Carbohydrates

Simple carbohydrates, often known as **simple sugars,** are the basic building blocks for carbohydrates. These simple sugars are technically known as **monosaccharides** and include glucose, fructose, and galactose. **Glucose** is the most important simple sugar in terms of optimal body functioning; it is the major energy-supplying molecule in the body. The brain and nervous system depend almost exclusively on glucose for nourishment, using almost two-thirds of the glucose needed by the body. When blood glucose levels fall below the necessary level, we become tired, irritable, and hungry. Appropriate blood-sugar levels are an important aspect of optimal functioning and high levels of wellness.

A second group of sugars, known as **disaccharides,** are molecules consisting of a combination of two simple sugars. Disaccharides include sucrose, maltose, and lactose.

Consumption of Sugar

It has been estimated that people in the U.S. eat an average of 133 pounds of sugar sweetener per person annually.[7] Of this, 76 percent consists of "invisible" sugars contained in processed foods and beverages prepared outside the home. The next time you go to the grocery store, examine food labels for sugar—not just in baked goods, candies, and other sweets, but in such food items as "fruit drinks," breakfast cereals, canned soups, prepared main dishes, and canned or frozen fruits. These processed foods, and many others, all contain hidden sugars.

The new food label will help you more easily identify how much sugar a product contains. However, the label does not distinguish between "naturally occurring" sugar, such as that found in fresh fruit, and "added sugar." The term "added sugar" is used to indicate that sugar was added during the manufacturing process. You can look for added sugar on a product's ingredients list. Watch for "code names" for added sugar such as invert sugar, corn syrup, honey, molasses, dextrose, sucrose, fructose, lactose, maltose, galactose, and fruit juice concentrate.

Carbohydrates: a nutrient composed of carbon, hydrogen, and oxygen, which is the body's preferred form of energy, supplying four calories per gram.

Glucose: a form of carbohydrate (simple sugar) that is a major energy-supplying molecule in the body, used to convert energy in metabolic reactions.

3-10

The New Food Label at a Glance

Claims: While descriptive terms like "low," "good source," and "free" have long been used on food labels, their meaning — and their usefulness in helping consumers plan a healthy diet — have been murky. Now FDA has set specific definitions for these terms, assuring shoppers that they can believe what they read on the package.

Health Claims: For the first time, food labels will be allowed to carry information about the link between certain nutrients and specific diseases. For such a "health claim" to be made on a package, FDA must first determine that the diet-disease link is supported by scientific evidence.

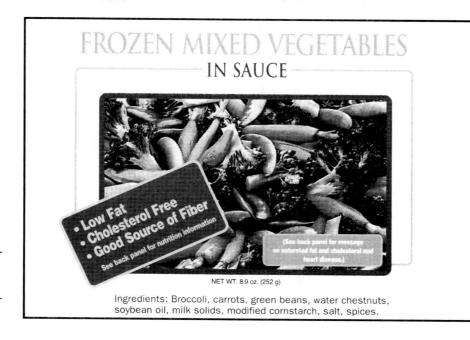

NET WT. 8.9 oz. (252 g)

Ingredients: Broccoli, carrots, green beans, water chestnuts, soybean oil, milk solids, modified cornstarch, salt, spices.

Ingredients still will be listed in descending order by weight, and now the list will be required on almost all foods, even standardized ones like mayonnaise and bread.

"While many factors affect heart disease, diets low in saturated fat and cholesterol may reduce the risk of this disease."

Health claim message referred to on the front panel is shown here.

Figure 3.2: The new food label at a glance

Refined and processed sugars represent 11 percent of the calories in the typical U.S. diet.[8] This level of sugar consumption is highly undesirable in several ways. First, sugar is a pure carbohydrate. Although it is a ready source of calories, it contains none of the other important nutrients such as vitamins, minerals, or protein. This is why sugar is often referred to as "empty calories." People who get 11 percent of their calories daily from sugar must rely on the other 89 percent of their diets to supply 100 percent of the nutrients necessary for optimal body functioning. This may be extremely difficult for the many people on low-calorie weight-reduction diets. Such individuals may be deficient in one or more of the nutrients vital for high levels of wellness.

Many books and articles have appeared in recent years linking sugar consumption with almost every noninfectious disease known today. Most medical and nutritional experts see little support in the research literature for these often simplistic claims. One disease, however, has been unquestionably linked to sugar consumption—tooth decay.[9]

It has been estimated that 70 percent of children in the U.S. have some tooth decay, although the rate has decreased 40 to 60 percent in the last twenty years. This reduction is largely attributed to the widespread increase of fluoride in toothpaste, mouth rinses, drinking water, and topical application.[10] **Dental caries** (tooth decay) begin with **dental plaque,** a sticky, colorless film containing colonies of bacteria that are constantly forming in the mouth. These bacteria break down carbohydrates—especially sugar—changing it to an acid. The sticky plaque then holds this acid to your teeth, allowing it to attack the tooth enamel.

Dental caries: the process through which teeth decay. Commonly known as cavities.

Dental plaque: a gummy mass of microorganisms on the crown of teeth, spreading to the roots, that makes teeth susceptible to decay.

Whether or not this attack will cause cavities depends on three factors: (1) the hardness of your tooth enamel; (2) the strength of the acids; and (3) the length of time the acid is on your teeth. Acids usually work on the tooth enamel for about fifteen to twenty minutes after sugary foods are eaten. If the teeth are not brushed immediately following each meal, three meals a day add up to an hour of acid attack per day. Snacking—especially on sugary foods—increases your acid exposure. Changing your diet and dental-health habits may halt the decay process before a true cavity appears. Dental-health guidelines include the following:

1. Reduce consumption of sugars and foods high in sugar.
2. Avoid between-meal snacks of sweet or sticky foods. Replace with foods such as nuts, fresh fruits, raw vegetables, and milk.
3. Brush and floss teeth or rinse your mouth after meals and snacks—particularly after eating sweet or sticky foods (see Activity for Wellness 3.2).
4. Use a toothpaste that contains fluoride. Fluoride helps in reducing cavities by increasing the return of minerals to the teeth before substantial decay can occur.[11]

Reducing Your Intake of Refined and Processed Sugars

Decreasing your intake of refined and processed sugars can be a challenge. The following suggestions will help you in your attempt to cut down on the added sugar in your diet.

1. Limit your intake of soft drinks containing sugar. This would bring many of us halfway to our goal, since soft drinks are the single greatest contributor of sugar to the typical U.S. diet. Just one twelve-ounce soft drink contains eight to ten teaspoons of sugar. Substitute fruit juices or plain water for your daily beverages.
2. Processed baked goods, such as cakes, pies, cookies, and doughnuts, are estimated to be the second greatest source of added sugar in the U.S. diet. Instead of eating sugary desserts, occasionally top off your meal with fresh fruit, which will satisfy your desire for something sweet while supplying valuable nutrients.
3. Many cereals are presweetened. Check the labels next time you shop and choose the unsweetened variety so that you can control the amount of sugar added.
4. If you add sugar to foods, such as coffee, tea, or cereal, gradually reduce the amount you use each time until you feel comfortable doing without it.
5. Begin to experiment with reducing the amount of sugar you add to foods prepared at home. Be prepared for foods to look and taste different.

Complex Carbohydrates

Complex carbohydrates (polysaccharides) consist of three or more simple-sugar molecules bonded together in varying patterns. The three most common types of complex carbohydrates are starch, fiber, and glycogen.

Starch

Starch is a plant source of complex carbohydrates and may consist of 300 to 400 glucose molecules joined together. Common plant sources of starches include whole-grain foods, potatoes, rice, beans, and vegetables. Carbohydrates should provide the major portion of calories (energy) to our diets. Starch is the most important carbohydrate food source, supplying us with valuable vitamins, minerals, and protein in addition to calories. Wheat, corn, oats, and rice products such as bread, cereal, spaghetti, macaroni, and grits are especially good sources of nutritious starch. So are potatoes, peas, beans, nuts, and soybeans (see figure 3.3).

Fiber

Many of these nutritious sources of starch are also rich in fiber. **Dietary fiber** is commonly defined as the part of food that is not digested by enzymes in the small intestine, where most other foods are digested and absorbed into the bloodstream. There are two major types of dietary fiber—insoluble and soluble. Both play important, though somewhat different, roles in our nutritional health and wellness.

Insoluble fibers, including cellulose, hemicellulose, and lignin, come from the cell walls of plants and are not digested by the body. Whole grains and beans are good sources of insoluble fiber, but wheat bran is by far the richest source. Insoluble fiber speeds up the movement of food through the

How to Brush and Floss

Brushing

For general adult usage, a straight-handled brush with soft polished nylon bristles is best. Whichever type of toothbrush is used, one should use it to brush at least twice a day, but preferably after every meal and at bedtime for maximum effect. The toothbrush is seldom used alone; most individuals use a commercial dentifrice (toothpaste, dental gel, or toothpowder) with their brush. Since all toothpastes and gels are similar, can one be better than another? Yes! How abrasive a dentifrice is and if it contains an acceptable fluoride should be the major concerns. One effective method of brushing follows:

1. Start by brushing along the gum line, moving the brush back and forth with short, gentle strokes.
2. Brush the outer and inner surface of each tooth, upper and lower.
3. Brush the chewing surface of each tooth, upper and lower.
4. Brush your tongue to complete the process.

Flossing

A second method of disrupting the buildup of bacteria on the teeth is by using dental floss. Toothbrush bristles cannot reach plaque and small food particles caught between teeth. The following is a good technique for using floss correctly:*

1. Break off a piece of floss about eighteen inches long.
2. Wind each end of the floss two or three times around the middle finger on each hand. If you are just beginning or have trouble manipulating the floss in the traditional way, try tying it in a loop and holding the loop between your two middle fingers. You should have about two inches of floss between your hands.
3. Hold the floss taut. Use your thumbs and forefingers to guide the floss gently between your teeth.
4. Keep the floss pressed against the surface of your tooth as you move it back and forth and toward the gum. Slide the floss just below the gum margin.
5. Use a straight up-and-down cleaning motion to get rid of plaque that has settled between your teeth.

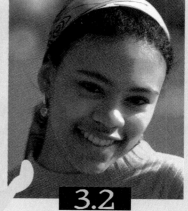

3.2
Activity for Wellness

6. When the floss gets soiled, move to a new section until you have finished flossing all your teeth. Make sure that you get the area behind your back molars, too.

*Brent Q. Hafen, *The Self-Health Handbook.* Copyright ©1980 Prentice-Hall, Englewood Cliffs, N.J.

Source: Adapted from James H. Price et al., *Consumer Health: Contemporary Issues and Choices,* 1985 Wm. C. Brown Communications, Inc., Dubuque, Iowa.

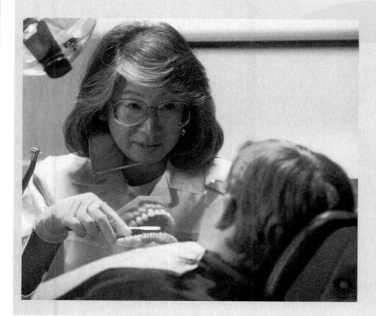

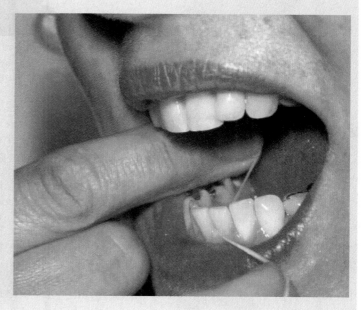

Figure 3.3: What Do You Think?

1. Starches, a plant source of complex carbohydrates, supply valuable vitamins, minerals, and protein. How many servings of complex carbohydrates do you eat each day? Does your diet meet the six or more servings daily recommended by the National Research Council?
2. What are six food items high in complex carbohydrates that you would be likely to consume today?

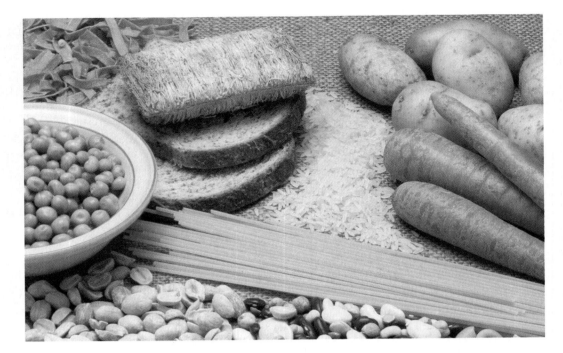

Diverticular disease: a disease characterized by the formation and inflammation of sacs opening off of the colon.

Carcinogens: substances capable of causing cancer.

Diabetes: a chronic disease of the pancreas in which the body is unable to utilize sugars and other carbohydrates normally.

Hypoglycemia: an abnormally low blood glucose level (sometimes referred to as low blood sugar).

Blood cholesterol: the amount of cholesterol circulating in one's blood. It is high blood cholesterol levels that constitute a major risk factor for coronary artery disease.

digestive tract, absorbing water as it passes through. Insoluble fiber increases fecal bulk and contributes to regularity; it may thus play an important role in preventing constipation and **diverticular disease.**

In recent years a number of epidemiological studies have shown that people who eat a diet high in fiber have lower rates of colon cancer.[12] Scientists have yet to explain why fiber seems to decrease the risk of colon cancer; however, several theories are currently being tested. Because insoluble fiber speeds wastes through the colon, it is believed that this may decrease the time that cancer-causing substances are in contact with the colon. Additionally, by increasing stool size, insoluble fiber may reduce the concentration of **carcinogens.**[13] Finally, scientists are investigating whether specific chemical components of fiber, called phytates, may be responsible for inhibiting cancer formation.[14]

Soluble fibers, such as gums, pectins, and storage polysaccharides, are those fibers that, while remaining undigested in the small intestine, are digested and absorbed in the large intestine. Good sources of soluble fiber include oat bran, beans, and fruit, although most plant foods usually contain both soluble and insoluble fiber. Soluble fiber may play an important role in pacing the absorption of carbohydrates into the bloodstream. Because these fibers tend to form gels, the nutrients in high-fiber foods are absorbed slowly over the entire length of the small intestine. This prevents dramatic swings in blood-sugar levels. Some believe soluble fiber may thus be important in controlling **diabetes** and **hypoglycemia.**[15]

For several years, soluble fiber and its role in decreasing **blood cholesterol** levels has been "in the news." Many studies now provide evidence that eating foods high in soluble fiber, especially oat bran and oatmeal, helps to reduce an individual's total blood cholesterol level.[16] Oat bran and its relationship to cholesterol are discussed in greater detail later in this chapter.

People in the U.S. currently eat about 15 grams of fiber daily. The National Cancer Institute (NCI) recommends doubling this amount to between 20 and 30 grams of fiber daily.[17] The NCI cautions against consuming over 35 grams of fiber daily because of the possibility of adverse effects. It is best to consume fiber from a variety of food sources rather than by supplements. The fiber content of many common foods is highlighted in table 3.5. This information, and information available to you on food labels, will help you learn to select foods high in fiber.

Glycogen

Glycogen, the third major complex carbohydrate, is formed in the body by a process that binds glucose molecules. Glycogen is the principal way the body stores sugar for energy needs. Glycogen is stored

TABLE 3.5

Dietary Fiber Content of Selected Foods

Vegetables	Serving size (*½ cup cooked unless otherwise marked)	Total fiber (grams)	Soluble fiber (grams)	Insoluble fiber (grams)
Peas	*	5.2	2.0	3.2
Parsnip	*	4.4	0.4	4.0
Potato	1 small	3.8	2.2	1.6
Broccoli	*	2.6	1.6	1.0
Zucchini	*	2.5	1.1	1.4
Squash, summer	*	2.3	1.1	1.2
Carrot	*	2.2	1.5	0.7
Tomato	*	2.0	0.6	1.4
Brussels sprouts	*	1.8	0.7	1.1
Beans, string	*	1.7	0.6	1.1
Onion	*	1.6	0.8	0.8
Rutabaga	*	1.6	0.7	0.9
Beet	*	1.5	0.6	0.9

Fruits	Serving size (raw)	Total fiber (grams)	Soluble fiber (grams)	Insoluble fiber (grams)
Apple	1 small	3.9	2.3	1.6
Blackberries	1/2 cup	3.7	0.7	3.0
Pear	1 small	2.5	0.6	1.9
Strawberries	3/4 cup	2.4	0.9	1.5
Plums	2 med.	2.3	1.3	1.0
Tangerine	1 med.	1.8	1.4	0.4

Breads, cereals	Serving size (*½ cup cooked unless otherwise indicated)	Total fiber (grams)	Soluble fiber (grams)	Insoluble fiber (grams)
Bran (100 percent) cereal#	*	10.0	0.3	9.7
Popcorn	3 cups	2.8	0.8	2.0
Rye bread#	1 slice	2.7	0.8	1.9
Whole-grain bread#	1 slice	2.7	0.08	2.6
Rye wafers#	3	2.3	0.06	2.2
Corn grits	*	1.9	0.6	1.3
Oats, whole	*	1.6	0.5	1.1

Legumes				
Kidney beans#	*	4.5	0.5	4.0
White beans#	*	4.2	0.4	3.8
Pinto beans	*	3.0	0.3	2.7

Currently, researchers use different methods to analyze dietary fiber content in foods. Until a single testing protocol is adopted, precise fiber totals will vary from laboratory to laboratory.

Meats, milk products, eggs, and fats and oils are not listed in this food-fiber survey because they are virtually devoid of fiber content.

This symbol, (#), indicates that the fiber analysis was carried out on cooked food, rather than raw food.

mainly in the liver and voluntary skeletal muscles. It can be called on in stressful situations as a source of ready energy. During a stressful situation, the fight-or-flight response triggers the breakdown of glycogen into glucose, and it is then released into the bloodstream to be used for quick energy.

Achieving the Dietary Recommendations

Increasing your consumption of complex carbohydrates and "naturally occurring" sugars may present a challenge. The following suggestions will help you in your attempt to increase your intake of complex carbohydrates.

1. Include more fruits and vegetables in your meals. According to the National Research Council, you should try to eat at least five servings of a combination of fruits and vegetables each day.

2. Whenever possible buy fresh fruits and vegetables. They are likely to have greater amounts of vitamins and minerals than processed varieties. When fresh fruits and vegetables are not available, frozen produce is preferable to canned because it retains more nutrient value.

3. Increase your consumption of whole-grain products, such as whole-wheat bread, whole-grain (wheat, rye, or oat) cereal, legumes, and brown rice to at least six servings each day. Refined-grain products, such as white bread, white enriched or instant rice, macaroni, egg noodles, and the like, have undergone processing that removes valuable nutrients and fiber. Some of these lost nutrients are replaced in products labeled as "enriched," but there is a danger that nutrients, both known and unknown, have been removed or altered in ways not currently understood.

Fats

Fats, also known as **lipids,** are a group of chemical compounds that, like carbohydrates, are composed of carbon, hydrogen, and oxygen atoms linked together in specific ways. Fat is the second major source of energy for the body, supplying nine calories for every gram of fat consumed. Because a gram of fat is a condensed source of energy, that is, it contains more than twice the amount of calories contained in 1 gram of protein or

carbohydrate, it is a perfect way for the body to store energy. Body fat stores energy (calories) in **adipose** (fat) **cells** for the times you will need more energy than your diet supplies. Your adipose tissue also serves as padding to protect vital organs of the body and helps insulate the body from extremely cold weather. Fat molecules also form the chemical core of certain hormones and help transport and store certain vitamins. Fats are a popular food component because they add flavor and texture to our foods. Fats also contribute to a feeling of satisfaction after eating because they slow down the rate at which food is emptied from the stomach.

Saturated and Unsaturated Fats

There are three major types of fat in the body: triglycerides, phospholipids, and steroids. **Triglycerides** are the major dietary source of fat; 95 percent of all fat consumed in food consists of triglycerides. Triglycerides are composed of two different clusters of atoms—glycerol and fatty acids. Each triglyceride consists of three fatty-acid molecules attached to a glycerol molecule.

Some triglycerides are a major source of dietary concern because of the type of fatty acid they contain. Fatty acids consist of a chain of carbon and hydrogen atoms with a few oxygen atoms on the side. If all of the carbon atoms are linked together with single bonds, it allows the maximum number of hydrogen atoms to bond to the molecule. Thus, it is said to be **saturated** with hydrogen. Some fatty-acid molecules have one double bond between their carbon atoms and therefore cannot carry the maximum hydrogen atoms. This type of fatty acid is said to be **monounsaturated.** In still other fatty acids there are two or more double bonds between the carbon atoms making these fatty acids **polyunsaturated** (see figure 3.4).

Animal fats generally contain greater proportions of saturated fatty acids; plant fats usually contain monounsaturated or polyunsaturated fatty acids (see figure 3.5). Additionally, saturated fats are usually solid at room temperature while unsaturated fats tend to be liquid at room temperature. There is a major exception to these generalities: coconut oil, palm oil, and palm kernel oil, often called **"tropical oils,"** are highly saturated fats.

Diets high in fat, especially saturated fat, have been linked with many of the chronic

Lipids: a fat compound that usually has fatty acids as a part of its structure.

Triglycerides: a lipid that consists of three fatty acid molecules attached to a glycerol molecule. Triglycerides are stored in fat cells; elevated blood triglyceride levels are associated with an increased risk of cardiovascular disease.

Saturated fat: a type of fatty acid with all carbon atoms joined by single bonds, allowing the maximum number of hydrogen atoms to bond to the molecule. Often found in animal sources, saturated fats are usually solid at room temperature. Consumption of foods containing saturated fats increases one's total and LDL blood cholesterol, increasing the risk of cardiovascular disease.

Tropical oils: highly saturated fats that come from certain tropical plants. The term refers primarily to coconut oil, palm oil, and palm kernel oil.

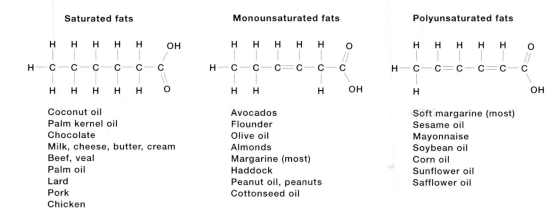

Saturated fats

Coconut oil
Palm kernel oil
Chocolate
Milk, cheese, butter, cream
Beef, veal
Palm oil
Lard
Pork
Chicken

Monounsaturated fats

Avocados
Flounder
Olive oil
Almonds
Margarine (most)
Haddock
Peanut oil, peanuts
Cottonseed oil

Polyunsaturated fats

Soft margarine (most)
Sesame oil
Mayonnaise
Soybean oil
Corn oil
Sunflower oil
Safflower oil

Figure 3.4:
Structure of saturated,
monounsaturated, and
polyunsaturated fats

and degenerative diseases prevalent today. The link appears to be strongest between saturated fat, cholesterol, and **coronary artery disease.**[18] Food rich in saturated fats, such as beef, whole milk, cheese, coconut oil, and palm oil, have been shown to cause elevations in the blood-cholesterol levels of humans. Monounsaturated fats and polyunsaturated fats appear to lower total blood cholesterol.[19]

The National Research Council recommendations, outlined at the beginning of this chapter, suggest that people should consume 30 percent *or less* of their total calories from fat daily. This does *not* mean that you should eat only foods with less than 30 percent of their calories from fat. Rather, you should balance your diet so that your *total daily food intake* has less than 30 percent fat calories. For instance, if you eat a food, such as a piece of cake, that has 45 percent of its calories from fat, you can balance your diet that day by eating other foods that are low in fat. For a 2,000 calorie diet, 29 percent of calories from fat would equal about 65 grams of fat daily. The new food labels provide you with the number of grams of fat a product contains, so you can more easily track your daily fat intake.

In addition to total fat intake, the National Research Council recommends that *less than* 10 percent of your calories daily should come from saturated fat. Many scientists believe that the current fat guidelines are set too high. They suggest that a daily total fat intake of 20 to 25 percent of calories, with no more than 7–8 percent of calories from saturated fat, would be the ideal level for lowering the risk of coronary artery disease.[20]

Reading food labels to check whether or not a product contains saturated sources of fat will not always tell you the complete story.

Manufacturers commonly use a technique called **hydrogenation** in which they add hydrogen to polyunsaturated or monounsaturated fats. This process changes the consistency of oil, making it a harder, more spreadable form of fat. For instance, corn oil can be hydrogenized to form margarine, an unsaturated, spreadable fat. Margarine and butter have the same number of calories per gram (nine), but margarine does not contain as much saturated fat (see figure 3.5).

Consuming a product with hydrogenated corn oil is not the same as consuming one with plain corn oil. Even though both oils are from a plant source, the process of hydrogenation will cause the corn oil to become more saturated. Additionally, during the process of hydrogenation, some of the fatty acid molecules become rearranged into a form known as **trans-fatty acids,** sometimes referred to as transfat (see figure 3.6). A study reported in the *New England Journal of Medicine* in 1990 found that a diet high in transfats caused a rise in **LDL** cholesterol to a level similar to that associated with a diet high in saturated fat.[21] High blood levels of LDL cholesterol are strongly associated with an increased risk of coronary artery disease. Even more distressing was the finding that, unlike a diet high in saturated fat, the diet high in transfats decreased the amount of **HDL** cholesterol in the blood (the kind of cholesterol thought to lower one's risk of coronary artery disease.)

Epidemiological studies have found additional evidence of an important relationship between diets high in transfats and the risk of coronary artery disease. As far back as 1983, a study reported in the *Journal of Epidemiology and Community Health* found higher levels of trans-fatty acids in the fat

Coronary artery disease: a chronic disease condition in which the normal flow of blood through the coronary arteries is reduced or impaired.

Hydrogenation: a manufacturing technique whereby hydrogen is added to unsaturated fats, thus making them more saturated (with hydrogen) than they would be naturally.

Trans-fatty acids: a form of fatty acids derived from the process of hydrogenation. These fatty acids, when consumed in foods, are believed to increase total and LDL blood cholesterol, and decrease HDL cholesterol, thus increasing a person's risk for coronary artery disease.

LDL: low density lipoprotein; a type of lipoprotein that carries cholesterol from the digestive tract to other body cells. High blood levels of LDL are associated with an increased risk of coronary artery disease.

HDL: high density lipoprotein; a type of lipoprotein that carries cholesterol from the bloodstream to the liver, where it can be excreted from the body. High blood HDL levels may help protect individuals against coronary artery disease.

Figure 3.5: The fat family weighs in.

Every fat or oil is made up of a combination of saturated, monounsaturated, and polyunsaturated fatty acids. In general, the less saturated fat and the more monounsaturated fat, the better. We've ranked the fats and oils from lowest amount of saturated fat to highest.

From *Nutrition Action Healthletter,* March 1994, Center for Science in the Public Interest, Washington, D.C.

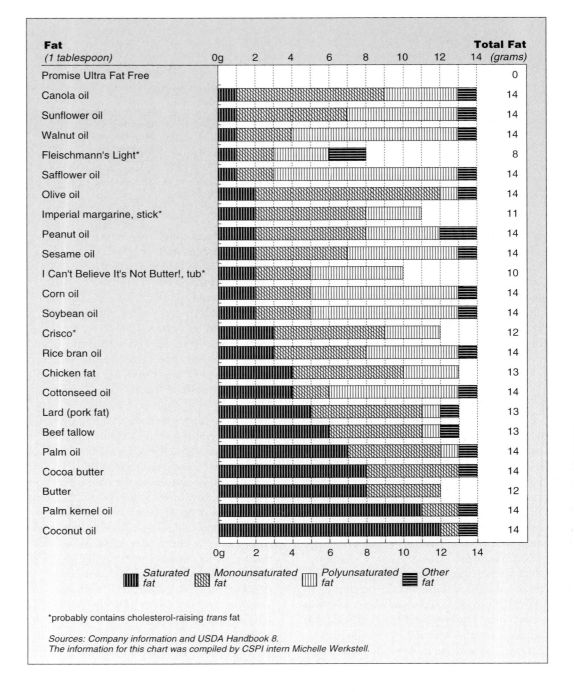

Fat (1 tablespoon) — Total Fat (grams)

Fat	Total Fat (grams)
Promise Ultra Fat Free	0
Canola oil	14
Sunflower oil	14
Walnut oil	14
Fleischmann's Light*	8
Safflower oil	14
Olive oil	14
Imperial margarine, stick*	11
Peanut oil	14
Sesame oil	14
I Can't Believe It's Not Butter!, tub*	10
Corn oil	14
Soybean oil	14
Crisco*	12
Rice bran oil	14
Chicken fat	13
Cottonseed oil	14
Lard (pork fat)	13
Beef tallow	13
Palm oil	14
Cocoa butter	14
Butter	12
Palm kernel oil	14
Coconut oil	14

Saturated fat   Monounsaturated fat   Polyunsaturated fat   Other fat

*probably contains cholesterol-raising *trans* fat

Sources: Company information and USDA Handbook 8.
The information for this chart was compiled by CSPI intern Michelle Werkstell.

---

tissue of persons who had died from heart attacks, as compared with persons who had died from other causes.[22] More recent studies confirm the relationship between transfats consumption and the risk of a heart attack. An article published in 1993 in the British medical journal *Lancet* described the results of a study that followed nearly 90,000 female nurses for eight years. The results confirmed concerns about transfats; women in the study who consumed diets highest in transfats had a 50 percent higher risk of heart attack than those women in the study who consumed the least amount of transfats.[23] Another study recently reported in the *American Journal of Cardiology*[24] found that people with documented coronary artery disease had higher levels of trans-fatty acids in their blood.

The body of research now available has led some researchers to the conclusion that a diet high in transfats may have a greater impact on risk for coronary artery disease than saturated fats.[25] While further research is needed to verify the results of these

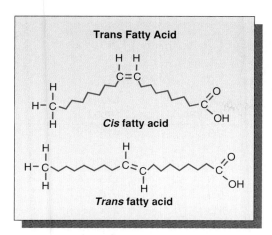

Figure 3.6: A trans-fatty acid
Partially hydrogenated oils stay solid at room temperature and won't go rancid as quickly as polyunsaturated oils. However, with hydrogenated oil, some of its fats are converted from a *cis* structure (which occurs naturally) to a *trans* structure. *Cis* fats have a "bend" in their chain of carbon atoms, whereas *trans*fats are straight—making them solid at room temperature.

metabolic and epidemiological studies, it would be prudent to cut down on your intake of foods high in transfats. Margarine is thought to be the food item containing the greatest amount of transfats. However, food products such as frozen cakes, bran muffins, Danish pastry, doughnuts, imitation cheese, candies, frozen fish sticks, French fries, and ready-made frostings, often contain partially hydrogenated vegetable oils or fats and may therefore be high in transfats.

Reading the Nutrition Facts label on a food product will not help you identify transfats in foods. The FDA currently requires reporting of only total fat and saturated fat. However, reading the product ingredients list will help you identify food items with partially hydrogenated oils or fats. If you eat often at fast-food restaurants it will be even more difficult to monitor your transfat intake, as there is no food labeling requirement for fast-food restaurants, and many of them use hydrogenated oils high in transfats. Limiting your intake of total fat, as well as products containing partially hydrogenated fats, may help reduce your risk of coronary artery disease through an effect on levels of blood cholesterol.

The Cholesterol Controversy

Cholesterol, the subject of great nutritional controversy, is a fatlike waxy material found in animal tissues. It is technically classified as a steroid. Cholesterol plays an important role in many body functions. It is a major constituent of cell membranes and the covering that protects nerve fibers. Cholesterol also aids in the formation of vitamin D and the sex hormones androgen, estrogen, and progesterone. Cholesterol is also used by the body to produce **bile salts,** which in turn aid in digesting fat.

The body receives cholesterol from two major sources. Cholesterol is present in the animal products we consume, and it is manufactured by the body itself in the liver. The term **dietary cholesterol** is used to refer to the cholesterol we consume in food. The National Research Council recommends that we limit our dietary cholesterol intake to *less than* 300 mg daily. This recommendation is aimed at helping to keep our blood-cholesterol levels at a healthy level. It is high levels of blood cholesterol that constitutes one of the major risk factors of coronary artery disease. Remember that foods high in cholesterol, such as eggs and liver, are not the only foods that can raise your blood-cholesterol level. As we discussed previously, foods high in saturated fats and transfats have the greatest effect on raising total and LDL blood-cholesterol levels (see table 3.6).

Large population studies in the United States have shown that a high level of LDL cholesterol in the bloodstream is associated with an increased risk of coronary artery disease.[26] (Heart disease and cholesterol screening are discussed in greater detail in chapter 10.)

HDLs also carry cholesterol in the bloodstream; however, they pick up cholesterol and carry it back to the liver where it is used to produce bile salts. High levels of HDL in the bloodstream ($\geq$60 mg/dl) are thought to be protective against coronary artery disease. Additionally, new evidence indicates that a low level of HDL (<35 mg/dl) increases the risk for coronary artery disease even when total cholesterol and LDL cholesterol levels are normal.[27]

The major controversy surrounding cholesterol pertains to its relationship to coronary artery disease. Most experts agree that a high blood cholesterol level, especially a high LDL level, is a major risk factor for coronary artery disease.

In 1984 the first definitive study linking a reduction in blood cholesterol to a reduction in deaths from coronary artery

Dietary cholesterol: cholesterol that is consumed in food products. Some foods such as liver, egg yolks, cheesecake, and soft serve ice cream are high in cholesterol. The American Heart Association and the U.S. Daily Reference Value recommend that people consume less than 300 mg of cholesterol daily.

Bile salts: a major component of bile, these molecules aid in the digestion and absorption of fats.

TABLE 3.6 — Dietary Sources of Fat, Saturated Fat, and Cholesterol

Food	Total Fat (gm.)	Saturated Fat (gm.)	Cholesterol (mg.)
Liver, fried, sliced (3 oz)	7	2.5	410
Egg, (1)			
raw, whole	5	1.6	213
raw, yolk only	5	1.6	213
raw, white only	0	0.0	0
whole, fried in margarine	7	1.9	211
Cheesecake (1 piece)	18	9.9	170
Ice cream (vanilla) (1 cup)			
soft serve (frozen custard)	23	13.5	153
regular, hardened	14	8.9	59
Eggnog (1 cup)	19	11.3	149
Lemon meringue pie (1 slice)	14	4.3	143
French toast (1 slice)	7	1.6	112
Bread stuffing (prepared from a mix) (1 cup)	26	5.3	67
Clams (canned, drained) (3 oz)	2	0.5	54
Tuna (water packed)			
solid white (3 oz)	1	0.3	48
Devil's Food Cake with chocolate frosting (1 piece)	8	3.5	37
Cheddar Cheese (1 oz)	9	6.0	30
Milk (1 cup)			
Whole	8	5.1	33
Skim	Trace	0.3	4
Butter (1 pat)	4	2.5	11
Mayonnaise (regular) (1 tbsp)	11	1.7	8

Source: Data from *USDA Nutritive Values of Food*. A copy of the entire food values document can be found in Appendix B, *Connections for Health Student Workbook*.

disease was released. Since that time, many other studies have also shown similar results.[28] Yet another question still remained: "Does lowering blood cholesterol levels really save lives?" For instance, some recent cholesterol lowering studies have found "an increase in the death rate among males from violent deaths, including suicide, accidents, and murder."[29] These increases in death rates from other causes, however, were very small and many researchers questioned their validity.

In November 1994 the British journal *Lancet* published the results of a five year prospective clinical intervention study that, for the first time, documented both a decrease in overall deaths as well as deaths from fatal heart attacks.[30] Scandinavian researchers studied over 4,000 men and women who had documented heart disease and high blood-cholesterol levels. One half of the subjects were randomly assigned to the treatment group and received a cholesterol-lowering drug; the control group received a placebo. After almost five years, the experimental group had, on average, a 35 percent drop in blood-cholesterol levels. They also had 42 percent fewer deaths from coronary artery disease, and *30 percent fewer deaths from all causes* when compared to the control group.

Based upon the evidence available to date, it appears that attempts to lower blood cholesterol may have large health payoffs. Therefore, it would be prudent for you to consider having your blood-cholesterol level checked and to begin to make changes in your lifestyle that will decrease LDL cholesterol and increase HDL cholesterol.

Achieving the Dietary Recommendations

The National Research Council recommends that people in the U.S. decrease their intake of fat to 30 percent *or less* of their total energy (caloric) intake. They should also reduce saturated-fat consumption to *less than* 10 percent of their total energy intake.

Monounsaturated and polyunsaturated fats should account for the remaining energy intake from fat. Dietary cholesterol consumption should be limited to *less than* 300 milligrams a day. The following suggestions should help you on your way to reducing fats and cholesterol in your diet.

1. Include more fruits (except avocados and olives), vegetables, breads, cereals, dry beans, and dry peas in your meals.

2. In the late 1980s several studies indicated that consuming oat bran may help to lower blood-cholesterol levels.[31] Then in 1990 a study was published in the *New England Journal of Medicine* that seemed to explain the cholesterol lowering effect of oat bran. This study found that people who ate more oat bran also ate less foods high in saturated fat—thus explaining the effects on blood-cholesterol levels. In April 1991, however, Michael Davidson and his colleagues at Rush-Presbyterian-St. Luke's Medical Center in Chicago published the results of a study that found oat bran and oatmeal have an independent effect on lowering blood-cholesterol levels.[32]

   Davidson's subjects (experimental and control) were already on a fat-modified diet, yet he found significant decreases in blood-cholesterol levels for subjects who consumed two ounces of oat bran or three ounces of oatmeal. No such changes were found in the control group who consumed farina instead of oats. Recently, other researchers have found similar results.[33]

   The final word is not in on oat bran. Yet consumed in moderation, it will help you increase complex carbohydrates in your diet, and may, in combination with a diet low in saturated fats, help control your blood-cholesterol level.

3. Cut down on fatty meats. These include regular ground beef, corned beef, spareribs, sausage, hot dogs, luncheon meat, and heavily marbled cuts, such as prime rib. Keep in mind that different grades of meat contain different amounts of fat. Remember that the new food labels will help you choose low-fat meals with their label designation of lean and extra lean.

4. Include more chicken and turkey in your diet. These foods are generally lower in fat content than many meats.

5. Include more fish in your diet. Recent scientific evidence indicates that eating two to three fish meals a week may help to prevent deaths due to heart attacks. It is believed that consuming a type of polyunsaturated fat found in some fish—**omega-3 fatty acids**—reduces the chance of developing artery-clogging blood clots and decreases blood-cholesterol levels. Fish oil supplements, however, are not recommended at this point because their potential benefits and harm have not been fully evaluated.

6. Limit nuts, peanuts, and peanut butter, which contain considerable amounts of fat.

7. Trim excess fat from meat before cooking.

8. Bake, broil, roast, stew, or barbecue foods using a rack for cooking so that fat will drain away from the food. Avoid fried foods.

9. Baste meats with wine, tomato juice, or the like, rather than using meat drippings.

10. Make stews and soups a day ahead. Chill them and scrape off the congealed fat before reheating.

11. Reduce the use of whole milk and whole-milk products, such as most cheeses and ice cream. Substitute skim or low-fat milks and their products, such as uncreamed cottage cheese, which are lower in fat content. Recently, several **fat substitutes** have been developed which are being marketed as products to help people achieve the dietary guidelines and still be able to consume ice cream and other formerly high-fat foods. One such substitute, *Simplesse,* marketed by the *Nutrasweet Company,* consists of blended egg whites and milk proteins. This creamy mixture tastes like fat, but has very few calories from fat. Many health claims are being made for the variety of fat substitutes currently being marketed. Of Special Interest 3.1 takes a more detailed look at a proposed health benefit of fat substitutes.

Omega-3 fatty acids: a type of fatty acid found mostly in the oils of cold-water fish such as salmon, halibut, mackerel, herring, and lake trout.

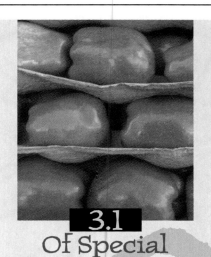

3.1

Of Special Interest

A Fat Substitute That Lowers Cholesterol

Walk down the aisles of your supermarket and you'll get a glimpse of the future: foods made with fat replacers. For instance, there are now dozens of ice-cream cones with the taste and texture of real ice cream, but with little or no fat. To approximate the creamy texture of ice cream (or salad dressing or mayonnaise), they use fat substitutes such as Simplesse (made from whey), as well as a variety of carbohydrate-based compounds, such as maltodextrin and polydextrose, which trap water and thus create a moist texture. Food manufacturers are constantly experimenting with these and other compounds to get a better imitation fat. One of the newest of these carbohydrate compounds is Oatrim (also called TrimChoice). Since it is made from oat flour, Oatrim has an advantage over other fat substitutes: it contains soluble fiber.

Developed by the USDA in 1993, Oatrim has been licensed to Quaker and ConAgra. It is already being used in several of ConAgra's Healthy Choice products, such as its cheeses and ground beef; it may be called "hydrolyzed oat flour" on the ingredients list. Smaller companies are using it in baked products such as cookies and muffins, and dozens of products are under development. Oatrim has received excellent reviews from food scientists, who have found that it is easy to incorporate into foods, that its gelling property adds a creamy fatlike texture, and that it is good in baking. One gram of Oatrim has just one calorie (compared to nine in a gram of fat). It contains the carbohydrate amylodextrin, along with beta glucan, the principal fiber in oats and barley. This fiber may help lower blood cholesterol and have other good effects. But like any type of fiber, large amounts may cause bloating and gas in people not used to it.

One recent USDA study found that twenty-four people with elevated cholesterol levels who consumed large amounts of Oatrim, disguised in foods, for five weeks experienced a 16 percent drop in cholesterol levels (but no drop in "good" HDL), an 8 percent drop in systolic blood pressure, and improved control of blood sugar. Oatrim should not be oversold, however, as oat bran was a few years ago. This study was small and used more Oatrim than people will normally eat. Still, like oats themselves, Oatrim seems to be a good food, and may have modest health benefits. One thing is sure: it is better for you than the fats it replaces.

What Do You Think?

1. Would you be willing to switch from high-fat desserts to desserts made with fat substitutes? What do you perceive to be the main benefits and risks of consuming fat substitutes?
2. Based on your knowledge of human behavior, why do you think some people who consume food containing fat substitutes may feel free to eat more of other high-fat foods? How might this affect their health?

Reprinted by permission of the *University of California at Berkeley Wellness Letter,* Health Letter Associates, 1994..

---

12. Select salad oils, cooking oils, and margarine, such as canola oil and olive oil (see figure 3.5) that are high in monounsaturated fats. Selecting fat-free salad dressings and mayonnaise would be even better. Avoid hydrogenated fats because they contain high amounts of transfats.
13. Egg yolks are very high in cholesterol (see table 3.6). Cut back your consumption of egg yolks to three per week. Try replacing breakfast eggs with high-fiber cereal. In recipes, try one of the many egg substitutes now on the market.
14. For desert, make low-fat choices such as angel food cake, sherbet, fat-free frozen yogurt, or fresh fruit (see figure 3.7).

Protein

Like carbohydrates and fat, **protein** is composed of carbon, hydrogen, and oxygen. Protein, however, has an important distinguishing element—nitrogen. Nitrogen gives protein the important function of growth, maintenance, and regulation of body tissues and processes. All proteins are formed from varying combinations of twenty-one specific nitrogen-containing chemicals called **amino acids.**[34] These amino acids are often referred to as the building blocks of protein because they string together to form an almost endless variety of protein molecules, much like we string together the letters of the alphabet in order to form different words.

Protein is a major component of almost every cell in the body. It helps build muscle, bone, skin, and blood. Protein is a major constituent of antibodies, an important part of our immune system, so it helps us fight infections. It also aids in the formation of hormones, such as **insulin** and **thyroxine,** which regulate our body's chemical processes,

Insulin: a hormone secretion of the pancreas necessary to convert carbohydrates into energy and sometimes used therapeutically to control diabetes.

Thyroxine: a hormone secretion of the thyroid gland that regulates the basal metabolic rate and increases the synthesis of protein in some organs of the body.

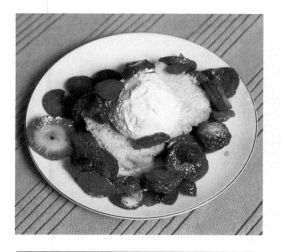

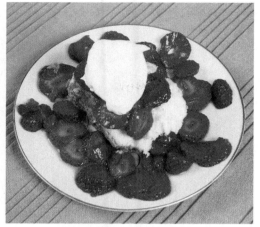

This slice of pound cake topped with vanilla ice cream and strawberries will give you approximately:

415	calories
19.6	grams of fat
72	milligrams of cholesterol

This slice of angel food cake topped with non-dairy lite whipped topping and strawberries will give you approximately:

211	calories
1.6	grams of fat
0	milligrams of cholesterol

Figure 3.7: What Do You Think?

1. As the two strawberry and cake desserts above illustrate, making just a few simple substitutions when eating can drastically reduce calories, fat, and cholesterol consumption, while still tasting great. How easy do you think it would be for you to make such substitutions in your diet?

2. How important do you think it is to make these substitutions at least some of the time?

known as **metabolism.** Protein plays an important role in forming enzymes, which control the speed of various chemical reactions. Protein also carries iron, oxygen, and nutrients to all the cells of the body. Next to water, protein is the major constituent of the human body.

In addition to its many tissue-building, maintenance, repair, and regulation functions, protein can also be used by the body as a source of energy. Protein, like carbohydrates, supplies the body with four calories per gram consumed. If your diet does not contain enough carbohydrates or fat to be used as energy, your body will use protein, even at the expense of building or maintaining your body tissue. On the other hand, if you consume more protein than your body needs for growth and maintenance, the extra protein is broken down to be used for calories or is converted into body fat and stored. Protein, however, is an expensive and inefficient source of calories for the body. When protein is broken down to be used for energy, not all of the protein molecule is used. The nitrogen is not needed and must therefore be excreted by the kidneys. As health writer Jane Brody wrote, "Americans excrete the most expensive urine in the world. If it were economical to collect and dry it, tons of nitrogen could be harvested from the nation's toilet bowls each day."[35]

In order to be used by the body, protein must first be broken down into amino acids. During this breakdown the human body can make many of the amino acids it needs for efficient building of body tissues. There are eight **essential amino acids,** however, which the body must consume from food. Any food containing all eight of these essential amino acids is known as a **complete protein.** It is important to consume complete or high-quality protein foods daily so that optimal growth and maintenance of body tissues is enhanced.

Achieving the Dietary Recommendations

It is relatively easy for most people in the U.S. to consume quality sources of protein daily. Meat, poultry, fish, and milk products are all good sources of complete protein. Many of these good sources of protein, however, are animal sources and thus are likely to be high in saturated fat, cholesterol, and calories. Choosing leaner cuts of red meat, trimming excess fat, and cooking with less fat can help greatly. Poultry, fish, and low-fat milk

Metabolism: the physical and chemical processes of the body that contribute to the growth, maintenance, repair, and breakdown of body tissues, as well as making energy available.

1. Mexican dinners typically feature beans and rice, two complex carbohydrates that together form a complete protein. What other plant sources of food do you combine in your diet during a typical week that together form complete proteins?

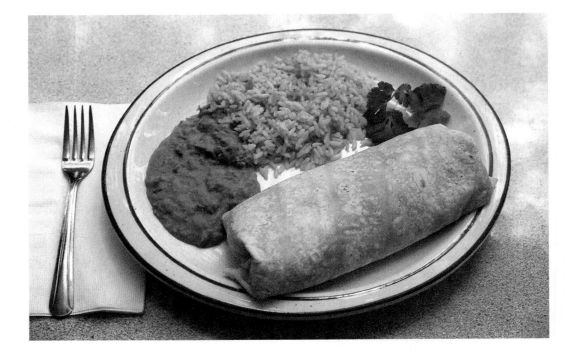

Megadose: referring to vitamins and minerals, doses in excess of ten times the RDA.

Antioxidants: substances that prevent the formation of free radicals, or atoms in which there is an unpaired electron. Free radicals are natural byproducts of the body burning oxygen (oxidation). By inhibiting the formation of free radicals, antioxidants are thought to decrease the risk of developing a variety of chronic diseases including heart disease and some cancers.

products also contain less fat, cholesterol, and calories without losing their protein value.

Many plant sources of protein are lacking in one or more of the essential amino acids. Plant foods, however, can be good sources of complete protein if two or more complementary sources are combined so that one food supplies the essential amino acids missing in the other (see figure 3.8). You have, no doubt, eaten such complementary protein pairs as peanut butter on whole-wheat bread, macaroni and cheese, or skim milk on cereal (see table 3.7).

Most people in the U.S. are getting adequate amounts of high-quality protein. The major change recommended for protein can be accomplished by eliminating some of our fatty sources of protein (animal products) and replacing them with complex-carbohydrate sources; however, we must be careful to remember to eat complementary sources of plant protein.

Vitamins

The body has a special need for small amounts of certain chemicals to help perform many complex chemical reactions. These chemicals are commonly referred to as **vitamins.** A substance is defined as a vitamin if it plays a vital role in human metabolism and a deficiency disease results when inadequate amounts are consumed.

Vitamins are commonly grouped into two categories: fat soluble and water soluble. **Fat-soluble vitamins** (A, D, E, and K) are transported and stored by the body's fat cells. Because the body stores these vitamins they can build up in the system and become toxic if great quantities (**megadoses**) are consumed. The **water-soluble vitamins** (eight B vitamins and vitamin C) are not stored by the body in any significant amount and therefore need to be consumed in adequate proportions in the diet daily. Table 3.8 describes these vitamins, including their food sources, functions, and the adult recommended dietary allowance (RDA).

Vitamin supplementation has long been a controversial subject. Health food enthusiasts have advocated taking large doses of vitamin supplements daily, often at megadose levels. Health scientists, on the other hand, have argued that scientific evidence for the benefits of megadoses of vitamin supplements was lacking and that some vitamins, especially those that are fat soluble, can be toxic at high levels. Recently, however, new and reputable scientific studies have begun to provide evidence that megadoses of *some* vitamins *may* provide protection from a variety of chronic diseases. One of the most widely publicized and controversial involves the class of vitamins known as **antioxidants.**

TABLE 3.7 How to Mix and Match Protein Pairs

To make protein-rich combinations, you can:

Number 1—Match vegetable proteins:
Mix foods from two or more groups in column A such as: peanut butter (a legume) and whole-wheat bread (a grain).

Number 2—Match vegetable and low-fat animal proteins:
Mix foods from any group(s) in column A with small amounts from any group(s) in column B such as: rice (a grain) and chicken (a low-fat meat).

A	B
Vegetable proteins ("*incompletes*")	*Low-fat animal proteins* ("*completes*")
Legumes:	**Low-fat dairy products:**
dry beans and peas—kidney, navy, lima, pinto, black, or soybeans black-eyed or split peas soybean curd (tofu) soy flour peanuts and peanut butter (use wisely, has medium fat level)	nonfat dry milk skim milk low-fat cottage cheese egg whites (where most of the egg protein lies)
Grains:	**Low-fat meats:**
whole grains—barley, oats, rice, rye, wheat (bulgur, cracked wheat) corn pasta—noodles, spaghetti, macaroni, lasagna	poultry fish lean cuts of red meat
Nuts and seeds:	
almonds, cashews, pecans, and walnuts sunflower seeds, pumpkin seeds, sesame seeds	

Source: From *Eaters Almanac*. National Heart, Lung, and Blood Institute, National Institutes of Health, Bethesda, MD.

Antioxidants

In the last few years evidence has pointed to the possibility that antioxidant vitamins, especially vitamins C, E, and beta-carotene (a plant form of vitamin A), may play an important role in preventing heart disease, certain types of cancer, **cataracts,** and other chronic diseases.[36] Antioxidants are thought to decrease the risk of chronic disease through their ability to deactivate free radicals. Free radicals are "activated" oxygen molecules that are a natural by-product of the body metabolizing or burning oxygen. Free radicals can damage body cells, eventually contributing to disease. Antioxidants are believed to intervene in this process, preventing cell damage.

Each of the antioxidant vitamins appear to play differing roles in chronic disease. A high intake of vitamin E, for instance, has been associated with a decreased risk of heart disease,[37] oral cancer,[38] and cataracts.[39] Vitamin C has been associated with both a decreased risk of **hypertension** and an increase in levels of HDL.[40] Additionally, vitamin C and beta-carotene may be synergistic with vitamin E in lowering the risk for coronary artery disease.[41]

Much of the evidence, however, has come from observational or epidemiological studies, where scientists compare the antioxidant vitamin intake levels of persons who have a specific chronic disease to those who don't. This type of study is less reliable

Cataracts: a common occurrence with aging in which the lens of the eye becomes increasingly opaque, resulting in obscured vision.

Hypertension: abnormally high arterial blood pressure of a chronic nature, generally identified in persons with a diastolic pressure above 90 mm Hg, or a systolic pressure above 140 mm Hg.

TABLE 3.8 Vitamins

Vitamin	Why needed	Important sources	Deficiency symptoms	Risks of megadose	Adult RDA
A	• Helps keep eyes healthy and able to see in dim light • Helps keep skin healthy and smooth • Helps keep lining of mouth, nose, throat, and digestive tract healthy and resistant to infection • Aids normal bone growth and tooth formation through proper utilization of calcium and phosphorous	Liver; butter; margarine; whole milk; vitamin-A fortified milk; cheddar cheese; deep yellow, green, or orange fruits and vegetables such as cantaloupe, apricots, carrots, spinach, collards, broccoli, kale, nectarines, mangoes, pumpkins, winter squash, turnip greens, sweet potatoes, and watermelon	• Night blindness; eye secretions cease; infection of mucous membranes; skin changes; stunted growth • Deficiency seldom seen in the U.S.	Headache; diarrhea; nausea; loss of appetite; dry, itching skin: elevated blood calcium; may cause birth defects if taken in excess during pregnancy	800 RE (8,000 IU), women; 1,000 RE (10,000 IU), men
D	• Helps promote normal growth • Helps body use calcium and phosphorus for the building and maintenance of strong bones and teeth	Fish-liver oils; vitamin-D fortified milk; liver; egg yolk; salmon; tuna; sunlight produces vitamin D from a form of cholesterol in the skin	• Rickets; a softening of the bones leading to bow legs and other bone abnormalities	Early stage: weakness, fatigue, headache, nausea, vomiting, diarrhea; later stage: kidney impairment, deposits of calcium salts in the kidney, osteoporosis of the bones, calcium deposits in soft body tissue	5 mcg. (micrograms) or 200 IU; 10 mcg or 400 IU before age 25
E	• Helps prevent red blood cell destruction • Helps prevent damage to cells from oxidation	Vegetables; vegetable oils; wheat germ; nuts; fortified ready-to-eat cereals; green leafy vegetables; shrimp; other seafood (including clams, salmon, and scallops); apples; apricots; and peaches	• Anemia due to increased red blood cell destruction • Nerve damage	May cause increased levels of blood cholesterol and lipids	8 mg. women; 10 mg. men
K	• Helps with blood clotting	Green leafy vegetables (including lettuce, spinach, kale and cabbage); liver; and produced by intestinal bacteria	• Severe bleeding, poor blood clotting	Natural forms: no known toxic effects Synthetic forms: anemia, jaundice	60–65 mcg. women; 70–80 mcg. men
C (ascorbic acid)	• Helps bind body cells together through the production of connective tissue • Aids normal bone and tooth formation, maintenance, and repair • Aids in healing wounds • Helps the body utilize iron • Helps resist infection	Citrus fruits and juices, tomatoes, green peppers, strawberries, cantaloupe, watermelon, cabbage, potatoes, broccoli, brussels sprouts, kale, collards, mustard greens	• Scurvy—degeneration of bones, teeth, and gums, anemia, rough skin, wounds that don't heal; increased susceptibility to infection	Diarrhea, nausea, abdominal cramps, kidney stones If large doses are taken during pregnancy the infant may develop scurvy after birth	60 mg.

Vitamin	Functions	Food Sources	Deficiency Symptoms	Toxicity	RDA
Folacin (folic acid)	• Aids in the formation of hemoglobin in the red blood cells • Necessary for the production of genetic material	Liver, green vegetables, dried beans and peas, nuts	• Anemia, diarrhea, smooth red tongue	None identified in humans to date. Has produced enlarged cells in the kidneys of laboratory animals.	180 mcg., women; 200 mcg., men (RDI = 0.4 mg.)
Pantothenic acid	• Helps release energy from carbohydrates, fat, and protein • Helps form hormones	Liver, whole-grain cereal and bread, green vegetables, eggs, nuts	• Nausea, headache, muscle cramps, low blood sugar	Increased need for thiamine	No RDA (RDI = 10 mg.)
Biotin	• Helps release energy from carbohydrates • Helps the body synthesize fatty acids	Liver, kidney, egg yolks, green beans	• None known under normal conditions	None known	No RDA (RDI = 0.3 mg.)
B$_1$ (thiamine)	• Helps the body change carbohydrate foods into energy • Promotes normal appetite and digestion • Helps to maintain a healthy nervous system	Pork, liver, dry beans and peas, whole-grain and enriched breads and cereals, nuts	• Beriberi—muscular weakness, mental confusion, cardiac abnormalities	Few cases of toxicity reported. Some people are hypersensitive to large doses resulting in cardiac abnormalities.	1–1.1 mg., women; 1.2–1.5 mg., men
B$_2$ (riboflavin)	• Helps release energy from carbohydrates, fat, and protein • Helps keep skin healthy	Milk, liver, eggs, green leafy vegetables, lean meats, dried beans and peas, enriched breads, cereals, and pasta	• Skin sores around the nose and lips, cracking of the corners of the mouth, eyes sensitive to light	None known	1.2–1.3 mg., women; 1.4–1.7 mg., men
B$_3$ (niacin)	• Helps release energy from carbohydrates, fat, and protein • Helps maintain all body tissues	Tuna, poultry, lean meat, fish, liver, peanuts, peas, whole-grain or fortified breads, cereals, and pasta	• Pellagra—diarrhea, mental disorders, skin rash, irritability	Skin rash, flushed skin, abnormal liver function, jaundice, blurred vision	13–19 mg.
B$_6$ (pyridoxine)	• Helps the body to use protein to build body tissue • Helps the body to use carbohydrates and fat for energy	Whole grains, meat, liver, fish, wheat germ, bananas, spinach, green leafy vegetables	• Skin disorders, mental depression, weakness, irritability	Dependency on high doses leading to deficiency symptoms when returned to normal doses	1.6 mg., women; 2 mg., men
B$_{12}$ (cyanocobalamin)	• Helps the body form red blood cells • Aids in normal function of all body cells	Lean meat, liver, eggs, milk, cheese (animal products)	• Pernicious anemia, nervous system malfunctions, soreness and weakness in arms and legs	None known	2 mcg.

than intervention studies or clinical trials, where a scientist randomly assigns subjects to two or more groups and gives an "experimental" group the antioxidant vitamin supplement while giving a "control" group a look-alike placebo. Intervention trials are now underway to study the role of antioxidants in preventing a variety of chronic diseases. It will be several years, however, before we know the results from many of these studies.[42]

One intervention study, however, has been completed and the results are cause for concern.[43] In April 1994, researchers from Finland and the U.S. National Cancer Institute published the results of an antioxidant intervention study in the *New England Journal of Medicine*. Researchers had randomly assigned male smokers to three experimental groups, and a control group (which received a placebo). The experimental groups received one of the following treatments: 20 milligrams of beta-carotene, 50 milligrams of vitamin E, or a combination of both the beta-carotene and vitamin E. After following these smokers for five to eight years, the researchers noted that smokers receiving the beta-carotene had an 18 percent higher incidence of lung cancer. They also saw preliminary evidence that beta-carotene may have increased the risk of heart disease in these smokers. The subjects who received the vitamin E appeared to have a lower risk for prostate cancer, but a higher risk for one type of stroke. While one study can never prove or disprove a hypothesis, it does suggest that caution should be taken regarding the use of antioxidant vitamin supplements until the results of other intervention studies are available.

In light of the controversial evidence available for antioxidant vitamins, the American Heart Association, the American Cancer Society, and the Center for Science in the Public Interest all believe that we should wait for the results of more clinical intervention studies before we regularly consume antioxidant vitamin supplements.[44] These organizations point out that more long-term studies are necessary to provide evidence of both the safety and effectiveness of antioxidant supplementation.[45]

Even though scientists recommend a wait-and-see attitude toward antioxidant supplementation, they *do* recommend that consumers make a concerted effort to eat foods, especially fruits and vegetables, that are good sources of antioxidant vitamins. Table 3.8 provides the RDA and major food sources for each of the antioxidant vitamins.

Antioxidants, however, are not the only vitamins being studied for their chronic disease prevention benefits. **Folic acid** is also receiving much attention from public health professionals.

Folic Acid

In 1992, the Centers for Disease Control and Prevention (CDC) published a recommendation that all women of childbearing age should consume 0.4 milligrams daily of folic acid, also known as folacin. Recent studies from the U.S. and other countries have shown that this daily dose of folic acid, if taken prior to conception and during the early weeks of pregnancy, would reduce the risk of having children born with **neural tube defects.**[46]

The most common neural tube defects include **spina bifida,** a condition in which infants are born with a spinal column that does not close completely, leaving the spinal cord exposed, and **anencephaly,** a condition in which an infant is born with little or no brain tissue. Infants born with anencephaly are stillborn or die shortly after birth. Those born with spina bifida survive to adulthood with a variety of disabilities even with treatment. It is estimated that approximately 2,500 infants are born each year with neural tube defects.[47] Researchers estimate that if women consumed the recommended daily intake of folic acid, 50 to 70 percent of neural tube defects could be prevented.[48]

Neural tube defects develop between the third and fourth weeks following conception. Often, a woman might not even know she was pregnant until the damage was already done. For this reason, the CDC recommends that any woman capable of having children should daily consume the current RDA for folic acid. Some of the foods rich in folic acid include lentils, sunflower seeds, spinach, peanuts, split peas, and orange juice. Many breakfast cereals are fortified with folic acid. Additionally, the FDA has proposed that folic acid be added to flour, breads, and other grain products. This recommendation is not without controversy. While folic acid

Folic acid: a B vitamin, also known as folacin, that aids in the formation of hemoglobin in the red blood cells and is necessary for the production of genetic material. Recently, daily consumption of 0.4 mg. of folic acid by pregnant women has been associated with a reduction in neural tube defects in newborns.

Neural tube defects: defects to the neural tube that occur during the embryonic period of human development. The embryonic neural tube eventually develops into the brain and spinal cord under normal conditions.

supplementation would help prevent neural tube defects, it might also put other people at risk. High folic acid intake can mask the signs of **pernicious anemia,** a vitamin B_{12} deficiency. The elderly and vegetarians who do not consume any animal products are the most susceptible to vitamin B_{12} deficiency. If vitamin B_{12} deficiency is not caught early enough it can result in permanent nerve damage. If grain products are fortified with folic acid it may result in certain vulnerable populations, such as the elderly, being exposed to too much folic acid.

While the new research on vitamins is promising, consumers are left in the position of having to decide how to use this, as yet incomplete, information.

Vitamin Consumption

Vitamins are big business in the United States. It is estimated that annual sales of dietary supplements exceed $3.3 billion per year.[49] One recent survey noted that 45 percent of women and 32 percent of men had taken a dietary supplement within two weeks previous to the survey.[50] Another study noted that sales of vitamin A/beta-carotene supplements increased by 45 percent and vitamin E supplements by 39 percent between 1992 and 1993.[51] It seems clear that many consumers are not taking a wait-and-see attitude toward vitamin supplementation.

While there is great controversy surrounding vitamin supplements, researchers do agree on one point. Vitamin supplements *cannot* substitute for a healthy diet. Food supplies much more than just vitamins, it is also an important source of minerals, protein, water, fiber, and many other elements that we have yet to discover.[52] The best advice remains unchanged: make healthy food choices so that you consume the RDA for all vitamins, including folic acid and antioxidants. The American Cancer Society recommends that people consume at least five servings of fruits and vegetables a day. Yet a recent study found that only 9 percent of people in the U.S. currently follow this recommendation.[53] Grain products, especially whole grains, are also good sources of vitamins. You should try to eat six to eleven servings of grains daily. (A serving size of grains equals one piece of bread, half a bagel, etc.) Currently, it is estimated that we consume only five servings of grains daily.[54]

Most individuals do *not* need to take a daily multivitamin supplement.[55] Exceptions to this include smokers, heavy alcohol drinkers, those with impaired immune systems, and some elderly people. Additionally, pregnant women will often be prescribed a special vitamin supplement by their physicians.

Vitamin supplementation is one area of health and wellness where quackery abounds. Some of the more prominent myths include the following:

Myth 1: If certain amounts of the various vitamins are good, more is always better. Our best research to date indicates that, for most vitamins, the RDA will supply appropriate amounts of vitamins for living a healthy life. Excess amounts of the water-soluble vitamins are flushed out of the body daily; therefore, consuming them in excess of need often leads to expensive urine rather than better health. Megadoses of some water-soluble vitamins can also be toxic. For instance, kidney stones have long been known to result from megadoses of vitamin C.[56] More recently, a study has indicated that, in men with a tendency to have excess stores of iron in the body, vitamin C interacts with the iron as a pro-oxidant.[57] In the 10 percent of men in the U.S. with this condition, high doses of vitamin C may increase their risk of heart disease.

The fat-soluble vitamins are stored and excesses often lead to toxic or harmful levels. For instance, high doses of vitamin A can result in headaches, diarrhea, nausea, loss of appetite, dry itching skin, and elevated blood calcium. Additionally, it may cause birth defects if taken in excess during pregnancy. Table 3.8 notes which vitamins are known to be toxic in high doses.

Sometimes a physician will recommend a vitamin supplement that contains amounts of certain vitamins that exceed the RDA. When vitamins are prescribed by a physician, they should be viewed as a drug necessary to treat a certain medical condition.

Myth 2: Natural vitamins are better than synthetic vitamins. Natural and synthetic vitamins are chemically identical and are used exactly the same way by the human body. The major distinction between natural and synthetic vitamins is their price—not their health benefits. The Center for Science in the Public Interest notes one exception to this

Pernicious anemia: a type of anemia (a decreased ability of the blood to carry oxygen) that results from a genetic defect that interferes with the body's ability to absorb vitamin B_{12}.

general rule. " 'Natural' vitamin E is the only vitamin that our bodies seem to utilize better than the synthetic form, according to some researchers. To find it, ignore 'natural' claims on labels. Look for 'd-alpha-tocopherol' (not 'dl-') as the only type of vitamin E listed."[58]

Vitamin Supplementation

Most people do *not* need to supplement their diet with a multipurpose vitamin supplement. If you do take a vitamin supplement, the following tips[59] will help you get the most benefit for your money.

1. *Find a supplement that supplies no more than 100 percent of the RDA for any vitamin included.* Remember that you will also be consuming a significant amount of vitamins in the food you eat.

2. *Read labels to make sure that any vitamin supplement you take will dissolve in less than one hour.* To do any good, a vitamin must dissolve in the digestive tract and be absorbed into the bloodstream. Not all vitamin supplements meet this criteria. The Center for Science in the Public Interest (CSPI) recommends buying supplements that meet new *voluntary* criteria set by the U.S. Pharmacopoeia (USP). CSPI suggests looking for a statement that reads "This product is specifically formulated to pass a rigid 45-minute laboratory dissolution test."

3. *Read labels for expiration dates.* The expiration date on a dietary supplement, however, does *not* mean the same thing as the expiration date on a drug. Expiration dates on drugs must be based on testing, while on dietary supplements these dates can mean whatever the manufacturer wants it to. CSPI suggests that consumers avoid dietary supplements with expiration dates within six to nine months of expiration.

4. *Price shop for your vitamins.* Name brand vitamins are not necessarily better than store brands. In fact, CSPI has investigated vitamin sources and found that all vitamin manufacturers buy most of their vitamins from the same small group of vitamin suppliers. CSPI recommends saving money by purchasing the cheaper store brand vitamins. They suggest, however, that you stick to large national retail store brands because of their reputation for quality.

Vitamin supplements are often combined with minerals, another important nutrient group.

Minerals

Minerals are inorganic substances vital to many body functions. Minerals are commonly divided into two groups: major minerals and trace elements. **Major minerals** are needed in large amounts (but not megadoses) by the body. Some of the known major minerals include calcium, phosphorus, magnesium, potassium, sulfur, sodium, and chloride. **Trace elements** serve an equally important role in body functioning but are needed in much smaller amounts. Minerals needed by the body in trace amounts include iron, zinc, manganese, copper, iodine, and cobalt. Table 3.9 presents a more detailed look at these important minerals including their common food sources, functions, and symptoms of deficiency.

Several minerals have recently been singled out by researchers and consumers alike because of their effects on health and wellness. One of the most prominent mineral controversies today surrounds the overconsumption of sodium in the typical U.S. diet.

Sodium Consumption

In appropriate amounts, **sodium** plays several vital roles in body functioning. Sodium is known to help regulate blood and other body fluids, to aid in nerve-impulse transmission and heat action, and even to facilitate the metabolism of carbohydrates and protein. As important as sodium is, however, your body needs very little. The basic human requirement for sodium is only 200 milligrams daily, or about one-tenth of a teaspoon of salt. Even those who lose sodium from sweating great amounts need only a maximum of 2,000 milligrams of sodium, or about one teaspoon of salt daily.

The average man in the U.S. eats 4,000 milligrams of sodium each day, while the average woman in the U.S. eats 3,000 milligrams.[60] Sodium is most often consumed in our diets in the form of salt (sodium chloride). Roughly 40 percent of table salt is sodium. In addition to our salt intake, we consume many additives in processed foods that contain sodium. Monosodium glutamate, sodium bicarbonate (baking soda), baking powder, disodium phosphate, sodium

Minerals: inorganic substances, found naturally in the earth, that play a vital role in human metabolism. Some minerals, such as iron and zinc, are needed in only small amounts and are known as trace elements. Other minerals, such as calcium and sodium, are required by the body in larger amounts and are called major minerals.

Mineral	Distribution	Functions	Sources
Calcium (Ca)	Mostly in the inorganic salts of bones and teeth	Structure of bones and teeth, essential for nerve-impulse conduction, muscle-fiber contraction, and blood coagulation, increases permeability of cell membranes, activates certain enzymes	Milk, milk products, leafy green vegetables
Phosphorus (P)	Mostly in the inorganic salts of bones and teeth	Structure of bones and teeth, component in nearly all metabolic reactions, constituent of nucleic acids, many proteins, some enzymes, and some vitamins, occurs in cell membrane, ATP, and phosphates of body fluids	Meats, poultry, fish, cheese, nuts, whole-grain cereals, milk, legumes
Potassium (K)	Widely distributed, tends to be concentrated inside cells	Helps maintain intracellular osmotic pressure and regulate pH, promotes metabolism, needed for nerve-impulse conduction and muscle-fiber contraction	Avocados, dried apricots, meats, nuts, potatoes, bananas
Sulfur (S)	Widely distributed	Essential part of various amino acids, thiamine, insulin, biotin, and mucopolysaccharides	Meats, milk, eggs, legumes
Sodium (Na)	Widely distributed, large proportion occurs in extracellular fluids and bonded to inorganic salts of bone	Helps maintain osmotic pressure of extracellular fluids and regulate water balance, needed for conduction of nerve impulses and contraction of muscle fibers, aids in regulation of pH and in transport of substances across cell membranes	Table salt, cured ham, sauerkraut, cheese, graham crackers
Chlorine (Cl)	Closely associated with sodium, most highly concentrated in cerebrospinal fluid and gastric juice	Helps maintain osmotic pressure of extracellular fluids, regulate pH, and maintain electrolyte balance, essential in formation of hydrochloric acid, aids transport of carbon dioxide by red blood cells	Same as for sodium
Magnesium (Mg)	Abundant in bones	Needed in metabolic reactions that occur in mitochondria and are associated with the production of ATP, plays role in conversion of ATP to ADP	Milk, dairy products, legumes, nuts, leafy green vegetables
Iron (Fe)	Primarily in blood stored in liver, spleen, and bone marrow	Part of hemoglobin molecule, catalyzes formation of vitamin A, incorporated into a number of enzymes	Liver, lean meats, dried apricots, raisins, enriched whole-grain cereals, legumes, molasses
Manganese (Mn)	Most concentrated in liver, kidneys, and pancreas	Occurs in enzymes needed for synthesis of fatty acids and cholesterol, formation of urea, and normal functioning of the nervous system	Nuts, legumes, whole-grain cereals, leafy green vegetables, fruits
Copper (Cu)	Most highly concentrated in liver, heart, and brain	Essential for synthesis of hemoglobin, development of bone, production of melanin, and formation of myelin	Liver, oysters, crabmeat, nuts, whole-grain cereals, legumes
Iodine (I)	Concentrated in thyroid gland	Essential component for synthesis of thyroid hormones	Food content varies with soil content in different geographic regions, iodized table salt
Cobalt (Co)	Widely distributed	Component of cyanocobalamin, needed for synthesis of several enzymes	Liver, lean meats, poultry, fish, milk
Zinc (Zn)	Most concentrated in liver, kidneys, and brain	Constituent of several enzymes involved in digestion, respiration, bone metabolism, liver metabolism, necessary for normal wound healing and maintaining integrity of the skin	Seafoods, meats, cereals, legumes, nuts, vegetables

From John W. Hole, Jr., *Human Anatomy and Physiology* 6th ed. Copyright © 1993 Wm. C. Brown Communications, Inc. Reprinted by permission of Times Mirror Higher Education Group, Inc., Dubuque, Iowa. All rights reserved.

alginate, sodium benzoate, sodium hydroxide, sodium propionate, sodium sulfite, and sodium saccharin are just a few sodium additives you may be consuming on a regular basis. The new food label will provide you with the exact number of milligrams of sodium in the food products you purchase.

Excess sodium in the diet is one of several risk factors associated with high blood pressure (hypertension).[61] High blood pressure is of great concern because of its causative link to stroke, coronary artery disease, congestive heart failure, and kidney failure. Although researchers are not completely sure of the mechanism behind the sodium-hypertension connection, many believe that certain individuals are sensitive to sodium and will develop high blood pressure when excess sodium is consumed. It is estimated that 50 million people in the U.S. are hypertensive:[62] About half of them are believed to be sodium sensitive.[63] Some individuals may be sodium-resistant, maintaining normal blood pressure no matter how much salt they ingest.

The sodium-sensitivity theory is largely responsible for the great controversy surrounding the dietary guideline for sodium. The new daily reference value (DRV) for sodium is 2,400 milligrams. For reference, one teaspoon of salt contains 2,132 milligrams of sodium. Food labels will tell you the percent of the sodium DRV per serving in food products you purchase.

Some people argue that since only a certain percentage of the population is sodium-sensitive, it doesn't make sense to recommend that all persons in the U.S. cut down on sodium and salt. Right now, however, we have no way to identify who is sensitive to salt and who is not.

There is no definitive proof that excess sodium "causes" hypertension or that lowering sodium intake will prevent hypertension. A recent cross-cultural study of salt and its relationship to hypertension, the Intersalt study, found only a small relationship between salt and hypertension.[64] Other risk factors for hypertension, such as race, potassium intake, and alcohol consumption were much more pronounced.

High sodium intake, however, is also associated with an increased risk for **osteoporosis.** Scientists believe the risk increases because calcium appears to be excreted from the body when sodium is

consumed. According to the Center for Science in the Public Interest, "on average, urinary calcium increases by about (23 mg) for every teaspoon of salt consumed. . . . An uncompensated calcium loss of 23 mg per day is enough to dissolve one percent of the skeleton annually—that is, 10 percent in a decade"![65]

Stomach cancer is also associated with a high sodium intake. Researchers believe that excess salt irritates the lining of the stomach, resulting in an increase in cell reproduction.[66] Observational studies have found higher levels of salt intake in people who have stomach cancer.[67]

In light of all the evidence linking high salt (sodium) intake to a variety of chronic diseases, health authorities such as the U.S. Surgeon General, the National Academy of Sciences, and the Center for Science in the Public Interest recommend that people consider controlling their salt and sodium intake.[68]

Achieving the Dietary Recommendations

There are many enjoyable and tasty ways to cut down on the amount of sodium and salt in our diets. Many people discover that foods have richer tastes without large amounts of salt. Controlling sodium intake will involve using your creativity in experimenting with new foods and condiments as well as cutting back on certain salty foods. The following suggestions should help you on your way to meeting the National Research Council's dietary recommendation of limiting daily intake of salt to 6 grams *or less*.

1. Increase your consumption of fresh or frozen fruit, fruit juices, and vegetables. Most of these foods will contain 35 milligrams or less of sodium. Many grocery stores voluntarily provide nutrition information about fresh fruits and vegetables in the produce department (see figure 3.9). Frozen vegetables that contain a sauce may have a higher sodium content (140 to 460 milligrams). Read food labels to determine milligrams and the percent daily value of sodium per serving.

2. Most grains are naturally low in sodium. Pasta and regular hot cereals cooked without salt usually contain 5 milligrams or less of sodium; white or whole-grain bread typically contains 110 to 150 milligrams.

Osteoporosis: a disease condition of the bone resulting from a decline in bone mineral content and predisposing it to injury and fracture.

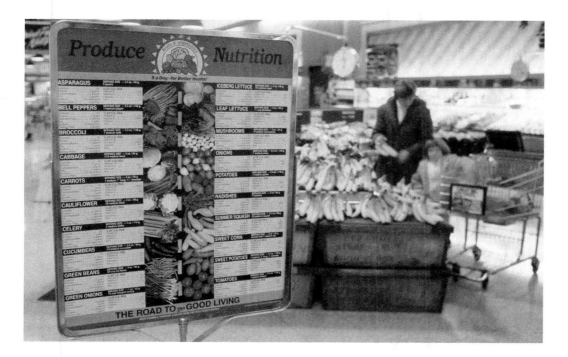

Figure 3.9: What Do You Think?

1. Under the new food labeling laws grocers must provide nutrition information for the 20 most popular raw vegetables. Many grocers have elected to use large posters placed in the produce section of their stores. Do you make use of the nutrition information now available to you when you shop for produce? If not, why?

3. Fresh meats, poultry, and fin fish usually range from 15 to 25 milligrams of sodium per ounce.

4. Cut down on your consumption of fast foods. Many items sold at fast-food restaurants are very high in sodium (see table 3.10).

5. Be creative in your cooking. A variety of alternatives will contribute to a tasty yet nutritious meal. You might try lemon or lime juice, wines, onion, garlic, ground pepper, horseradish, and herbs.

6. Experiment with tasting the natural flavor of foods. Cut down on the salt used in cooking and remove the salt shaker from the table.

7. Look for salt-free beverages. Club soda and soda water, as well as diet soft drinks containing saccharin (sodium saccharin), all contain sodium.

8. Cut down on foods prepared in brine, such as pickles, olives, and sauerkraut.

9. Use lesser amounts of salty or smoked meat, such as bologna, corned or chipped beef, frankfurters, ham, luncheon meats, salt pork, and sausage.

10. Eat sparingly such salty or smoked fish as anchovies, caviar, salted and dried cod, herring, sardines, and smoked salmon.

11. Limit snack items such as potato chips, salted pretzels, salted popcorn, salted nuts, and salted crackers. Replace them with snacks like fresh fruit, raw vegetables, unsalted nuts, unsalted pretzels, and unsalted unbuttered popcorn.

12. Avoid bouillon cubes, seasoned salts (including sea salt), soy sauce, Worcestershire sauce, and barbeque sauce.

Calcium Consumption

Another mineral that has received widespread attention in recent years is **calcium.** Calcium is the body's most abundant mineral and plays major roles in building strong bones and teeth, in regulating blood clotting, in the transmission of nerve impulses, in heart-muscle contraction, and in regulating the flow of fluids in and out of body cells.

The calcium RDA is currently 1,200 milligrams for people aged twelve through twenty-four, 800 milligrams for people aged twenty-five and older, and 1,200 milligrams for pregnant and lactating women. The Reference Daily Intake (RDI), or the value used on food labels, is 1,000 milligrams of calcium (or 1 gram). However, in June 1994, The National Institute of Health sponsored a consensus conference to determine the most up-to-date optimal calcium intake,

Calcium: a major mineral which is critical for bone growth, muscle contraction, and other metabolic functions; in its solid state it comprises about 85 percent of the mineral matter in bones.

TABLE 3.10   *Fast Foods High in Sodium*

Company/Product	Sodium (mg.)
Shoney's Reuben Sandwich	3,873
Shakey's Pizza potato wedges (15 pieces)	3,703
Chick-Fil-A Turkey Sandwich ('Club' 9.3 oz.)	2,890
Subway Submarine Sandwich (club Italian, on honey wheat roll, 12-inch)	2,776
Long John Silver's Combination entree with fish, shrimp, clams, fries, hushpuppies, coleslaw)	2,630
Captain D's Chicken Entree (with rice, green beans, breadstick, salad)	2,615
Subway Submarine Sandwich (turkey breast, on honey wheat roll, 12-inch)	2,520
Subway Submarine Sandwich (roast beef, on honey wheat roll, 12-inch)	2,347
Hardee's Big Country Breakfast (sausage)	2,240
Rax Smokin Sausage with chili	2,163
Captain D's Fish Dinner (orange roughy, with rice, green beans, breadstick, salad)	2,156
Shoney's Ham Sandwich Club, on whole wheat	2,105
Taco Bell Taco Platter, light	2,068
Arby's Italian Submarine Sandwich	2,062
Arby's Turkey Submarine Sandwich	2,033
Steak 'N Shake Breakfast Sandwich (ham, with egg)	1,850
Rax Ham and Cheese Sandwich (with Swiss cheese, 7.9 oz.)	1,737
Little Caesar's vegetable pizza with individual tossed salad	1,715
Shoney's Fish, baked Light Side'	1,641
Rally's Bacon Cheeseburger	1,629

Source: Data from A. Ulene, *The NutriBase Nutrition Facts Desk Reference,* Avery Publishing Group, Garden City Park, NY.

based on the most recent scientific evidence.[69] This panel agreed that optimal calcium intake should be higher for most age groups than either the RDA or the RDI recommends (see table 3.11). For instance, the consensus conference recommendation for children and young adults age eleven to twenty-four years ranges from 1,200 to 1,500 mg. The upper end of this range would increase calcium intake by 300 mg as compared with the RDA. The RDI of 1,000 mg calcium meets the consensus conference recommendation for only men age twenty-five to sixty-five and for women age twenty-five to fifty, or fifty plus years for women on estrogen replacement therapy. For all others, the RDI standard used for food labels is *less* than recommended by the NIH consensus panel.

Healthy People 2000 objectives for the nation recommends that people through age twenty-four, and pregnant and lactating women, consume three or more servings daily of foods rich in calcium (see table 3.12). Those people age twenty-five and older should consume two or more servings daily. Most people, however, take in much less. A study reported in a 1992 issue of the *Journal of the American Medical Association* found that the average calcium intake for the White, college-age women they studied was only 781 milligrams.[70]

Calcium deficiencies have been linked with several major diseases, the most notable to date being osteoporosis. Osteoporosis consists of a thinning of the bone materials, which leads to an actual loss of bone mass. This causes bone to become brittle and prone to breakage. It is estimated that 25 million people in the U.S. have some degree of osteoporosis.[71] Women especially seem susceptible to this disease. Osteoporosis is not

TABLE 3.11 — Optimal Calcium Recommendations, National Institutes of Health Consensus Panel, 1994

Age group	Recommended daily calcium intake (mg)
Infant	
birth–6 months	400
6 months–1 year	600
Children	
1–5 years	800
6–10 years	800–1200
Adolescents/young adults	
11–24 years	1200–1500
Men	
25–65 years	1000
Over 65 years	1500
Women	
25–50 years	1000
Over 50 years (postmenopausal)	
on estrogens	1000
not on estrogens	1500
Over 65 years	1500
Pregnant and nursing	1200–1500

Source: Data from the Office of Medical Applications of Research, National Institute of Health, Bethesda, MD.

just a disease of the elderly. Women as young as age twenty-five have been diagnosed with signs of significant bone loss.

It was long believed that our need for calcium decreased as we aged. It now seems likely that our need actually increases. Childhood is a time for major bone growth, but adults continue to develop bone mass until about age thirty-five. Peak adult bone mass, or the largest amount of bone the body ever contains, appears to play a vital role in the process of osteoporosis. It is very important that adults consume adequate amounts of calcium during the years of bone growth. (Osteoporosis is discussed in greater detail in chapter 18.)

Calcium can be increased in the diet by consuming more dairy products, fish, dark leafy greens, broccoli, tofu, and legumes (see table 3.12). Generally, it is best to consume the RDA of calcium through food sources, especially low-fat dairy products.[72] A balanced diet provides a variety of nutrients other than calcium, and allows the body to absorb small amounts of calcium at a time.

Women who do not eat enough foods high in calcium, however, may want to consider taking a calcium supplement. The Center for Science in the Public Interest (CSPI) suggests the following rule of thumb regarding calcium supplementation: "If you're a post menopausal woman and don't eat at least four daily servings of high-calcium foods—like milk, yogurt, or calcium-fortified bread or juice—consider a supplement. For teens, make that at least three servings. For everyone else, two daily servings is enough."[73] Additionally, it is recommended that anyone taking a calcium supplement choose one containing factory-made calcium carbonate (like Tums) and take it with meals, to increase absorption.[74] It is especially important to avoid supplements containing "natural source"

TABLE 3.12

Dietary Sources of Calcium

Food	Calcium
Whole milk, 1 cup	291 mg
Low-fat milk, 1 cup (2 percent)	297 mg
Skim milk, 1 cup	302 mg
Low-fat yogurt, 1 cup (plain)	415 mg
Low-fat yogurt, 1 cup (fruit-flavored)	345 mg
Swiss cheese, 1 oz.	272 mg
Cheddar cheese, 1 oz.	204 mg
Brick cheese, 1 oz.	191 mg
Pink salmon, 3 oz. (canned with bones)	167 mg
Sardines, 3 oz. (canned with bones)	372 mg
Kale, cooked, 1 cup	206 mg
Broccoli, cooked, 1 cup	136 mg

Source: Data from USDA Handbooks Nos. 8–1 and 456.

calcium from fossilized oyster shells, or from bonemeal. A recent study in the *American Journal of Public Health* reported that these supplements contain lead levels believed to be unsafe.[75]

Whether or not you take calcium supplements, you need to be aware of dietary factors that may affect your body's ability to absorb calcium. For instance, excess protein consumption increases the amount of calcium that is excreted from the body rather than being absorbed.[76] Recent research, however, suggests that the protein consumed in dairy products is offset by the surplus of calcium they contain. Similar results have been found in studies of caffeine consumption's effect on calcium absorption. Results to date indicate that young women who balance moderate caffeine intake with adequate calcium consumption do not experience deleterious effects.[77] Older women, however, appear to have more problems maintaining the appropriate calcium balance.

Preliminary studies suggest that a high intake of phosphates may also increase calcium excretion. Two prime sources of phosphates in the U.S. diet are cola drinks and meat. Substituting cola for milk is a practice of many young adults. A high phosphorus, low calcium diet may be detrimental to both building strong bones in youth as well as slowing the rate of bone loss as one ages.[78] As mentioned earlier in this chapter, sodium intake also affects the excretion rate of calcium.[79]

Some nutrients actually help the body absorb calcium. Vitamin D is one such nutrient. Most people get plenty of vitamin D through fortified milk and cereals. Additionally, exposure to the sun allows the body to make vitamin D.

As with vitamins, the U.S. Pharmacopeia (USP) has dissolution standards for calcium. If a product meets the USP standard, the supplement will dissolve in the body and increase the likelihood of calcium absorption. Some product labels will contain a statement that they meet the USP standard. Also, if a product label mentions that a calcium supplement helps decrease the risk of osteoporosis it must, by FDA regulation, meet the USP standard.

Water

Water is an essential nutrient. Humans can live approximately two weeks without food, but under optimal conditions can live only ten days without water. Even short-term losses of water can be life threatening due to dehydration. Approximately two-thirds of your body weight is water (65 to 70 percent water in males, and 55 to 65 percent water in females). The total amount of water in your body is directly related to the amount of lean tissue in your body rather than to your total body weight. This is because fat tissue contains less water than lean tissue. Females typically have a greater percentage of body fat related to their secondary sex characteristics, so they have a lesser amount of water than males.

Water is found in three major body compartments—inside your cells, outside your cells, and in your bloodstream. From these compartments, water performs a variety of functions. Water bathes all of our body cells, helping to transport oxygen and various nutrients to the cells and waste products out of the body. Water also plays an important role in regulating our body temperature by removing heat from the body during the evaporation of sweat.

Water is regulated in the body by a center in the brain that controls our thirst response. When the body needs more water, we become thirsty. When there is too much water in the body, the brain sends out signals to the kidney to get rid of more water in the urine. Under most conditions this thirst mechanism works well; however, during physical activity you may not become thirsty until you are severely dehydrated. During exercise or other forms of physical activity it is important to drink plenty of water before, during, and after the activity.

We get water from many dietary sources. In addition to tap water, many foods are plentiful sources of water. Apples, lettuce, watermelon, green beans, broccoli, and white potatoes are only a few examples of foods that are more than 80 percent water. Milk, fruit juices, and other beverages are additional sources of water.

Healthy Food Choices

The study of nutrients is quite complex. Yet we need to be able to translate the ongoing recommendations about nutrients—fat, carbohydrates, protein, vitamins, minerals, and water—into our daily food choices. In 1992 the U.S. Department of Agriculture (USDA) issued a public education tool to help consumers make wise food choices, called the Food Guide Pyramid. This pyramid is divided into six groups: 1) fats, oils, and sweets; 2) milk, yogurt, and cheese; 3) meat, poultry, fish, dry beans, eggs, and nuts; 4) vegetables; 5) fruits; and 6) bread, cereal, rice, and pasta. For each group, the USDA recommends a specific number of daily servings. Many health professionals have criticized the pyramid because it does not distinguish between foods in each group that should be eaten often and those that should be eaten sparingly. Keeping this criticism in mind, the Center for Science in the Public Interest has improved the food pyramid by listing food choices people should eat "anytime," "sometimes," or "seldom" (see figure 3.10). Additionally, CSPI recognized that many foods, such as lasagna and burritos, fall into several of the USDA pyramid's groups. The CSPI pyramid therefore includes a grouping called "mixed foods." The CSPI pyramid has been endorsed by a variety of professional organizations, including the American College of Preventive Medicine and the Association of Black Cardiologists, as well as individual health scientists. Study the CSPI Pyramid and rate your current diet according to its recommendations. Are you eating the recommended number of servings each day? How often are you eating foods from the seldom group? What specific improvements does the pyramid suggest for your diet?

Learning to select healthy foods is the first step in improving your health and well-being. However, this is only part of the diet and health picture. The safety of our food supply is a subject often debated these days. Will the food we buy at the grocery store and at restaurants help us in our quest for wellness, or will it lead us down the path to disease?

Food Safety

Food contamination is an issue currently raising concern among consumers and health scientists alike. According to the Centers for Disease Control and Prevention (CDC), no count of bacterial, viral, and parasitic food-borne infections has been taken since 1983, when such infections caused 6 million illnesses and 9000 deaths a year.[80] The sense is, however, that some types of food-borne infection are on the rise. For instance, the incidence of reported cases of **salmonella** appear to have leveled off over the past four to five years, however, they are still estimated to cause 800,000 to 4 million infections annually.[81] During that same time period, the incidence of food-borne *E. coli* O157:H7 infections has increased. The CDC estimates that there may be 20,000 cases of *E. coli* O157:H7 each year.[82] According to a recent report in the *Journal of the American Medical Association*, "the federal government currently estimates that national costs associated with food-borne illness from meat and poultry—including lost productivity—reach $4 billion annually."[83] Clearly, food-borne infection is a major public health problem in the United States today.

The U.S. Public Health Service believes that there are currently four major microbiological threats to our food supply: **campylobacter,** *E. coli* O157:H7, **listeria,** and **salmonella.** While there are many other sources of food-borne infection and food poisoning (see table 3.13), we will focus our attention on the major threats.

Campylobacter

Campylobacter infections occur two to ten days after consuming contaminated food,

CSPI's Healthy Eating Pyramid

Diets Low in:
- Fat, saturated fat, and cholesterol
- Sodium
- Sugar

Reduce Risk of:
- Heart disease, cancer, and obesity (which can lead to diabetes)
- High blood pressure and stroke
- Tooth decay

Diets High in:
- Fruits, vegetables, beans, and whole grains

Reduce Risk of:
- Cancer, constipation, and diverticulosis

The best diets are rich in whole grains, beans, and fresh vegetables and fruit. They include only modest portions of low-fat animal foods like skim or 1% fat milk, yogurt, cottage cheese, fish, and skinless chicken or turkey. (Vegetarians should replace meat with beans, peas, and lentils.) Here's how this pyramid can help you build a better diet.

Make **ANYTIME** foods the backbone of your diet. They're low in fat (except oily fish) and saturated fat and have no serious flaws.

Limit **SOMETIMES** foods to two or three a day or use small portions. Most contain moderate amounts of fat or saturated fat; a few are high in unsaturated fat. Others are high in sodium, cholesterol, or added sugar, or are made from white flour or white rice.

If you eat **SELDOM** foods, keep the portions small and/or limit them to two or three times a week. Most are high in fat and saturated fat. Others are moderate in fat but have at least one other major flaw.

SERVING SIZES: *Breads, Cereal, Rice, Pasta, & Baked Goods:* 2 slices bread; 1/2 cup dense cereals (like granola); 1 cup other cooked cereal or pasta; 3/4 cup cooked rice; 2 waffles; 3 pancakes; 1/10 cake; 1 oz. (2 to 3) cookies; 1/8 pie; 1/2 oz. (about 4) crackers; 1 oz. (about 14) chips. ***Vegetables & Beans:*** 1 cup lettuce; 1/2 cup cooked vegetables or beans. ***Fruit:*** 1 medium fruit; 1/2 cup canned fruit; 1 cup juice. ***Dairy Foods:*** 1 cup milk, yogurt, or ice cream; 1 oz. cheese; 1/2 cup cottage cheese. ***Fish, Poultry, Meat, Nuts, & Eggs:*** 4 oz. cooked meat, poultry, or seafood; 1.5 oz. shrimp; 3 oz. tuna; 2 oz. (2 slices) luncheon meat; 1 hot dog; 1 egg; 2 Tb. peanut butter; 1/4 cup nuts. ***Fats, Sweets, & Condiments:*** 1 Tb. margarine, butter, oil, catsup, mayonnaise, soy sauce, or jelly; 1 tsp. mustard; 2 Tb. salad dressing. ***Mixed Foods:*** 7 oz. (about 2 slices) pizza; 1 cup soup, cooked spaghetti, or chili.

Catsup
Olives
Mustard
Mayonnaise, *fat-free*
Salad dressing, *fat-free*
FATS, SWEETS, & CONDIMENTS

Buttermilk
Cheese, *fat-free*
Cottage cheese, *fat-free or low-fat*
Milk, *skim or 1% fat*
Plain yogurt, *non-fat*
DAIRY FOODS
(2 to 3 servings a day)

Seafood, *all*
Pork tenderloin
Tuna, *in water*
Egg white or substitute
Beef top or eye of round, *Select*
Turkey, except wing, *no skin*
Chicken breast or drumstick, *no skin*
FISH, POULTRY, MEAT, NUTS, & EGGS
(1 to 2 servings a day)(Trimmed; baked or roasted)

Vegetables, *fresh, frozen, or canned*
Vegetable juice, *no-salt or light*
Beans (eg., Black, Garbanzo, Pink, Pinto, Great northern, Kidney)
Split peas, Lentils, Black-eyed peas
VEGETABLES & BEANS
(4 to 6 servings a day)

Fruit, *fresh, frozen, dried, or canned with juice*
Fruit juice
FRUITS
(2 to 4 servings a day)

ANYTIME

Bread, English muffins, Rolls, Bagels, *whole wheat or whole grain*
Breakfast cereals, *cold, whole grain, low-sugar* (eg., bran flakes, Cheerios, Grape-Nuts, Life, Nutri-Grain, shredded wheat, Total, Weetabix, Wheaties)

Rice, brown
Corn tortillas
Bulgur
Pasta

Breakfast cereals, *hot, whole grain, low-sugar* (eg., oatmeal, Wheatena)
Crackers, *whole grain, low-fat* (eg., crispbread, Triscuits)
Popcorn, *air-popped*
Pretzels, *whole grain, unsalted*; Tortilla chips, *no-oil*
BREAD, CEREAL, RICE, PASTA, & BAKED GOODS *(6 to 11 servings a day)*

Bean burrito
Cheeseless pizza
Grilled chicken sandwich
Pork & beans

Garden salad w/chicken chunks & light dressing

Canned soup, *low-sodium*
Spaghetti w/tomato sauce

Vegetable pita sandwich
Stir-fried vegetables & rice w/ chicken or seafood
Turkey *(fresh-cooked)* sandwich
MIXED FOODS

SOMETIMES

FATS, SWEETS, & CONDIMENTS
Jelly
Sugar
Oils, Mayo.
Salad dressing
Salt, Soy sauce
Margarine, *diet, tub*

DAIRY FOODS
Milk, *2% fat*
Fruit yogurt, *non-fat or low-fat*
Sherbet, Ice milk
Ice cream, *non-fat*
Frozen yogurt, *all*
Cottage cheese, *4% fat*
Cheese, Cream cheese, Sour cream, *light*

FISH, POULTRY, MEAT, NUTS, & EGGS
(Trimmed; baked or roasted)
Turkey, *w/skin*
Turkey roll; Tuna, *in oil*
Chicken nuggets
Nuts, Peanut butter
Pork loin (except blade)
Beef round or sirloin steak
Chicken breast or drumstick, *w/skin*; thigh, *no skin*

VEGETABLES & BEANS
Avocado
Cole slaw
French fries
Guacamole
Hash browns
Potato chips
Corn chips
Potato salad
Soybeans
Tofu

FRUITS
V8 juice
Tomato juice, *canned*
Fruit, *canned in syrup*
Cranberry sauce, *canned*
Fruit "drinks," "blends," "cocktails," or "beverages"

BREAD, CEREAL, RICE, PASTA, & BAKED GOODS
Angelfood cake
Fig bars
Pancakes, Waffles
Oatmeal raisin cookies
Gingersnaps
Biscuits, Croissants
Cakes, Cookies,
Granola bars, *fat-free*
Breakfast cereals, *refined* (eg., corn flakes, Rice Krispies)
Bread, English muffins, Rolls, Bagels (eg., multi-grain, oatmeal, rye, pumpernickel, white)
Molasses cookies
Pretzels
Rice, white
Packaged rice mixes
Tortilla chips, *light*
Crackers, *refined* (eg., saltines, oyster)
Crackers, *not low-fat* (eg., cheese, Ritz)
Breakfast cereals, *heavily sweetened* (eg., Cap'n Crunch)

MIXED FOODS
Baked potato w/cheese
Beef or chicken burrito
Canned or dried soup
Cheese pizza
Chef salad w/light dressing
Chicken taco
Hummus w/pita
Lasagna w/meat
McLean Deluxe
Macaroni & cheese
Peanut butter & jelly sandwich
Roast beef sandwich
Spaghetti w/meatballs
Tuna or chicken salad sandwich

SELDOM

FATS, SWEETS, & CONDIMENTS
Chocolate
Butter
Margarine, *stick*

DAIRY FOODS
Milk, *whole*
Cheesecake
Cream cheese
Yogurt, *whole-milk*
Ice cream, *regular or gourmet*
Cheese (eg., cheddar, Swiss, American)

FISH, POULTRY, MEAT, NUTS, & EGGS
(Trimmed; baked or roasted)
Eggs, Ribs
Ham, Bologna
Red meat, *untrimmed*
Hot dog, *turkey or meat*
Chicken thigh or wing, *w/skin*
Beef steaks or roasts, most types, *Choice*
Ground beef, *regular or lean*

VEGETABLES & BEANS
Onion rings
Potatoes au gratin
Vegetables w/Hollandaise sauce

FRUITS
Coconut

BREAD, CEREAL, RICE, PASTA, & BAKED GOODS
Apple pie, *fried*
Bread stuffing from mix
Cake *(except fat-free)* w/frosting
Chocolate chip cookies
Danish
Cream pie
Doughnuts
Granola bars *(except fat-free)*
Chocolate sandwich cookies
Lemon meringue pie
Peanut butter cookies
Pecan pie
Shortbread cookies

MIXED FOODS
Bologna sandwich
Chef salad w/regular dressing
Double hamburger or Cheeseburger
Chili
French toast w/syrup
Grilled cheese sandwich
Ham & cheese sandwich
Hot dog on bun
Nachos w/cheese
Pizza, pepperoni or sausage
Quarter-pound hamburger or Cheeseburger
Beef taco
Taco salad

TABLE 3.13   *The Facts about Food Poisoning*

Type	Occurrence	Symptoms	Onset after eating	Foods found in	Preventive measures
Campylobacter	Common	Muscle pain, nausea, vomiting, fever, and cramps; occasionally bloody diarrhea	2 to 10 days	Meat, poultry, eggs, unpasteurized dairy products, fish, shellfish, and untreated water	Cook meat, poultry, & eggs thoroughly; wash hands & work surfaces before and after contact with raw animal products; don't drink unpasteurized milk or untreated water
Clostridium perfringens	Common	Diarrhea and cramps	9 to 15 hours	Meat & poultry	Keep cooked foods above 140° while serving; cook, cool, and reheat foods thoroughly
E. coli O157:H7	Common	Bloody diarrhea; cramps, low-grade fevers; complications include kidney failure, strokes, seizures, & brain damage	4 to 9 days	Undercooked hamburger & roast beef, raw milk, improperly processed cider, contaminated water; vegetables grown in cow manure	Cook meat, poultry, & fish to 160° F; don't drink raw milk; wash all fruits & vegetables before eating; consider buying pasteurized cider
Hepatitis A	Common	Fever, nausea, abdominal pain, and loss of appetite; after 3 to 10 days, dark urine and jaundice	15 to 50 days	Raw shellfish, untreated water and any food handled by contaminated people	Wash hands thoroughly and frequently; avoid raw shellfish
Salmonella	Common	Nausea, vomiting, diarrhea, cramps, fever, and headache	6 to 48 hours	Meat, poultry, eggs, and unpasteurized dairy products	Cook meat, poultry, and eggs thoroughly; wash hands & work surfaces before & after contact with raw animal products; don't let foods sit at room temperature for more than 2 hours; don't drink unpasteurized milk

most often unpasteurized dairy products, meat, poultry, fish and shellfish, and untreated water. The most common symptoms include muscle pain, nausea, vomiting, fever, and cramps. Recently, a survey of State health departments was conducted to determine the number of outbreaks of campylobacter infections between 1981 and 1990. The survey discovered twenty outbreaks involving 450 young people.[84] Most of the outbreaks involved elementary school field trips to dairy farms, where the children were allowed to drink raw milk.

Type	Occurrence	Symptoms	Onset after eating	Foods found in	Preventive measures
Staphylococcus	Common	Vomiting & diarrhea; occasionally weakness and dizziness	30 minutes to 8 hours	Cooked meat & poultry; meat, poultry, potato and egg salads; cream-filled pastries	Cooking does *not* inactivate the staph toxin; wash hands & utensils before preparing food; don't let food sit at room temperature for more than 2 hours
Scrombroid poisoning	Uncommon	Facial flushing, headache, dizziness, burning sensation in the throat, hives, nausea, vomiting, & abdominal pain	5 minutes to 1 hour	Mackerel, tuna, and bonito	Make sure fish is fresh; if it has a peppery taste, stop eating it.
Botulism	Rare	Double vision; difficulty speaking, breathing, and swallowing; nausea, vomiting, abdominal pain, and diarrhea	12 to 48 hours, sometimes as long as 8 days later	Improperly canned goods, and honey (for infants)	Follow established guidelines for home canning; don't buy damaged canned goods; cook & reheat foods thoroughly; don't eat cooked foods that have been left at room temperature for more than 2 hours; don't give infants honey
Listeria	Rare	Flu-like symptoms, including fever & chills; can cause spontaneous abortions and stillbirths, as well as severe illness in newborns & immune-suppressed people	2 to 4 weeks	Unpasteurized milk & cheese made from unpasteurized milk; processed meats	Avoid raw or undercooked animal products, especially if you're pregnant or immune-suppressed
Trichinosis	Rare	Fever, edema (swelling) of the eyelids, and muscle pain	1 to 2 days	Pork	Cook pork thoroughly (to an internal temperature of 160°)

Source: Adapted from the Centers for Disease Control and Prevention and The U.S. Department of Agriculture.

E. coli O157:H7

In January 1993, almost 500 people in Washington state were diagnosed with laboratory-confirmed *E. coli* O157:H7 infections.[85] Most of the infected had eaten undercooked hamburgers from a local Jack-in-the-Box fast-food restaurant. Three children died from their infection. It was this event that brought national attention to the problem of *E. coli* food-borne infection.

The U.S. Department of Agriculture estimates that between 7,700 and 20,448 people a year in the U.S. become infected with *E. coli*, with economic costs ranging from $229 million to over $600 million.[86]

E. coli is a bacterial type with many variants. Not all *E. coli* variants are harmful to humans. In fact, some are quite helpful. In healthy people, *E. coli* resides in the human intestines and reduces the chance that other harmful microorganisms will multiply in the intestines and cause illness.

In 1975 the CDC first isolated the *E. coli* variant known as O157:H7. Yet it was not until 1982 that *E. coli* O157:H7 was identified as a source of food-borne infection. This form of *E. coli* produces a toxin in the human intestines that damages the cells that line the intestines, causing them to bleed. Approximately four to nine days after eating food contaminated with *E. coli* O157:H7, an individual will experience diarrhea that is often bloody, as well as cramps and a low-grade fever. In 2 to 7 percent of cases, the *E. coli* toxin enters the bloodstream and can cause complications such as kidney failure, strokes, and seizures. Such complications result in death in about 3 to 5 percent of cases.

While *E. coli* O157:H7 can contaminate any food, most outbreaks in the U.S. have been traced to undercooked beef, especially hamburger. *E. coli* contamination of hamburger is especially dangerous because the bacterium does not stay on the outside of the meat where it is more easily killed by cooking. Rather, when the beef is ground, the *E. coli* becomes mixed throughout the meat. Thorough cooking of ground meat is therefore essential for protecting yourself against *E. coli* O157:H7 food-borne infection.

Recently, manure spread on soil to fertilize gardens has been identified as a source of *E. coli*.[87] To avoid food-borne infection from manure, individuals are warned to be careful when handling manure, to use thorough hand washing techniques, and to carefully wash all garden produce. Additionally, *E. coli* can be passed from an infected person to an uninfected person. Most often feces from an infected person comes in contact with another person because of improper hand washing after using the toilet or changing a baby's diaper. Careful hand washing, using soap and warm water, is an important preventive measure.

Listeria

Listeria, caused by the bacterium listeria monocytogenes, is a rare but potentially fatal type of food-borne infection. According to the CDC, approximately seven cases of listeria per million people occur each year in the U.S.[88] About 23 percent of cases have resulted in death. As with most food-borne infections, pregnant women and people with impaired immune systems are most susceptible to listeria infection.

The most common sources of listeria contaminated foods include unpasteurized dairy products and processed meats. One recent study, reported in the journal *Nutrition Week*, found that 17 percent of major hot dog brands were contaminated with listeria.[89] The CDC notes that Mexican-style cheese, feta cheese, undercooked chicken, and "deli" counter food items were the foods most likely to be associated with listeria infection in the U.S.[90] Approximately two to four weeks after eating listeria-contaminated foods, an individual will usually experience flu-like symptoms. In pregnant women, listeria infection can cause miscarriages and stillbirths. The CDC recommends that pregnant women, people older than sixty, people who have cancer or AIDS, and people who have either had an organ transplant or are currently taking **corticosteroids** take special precautions to prevent listeria food-borne infection.[91] These high-risk individuals should avoid eating raw or undercooked meat and poultry, delicatessen foods, and soft cheeses, such as Mexican-style, feta, brie, Camembert, and Roquefort. (Hard cheeses, cottage cheese, and cream cheese are not a problem.) Additionally, they should heat leftovers and ready-to-eat foods, like hot dogs, until steaming hot.

Salmonella

Salmonella is the most commonly reported cause of food-borne infection in the United States. The CDC notes that about 40,000 cases of salmonella infection are reported to them each year.[92] It is believed that more than a million cases go unreported annually, often misdiagnosed as the flu. Salmonella infection, which results in severe diarrhea, vomiting, cramps, fever, headache, and sometimes death, is particularly dangerous for infants, the elderly, and people with weakened immune systems (such as persons with AIDS and cancer).

Many foods are susceptible to contamination; however, poultry is the food item most often found to contain disease-causing salmonella. At least 25 percent of chickens

Corticosteroids: steroid hormones secreted by the adrenal cortex, including hydrocortisone and aldosterone. These hormones are sometimes used as a prescription medication to treat a variety of conditions.

leave the processing plant with detectable levels of salmonella bacteria.[93] Eggs, too, may be contaminated, whether or not their shells are cracked. However, a recent USDA survey found that only 0.02 percent of eggs nationwide were contaminated with salmonella.[94]

Approximately six to forty-eight hours after eating salmonella-contaminated food, an infected individual will experience nausea, vomiting, cramps, and diarrhea. Sometimes a fever or headache may also occur.

Even though poultry, eggs, and other food items may be contaminated with salmonella, how we handle, store, and cook these foods can have a dramatic influence on whether we will become the next victim of a salmonella infection. Heat kills the salmonella bacteria, preventing infection. It is important that foods suspected of salmonella contamination be thoroughly cooked. Eggs, for instance, should be cooked until both the yolk and white are firm, not runny. Foods containing raw eggs, such as Caesar salad, Hollandaise sauce, homemade ice cream, homemade eggnog, and homemade mayonnaise may be contaminated with salmonella. It is best to avoid these foods *unless* you can be sure that pasteurized (heat treated) eggs were used in place of raw eggs. Beef and poultry should also be thoroughly cooked. If it is still pink inside, it is not ready to eat.

Preventing Food-Borne Infections

Food-handling techniques are one important ingredient in preventing food-borne illness. As the old saying goes, "cleanliness counts." When cooking, always wash your hands both before and after you handle raw meat or poultry. If you have any open cuts or sores on your hands, make sure they are completely covered. If the cut or sore is infected, you should avoid being the cook.

Clean cooking utensils are also important. Wash utensils and cutting boards between use with different foods. For instance, when making a salad, do not use the cutting board you just used to cut up the chicken, unless you wash it first in hot soapy water. Otherwise, it would be very possible for you to contaminate your salad with salmonella bacteria. Even if you thoroughly cooked your chicken, killing the salmonella bacteria, you could become infected by consuming the contaminated salad.

Recently there has been some debate as to whether it is best to use a plastic or glass cutting board rather than wood.[95] For some

time, the USDA has been recommending that consumers use plastic cutting boards because wooden cutting boards receive small cuts that may harbor bacteria. However, in 1993 an article was published in the journal *Science News* that indicated wooden cutting boards may be better than we had previously thought.[96] Researchers contaminated both wooden and plastic cutting boards with salmonella, listeria, and other bacteria. After just three hours the wooden cutting boards were virtually free of bacteria, while the bacteria on the plastic boards actually multiplied over a period of several days. No one is sure why the wooden boards appeared to kill the bacteria so quickly; more studies are needed to determine if wooden boards are a better choice. Until the results of these studies are available, the USDA continues to recommend the use of plastic or glass cutting boards. However, they have issued additional guidelines for cleaning cutting boards. Consumers should wash any cutting board with hot soapy water and let it air dry after each use. Plastic, glass, and solid wood cutting boards can be safely washed in a dishwasher. Additionally, the USDA recommends that cutting boards be sanitized once a week, using two teaspoons of chlorine bleach mixed with one quart of water. The surface of the cutting board should be flushed with the chlorine solution and left to stand for a few minutes. Following this, the board should be rinsed in clean water and air dried. Once a plastic cutting board becomes excessively cut up, the USDA recommends that it be replaced. Also, if a wooden cutting board is used for meat and poultry, it should *not* be used for other food items, even after washing.

When your meat or poultry is cooked, it is important to serve it on a clean plate. If you put it back on the plate that held the raw meat, you could recontaminate it.

It is essential that consumers take a greater interest in food safety. Lobbying your congressional representatives for legal solutions to the problem of initial food contamination is one important and appropriate disease prevention action. Additionally, careful handling of potentially contaminated food items is essential to food safety.

Nutritional Needs of Special Populations

The basic nutritional guidelines we have discussed so far apply to normal, healthy U.S.

adults. Certain groups of people, such as vegetarians, athletes, pregnant women, and the elderly, have special needs that may differ from or exceed the general guidelines.

Vegetarians

Vegetarians choose to consume the majority of their calories from plant foods. Vegetarianism appears to be an increasingly popular lifestyle in the U.S., especially among young adults.

There are many types of vegetarians, however, the more common types include **vegans,** who eat no animal foods, and **lacto-ovo-vegetarians,** who eat dairy foods and eggs but no animal flesh. Additionally, the Institute of Food Technologists has identified four other types of vegetarians: 1) **lacto-vegetarians,** who eat dairy food but not eggs or animal flesh; 2) **ovo-vegetarians,** who eat eggs but no other dairy foods or animals, 3) **pesco-vegetarians,** who eat dairy foods, eggs, and fish but no other animal flesh; and 4) **semi-vegetarians,** who eat dairy foods, eggs, chicken, and fish, but no other animal flesh.[97]

A vegetarian lifestyle can provide an enjoyable and nutritious diet. Although research continues, there appear to be several health benefits associated with vegetarian diets. Vegetarians have been shown to have lower weights, less constipation, lower total and LDL blood-cholesterol levels, and lower blood pressure levels.[98] Additionally, vegetarians appear to have lower rates of certain cancers, alcoholism, **type II diabetes, gallstones,** and coronary artery disease.[99] Researchers are not sure, however, how much of these health benefits are due to dietary patterns and how much may be due to other more healthy lifestyle habits often practiced by vegetarians.

Although there appear to be major benefits from a vegetarian lifestyle, there are also several important dietary risks. Those of greatest concern relate to vitamins B_2, B_{12}, and D, as well as certain minerals, such as calcium, iron, and zinc.[100] Vegans are at special risk for these deficiencies as they avoid consuming all animal food sources and dairy products. Vitamins B_{12} and D are found only in animal products. Therefore, it is recommended that all vegans select fortified B_{12} products such as soy milk and nutritional or food yeast, or take a vitamin B_{12} supplement equivalent to the RDA. With adequate exposure to the sun the body can make vitamin D so the prevalence of

deficiencies is small. However, if exposure to sunlight is infrequent, such as in northern climates during the winter, a vitamin D supplement equivalent to the RDA may be needed. Careful planning of food choices will ensure that vegetarians consume adequate amounts of vitamin B_2, calcium, iron, and zinc.

Receiving enough high-quality protein (complete proteins) is a problem for all vegetarians but especially for vegans and children vegetarians. Following the complementary protein guidelines suggested earlier in this chapter can help all vegetarians to meet their protein needs.

If you want to eat a vegetarian diet, it is helpful to keep the following recommendations in mind:

1. Eat a variety of foods. This will help to insure that you are getting adequate amounts of the essential nutrients.

2. Pay attention to matching your plant protein sources so that you eat complementary pairs. This will help you to take in enough complete proteins, which are essential to building and maintaining your body.

3. If dairy products are a major part of your vegetarian diet, try to select low-fat dairy products such as 1 percent or skim milk and low-fat cheeses.

Athletes

Optimal nutrition is of great importance to athletes in obtaining peak performance in their chosen sport or activity. Most of the nutritional requirements, however, are easily met by eating a large variety of foods in the proportions suggested by the CSPI's Healthy Eating Pyramid (see figure 3.10). Athletes and their coaches are often misinformed regarding nutrition and are therefore prone to health fads and quackery that, at the least, provide no additional benefits and may in fact be harmful.

Every athlete needs to take in enough calories to meet the extra energy demands of training and competition. Caloric requirements will vary from person to person depending on age, sex, body size, and level of activity. It is not uncommon for athletes to consume between 3,000 and 6,000 calories a day. Athletes should select their diet carefully so that 60 to 70 percent of the calories are from carbohydrates (with an emphasis on complex carbohydrates), 12 to

Vegetarians: individuals who consume the majority of their calories from plant foods. Some vegetarians eat only plant foods, while others may consume a combination of plant foods and dairy products, fish, or poultry.

Type II diabetes: diabetes arising from changes in insulin secretion or sensitivity of the body to insulin.

Gallstones: cholesterol crystals hardened by inorganic salts that may form in the gallbladder, producing pain.

15 percent of calories are from protein, and less than 25 to 30 percent are from fats.[101] Additionally, athletes should follow the general recommendation to eat at last five daily servings of fruits and vegetables. If such a diet is consumed regularly, vitamin and mineral supplementation is unnecessary. Many athletes believe that supplementation enhances performance, but this is not supported by research findings.[102]

Some athletes, especially those participating in endurance activities such as distance running and distance swimming, participate in a nutritional regimen known as carbohydrate loading. **Carbohydrate loading** consists of depleting body stores of carbohydrate (glycogen) by exercise, followed by several days of dietary carbohydrate restriction and then by several days of high dietary carbohydrate intake. This regimen has been shown to double the glycogen stores in the liver and large skeletal muscles of some athletes.[103] Long-term effects of repeated carbohydrate loading are not known at this time, and many sports nutritionists and exercise physiologists therefore caution against its use. Recent evidence has indicated that increased glycogen stores can be attained by simply resting several days before competition and consuming a high-carbohydrate diet.[104] The benefits of building up extra glycogen stores has recently been questioned. Preliminary studies have indicated that the higher levels of muscle glycogen achieved through carbohydrate loading do not appear to provide any advantage to athletes.[105]

A common nutritional myth endorsed by many athletes is the belief that a substantial amount of protein is needed in order to build muscle mass, meet energy needs, and increase athletic performance. Weight lifters are especially vulnerable to protein myths. While it is true that athletes need more energy than their sedentary peers, the most efficient source of energy is complex carbohydrates and fats. Additionally, there is no sound evidence that a high-protein intake (more than 12 to 15 percent of daily caloric intake) builds more muscle or increases performance.[106] Additionally, there is no scientifically proven rationale for athletes to use **amino acid supplements.** In fact, even though amino acids are currently available to consumers at health-food stores, it has been technically illegal to sell them as dietary

supplements since the early 1970s when the FDA took them off their "generally recognized as safe" list. This was due to the lack of information regarding the safe use of amino acid supplements in humans.[107] In 1992 the FDA released a report from the Federation of American Societies for Experimental Biology that pointed out a continued lack of human safety studies. Amino acid studies conducted on laboratory animals, however, have pointed to many potential dangers including brain chemistry changes and abnormally small brains in the offspring of animals that consumed amino acids.[108]

Fluid replacement is a very important component of optimal athletic performance. During prolonged exercise it is possible for the athlete to lose as much as six to eight pounds of body weight due to sweating. It is recommended that athletes consume proper amounts of fluids, prior to, during, and after athletic competition. Water is the best fluid-replacement choice prior to and during an athletic event. Experts recommend drinking "at least 16 to 20 ounces of fluid two hours before exercising and another 8 ounces 15 to 30 minutes before. While you exercise sip 4 to 6 ounces every 15 to 20 minutes."[109] After exercise, it is important to replace the fluids lost from sweating.

Some athletes choose to consume commercial beverages during their event because they supply sugar. If these beverages are consumed, you should be certain that they don't contain more than 10 percent sugar,[110] or they may slow down the fluid's absorption time resulting in some degree of dehydration. Sodium and chloride losses from sweating are easily replaced by normal food intake after the competition. Salt tablets are not recommended, as they can cause nausea and vomiting and lead to greater dehydration of fluid within the cells.

Pregnant and Lactating Women

Pregnant women and those breast-feeding their infant (lactating) have an increased need for energy and nutrients. As detailed in the Appendix, the RDA for pregnant and lactating women increases for most nutrients. Energy requirements increase by 300 calories during the second and third trimesters of pregnancy, and increase 500 calories for women who breast-feed. Vitamin and mineral needs also increase during this time; however, most of these needs can be met by consuming

Amino acid supplements: a product sold in many health-food stores that contains amino acids. Often in tablet or powder form, these supplements are touted as having the ability to increase muscle mass, and thus athletic performance. Scientific evidence does not support these claims, and there are dangers in taking these supplements in high doses.

an adequate diet. The recommendation to take an iron supplement during pregnancy has been a standard procedure for years. Because the increased need for iron is difficult to meet through diet alone, it is usually recommended that pregnant women take a supplement of 30 milligrams of iron daily during the second and third trimesters of pregnancy.[111]

Recent scientific studies have provided convincing evidence that daily consumption of 0.4 milligrams of folate, both before and during pregnancy, may prevent neural tube defects. As discussed previously in this chapter, the FDA is considering fortifying food substances, such as cereal and grain products, to ensure that women of childbearing age consume the recommended amount of folate. Nutritional concerns of pregnancy are described in greater detail in chapter 7.

The Elderly

Every day more people enter old age than leave it. Currently 12 percent of the United States population is estimated to be over the age of sixty-five. As more people are living longer, researchers have become interested in nutritional aspects of the aging process. Careful research into nutritional requirements for the elderly, however, is still in its infancy. This leaves much room for speculation about what constitutes the best diet for our aging population.

Researchers do, however, seem to be in agreement on several aspects of nutrition and aging.

1. The basic principles of good nutrition remain the same for older as for younger people. Modifying our diets toward the dietary guidelines is recommended for people of all ages.

2. Obesity may be a serious problem for older people who remain on their own. This relates directly to the decreasing energy needs of older people due to a slowing down of their metabolism. The older we get, the fewer daily calories we require to remain at optimal weight. Monitoring caloric intake and increasing activity levels is important to counteract a decreasing metabolism as we age.

3. Recent studies have indicated that many elderly people may be consuming diets deficient in a number of important nutrients. In one study, 38 percent of subjects seventy years and older consumed less than 75 percent of the RDA for three or more nutrients.[112] This same study also found that eating more than the recommended amounts of fat and cholesterol is also a problem for many older adults.

Other studies have found that a significant number of older adults report eating less calories than recommended for their age. This makes it difficult for them to get the recommended amounts of vitamins and minerals from food.[113] In a recent study of **Medicare** recipients, 33 percent were underweight.

Many nutritional problems of the elderly are thought to result from several sociodemographic factors. Living alone, having low and fixed incomes, and having low educational levels may increase the chances that elderly people will consume nutrient-poor diets. Additionally, chronic diseases and physiological aspects of aging may contribute to nutritional risk. For instance, many older people experience declining motor skills due to **arthritis** and other chronic diseases. This may make it difficult for them to shop for foods, as well as cook them.[114] Many elderly people also have declining senses of taste and smell that make eating less enjoyable. Medications can also cause declines in taste and smell.

Health scientists believe that the elderly should be routinely screened for nutritional status. Additionally, community health programs should provide social support for elderly people, especially those who are disabled or live alone. Many communities have these programs, including Meals on Wheels, where meals are delivered to elderly people in need, and recreational centers where the elderly can socialize and eat meals together.[115]

4. There appears to be an increasing need for calcium as we age in order to combat osteoporosis. Older women in particular need to increase their calcium intake. Currently, it is estimated that 1,000 milligrams of calcium each day would meet the increased needs of post menopausal women who are being treated with **estrogen,** while 1500 milligrams of calcium is needed for post menopausal women not taking estrogen supplements.[116] This is roughly

Medicare: a federally funded program that assists in the payment of health expenses for persons sixty-five years and older who are entitled to Social Security benefits.

Arthritis: a general term referring to an inflammation of the joints.

Estrogen: the primary female sex hormone that stimulates the development of a female physique and reproductive organs. Estrogen also stimulates the female reproductive cycle and maintains the adult female reproductive organs.

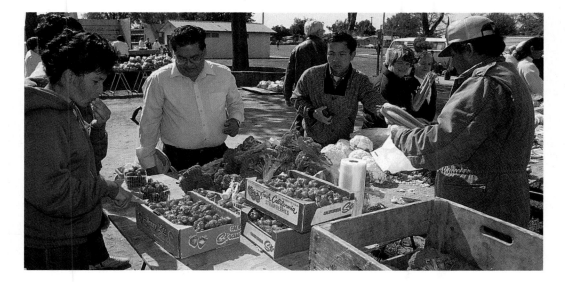

Figure 3.11: What Do You Think?

1. It is possible to buy high-quality produce at inexpensive prices from the growers themselves. Have you ever been to a farmers' market similar to the one pictured here? If so, what benefits did you receive from shopping there?
2. Where is the nearest farmers' market in your community? What hours are they open? What types of produce do they sell?

equivalent to three or four glasses of milk daily. Some experts recommend that low-fat dairy products be consumed as sources for calcium.

Personal and Social Influences

When it comes to eating, most of us are influenced by many factors other than our knowledge of the nutrients essential for optimal health. Cost, convenience, cultural influences, personal tastes and preferences, and habit are just a few of the many factors that interact and contribute to our food choices and ultimately to our level of wellness.

Cost

Everyone is concerned with today's high cost of food. We all want to get the best nutrition for the least amount of money. Fortunately, for many people this is not as difficult as it may sound. Foods that are high in cholesterol, fat, and sugar are not the best buys in terms of money or health. Generally, a diet closer to the dietary guidelines will tend to lower food costs. Fresh fruit and vegetables in season are usually good buys, especially if you get them at a local farmers' market where you can bypass many of the costs of processing and transportation (see figure 3.11). Other complex carbohydrates, such as whole-grain cereals, breads, and pasta, are also cheaper and healthier food options. With a little planning on your part, it is generally easy to prepare enjoyable and inexpensive foods that make a major contribution to optimal well-being (see Activity for Wellness 3.3).

According to the U.S. Census Bureau, 5.4 million people have been added to the ranks of the poor in the U.S. since 1989.[117] In 1993, this meant that more than 37 million people in the U.S. met the official poverty guidelines of $6,970 or less annual income for an individual, or $14,350 or less for a family of four. Minorities and children are hardest hit by poverty in the U.S. (see figure 3.12).

One of the many problems faced by the poor is hunger. Although the U.S. has a number of federal and state nutrition programs for the poor, they are often underfunded, leaving many poor families unserved. For instance, the 1993 federal appropriation for the Special Supplemental Food Program for Women, Infants, and Children (WIC) provided only enough funds to serve about 55 percent of those eligible for the program.[118] Thomas Moore, a researcher at the Graduate Institute for Policy Research at George Washington University believes that the U.S. has one of the lowest life expectancy rates of any of the countries with well-developed, modernized economies because people in the U.S. tolerate such high levels of poverty. Moore states "The countries that have higher life expectancies than we do do not have large poor populations living in dismal circumstances."[119] Hunger and poverty are important public health problems in the United States, and everyone must play a role in solving them (see A Social Perspective 3.1).

Cultural Influences

Food choices are often based on cultural traditions and preferences. These cultural

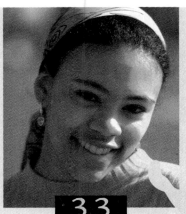

3.3
Activity for Wellness

Ways to Boost Your Buying Power

1. Remove the excess fat from regular ground beef by breaking up, cooking, and draining the meat. Lean and extra-lean ground beef cost more than regular ground beef. After breaking up, cooking, and draining, the fat content in regular, lean, and extra-lean ground beef is about the same. So considering the meat that's left, ounce for ounce, well-drained regular ground beef (broken up) can be a cheaper, low-fat buy. But whatever type of ground beef you choose, remember to drain off the extra fat after cooking.

2. Combine vegetable proteins to help stretch your protein dollar. Many vegetable protein combinations, like rice and beans, can be combined to give you protein just as good as that in meat, but with less-saturated fats and no cholesterol. Vegetable proteins can also be paired with low-fat dairy products or small amounts of lean meats, poultry, or fish to help stretch your protein dollar.

3. Stretch your meat dollar with vegetables and starchy foods. For a tasty, more economical meat dish, try adding tomatoes, macaroni, and chili seasoning to ground beef. The Chinese stir-fry cooking style also helps cut down on fat.

4. Change gradually to low-fat dairy products. If you're buying whole milk now, try one step over to 2 percent fat milk. It has almost half as much fat, and it's hard to taste the difference. As you work your way down to skim milk, you will be saving dollars, too. You can use nonfat milk in your cooking right away and you won't notice the difference in taste.

5. Prepare more foods yourself, instead of buying more expensive convenience foods. By buying more basic foods yourself, you can use your favorite ingredients such as spices and seasonings to suit your family's tastes. You can control the amount of meat and fat in your dishes as well. Convenience foods can be high in fats and calories. They usually cost more as well. Some convenience foods are also very salty or high in sugar.

6. Choose fresh fruits and vegetables in season when there's more variety, lower prices, and better quality. Fresh fruits and vegetables have a lot more to offer: They're low in saturated fats and calories, with no cholesterol, and high in vitamins and minerals. They also give you a variety of colors and texture and are easy to prepare.

7. Use unit-pricing labels to compare similar products. Unit-pricing labels show the cost of the product per unit—such as the cost per pound or quart. If your store has unit-pricing labels, use them to compare the costs of different varieties, brands, or sizes of a particular product.

Source: From *Eaters Almanac*, National Heart, Lung, and Blood Institute, National Institutes of Health, Bethesda, MD.

Figure 3.12: What Do You Think?

1. Which population group depicted at right has the highest poverty rate in the U.S.?
2. Do Whites in the U.S. have a poverty problem? Remember that this graph shows the *percent* of persons at or below the poverty level, not the actual *number* of people affected in each group.

Source: Data from the U.S. Census Bureau.

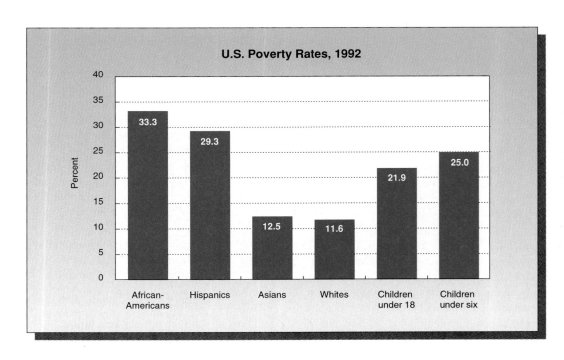

U.S. Poverty Rates, 1992

Group	Percent
African-Americans	33.3
Hispanics	29.3
Asians	12.5
Whites	11.6
Children under 18	21.9
Children under six	25.0

The Entire Community Has a Role in Anti-Hunger Efforts

What Individuals Can Do

Everyone needs to be well-informed. Reading articles about hunger, volunteering to serve food in a local soup kitchen or provide food baskets at a pantry, and joining a hunger task force are important steps.

Once people understand and can speak knowledgeably about the problem, then they can start influencing others. They become advocates who make fighting local hunger a personal priority. Being an advocate doesn't necessarily mean being vocal, but it does mean voting for legislation that benefits hungry people and for politicians who have demonstrated a commitment to ending hunger.

Individuals can pledge to donate even more food, more money, and more time to local food programs. These programs are straining to serve everyone who comes to them for assistance; they need all the help they can get.

Lastly, individuals can seek out and listen to those in need. All too often, people who are hungry and homeless are shunned; we try to pretend that they don't exist. Yet a face-to-face encounter with someone who is poor can lead to a better understanding of why people are in need, what problems they face, and what can be done to improve their situation.

What Religious Groups Can Do

Members of a church or synagogue or mosque can ensure that the mission of serving others is central to their activities. This means inviting representatives from local hunger-relief agencies to speak to the congregation, featuring the work of local agencies in religious bulletins and newsletters, and discussing in sermons and youth classes the importance of sharing our bounty with others who are less fortunate.

Many religious groups already contribute financial support through pre-arranged gifts and special collections, and this needs to continue. Religious groups have played a central role in organizing volunteers to staff food pantries and soup kitchens, which is important too.

What Community Agencies Can Do

As a service provider, it is all too easy to be consumed by the day-to-day fight against hunger. Community agencies need to step back sometimes, however, and look at their role in the context of the larger problem. They should decide to devote at least a small percentage of their time to action that addresses root causes of hunger. In this way they are working to cure hunger, as well as providing a temporary "band-aid."

Agencies need to get out into the community and tell people why they exist, what they are doing, and who they are serving. It is not enough to do good work, otherwise hunger will remain largely hidden.

What Business Can Do

In 1979, a minimum-wage salary was adequate to support a family of three above the poverty line. Today, a minimum-wage salary leaves a three-person family $2,300 *below* the federal poverty line. Companies have a responsibility to pay employees fair salaries that keep them out of poverty. Employees need to earn wages that make it possible for them to be self-sufficient.

What Government Can Do

Government can and should make food security for all a national priority. This means increasing funding for those programs that have proven to be successful in fighting hunger. The WIC program, in particular, should be supported so that everyone who is eligible is served. Local government, as well as business, community agencies, and private individuals, should advocate for WIC at the state and federal level.

Other necessary steps to reducing hunger include raising the minimum wage to at least the poverty level for a family of three, sponsoring job-training programs that lift workers out of poverty, and providing

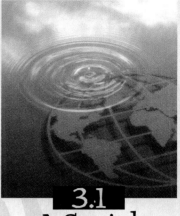

3.1 A Social Perspective

health-care coverage for all citizens. All of this requires a restructuring of priorities and massive shifts in spending. If the goal is justice and not charity, only government can fill the need in the long run.

What Everyone Can Do

To solve the problem of hunger requires the participation of the entire community from government and businesses to concerned citizens and people who are hungry. It's an enormous challenge, but a solution is possible. In the midst of affluence, no one should go hungry.

This call to action is taken from the Contra Costa County (Calif.) Hunger Task Force's recent report *Hunger in the Midst of Affluence,* as adapted from *Nutrition Week,* 1993, (20): 4–5, the publication of the Community Nutrition Institute, Washington, D.C. Reprinted by permission.

What Do You Think?

1. What priority should the U.S. give to helping reduce the number of hungry people in the U.S. and throughout the world?
2. Referring to Maslow's hierarchy of needs (discussed in chapter 1), how does hunger impact on an individual's, a community's, a nation's, and the world's level of wellness?

TABLE 3.14   *World's Fare: How to Savor the Flavors Without the Fat*

	Fine any time	Go easy on
Cajun	Red beans and rice (without sausage); greens, meaning kale, mustard greens, or okra; cornbread; shrimp creole (in a tomato sauce over rice); jambalaya or gumbo (order the poultry or seafood versions); blackened fish (heavily seasoned and cooked quickly with very little oil); boiled seafood dishes	Hush puppies (fried cornbread); dirty rice (fried rice with fatty meats); sausage dishes including *boudin* or *andouille;* rich soups or stews like bisque (cream broth) and *etouffé* (lots of butter); batter-fried seafoods
Chinese	Hot-and-sour or wonton soup; steamed dumplings; steamed or braised whole fish or scallops with black bean sauce; chicken or eggplant steamed or braised; stir-fried dishes (ask the cook to go easy on the oil or to use broth instead); dishes made with sliced meat rather than diced (often hides a fatty cut)	Fried egg rolls and dumplings; sesame noodles; fried rice; Peking duck; anything "crispy" or "batter-coated" (both terms indicate deep-frying); dishes heavy on nuts, such as *kung pao* chicken
Italian	Vegetable antipasto (roasted peppers and zucchini, grilled mushrooms,caponata); salads such as *panzanella* (with tomatoes and bread); pasta with tomato- or wine-based sauce; linguine with clam sauce; *pasta e fagioli* (shells and beans); *ribollito,* the thick vegetarian stew; grilled game, veal, and fish; chicken cacciatore; snapper in *cartoccio* (baked in parchment); marinated calamari	Meat and cheese antipasto; *fritto misto* (the "fired mixed" seafood, meat, or vegetable platter); cannelloni, lasagna, and other cheese-filled pasta; pesto and pasta with cream sauces, including carbonara and *alfredo;* risotto (heavy with butter and cheese); cheesy eggplant or veal parmigiana; veal *piccata* and marsala
Mexican-Southwestern	Mesquite-grilled chicken, seafood, or lean cuts of beef or pork, especially with fresh salsa; fajitas or tacos *al carbon,* especially seafood (hold the sour cream); bean or vegetable burritos; soft tacos	Tortilla chips and nachos; gaucamole; fried dishes such as chimichangas, hard-shell tacos, *flautas, taquitos;* tamales, quesadillas, cheese enchiladas, and chile *con queso;* dishes with *poblano* aioli (chill mayonnaise) or cilantro pesto (nuts and oil); refried beans (ask for whole ones)
Middle Eastern	*Hummus* (mashed chick-peas); *baba ghanoush* (mashed eggplant); pita bread; *ful medames* (fava beans and chick-peas); any of the salads, such as tabouleh or *fattoush;* lentil soup; rice pilaf; shish kebab; kibbe (baked meat with wheat, onions, and pine nuts); kofta grilled ground beef with parsley and onions)	*Saganaki* (contains fried cheese and butter); falafel (deep-fried); *kasseri* (cheese and butter casserole)

Researched by John Hastings, "World's Fare: How to Savor the Flavors Without the Fat." Excerpted from *Health* 7 (5): 44–45, © 1993.

food preferences, in turn, are usually based on the availability of foods in different regions of the world. For instance, traditional Middle Eastern food preferences include a heavy reliance on plant food sources widely available in Middle Eastern countries, such as wheat, legumes, olives, and a variety of fresh fruits and vegetables.[120] Similarly, traditional Mexican food preferences are based upon foods commonly available in Mexico, such as corn, beans, rice, meats, eggs, and cheese.[121]

Over the years, immigrants to the United States have brought their traditional food preferences with them, sharing their specialty dishes with people from other cultural backgrounds. Many of these "ethnic foods" have become quite popular in the U.S. Ethnic restaurants abound, as do ethnic cookbooks. Even supermarkets commonly carry sauces, spices, and other food products needed to prepare a variety of ethnic foods, from Chinese to Mexican, Italian, Greek, and many others.

Trying new foods, especially ethnic foods, can enhance our well-being and enjoyment of eating. New smells and tastes can make eating an adventure. However, just as the traditional U.S. diet has both nutritional strengths and weaknesses, so do the many ethnic foods available. For instance, many health scientists are currently focusing on the health benefits of eating a traditional Mediterranean diet.[122] This diet relies heavily on semi-vegetarian food choices such as fresh fruits and vegetables, grains, legumes, fish, and olive oil, rather than butter and red meats. Yet, there are some food choices within a Mediterranean diet that are better than others in terms of decreasing the risk of heart disease and other chronic diseases discussed earlier in this chapter. For instance, when eating Italian food, vegetable antipasto would be a lower fat choice than a meat and cheese antipasto, and pasta with a tomato or wine based sauce would be a lower fat choice than pasta in a heavy cream sauce like an *alfredo* or carbonara. Table 3.14 provides you with advice on low fat choices for a variety of ethnic foods.

TABLE 3.15   *How Fat Is Fast Food?*

High in Fat		Low in Fat	
Company/Product	Fat (grams)	Company/Product	Fat (grams)
Shakey's Pizza chicken entree 5 pieces fried, with potatoes	90	McDonald's Apple Bran Muffin	0
		Roy Roger's Plain Baked Potato	0
Perkins Granny's country omelette, with 9 oz. hash browns	89.2	Wendy's Plain Baked Potato	trace
Jack-in-the-Box Ultimate Hamburger	69	Carl's Jr. Old-Fashioned Chicken Noodle Soup	1
Long John Silver's 6-Piece Homestyle Fish Dinner	64	Kentucky Fried Chicken Mashed Potatoes and Gravy	1
Chick-Fil-A Chicken entree, salad plate	63	McDonald's Strawberry Low-fat Frozen Yogurt Sundae	1
Burger King Double Whopper with Cheese	61	McDonald's Vanilla Low-fat Cone	1
Taco Bell Taco Salad	61	McDonald's Side Salad with 1 tbsp. Vinaigrette Dressing	1.5
Hardee's Big Country Breakfast (Sausage)	61	Arby's Plain Baked Potato	1.9

Source: Data from A. Ulene, *The NutriBase Nutrition Facts Desk Reference,* 1995, Avery Publishing Group, Garden City Park, NY.

Convenience

The college years are a busy time for most people. In addition to the many hours of study, work responsibilities and social activities abound. Students seldom have elaborate cooking facilities. All of these factors contribute to the appeal of convenient and attractive fast foods. In the U.S., according to the Department of Agriculture, almost $5 out of every $10 spent on restaurant foods goes to fast-food establishments. Additionally, it has been estimated that each person spends an average of $200 a year on fast foods.[123]

Many consumers are beginning to wonder about the nutritional value of their fast-food diets. In response to consumer demand, many fast-food chains have contracted to have their food analyzed and are beginning to make this analysis public. Results indicate that most fast foods are high in calories, sodium, and fat. Additionally, they appear to have a moderate amount of carbohydrate; however, it is not clear how much is sugar and how much is starch. Most fast foods are low in fiber and vitamins but supply adequate amounts of protein, iron, and calcium. More research needs to be done in the area of trace minerals.

The calorie content of a fast-food meal is generally between 900 and 1,800 calories. This equals 33 to 66 percent of the total daily recommended calories for young men and 45 to 90 percent of the total daily recommended calories for young women. It is not uncommon for 50 percent of these calories to be from fat. Fast-food meals could thus help to contribute to the problem of obesity for many people (see table 3.15).

Be sure to moderate the number of fast-food meals you consume; however, it is possible to enjoy the convenience of fast foods and still maintain a good diet. To accomplish this you must take stock of other foods eaten on the same day. Be certain to include dairy products for additional calcium and fresh fruits and vegetables for vitamins A and C. These vegetables, in addition to whole-grain products, will also help you get needed sources of fiber. If you plan to eat more meat that day, select poultry or fish in order to cut down on total calories from fat. Many fast-food restaurants now provide salad bars that will allow you to include fresh vegetables with your other selections. Take advantage of salad bars, but watch the amount and type of salad dressing you add.

Making changes in your diet is not an easy process. You will probably find that you go through a series of steps, like those listed below, each time you try to make healthy changes in your behavior. Whether you want to decrease the amount of fat you eat, or increase your consumption of foods high in antioxidant vitamins, the following tips will help you as you progress through the stages of change* for a healthy diet.

Precontemplation → Contemplation

If you have never thought about making healthy changes in your diet or you do not intend to make any changes within the next six months you might want to consider:

- assessing your current dietary patterns by completing and carefully evaluating your responses to Activity for Wellness 3.1 "How's Your Diet?"
- choosing to read one or more of the recommended readings at the end of this chapter to increase your knowledge of healthy food choices.

Contemplation → Preparation

If you have been seriously considering making some changes in your food choices, but have not yet attempted any changes, try to thoughtfully answer the following questions:

- How do I think or feel about eating foods that may put me at risk for coronary artery disease, or other chronic, degenerative diseases?
- How do I think or feel about eating foods that may help me to have more energy, attain my optimal body weight and shape, and increase my level of well-being?

Preparation → Action

If you are ready to make some definite plans for making healthy food choices during the next month, or if you have already made small changes in the past but were not able

to maintain those changes as a permanent part of your lifestyle, consider the following actions:

- Make a resolution to yourself to begin a certain change in your diet on a certain date; for instance, make a commitment to yourself that "starting Monday I will read food labels and choose more foods that contain low- or no-grams of fat."
- Set measurable objectives for your behavior change, for instance, "I will consume no more than the U.S. Daily Reference Value of fat each day."

Action → Maintenance

If you have recently started to make some healthy changes in how you select the food you eat, the following tips will help you continue on this healthy path:

- Write a behavior change contract, such as that found in chapter 1, and find a support person who will help you keep with your plan; have a support person sign your contract.
- Give yourself rewards *often* for meeting your goals and objectives; rewards should be things you really enjoy, but that you are willing to do without if you do not meet your goal.

Maintenance

If you have made important changes in your dietary habits that you have practiced for six months or longer you now need to focus on maintaining your healthy choices every day:

- Rehearse situations in your mind that may tempt you to relapse on your new eating habits; for instance, if you are trying to cut down on fatty foods imagine situations where you may be tempted to eat too much of high fat foods—think about how you will choose to balance your intake of higher fat foods with lower fat foods.
- If you have a day where you do not follow your new eating habits, learn to view this as a lapse, rather than a catastrophe—then go back to following your new behavior patterns.

*Based on Prochaska, Norcross and DiClemente's transtheoretical model. See Prochaska, J. O., Norcross, J. C., & DiClemente, C. C. (1994). *Changing for Good.* New York: William Morrow and Company, Inc.

Personal and social food preferences can act to enhance our nutritional needs or serve as major barriers. An understanding of the basic nutrients and their functions is a sound foundation on which to build a diet that emphasizes the good preferences and minimizes the barriers. Table 3.16 will give you suggestions on how to make healthy changes in your diet. Eating for health can be an adventure you don't want to miss.

Summary

1. Today's typical U.S. diet is too high in fats, refined and processed sugar, salt, cholesterol, and calories. Many researchers believe that this typical diet is strongly associated with many of the chronic and degenerative diseases so common in the U.S.

2. The National Research Council has issued dietary recommendations for people in the U.S. These guidelines suggest that we eat more like our grandparents did. Specifically, we should consume a greater percentage of our calories as complex carbohydrates, such as fresh fruits and vegetables and whole grain products.

3. The new food labels can provide invaluable assistance to consumers who are trying to follow the recommendations of the National Research Council and the *Healthy People 2000* Objectives. The new labels make it especially easy to monitor your intake of fat, saturated fat, calories, cholesterol, sodium, total carbohydrate, dietary fiber, sugars, protein, vitamins A and C, calcium, and iron.

4. Three of the six major nutrients—carbohydrates, fats, and protein—supply us with calories or energy. The other three nutrients—vitamins, minerals, and water—assist in utilizing this energy.

5. Carbohydrates are the body's preferred form of energy and supply us with four calories per gram—less than one-half the calories supplied by a gram of fat. Complex carbohydrates are a rich source of important vitamins, minerals, and water. Many complex carbohydrates are also rich in fiber, which may help prevent a variety of chronic diseases.

6. Foods high in processed and refined sugars, such as table sugar, are often labeled "empty calories"; they contain few of the important nutrients such as vitamins, minerals, and protein. These foods add only calories to our diet and increase the risk of developing tooth decay.

7. Fats supply us with nine calories per gram and thus are a condensed source of energy and a perfect energy-storage vehicle for the body.

8. A diet high in saturated fats has been strongly linked to coronary artery disease.

9. Scientists have distinguished several types of cholesterol. HDL cholesterol may be protective against coronary heart disease, while LDL cholesterol seems to increase the risk of this disease. Additionally, trans-fatty acids, produced during hydrogenation of unsaturated fats, are believed to increase one's risk of coronary artery disease.

10. New substances called fat substitutes are now on the market to help consumers decrease their fat intake. These substitutes have the consistency of fat and are used in products, like mayonnaise, in place of fats.

11. The major function of protein is for growth, maintenance, and repair of body tissues. Protein can also be used as a source of energy, if sufficient carbohydrates and fats are lacking in the diet.

12. Protein is composed of amino acids, eight of which must be taken into the body from food. These are known as the essential amino acids and are vital to tissue growth. Foods that contain all eight essential amino acids are called complete proteins. Individual plant foods are often lacking in the complete eight amino acids. However, when you combine several plant foods, like rice and beans, you create a complete protein.

13. Vitamins are either water soluble or fat soluble. The water-soluble vitamins (B-complex and C) are not stored by the body and must be consumed daily. Fat-soluble vitamins (A, D, E, K) are stored by the body and can be toxic in large doses. The best source of vitamins is a well-balanced diet.

14. Recently, a group of vitamins known as antioxidants have been studied for their proposed benefits in preventing a variety of chronic diseases. Some studies have shown promising evidence of a protective effect for coronary heart disease, certain cancers, and cataracts. A recent intervention study, however, found that risk for certain cancers increased when subjects were given antioxidant supplements. Scientists currently recommend eating foods high in antioxidant vitamins, but waiting for more scientific evidence before consuming antioxidant supplements.

15. Minerals are inorganic substances that, in correct amounts, are vital to bodily functions. Excess or deficiency levels of minerals are considered to be health risks. For instance, excess sodium consumption is considered a major risk factor for high blood pressure, as well as for osteoporosis and stomach cancer. Calcium deficiencies are believed to be a risk factor for osteoporosis.

16. The Food and Drug Administration has created a food guide called the Food Pyramid, that recommends daily numbers of servings for a variety of food groups. The Center for Science in the Public Interest has expanded on this concept and provides examples of foods within each pyramid food group that you should eat anytime, sometimes, or seldom.

17. Food-borne infections are an increasingly important health concern in the U.S. The four major sources of food poisoning, according to the Centers for Disease Control and Prevention, include *campylobacter*, *E. coli* O157:H7, *listeria*, and *salmonella*. With proper food handling and cooking techniques, you can prevent most cases of food poisoning.

18. Certain groupings of people in the U.S., such as athletes, vegetarians, pregnant and breast-feeding women, and the elderly, have special nutritional needs. An awareness of these needs and several minor diet changes will help these groups achieve their quest for wellness.

19. Many variables, such as cost, cultural influences, convenience, and taste contribute to our choice of foods.

Being aware of these factors and using them to your advantage will help you achieve higher levels of wellness.

20. Hunger is an important health problem for many people. There are a variety of things that communities could do to ease this problem. Your community needs your help in solving the problem of hunger.

Recommended Readings

Jacobson, Michael F., Lisa Y. Lefferts, and Anne Witte Garland. *Safe Food: Eating Wisely in a Risky World.* Los Angeles: 1991, Living Planet Press.

In recent years public concern over food-safety issues has intensified. Jacobson, Lefferts, and Garland evaluate food-safety risks and provide the information necessary to help consumers make safer food choices.

Nutrition Action Healthletter
This highly regarded newsletter carries articles on a variety of nutrition-related topics. The *Nutrition Action Healthletter*, is published by the Center for Science in the Public Interest (CSPI), a nonprofit membership organization that advocates for improved health and nutrition policies that are in the public interest. Subscription information is available by writing: Center for Science in the Public Interest, 1875 Connecticut Ave., N.W., Suite 300, Washington, D.C. 20009–5728; or by calling (202) 332–9110.

Schrambling, Regina. "Ethnic light." *Health* 7.5 (1993): 39–51.

This well-written article provides tips for consumers on the most healthy choices for a wide variety of ethnic diets, including Cajun, Caribbean, Chinese, Eastern European, French, Greek, Indian, Indonesian, Italian, Japanese, Korean, Mexican-Southwestern, Middle Eastern, Spanish, and Thai. Additionally, Schrambling provides sample recipes and ingredients to stock in your kitchen for cooking Italian, French, Mexican, Chinese, and Greek cuisine.

References

1. "Are you eating right?" (1992) *Consumer Reports* (October): 644–653; "Research notes healthy diets." (1993) *Nutrition Week XXIII* (25): 8; Welsh, S., Davis, C., and Shaw, A. (1992) "A brief history of food guides in the United States." *Nutrition Today* 27 (6): 10; "Pulsepoints: Americans are consuming less fat." (1994) *American Health* XIII (4): 6.

2. U.S. Department of Health and Human Services. (1988) *The Surgeon General's Report on Nutrition and Health.* Rocklin, CA: Prima Publishing and Communication.

3. Hegsted, D. M. (1993) "Nutrition standards for today." *Nutrition Today* 28 (2): 34–36.

4. Liebman, B. (1993) "Baby 'label' arrives." *Nutrition Action Healthletter.* March: 7.

5. Liebman, "Baby 'label' arrives."

6. Liebman, "Baby 'label' arrives."

7. Liebman, B. (1990) "The changing American diet." *Nutrition Action Healthletter* (May): 8–9.

8. "Are you eating right?"

9. "Are you eating right?"

10. *Surgeon General's Report on Nutrition and Health.*

11. Mandel, I. D. (1994) "Who needs fluoride?" *Consumer Reports on Health* 6 (4): 47.

12. "Cutting your risk of colon cancer." (1994) *Consumer Report on Health* 6 (5): 55–58.

13. Maryce M. Jacobs. (1993) "Diet, nutrition, and cancer research: An Overview." *Nutrition Today* 28 (3): 19–23.

14. "Research Notes: Cancer." (1993) *Nutrition Week XXIII* (17): 7.

15. *Surgeon General's Report on Nutrition and Health,* 260.

16. Napier, Kristine. (1993) "Understanding cholesterol once and for all." *American Health* XII (9): 42–47.

17. Allison, Kathleen Cahill. (1993) "Eat to beat cancer." *American Health* XXII (8): 72–77.

18. "The new thinking about fats." (1993) *UC Berkeley Wellness Letter* 9 (12), 4–6.

19. "The new thinking about fats."

20. Hegsted, D. M. (1993) "Nutrition standards for today." *Nutrition Today* 28 (2): 34–36; "The new thinking about fats"; Napier, Kristine "Understanding cholesterol . . . ."

21. Mensind, R. P. M., and Katan, M. B. (1990) "Effect of dietary trans-fatty acids on high-density and low-density lipoprotein cholesterol levels in healthy subjects." *New England Journal of Medicine* 323: 439–445; "The trouble with margarine," (March 1991) *Consumer Reports:* 197.

22. Thomas, L. H., Winter, J. A., and Scott, R. G. (1983) "Concentration of 18:1 and 16:1 *trans*unsaturated fatty acids in the adipose body tissue of decedents dying of ischaemic heart disease compared with controls: analysis by gas liquid chromatography." *Journal of Epidemiology and Community Health* 37: 16–21.

23. Willett, W. C., Stampfer, M. J., Manson, J. E., et al. (1993) "*Trans*-fatty acid intake in relation to risk of coronary heart disease among women." *Lancet* 341: 581–585.

24. Siguel, E. N., and Lerman, R. H. (1993) "*Trans*-fatty acid patterns in patients with angiographically documented coronary artery disease." *American Journal of Cardiology* 71: 916–920.

25. Willett, Walter C., and Ascherio, Albert. (1994) "*Trans* Fatty Acids: Are the effects only marginal?" *American Journal of Public Health* 84 (5): 722–724.

26. Creager, Joan G. (1992) *Human Anatomy and Physiology* (Dubuque, Iowa: Wm. C. Brown Publishers), p. 707.

27. "HDL: 'Good' cholesterol looks even better." (1994) *Consumer Reports on Health* 6 (3): 28–30; "New national cholesterol education program (NCEP) guidelines." (1993) *Nutrition Today* 28 (4): 4.

28. "Powerful new evidence: lowering cholesterol does save lives." (1995) *UC Berkeley Wellness Letter* 11 (5): 1.

29. Leonard, Rodney E. (1993) "Federal dietary advice weakens health reforms." *Nutrition Week* XXIII (15): 4–5.

30. "Cutting cholesterol: more vital than ever." (1995) *Consumer Reports on Health* 7 (2): 13–14.

31. Blumenthal, Dale. (1990) "Making sense of the cholesterol controversy." *FDA Consumer* 24 (5): 14.

32. Davidson, Michael, et al. (1991) "The hypocholesterolemic effects of β-glucan in oatmeal and oat bran: A dose-controlled study." *JAMA* 265 (14): 1833–39.

33. Anderson, James W., Thomas F. Garrity, Constance L. Wood, Sarah E. Whitis, Belinda M. Smith, and Peter R. Oeltgen. (1992) *American Journal of Clinical Nutrition* 56 (5): 887–894; Keenan, Joseph M., Joyce B. Wenz, Shepherd Myers, Cynthia Ripsin, Zhiquan and Huang. (1991) *The Journal of Family Practice* 33 (6): 600–608.

34. Hole, John W., Jr. (1993) *Human Anatomy and Physiology* (Dubuque, Iowa: Wm. C. Brown Publishers).

35. Brody, Jane. (1987) *Jane Brody's Nutrition Book* (New York: Bantam Books), p. 34.

36. "Our vitamin prescription: The big four." (1994) *UC Berkeley Wellness Letter* 10 (4): 1–2.

37. Liebman, Bonnie. (1994) "The heart health-E vitamin?" *Nutrition Action Healthletter* 21 (1): 8–10; Russell, Robert M. (1993) "Nutrition." *JAMA* 270 (2): 233.

38. "E: the evidence grows stronger." (1993) *UC Berkeley Wellness Letter* 9 (5): 2–3.

39. "Our vitamin prescription."

40. Kritchevsky, David. (1992) "Antioxidant vitamins in the prevention of cardiovascular disease." *Nutrition Today* 27 (1): 30–33; "Can vitamin C save your life?" (1994) *Consumer Reports on Health* 6 (3): 25–27.

41. Russell, "Nutrition."

42. Liebman, "The heart health-E vitamin?"

43. Liebman, Bonnie. (1994) "Antioxidants: Surprise, surprise." *Nutrition Action Healthletter* 21 (5): 4.

44. "Antioxidants: Antidote to aging?" (1993) *Food Insight: Current Topics in Food Safety and Nutrition* (November-December): 1, 4; Liebman, "Antioxidants."

45. "Vitamin E megadoses." (1993) *Nutrition Week* XXIII (19): 3.

46. Herbert, Victor. "Folate and neural tube defects." (1993) *Nutrition Today* 27 (6): 30–33.

47. "FDA proposes to add folic acid to food supply." (1993) *Nutrition Week* XXIII (37): 2.

48. McBride, Gail. (1994) "Fantastic folic acid." *American Health* XIII (3): 11–13.

49. "Supplements don't extend lifespan, say researchers." (1993) *Nutrition Week* XXIII (19): 3.

50. Kim, Insun, David F. Williamson, Tim Byers, and Jeffrey P. Koplan. (1993) *American Journal of Public Health* 83 (4): 546–550.

51. "Supplements." (1994) *Nutrition Week* XXIV (10): 7.

52. "Our vitamin prescription."

53. "Our vitamin prescription."

54. "Eating right?" (1994) *Nutrition Week* XXIV (10): 7.

55. "Vitamins: Charting your course." (1994) *UC Berkeley Wellness Letter* 10 (4): 4–5.

56. Zimmerman, David R. (1994) "The truth about vitamins." *Consumers Digest* 33 (4): 24–30.

57. Herbert, Victor. (1993) "Viewpoint does mega-C do more good than harm, or more harm than good?" *Nutrition Today* 28 (1): 28–32.

58. Schardt, David. (1993) "Vitamins 101: How to buy them." *Nutrition Action Healthletter* 20 (1): 5–6.

59. Schardt, "Vitamins 101."

60. Liebman, Bonnie. (1994) "The salt shakeout." *Nutrition Action Healthletter* 21 (2): 1, 5–7.

61. Liebman, "The salt shakeout."

62. Liebman, "The salt shakeout."

63. "Stress, salt, and blood pressure." (1993) *UC Berkeley Wellness Letter* 9 (7): 7.

64. Liebman, "The salt shakeout."

65. Liebman, "The salt shakeout."

66. Liebman, "The salt shakeout."

67. Liebman, "The salt shakeout."

68. Liebman, "The salt shakeout."

69. NIH Consensus Development Panel on Optimal Calcium Intake. (1994) *JAMA* 272 (24): 1942–1948.

70. Recker, Robert R., Michael Davies, Sharilyn M. Hinders, Robert P. Heaney, Mary Ruth Stegman, and Donald B. Kimmel. (1992) "Bone gain in young adult women." *JAMA* 268 (17): 2403–2408.

71. Liebman, Bonnie. (1994) "Calcium: After the craze." *Nutrition Action Healthletter* 21 (5): 1, 5–7.

72. Tolstoi, Linda G., and Robert M. Levin. (1992) "Osteoporosis—The treatment controversy." *Nutrition Today* 27 (4): 6–12.

73. Liebman, Bonnie. (1994) "Just the calcium facts." *Nutrition Action Healthletter* 21 (5): 8.

74. Tolstoi and Levin, "Osteoporosis"; Liebman, "Just the calcium facts."

75. Bourgoin, Bernard P., Douglas R. Evans, Jack R. Cornett, Susanne M. Lingard, and Alfredo J. Quattrone. (1993) *American Journal of Public Health* 83 (8): 1155–1160.

76. Schardt, David. (1993) "The problem with protein." *Nutrition Action Healthletter* 20 (5): 1, 5–7.

77. Massey, L. K., and S. J. Whiting. (1993) "Caffeine, urinary calcium metabolism and bone." *The Journal of Nutrition* 123: 1611–1614.

78. Calvo, M. S. (1993) "Dietary phosphorus, calcium metabolism and bone." *The Journal of Nutrition* 123: 1627–1633.

79. Nordin, B. E. C., A. G. Need, H. A. Morris, and M. Horowitz. (1993) "The nature and significance of the relationship between urinary sodium and urinary calcium in women." *The Journal of Nutrition* 123: 1615–1622.

80. Voelker, Rebecca. (1994) "Food-borne illness problems more than enteric." *JAMA* 271 (1): 8–9, 11.

81. Voelker, "Food-borne illness problems more than enteric."

82. Gantz, Herb. (1993) "Answering your questions on E. coli." *Food News for Consumers* 10 (3): 4–5.

83. Voelker, "Food-borne illness problems more than enteric."

84. Liebman, Bonnie. (1993) "Unsafe food." *Nutrition Action Healthletter* 20 (3): 4.

85. Foulke, Judith E. (1994) "How to outsmart dangerous E. Coli strain." *FDA Consumer* 28 (1): 7–11.

86. "As E. coli infections hit home, parents mount meat safety campaign." (1993) *Nutrition Week* XXIII (31): 1–2.

87. "E. coli." (1994) *Nutrition Week* XXIV (3): 8.

88. Liebman, Bonnie. (1992) "Don't get Listerical." *Nutrition Action Healthletter* 19 (6): 4.

89. "LA Times finds hot dog contamination widespread." (1993) *Nutrition Week* XXIII (27): 7.

90. Liebman, "Don't get Listerical."

91. Liebman, "Don't get Listerical."

92. Soucie, Gary. (1994) "Good eggs." *Health* 8 (3): 26, 28; Kuznik, Frank. (1992) "Animal feed render unto Salmonella." *Nutrition Action Healthletter* 19 (3): 8–9.

93. Troiano, Joan. (1993) "Trisodium phosphate—new tool for reducing bacteria on chicken." *Food News for Consumers,* 10 (1–2): 15.

94. Soucie, "Good eggs."

95. Conley, Susan, and CiCi Williamson. (1993) "No conclusive evidence on cutting boards yet." *Food News for Consumers* 10 (3): 11.

96. "Food safety." (1993) *Nutrition Week* XXIII (10): 7.

97. Farley, Dixie. (1992) "Vegetarian varieties." *FDA Consumer* 26 (4): 22.

98. "The new vegetarianism." (1993) *The UC Berkeley Wellness Letter* 9 (6): 4–5.

99. Farley, Dixie. (1992) "Vegetarian diets: the pluses and the pitfalls." *FDA Consumer* 26 (4): 21–24.

100. Farley, "Vegetarian diets."

101. "Nutrition and exercise: What your body needs." (1993) *UC Berkeley Wellness Letter* 9 (8): 4–5.

102. "Nutrition and exercise."

103. Kris-Etherton, P. M. (1990) "Nutrition and Athletic Performance." *Nutrition Today* 24 (5): 35–37.

104. Simopoulos, Artemis P. (1992) "Nutrition and fitness: A conference report." *Nutrition Today* 27 (6): 24–29.

105. "Athletics." (1993) *Nutrition Week* XXIII (22): 7.

106. Houston, Michael. (1992) "Protein and amino acid needs of athletes." *Nutrition Today* 27 (5): 36–38.

107. Long, Patricia. (1993) "The vitamin wars." *Health* 7 (3): 44–54.

108. Nightingale, Stuart L. (1993) "From the Food and Drug Administration: Regulation of dietary supplements." *JAMA* 270 (6): 693.

109. "Drink to win." (1993) *UC Berkeley Wellness Letter* 9 (8): 6.

110. "Drink to win."

111. "Which supplements should you take?" (1991) *American Health* X (2): 40.

112. Posner, Barbara Millen, Alan M. Jette, Kevin W. Smith, and Donald R. Miller. (1993) "Nutrition and health risks in the elderly: The Nutrition Screening Initiative." *American Journal of Public Health* 83 (7): 972–978.

113. Liebman, Bonnie. (1993) "Older eaters." *Nutrition Action Healthletter* 20 (2): 4.

114. Posner et al., "Nutrition and health risks in the elderly"; "Tasteful solutions to elderly malnutrition." (1993) *Food Insight* (May/June): 5.

115. "Initiative targets malnutrition among the elderly." (1991) *Food Insight* (July/August): 6.

116. Blumberg, Jeffrey B. (1992) "Changing nutrient requirement in older adults." *Nutrition Today* 27 (5): 15–20.

117. "American's grow poorer, lack health insurance, despite recession's end." (1993) *Nutrition Week* XXIII (37): 1–2.

118. "WIC bill would mandate full funding by 1996." (1993) *Nutrition Week* XXIII (12): 7.

119. "Diet not major factor in average life expectancy." (1992) *Nutrition Week* XXII (6): 4–5.

120. Packard, Diane P., and Margaret McWilliams. (1993) "Cultural foods heritage of Middle Eastern immigrants." *Nutrition Today* 28 (3): 6–12.

121. Romero-Gwynn, Eunice, Douglas Gwynn, Louis Grivetti, Roger McDonald, Gwendolyn Stanford, Barbara Turner, Estella West, and Eunice Williamson. (1993) "Dietary acculturation among Latinos of Mexican descent." *Nutrition Today* 28 (4): 6–12.

122. "Importing the Pacific Rim diet." (1993) *UC Berkeley Wellness Letter* 10 (2): 1–2.

123. Franz, Marion J. (1990) *Fast Food Facts* (Wayzata, Minn.: DCI Publishing): 1.

Weight Management: A Lifelong Challenge

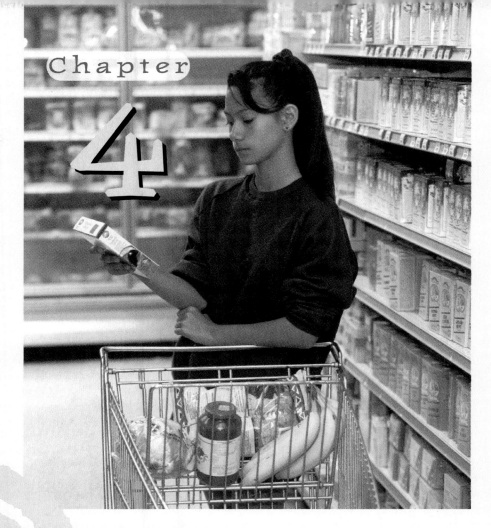

Chapter

4

Student Learning Objectives

Upon completion of this chapter, you should be able to:

1. evaluate the weight management concerns of a variety of people, considering both sex and race/ethnicity;

2. explain the difference between being overweight and obese;

3. explain and critique various methods of assessing body fat;

4. explain two common methods of assessing body weight, evaluating their relevance as measures of obesity;

5. determine your body mass index and waist-to-hip ratio;

6. compare the six major theories that describe possible causes of obesity;

7. discuss various categories of obesity and health problems that may be associated with each;

8. describe possible bodily reactions to weight-loss attempts using low-calorie diets;

9. analyze the relationship between aerobic exercise and weight loss;

10. calculate the calories expended for a variety of aerobic exercises;

11. explain the role of a low-fat diet in lifelong weight management;

12. describe the four phases of a behavior modification program, specifying why each phase is important for behavior change;

13. discuss the problems associated with maintenance of weight loss, and describe at least three relapse prevention strategies;

14. describe and evaluate the social prejudice experienced by many obese people;

15. present two lifestyle barriers that may hinder efforts at weight management and two lifestyle assets that may enhance weight-management efforts;

16. compare characteristics common to fad diets with safe, sensible weight reduction diets;

17. describe the two most common eating disorders and what you should do if you know someone with signs and symptoms of them.

Maintaining optimal body weight (and fat) is a key component of wellness. People in good physical shape feel better about themselves and this in turn affects how they interact with others. Additionally, they are energetic and enjoy the many activities awaiting them each day. For people in good physical shape, weight control is a part of a general style of living that is both beneficial and enjoyable.

Unfortunately, the weight of people in the U.S. is on the rise. Between 1986 and 1993 the average weight of young adults eighteen- to thirty-years old increased by about ten pounds.[1] In light of these findings, weight control during the college years takes on added significance. Learning to maintain your optimal body weight now will help enhance both your current and future well-being.

Healthy weight control involves more than just sporadic "crash" dieting. Yet for many people, yo-yo dieting is the rule, not the exception. It is estimated that over a third of adult women and almost a quarter of adult men are trying to lose weight.[2] However, according to recent studies, only 10 percent of them are likely to be successful in maintaining their weight losses.[3] One major reason for this high failure rate is that most people who attempt to lose weight do not establish new eating and activity habits that become part of their wellness lifestyles.

Your lifestyle can enhance your ability to maintain optimal body weight and composition. This chapter will help you evaluate the many weight-control options available today, as well as the known social supports and barriers to maintaining optimal weight and body composition.

Overweight People in the U.S.: A Status Report

People in the U.S. are heavier, on average, than we were at the turn of the century, and our weight continues to climb as we approach the next century. In 1900 about 5 percent of the population was overweight.[4] Recent studies estimate that 31 percent of adult men and 35 percent of adult women in the U.S.

are overweight.[5] Additionally, 21 percent of adolescents, aged twelve through nineteen, are considered to be overweight.[6] Several factors are believed to account for this increase in overweight, including more sedentary lifestyles and the widespread availability of fast foods that are both high in calories and fat.[7]

The prevalence of overweight in the U.S. population increases with age until age seventy for men and age sixty for women.[8] Thus, many of us are faced with the problem of creeping obesity: as we age we get heavier and fatter.

Recognizing the importance of decreasing the number of overweight people, the U.S. Public Health Service has set a goal to reduce overweight in the U.S. to a level of no more than 20 percent overweight by the year 2000 (see table 4.1). While being overweight is a significant health concern for people in general, it is of special concern to women, certain minority groups, people with disabilities, and people with high blood pressure. As you can see in table 4.1, each of these groups has been identified by the *Healthy People 2000* report as a special target population for weight-reduction efforts. Unfortunately, the U.S. population appears to be moving away from the *Healthy People 2000* goal. In recent years the prevalence of overweight has increased for both men and women of all racial and ethnic groups (see figure 4.1).

Special Target Populations

One factor associated with obesity in the U.S. is poverty. As figures 4.2 a and b illustrate, women with income levels below poverty have an exceptionally high prevalence of overweight. A recent study found that 37 percent of women below poverty level were overweight compared with only 25 percent of women with incomes above the poverty level.[9]

Certain minority groups are disproportionately affected by overweight in the U.S. Overweight is more common in Black and Mexican-American men than among White men[10] (see figure 4.1). Minority women, particularly Mexican-American women and Black women, have the highest prevalence of overweight of any other group

1. **Reduce overweight to a prevalence of no more than 20 percent among people aged 20 and older and no more than 15 percent among adolescents aged 12 through 19.** (Update: 33 percent for people aged 20 and older in 1988–91; 21 percent for adolescents aged 12 through 19 in 1988–91) (Special target populations: low-income women aged 20 and older; Black women aged 20 and older; Hispanic women—Mexican American, Cuban, and Puerto Rican—aged 20 and older; American Indians/Alaska natives; people with disabilities; women with high blood pressure; and men with high blood pressure).

2. **Increase to at least 50 percent the proportion of overweight people aged 12 and older who have adopted sound dietary practices combined with regular physical activity to attain an appropriate body weight.** (Update: 22 percent of overweight women and 19 percent of overweight men for people aged 18 and older in 1991, down from 30 percent and 25 percent respectively in 1985).

3. **Increase to at least 90 percent the proportion of restaurants and institutional food service operations that offer identifiable low-fat, low-calorie food choices, consistent with the *Dietary Guidelines for Americans.*** (Update: 75 percent in 1990, up from 70 percent in 1989–90).

4. **Increase to at least 50 percent the proportion of work sites with fifty or more employees that offer nutrition education and/or weight management programs for employees.** (Update: 31 percent offered nutrition education activities and 24 percent offered weight control activities in 1991, up from 17 percent and 15 percent respectively in 1985).

5. **Increase to at least 30 percent the proportion of people aged six and older who engage regularly, preferably daily, in light to moderate physical activity for at least thirty minutes per day.** (Update: 24 percent 5 or more times per week and 17 percent 7 or more times per week for people 18 to 74 years in 1991, up from 22 percent and 12 percent respectively in 1985).

Source: Data from *Healthy People 2000 National Health Promotion and Disease Prevention Objectives.* Department of Health and Human Services, Washington, D.C., 1991; *Healthy People 2000 Review 1993.* Department of Health and Human Services, Washington, D.C., 1994; Prevalence of Overweight Among Adolescents—United States, 1988–91. *MMWR, 43:*818–821, 1994.

of men or women, with almost half of these minority women being overweight.[11] Black and Mexican-American women are also more likely to have **upper-body obesity,** as compared to White women, which may put them at increased risk for deaths from cardiovascular disease, **diabetes,** and cancer.[12]

Native Americans also have a higher rate of overweight. It is estimated that 34 percent of Native American men and 40 percent of Native American women are overweight.[13] In Native Americans, upper body obesity is quite prevalent in men, while less common in women.[14] A higher rate of diabetes in Native Americans—ten times the rate in Whites—has been documented as well.[15] Again, it is believed that obesity is one of the risk factors accounting for such high rates of diabetes.

Certain Asian Pacific Americans also have high rates of obesity. Samoans and Native Hawaiians have particularly high rates. For instance, it is estimated that for Native Hawaiians between the ages of forty and forty-nine years, 68 percent of men and 71 percent of women are obese.[16]

Researchers are actively pursuing the question of why some groups have higher levels of obesity than others. A genetic basis is being carefully examined, in conjunction with the environmental influences of the western world. It is hypothesized that adopting the sedentary routines, high fat diet, and stressful existence of a western lifestyle may interact with genetic potential for obesity.

Overweight versus Obesity

Our body tissue can be divided into two major categories: **fat** and **lean.** Body fat has several very important functions. As we saw in chapter 3, fat helps store and transport the

Upper-body obesity: a type of obesity characterized by greater fat stores in the abdominal area. These fat cells are believed to be larger and to store the fat in a manner that is easily mobilized. It is this form of obesity that is associated with a greater risk of several chronic diseases.

Diabetes: a chronic disease of the pancreas in which the body is unable to utilize sugars and other carbohydrates normally.

Fat: a body tissue, sometimes called adipose tissue, composed of fat cells. Fat cells contain stored fat in the form of triglycerides.

Lean: all body tissues other than fat, sometimes called fat-free tissue.

1. Looking at the data presented in this figure, what trend do you see regarding prevalence of overweight adults in the U.S.?
2. Which group (sex and race/ethnic specific) has the highest prevalence of overweight in the United States, according to the 1988–1991 data?
3. Which group had the largest increase in prevalence of overweight between the time periods compared in this figure?
4. What factors do you think account for the trends in prevalence of overweight illustrated here?

Source: Data from the Division of Health Examination Statistics, National Center for Health Statistics, Centers for Disease Control and Prevention, Atlanta, GA.

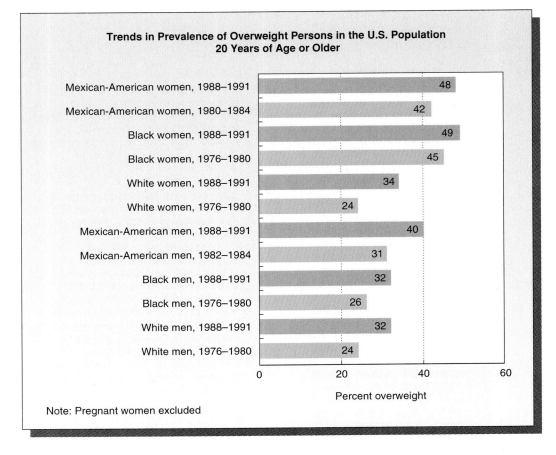

Trends in Prevalence of Overweight Persons in the U.S. Population 20 Years of Age or Older

Group	Percent overweight
Mexican-American women, 1988–1991	48
Mexican-American women, 1980–1984	42
Black women, 1988–1991	49
Black women, 1976–1980	45
White women, 1988–1991	34
White women, 1976–1980	24
Mexican-American men, 1988–1991	40
Mexican-American men, 1982–1984	31
Black men, 1988–1991	32
Black men, 1976–1980	26
White men, 1988–1991	32
White men, 1976–1980	24

Note: Pregnant women excluded

Obesity: a condition whereby too great a proportion of the body tissue is fat. A variety of standards for obesity exist including body weight, body mass index, and percent body fat. Values considered as obese vary by sex, and sometimes by age.

fat-soluble vitamins, protects and pads vital body organs, forms the chemical core of certain hormones, and helps insulate the body from extremely cold temperatures. Only small amounts of body fat, however, are needed to perform these important functions. Lean cells make up the remainder of our body weight and include tissues such as muscle and bone and body fluids.

Our body fat can be divided into two major categories: essential fat and storage fat. **Essential fat** is that amount of fat that is necessary for normal, healthy functioning of the human body. Essential fat is stored in major body organs and tissues such as bone, muscle, heart, lungs, liver, spleen, kidneys, intestines, and the central nervous system. Typically, essential fat comprises about 3 percent of body weight for men and about 10 to 12 percent of body weight for women. Women tend to have greater amounts of essential fat in order to maintain hormonal and reproductive functions specific to females. Most of us carry around considerably more body fat than this essential level. Extra fat is called **storage fat;** it tends to accumulate around the abdomen, upper and

lower back, upper arms, and buttocks in men and in the thighs, hips, buttocks, and breasts in women. Storage fat is fat that accumulates in **adipose cells,** or fat cells. The fat cells of our body are very elastic and contain fat droplets (**triglycerides**) of varying size. Some storage fat is needed as it is this type of fat that protects and pads the internal organs and insulates the body during extreme cold.

Assessing Body Fat

All too often the concepts of **overweight** and **obesity** (overfat) are used interchangeably. A prime example of this is using a scale to determine your weight and then comparing that weight to the standard height/weight tables in order to determine how "fat" you are. A scale, which measures body weight in pounds or kilograms, can only tell you how much you weigh. It has no mechanism to allow it to tell you how much of that weight is fat versus how much is lean. As a general rule, most people who are "overweight" according to the height/weight tables are also "overfat," but there are exceptions to this rule. Take the case of many football players or body builders. They typically weigh more

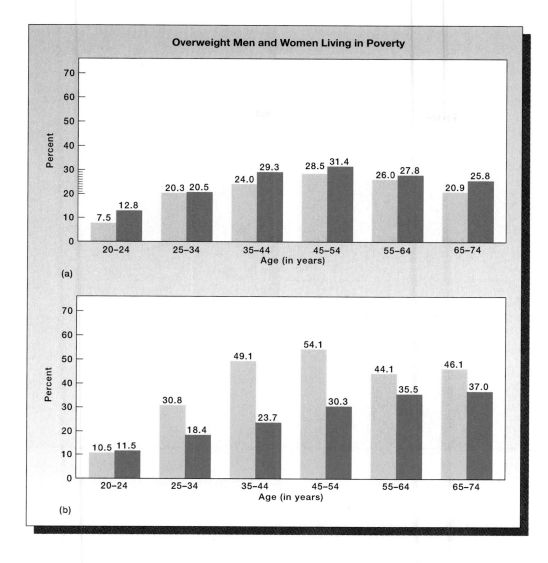

(a)

(b)

Figure 4.2:
(*a*) Percentage of men overweight by poverty status and age. (Yellow bars indicate poverty, and orange bars indicate nonpoverty.)
(*b*) Percentage of nonpregnant women overweight by poverty status and age. (Yellow bars indicate poverty, and orange bars indicate nonpoverty.)

What Do You Think?

1. Comparing the data on the percentage of overweight men living in poverty (figure a) and the percentage of overweight women living in poverty (figure b), which sex has the most significant problem?
2. Why do you think that there are such pronounced sex differences for overweight adults living in poverty?

Reproduced with permission, from TV Van Italie, Annals of Internal Medicine, 1985, 103: 983–988. American College of Physicians, Philadelphia, PA.

than recommended by the height/weight tables, yet most of this weight is muscle tissue, which actually weighs more than fat (see figure 4.3). At the other extreme, some people can be considered underweight according to such tables and still be fat—that is, they maintain too great a percentage of their body weight as fat rather than lean tissue. As you can see, using a scale and height/weight tables to measure fatness or obesity may lead some people to assume they have a fat problem when they do not and it may lead others to assume they are healthy and lean when in fact they may have a problem with excess fat.

There are several good ways to measure your **percentage of body fat.** One of the best ways is called hydrostatic (or underwater) weighing; it involves submersion in a tank of water in order to measure weight in water. A person's weight in water is a function of

individual body density. Muscle has a greater density than fat and therefore sinks in water; fat, which is less dense, floats. Thus, the leaner you are, the more you will weigh underwater, reflecting the density of your body weight. The density figure calculated by underwater weighing is then used in an algebraic equation to estimate your percentage of body fat.

Underwater weighing is one of the most accurate ways to determine percentage of body fat; however, it is also a complicated technique that requires special equipment and facilities not always readily available to the average consumer (see figure 4.4). Fortunately, there are several other less-complicated techniques that produce reliable measures of percentage of body fat (highly correlated with underwater weighing figures).

One such measure is the skin-fold technique. Approximately one-half of the

Percentage of body fat: the proportion of one's body tissue that is fat or adipose tissue.

Figure 4.3: What Do You Think

1. These photos illustrate the difference between overweight due to too much fat (a) versus overweight due to enlarged muscle mass (b). Are both types of overweight a health risk?
2. In the U.S., do you think it is more common for overweight to be due to excess fat or excess muscle mass? What evidence did you rely on to answer this question?

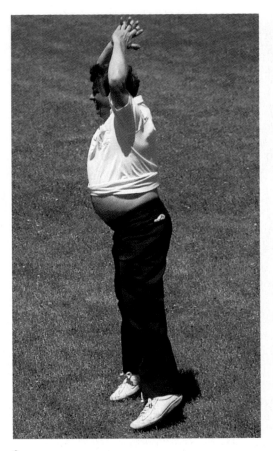

a.

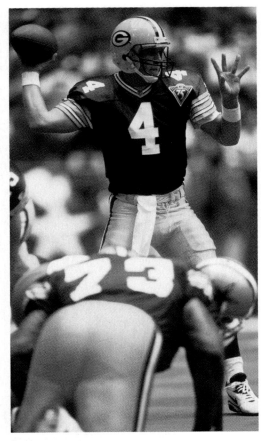

b.

Figure 4.4: What Do You Think?

1. Underwater weighing is one of the most accurate ways to measure the percentage of body fat, although it may be expensive and time consuming. Have you or anyone you know been underwater weighed?
2. Does your campus have facilities for underwater weighing? If so, who is able to access this service and at what cost?

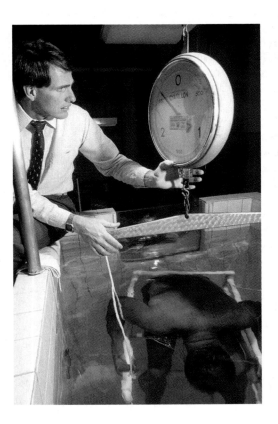

body's fat is stored beneath the skin and is referred to as **subcutaneous fat.** The skin-fold technique measures this subcutaneous fat at various body sites. These measurements are then used to estimate percentage of body fat. Special calipers measure a fold of skin and fat that is grasped firmly between the thumb and forefinger while the skin and fat are pulled away from the underlying muscle (see figure 4.5). The recommended sites for skin-fold measurement of women include the back of the right upper arm (triceps), just above the hipbone (suprailium), and on the abdomen an inch to the right of the naval; and for men the chest, the triceps, and just below the tip of the right shoulder blade (scapula).[17] The accuracy of this method is dependent, however, on the skill and experience level of the technician measuring the skin folds. Additionally, the equipment and skilled technicians are not readily available in many community settings.

Several other body-fat measurement techniques are currently used, often in laboratories for body-composition research.

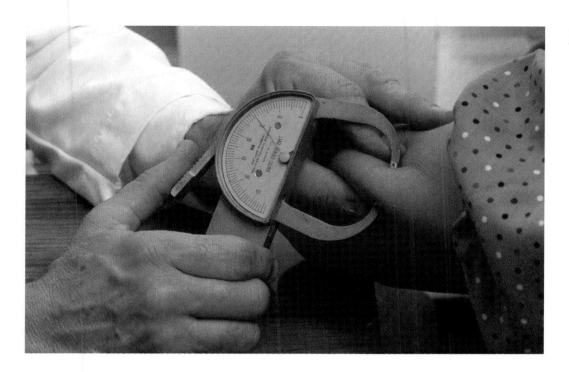

Figure 4.5: What Do You Think?

1. Measuring subcutaneous fat by the skin-fold technique is another valid way to gauge your percentage of body fat. Have you or anyone you know had their body fat measured using the skin-fold technique?

2. Does your campus have facilities and technicians available for skin-fold measurements? If so, who is able to access this service and at what cost?

These include ultrasound, X ray, nuclear magnetic resonance (NMR), near-infrared interactance (NIR), and bioelectrical impedance analysis (BIA). There is some question as to the validity of both **near-infrared interactance** and **bioelectrical impedance analysis,**[18] which have become popular in health screening fairs and fitness centers because of the quickness and portability of these measures. A recent study of body composition measurement concluded that skin-fold thickness and body mass index measurements were the most precise ways to measure body fat levels.[19] Body mass index is discussed later in this chapter.

Many scientists have suggested standards for what percentage of our body weight should be fat. Most of these standards are based on population norms. But because many of us tend to carry excess fat, the average level of fat found in people in the U.S. may not be the goal we want to set for our wellness lifestyle. Table 4.2 presents a set of body-fat standards directed at fat levels for optimal functioning and well-being. According to these standards, women are described as fat when their percentage of body fat reaches 27 percent or higher, with obesity starting at 30 percent body fat. For men these levels are much lower; 20 to 25 percent body fat is described as fat with above 25 percent described as obese.

Assessing Body Weight

The usual method for measuring body weight is to use a scale that determines weight in pounds or kilograms. Typically, health professionals and the general public have turned to the Metropolitan Life Insurance Company's chart of ideal weights to interpret individual weight measures. There is growing controversy over the appropriateness of these tables for the general public. These ideal-weight charts are based on death rates of people who purchase life insurance policies and are not necessarily appropriate standards for all people. Adding to the controversy, in 1983 the Metropolitan Life Insurance Company revised their ideal-weight charts, increasing the "ideal weights." This increase related directly to life insurance studies that indicated that their life insurance policy holders who had the lowest weight had higher mortality rates compared with their policy holders that had somewhat higher weights. Thus, the new charts encourage many to maintain higher weights and, probably for most, higher levels of body fat. At the 1983 annual meeting of the American Heart Association, Dr. William P. Castelli, chief of the Framingham heart-disease study, stated that "recent moves toward upward revision of 'ideal' weights on standard charts are based on a misreading of mortality data and are a disservice to Americans who are

Bioelectrical impedance analysis (BIA): a method of estimating body composition using a painless electrical current introduced into the body that measures the conductivity of lean body mass. The validity of this body fat measurement technique is uncertain.

Near-infrared interactance (NIA): a method of estimating body composition using a painless infrared light beam introduced into the body that measures the degree of infrared energy absorption as it passes through the body. The validity of this body fat measurement technique is uncertain.

TABLE 4.2 — Guidelines for Evaluating Percent Body Fat

Relative Body Fat Level	Women	Men
Very low fat	14–17%	7–10%
Low fat	17–20%	10–13%
Ideal fat	20–24%	13–17%
Above ideal fat	24–27%	17–20%
Very high fat	27–30%	20–25%
Obese	Above 30%	Above 25%

*Norms for female athletes are 13–20%, with an absolute minimum of 10%; for male athletes, norms are 4–12%, with an absolute minimum of 3%.
Used with permission from "Procedures for Your Practice: Skinfold Measurements." *Patient Care*, July 15, 1987; 21 (12):189–196. Copyright 1987 *Patient Care*.

'too fat as it is'. . . . What is a good risk for the insurance companies is not necessarily a good risk for the individual who is deciding to eat more or to eat less."[20]

Recent literature reviews have pointed to two important factors that may account for this "misreading" of life insurance mortality data.[21] Cigarette smoking and illness are factors correlated highly with both lower body weight and higher mortality rates. Studies upon which the standard weight charts are based did not control for cigarette smoking or disease-induced weight loss. This is important because the low weights of policy holders who had died could have been due to illness, which often causes weight loss prior to death. Thus, it is not "leanness" itself that increases one's risk of premature death, nor is it likely that being above-average weight will be protective. In fact, several recent studies have confirmed that "increased levels of adiposity over that associated with an optimal weight range (a body mass index of 21 to 25 . . .) is associated with a significantly increased risk of developing coronary heart disease, hypertension, Type II diabetes, and other obesity-associated diseases."[22]

Many people, however, are now using height/weight tables endorsed by the U.S. Department of Agriculture, that define suggested weight levels even higher than those in the 1983 Metropolitan Life tables. Tony, for instance, is a thirty-five-year-old man who is 5′10″ and weighs 175 pounds. If Tony looked at the 1959 Metropolitan Life height/weight tables he would be told that the recommended weight for a man his height is between 137–172 pounds. Therefore, he would be considered overweight. Yet, if he looked at the 1983 Metropolitan Life height/weight tables the suggested weight range is 141–179 pounds; Tony would be within his ideal weight range. If Tony used the 1990 USDA height/weight tables his suggested weight range would be even higher—146 to 188 pounds. Yet, according to a recent study published in the *Journal of the American Medical Association*, men of Tony's height and age who were at the lowest risk of death weighed less than 157 pounds.[23] As you can see, using height/weight charts for advice on how much you should weigh to enhance your health can be confusing.

Another, better method exists to estimate body fat using height and weight measures. This technique, called the **Body Mass Index (BMI)**, is calculated by taking your body weight in kilograms and dividing it by the square of your height in meters. BMI is highly correlated with other estimates of fatness and is considered to be a good proxy measure for obesity.[24] You can easily determine your BMI and category of body composition (underweight, desirable, increased health risks, obese, or extremely obese) by using table 4.3. There is general agreement that a BMI of 26 or greater increases your risk of developing obesity-related health problems, as well as your risk of dying prematurely.[25]

What Causes Obesity?

In past years, many health professionals believed that the major cause of obesity

Body Mass Index (BMI): a measure of body composition that is highly correlated with percent body fat measures. To calculate BMI, you divide weight (in kilograms) by body height (in meters) squared.

TABLE 4.3   BMI Chart

Height (in.)	49	51	53	55	57	59	61	63	65	67	69	71	73	75	77	79	81	83
Weight (lb)																		
66	19	18	16	15	14	13	12	12	11	10	10	9	9	8	8	8	7	7
70	20	19	18	16	15	14	13	13	12	11	10	10	9	9	8	8	8	7
75	22	20	19	17	16	15	14	13	12	12	11	10	10	9	9	9	8	8
79	23	21	20	18	17	16	15	14	13	12	12	11	11	10	9	9	9	8
84	24	22	21	19	18	17	16	15	14	13	12	12	11	11	10	10	9	9
88	26	24	22	20	19	18	17	16	15	14	13	12	12	11	11	10	10	9
92	27	25	23	21	20	19	17	16	15	15	14	13	12	12	11	11	10	10
97	28	26	24	22	21	20	18	17	16	15	14	14	13	12	12	11	10	10
101	29	27	25	23	22	20	19	18	17	16	15	14	13	13	12	12	11	10
106	31	28	26	24	23	21	20	19	18	17	16	15	14	13	13	12	11	11
110	32	30	27	26	24	22	21	20	18	17	16	15	15	14	13	13	11	11
114	33	31	29	27	25	23	22	20	19	18	17	16	15	14	14	13	12	12
119	35	32	30	28	26	24	22	21	20	19	18	17	16	15	14	14	13	12
123	36	33	31	29	27	25	23	22	21	19	18	17	16	16	15	14	13	13
128	37	34	32	30	28	26	24	23	21	20	19	18	17	16	15	15	14	13
132	38	36	33	31	29	27	25	23	22	21	20	19	18	17	16	15	14	14
136	40	37	34	32	29	28	26	24	23	21	20	19	18	17	16	16	15	14
141	41	38	35	33	30	28	27	25	24	22	21	20	19	18	17	16	15	15
145	42	39	36	34	31	29	27	26	24	23	22	20	19	18	17	17	16	15
150	44	40	37	35	32	30	28	27	25	24	22	21	20	19	18	17	16	15
154	45	41	38	36	33	31	29	27	26	24	23	22	20	19	18	18	17	16
158	46	43	40	37	34	32	30	28	26	25	24	22	21	20	19	18	17	16
163	47	44	41	38	35	33	31	29	27	26	24	23	22	20	19	19	18	17
167	49	45	42	39	36	34	32	30	28	26	25	23	22	21	20	19	18	17
172	50	46	43	40	37	35	32	30	29	27	25	24	23	22	21	20	19	18
176	51	47	44	41	38	36	33	31	29	28	26	25	23	22	21	20	19	18
180	52	49	45	42	39	36	34	32	30	28	27	25	24	23	22	21	20	19
185	54	50	46	43	40	37	35	33	31	29	27	26	25	23	22	21	20	19
189	55	51	47	44	41	38	36	34	32	30	28	27	25	24	23	22	20	20
194	56	52	48	45	42	39	37	34	32	30	29	27	26	24	23	22	21	20
198	58	53	49	46	43	40	37	35	33	31	29	28	26	25	24	23	21	20
202	59	54	50	47	44	41	38	36	34	32	30	28	27	25	24	23	22	21
207	60	56	52	48	45	42	39	37	35	33	31	29	27	26	25	24	22	21
211	61	57	53	49	46	43	40	38	35	33	31	30	28	27	25	24	23	22
216	63	58	54	50	47	44	41	38	36	34	32	30	29	27	26	25	23	22
220	64	59	55	51	48	44	42	39	37	35	33	31	29	28	26	25	24	23
224	65	60	56	52	49	45	42	40	37	35	33	31	30	28	27	26	24	23
229	67	62	57	53	49	46	43	41	38	36	34	32	30	29	27	26	25	24
233	68	63	58	54	50	47	44	41	39	37	35	33	31	29	28	27	25	24
238	69	64	59	55	51	48	45	42	40	37	35	33	32	30	28	27	26	24
242	70	65	60	56	52	49	46	43	40	38	36	34	32	30	29	28	26	25
246	72	66	61	57	53	50	47	44	41	39	37	35	33	31	29	28	27	25
251	73	67	63	58	54	51	47	45	42	39	37	35	33	32	30	29	27	26
255	74	69	64	59	55	52	48	45	43	40	38	36	34	32	31	29	28	26
260	76	70	65	60	56	52	49	46	43	41	39	36	34	33	31	30	28	27
264	77	71	66	61	57	53	50	47	44	42	39	37	35	33	32	30	29	27
268	78	72	67	62	58	54	51	48	45	42	40	38	36	34	32	31	29	28
273	79	73	68	63	59	55	52	48	46	43	40	38	36	34	33	31	30	28
277	81	75	69	64	60	56	52	49	46	44	41	39	37	35	33	32	30	29
282	82	76	70	65	61	57	53	50	47	44	42	40	37	35	34	32	30	29
286	83	77	71	66	62	58	54	51	48	45	42	40	38	36	34	33	31	29
290	84	78	72	67	63	59	55	52	48	46	43	41	39	37	35	33	31	30
295	86	79	74	68	64	60	56	52	49	46	44	41	39	37	35	34	32	30
299	87	80	75	69	65	60	57	53	50	47	44	42	40	38	36	34	32	31
304	88	82	76	70	66	61	57	54	51	48	45	43	40	38	36	35	33	31
308	90	83	77	71	67	62	58	55	51	48	46	43	41	39	37	35	33	32
312	91	84	78	72	68	63	59	55	52	49	46	44	41	39	37	36	34	32

Legend: Extremely obese · Obese · Increased health risks · Desirable · Underweight

Note: Categories are based on value published by the Panel on Energy, Obesity, and Body Weight Standards, 1987. *American Journal of Clinical Nutrition,* 45, p. 1035.

From the Panel on Energy, Obesity, and Body Weight Standards, 1987, © *American Journal of Clinical Nutrition,* American Society for Clinical Nutrition, Bethesda, MD.

(overfat) was overeating. Recently, however, we have come to recognize that the number of calories consumed is only one part of the complex puzzle of obesity. There are currently several important theories that attempt to explain the causes of obesity. These include the energy-balance equation, the fat-cell theory, the set-point theory, the insulin theory, the dietary fat theory, and the genetic theory.

The Energy-Balance Equation

The **energy-balance equation** theory tells us that a calorie is a calorie. There is no magic way to lose weight. When you take in the same number of calories that your body needs for its daily activities you will maintain your current body weight. If you happen to take in more calories daily than your body needs for its activities, you will tend to gain weight over a period of time. If you eat fewer calories than your body needs daily for activity you will, over time, tend to lose weight.

One pound of body fat contains approximately 3,500 calories. According to the energy-balance equation, each time you consume an excess of 3,500 calories you will gain a pound of fat. Each time your body experiences a deficit of 3,500 calories you will lose a pound of fat. It would seem obvious, based on this theory, that there are three major ways to reduce body weight. These would include decreasing caloric intake, increasing energy expenditure, or a combination of the two.

Let's look at the case of Maria, a nineteen-year-old college sophomore who weighs 155 pounds, has a percent body fat of 27, and a BMI of 26. Maria wants to lose 20 pounds to achieve a weight of 135 pounds and a BMI of 23. Maria takes in an average of 2,325 calories daily to maintain her current weight of 155 pounds (your weight × 15 = your daily caloric intake to maintain current weight). According to the energy-balance equation, Maria needs a deficit 7,000 calories weekly in order to lose 2 pounds of fat in that week. (Remember, each pound of fat contains 3,500 calories.) If Maria chooses to diet only, she will need to cut her daily intake of calories to 1,325. Such a drastic reduction in food may be difficult for Maria. If Maria decided to try weight loss by exercise alone she would lose an estimated one-half pound weekly by exercising four to five times per week. For instance, Maria would burn 1,740 calories per week by adding a one-hour brisk walk, five days a week, to her schedule. If, however, Maria chose to combine diet and exercise she would

need to cut her calories by only 5,260 calories a week in addition to her five-day walking program. This means she could consume 1,574 calories daily—249 calories more a day than if she chose not to exercise. Maria could safely lose the 20 pounds even more slowly with much less change in her lifestyle by decreasing her daily caloric intake by 100 calories and increasing her daily caloric expenditure by 100 calories. Specifically, Maria might forgo dessert or a soft drink each day and walk briskly for fifteen to seventeen minutes. At this rate she would lose about 1¾ pounds per month or the 20 pounds in about 12 months.

These calculations work out well on paper, but in recent years experts have found that there are factors other than the simple balancing of energy intake with energy output that may have dramatic influences on weight gain and loss in humans. The following theories present other pieces in the puzzle of obesity.

The Fat-Cell Theory

Many experts believe that obesity is related to both the size and number of fat cells in the human body. The **fat-cell theory** states that the human body increases fat storage in two ways. The first involves fat increases in already existing fat cells; the second involves an actual increase in the number of fat cells.

Research has indicated that a major difference in the composition of fat tissue between obese and nonobese people is the number of fat cells. As a general guideline, an average nonobese individual has about 25 billion fat cells, while an obese person has 60–80 billion.[26] Studies indicate that fat cells increase significantly in number throughout the childhood growth years.[27] Additionally, studies have demonstrated that adults with large amounts of fat can increase the number of fat cells when their existing fat cells reach their maximum storage capacity.[28]

Studies indicate that weight-reduction efforts can cause a reduction in the size of fat cells but not a decrease in their number. People who gain large numbers of fat cells during childhood may be predisposed to obesity. They can reduce the amount of fat in their fat cells, but the large numbers of fat cells remain, waiting to be filled once again. This may partially explain why many people are able to lose fat weight but so easily gain it back (see figure 4.6).

The size and location of fat cells may be more important than the sheer number of fat cells. It is known that obese men tend to store

Energy-balance equation: a theory of obesity causation that suggests that obesity results, over a period of time, from consuming more calories than one expends.

Fat-cell theory: a theory of obesity causation that suggests that people gain fat cells primarily in youth. As adults, fat weight gain or loss is usually a result of expanding or contracting fat cells, rather than adding or subtracting fat cells.

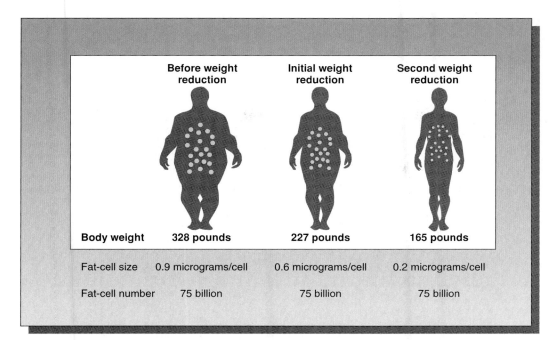

Before weight reduction

Initial weight reduction

Second weight reduction

Body weight	328 pounds	227 pounds	165 pounds
Fat-cell size	0.9 micrograms/cell	0.6 micrograms/cell	0.2 micrograms/cell
Fat-cell number	75 billion	75 billion	75 billion

Figure 4.6:
Changes in adipose cellularity with weight reduction in obese subjects

Source: Data from I. Katch & Wm. D. McArdle, *Nutrition, Weight Control and Exercise,* 3rd edition, 1988, Lea & Febiger, Malvern, PA.

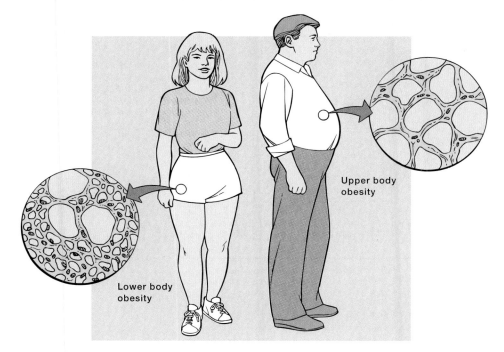

Upper body obesity

Lower body obesity

Figure 4.7:
Different patterns of fat distribution

Estrogen: the primary female sex hormone. This hormone stimulates the development of a female physique and reproductive organs. It also stimulates the female reproductive cycle and maintains the adult female reproductive cycle.

Progesterone: a steroid hormone responsible for the preparation of the inner lining of the uterus for possible pregnancy. If pregnancy occurs, it maintains the uterus and prevents ovulation.

Testosterone: the primary male sex hormone. This hormone stimulates the development of male reproductive organs and secondary sex characteristics such as muscle development and beard growth. It also stimulates the female reproductive cycle and maintains the adult female reproductive cycle.

Lower-body obesity: a type of obesity characterized by greater fat stores in areas of the body such as the thighs, hips, and buttocks.

greater amounts of excess fat on the upper body (the abdomen), while premenopausal obese women tend to store greater amounts of fat on the lower body, especially on the thighs, hips, and buttocks. After menopause women too begin to store more fat in the abdominal area. Thus, distribution of fat appears to be influenced by hormones such as **estrogen, progesterone,** and **testosterone.**[29] Researchers have noted that it is upper-body obesity that carries the greater risk for diabetes, heart disease, and for women, uterine and breast cancer.[30] It is not currently known exactly why upper-body obesity is associated with greater disease risk. Preliminary results, however, indicate that upper-body obesity is characterized by larger adipose cells, which store fat in a manner whereby it is easily mobilized (released into the bloodstream). **Lower-body obesity,** on the other hand, is characterized by a greater number of fat cells that store fat in a more stable, "captive" manner (see figure 4.7).[31] This

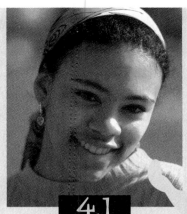

4.1

Activity for Wellness

Nomograph for Waist-to-Hip Ratio (WHR)

Find your waist-to-hip ratio (WHR) by measuring your waist circumference just above the pelvic bone on the side of your torso, and your hip circumference around the most prominent area of your buttocks and hips. Then lay a straight edge across the corresponding points on the two side lines of this nomograph. The straight edge will intersect the WHR line at your waist-to-hip ratio.

From G. S. Bray and D. S. Gray, "Obesity: Pathogenesis" in *Western Journal of Medicine,* vol. 149, pp. 429–441. Copyright © 1988 California Medical Association.

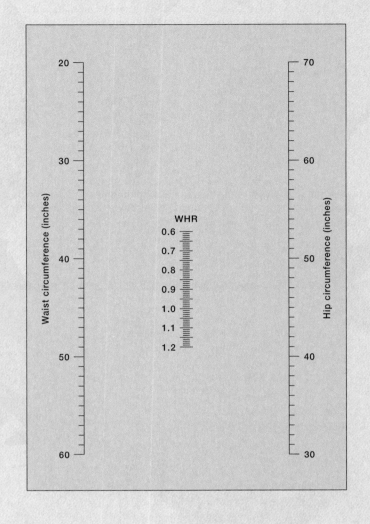

leads to difficulty in losing fat for those people (usually women) with large amounts of lower-body fat but a greater risk of disease for those people with excess upper-body fat.

In light of the research on fat-cell distribution, it has been suggested that an important measure of risk due to obesity may be the ratio of the abdominal to hip circumference. The risk of diabetes, heart disease, and uterine and breast cancer increases dramatically when the circumference of the waist starts to exceed that of the hips. Activity for Wellness 4.1

will help you assess your waist-to-hip ratio (WHR). For men, a WHR below 0.95 is desirable; for women, it is best to stay below 0.80 to avoid increased risk of disease.[32]

The Set-Point Theory

Another interesting theory of obesity postulates that the human body maintains a **set point** for fat storage. This set point acts like a thermostat, dictating how much fat a person should carry.[33] If fat levels fall below the set point, the body will undergo certain changes designed to return the body to its set level of fat. Body metabolism will decrease, causing calories to be burned at a much slower rate, thus conserving remaining fat stores and slowing down weight loss. Additionally, the brain will send out signals to increase hunger. This theory may explain the typical dieter's plateau—the point in a diet where, even with severe caloric restriction, weight loss seems to come to a standstill. Weight control by diet alone is a difficult and often an unsuccessful ordeal because it amounts to a battle against your set point.

It is believed that some people have high set points, causing them to maintain higher levels of body fat, while others seem to have low set points. Heredity may play an important role in determining variations in individual set points. Practically speaking, the body weight at which you tend to stabilize when not dieting is currently the best way to estimate your personal set point.

It is not well understood exactly how the set-point mechanism works. One theory suggests that signals are given off by the body's fat cells, reflecting the amount of fat currently being stored. This signal is then thought to be interpreted by a center in the brain (possibly the hypothalamus). The brain considers input from fat cells, along with other environmental stimuli, and determines what the body's set point should be. These same signals are used to maintain fat levels.

Various factors can influence set point. The taste and smell of food high in sugar and fat, as well as access to a wide variety of food, seem to increase the body's set point. Artificial sweeteners may also tend to raise set point. We have all heard people state that they can put on fat just from looking at food. According to the set-point theory this may be close to the truth. Although looking doesn't actually add calories to the diet, it may cause metabolism to slow down and hunger to increase, all in an effort to increase body fat. This tendency to increase set point would have been very important for our ancient ancestors who lived with frequent food shortages. When good foods were available their set points would rise. Thus, they would consume larger amounts of food and increase fat stores, all as a protection against times of shortage when high levels of body fat would mean survival.

Several factors are thought to decrease set point, including the drugs amphetamine and nicotine and regular exercise. **Amphetamine** and **nicotine,** however, are *not* considered healthy ways to lower set point. The effects of these two drugs on set point last only as long as the drug is taken regularly. Both amphetamine and nicotine have numerous and well-documented harmful effects on the body with long-term use. (These drugs are discussed in detail in chapters 14 and 15.) Exercise, on the other hand, may be one of the best ways to lose fat weight. By lowering set point, exercise marshals the body to help in the attempt to lose fat, rather than fighting against itself.

The kinds of food you eat can have dramatic effects on both your appetite and your ability to lose weight. The insulin and the dietary fat theories attempt to explain the effects of diets high in sugar and fat on obesity.

The Insulin Theory

Insulin is a hormone produced by the body to help guide sugar and fat from the bloodstream into various body cells where it is then used for energy or is stored as fat. Typically, when we eat foods high in sugar our blood-sugar level rises. The body reacts to this by secreting more insulin. Additionally, eating one or two large meals daily also increases your blood-insulin level. This increased secretion of blood-insulin lowers our blood-sugar level; however, it often leaves us with high blood-insulin levels for several hours. Eating more small meals throughout the day will usually help keep blood-insulin levels more stable.

High blood-insulin levels make us hungry. Additionally, it causes an increase in the secretion of an enzyme that, in turn, increases the amount of fats taken from the bloodstream and deposited into fat cells for storage. High blood-insulin levels also direct fats in the blood into fat cells in your upper body, increasing the chances of upper-body obesity.[34]

Being fat can contribute to a cycle of excess insulin secretion. As you gain weight, your body cells become less sensitive to insulin. Your body must then compensate by producing more insulin to accomplish the same function. It is believed that this extra insulin can increase fat tissue as well as keep you hungry. Aerobic exercise tends to have the exact opposite effect, actually increasing the body's sensitivity to insulin.

Amphetamine: a class of drugs that stimulates the central nervous system and promotes wakefulness and arousal. Tolerance develops rapidly, requiring ever increasing doses to maintain its effects. Prolonged use may lead to dependence.

Nicotine: the active ingredient in tobacco with addictive potential. Nicotine acts as a potent central nervous system stimulant and is considered to be a drug.

Insulin: a hormone secretion of the pancreas necessary to convert carbohydrates into energy and to help store fat; sometimes used therapeutically to control diabetes.

The Dietary Fat Theory

Some researchers now believe that obesity and overweight result from the type of food you eat, more than from the number of calories consumed.[35] Specifically, consuming a diet high in fat has been found to be significantly correlated with high body fat levels in both men and women.[36]

According to proponents of the dietary fat theory, calories consumed as fat are different from calories consumed as protein or carbohydrates. Dr. Dean Ornish, in his book *Eat More, Weigh Less*, points out that

> One hundred fat calories can be stored as body fat by expending only 2.5 calories, whereas your body must spend twenty-three calories—almost ten times as much—to convert one hundred calories of dietary protein or carbohydrate into body fat. Only about 1 percent of dietary protein and carbohydrate end up as body fat, because your body would rather use them up right away than waste energy to store them.[37]

Several weight-control intervention studies that have focused on a *low-fat diet,* rather than a low-calorie diet, have found promising results. One study put women on a twenty-week diet that contained 20 percent of its calories from fat.[38] During that time the women lost an average of four to five pounds. This weight loss occurred even though the women actually consumed *more* calories than they had before the diet.

Another sixteen-week program that restricted dietary fat to an average of 23 percent of calories, but did not restrict total calorie intake, found similar results.[39] The women in this study lost an average of thirteen pounds and decreased their percent of body fat by 3.7 percent. While total calorie intake was not restricted in this diet, the women did eat fewer calories as well as less dietary fat.

Dr. Dean Ornish, one of the pioneer researchers of the effects of a low-fat diet on heart disease, has also found very promising results. After following Dr. Ornish's program for one year, patients lost an average of twenty-two pounds.[40] Dr. Ornish's patients were eating *more calories* than before, but *less than 10 percent* of those calories *came from fat.* Additionally, Dr. Ornish's program involved regular exercise and stress-management techniques. Some health professionals have criticized the results of Ornish's work, claiming that a diet with only 10 percent of its calories from fat is so strict that the average person will not be able to comply with it. Ornish responds to this criticism in the following manner:[41]

> If you really want to be able to eat as much as you want until you are full and still lose weight, then you need to reduce fat down to below 10 percent of calories. . . . To the best of my knowledge, our study is the only one to demonstrate that it really is possible for many people to maintain comprehensive changes in diet and lifestyle for several years. . . . Before joining our study, many of the research participants had been on and off diets for many years without much success. I asked them why they were able to follow our program so successfully, and for so long. Here's what I learned from them:
>
> - Most diets are too complex to follow for very long; the food doesn't taste good; and you feel hungry and deprived.
> - Comprehensive changes are easier to make than moderate ones because you feel healthier and so much more energetic so quickly— instant gratification.
> - Joy is a more powerful motivator than fear—change to feel better, not just to live longer.

For more information on Dr. Ornish's weight loss plan, refer to the recommended readings at the end of this chapter.

While the effects of diet and exercise play an important role in determining body weight and composition, many researchers now recognize that these factors play themselves out against a backdrop of genetic predisposition.

The Genetic Theory

Scientists have long wondered whether obesity is caused by an obesity gene passed on from parent to child, or from the environmental influences of dietary and exercise lifestyle habits passed on from parent to child. Studies of adoptees and twins have shed some light on the genetic piece of the obesity puzzle.

In a study of adoptees conducted by Albert Stunkard, a leading researcher on the causes and treatment of obesity, the weights of adults who had been adopted were evaluated to determine whether inherited or environmental influences were predominant.[42] Stunkard found that the weights of the adoptees as adults were more like the weights of their biological parents than the weights of the parents who raised them.

In another study of identical twins, Pennsylvania researchers compared the BMI of pairs of twins raised apart from each other. They found high correlations (.70 for men and .66 for women) within pairs of identical twins. It was concluded that childhood environmental influences had little or no influence on BMI, while genetic influences accounted for 70 percent of the variance.[43]

Another twin study, The National Heart, Lung and Blood Institute Twin Study,[44] followed male twins in the U.S. from the time they signed up for military service in 1943 (at an average age of twenty) through 1986, when the twins reached an average age of sixty-three years. The researchers found that the total BMI gained over the forty-three years of the study, as well as the trends in weight gain through the adult life cycle, were "under significant genetic control." The results also confirmed the results from the Stunkard twin study, with 70 percent of the variability in total BMI determined by genetics. Studies such as these have helped to establish a clear link between obesity and genetics.

Recently, researchers at New York City's Rockefeller University released the results of a study on rats that indicated that the presence of a genetic mutation in the rats was associated with obesity. Researchers theorize that the mutation slows metabolism and prevents the brain from realizing that the stomach is full. Although the results of this study were greeted by great media fanfare, the application of these findings to human obesity has yet to be studied.

A genetic predisposition, however, does not guarantee that an individual will be overweight or obese. In fact, obesity researchers believe that environmental factors, such as exposure to foods high in fat and a sedentary lifestyle, interact with a genetic predisposition in a complex manner. Some of the obesity-related characteristics that are currently being studied as genetically inherited include a low level of physical activity, an increase in insulin sensitivity prior to obesity, an impairment of one's ability to use one's own storage fat, a low resting metabolic rate, a propensity to gain weight in the form of storage fat, and various hormonal imbalances.[45]

Our current understanding of the factors related to body composition lead us to the realization that the puzzle of obesity and overweight is quite complex. Some people might think that the problem is so complex that there is nothing they can do about being overweight. Yet there are many important reasons to adopt lifestyle habits that will contribute to a more healthy body composition and potentially, higher levels of wellness.

Why Maintain Optimal Body Composition?

Many of the enjoyable activities in life require some movement on our part. Bicycling, swimming, or playing tennis or racquetball all require some level of movement. Other daily activities, such as running to catch a bus, carrying a heavy bag of groceries, or even climbing a few flights of stairs, call on us to use our muscles in an efficient manner. Our muscles support our desire and our need to be active. Much of our body fat, on the other hand, serves only as an extra burden. The more excess fat we carry, the less efficiently our bodies can move. Think about how much more difficult it is to climb three flights of stairs carrying twenty pounds of books, compared to carrying nothing as you climb. Having twenty extra pounds of fat to carry around with you daily creates a comparable workload. Maintaining an ideal level of body fat allows your body to function actively in an efficient manner, lending a valued boost to your quality of life and level of wellness (see figure 4.8).

Research studies over the years have linked many diseases with the risk factor of obesity. Health professionals often distinguish between two types of obesity—moderate and morbid. **Moderate obesity** is currently defined as 20 to 50 percent overweight according to height/weight tables, while **morbid obesity** is considered anything above 50 percent over normal weight. Once again, common definitions of obesity confuse the concept of

Figure 4.8: What Do You Think?

1. Ideal levels of body fat allow our bodies to function efficiently and actively. Does your body composition currently enhance or act as a barrier to physical activity?

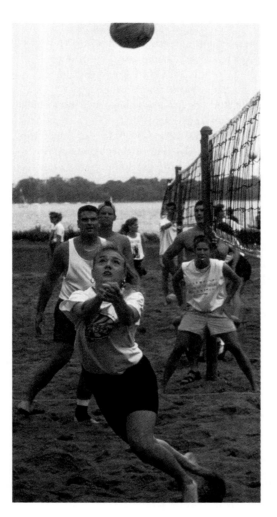

weight (which includes lean and fat weight) with the concept of overfat (see figures 4.9 and 4.10). The BMI ratings presented earlier in this chapter suggest standards for these classifications which are highly correlated with body-fat measures.

According to the standards presented in table 4.3, the "desirable" category of BMI would give you the most efficient level of fat for an enhanced work/play capacity, enhancing well-being. A BMI between 26 and 29 falls in the "increased health risks" category. Elevated blood cholesterol, blood glucose, and blood insulin levels, as well as hypertension, commonly accompany this level of body fat.[46] Recent studies have shown that the risk of heart disease and noninsulin-dependent diabetes mellitus also increases.[47] The BMI categories labeled "obese" and "extremely obese" are of special concern in terms of risk for a variety of chronic diseases. Studies have indicated that at this extreme level of body fat, premature death and debilitating diseases such as coronary artery disease, diabetes, and cancer occur at very high rates.[48]

People who fall into the BMI categories of "increased health risks," "obese," and "extremely obese" should make a concerted attempt to lose this excess fat. Many people with diabetes and hypertension benefit greatly by reducing their weight and fat levels.[49] Many obese hypertensives return to a normal blood pressure range with fat loss. Obese adult-onset diabetics can often be taken off insulin medication with a loss of fat. Reductions in total blood cholesterol levels have also been documented in obese subjects after fat loss. Additionally, people with upper-body obesity, especially if the waist circumference is larger than the hip circumference, are at a greater risk of cardiovascular disease and should make a concerted effort to reduce their levels of body fat.

Body Composition and Lifestyle Change

When you go on a low-calorie diet your body reacts in several predictable ways. Your body's preferred form of energy is carbohydrates. When you restrict your food intake your body will use the glycogen (a carbohydrate) stored in your muscles and liver for energy. Carbohydrates are stored with water in a 1:3 ratio (1 gram of carbohydrate for each 3 grams of water). As you use glycogen for energy you also tend to lose water. It is estimated that 70 percent of the weight lost during the first few days of a diet is due to water loss.[50] By the end of the third week of dieting, water losses are minimal.

As you continue on a low-calorie diet, your body begins to use up its second form of preferred energy—fat. Triglycerides, which have been stored in your adipose cells, begin to break down into fatty acids and glycerol and are secreted into the bloodstream. The glycerol is taken to the liver and converted into glucose to be used by body cells, especially the brain. The fatty acids, however, can be taken up and used immediately by the muscles for fuel.

When you attempt fat loss solely by restricting caloric intake your body will use protein, in addition to the carbohydrates and

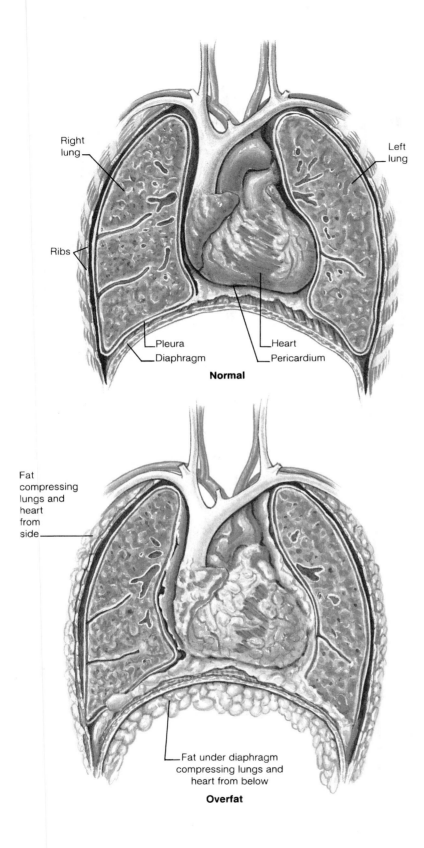

Right lung

Left lung

Ribs

Pleura
Diaphragm

Heart
Pericardium

Normal

Fat compressing lungs and heart from side

Fat under diaphragm compressing lungs and heart from below

Overfat

Figure 4.9:
Shortness of breath may be a first sign of pulmonary distress and heart strain caused by obesity, which increases the heart's workload and contributes to premature death. Fat enlarges the capillary bed (tiny connective blood vessels in an area or organ of your body), which increases the amount of tissue to be nourished by the blood and through which the blood must be pumped by your heart. Some very fat people can't sit, because if they do, there's no space for their lungs to operate in, as the fat invades the chest. These people have to stand up or lie down all the time. And again a breathing problem—overfat people can't take anesthesia as well as people with ideal fat levels.

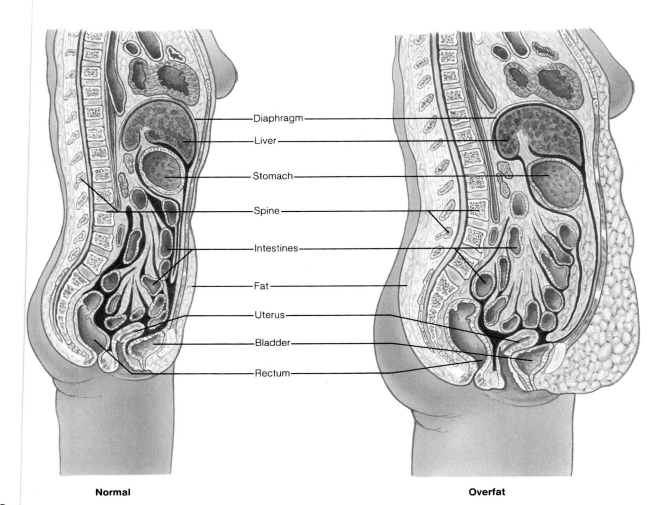

Normal   **Overfat**

Labels: Diaphragm, Liver, Stomach, Spine, Intestines, Fat, Uterus, Bladder, Rectum

Figure 4.10:
Fat infiltrates the liver and other organs. It's a squeeze process, an invasion. Fat compresses the heart, decreases the blood supply to the intestines, and so on. Along with all this, excessively heavy people—and even moderately overfat persons—are putting an extra burden on their backs and legs (the weight-bearing joints), which causes or increases arthritic problems. Complications following surgery occur more frequently in fat people versus thin. Wounds don't heal as well or as fast.

From "Facts About Fat, Take a Look at the Inside . . ." from *Medical Times* Patient Education Chart. Reprinted by permission of Romaine Pierson Publishers, Inc., Port Washington, NY.

fats, as a source of energy. This translates into a significant loss of muscle mass, as muscle cells are broken down to be used for fueling the body.

When you go on a low-calorie diet, your body interprets these signals as starvation and reacts, within twenty-four to forty-eight hours, by slowing down your metabolism as much as 15 to 30 percent. This causes you to conserve energy by burning fewer calories for your daily activities and also makes fat loss more difficult.

Charlatans have found fat control to be a big moneymaker. Consumers spend over $30 billion annually on weight-reduction gimmicks and fad diets.[51] Only 5 to 10 percent or so of those who lose weight from such diets are able to maintain their weight losses.[52] The various theories of obesity give us many plausible explanations for such failures. Too many fat cells, a low metabolism, a high set point, a high-fat diet, genetic tendencies, and a lack of exercise may all play a role. Together, however, these theories direct us to an important realization. Optimal body composition is a result of lifestyle changes; it does not result from isolated bouts of exercise or caloric restriction.

Research studies based on our best theories continually point to three basic approaches to fat control—aerobic exercise, a healthy low-fat diet, and behavior-modification techniques. A healthy change in lifestyle, leading to optimal body composition and higher levels of wellness, would probably include an integration of all three of these approaches.

The Need for Exercise

People have become ingenious in their inventions to avoid muscle movement. Electric can openers, electric toothbrushes, electric garage-door openers, and the automobile are only a few of the "time-saving" and "energy-saving" devices developed to increase our abilities to be sedentary. As we "save" our energy with these devices and fill our leisure time watching others exercise, we tend to throw our energy balance out of kilter.

Inactivity has been cited as a major cause of obesity; however, some experts have posed a question as to whether inactivity is a consequence of obesity rather than a cause. We know that the more excess fat we carry, the less efficiently our bodies move and the greater the number of calories we burn for a given activity. Thus, it would not be surprising to find that becoming overfat slows people down.

Regardless of whether inactivity is a cause or a consequence of obesity, exercise is one of the primary techniques recommended by experts for losing weight and changing body composition. There are many benefits to be achieved by a regular exercise program that will aid in an attempt to lose body fat.

1. *Exercise increases metabolism*. Exercise increases the rate at which you burn calories. Extra calories are needed for any activity. Overfat people will actually burn more calories for any given activity than their leaner counterparts. It has been estimated that a 100-pound person will burn an extra 70 calories when jogging one mile. A person weighing 200 pounds, however, will burn up to an extra 140 calories jogging the same mile. Some people become discouraged when they realize that such strenuous exercise as jogging a mile burns so few calories. We must remember, however, that successful fat control involves a slow change in lifestyle habits. People don't put on twenty pounds of excess fat overnight, nor should they expect to take it off at that rate. Most weight-control experts recommend that for a safe and healthy fat loss, a person should attempt to lose *no more than* two pounds of fat per week. When we look at fat control as a

long-term improvement in lifestyle, the energy-expenditure benefits of exercise become clearer. For instance, a daily thirty-minute brisk walk would consume about 55,000 calories in one year, the equivalent of almost fifteen pounds. Additionally, it has been suggested that our bodies continue to burn an extra 30 to 50 calories per hour for six to eight hours or longer after a strenuous workout. This would add at least an extra 180 to 400 calories to the total energy cost of each exercise session. This increase in metabolism is also believed by many to offset the body's natural decrease in metabolism when dieting. You can easily calculate the calories you expend (or *would* expend) from engaging in a variety of aerobic activities by completing Activity for Wellness 4.2.

2. *Exercise may lower your set point.* Proponents of the set-point theory of obesity believe that exercise may be the most healthy and natural way to lower the thermostat in the body that dictates the amount of fat your body carries. A lowering of the set point is thought to cause an adjustment of food intake as well as increasing the rate at which calories are burned. A study of middle-aged men conducted at Stanford University illustrates the effect of exercise on set point. Peter Wood, a biochemist at Stanford, compared forty-eight middle-aged men involved in an aerobic exercise program with a control group that remained sedentary over the course of the year they were studied. The results of this study showed that the men in the exercise group who ran only a few miles a week ate less food than the sedentary controls. The exercisers' set points may have been lowered, leading to decreased food intake. The men in the exercise group who ran more than twenty-five miles each week increased their food intake in direct proportion to their increase in activity.[53] These men, however, also lost the most body fat. Activity may thus be more important than food intake for fat loss. In this experiment the men who lost the most fat were those who ate the most. It may well be that their set points were lowered by exercise, allowing them to eat more food without adding fat.

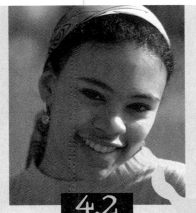

Activity for Wellness

Gross Energy Cost for a Selected Group of Aerobic Activities

Energy expenditure is computed as the number of minutes of participation multiplied by the calorie value in the appropriate body weight column. For example, the caloric cost of one hour of tennis for a person weighing 150 pounds is 444 calories (7.4 calories × 60 minutes).

The caloric cost of _____ minutes of _____ activity, at my body weight of _____ pounds = _____ ×

(calories from chart)

_____ = _____

(minutes of participation)   (total calories)

Activity	110 lb.	117 lb.	123 lb.	130 lb.	137 lb.
Cycling:					
Leisure, 5.5 mph	3.2	3.4	3.6	3.8	4.0
Leisure, 9.4 mph	5.0	5.3	5.6	5.9	6.2
Dancing:					
Aerobic, medium	5.2	5.5	5.8	6.1	6.4
Aerobic, intense	6.7	7.1	7.5	7.9	8.3
"Twist," "wiggle"	5.2	5.5	5.8	6.1	6.4
Jumping rope:					
70 per minute	8.1	8.6	9.1	9.6	10.0
125 per minute	8.9	9.4	9.9	10.4	11.0
Racquetball:	8.9	9.4	10.0	10.5	11.0
Running:					
9 minutes per mile	9.7	10.2	10.8	11.4	12.0
8 minutes per mile	10.8	11.3	11.9	12.5	13.1
7 minutes per mile	12.2	12.7	13.3	13.9	14.5
Skiing, hard snow:					
Level, moderate speed	6.0	6.3	6.7	7.0	7.4
Level, walking	7.2	7.6	8.0	8.4	8.9
Uphill, maximum speed	13.7	14.5	15.3	16.2	17.0
Swimming:					
Backstroke	8.5	9.0	9.5	10.0	10.5
Breaststroke	8.1	8.6	9.1	9.6	10.0
Crawl, fast	7.8	8.3	8.7	9.2	9.7
Crawl, slow	6.4	6.8	7.2	7.6	7.9
Tennis:	5.5	5.8	6.1	6.4	6.8
Walking, normal pace:					
Asphalt road	4.0	4.2	4.5	4.7	5.0
Fields and hillsides	4.1	4.3	4.6	4.8	5.1

3. _Exercise decreases loss of muscle tissue during weight loss._ Studies have shown that people who diet and do not exercise lose significant amounts of lean body tissue (muscle). Aerobic exercise, however, either alone or in combination with dieting, protects against this loss of muscle. This is due, in part, to an enhanced breakdown of fat for the body's energy supply and to the increase in the rate of protein buildup in skeletal muscles. In one study three groups of adult women were put on a weight-loss program designed to give them a 500-calorie deficit daily. One group of women was put on a diet that cut 500 calories daily from their normal food intake. Another group was prescribed an exercise program that caused them to expend an extra 500 calories daily. The third group used a combination of both diet and exercise to attain their 500-calorie deficit. There was little difference in the total number of pounds lost on these three weight-control programs (see table 4.4). Notice, however, that 2.4 pounds of the weight lost by the diet-only group consisted of muscle loss, while neither of the groups that included exercise in their routine lost lean body tissue.

143 lb.	150 lb.	157 lb.	163 lb.	170 lb.	176 lb.	183 lb.	190 lb.	196 lb.	203 lb.	209 lb.	216 lb.
4.2	4.4	4.5	4.7	4.9	5.1	5.3	5.5	5.7	5.9	6.1	6.3
6.5	6.8	7.1	7.4	7.7	8.0	8.3	8.6	8.9	9.2	9.5	9.8
6.7	7.0	7.3	7.6	7.9	8.2	8.5	8.9	9.2	9.5	9.8	10.1
8.7	9.2	9.3	10.0	10.4	10.8	11.2	11.6	12.0	12.4	12.8	13.2
6.7	7.0	7.3	7.6	7.9	8.2	8.5	8.9	9.2	9.5	9.8	10.1
10.5	11.0	11.5	12.0	12.5	13.0	13.4	13.9	14.4	14.9	15.4	15.9
11.5	12.0	12.6	13.1	13.6	14.2	14.7	15.2	15.8	16.3	16.8	17.3
11.6	12.1	12.6	13.2	13.7	14.2	14.8	15.3	15.8	16.4	16.9	17.4
12.5	13.1	13.7	14.3	14.9	15.4	16.0	16.6	17.2	17.8	18.3	18.9
13.6	14.2	14.8	15.4	16.0	16.5	17.1	17.7	18.3	18.9	19.4	20.0
15.0	15.6	16.2	16.8	17.4	17.9	18.5	19.1	19.7	20.3	20.8	21.4
7.7	8.1	8.4	8.8	9.2	9.5	9.9	10.2	10.6	10.9	11.3	11.7
9.3	9.7	10.2	10.6	11.0	11.4	11.9	12.3	12.7	13.2	13.6	14.0
17.8	18.6	19.5	20.3	21.1	21.9	22.7	23.6	24.4	25.2	26.0	26.9
11.0	11.5	12.0	12.5	13.0	13.5	14.0	14.5	15.0	15.5	16.1	16.6
10.5	11.0	11.5	12.0	12.5	13.0	13.4	13.9	14.4	14.9	15.4	15.9
10.1	10.6	11.1	11.5	12.0	12.5	12.9	13.4	13.9	14.4	14.8	15.3
8.3	8.7	9.1	9.5	9.9	10.2	10.6	11.0	11.4	11.8	12.2	12.5
7.1	7.4	7.7	8.1	8.4	8.7	9.0	9.4	9.7	10.0	10.4	10.7
5.2	5.4	5.7	5.9	6.2	6.4	6.6	6.9	7.1	7.4	7.6	7.8
5.3	5.6	5.8	6.1	6.3	6.6	6.8	7.1	7.3	7.5	7.8	8.0

Data from Frank I. Katch and William D. McArdle, *Nutrition, Weight Control, and Exercise*, 3d edition, 1988, Lea & Febiger, Philadelphia, PA.

4. *Exercise suppresses appetite.* Many people mistakenly believe that they should not exercise when they diet because it will increase their appetites and their food intake. Most research to date, however, points to the opposite conclusion. Studies indicate that when obese or sedentary people begin a moderate exercise program, appetite does not seem to increase.[54]

5. *Exercise changes how your body handles fat.* Obesity is associated with high levels of **triglycerides** and with low levels of **HDL cholesterol.** Both of these factors are, in turn, related to coronary heart disease.

Plasma triglycerides have been shown to decrease dramatically with physical training, especially in those people who have high levels initially. Additionally, exercise can increase the levels of HDL cholesterol (the good cholesterol). Many weight-control experts believe that these changes in **lipids** (fats) may benefit the obese by lowering their risk of coronary heart disease.

Proponents of the insulin theory believe that exercise may benefit people who are overfat by its effects on plasma-insulin levels. One of the major functions of insulin is to guide blood fats

Triglycerides: a lipid that consists of three fatty acid molecules attached to a glycerol molecule. Triglycerides are stored in fat cells; elevated blood triglyceride levels are associated with an increased risk of cardiovascular disease.

HDL cholesterol: a type of lipoprotein that carries cholesterol from the bloodstream to the liver, where it can be excreted from the body. High blood HDL levels may help protect individuals against coronary artery disease.

Lipids: a fat compound that usually has fatty acids as a part of its structure.

TABLE 4.4	Pounds of Lean and Fat Body Weight Lost on Three Different 500-Calorie Deficit Weight-Loss Programs		
	Lost Body Weight	Lost Body Fat	Lost or Gained Lean Body Tissue
Diet group	−11.7	− 9.3	−2.4
Exercise group	−10.6	−12.6	+2.0
Exercise-diet group	−12.0	−13.0	+1.0

Source: From W. B. Zuti, "Effects of Diet and Exercise on Body Composition of Adult Women during Weight Reduction," in *Physical Fitness Research Digest*, 5(2), April 1975, President's Council on Physical Fitness, Washington D.C.

into adipose cells for storage. High levels of plasma insulin seem to increase the amount of fat your body will store. One of the earliest changes seen in people who undertake physical training is a decrease in their plasma-insulin levels. This decrease is seen even after a single bout of exercise; therefore, experts believe that lowered insulin is a result of the exercise itself, rather than from a secondary effect of weight loss. There is also evidence that exercise increases the insulin sensitivity of muscle tissue. This would seem to help in regulating the amount of insulin needed by the body for optimal functioning.

6. *Exercise may lower risk even without weight loss.* Several of the beneficial effects of exercise have been shown to occur even when weight loss does not accompany the exercise program. Blood lipids, such as triglycerides and HDL cholesterol, change favorably even without weight loss, as do plasma-insulin levels. Additionally, exercise has been shown to lower blood-pressure levels, especially in those people who had high blood pressure before beginning a regular exercise program. Exercise of an aerobic nature will also increase cardiovascular functioning in general. Resting heart rate will decrease, exercise tolerance will improve, and heart rhythm abnormalities will decrease. For people who fit the obese category, exercise may contribute in a significant way to a reduction in cardiovascular risk, even if weight is not lost. Even those in the "acceptable" range will benefit from regular exercise through an increase in their work/play capacities. They would be able to be more active with greater efficiency and less physical discomfort.

An Exercise Program for Obesity

Our muscles depend on two different types of fuel to power them—glycogen and fatty acids. The type of activity that burns fat is commonly known as **aerobic exercise.** The word aerobic means "with air," or exercise that uses oxygen. Exercises such as sprinting or weight lifting that call for a short, intense effort rapidly break down the glycogen through a process that does not need oxygen. This type of activity is called **anaerobic.** Glycogen, or stored sugar, is found in the large skeletal muscles and the liver and is used for short bursts of work. Your muscles can rely solely on glycogen for fuel for as long as sixty seconds. This anaerobic energy system is not very efficient in the long run for two major reasons. First, glycogen is a bulky way to store energy. Each gram of glycogen contains only four calories of energy. Second, when glycogen is used for fuel a waste product known as lactic acid will build up in the muscles. This waste must be removed from the muscles or it will injure them. Our bodies, however, have a built-in mechanism for safeguarding our muscles. There is a limited amount of time we are capable of such an all-out effort before we must stop and recover.

Aerobic exercise, on the other hand, allows us to work somewhat below our maximum level for a longer and sustained period of time. Some examples of aerobic exercise include jogging, swimming, bicycling, and brisk walking. Aerobic exercise uses the fatty acids released from the fat tissue for its fuel source. The fatty acids are combined with oxygen to give us a steady supply of needed energy. Fat is a very efficient source of fuel, containing about 9 calories per gram.

If you want to lose fat, aerobic exercise is the type of activity to choose. For those people in the "above ideal fat" and the "very

Aerobic exercise: activities that cause a sustained increase in heart rate and use the large muscles of the body continuously for an extended period of time.

Anaerobic exercise: activities requiring an intense, maximum burst of energy and which are done for short time intervals (ten to ninety seconds).

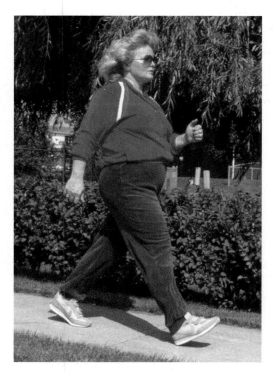

Figure 4.11: What Do You Think?

1. Walking briskly is a good way to work aerobics into your lifestyle and help you achieve or maintain a healthier body composition. Do you participate in aerobic activity four to five days a week for 40 to 60 minutes? If not, what type of aerobic activity would you be willing to add to your daily routine?

high fat" categories, and for those who dislike jogging or bicycling, many fat-control experts recommend a walking program (see figure 4.11). A brisk walk can be very effective as a physical conditioning and fat-loss program. Whichever aerobic exercise you choose, it is recommended that you exercise moderately *at least* four to five days a week for forty to sixty minutes per session.[55]

In addition to a regularly scheduled exercise program, it is important for overfat people to fit more routine activities into their lifestyles. These might include such activities as using stairs rather than escalators and elevators or parking the car a few blocks from your destination and walking the rest of the way.

One of the most popular misconceptions regarding exercise and fat control is the notion of "spot reducing." Strength exercises such as weight lifting and calisthenics will strengthen specific muscle groups, depending on the particular exercise. They do not, however, burn off fat from any particular area of the body. Remember that these activities are for the most part anaerobic and use glycogen rather than fat for their fuel source.

Aerobic exercise, on the other hand, will gradually shrink existing fat cells from all sites on the body as it uses the fat for energy.

While anaerobic exercises, such as weight lifting and calisthenics, will not use fat as a fuel source, they will help you build muscle mass. This is important for two reasons.[56] First, muscle is more metabolically active than fat tissue, thus it burns more calories, even at rest. Additionally, building muscle mass will help counteract the effects of dieting, which reduces fat-free, or lean, tissue.

Aerobic activities should be used to reduce levels of fat on the total body. Anaerobic strength exercises can then be used in a complementary manner to tone up and strengthen specific muscle groups. Aerobic exercise and anaerobic exercise are explained in greater detail in chapter 5.

The Role of Diet

Low-calorie diets have long been a mainstay of weight-control regimens. Decreasing your intake of food seems like a common sense option for balancing your energy (calorie) intake and output. But is decreasing your calorie intake the best way to lose weight and maintain that weight loss, as well as change your body composition?

Controlling the amount of food you eat is considered by most experts to be an important component of a sound and healthy fat-loss program. The level of caloric restriction, however, is very important, as well as the types of foods you consume. In order to meet your daily nutritional needs for protein, carbohydrates, vitamins, and minerals, most experts believe that women must consume a *minimum* of 1,200 calories a day, and men a *minimum* of 1,800 calories daily.[57] Below this caloric level it becomes almost impossible for most people to meet the **Recommended Dietary Allowances (RDA)**. Remember, too, that your body will interpret very-low calorie diets as starvation and begin almost immediately to slow down your metabolism to counteract the decrease in food.

If the set-point theorists are correct, simply dieting may be of little help in adjusting your set point. In fact, it may begin a chain of events that will make life very unpleasant due to a continuous state of hunger and a decreased metabolism. This, in turn, may make it almost impossible to lose significant amounts of fat.

Recommended Dietary Allowances (RDA): the amount of various nutrients, recommended by the Food and Nutrition Board of the National Research Council, considered to be adequate for the maintenance of good nutrition in most healthy persons in the U.S.

Proponents of the insulin theory believe that controlling the intake of those foods that cause sudden increases in blood-glucose levels, such as foods high in sugar, may be an important adjunct to a fat-loss diet because this will help maintain steady levels of both blood glucose and insulin. This may then help to control excess hunger and excess fat storage.

Proponents of the dietary fat theory believe that eating a diet low in fat and sugar, and high in complex carbohydrates will lead to substantial weight loss, even *without* major restrictions in calories.

Proponents of the genetic theory believe that individuals have a predisposition to store calories as either fat or fat-free tissue. Yet, even these researchers point out that it is genetic interaction with an environment that promotes high-fat diets and a sedentary lifestyle that results in obesity.

A Low-Fat, High-Carbohydrate Diet for Fat/Weight Control

A diet that seems to combine the best components of the major theories of obesity is a low-fat, high-carbohydrate diet. Dr. Dean Ornish, in his book *Eat More, Weigh Less*, gives important guidelines for individuals who want to lose weight following a sensible low-fat diet.[58] Dr. Ornish recommends that people trying to lose weight focus on eating beans and legumes, fruits, grains, and vegetables whenever they feel hungry. However, they should stop eating when they feel full, taking care not to reach the point where they feel "stuffed." Other foods should be eaten in moderation. These include *nonfat* dairy products, and *nonfat* or *very low-fat* products such as nonfat mayonnaise, and fat-free baked goods. The new food labels, discussed in chapter 3, will help consumers track just how much fat a food contains per serving size.

Dr. Ornish also recommends that people avoid certain foods as much as possible. These foods include meats, oils, avocados, olives, nuts and seeds, high-fat or low-fat dairy products, simple sugars, alcohol, and any commercially prepared food with greater than 2 grams of fat per serving. Basically, Dr. Ornish's diet is a semi-vegetarian diet that gets 10 percent or less of its calories from fat. Studies of the effectiveness of this diet are impressive, with both reported weight loss and reversal of coronary artery disease.

However, to get the best results, Dr. Ornish recommends a moderate aerobic exercise program along with the regular practice of stress-management techniques. (For more information on Dr. Ornish's diet see the recommended readings at the end of this chapter.)

Remember that the best combination for fat loss is aerobic exercise and a healthy, low-fat, high complex carbohydrate diet. This combination promotes the greatest amount of fat loss without losing muscle tissue at the same time. Chapter 3 provides important information about how to eat a low fat, high carbohydrate, nutritiously balanced diet. Chapter 5 will describe, in detail, how to become more physically active through aerobic activities.

Modifying Eating and Exercise Behaviors

Often we need help in learning new behavior patterns, such as beginning an exercise program or changing our eating habits. Psychologists have had some measure of success in helping people lose fat with a technique called **behavior modification.** Behavior modification includes four distinct phases: (1) describing the behavior to be modified; (2) replacing the established behaviors with more desirable behaviors; (3) developing techniques to control behaviors; and (4) using positive reinforcements or rewards for successful behavior changes.

Modifying Eating Behaviors

The first step in modifying eating behaviors is to determine the behaviors to be modified. This is usually accomplished by keeping a detailed food diary that describes the type and quantity of food you consume, the time of day you consume it, how you feel while eating, any activities you are involved with while eating, how long you spend eating, where you eat, and how hungry you were before eating. This food diary should be kept for a minimum of three days and may be used for several weeks in order to get an adequate picture of your dietary habits (see figure 4.12). Usually when people analyze their food diaries, they find that they have very predictable behavior patterns regarding food. Possibly you might notice that you eat every time you turn on the television, or that you always eat when certain people are

180 Calories

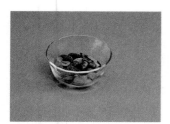

1 oz.
mixed nuts,
17 g fat

2 oz. unbuttered
microwave
popcorn,
2 g fat

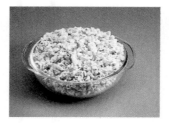

Same Calories, Different Foods: What Do You Think?

When you switch from high-fat to low-fat foods, you can actually eat more food for the same number of calories, as the examples shown demonstrate. Have you incorporated low-fat food choices into your current diet? Would you be willing to make some of the switches illustrated here?

500 Calories

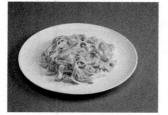

Fettucine
Alfredo,
28 g fat

Fettucine with
marinara
sauce,
10 g fat

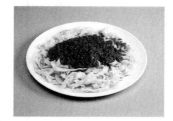

370 Calories

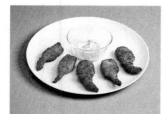

Fried shrimp
with tartar
sauce,
27 g fat

Boiled shrimp
with cocktail
sauce,
3 g fat

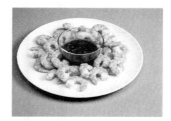

250 Calories

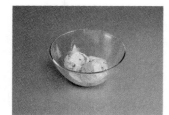

Strawberry
premium ice
cream,
15 g fat

Strawberry
sorbet,
0 g fat

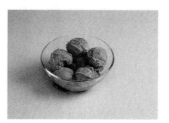

Food diary

Day of the week _____

Time	Food type and quantity	Feeling while eating	Activity while eating	Minutes spent eating	Degree of hunger	Location of eating
6:00– 11:00 A.M.						
11:00 A.M.– 4:00 P.M.						
4:00– 9:00 P.M.						
9:00 P.M.– 6:00 A.M.						

Figure 4.12:
A detailed food diary is essential to succcessful weight control.

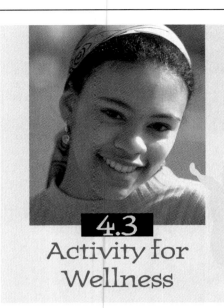

4.3
Activity for Wellness

Strategies to Help Control the Act of Eating

There are many useful strategies to gain control over eating habits once you have identified undesirable environmental cues. How many of the following techniques do you use? Check the items you have tried. Are you willing to try a new strategy to change your eating pattern?

❑ *Make a ritual out of eating.* Each time you eat, even snacks, follow a specific routine. For instance, set the table with a place mat, silverware, and nice dishes every time you eat.

❑ *Eat slowly.* Cut your food into small pieces and chew each piece thoroughly before swallowing. Enjoy the taste and texture of the food as you chew it. Learn to put your knife, fork, or spoon down between bites, and wait a minute or so before taking another bite. Eating slowly can enhance your enjoyment of food as well as helping you to eat less.

❑ *Use small dishes.* You may have been taught that it is very important to "clean up your plate" at every meal. Using smaller dishes will give you the satisfaction of cleaning your plate without having to eat as much food.

---

with you. Some people find that their food consumption is tied to an emotional state such as feeling angry, sad, bored, or lonely. Others may typically binge on sweets after an argument with their boyfriend or girlfriend. In behavior-modification terms, these moods, activities, or even certain people are considered to be **cues to eating.**

Once your cues to eating have been documented, they can be replaced with more acceptable and healthy behavior patterns. For instance, if you find that you always eat ice cream after an argument with your boyfriend or girlfriend, you could choose to go for a brisk walk after an argument instead. If you find that you usually eat a candy bar in the morning on your drive to campus, try and sing along with the radio instead. The possibilities for acceptable alternatives are endless and are bound only by your creativity. Your goal is to establish new behaviors for the environmental cues you receive. It is also helpful to establish some techniques you can use to control the act of eating (see Activity for Wellness 4.3).

Finally, it is important to reward yourself for short-term goals you have successfully accomplished. Your rewards should be things other than food that you would not have given yourself if you hadn't completed the short-term goal you set. Buying some new clothes, going to a movie, or taking a trip are all good options for rewards. Keeping charts

and records of your fat loss and behavior change is also a motivating and reinforcing technique that is helpful for many people.

Modifying Exercise Behaviors

The process for modifying your exercise behaviors parallels that of modifying eating behaviors. The first step is to identify what behaviors need to be modified. This is done by keeping a diary of your activities for a period of time ranging from several days to several weeks. An analysis of your diary will indicate how active you really are and where you could make realistic changes in your exercise routines.

Adding exercise and activity to your lifestyle doesn't have to be considered solely in terms of a regularly scheduled "exercise session." Although this is extremely helpful, it is also useful to consider more routine ways in which you could fit more activity into your daily life (see Activity for Wellness 4.4).

Rewarding and reinforcing yourself for successfully adding more activity to your life is very important. Many people make their exercise session a social occasion by exercising with a group of friends. You could also try running in fun runs, keeping charts to record your progress, or plotting the miles you cover through walking, running, bicycling, or swimming on a map route leading to some faraway destination. Again, the possibilities are endless—being creative in your reward system is part of the fun!

Cues to eating: a behavior modification term describing activities or events associated with initiation of food consumption.

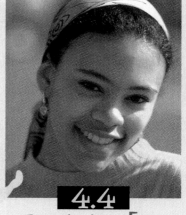
Preventing an Eating or Activity Relapse

Once you have changed your eating patterns to a low-fat, high complex carbohydrate, nutritious diet, and learned to fit aerobic activity into your daily routine, you are only half way to your goal. Weight management and wellness are life-long goals, and maintaining your new habits for a lifetime is essential to attaining these goals.

Switching to a low-fat, high carbohydrate diet will not be easy at the beginning. Cravings for high-fat foods like a cheeseburger may be strong. Learning to deal with food cravings and small lapses in your healthy eating and activity pattern is critical to successful weight management. Kelly Brownell, a well-known obesity researcher from Yale University, likens food cravings to "waves that build, crest, but quickly subside."[59] Brownell suggests that when a food craving hits you imagine yourself riding that wave until it passes. Becoming involved in an absorbing activity, such as reading a good book or taking a scenic walk, is also very helpful.

If you find that you have given in to a food craving or have gone several days without aerobic activity, you have experienced a "lapse" in your plan. Brownell cautions that a lapse is not a catastrophe and should not be viewed as such. Rather, it should be viewed as a temporary and minor mistake that can be easily remedied by returning to your healthy lifestyle.

Certain situations in life are high risk for cravings and lapses. If you can anticipate these high-risk situations before they occur, you can plan in advance how to deal with them. For instance, if you are going to a party at a friends and you know there will be many high-fat snacks, devise a plan for how you will cope with this. Maybe you could volunteer to make a snack to take to the party and bring a tasty but low-fat snack. Chances are good that others at the party will appreciate having a low-fat alternative as well. You could also rehearse, in your mind, staying out of the kitchen and dining room where the food will be kept. Plan on socializing and dancing to help you keep your snack consumption at a reasonable level. Remember, a healthy diet does not have to mean that you can never have a high-fat snack. It does require moderation in fat consumption.

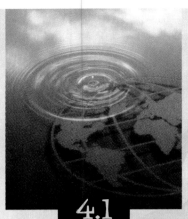

4.1
A Social Perspective

Consequences of Obesity

Obesity takes a social and economic toll on young adults, according to researchers from Harvard and the New England Medical Center. The consequences particularly affect women, claim the researchers, who published their data in *The New England Journal of Medicine* in October, 1993.

According to the study, obese women were 20 percent less likely than slimmer women to marry, and had annual household incomes that were $6,710 lower, on average. Obese women were 10 percent more likely to be living in poverty.

The effects of obesity on men were less marked. Obese men were only eleven times less likely to marry, and were also less likely to suffer economic consequences than women. But men were more likely than women to be hurt by shortness. The researchers associated a one foot decline in height with a drop in annual income of $3,037. Shorter men were 10 percent more likely to live in poverty.

In 1981, the researchers randomly chose 10,039 people between the ages of sixteen and twenty-four. At the time, 307 of the subjects were classified as obese, where obesity was defined as weighing more than 95 percent of individuals of the same age, sex, and height. On average, obese women in the study weighed 200 pounds and were 5 feet 3 inches tall. The average obese man weighed 225 pounds and was 5 feet 9 inches tall.

Between 1981 and 1988, the study followed all participants, and found that those people classified as obese fared worse in social and economic terms— even when subjects were examined independently of their initial social and economic status.

A significant body of research has demonstrated that obesity is associated with lower incomes, without demonstrating whether a lower income causes obesity or vice versa. But since researchers in the new study controlled for factors that might cause lower incomes, such as chronic medical conditions, they suggest that their study may indicate that obesity does indeed play a causal role in lowered incomes and social opportunities.

What Do You Think?

1. What examples of the social stigma of obesity have you personally experienced or witnessed?
2. Why do you think that people and organizations discriminate against people based on their weight?
3. What can be done to decrease discrimination based on weight or fat?

From "Consequences of Obesity," 1993, *Nutrition Week* (37): 3, the publication of the Community Nutrition Institute, Washington, D.C.

Finally, the best technique for preventing lapses and coping with cravings may be to ask your friends and family for help. Social support and a shared lifestyle can make your dietary and activity changes even more enjoyable.

Personal and Social Influences

Our society supports many notions and activities that may serve as barriers to attaining an optimal level of body fat. Many of these barriers involve support and reinforcement for lifestyle factors that oppose wellness. Others involve the widespread availability of fad diets and weight-control quackery. Additionally, there exists a bias in the U.S. against obesity, the results of which range from blatant discrimination to a high incidence of anorexia nervosa and bulimia in young people. To succeed in reaching your goals regarding body composition, it is helpful to have some insight into these potential barriers.

Lifestyle Barriers

Our culture and social-support systems often reward us for living a sedentary lifestyle. New technological innovations at work and in the home "save" us energy. What do we do with this saved energy? Too many of us choose to store it by sitting in front of the television and watching other people exercise. Additionally, some nutrition experts now believe that prime-time television shows are sending implicit messages to viewers that over-eating and indulging in junk food and alcohol are harmless. During a typical week's prime-time programming, characters eat an average of eight times an hour.[60] A study completed at the University of Minnesota School of Public Health[61] noted that 60 percent of all food references on prime-time television were for sweets, and low-nutrient beverages such as coffee, alcohol, and soft drinks. Foods were usually consumed as snacks rather than meals. Only 3 percent of snacks were fruits and only 6 percent

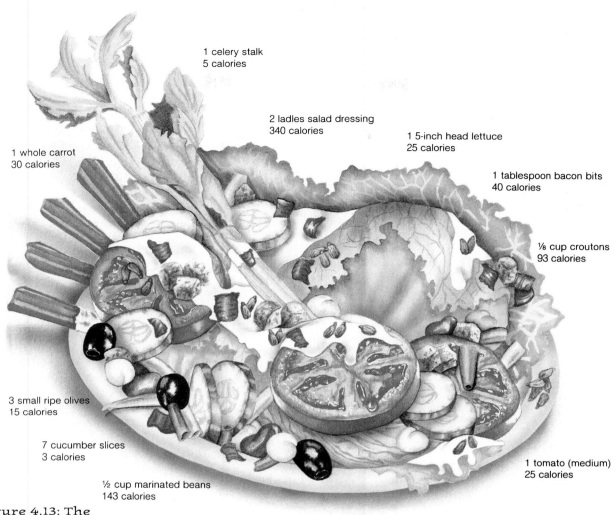

1 celery stalk
5 calories

2 ladles salad dressing
340 calories

1 5-inch head lettuce
25 calories

1 whole carrot
30 calories

1 tablespoon bacon bits
40 calories

⅛ cup croutons
93 calories

3 small ripe olives
15 calories

7 cucumber slices
3 calories

1 tomato (medium)
25 calories

½ cup marinated beans
143 calories

Figure 4.13: The 884-calorie salad

Source: Data from *Independence Health Plan Newsletter*, July 1981, SHAPE, a division of United Health Care Corporation.

½ cup garbanzo beans
113 calories

1 tablespoon sunflower seeds
50 calories

vegetables. These researchers point out that people spend more time watching television than they spend doing any other activity except sleeping and working. Television viewing could indeed be fattening, due to its reinforcement of a sedentary lifestyle and overconsumption of a variety of nonnutritious foods. This problem may be especially prevalent among adolescents. Recent estimates indicate that obesity in children has increased by approximately 54 percent in the United States.[62] Studies suggest that in children twelve to seventeen years of age, the prevalence of obesity increases by 2 percent for each additional hour of television watched.[63]

Many of us carry with us and practice mistaken notions about "diet foods." The

salad bar is one notorious example. How many times have you elected to eat only the salad bar for lunch or dinner, telling yourself the reason for this was because you were on a diet? Salads *can* be a healthy low-calorie choice. However, as figure 4.13 so graphically illustrates, the typical salad could also have as many calories, and possibly even more, than the typical luncheon entree. Hidden fats and refined sugar have even infiltrated the salad bar. Study figure 4.13 and learn to make healthy choices when making a salad.

No one food in and of itself is "fattening." The overall selection of a reasonable amount of nutritious food and a physically active lifestyle seem to correlate best with optimal body composition and high levels of wellness.

Fad Diets and Diet Quackery

Pick up any current issue of a popular magazine, or even the Sunday newspaper, and you are likely to find dozens of advertisements for weight-loss products. Estimates indicate that consumers may spend as much as $30 billion a year for diets, gadgets, pills, and potions promising to take off those ugly pounds *fast*. Advertisements for fad diets have several common characteristics:[64]

1. *The promise of a quick fix.* Many diets will promise a magical loss of weight (but not fat) within a matter of hours or days. Beware the advertisement that promises weight losses of over two to four pounds per week. The weight lost on these "quick" diets will most often be water weight. Remember that carbohydrates retain three times their weight in water. When you consume less than 60 grams of carbohydrates your body will start to lose water. This water weight is quickly replaced as soon as you return to your regular diet or consume fluids.

2. *A strong sexual overlay.* Most of the models in weight-loss advertisements are beautiful, curvaceous women or handsome, muscular men. The only "fat" people are those in the "before" photographs. These ads often blatantly suggest that love is available only to thin, beautiful people.

3. *No pain, no strain.* Many fad diets promise pounds off fast with no exercise and no restrictions on food intake. By using their magic lotion, belt, pills, and the like, you can help your body "melt away unwanted fat."

4. *Testimonials.* Most fad diets rely on testimonials from "the person on the street" who has tried this great diet. Often the weight losses reported are incredible—sixty pounds or more. Some of these testimonials have been attained by paid solicitation.

5. *The imprimatur of experts.* Fad diet advertisements are almost all based on the research or beliefs of "scientists," "doctors," and "medical experts" from "medical schools" or "medical laboratories" across the U.S. Few of these experts or institutions are ever identified by name.

6. *Figments and fragments of science.* Many diets use medical jargon to persuade the consumer. For example, one diet promises a "hypocaloric effect" (medical jargon for calorie restriction) and states that on their diet the food will be metabolized and oxidized in as little as two to three hours after eating (this is the normal physiological time frame).

Health Hazards of Fad Diets

Many fad diets provide either too few calories (less than 1,200–1,800 a day), inadequate nutrients (less than the RDA), or both. Under these conditions many complications detrimental to health can occur.[65] Some of the most common complications include dizziness, weakness, and muscle cramps. These are often due to loss of body water and salt. Remember that on a low-calorie diet the body will use stored carbohydrate (glycogen) as a fuel source, resulting in water and salt loss. **Depression** and irritability are also common results of fad dieting. Some fad dieters report hair loss as a side effect. This results from major changes in metabolism during weight loss and is temporary in most cases. Losing weight slowly helps in avoiding this side effect. Some women report skipped menstrual periods with major weight loss; this side effect is also usually temporary. Gall bladder disease is a more serious complication of low-calorie dieting. Usually associated with very-low-calorie diets (400–800 calories daily), gall bladder disease requires prompt medical attention. Any severe abdominal pain should be reported to a physician immediately. While not common, deaths have also been linked to fad diets. At least six deaths were associated with the Cambridge Diet and over forty deaths with the old over-the-counter liquid-protein diets. Both of these diets were popular in the 1970s and early 1980s.

Fad diets appear with a frequency so great that it is almost impossible to keep up with them. When analyzing any popular new diet there are several major questions you should use to test its effectiveness and safety.[66]

1. Is the diet nutritionally well balanced, including an adequate number of calories?

2. Is the person or organization promoting the diet well-respected and knowledgeable about nutrition and fat loss?

3. Does the diet represent and follow the recommendations of the best fat-loss authorities?

Depression: a state of altered mood ranging in severity and duration; in its mild form, it consists of sadness and discouragement, usually of a brief duration. In more serious forms, called clinical depression, it consists of prolonged or recurrent mental incapacitation, possibly with thoughts of self-destruction or death.

4. Does the diet allow for individual preferences, practices, and taste?
5. Could you live on this diet for the rest of your life?

If your answers to these questions are affirmative it is likely that the diet is sound and will help you on your journey to optimal body composition. Many people, however, do not go on a diet alone. They join a weight-loss clinic's program thinking that experts there will help them lose weight quickly and safely. Some weight-loss clinics may provide safe and effective weight-management programs. Yet many of these clinics are not professional sources of help; rather they are scams preying on overweight people. In 1993, New York City (NYC) became the first city to regulate weight-loss centers within the city limits.[67] NYC now requires that weight-loss clinics let consumers know both the health risks and costs of their particular program, as well as their staff's qualifications. Additionally, the clinics must warn consumers about the dangers of rapid weight loss. If you do not live in NYC, however, Activity for Wellness 4.5 will help you evaluate weight loss clinics *before* you spend your money and risk your health.

Most people who want to lose weight want to lose it quickly. Even though they may know this is dangerous, they look for any product or person who will help them lose weight *fast* and with a minimum amount of effort. This leads many consumers to try over-the-counter weight loss drugs, which they assume are not dangerous because they are sold without a prescription. This assumption, however, is not accurate. The truth is that many OTC diet pills can be very dangerous, especially for individuals with high blood pressure, heart disease, diabetes, or thyroid disease (see Of Special Interest 4.1). Current research on weight management tells us that permanent weight loss is the result of a slow process that incorporates aerobic physical activity and a low-fat diet into a permanent lifestyle change. Pills and potions will not, by themselves, help you to safely reach your weight goals.

Many people are not satisfied with their current weights and the images they have of their bodies. This is often reinforced by our society, where images of thin athletic people are continuously displayed as the ideal weight that leads to happiness, success, and love. When people act on this ideal body image goal by practicing drastic weight reduction techniques it can lead to conditions known as eating disorders.

Eating Disorders

The two most common eating disorders in the U.S. today are **anorexia nervosa** and **bulimia nervosa.** Anorexia nervosa and bulimia nervosa are not new diseases. Accounts of anorexia can be found in the medical literature dating back to the Middle Ages.[68] Over the past thirty years the prevalence of eating disorders has increased twofold to fourfold in the U.S.[69] Studies suggest that anorexia and bulimia affect 10 to 15 percent of adolescent girls and young women. When looking at college women specifically, it is noted that as many as 19 percent may be bulimic.[70]

It is estimated that over 90 percent of eating disorders occur in women. Some researchers suggest that this unequal distribution exists because thinness in women is associated, in our society, with femininity and attractiveness. Thus, some women will seek thinness at any cost. Our socially accepted weight norm emphasizes a thin, physically fit body shape. Yet, the most recent trend in actual body shape in the U.S. is toward greater body weight. In young women who may be psychologically vulnerable to anorexia and bulimia, this dissonance between actual and socially acceptable body size may put them at an increased risk. In fact, the medical literature confirms that "anorexia nervosa appears most commonly in the vulnerable population of teenage girls and young women who are often extremely conscious of their appearance and preoccupied with dieting and slimness."[71] Women who become involved in professions that have weight requirements, such as modeling, dancing, acting, and athletics, have been shown to have a higher incidence of eating disorders.

Eating disorders can occur in males as well, although it is certainly rare compared to the prevalence in women. Male athletes, such as wrestlers who have to maintain a certain weight in order to compete, may be at a higher risk than the general male population.[72]

Anorexia Nervosa

Anorexia occurs most commonly in young adolescent girls. While anorexics are often successful with academic achievements, they also suffer from a low self-esteem. A distorted body image is extremely common with anorexics. They often interpret the normal growth and development pattern of increasing hip and breast size as signs of obesity. In response to their dismay over their

Anorexia nervosa: an eating disorder characterized by a loss of at least 25 percent of original body weight, preoccupation with food, preoccupation with diet and body image, fear of fat, reduced sexual activity, loss of menstrual periods, and hyperactivity.

Bulimia nervosa: an eating disorder characterized by binge eating, often followed by self-induced vomiting or purging through the use of laxatives.

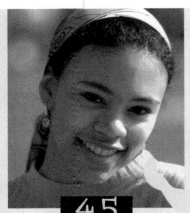

4.5
Activity for Wellness

Evaluating Weight Management Clinics

Use this quiz as a guide to evaluate any program you are thinking about joining. If you are going to pay money to get help with weight management, you have a right to make sure the program meets the highest standards. Take this quiz to the clinic you are investigating and go over each item carefully. Mark each item as either *P* for pass or *F* for fail. Don't talk to a salesperson; get your questions answered by a health professional.

1. Does the weight-management clinic provide for medical and psychological screening? P F
2. Does the clinic help you with out-of-control binge eating? P F
3. Is an assessment of your body composition (percent body fat) done? P F
4. Is counseling provided by persons licensed to practice? P F

5. Is nutrition taught by registered dietitians (RD)? P F
6. Is exercise instructed by certified persons (e.g., by the American College of Sports Medicine)? P F
7. Is medical supervision done by licensed physicians who are present at the clinic for more than quick visits? P F
8. Do you get a written estimate of the total costs to you and the schedule of treatment and follow-up classes recommended for you? P F
9. Do you get a written, informed consent form which states the benefits and risks to you; how much you can expect to lose; what the drop out rate is for the clinic's clients; and what the success rate is for this clinic? P F
10. Is the goal-weight recommended for you based on family history of obesity, your body composition and weight-loss history, and not on charts? P F
11. Is the emphasis in treatment on achieving optimal physical and mental health? P F
12. Is the rate of weight loss one pound per week or less (unless medically-supervised very-low-calorie diet)? P F
13. Does the program encourage you to get the recommended dietary allowance (RDA) of vitamins and minerals, no less and not much more? P F
14. Does the medical exam include an evaluation for exercise? P F
15. Does the exercise-program goal recommend a gradual increase to about four hours of physical activity each week, based on how much you can do and still feel comfortable and energetic? P F

16. Does the psychological component teach behavior modification techniques for changing eating and physical activity patterns, with a strong emphasis on social support in groups? P F
17. Does the psychological component emphasize the cultural pressures to be thin, how self-esteem is often linked with body image, and how to develop a better self-image regardless of appearance? P F
18. Does the clinic rely on appetite suppressant medications? P F
19. Does the clinic provide a maintenance follow-up program which you can attend indefinitely for continuing support? P F
20. Does the clinic give you copies of the scientific research published by others in scientific journals showing the results of the methods used? P F
21. If you pay in advance for maintenance classes, does the contract specify that your money will be refunded to a charity rather than kept by the clinic if you decide to drop out? P F
22. Can the clinic address your special ethnic needs? P F

Answers to Program Quiz
1. Careful screening is needed to tailor a program to your individual case. For example, you may already be exercising but need help with reducing fat in your diet.
2. If your dietary behavior involves binge eating, and you feel that you really are unable to control your intake of food, the program should provide counseling to help you understand how binge eating habits get started, and how to reduce out-of-control overeating. This will require

---

"growing" body, these young women may go on extremely low-calorie diets (less than 600 calories a day) or fast, in combination with a strenuous exercise program. Some anorexics will exhibit bulimic behaviors (self-induced vomiting and excessive use of laxatives) as well (see table 4.5). Even with excessive weight loss, anorexics continue to view themselves as fat.

This distorted body image motivates them to continue the dangerous cycle of extreme diet and exercise followed by dangerous, life-threatening weight loss.

Bulimia Nervosa
Bulimia nervosa is a disturbed eating pattern that consists of binge eating (often

group therapy to provide the kind of social support needed. The counseling should include a psychological evaluation with interviews and/or tests to determine your level of depression, anxiety, relationship problems, and symptoms of eating disorders such as binges, purges, and excessive feelings of shame over being unable to control eating. If you feel extremely uncomfortable in groups, you may want to try individual counseling first. One of the goals of this counseling would be to try to make you feel more at ease with others, since the ability to give and receive social support is a key to success and emotional well-being in general.

3. The amount of fat you have may determine your realistic goal weight. If you have lots of muscle, you can't expect to lose a lot of muscle healthfully in order to lose weight. Also, if you have a very high percentage of body fat, this may indicate that you have an overabundance of fat cells. These cells have a lower limit in size which may restrict how much you can reduce in body size.

4. Don't turn your personal and weight-management problems over to someone who hasn't the proper training and experience. Licensed counselors will at a minimum have masters degrees and supervised experience, and are required to adhere to a professional code of ethics which inhibits them from exploiting you or from using untested methods.

5. There have been so many weird ideas about weight management and nutrition that it can really pay to make sure that your nutrition consultant is a registered dietitian who has training in the scientifically valid approaches to sound nutrition and sensible weight control.

6. Certified exercise instructors are required to keep your physical activity program safe.

7. Some programs advertise medical supervision by licensed physicians, but the M.D. only spends a few minutes a week at the clinic checking records.

8. Get everything in writing before you spend money. You are entering into a business contract. Read the fine print.

9. The risks and benefits of the program, the predicted realistic weight outcome for you, and the success rate for the clinic should be made known before you pay.

10. Your goal weight probably should be about halfway between what you weigh now and your ideal weight from height/weight charts.

11. The way to optimal mental and physical health for the overweight person involves increasing physical activity, reducing fat in the diet, and accepting the weight you achieve after you have adopted healthful lifestyle changes. In other words, the clinic should not appeal to your vanity, but strive to help you be healthier and more self-accepting.

12. Faster rates of loss may cause you to relapse or become ill.

13. There is no evidence that excessive supplementation of any vitamins or minerals will have a beneficial effect on weight loss or maintenance.

14. A physician should go through a checklist to make sure you are not at a high level of risk to suffer injuries to legs or feet, or to damage your heart.

15. The physical activity program should be gradual, based on how you respond to exercise, so that physical pain can be minimized, and maximum enjoyment obtained from exercise.

16. Behavior modification is the best way to learn to change your eating and physical activity habits. Social support should be used to help you through crises.

17. The cultural pressures to be thin are thought to be among the primary causes of eating disorders. Some overweight persons may have low self-esteem because of their perceived inability to control weight, and because of the prejudices against the obese which they experience. Dealing with these feelings and prejudices should be an important part of any program.

18. Appetite suppressants are only effective for relatively short periods of time, and may cause harmful physical and psychological side effects if used for longer periods.

19. Long-term support through counseling or groups seems to be needed for many to help them maintain new eating and physical activity habits.

20. There have been so many fraudulent weight-loss treatments that you can't be too careful.

21. The incentive for both you and the clinic should be to keep you in the program.

22. The cultural and family rules you live with may influence your eating and exercise. If your spouse wants you to stay overweight, or if all your friends are overweight and not concerned about reducing, your weight-management clinic should be able to provide some help in how to deal with resistance from others. If your cultural heritage requires you to prepare high-fat ethnic foods, your clinic's dietitian should be able to work with you to develop similar, lower-fat recipes which should help to satisfy your family.

Adapted from John P. Foreyt & G. Ken Goodrick, (1994), *Living Without Dieting*. Warner Books, New York, NY.

consuming more than 3,400 calories in 1¼ hours[73]) followed by self-induced vomiting or purging by excessive laxative use. Bulimia appears to be most common among young women in their teens or early twenties; however, some women successfully hide bulimia until they reach their thirties or forties. This may be explained by the fact that most bulimics maintain a more normal appearance, with weight losses and gains fluctuating around 10 to 15 percent above and below their ideal weight. Another reason that bulimics may go undiagnosed is their tendency to binge and purge in secret. Bulimics usually recognize that their eating behaviors are not normal, so they often hide

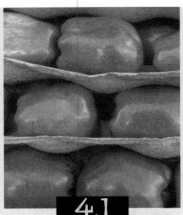

4.1
Of Special Interest

Over-the-Counter Drugs to Lose Weight

U.S. drug manufacturers have been quick to capitalize on—and to promote—public preoccupation with weight loss by filling neighborhood drugstores with prominent displays of diet aids of every description. Consumers, mostly women, have literally eaten it up, to the tune of $314 million in 1988.

Over the past few decades, a parade of diet products has been placed on the market and disappeared unnoticed, while others have risen to take their place. For years a variety of capsules, tablets, powders, liquids, gums, candies, and canned low-cal meals, often with fantastic claims and prices to match, have been available to U.S. consumers.

In 1982, a Food and Drug Administration (FDA) advisory panel proposed marketing rules for over-the-counter weight control drug products. The only two ingredients approved for use in weight control were phenylpropanolamine hydrochloride (PPA) and benzocaine. All other drug products touted in any way for weight control lack evidence of safety, effectiveness, or both. In the dozen years since this report, the FDA has taken no further action in regulating this widely abused and misrepresented class of drugs.

Phenylpropanolamine-containing Products

Today, the most tempting items are those flat little boxes that dangle enticingly from drug store and supermarket shelves and promise "Fast Weight Loss." These are the current stars of the profitable diet world: products containing PPA. This chemical is very similar to amphetamines—"speed" or "uppers." Originally marketed as a nasal decongestant, PPA is now the leading over-the-counter diet aid, accounting for most sales in this category. Products such as Dexatrim (the sales leader), Acutrim, Control, Dietac, Permathene, Prolamine, and Thinz-span all contain PPA.

PPA was rated safe and effective by the FDA advisory panel for use as an anorectic (appetite suppressant) in weight control. Despite the panel's decision, it is our opinion that this chemical poses a substantial hazard to users, and has not succeeded in proving long-term effectiveness. For this reason, *we recommend strongly against the use of all phenylpropanolamine-containing products in weight-loss programs.*

No well-controlled study has shown PPA to be effective as an aid in long-term weight control. It may help you lose weight for a few days, but you gain the pounds back when you stop taking it, and it doesn't help in making the lifestyle changes that are needed to keep unwanted pounds from coming back.

Not only are there significant questions about PPA's effectiveness, but also serious doubts about its safety. PPA can cause hypertension (high blood pressure), even in young, healthy adults given amounts within the recommended dosage.

The FDA acknowledges that PPA can be hazardous to a significant portion—at least 20 percent—of the population. People who *must* avoid PPA include anyone with hypertension, heart disease, diabetes, or thyroid disease. The issue is made more serious by the fact that overweight individuals (the people who use PPA as an anorectic) are more likely than normal-weight people to suffer from all of these disorders. Additionally, it is estimated that 40 percent of all diabetics and 30 percent of all hypertensives are not aware of their disorders; for them PPA-containing products pose an unsuspected but significant risk. There have been cases of fatal cardiovascular problems, kidney disease, and muscle damage associated with the use of phenylpropanolamine-containing products, although these effects have yet to be clearly shown in healthy subjects taking the recommended doses.

There have also been reports of amphetamine ("speed")-like adverse reactions to PPA-containing products. These include accelerated pulse rate, tremor, restlessness, agitation, anxiety, dizziness, and hallucinations. These reactions may be aggravated by the presence of caffeine in many of these products.

As mentioned earlier, adverse reactions can occur with the PPA products at "recommended" dose levels. Reactions are often more severe or even life-threatening when these products are abused and overused. OTC diet aids consistently appear prominently in official statistics of drug abuse problems reported from hospital emergency rooms. This fact, along with the hazards and ineffectiveness of these products in weight control, raises serious questions about the wisdom of making them available at all.

What Do You Think?

1. Do you know anyone who has taken over-the-counter (OTC) diet pills containing PPA? Did they realize the risk they were taking by using this drug?
2. Do you think that OTC drugs containing PPA should be removed from the market by the FDA? Explain your rationale.

From "Losing Weight: The Truth is Hard to Swallow" in *Public Citizen Health Research Group Health Letter, 10* (4): 6, 1994. Public Citizen Foundation, Washington, D.C. Reprinted by permission.

high-calorie foods, waiting to consume them in private and in great quantities. Such bingeing, however, is followed by a purge in order to rid the body of the calories in an attempt to maintain their desired weight.

The purging bulimics routinely perform carries great health risk. Body chemicals, such as the electrolytes sodium and potassium, can become out of balance resulting in fatigue, seizures, heart palpitations, and thin bones.

TABLE 4.5 — Characteristics of Anorexia Nervosa and Bulimia Nervosa

According to the American Psychiatric Association, a person diagnosed as bulimic or anorectic must have all of that disorder's specific symptoms:

Anorexia Nervosa

- refusal to maintain weight that's over the lowest weight considered normal for age and height
- intense fear of gaining weight or becoming fat, even though underweight
- distorted body image
- in women, three consecutive missed menstrual periods without pregnancy

Bulimia Nervosa

- recurrent episodes of binge eating (minimum average of two binge-eating episodes a week for at least three months)
- a feeling of lack of control over eating during the binges
- regular use of one or more of the following to prevent weight gain: self-induced vomiting; use of laxatives or diuretics; strict dieting or fasting; vigorous exercise
- persistent over-concern with body shape and weight

Source: Data from D. Farley, "Eating Disorders Require Medical Attention" in *FDA Consumer*, 26:28. U.S. Food and Drug Administration.

TABLE 4.6 — Where to Get More Information on Eating Disorders

American Anorexia/Bulimia Association Inc., 418 E. 76th St., New York, N.Y. 10021, (212) 734–1114. AABA functions as an information and referral service for anorexics, bulimics, and members of their immediate families.

American College of Sport Medicine, P.O. Box 1440, Indianapolis, Ind. 46206–1440, (317) 637–9200. This professional organization has devoted increasing attention in recent years to eating disorders among female athletes.

National Association of Anorexia Nervosa and Associated Disorders, Box 7, Highland Park, Ill. 60035, (708) 831–3438. ANAD, the oldest U.S. organization of its kind, sponsors support groups.

From "Eating Disorders" in *CQ Researcher*, 2:1114, 1992. Reprinted by permission of Congressional Quarterly, Inc., Washington, D.C.

Vomiting excessively can damage the esophagus and stomach, as well as the gums and teeth. Using drugs to induce vomiting can be extremely dangerous. Karen Carpenter, a well-known recording artist, died from heart damage caused by excessive use of syrup of ipecac, a drug used to induce vomiting.

Getting Help for Eating Disorders

Eating disorders can become untreatable and life threatening if they continue for extended periods of time. Therefore, early recognition and professional treatment is essential. If someone you know has signs and symptoms of an eating disorder, talk to them in a caring way about the behaviors you have observed and encourage them to seek medical help from their family physician or another health care professional that they trust. Table 4.6 lists a variety of organizations that will provide additional information on eating disorders. The most important point to remember is that professional help must be received as soon as possible when an eating disorder is suspected.

Therapy for eating disorders often involves a variety of treatments including psychotherapy, nutrition counseling, self-help groups, and behavior modification.[74] With medical help, many people with eating disorders are able to attain healthier weight, eating habits, and body image.

Making Healthy Choices for Fat and Weight Management

Our weight and body fat levels are influenced by many factors, especially genetics and

TABLE 4.7 — Tips for Making Healthy Changes in Your Weight

Making changes in your body weight and fat is not an easy process. You will probably find that you go through a series of steps, like those listed below, each time you try to make healthy changes in your behavior. To decrease your total weight and percent body fat you will need to consider changing to a low-fat, high-carbohydrate diet, as well as adding more exercise and activity to your lifestyle. The following tips will help you as you progress through the stages of behavior change.*

Precontemplation → Contemplation

If you have never thought about making healthy changes in your weight and body fat or you do not intend to make any changes within the next six months you might want to consider:

- assessing your current body mass index (table 4.3) and waist-to-hip ratio (Activity for Wellness 4.1) to determine if you need to lose fat or weight.
- assessing your current dietary patterns by completing and carefully evaluating your responses to Activity for Wellness 3.1 "How's Your Diet?" (see chapter 3) paying special attention to your responses regarding foods high in fat and low in complex carbohydrates.

Contemplation → Preparation

If you have been seriously considering making some changes in your weight or body fat level, but have not yet attempted any changes, try to thoughtfully answer the following questions:

- How do I think or feel about striving for a more optimal level of body fat that may help me to have more energy, attain my desired body weight and shape, and increase my level of well-being both now and in the future? Am I willing to change my lifestyle permanently to achieve this goal safely?

Preparation → Action

If you are ready to make some definite plans for making low-fat food choices and beginning an exercise routine during the next month, or if you have already made small changes in the past but were not able to maintain those changes as a permanent part of your lifestyle, consider the following actions:

- Make a resolution to yourself to begin a certain change in your diet and exercise habits; for instance, make a commitment to yourself to begin to choose more low-fat or fat-free foods each day or to become more active.
- Set a specific date to begin your new behavior, for example "starting Monday I will walk with my friend Jill for 45 minutes, five days a week, at a brisk yet comfortable pace."

Action → Maintenance

If you have recently started to make some healthy changes in how you select the food you eat, and your activity level, the following tips will help you continue on this healthy path:

- Write a behavior change contract, such as found in chapter 1, and find a support person who will help you keep with your plan; have your support person sign your contract.
- Give yourself rewards *often* for meeting your goals and objectives; rewards should be things other than food that you really enjoy, but that you are willing to do without if you do not meet your goal.

Maintenance

You have made important changes in your dietary and exercise habits that you have practiced for six months or longer; now you need to focus on maintaining your healthy choices every day:

- Try to predict situations where you will be tempted to eat too much high-fat food or skip your regular physical activity routine. Develop a plan for how to deal with these situations before they occur so that they do not take you by surprise.
- Ask your friends or family to join you in your new lifestyle changes. Social support is very powerful!

*Based on Prochaska, Norcross and DiClemente's transtheoretical model. See Prochaska, J. O., Norcross, J. C. & DiClemente, C. C. (1994). *Changing for Good.* New York: William Morrow and Company, Inc.

environmental factors, such as exposure to an abundance of high-fat foods and a sedentary lifestyle. Yet we can make many choices each day that will make the most of our genetic potential by controlling our environment and our lifestyle. George Blackburn, an obesity researcher from Harvard Medical School, sums up an optimal weight-management plan like this:[75]

- Strive for weight loss you can maintain, not what weight tables define as ideal.

- Stick to a modest rate of loss—about 2 to 4 pounds per month.
- Eat less fat, not less food.
- The best way to keep weight off is through regular exercise.

Developing a lifestyle of sound dietary practices and activity can be approached as an adventure. Seek out new activities and new and nutritious foods. Table 4.7 offers suggestions on making healthy behavior changes that will help you achieve the body weight and composition that is right for you. These changes will help you in your quest for wellness.

Summary

1. Body weight is composed of fat cells and lean cells. The fat cells are elastic and store fat deposits. The lean cells make up all other body cells, such as bone, blood, muscle, and organs.

2. Fat can be divided into two categories: essential fat and storage fat. Essential fat is necessary for normal body functioning. Some storage fat is necessary to pad vital organs and insulate the body. The rest of storage fat is used to store energy or calories.

3. Scales and height/weight tables are *not* good ways to measure body fat. They have no mechanism to differentiate fat weight from lean body weight. The skin-fold technique and underwater weighing are better methods for fat measurement because they are able to estimate percentage of body fat. They do, however, rely on special equipment and trained personnel that may not be available to all people who want to know whether they are "overweight" or "obese."

4. The BMI (Body Mass Index) is an easily calculated measure of obesity. Until more direct methods of measuring percent body fat are perfected and made more readily available to the general public, weight management researchers recommend the use of BMI as a proxy measure of obesity.

5. There are several good theories that attempt to explain the cause of obesity. The energy-balance equation theory, the fat-cell theory, the set-point theory, the insulin theory, the dietary fat theory, and the genetic theory all add important pieces to the puzzle of obesity causation.

6. Maintaining optimal levels of body fat helps to facilitate optimal and efficient body function. This lends a valuable boost to your wellness lifestyle.

7. Body-composition experts suggest that people who are moderately to morbidly overweight, especially those with upper-body obesity, are at risk for hypertension, diabetes, elevated blood cholesterol, and coronary artery disease. These people would benefit from a disease prevention program aimed at reducing percentage of body fat.

8. Dieting, by itself, causes water and protein loss, as well as fat loss. Additionally, body metabolism slows down by as much as 15 to 30 percent.

9. The optimal way to lose body fat is to combine aerobic physical activity with a nutritionally well-balanced, low-fat diet.

10. New research indicates that, in terms of diet, it may be more important to decrease the percentage of calories you consume from fat than to decrease the total number of calories you consume. The low-fat diets that have shown the greatest success in terms of weight loss are those in which the subjects decreased the amount of fat they consumed while eating the same number of calories; complex carbohydrates were substituted for fatty foods. Aerobic activity was also an important aspect of these programs.

11. Exercise increases metabolism, lowers the set point, decreases muscle loss, suppresses appetite, and changes how your body handles fat. All of these contribute to safe and effective fat loss.

12. Aerobic exercise uses fatty acids for its energy source and is thus the best type of fat-loss exercise.

13. Behavior-modification techniques can help people learn new food and exercise habits. Three steps are involved with behavior modification: assessing eating and exercise cues, modifying diet and exercise habits, and reinforcing positive changes.

14. There are many barriers to attaining and maintaining optimal body composition. Factors that support sedentary lifestyles and overindulgence in food are primary barriers. The abundance of fad diets and weight-control quackery, as well as social norms that may increase the incidence of anorexia and bulimia in young women are additional barriers.

15. Optimal body composition involves lifestyle changes that can add to life's adventure. Begin to explore new activities and taste new lower-fat food. Try to view your fat-control effort as adding a new, positive direction to your life.

Recommended Readings

Bennion, L. J., E. L. Bierman, J. M. Ferguson, and the Editors of Consumer Reports Books. (1991) *Straight Talk About Weight Control: Taking the Pounds Off and Keeping Them Off.* (Yonkers, N.Y.: Consumers Union.)

Straight Talk About Weight Control provides the reader with a comprehensive review of weight control including theories of obesity, eating disorders, and treatment of obesity. The treatment section is especially valuable, covering diet, exercise, pills, potions, shots, surgery, and behavior modification.

"Eating disorders: Is there too much pressure on women to be slim?" (1992) *CQ Researcher* 2(47): 1097–1120.

A comprehensive review of eating disorders, this article describes the cultural pressure on women to be thin as well as the signs and symptoms, health effects and treatment of eating disorders. Especially interesting is the point/counterpoint on whether or not women in the U.S. are hampered by a cultural edict to be beautiful.

Ornish, Dean. (1993) *Eat More, Weigh Less: Dr. Dean Ornish's Life Choice Program for Losing Weight Safely While Eating Abundantly.* (New York: Harper Collins Publishers.)

Eat More, Weigh Less clearly describes how to change your diet to one low in fat and sugar, and high in complex carbohydrates, so that you can eat more food and lose weight. Over one half of this book contains recipes created by gourmet chefs from across the United States. Additionally, Dr. Ornish provides chapters on adding exercise and stress-management strategies to help with weight loss.

References

1. Chrebet, Jennifer. (1994) "Pulse points: The average weight of men and women.' *American Health* XIII (6): 8.

2. "Weight management: Making the leap to a healthy life." (July/August, 1992) *Food Insight* 1, 4–5.

3. "Heavy news." (1994) *UC Berkeley Wellness Letter* 10 (5): 2.

4. Bennion, L. J., E. L. Bierman, and J. M. Ferguson. (1991) *Straight Talk About Weight Control: Taking Pounds Off and Keeping Them Off* (Yonkers, N.Y.: Consumers Union), 14.

5. Kuczmarski, Robert J., Katherine M. Flegal, Stephen M. Campbell, & Clifford L. Johnson. (1994) "Increasing prevalence of overweight among U.S. adults: The National Health and Nutrition Examination Surveys, 1960 to 1991". JAMA 272: 205–211.

6. "Prevalence of overweight among adolescents—United States, 1988–1991." (1994) JAMA 272: 1737.

7. Pi-Sunyer, F. Xavier. (1994) "The fattening of America." JAMA 272: 238–239.

8. Kuczmarski et al., "Increasing prevalence of overweight among U.S. adults," 207.

9. U.S. Department of Health and Human Services, (1991) *Healthy People 2000 Health Promotion and Disease Prevention Objectives for the Nation,* Washington, D.C., 115.

10. Kuczmarski et al., "Increasing prevalence of overweight among U.S. adults." 207.

11. Kuczmarski et al., "Increasing prevalence of overweight among U.S. adults." 207.

12. Kanders, Beatrice S., Patrice Ullman-Joy, John P. Foreyt, Steven B. Heymsfield, David Heber, Robert M. Elashoff, Judith M. Ashley, Rebecca S. Reeves, and George Blackburn. (1994) "The Black American Lifestyle Intervention (BALI): The design of a weight loss program for working-class African-American women." *Journal of the American Dietetic Association* 94 (3): 310–312; Centers for Disease Control. (1990) "Prevalence of overweight for Hispanics—United States, 1982–1984." JAMA 263: 631–632.

13. Young, T. Kue. (1994) *The Health of Native Americans* (New York: Oxford University Press), 141.

14. Young, *The Health of Native Americans,* 143.

15. U.S. Department of Health and Human Services, Public Health Service, Office of Minority Health. (Undated) *Closing the Gap: Diabetes and Minorities* (Office of Minority Health Resource Center).

16. Crews, Douglas E. (1994) Obesity and Diabetes. In *Confronting Critical Health Issues of Asian and Pacific Islander Americans.* Nolan W. S. Zane, David T. Takeuchi, and Kathleen N. J. Young Editors, (Thousand Oaks, CA: SAGE Publications).

17. Powers, Scott K., and Edward T. Howley. (1994) *Exercise Physiology: Theory and Application to Fitness and Performance* (Dubuque, Iowa: Brown & Benchmark Publishers), 391.

18. Winett, Liana B., and Wesley F. Alles. (1993) "Questioning the use of body fat analysis as a stand-alone screening device." *American Journal of Health Promotion* 8 (1): 12–14.

19. Jebb, S. A., P. R. Murgatroyd, G. R. Goldberg, A. M. Prentice, and W. A. Coward. (1993) "In vivo measurement of changes in body composition: Description of methods and their validation against 12-day continuous whole-body calorimetry." *The American Journal of Clinical Nutrition* 58: 455–462.

20. International Medical News Service. (1983) "Raising of 'ideal' weights held a disservice." *Family Practice News* 13 (2): 2, 85.

21. Bennion, Bierman, and Ferguson, *Straight Talk About Weight Control,* 129–130.

22. "Science advisor dodges body weight controversy." (1993) *Nutrition Week* XXIII (34): 3.

23. "Leanest men live longer, Harvard study indicates." (1993) *Nutrition Week* XXIII (48): 3.

24. Jebb et al., "In vivo measurement of changes in body composition:."

25. Schardt, David. "Science advisor dodges body weight controversy", (1994) "Lifting weight myths" *Nutrition Action Healthletter* 20 (8): 8–9.

26. Powers and Howley, *Exercise Physiology,* 394.

27. Powers and Howley, *Exercise Physiology,* 394.

28. Bennion, Bierman, and Ferguson, *Straight Talk About Weight Control,* 142.

29. Bennion, Bierman, and Ferguson, *Straight Talk About Weight Control,* 142; Emery, Eileen M., Thomas L. Schmid, Henry S. Kahn, and Peter P. Filozof. (1993) "A review of the association between abdominal fat distribution, health outcome measures, and modifiable risk factors." *American Journal of Health Promotion* 7 (5): 342–353.

30. Ornish, Dean. (1993) *Eat More, Weigh Less* (New York: Harper Collins Publishers), 27.

31. Stamford, Bryant. (1991) "Apples and pears: Where you 'wear' your fat can affect your health." *The Physician and Sports Medicine* 19 (1): 123–124.

32. "Where's the fat?" (1993) *American Health* XII (5): 100, 102.

33. Powers and Howley, *Exercise Physiology,* 396.

34. Ornish, *Eat More, Weigh Less,* 27.

35. Miller, Wayne C. (1991) "Diet composition, energy intake, and nutritional status in relation to obesity in men and women." *Medicine and Science in Sports and Exercise* 23 (3): 280–284.

36. Miller, Wayne C., A. K. Lindeman, J. Wallace, and M. Niederpruem. (1990) "Diet composition, energy

intake, and exercise in relation to body fatness in men and women." *American Journal of Clinical Nutrition* 52: 426–430.

37. Ornish, *Eat More, Weigh Less*, 20.

38. "Losing weight: What works, what doesn't." (1993) *Consumer Reports* 58 (6): 347–352.

39. Miller, "Diet composition, energy intake, and nutritional status . . . ," 283.

40. Ornish, *Eat More, Weigh Less*, 8.

41. Ornish, *Eat More, Weigh Less*, 34, 54–55.

42. Stunkard, A. J., T. I. A. Sorensen, C. Hanis, T. W. Teasdale, R. Chakraborty, W. J. Schull, & F. Schulsinger. (1986) "An adoption study of human obesity." *New England Journal of Medicine* 314: 193–198.

43. Stunkard, A. J., J. R. Harris, N. L. Pedersen, & G. E. McLearn. (1990) "The body mass index of twins who have been reared apart." *New England Journal of Medicine* 322: 1483–1487.

44. Fabsitz, R. R., P. Sholinsky, & D. Carmelli. (1994) "Genetic influences on adult weight gain and maximum body mass index in male twins." *American Journal of Epidemiology* 140: 711–720.

45. Schardt, David. (1993) "Lifting weight myths." *Nutrition Action Healthletter* 20 (8): 8–9.

46. Schardt, "Lifting weight myths," 9.

47. "Science advisor dodges body weight controversy." (1993) *Nutrition Week* XXIII (34): 3.

48. Schardt, "Lifting weight myths," 9.

49. Bennion, Bierman, and Ferguson, *Straight Talk About Weight Control*, 103.

50. Katch, Frank I., and William D. McArdle. (1993) *Introduction to Nutrition, Exercise and Health.* 4th ed. (Philadelphia: Lea & Febiger), 295.

51. Russell, Robert M. (1993) "Nutrition." *JAMA* 270 (2): 233–234.

52. "Heavy news." (1994) *UC Berkeley Wellness Letter* 10 (5): 2.

53. Bennett, William, and Joel Gurin. (1982) "Book bonus: How the body outwits the dieter." *American Health* 1 (2): 44–51.

54. Powers and Howley, *Exercise Physiology*, 404.

55. "Which exercise is best for you?" (1994) *Consumer Reports on Health* 6 (4): 37–40; Ballor, Douglas L., and Eric T. Poehlman (1994) "Exercise-training enhances fat-free mass preservation during diet-induced weight loss: A meta-analytical finding." *International Journal of Obesity* 18 (1): 35–40.

56. "Which exercise is best for you?" 39–40.

57. Hawks, S. R., & P. Richins. (1994) "Toward a new paradigm for the management of obesity." *Journal of Health Education* 25: 147–153.

58. Ornish, *Eat More, Weigh Less*.

59. Brownell, K. (1988) "Heart attack risk? The yo-yo trap." *American Health*.

60. Story, Mary, and Patricia Faulkner. (1990) "The prime time diet: A content analysis of eating behavior and food messages in television program content and commercials." *AJPH* 80 (6): 738–740.

61. Story and Faulkner, "The prime time diet," 739–740.

62. "TV may greatly increase risk of obesity in children." (1993) *Nutrition Week* XXIII (8): 3.

63. "TV may greatly increase risk of obesity in children," 3.

64. Fitzgerald, Faith T. (1984) "Weight reduction: Science vs. scam." *National Forum* LXIV (1): 31–33.

65. Bennion, Bierman, and Ferguson, *Straight Talk About Weight Control*, 234–239.

66. Berland, Theodore. (1983) *Rating the Diets* (New York: Signet Books).

67. "New York City regulates weight loss centers." (1993) *Nutrition Today* 28 (4): 5.

68. Strober, Michael. (1986) "Anorexia nervosa: History and psychological concepts," in *Handbook of Eating Disorders: Physiology, Psychology, and Treatment of Obesity, Anorexia, and Bulimia*, eds. Kelly D. Brownell and John P. Foreyt (New York: Basic Books), 231–246.

69. Yager, Joel. (1991) "Common eating disorders." *Hospital Medicine* 27 (2): 76; Bennion, Bierman, and Ferguson, *Straight Talk About Weight Control*, 46.

70. Bennion, Bierman, and Ferguson, *Straight Talk About Weight Control*, 54–55.

71. Lucas, Alexander R. (1986) "Anorexia nervosa." *Hospital Medicine* 22 (3): 127–149.

72. "Eating disorders." (1992) *CQ Researcher* 2: 1111.

73. Farley, D. (1992) "Eating disorders require medical attention." *FDA Consumer* 26 (2): 28.

74. Yager, "Common eating disorders," 85.

75. "Lose a little, win big." (1994) *Consumer Reports on Health* 6: 69.

Fitness Potentials: Discovering Your Play

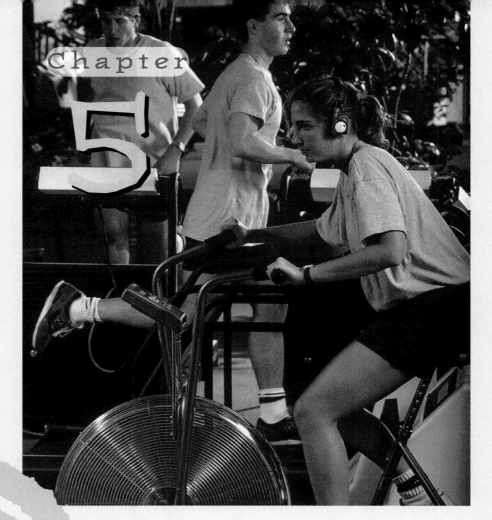

Chapter 5

Student Learning Objectives

Upon completion of this chapter, you should be able to:

1. describe what is meant by the phrase "playful physical activity";
2. identify at least eight benefits of physical activity;
3. define fitness;
4. list and describe the four major classifications of physical activities that contribute to wellness;
5. discuss the four accepted principles of fitness;
6. define and give three examples of aerobic exercise;
7. describe two major goals of aerobic exercise;
8. define and give three examples of anaerobic exercise;
9. describe two methods of determining levels of aerobic fitness;
10. list and describe the F.I.T. Guidelines;
11. compare the recommended frequency, intensity, and duration of physical activity to gain health promotion benefits with physical activity to gain physical fitness;
12. describe the differences between resting, target, and maximum heart rates;
13. calculate your target heart rate;
14. demonstrate how to measure resting and target heart rates;
15. demonstrate five stretching exercises that contribute to one's flexibility;
16. demonstrate three strengthening exercises that enhance participation in vigorous activities;
17. evaluate the safety of health and fitness clubs;
18. list and describe the three stages of progress for an aerobic exercise program;
19. discuss common barriers to establishing and maintaining an exercise program and possible strategies for eliminating these barriers.

One of the most visible wellness trends in the U.S. today is a growing interest in physical fitness. Health spas and fitness centers are springing up in most communities to cater to this thriving interest in fitness. Newsstands, too, mirror public interest with a variety of fitness magazines.

Most college campuses offer a variety of opportunities to students that could enhance physical fitness and well-being. Student recreation center programs, intramural sports, and physical activity courses are just a few of the many fitness activities students can participate in during their college years.

Most people in the U.S., including college students, do not engage in *regular* physical activity. However, at least 70 percent of adults do participate in some type of leisure-time physical activity and may be interested in becoming more physically fit. While the *interest* in fitness among people is high, this does not necessarily translate into beneficial and safe exercise programs. Unfortunately, there are many charlatans eager to capitalize on our lack of knowledge and high interest in becoming more physically fit. This chapter introduces you to the concept of fitness and its various dimensions. Additionally, it helps you learn how to set up safe, beneficial, and enjoyable fitness activities. Becoming more active will help you in your quest for wellness.

How Physically Fit Are People in the U.S.?

People in the U.S. are generally more adept at watching physical activity than at participating in an active way. It is estimated that only 24 percent of adults participate in *moderate* physical activity five or more times each week.[1] Activities such as swimming, cycling, dancing, gardening, and yard work may fit this classification, depending on the intensity at which they are done. The number of people who exercise *vigorously* on a regular basis is even smaller. Only 12 percent of people aged eighteen and older report participating in aerobic activities three or more days a week for twenty or more minutes each occasion.[2] The Centers for Disease Control and Prevention estimates that 58 percent of people in the U.S. are sedentary, participating in infrequent or no leisure-time activity.[3]

Little has been published in the research literature about differences in physical activity patterns in various racial or ethnic groups. One study looked at the caloric expenditures of African-American and White college women.[4] Their results indicate that African-American college women may have significantly lower levels of physical activity than White college women. The African-American college women expended an average of 1,561 calories a week, while the White women averaged an expenditure of 2,834 calories weekly. This study must be interpreted with caution, however, due to the small number of subjects (only 116).

Cora Lewis and her colleagues at the University of Alabama surveyed residents of seven predominantly African-American public housing communities, in Birmingham, to investigate physical activity levels of African-Americans of low socioeconomic status.[5] They found that levels of physical activity were lower in these African-American communities, as compared to White, middle-class samples from other studies. Approximately 30 percent of the African-American subjects reported that they did not participate in any of the physical activities being studied. Walking and hiking were the activities with the greatest participation levels; 17 percent of subjects stated that they walked to work or school and 12 percent reported walking to food stores. Additionally, men in this study reported higher levels of physical activity than women, and younger people were more active than older people.

Researchers at the University of Washington in Seattle recently interviewed Native Americans between the ages of eighteen to forty-nine on an American Indian reservation in the Plains region of the western United States.[6] While their overall health status was lower than the studies comparison group, a random selection of almost 9,000 people from three other Plains states, the Native Americans reported higher levels of physical activity. Only 29.3 percent of the

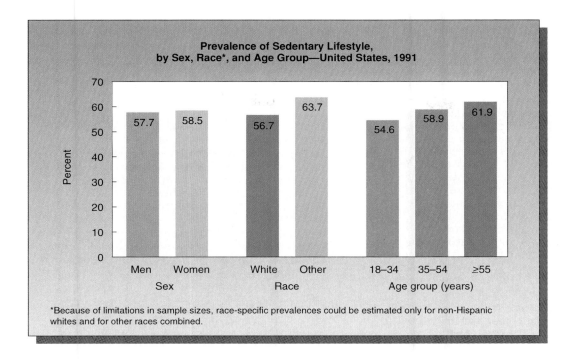

**Prevalence of Sedentary Lifestyle,
by Sex, Race*, and Age Group—United States, 1991**

Men 57.7 · Women 58.5 (Sex)

White 56.7 · Other 63.7 (Race)

18–34 54.6 · 35–54 58.9 · ≥55 61.9 (Age group (years))

*Because of limitations in sample sizes, race-specific prevalences could be estimated only for non-Hispanic whites and for other races combined.

Figure 5.1: What Do You Think?

1. According to this data, is there a significant difference in the level of sedentary lifestyle reported by men and women in the United States? Is there a significant difference according to race or age?
2. What factors might explain the findings that over one half of adults in the United States report no or irregular leisure-time activity? What factors may explain the racial and age differences in rates of participation in leisure-time activity?

Source: From "Prevalence of Sedentary Lifestyle—Behavioral Risk Factor Surveillance System," United States, 1991, MMWR, (1993) 42 (29), fig. 1, p. 577, Centers for Disease Control, U.S. Government Printing Office.

Native American subjects reported no frequent exercise, compared to over 47 percent in the control group. The Native American men reported less sedentary living than the females, 19.5 percent and 35.9 percent respectively.

In 1991, The Centers for Disease Control and Prevention surveyed 87,433 people in the U.S. to determine the frequency, intensity, and duration of their physical activity.[7] As figure 5.1 illustrates, the White respondents reported a higher level of physical activity than respondents from other races; 56.7 percent of Whites reported participating in little or no regular physical activity compared to 63.7 percent of other races combined. This study, however, had several limitations. First, it relied on individuals accurately reporting their level of leisure-time physical activity. Additionally, occupational activity levels were not measured. Further research is needed to clarify exercise patterns of ethnic and racial groups.

Health and exercise specialists are deeply concerned about the low level of physical activity in the U.S. In recognition of the magnitude of the problem of sedentary living in this country, the U.S. Public Health Service has included physical activity and fitness as one of their priority target areas for the year 2000 objectives for the nation (see table 5.1).

Discovering Your Play

According to Dr. George Sheehan, cardiologist and author of numerous exercise articles and books, the key to enhancing your level of wellness through activity is to find your play.[8] We should ask ourselves: What activities bring joy and creativity into our lives? and What activities do we consider to be fun?

Play is an attitude that can transform any activity into a joyful, rewarding experience. As children, we looked forward to the moment we were set loose for recess or the end of the school day. We couldn't wait to get outside to run, play tag, climb in trees or on monkey bars, ride bikes, roller skate, or jump rope. We called this play! What has happened in our transition to adulthood that turned so many of these activities into work? Why do so many of us now finish a day at school or the office and rush home, only to turn on the television set and watch others play for us? What have we done with our play?

One of the best motivations for physical activity is enjoyment. As you contemplate ways to become physically fit, keep in mind that you are looking for "play" as much as for a "workout." Experiment with many different activities until you find those that truly enhance your life and well-being (see Of Special Interest 5.1).

1. **Increase to at least 30 percent the proportion of people aged six and older who engage regularly, preferably daily, in light to moderate physical activity for at least thirty minutes per day.** Light to moderate physical activity requires sustained, rhythmic muscular movements, is at least equivalent to sustained walking, and is performed at less than 60 percent of maximum heart rate for age. Examples may include walking, swimming, cycling, dancing, gardening and yard work, various domestic and occupational activities, and games and other childhood pursuits. (Update: 24 percent of people aged 18 and older were active for at least 30 minutes 5 or more times per week and 17 percent were active 7 or more times per week in 1991, up from 22 percent and 12 percent respectively in 1985.)

2. **Increase to at least 20 percent the proportion of people aged eighteen and older and to at least 75 percent the proportion of children and adolescents aged six through seventeen who engage in vigorous physical activity that promotes the development and maintenance of cardiorespiratory fitness three or more days per week for twenty or more minutes per occasion.** Vigorous physical activities are rhythmic, repetitive physical activities that use large muscle groups at 60 percent or more of maximal heart rate for age. . . . (Update: 14 percent for people aged 18 and older in 1991, up from 12 percent in 1985.) (Baseline: 66 percent for youth aged 10 through 17 in 1984.) (Special Target Population: lower income people aged 18 and older—annual family income < $20,000.)

3. **Reduce to no more than 15 percent the proportion of people aged six and older who engage in no leisure-time physical activity.** (Update: 24 percent for people aged 18 and older in 1991, remaining unchanged from 1985.) (Special Target Populations: people aged 65 and older; people with disabilities; lower income people—annual family income < $20,000.)

4. **Increase to at least 40 percent the proportion of people aged six and older who regularly perform physical activities that enhance and maintain muscular strength, muscular endurance, and flexibility.** (Update: For students in 9th–12th grade, 43 percent stretch 4 or more times per week and 37 percent do strengthening activities 4 or more times per week in 1991; 16 percent of people 18–64 years lift weights in 1991, up from 11 percent in 1990.)

5. **Increase to at least 50 percent the proportion of children and adolescents in first through twelfth grades who participate in daily school physical education.** (Baseline: 36 percent of 1st–12th grade students in 1984–86, 42 percent of 9th–12th grade students in 1991.)

6. **Increase to at least 50 percent the proportion of school physical education class time that students spend being physically active, preferably engaged in lifetime physical activities.** Lifetime activities are activities such as swimming, bicycling, jogging, racquet sports, and vigorous social activities such as dancing, which may be readily carried into adulthood because they generally need only one or two people. (Baseline: 49 percent of students in 9th–12th grade exercised 30 or more minutes in physical education class 1 or more times per week in 1991.)

7. **Increase the proportion of worksites offering employer-sponsored physical activity and fitness programs as follows: 20 percent of worksites with 50–99 employees, 35 percent of worksites with 100–249 employees, 50 percent of worksites with 250–749 employees, and 80 percent of worksites with 750 or more employees.** (Update: 33 percent of worksites with 50–99 employees, 47 percent of worksites with 100–249 employees, 66 percent of worksites with 250–749 employees, and 83 percent of worksites with 750 or more employees in 1992, up from 14 percent, 23 percent, 32 percent, and 54 percent respectively in 1985.)

8. **Increase community availability and accessibility of physical activity and fitness facilities as follows: Hiking, biking, and fitness trail miles: 1 per 10,000 people; Public swimming pools: 1 per 25,000 people; Acres of park and recreation open space: 4 per 1,000 people (250 people per managed acre).** (Baseline: 1 hiking, biking, and fitness trail mile per 71,000 people, 1 public swimming pool per 53,000 people, and 1.8 acres of park and recreation open space per 1,000 people in 1986.)

Source: From *Healthy People 2000 National Health Promotion and Disease Prevention Objectives.* Department of Health and Human Services, Washington, D.C., 1991; *Healthy People 2000 Review 1993.* Department of Health and Human Services, Washington, D.C., 1994.

Benefits of Physical Activity

Many people are physically active because of the benefits they experience as a result of choosing this lifestyle. Benefits of physical activity thus serve as incentives and motivators. What are the benefits of regular, physical activity?

Psychological Benefits

Regular physical activity can lead to improvements in perception of body image, a more positive self-concept, and decreases in levels of both anxiety and depression[9] (see table 5.2). All of these changes have been linked to the state that habitual exercisers refer to as "the feeling-better sensation."

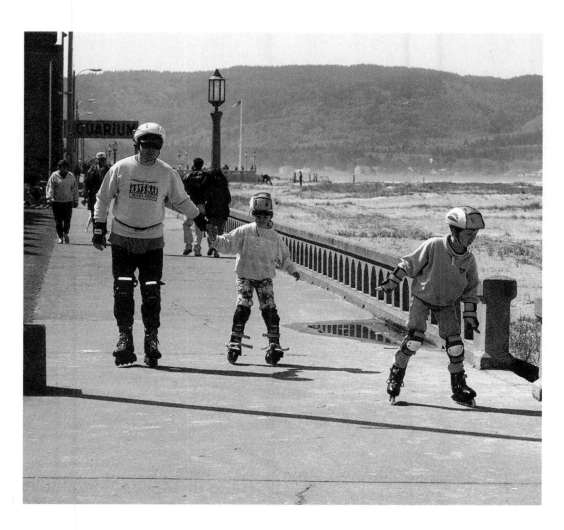

What Do You Think?

1. It is important for both adults and children to find playful physical activity. What types of physical activity did you enjoy as a child? Do you still participate in those activities? What factors do you think account for your answers?

Many people use exercise as one of their primary stress-coping skills. The stress response, often called the "fight or flight" response, prepares the body for physical action. Thus, physical activity allows us to follow a natural pathway for the relief of stress. Additionally, many people believe that a regular exercise program helps them to prevent the stress response from occurring, or at least decreases its intensity. As Daniel Girdano and his colleagues point out in their book *Controlling Stress and Tension,* "About ninety minutes after a good physical bout of exercise there occurs a feeling of deep relaxation. If you are a consistent exerciser, you know that feeling and perhaps are aware of its lasting effects throughout the day. . . . The step is a little lighter, the attitude more positive, and it takes more to get upset."[10]

Many runners have reported experiencing positive psychological states during long-distance runs, which they have labeled "exercise highs." Some researchers have proposed that an increase of a substance known as **beta-endorphin,** a morphine-like chemical produced by the body, may be responsible for this elevated mood.[11] More research is needed to aid in our understanding of this phenomenon, as well as other psychological benefits of physical activity.

Cardiovascular Benefits

Physically active individuals may experience a cardiovascular conditioning, or **training effect.** Regular *vigorous* activity helps to strengthen the heart muscle. The walls of the heart become thicker and stronger, allowing it to pump more blood per beat than an untrained heart. This, in turn, helps the heart to work more efficiently, both during exercise and at rest. One measure of the heart's efficiency is the resting heart rate. Normal resting heart rates for adults vary between sixty and eighty beats per minute. It is not uncommon to see resting heart rates of forty-five to fifty-five beats per minute in

Beta-endorphin: a chemical occurring in the brain that appears to have a pain-suppressing action, and which may be responsible for the "high" reported by some long-distance runners.

Training effect: cardiovascular conditioning from an aerobic exercise program designed to build a thicker and stronger heart muscle that can pump more blood per beat than an untrained heart. A cardiovascular training effect results from regular, vigorous aerobic activity.

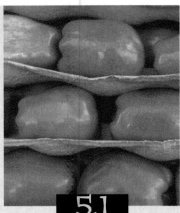

5.1

Of Special Interest

If the Spirit Is Willing, the Flesh Will Follow

On a recent radio show I discussed exercise with a woman who did not exercise. "The spirit is willing," she told me, "but the flesh is weak."

I had, of course, heard that excuse many times before. But for the first time, it occurred to me that the opposite was true.

The flesh is willing. It is the spirit that is weak. Our bodies are capable of the most astounding feats, but the horizons of our spirits do not reach beyond the television, the stereo, and the car.

The flesh is not only willing, it is wanting and waiting to be put into action. The flesh is filled with everything the spirit lacks: grit, pluck, nerve, and determination. We come from a breed that crossed continents on foot and trekked from pole to pole. And even now we see teachers running marathons, stockbrokers in Outward Bound, retired executives climbing Everest.

Our flesh asks for more challenges and seeks new frontiers. What is missing is not physical energy. Physical energy is there for the using. The fuel is there. It is waiting to be ignited. We need something to light the fire, something to get us into action.

This can be seen from the moment we wake up. We lie abed waiting the third, and last, and now frantic call. The alarm clock, the radio, and the family have taken turns trying to get us up. Still we lie immobile until the last possible minute.

Survey this scene and tell me that the spirit is willing but the flesh is weak. How many calories does it take to get out of bed? Whose bodies are so exhausted that they can't get their feet on the floor?

I can plead that I'm in a semicoma, not yet ready for coordinated action, but the same inertia happens again and again throughout the day. The body is ready and willing and able, but the spirit is becalmed. Where there is no emotion, there is no motion, either.

What is missing is the spiritual energy, what the Greeks called "enthusiasm." There are, of course, many other desirable qualities missing as well, but enthusiasm is the key.

It is from lack of enthusiasm that the failures of the spirit multiply during the day. We must, as the word implies, be filled with and possessed and inspired by a divine power or spirit.

When we are enthusiastic, we take on the qualities that go with it. We develop a determination to equal the endurance of our muscles, a fortitude to match the courage of our hearts, and a passion to join with the animal strengths of our bodies.

To succeed at anything, you need passion. You have to be a bit of a fanatic. If you want to move anyone to act, you must first be moved yourself. To instigate, said Emerson, you must first be instigated. I am aware of this every time I lecture. For an hour before the talk, I can be seen walking alone, muttering to myself, gradually building myself to a fever pitch.

But the spirit has more to offer than just this excitement. It gives us motivation and incentive when the excitement is missing. This spirit is what gets us through when everything else fails. In his paper on "Factors in Human Endurance," Oxford professor Ralph Johnson states that a man's ability to survive depends on the qualities of his personality.

This thought is particularly striking in the accounts of explorers and mountain climbers, people stretched to their limits and beyond. The explorer Captain Scott, writing of one of his men, said, "Browers came through the best. Never was there such a sturdy, active, undefeated man." Of Scott himself one of his companions wrote, "Scott was the strongest combination of a strong man in a strong body that I have ever known. And this because he was weak. He conquered his weaker self and became the strong leader we went to follow and came to love."

So behind the enthusiasm, behind the inspiration, behind the passion, there must be the will. What finally and irrevocably separates us from the rest of the world is our will.

We can choose. We can decide. We can will to do it our way. And when we do, nothing can prevail against us.

From George Sheehan, M.D., "If the Spirit Is Willing, the Flesh Will Follow," in *The Physician and Sportsmedicine* 7(3):39, March 1979. Reprinted by permission of George Sheehan, Jr.

What Do You Think?

1. Do you agree with Dr. Sheehan's statement, "the flesh is willing. It is the spirit that is weak?"
2. What could (or does) motivate you to exercise? Try to list at least three motivators.
3. What activities do you consider to be play? How does this label of "play" affect your willingness to participate?

individuals who regularly participate in *vigorous* activity. This indicates that the heart is able to pump enough blood to meet the body's needs by doing less work. Another sign of the heart's efficiency is the heart-rate level during and immediately following physical activity. During an exercise session, the trained heart will be able to pump more blood per beat than the untrained heart; therefore, the trained heart-rate response will be lower for any given exercise intensity. After the activity, the trained heart will return more quickly to a normal heart rate—it recovers faster.

TABLE 5.2

Some Proposed Psychological Benefits of Exercise

Increases	Decreases
Academic performance	Absenteeism at work
Assertiveness	Alcohol abuse
Confidence	Anger
Emotional stability	Anxiety
Independence	Confusion
Intellectual functioning	Depression
Internal locus of control	Dysmenorrhea
Memory	Headaches
Mood	Hostility
Perception	Phobias
Popularity	Psychotic behavior
Positive body image	Stress response
Self-control	Tension
Sexual satisfaction	Type A behavior
Well-being	Work errors
Work efficiency	

Source: Data from *Public Health Reports*, 100 (2), 1985.

Cardiovascular training also leads to improvements in an individual's ability to utilize oxygen during physical activity. Increases in both the amount of blood pumped per minute and changes in the body's ability to extract and utilize oxygen carried in the bloodstream lead to an increased consumption of oxygen. Meanwhile, the lungs are also increasing their capacity to bring more oxygen into the system to be carried in the bloodstream of the exerciser (see figure 5.2). These changes translate into the ability to perform an activity more strenuously or for a longer period of time than could a person whose cardiovascular system is untrained.

Contributions to Effective Weight Control

Exercise contributes to the maintenance of ideal body composition in many ways. Exercise can increase metabolism, which results in a greater number of calories burned during and after regular activity. Additionally, regular exercise increases the amount of muscle tissue an individual has. Muscle tissue is more metabolically active; therefore, the more muscle tissue you have the greater number of calories you expend doing any activity. Physical activity may also lower the amount of fat our body needs to store through its action on the body's set point. Additionally, exercise decreases the loss of muscle tissue during weight-loss attempts and helps to suppress appetite (especially for those of us who are inactive or obese). Physical activity also changes the way our bodies handle fat. **Insulin,** which is responsible for guiding fat into body cells for storage, decreases in the bloodstream after just one bout of exercise. Muscle tissue also becomes more sensitive to the insulin. All these changes are thought to help regulate the amount of insulin circulating in the bloodstream. We discussed these benefits in more detail in chapter 4.

Disease Prevention

Regular physical activity is believed to reduce the risk of several chronic disease conditions. One such disease is **osteoporosis,** a chronic disease that involves the thinning of bone materials, such as calcium, leading to an actual loss of bone mass. White and Asian women seem to be especially susceptible to this problem. African-American women have a lower incidence of osteoporosis. This is attributed to the greater bone density found in African-Americans.[12]

Exercise programs have been studied as a possible preventive measure. The exact mechanism for the protective effects of vigorous activity are still unknown; however, it has been suggested that vigorous activity, in combination with adequate amounts of dietary calcium, either increase the mineral content and size of bones in the limbs used for the activity[13] or decrease the loss of calcium from bones during the aging process.[14] Studies indicate that, in order to benefit bone density, weight-bearing exercises must be engaged in regularly. Nonweight-bearing activities, such as swimming, appear to be of little value in reducing the bone mass loss characteristic of osteoporosis. Osteoporosis is discussed in greater detail in chapter 19.

Heart disease is another chronic condition for which exercise has been suggested as a preventive measure. Recent studies have indicated that regular *moderate* aerobic exercise, such as brisk walking,

Insulin: a hormone secretion of the pancreas necessary to convert carbohydrates into energy and sometimes used therapeutically to control diabetes.

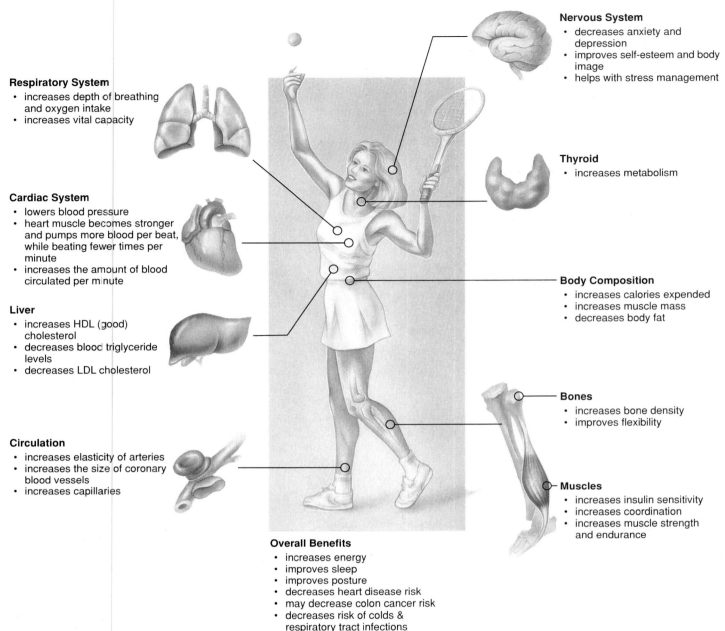

Respiratory System
- increases depth of breathing and oxygen intake
- increases vital capacity

Cardiac System
- lowers blood pressure
- heart muscle becomes stronger and pumps more blood per beat, while beating fewer times per minute
- increases the amount of blood circulated per minute

Liver
- increases HDL (good) cholesterol
- decreases blood triglyceride levels
- decreases LDL cholesterol

Circulation
- increases elasticity of arteries
- increases the size of coronary blood vessels
- increases capillaries

Nervous System
- decreases anxiety and depression
- improves self-esteem and body image
- helps with stress management

Thyroid
- increases metabolism

Body Composition
- increases calories expended
- increases muscle mass
- decreases body fat

Bones
- increases bone density
- improves flexibility

Muscles
- increases insulin sensitivity
- increases coordination
- increases muscle strength and endurance

Overall Benefits
- increases energy
- improves sleep
- improves posture
- decreases heart disease risk
- may decrease colon cancer risk
- decreases risk of colds & respiratory tract infections
- decreases risk of diabetes
- decreases risk of osteoporosis

Figure 5.2: Some benefits of exercise

swimming, or tennis, result in a reduced risk of coronary artery disease and decreased overall death rates. Dr. Ralph Paffenbarger reported the results of a study he conducted on over 10,000 male Harvard graduates over a period of twenty years.[15] He concluded that the sedentary alumni had a 25 percent higher risk of death from all causes, and a 36 percent higher risk of death from coronary heart disease. Comparing alumni who were sedentary to those who participated in regular yet moderately vigorous activity, Paffenbarger found a 41 percent lower risk of coronary heart disease.

One of the major risk factors for coronary artery disease is a high blood-cholesterol level. We discussed the relationship between diet, cholesterol, and heart disease in chapter 3. To review, high blood levels of LDL cholesterol have been linked with an increased risk of coronary artery disease; high blood levels of HDL cholesterol may actually protect us from this disease. *Vigorous* physical activity has been associated with lower blood levels of LDL cholesterol and higher blood levels of HDL cholesterol.[16] Both of these changes reduce the risk for coronary artery disease. Additionally, the results from a recent study of sedentary women, conducted at the Cooper Institute for Aerobic Research in Dallas, found that even *moderate* regular exercise like brisk walking significantly increased blood levels of HDL cholesterol.[17] Moderate to vigorous aerobic exercise has also been shown to exert a beneficial influence by helping control high blood pressure (hypertension).[18] These factors in combination are likely responsible for a large portion of the cardiovascular preventive benefits of regular aerobic exercise. Coronary heart disease and its many risk factors are discussed in greater detail in chapter 10.

Non-insulin dependent diabetes, sometimes called adult-onset diabetes, is another chronic disease that appears to be more common in sedentary individuals. The results of several large scale prospective studies have recently provided evidence that regular aerobic exercise of *moderate* intensity, such as walking, bicycling, and dancing, significantly decreases the risk for developing non-insulin dependent diabetes.[19] Researchers speculate that exercise increases cell sensitivity to insulin and helps to decrease abdominal fat stores, thus decreasing two risk factors for non-insulin dependent diabetes.[20]

What Is Fitness?

Fitness means different things to different people. Is the person who plays baseball every Saturday afternoon physically fit? What about the avid golfer or the weight lifter? Exactly what do we mean when we talk about physical fitness? (See figure 5.3.)

Exercise specialists commonly describe **physical fitness** as the ability to function efficiently. The American College of Sports Medicine has delineated four major classifications of activities that contribute to fitness: (1) cardiorespiratory endurance; (2) muscular fitness; (3) flexibility; and (4) body composition.

Cardiorespiratory endurance, or aerobic capacity, refers to the body's ability to sustain strenuous activities for long periods of time. Cardiorespiratory endurance relies on the ability of the circulatory and respiratory systems to supply the necessary oxygen for this sustained activity.

Muscular fitness includes both the strength and the endurance capability of your muscles. **Muscular strength** is described as the maximum amount of force that can be exerted by a muscle in a single effort. **Muscular endurance** is defined as the ability of specific muscles to sustain effort over a long period of time.

Flexibility refers to the ability of a specific joint to move through its entire range of motion without pain. The final component of fitness—**body composition**—refers to the amount of your body that is fat versus fat-free tissue. (Body composition was discussed in some detail in chapter 4.) Each of the four components make unique and important contributions to our level of physical fitness. Some activities make their major contribution to one aspect of fitness, while others give a broader range of benefits. Table 5.3 presents a list of physical activities and their contribution to the major components of fitness.

Principles of Fitness

There are four principles of fitness that apply to cardiorespiratory endurance, as well as to the flexibility and muscular strength/endurance activities. The four principles are overload, specificity, individual differences, and reversibility.

Overload

The first principle of fitness is **overload.** The whole concept of fitness is based on physiological adaptations that our bodies make in response to certain activities. In order for these adaptations to occur an individual must exercise the body at a level of activity greater than that to which it is accustomed. We can carry out the principle of overload in three ways: (1) we can increase the number of days that we exercise (**frequency**); (2) we can increase how strenuously we exercise for a given time period (**intensity**); or (3) we can increase the length of the exercise session at a given intensity (**time**).

For an illustration of the concept of overload, let's examine the fitness program of Jose, a college sophomore. Jose has developed a fitness program for himself that consists of swimming at a local pool three days a week for thirty minutes each session. Jose has followed this routine for about six months and has just noticed that his fitness potential is not improving as it had been in the beginning of the program. Jose could continue to improve his fitness level by implementing the principle of overload. He

Non-insulin dependent diabetes: sometimes referred to as Type II or adult-onset diabetes, this form of diabetes is usually diagnosed in persons over age forty; in this type of diabetes the body does not make enough insulin, the cells are not as sensitive to the insulin, or both.

Muscular strength: the amount of weight that an individual can safely lift in one all-out effort. For weight training, this would be high weight with few repetitions.

Muscular endurance: the ability to lift light to moderate amounts of weight repeatedly over a period of time. In weight training, this would be many repetitions with less weight.

Overload: exercising the body at a level of activity greater than that to which it is accustomed, as a way to increase physical fitness.

1. What is fitness? Can you participate
   in only one of these types of
   physical activities and achieve
   physical fitness?

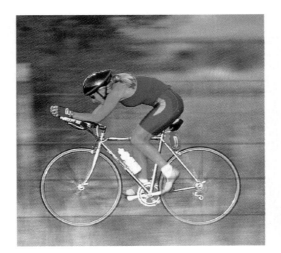

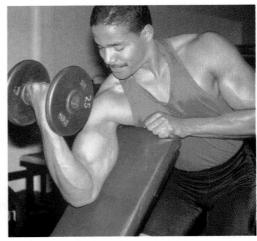

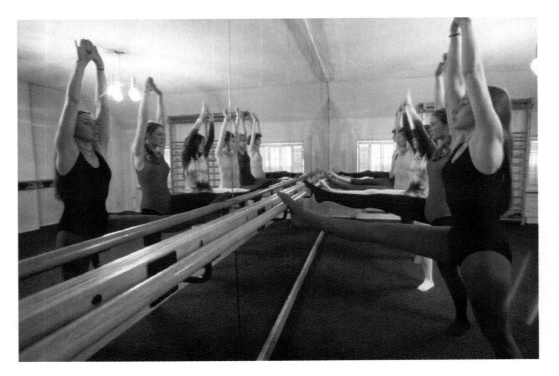

could, for instance, swim four days a week
rather than three. Or, if three days were all Jose
could fit into his schedule this semester, he
could choose instead to swim faster (and thus
farther) during his thirty-minute sessions. If, for
some reason, Jose did not want to alter his
pace, he could swim at his normal speed and
distance but for forty minutes each time. All of
these would place Jose in a state of overload
and gradually increase his level of fitness.

Specificity

Another important principle of fitness is
called the principle of **specificity.**
Physiological adaptations to activity are
specific to the type of activity and overload.
Let's look again at Jose's fitness program. Jose
swims as his major fitness activity; after six
months he has developed a good level of
physical fitness. Many of the fitness
adaptations his body has made, however, are
specific to swimming. This became very
obvious to Jose when he decided he would go
on a twenty-five-mile bicycle trip with
several of his friends. He found that he had
great difficulty keeping up with the pace set
by his friends. Additionally, he had some very
sore muscles when the trip was over. As the
principle of specificity points out, many of
the muscles needed for bicycling had not
been trained by Jose's swimming program.

TABLE 5.3   *What Some Activities Do for You*

	Cardiovascular endurance	Muscle endurance	Muscle strength	Flexibility	Body composition
Aerobic dance (low impact)	✓	✓		✓	✓
Bicycling	✓	✓	✓		✓
Cross-country skiing	✓	✓	✓		✓
Gardening		✓			✓
Golf (18 holes, with hand cart)	✓	✓			
Handball/racquetball	✓	✓	✓	✓	✓
Hiking	✓	✓	✓		✓
Jogging	✓	✓			✓
Square dancing	✓	✓			✓
Swimming	✓	✓		✓	
Tennis (singles)	✓	✓	✓	✓	✓
Step aerobics (moderate)	✓	✓	✓	✓	✓
Strength training (high weight, few repetitions)			✓		•
Strength training (low weight, many repetitions)		✓	✓		•
Walking (briskly)	✓				✓

• Strength training contributes to body composition by increasing muscle mass, thus increasing fat-free tissue and metabolism

Individual Differences

The third principle of fitness is the principle of **individual differences.** This principle tells us that individuals attain the many fitness benefits at varying rates. One of the biggest determinants of fitness gains is an individual's relative level of fitness at the start of a program. People who begin with low levels of fitness often see more dramatic improvements early in their fitness programs. The principle of individual differences is one of the major reasons that exercise specialists like to give individualized fitness prescriptions. These prescriptions will be discussed later in this chapter.

Reversibility

The fourth principle of fitness is that of **reversibility.** This principle is best summed up by the maxim "use it or lose it." Once you have trained your body and started to receive the benefits of regular exercise, you must continue to keep physically active or you will begin to lose those benefits. The capacity of the heart to pump blood during *strenuous*

activity will begin to decline. Generally, it is safe to say that there is no major loss of cardiovascular exercise benefits for the first five to seven days of missed physical activity.

Keeping these four general principles in mind, let's investigate cardiorespiratory endurance, the component many experts believe to be the most important fitness key to wellness.

Cardiorespiratory Endurance

Cardiorespiratory endurance activities, more commonly known as **aerobic exercises,** are activities that cause a sustained increase in heart rate and use the large muscles of the body continuously for an extended period of time (see figure 5.4). Many experts believe that cardiorespiratory endurance is the most important component of physical fitness.

Aerobic Exercises

Aerobic exercises have two major goals. The first goal is to improve the general circulatory

1. Step aerobics is a good form of vigorous aerobic exercise; the large muscles in both the legs and arms are used continuously. What other types of physical activity would be considered *vigorous* aerobic activity?
2. Do you regularly participate in any type of vigorous aerobic activity? If so, what motivates you to participate? If not, what are the barriers to your participation?

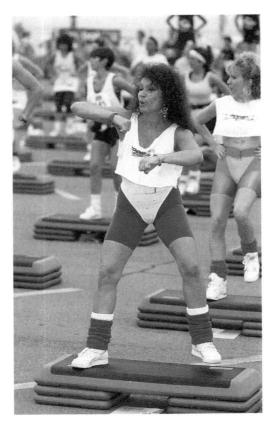

Fatty acid: an organic substance that serves as a building block for fat molecules.

Stress test: an aerobic exercise test that stresses the cardiorespiratory system. This test can be used, in conjunction with other tests, to diagnose coronary artery disease. It can also be used functionally to determine an individual's maximum heart rate during exercise, which is then used to guide a person in how strenuously they may safely exercise aerobically.

system (heart and lungs) so that greater amounts of blood and oxygen can be circulated throughout the body. The second goal is to improve the ability of specific muscles to consume greater amounts of oxygen. The particular muscles used for a given activity will be those targeted for aerobic improvements. If you are a runner, for instance, the muscles of your legs will increase their ability to use more oxygen, while your lungs increase the oxygen to the bloodstream and your heart adapts to pump greater amounts of blood each minute.

The key to aerobic exercise is oxygen (the word aerobic literally means "with oxygen"). Aerobic activities rely on oxygen in order to use **fatty acids** as their prime source of energy. Running, stationary cycling, jumping rope, and cross-country skiing are some of the better aerobic activities.

Anaerobic Exercises

Anaerobic exercise, on the other hand, is exercise that does not rely on oxygen. Anaerobic exercises use **glycogen** stored in the liver and skeletal muscles for its energy source. Glycogen can be broken down into

glucose without the presence of oxygen. Glycogen stores, however, are rapidly depleted. This means that after a very short time of maximal effort an individual must stop in order to take in enough oxygen to be able to use the more plentiful fatty acids as an energy source. Anaerobic activities are described as those requiring an intense, maximum burst of energy. Activities such as the 100-yard dash or the tennis serve would be considered anaerobic. During these activities, which require intense, short bursts of energy, waste products build up in the muscles and an oxygen debt occurs. By slowing down, or stopping, the body is able to take in needed oxygen and remove waste products from the muscles.

Designing an Aerobics Program

Before you begin an individualized aerobic activity program you will need to assess your present level of cardiorespiratory endurance.

Aerobics Fitness Testing

Currently the most accurate way to test cardiorespiratory endurance is to take what is known as a **stress test.** This test involves running on a treadmill or riding a stationary bicycle while trained medical and fitness personnel monitor the response of heart rate and blood pressure to *strenuous* exercise (see figure 5.5). Although it is a fairly accurate measure of aerobic fitness, it can be fairly expensive. The American Heart Association has issued exercise guidelines that recommend an exercise stress test for people over the age of forty, prior to beginning an exercise program.[21] Additionally, healthy adults under the age of forty who have two or more of the major risk factors for coronary artery disease (blood-cholesterol >200 mg/dl, cigarette smoking, or hypertension) should also have an exercise stress test.[22]

Dr. Kenneth Cooper, a well-known aerobics researcher, has developed several fitness tests that are more easily completed by the average person and are highly correlated with results obtained from a stress test. One of these tests is the one-mile walk test. To complete this fitness test you walk as quickly as you can, without straining, for one mile. At the end of the mile you measure your heart rate and record the time it took you to walk the mile. As illustrated in Activity for Wellness 5.1, you compare your time and

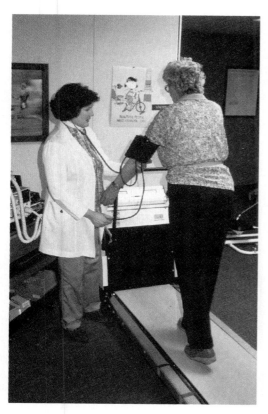

Figure 5.5: What Do You Think?

1. A stress test is one of the more accurate ways to measure aerobic fitness. What are the strengths and weaknesses of this form of aerobic testing?

heart rate to sex-based charts to determine your fitness level. As an example, let's analyze Jose's one-mile walk test results. Jose is twenty years old and weighs 175 pounds. After walking one mile in 16:10 (16 minutes and 10 seconds) his pulse rate was 140 beats per minute. Looking at the men's chart in Activity for Wellness 5.1, Jose determines that he is in the medium fitness category.

Before taking this fitness test, it is important that you take adequate precautions, especially if you have been sedentary for a while. Cooper recommends that males over the age of forty and females over the age of fifty, who are unaccustomed to regular exercise, should see their physician for a health screening before taking the one-mile walk test. Additionally, Cooper recommends the following safety precautions:

1. If you experience any unusual signs or symptoms such as shortness of breath, nausea, or light headedness while taking the test, STOP IMMEDIATELY and consult your physician.

2. Wait one to two hours after a meal before you begin the walk test.

3. Wear comfortable, loose clothing and comfortable, well-padded shoes suitable for walking.

4. Perform warm-up exercises, including walking and stretching, before taking the test. (Activities for Wellness 5.4 and 5.5 provide examples of good stretching and strengthening warm-up exercises.)

5. If you will be taking the test outdoors in extremely hot weather, it is best to do it during the morning or late afternoon hours to avoid the heat.

6. Do not take the walk test outdoors on days that are extremely cold or windy.

7. Do not drink caffeinated beverages for at least three hours before the test.

8. Do not take the walk test if you are taking any of the medications listed in Activity for Wellness 5.1.

Once you have determined your current level of aerobic fitness you are ready to design your aerobics program. In designing your program, you must keep in mind three major components. These components are easily remembered as the F.I.T. Guidelines: frequency, intensity, and time.

In 1995, the Centers for Disease Control and Prevention (CDC) and the American College of Sports Medicine (ACSM) announced new physical activity guidelines for health promotion that differ from guidelines recommended for those who want to improve their level of physical fitness as measured by improved aerobic capacity and body composition.[24] The new guidelines are quite simple in terms of frequency, intensity, and time, yet they are based on the results of numerous studies over the past ten years that have shown that health benefits, such as a reduced risk for the variety of chronic diseases discussed previously, can be achieved through *regular moderate* exercise. The CDC/ACSM exercise guidelines for health promotion recommend that *"every U.S. adult should accumulate thirty minutes or more of moderate-intensity physical activity on most, preferably all, days of the week."*[25] The half an hour of activity each day can be accumulated over the course of the day, rather than all at one time. For instance, you could walk for ten minutes in the morning, work in your garden for ten minutes in the afternoon, and ride

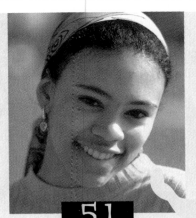

5.1
Activity for Wellness

One-Mile Walking Test

Purpose: To measure the efficiency with which the heart and lungs can take in and deliver oxygen to the body during exercise.

Equipment: Watch with a second hand, walking shoes.

Special Considerations:

1. Don't drink caffeinated beverages for at least three hours before the test. Caffeine elevates the pulse rate and would affect the validity of the test.

2. If you're taking blood pressure or other medication that prevents the heart rate from increasing during exercise or causes it to increase higher than normal, this test would be invalid for you. Don't take this test if you're currently using any of these types of medications: Alpha blockers, Beta blockers, Calcium channel blockers, Nitrates, Combined alpha and beta blockers, Centrally acting adrenergic inhibitors, Non-adrenergic peripheral vasodilators, Peripheral acting adrenergic inhibitors, Bronchodilators, Cold medications, Tricyclic antidepressants, Major tranquilizers, Diet medications, Thyroid medications.

Procedures:

1. Find a smooth, level surface where you can accurately measure a one-mile distance. A track at a school, a walking course in a park, a shopping mall or even your neighborhood streets. If you plan to walk on the street, avoid stoplights and heavy traffic areas.

2. Warm up for several minutes by stretching or walking briskly.

3. Walk (do not run) one mile as quickly as you can without straining. Maintain a constant pace.

4. After you finish the one-mile walk, keep moving while immediately taking your pulse for 15 seconds. Convert your 15-second heart rate to beats per minute by multiplying by 4. Example, if your 15-second count was 32 beats, your pulse rate was 128 beats per minute. Record your one-minute pulse rate.

5. Record the time it took to walk the one-mile distance in minutes and seconds. Most people take between 10 and 20 minutes to walk one mile.

6. Continue to walk slowly for at least five minutes to allow your heart rate and blood pressure to return to normal levels.

7. Use the charts that follow to interpret your test results.

Your Results:

My one-minute heart rate
equals _____
                    beats per minute

I walked one mile in

_____:_____
      minutes   seconds

My fitness category is: _____

From the Cooper Institute for Aerobics Research, *The Strength Connection: How to Build Strength and Improve the Quality of Your Life,* 94–95, 117–120, 1990. Reprinted by permission of The Cooper Institute for Aerobics Research, Dallas, TX.

One-Mile Walking Test—Men

On the left side of this chart, find your age category and pulse rate. If your exact pulse rate isn't shown, round it off. To the right of this value are the one-mile walk times for "Low," "Medium" and "High" fitness levels. *You may need to make an adjustment if your weight differs from the specified weight of 175 pounds. For every 10 lbs. over 175 lbs., men must walk 15 seconds faster to qualify for a fitness category. For every 10 lbs. under 175 lbs., men can walk 15 seconds slower to qualify for a fitness category.*

Age	Heart rate	Low fitness	Medium fitness	High fitness
20–29	110	>19:36	17:06–19:36	<17:06
	120	>19:10	16:36–19:10	<16:36
	130	>18:35	16:06–18:35	<16:06
	140	>18:06	15:36–18:06	<15:36
	150	>17:36	15:10–17:36	<15:10
	160	>17:09	14:42–17:09	<14:42
	170	>16:39	14:12–16:39	<14:12
30–39	110	>18:21	15:54–18:21	<15:54
	120	>17:52	15:24–17:52	<15:24
	130	>17:22	14:54–17:22	<14:54
	140	>16:54	14:30–16:54	<14:30
	150	>16:26	14:00–16:26	<14:00
	160	>15:58	13:30–15:58	<13:30
	170	>15:28	13:01–15:28	<13:01
40–49	110	>18:05	15:38–18:05	<15:38
	120	>17:36	15:09–17:36	<15:09
	130	>17:07	14:41–17:07	<14:41
	140	>16:38	14:12–16:38	<14:12
	150	>16:09	13:42–16:09	<13:42
	160	>15:42	13:15–15:42	<13:15
	170	>15:12	12:45–15:12	<12:45
50–59	110	>17:49	15:22–17:49	<15:22
	120	>17:20	14:53–17:20	<14:53
	130	>16:51	14:24–16:51	<14:24
	140	>16:22	13:51–16:22	<13:51
	150	>15:53	13:26–15:53	<13:26
	160	>15:26	12:59–15:26	<12:59
	170	>14:56	12:30–14:56	<12:30
60+	110	>17:55	15:33–17:55	<15:33
	120	>17:24	15:04–17:24	<15:04
	130	>16:57	14:36–16:57	<14:36
	140	>16:28	14:07–16:28	<14:07
	150	>15:59	13:39–15:59	<13:39
	160	>15:30	13:10–15:30	<13:10
	170	>15:04	12:42–15:04	<12:42

> means greater than; < means less than

One-Mile Walking Test—Women

On the left side of this chart, find your age category and pulse rate. If your exact pulse rate isn't shown, round it off. To the right of this value are the one-mile walk times for "Low," "Medium" and "High" fitness levels. *You may need to make an adjustment if your weight differs from the specified weight of 125 pounds. For every 10 lbs. over 125 lbs., women must walk 15 seconds faster to qualify for a fitness category. For every 10 lbs. under 125 lbs., women can walk 15 seconds slower to qualify for a fitness category.*

Age	Heart rate	Low fitness	Medium fitness	High fitness
20–29	110	>20:57	19:08–20:57	<19:08
	120	>20:27	18:38–20:27	<18:38
	130	>20:00	18:12–20:00	<18:12
	140	>19:30	17:42–19:30	<17:42
	150	>19:00	17:12–19:00	<17:12
	160	>18:30	16:42–18:30	<16:42
	170	>18:00	16:12–18:00	<16:12
30–39	110	>19:46	17:52–19:46	<17:52
	120	>19:18	17:24–19:18	<17:24
	130	>18:48	16:54–18:48	<16:54
	140	>18:18	16:24–18:18	<16:24
	150	>17:48	15:54–17:48	<15:54
	160	>17:18	15:24–17:18	<15:24
	170	>16:54	14:55–16:54	<14:55
40–49	110	>19:15	17:20–19:15	<17:20
	120	>18:45	16:50–18:45	<16:50
	130	>18:18	16:24–18:18	<16:24
	140	>17:48	15:54–17:48	<15:54
	150	>17:18	15:24–17:18	<15:24
	160	>16:48	14:54–16:48	<14:54
	170	>16:18	14:25–16:18	<14:25
50–59	110	>18:40	17:04–18:40	<17:04
	120	>18:12	16:36–18:12	<16:36
	130	>17:42	16:06–17:42	<16:06
	140	>17:18	15:36–17:18	<15:36
	150	>16:48	15:06–16:48	<15:06
	160	>16:18	14:36–16:18	<14:36
	170	>15:48	14:06–15:48	<14:06
60+	110	>18:00	16:36–18:00	<16:36
	120	>17:30	16:06–17:30	<16:06
	130	>17:01	15:37–17:01	<15:37
	140	>16:31	15:09–16:31	<15:09
	150	>16:02	14:39–16:02	<14:39
	160	>15:32	14:12–15:32	<14:12
	170	>15:04	13:42–15:04	<13:42

> means greater than; < means less than

PAR Q & YOU

PAR-Q is designed to help you help yourself. Many health benefits are associated with regular exercise, and the completion of PAR-Q is a sensible first step to take if you are planning to increase the amount of physical activity in your life.

For most people physical activity should not pose any problem or hazard. PAR-Q has been designed to identify the small number of adults for whom physical activity might be inappropriate or those who should have medical advice concerning the type of activity most suitable for them.

Common sense is your best guide in answering these few questions. Please read them carefully and check the ☑ YES or NO opposite the question if it applies to you.

YES NO

☐ ☐ 1. Has a doctor ever said that you have a heart condition and recommended only medically supervised activity?

☐ ☐ 2. Do you have chest pain brought on by physical activity?

☐ ☐ 3. Have you developed chest pain in the past month?

☐ ☐ 4. Do you tend to lose consciousness or fall over as a result of dizziness?

☐ ☐ 5. Do you have a bone or joint problem that could be aggravated by the proposed physical activity?

☐ ☐ 6. Has a doctor ever recommended medication for your blood pressure or a heart condition?

☐ ☐ 7. Are you aware through your own experience, or a doctor's advice, of any other physical reason against your exercising without medical supervision?

Note: If you have a temporary illness, such as a common cold, or are not feeling well at this time—**Postpone**

If You Answered

YES to one or more questions

If you have not recently done so, consult with your personal physician by telephone or in person BEFORE increasing your physical activity and/or taking a fitness test. Tell him what questions you answered YES on PAR-Q, or show him your copy.

programs

After medical evaluation, seek advice from your physician as to your suitability for:
• unrestricted physical activity, probably on a gradually increasing basis.
• restricted or supervised activity to meet your specific needs, at least on an initial basis. Check in your community for special programs or services.

NO to all questions

If you answered PAR-Q accurately, you have reasonable assurance of your present suitability for:
• A GRADUATED EXERCISE PROGRAM— A gradual increase in proper exercise promotes good fitness development while minimizing or eliminating discomfort.
• AN EXERCISE TEST—Simple tests of fitness (such as the Canadian Home Fitness Test) or more complex types may be undertaken if you so desire.

postpone

If you have a temporary minor illness, such as a common cold.

*Developed by the British Columbia Ministry of Health, Revised, 1991.

Reference: PAR-Q Validation Report, British Columbia Ministry of Health, May, 1978.

Produced by the British Columbia Ministry of Health and the Department of National Health & Welfare.

*Note: It is important that you answer all questions honestly. The PAR-Q is a scientifically and medically researched preexercise selection device. It complements exercise programs, exercise testing procedures, and the liability considerations attendant with such programs and testing procedures. PAR-Q, like any other preexercise screening device, will misclassify a small percentage of prospective participants, but no preexercise screening method can entirely avoid the problem.

TABLE 5.4

Examples of Common Physical Activities for Healthy U.S. Adults, by Intensity of Effort

Light Intensity	Moderate Intensity	Vigorous Intensity
Walking, slowly (strolling) (1–2 mph)	Walking, briskly (3–4 mph)	Walking, briskly uphill or with a load
Cycling, stationary (<50 W)	Cycling for pleasure or transportation (≤ 10 mph)	Cycling, fast or racing (>10 mph)
Swimming, slow treading	Swimming, moderate effort	Swimming, fast treading or crawl
Conditioning exercise, light stretching	Conditioning exercise, general calisthenics	Conditioning exercise, stair ergometer, ski machine
...	Racket sports, table tennis	Racket sports, singles tennis, racquetball
Golf, power cart	Golf, pulling cart or carrying clubs	...
Bowling	...	...
Fishing, sitting	Fishing, standing/casting	Fishing in stream
Boating, power	Canoeing, leisurely (2.0–3.9 mph)	Canoeing, rapidly (≥4 mph)
Home care, carpet sweeping	Home care, general cleaning	Moving furniture
Mowing lawn, riding mower	Mowing lawn, power mower	Mowing lawn, hand mower
Home repair, carpentry	Home repair, painting	...

From Pate et al., "Physical Activity and Public Health" in *JAMA* 273:402–407, 1995. Copyright © 1995 American Medical Association, Chicago, IL. Reprinted by permission.

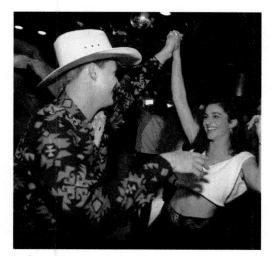

What Do You Think?

1. Dancing is a good way to include 30 minutes of moderate, and sometimes vigorous, physical activity into your lifestyle. Do you like to dance? How often do you dance each week?
2. The new physical activity guidelines for U.S. citizens recommend 30 minutes of moderate physical activity every day. What other physical activities would you enjoy making a regular part of your weekly lifestyle? When was the last time you participated in these activities?

your bicycle for ten minutes in the early evening, accumulating your thirty minutes of activity gradually. Moderate activities refer to the intensity of the activity; walking, mowing the lawn, and cycling are good examples of activities that, when done at a moderate intensity, result in important health benefits (see table 5.4).

For individuals who want to *optimally* improve their *physical fitness* level, including improving their muscular strength and endurance, cardiovascular endurance, flexibility, and body composition, the 1991 ACSM exercise guidelines still apply. These F.I.T. Guidelines are more involved than the health promotion activity guidelines just outlined, and are therefore explained here in some detail.

Frequency

The first F.I.T. Guideline is frequency. The American College of Sports Medicine suggests that, in order to receive optimal fitness benefits, you should exercise

1. Learning how to take your exercise
heart rate will help you to monitor
your exercise intensity. Do you
currently take your pulse several
times during an aerobic exercise
session? If so, do you adjust your
exercise intensity based upon your
exercise heart rate?

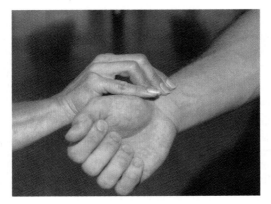

a.

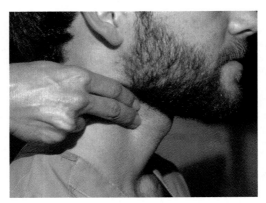

b.

vigorously three to five times each week.[26]
If you choose to exercise only three days
each week you will find that exercising
vigorously every other day will lead to the
greatest benefits and to a decreased risk of
muscle injury. Additionally, there should
not be more than two days of rest between
each exercise session or benefits will begin
to be lost.

Some people enjoy aerobics so much that
they participate six or seven days each week.
Exercising strenuously this frequently may
increase the likelihood of muscle, bone, and
joint injury.[27] If you decide to participate
more than four days a week you can lower the
risk of injury by slowing your pace every other
day or by alternating daily the muscle groups
you use by changing the type of aerobic
activity. Tami, for instance, is an avid jogger;
her day isn't complete without at least a short
run. Tami runs four miles every other day on
a scenic trail through the park near her
apartment. The other days, however, she runs
at a slightly slower pace and limits herself to
two miles. Larry runs with Tami on her four-
mile runs but chooses to swim on the
alternate days. In this way Larry can train his

Target heart rate: a measure of the
recommended intensity of an aerobic
exercise. The American College of
Sports Medicine recommends that an
individual's target heart rate be between
60 percent and 90 percent of their
estimated maximum heart rate.

Carotid arteries: arteries, located
along the side of the neck, that supply
blood to various structures in the neck,
face, jaw, scalp, and to the brain.

upper-body muscles with swimming, while
jogging increases the aerobic capacity of his
lower-body muscles.

Intensity

The second F.I.T. Guideline is intensity. An
important key to accruing aerobic benefits is the
"pace" you maintain during the activity you
choose. If the intensity is too low you will
receive little or no aerobic benefits, but if the
intensity is too great it may be too stressful for
the heart. One general guideline that you can
use to gauge the intensity of your aerobic
activity is the *talk test*. You should exercise at a
pace that allows you to talk to a fellow exerciser.
If huffing and puffing stop you from conversing
with someone, you should slow down.

A more scientific method of monitoring
your intensity is to calculate your **target heart
rate.** The target heart rate is the range you
should aim for when exercising and will vary
from person to person. This is one part of the
exercise prescription where the principle of
individual differences is clearly seen.

The target heart rate depends on the
individual's **maximal heart rate,** or the
highest heart rate reached during an all-out
aerobic effort. The best way to measure
maximal heart rate is to take a stress test and
measure the heart rate immediately at the
end of the test, but there are other ways to
estimate your maximal heart rate. Generally,
we know that the maximal heart rate
decreases as we age. By subtracting your age
from 220 you can get a rough estimate of your
maximal heart rate. The target heart-rate
range is then calculated by taking a
percentage of the estimated maximal heart
rate. For beginners the percentages range
between 60 percent and 80 percent of
maximal heart rate, while more advanced
participants may have a target range between
75 percent and 90 percent. Activity for
Wellness 5.3 will help you determine your
target heart-rate range.

In order to use your target heart-rate
prescription you will need to know how to
take your heart rate or pulse (see figure 5.6).
When you stop exercising you must quickly
locate your pulse. Your heart rate will drop
rapidly once you stop exercising. One place
to take an exercise heart rate is over the
blood vessels on your neck (the **carotid
arteries**), which are located directly to the
left or right of your Adam's apple. A better
place to take an exercise heart rate is over the

Target Heart Rate: Determining Exercise Intensity

It is important to exercise at an intensity level that is safe and appropriate. Intensity is measured by taking your heart rate or pulse. Below is an example of an exercise target heart-rate prescription for Jose, a twenty-year-old college sophomore, and blanks for you to use in determining your target heart-rate range.

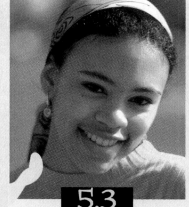

5.3 Activity for Wellness

1. Maximum heart rate (MHR) (estimated) = 220 − your age

JOSE 220 − *20 years* = *200 beats per minute*

YOU 220 − _____ = _____ beats per minute
          age   (MHR)

2. Target heart rate (THR) = 60 percent to 90 percent of MHR

JOSE (Jose is just beginning an aerobic exercise program so he will have a target heart-rate range of 60 percent to 80 percent of his maximum heart rate.)

$$\frac{200}{\text{(MHR)}} \times .60 = \frac{120 \text{ beats per minute}}{\text{(THR)}}$$

$$\frac{200}{\text{(MHR)}} \times .80 = \frac{160 \text{ beats per minute}}{\text{(THR)}}$$

Jose's target heart-rate range is 120–160 beats per minute. This is the rate he should aim for when exercising aerobically.

YOU (If you are beginning an aerobic exercise program use part A; if you have been participating in aerobic exercise at least three days per week for six or more continuous weeks, you may want to use part B to determine your target heart-rate range.)

Part A: (beginners) _____ × .60 = _____ beats per minute
               (MHR)   (THR)

                      _____ × .80 = _____ beats per minute
               (MHR)   (THR)

Part B: (advanced) _____ × .75 = _____ beats per minute
               (MHR)   (THR)

                      _____ × .90 = _____ beats per minute
               (MHR)   (THR)

HINT: To find out if you are exercising within your THR range, *immediately* after stopping your exercise count your pulse (radial or carotid) for ten seconds. Then multiply your ten second pulse count by six.

---

artery on the inside of your wrist just below the base of your thumb (the **radial artery**). Lightly place your index and middle finger over one of these arteries. As soon as you find your pulse, count the beats for ten seconds starting with zero as the first count. Multiply your ten-second count by six to determine if you are in your target range. If your heart rate is too high, you need to slow down. If it is too low, you will need to increase your pace in order to receive the optimal aerobic benefits.

A prime determinant of the amount of cardiorespiratory benefit that an activity will contribute to your *fitness level* is its ability to raise your heart rate into the target zone for a continuous period of time. Some exercises,

such as running, jumping rope, and stationary cycling, easily maintain the heart rate in the target zone for continuous lengths of time. This qualifies them as the best aerobic activities, or those that give the most cardiorespiratory benefits for the least amount of time invested. Other activities are more "stop and go" and therefore do not maintain the heart rate in the training range the entire time. Tennis is a good example of a moderately aerobic activity. During tennis rallies there is a level of intensity that will raise your heart rate to its training zone. Between rallies, however, there are many pauses that allow your heart rate to drop below the training zone. In general, to get

Radial arteries: arteries that travel along the thumb side of the arm from the forearm to the wrist.

TABLE 5.5

Cardiorespiratory Fitness Benefits of Various Exercises

A Do Condition Heart and Lungs	B Can Condition Heart and Lungs	C Do Not Condition Heart and Lungs
cross-country skiing	bicycling	baseball
hiking (uphill)	downhill skiing	bowling
ice hockey	basketball	football
jogging	calisthenics	golf (by cart)
jumping rope	field hockey	softball
rowing	handball	volleyball
running in place	racquetball	weight lifting
stationary bicycling	soccer	
	squash	
	swimming	
	tennis (singles)	
	walking	

Source: From *Exercise and Your Heart*, no. 81–1677: 34–35, May 1981, National Heart, Lung, and Blood Institute, National Institutes of Health, Bethesda, MD.

optimal cardiorespiratory benefits from moderately aerobic activities such as singles tennis, basketball, and racquetball, you should plan on spending twice the amount of time each session that you would for a more vigorous aerobic activity. Table 5.5 presents various types of activities and how they contribute to your cardiorespiratory endurance.

Time

The third F.I.T. Guideline considers the amount of time you need to devote to each exercise session. The American College of Sports Medicine has determined that for vigorous aerobic activities (column A in table 5.5) you will receive optimal aerobic benefits if you exercise in your target heart-rate zone for twenty to thirty minutes. For the more moderate aerobic exercises you will need to devote a little more time because of their "stop-and-go" nature. You should aim for a range of forty to sixty minutes each time for moderate aerobic exercises such as those listed in column B in table 5.5.

Putting It All Together

Now that you have determined your exercise prescription (frequency, intensity, and time) you are ready to begin your program. Before you start each exercise session it is very important to **warm up.** A general warm-up

before exercise will gradually increase the amount of blood your heart pumps each minute, the blood flow to active muscles, and your internal body temperature. This gradual increase is thought to aid in preventing injuries. Good activities for the beginning of a warm-up include brisk walking, or for those with a good fitness level, a slow jog. Once you have gradually increased circulation to the active muscles, you should engage in some limited stretching activities (see Activity for Wellness 5.4). Stretching activities will also contribute to your total fitness by improving your flexibility. Muscular strengthening activities are another important component of a general warm-up. Adequate strength will help to ensure that you can safely participate in aerobic activities, moving your body in a rapid yet controlled manner (see Activity for Wellness 5.5).

Just as it is important to warm up properly before you exercise, it is equally important to **cool down** after you exercise. The activities that make up a good cooldown are the same as those described for the warm-up. Generally, you should keep moving once you finish your aerobic activity. Walk slowly to keep the blood circulating and prevent it from pooling in the legs. This may also help remove waste products that have accumulated in the muscles during the exercise. It is important to let your heart rate

Cooldown: gradually slowing down at the end of an exercise session in order to keep blood from pooling in the lower extremities and to aid in the removal of waste products that may have built up in muscles during exercise.

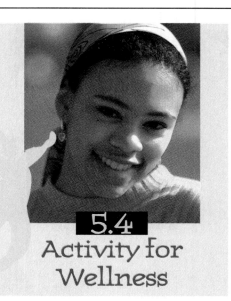
Recommended Stretching Exercises

Stretching

It is important that all major joints in your body allow you the full range of movement involved in any aerobic activity. Tight muscles can be damaged if they are forcibly stretched beyond their normal length. Again, limited range of joint motion and tight muscles may force you to perform in clumsy, stressful, and inefficient ways. That's why inflexible people are more prone to injury.

Guidelines for Stretching

• Wear comfortable, nonrestrictive clothing. Before you begin, warm up your body with a gentle activity. Try a three-to-five-minute walk.

• Hold each stretch at the point of tightness. (*Never bounce!*)

• Hold each stretch fifteen to thirty seconds.

• Try to *relax* the rest of your body while you stretch.

• Breathe normally during each stretch. (Do not hold your breath!)

• For best results, stretch every day.

• Discontinue any stretch if you experience pain.

Continued

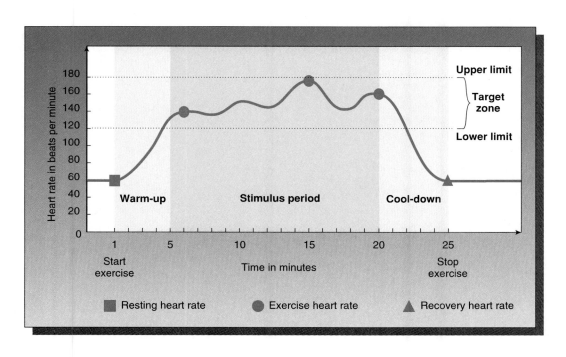

Figure 5.7
A typical exercise session is presented in this graph for Shelley, a college sophomore. Note the various times that the heart rate is measured, and the expected range the heart rate should be in during these times. For example, Shelley took an exercise heart rate at approximately 15 minutes into her exercise session. She noted that her pulse was in the "training range" at 179, but at the upper end of that range; therefore she cut back slightly on how hard she was exercising. At her 20 minute pulse check her pulse was 160, indicating that she had decreased her heart rate some but had still exercised at a level that would provide the benefits of vigorous aerobic activity.

drop gradually from the training zone toward a resting rate. The best time to do stretching activities is probably during the cooldown from aerobic exercise. At this time your muscles are warmed up and are less likely to be injured. Figure 5.7 illustrates how the whole pattern of aerobic exercise fits together. It shows the progression from warm-up, to a period of twenty to thirty minutes of aerobic activity in your target heart-rate range, and finally, to cooldown and recovery.

Starting Your Personal Exercise Program

Many consumers consider joining a fitness or health club to be the first step toward fitness; however, it is *not* necessary to join an exercise establishment in order to begin a safe and effective fitness program. Many aerobic, flexibility, and strengthening activities can be done with little or no equipment. Walking, running, bicycling, calisthenics, and stretching exercises are just a few of the many

Activity for Wellness—Continued

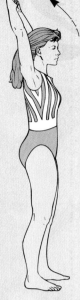

Shoulders: Stand with your feet shoulder-width apart, knees relaxed, chest up and shoulders back. Grasp your hands above your head. Gently push your arms backward until you experience mild tightness. *Do not* arch the back.

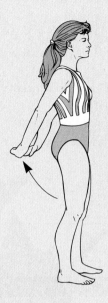

Chest: Stand with your feet shoulder-width apart, knees relaxed, chest up and shoulders back. Gently push your arms upward until you experience mild tightness. *Do not* bend at the waist or round the shoulders.

Back of Upper Arm: Place your hand behind your head on the opposite shoulder blade. Gently push on the raised elbow with the other hand, pressing downward to the point of mild tightness.

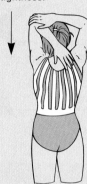

Lower Back: Lie flat on your back, head on the floor. Pull both knees up toward your chest.

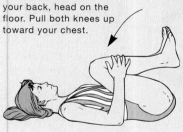

Lower Back: Lie flat on your back, head on the floor. Pull one knee up toward your chest, keeping the other leg straight.

Back of Thighs: Lie flat on your back, head and shoulders down on the floor. Bend one knee to the chest and extend the other leg straight upward. Slowly pull the extended leg toward your chest until you experience mild tightness.

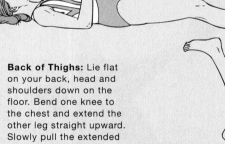

Hips: Stand with one foot in front of the other, chest up and shoulders back. Slowly flatten your lower back by tilting your pelvis backward until you feel mild tightness in the front of the hip region of your *rear* leg.

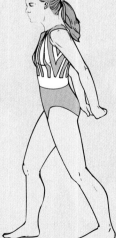

Back of Thighs: Lie flat on your back, head and shoulders down on the floor. Keep one foot on the floor, knee bent. Pull the other knee to the chest and gently attempt to straighten the leg until you experience mild tightness.

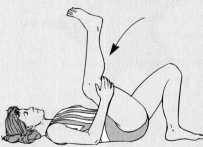

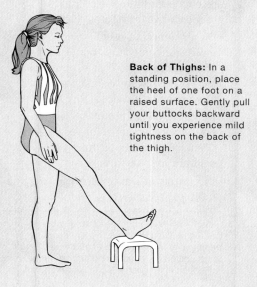

Back of Thighs: In a standing position, place the heel of one foot on a raised surface. Gently pull your buttocks backward until you experience mild tightness on the back of the thigh.

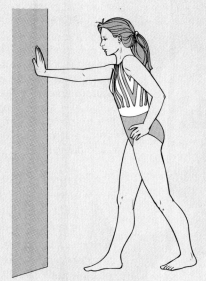

Calf: Lean against a wall or steady chair, placing one foot behind the other. Keep the rear heel in contact with the floor, toes pointing forward. Slowly lean forward at the hips until you experience mild tightness in the calf region of the back leg. Keep both knees relaxed.

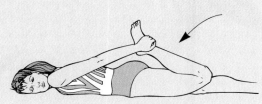

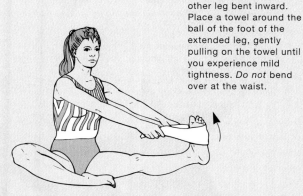

Calf: Sit on the floor with one leg extended, the other leg bent inward. Place a towel around the ball of the foot of the extended leg, gently pulling on the towel until you experience mild tightness. *Do not* bend over at the waist.

Front of Thighs: Lie flat on your stomach, head and shoulders on the floor. Grasp the outside of the ankle with your hand (same side hand as foot). Gently pull the foot toward your buttocks until you experience mild tightness. Keep the knee in line with the shoulder. *Do not* do this exercise if it hurts your knees. If you cannot reach your foot with your hand, loop a towel around your ankle and gently pull on the towel.

or

In a standing position hold onto a wall or other sturdy object. Pull the foot toward the buttocks, keeping the knee pointing straight down.

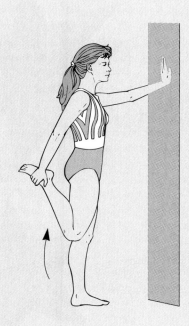

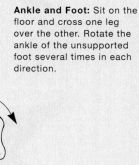

Ankle and Foot: Sit on the floor and cross one leg over the other. Rotate the ankle of the unsupported foot several times in each direction.

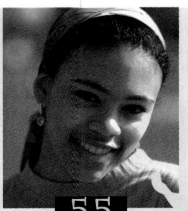

5.5
Activity for Wellness

Recommended Strengthening Exercises

Strengthening

Adequate strength is a prerequisite for participation in any vigorous activity. Strength allows you to move your body rapidly, and with control. The correct posture must also be maintained. Weak postural muscles make that impossible. For safety sake, opposing muscles should have approximately equal strength so that your joints are both flexible and balanced.

Guidelines for Strengthening

- Warm up with two to three minutes of comfortable walking, then gently stretch all of the muscles to be strengthened.

- Perform each exercise exactly as described. Make sure all movements are slow and controlled.

- Perform about ten to fifteen repetitions of each exercise, if you can. Discontinue the exercise if you feel pain or discomfort.

- When you have completed the recommended exercises, repeat the whole sequence two more times, if you can.

- Do not perform strengthening exercises more than three times per week, or on consecutive days. That is, you should always have a day of rest between strengthening sessions.

- Do not hold your breath while performing strengthening exercises. Get into the habit of exhaling as you contract your muscles.

- Discontinue any strengthening exercise if you experience pain.

From "The Pre-Aerobic Exercise Program" created by Drs. Lorna and Peter Francis, Department of Physical Education, San Diego State University, 1986. Reprinted by permission of Reebok International Ltd., Stoughton, MA.

Abdominals: Lie on your back, feet in the air or supported on a chair. Cross your arms over your chest. Slowly curl up, raising the shoulders and upper back off the floor. Slowly curl back down again. *Do not* allow the lower back to come off the floor. (If you experience tension in your neck, support your head with your hands as you lower your head.)

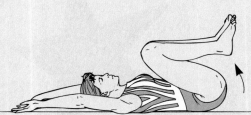

or

Lie flat on your back with knees up to your chest, hands resting comfortably above your head. Pull your buttocks toward your chest without swinging the legs.

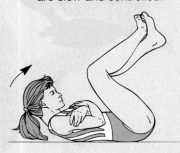

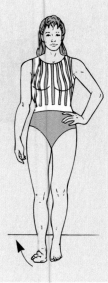

Front of Shins: This exercise is especially important in preparation for running or aerobic dancing. In a standing position, tap the toes up and down, each time pulling the toes up as high as possible. Or walk around on your heels, pulling the toes up as high as possible. *Do not* lock your knees.

Back of Shoulders: Lie flat on your stomach, both arms stretched out to your sides. Gently raise your arms as far as you can above the floor. Keep your head and shoulders on the floor.

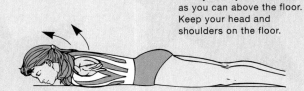

activities that can be done in your own home or around your neighborhood at little or no cost. Directions for several of these activities are provided in this chapter.

Simply joining a health club does not ensure that you will really begin or maintain an exercise program. Most health and fitness clubs can sell many more memberships than they can actually service, because they know that half or more of the members will drop out of their exercise program very soon after starting. Thus, many consumers continue to pay the health club but do not make use of their memberships. The only one benefiting from this relationship is the health club. If, however, you have the money to spend and want a more social atmosphere to exercise in, or if the sport you are interested in requires expensive equipment, such as a pool or a racquetball court, a fitness club may suit your needs.

Not all fitness and health clubs provide convenient, safe, and effective equipment and instruction for their clients. It is important that you investigate clubs thoroughly *before* you join. For instance, is the club in a convenient location, near your home or work? Research has shown that this is an important factor in both adopting and maintaining an exercise program. Activity for Wellness 5.6 will help you evaluate health clubs for both their safety and effectiveness.

Whether you join a health club, or begin an exercise program in the privacy of your own home, one of the most important things to remember is to *start slow*. Proceeding gradually to your fitness goals will help make your activities more enjoyable and make you less prone to injury. The American College of Sports Medicine has delineated three stages of progress for strenuous aerobic exercise.[28] The three stages are the initial-conditioning stage, the improvement-conditioning stage, and the maintenance stage.

Initial-Conditioning Stage

The **initial-conditioning stage** consists of low-level aerobic exercises, some mild stretching, and light calisthenics. The beginning exerciser with a low level of fitness should begin with twelve minutes for each exercise session and gradually increase toward the goal of twenty minutes. For many beginners this phase may last four to

six weeks. Monitor your heart-rate response to exercise to determine when to progress to the next stage. As the heart becomes trained it becomes stronger and thus pumps fewer times each minute in order to do the same amount of exercise. As you become more fit, you will need to increase your pace and the amount of time you spend each session in order to stay in your target heart-rate zone.

Improvement-Conditioning Stage

The second stage of progression is called the **improvement-conditioning stage.** During this stage you will advance more rapidly. You should be able to increase the duration of your exercise session every two to three weeks, eventually reaching your goal of thirty minutes. Additionally, during this stage your target heart rate will be raised to 75 to 85 percent of your estimated maximal heart rate. This is the stage where many of the cardiorespiratory benefits we discussed earlier in this chapter are experienced.

Maintenance Stage

The final stage of conditioning is the **maintenance stage.** This stage typically begins about six months into a regular aerobic fitness program. Many people reach a point in their aerobics program where they are completely satisfied with the level of cardiorespiratory endurance they have attained. At this point they are interested in maintaining the benefits of their program rather than continuing to improve. This is accomplished by maintaining the program they have established during the improvement-conditioning stage. For most people this will consist of twenty to thirty minutes of aerobic exercise at the target heart-rate range for three to five days each week.

In selecting an aerobic exercise it is important to consider your needs, interests, and lifestyle (see table 5.6). If you like social gatherings you might enjoy joining an aerobic dance class were you would meet other people who share your interest in exercise. If you are really out of shape you might want to consider beginning with a walking program, at least for the initial conditioning stage. If you have a very competitive nature you might enjoy a game such as racquetball. Remember,

Initial-conditioning stage: the beginning stage of progress for individuals starting a vigorous aerobic exercise program. This stage usually lasts from four to six weeks and gradually prepares an individual to safely participate in more strenuous physical activity.

Improvement-conditioning stage: the second stage of progress for individuals who want to improve their cardiovascular endurance. Duration of exercise sessions and target heart rate are both systematically increased during this phase, creating a state of overload that leads to a cardiovascular training effect.

Maintenance stage: the final stage of progress for individuals participating in a vigorous aerobic exercise program. During this stage the individual continues at a frequency, intensity, and duration of aerobic exercise that they have become accustomed to in the improvement-conditioning stage. They do not continue to overload for improvement, but rather maintain the level of physical fitness attained.

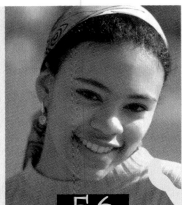

5.6
Activity for Wellness

How Fit Is Your Health Club?

You don't need to join a health club to be healthy, of course. But many people do spend lots of money on memberships to fitness centers—from neighborhood Ys and aerobics studios to hightech gyms. Some of them find that going to a health club helps motivate them and teaches them better ways to exercise. But just as many people who join end up not going regularly—or ever. Here are tips to help choose a facility that will help make your fitness plan rewarding and successful. Check the box next to each tip if your health club meets the standard.

❑ 1. **Get a one-day pass to sample the facility, and visit it during the hours you plan to use it.** If you intend to go after work and it's packed then, you'll waste time waiting in line for equipment and have to face overcrowded classes. Try out classes. Make sure instructors are enthusiastic and encouraging and that they address the different needs and ability levels of the participants. Talk to members—ask them if they're satisfied.

❑ 2. **Is it the right place for what you plan to do?** Fitness centers in the U.S. have diversified and matured. Many facilities today combine what used to be called "the gym" (push-ups, barbells, etc.) with features of the 1980s (aerobics classes and newfangled weight machines). They are likely to offer a variety of classes, from ballroom dancing and karate to bench-step aerobics (combining stair climbing and aerobic dance) and cardio-fitness classes.

❑ 3. **Judging the equipment.** Check the studios and workout rooms; they should be spacious, clean, well-lit, and well ventilated (especially in hot weather). Floors should be of appropriate materials (sprung wood floors for dance/exercise studios, resilient surfaces for weight-training areas). Class size should be limited to allow sufficient space for safe, comfortable movement, and to allow the teacher to observe everyone in the room. Equipment should be up-to-date and well-maintained (broken machines are a common problem at many gyms). If there's a variety of equipment, you'll be able to cross-train—that is, alternate different kinds of workouts during the week. There should be enough free weights to allow several people to work out simultaneously. A staff member should be present at all times. Check to see if showers, dressing rooms, saunas, and steam rooms are clean.

❑ 4. **Does the club require a stress test before you start your new program?** This is a good sign—and is especially important if you are over forty-five, overweight, at risk for heart disease, disabled, or have other health problems. If you fit one of these categories, have an exam by your doctor before starting any exercise program, whether the club requires one or not.

❑ 5. **Does the facility hire only qualified, certified personnel?** Certification—though not mandated by law—can come from a number of reputable organizations, including the American College of Sports Medicine, International Dance Exercise Association, Aerobics and Fitness Association of America, and the Institute of Aerobics Research. What type of in-house training does the club require of its teachers? The YMCA, for instance, has its own training program for instructors. Ideally, instructors should have degrees in exercise-related fields, such as exercise physiology, kinesiology, or physical education; they (or other staff members) should be trained in first aid and CPR. The club should also offer CPR training to members.

Caveat Emptor

Turn a deaf ear to a "today-only" sale price; you should be able to think it over for a few days. Most states require clubs to offer a three-day "cooling-off period" so you can change your mind even after signing up. It should also be possible to sign on for a short-term membership before you commit to joining for a year or more, and to freeze your membership temporarily in case of illness, injury, or travel. Read the contract carefully.

From the *Berkeley Wellness Letter,* "How Fit is Your Health Club," Novermber 1990. Reprinted by permission of the *University of California at Berkeley Wellness Letter,* © Health Letter Associates, 1990.

however, that if you select a moderately aerobic game such as racquetball or tennis you will need to invest a greater amount of time in order to achieve *optimal aerobic* benefits. It also helps to select a partner whose skill and fitness levels are similar to your own because the amount of time you will spend in your target range will probably increase. One study showed that in racquetball games where opponents were equally skilled and fit the typical match lasted fifty minutes rather than the average thirty-four minutes between opponents of varying abilities and fitness levels.[29]

Trouble Spots

Injuries happen to every kind of athlete, from beginners who try to do too much too fast to veterans who push too hard. Women, who tend to have proportionally wider hips than men, have more problems with knees and ankles because of the way their leg muscles are aligned. Since men tend to favor sports requiring upper-body strength, they often have more shoulder injuries.

1 Neck
Injury: Tightness and soreness.
Cause: Tension in overworked muscles, especially in bikers.
Treatment: Rotate and stretch neck to loosen muscles.
Prevention: Stretch before and after biking; make sure heights of seat and handlebar are correct.

2 Elbow
Injury: Soreness at the joint—often called tennis elbow.
Cause: Inflamed tendons due to overuse and poor technique, especially in racquet sports.
Treatment: Rest; use aspirin or ibuprofen to reduce swelling.
Prevention: Gradually work up to high-intensity sessions; take lessons to improve technique.

3 Thigh
Injury: Pulled hamstring muscle.
Cause: Inadequate warm up; sudden starts or stops; sprinting too fast. Occurs in stop-and-go activities such as football, soccer, and racquet sports.
Treatment: Apply ice to stop swelling. Most important, begin with gentle stretching as soon as possible, and continue stretching through recovery; the muscle tends to shorten as it heals.
Prevention: Warm up before exercising by stretching gently.

4 Foot
Injury: Blisters, strained tendons, microfracture in bones.
Cause: Overuse or sudden increase in exercise intensity, especially in running and sports involving jumping. A fracture can become larger if ignored.
Treatment: Blisters should be drained and covered with moleskin. Rest is best for strains in muscles and bones. Switch to a sport in which the feet are not under stress, such as swimming or bicycling, until the pain stops.
Prevention: Increase workouts gradually; make sure shoes fit.

5 Calf
Injury: Pain in front of lower leg (shinsplints), strain in calf muscle, Achilles' tendon.
Cause: Overuse, especially in runners.
Treatment: Rest or substitute a nonimpact sport such as swimming or bicycling until the injury heals. Healing will generally take as long as the original pain lasts; if you hurt for two weeks, figure two more to heal.
Prevention: Strengthen calf muscles by weight lifting or exercising with resistance bands. Stretch before and after you work out. Run on softer surfaces.

6 Ankle
Injury: Twists and sprains.
Cause: They often plague beginners, who insist on doing too much in one exercise session, especially in racquet sports, volleyball, and basketball. The ankle is more prone to rolling over during a sudden stop when the legs are tired.
Treatment: Treatment should be immediate, since reducing the swelling means a quicker recovery. Apply ice, wrap with a bandage, and elevate. Ice should be applied for about thirty minutes every two hours.
Prevention: Use resistance bands to strengthen ankles.

7 Knee (front view)
Injury: Sore kneecap, stiffness, inability to sit with the leg bent for a long time. Often called runner's knee, it also occurs in hikers, dancers, and gymnasts.
Cause: A change in workout—changing shoes or running on unfamiliar terrain. The kneecap moves too freely and rubs against bone, irritating it.
Treatment: Rest or switch to swimming. If pain continues, see a doctor.
Prevention: Build thigh muscles by cycling or weight lifting.

8 Hip, Groin
Injury: Soreness in hip joint, pulled muscle in buttocks or in groin.
Cause: Overuse, new stresses on legs due to change in exercise routine.
Treatment: Rest, run on softer surfaces, switch to low-impact activity such as swimming.
Prevention: Stretch, strengthen thigh muscles.

9 Back
Injury: Strain, soreness, muscle spasms.
Cause: Sudden lunges or twists when tired, such as in racquet sports or soccer; overdoing in impact sports like running.
Treatment: Stretch; apply heat. See a doctor if pain persists.
Prevention: Strengthen abdominal muscles and stretch before exercising.

10 Shoulder
Injury: Joint soreness.
Cause: Overuse, particularly in swimming, tennis, or sports that involve throwing, such as baseball and softball.
Treatment: Rest until the pain goes away, and switch activities temporarily.
Prevention: Exercise shoulders with stretching and weights.

If it hurts: How to treat injuries—and keep them from happening

Copyright, July 18, 1988, *U.S. News & World Report*

TABLE 5.6 Choosing Aerobic Exercises

Choose an aerobic exercise that fits!

The following chart is a general guide that can help you choose an aerobic exercise (or a combination of exercises) that fits your needs, interests, and lifestyle.

	aerobic dance	aerobicize	basketball	bicycling (indoors)	bicycling (outdoors)	cross-country skiing	handball, racquetball	jogging	jumping rope	mini-trampoline	rowing (indoor)	skating (ice or roller)	soccer	swimming indoor laps	tennis singles	walking
if you're out of shape	•			•	•					•	•	•		•		•
if you're in *great* shape	•	•	•	•	•	•	•	•	•	•		•	•	•	•	
if you want to be alone				•	•			•		•		•		•	•	•
if you like company	•	•	•				•					•	•		•	•
if you hate to sweat														•		
if you love the indoors	•	•		•			•			•	•	•		•		
if you love the outdoors					•	•		•				•			•	•
if you have joint problems				•						•				•		•
if you don't have much time				•					•	•	•	•				
if you're *easily* bored	•	•	•		•	•	•	•				•	•		•	
if you're competitive				•			•	•	•			•	•	•	•	
if you can't spend much			•						•					•		•
if you want to be flexible			•			•	•	•				•			•	•
if shorts are too revealing				•	•	•				•	•					•

From *The Hope Healthletter*, published by the Hope Heart Institute, Seattle, WA. Reprinted with permission.

Personal and Social Influences on Activity

One of the largest barriers to an active lifestyle is our own attitudes. The list of excuses for our inactivity is almost endless. We don't have the time, or exercise is boring, or we don't have the right equipment and clothes. What excuses do you use?

Exercise scientists have estimated that only half of those beginning an exercise program will still be exercising regularly by the end of a year. Because the benefits of exercise are accrued by consistent participation, the

TABLE 5.7 — Factors That Improve Adoption and Maintenance of Exercise

Adoption		Maintenance	
Personal factors	Situational factors	Personal factors	Situational factors
High income and educational levels	Convenience of facility	Nonsmoking	Social support
Young age		Normal weight	Convenience of facility
Male gender		White-collar occupation	Low-intensity or moderately vigorous exercise
Childhood sports participation		Self-motivation	
Expectation of health and other benefits		Perceived ability to find time	
		No medical contraindications	

Source: Data from James F. Sallis, "Exercise Adherence and Motivation" in *Focal Points,* 2:3, 1986.

adoption and maintenance of regular exercise has been the focus of much needed research. Preliminary results indicate that a variety of personal and social characteristics are predictive of adoption and maintenance of exercise programs (see table 5.7). One recent study, conducted on 120 employees of Michigan State University (MSU), used a combination of incentives, including monetary rewards, peer support, and written exercise contracts, to help people maintain an exercise program.[30] At the end of six months, the researchers found that 97 percent of the incentives program participants were still exercising regularly, while only 25 percent of the control group were regular exercisers. These researchers believe the key to their success was the use of a *combination* of incentives.

The MSU exercise program staff offer the following suggestions to help you learn to make exercise a routine part of your lifestyle.

1. Construct a written exercise contract, similar to the sample contract found in chapter 1 of this text. The contract should be very specific in terms of detailed and measurable objectives, as well as a weekly exercise schedule indicating the days and times you plan to exercise.

2. A support person should sign the contract indicating his or her willingness to help you with your plan. Finding several people to exercise with is often the best support.

3. Decide in advance the incentives and punishments that you will use for motivation. The incentives should be things that you really enjoy or find meaningful. Many people treat themselves to a new item of clothing or a new CD. Others choose to put away a certain amount of money for each week that they follow their plan, saving the money for a special vacation. Punishments, on the other hand, are unpleasant tasks or consequences, such as agreeing to wash your support person's car each week that you miss an exercise session.

Time is a valued commodity for most of us. When it comes to physical activity we just can't seem to "find" the time. To overcome this hurdle, you need to realize that you will never "find" the time. You must learn to "make" the time. Fortunately that won't be as difficult as it sounds.

Some people find that writing in the word "exercise" on their daily calendar helps in fitting physical activity into their day. It can also serve as a memory jogger to those who are forgetful.

Another way to make the time is to cut down on the number of hours you watch television. If you are like the typical person in the U.S., you may, on average, watch up to seven hours of television each day.[31] By carefully selecting the programs you watch on television you should be able to free up at least thirty

TABLE 5.8   *Squeezing Exercise into a Too-Tight Schedule*

You might as well give up trying to *find* the time to exercise. For most of us, time to exercise can't be *found;* it has to be *made.*

The good news is that getting regular exercise doesn't have to be a big deal and doesn't have to take much time. Studies have shown that getting (and staying) in shape need not take more than thirty minutes, three times a week (every other day).

So when's the best time to exercise? That depends on you and your lifestyle. The important thing is not *when* you exercise, but *whether.* . . .

Exercise Time	Possible Disadvantages	Possible Advantages
Morning (before breakfast)	• Sometimes hard to get out of the sack.	• Clears the fog so you can begin your day refreshed and alert. • You have to take a shower anyway. • Outside exercisers can enjoy the peace and quiet of their sleepy neighborhood. • Done in the morning, it's "out of the way."
Noon (before lunch)	• This is not possible if you have a short lunch period, or if showers are not available at work or school.	• Enables you to work off morning tensions. • Can help curb lunch appetite. • Refreshes you to meet afternoon demands.
Early evening (before dinner)	• Easy to postpone exercise due to coming home from work late feeling "too tired," etc.	• Clears day's tensions. • Helps you avoid "just home from the office" bingeing/snacking. • Can help curb dinner appetite. • Refreshes you for evening activities.
Late evening (before bed) • Note: if you have problems sleeping, do *not* exercise strenuously within two hours of bedtime.	• Easy to postpone exercise due to eating late, wanting to watch a good television program, telling yourself you'll get up early the next morning to do it, etc. • Necessary to wait an hour or so after a heavy meal.	• Can help you relax and clear your mind of the day's problems so you can sleep more soundly.

From *The Hope Health!etter,* published by the Hope Heart Institute, Seattle, WA. Reprinted with permission.

minutes a day, three days a week that you could use for experimenting with aerobic activity.

The time of day you select to participate in your physical activity will also present potential barriers and benefits (see table 5.8). For instance, you may want to exercise in the middle of the day in order to break up your work schedule. You may also find that it helps you to eat less when you go to lunch after exercising. While going to school this schedule may work very well for you. When you graduate and become employed, however, it may be more inconvenient, especially if your employer does not value exercise and provide appropriate facilities for your use. Fortunately, many companies are discovering that physically fit employees are good for the "bottom line."

Find Your Play

Many of us have developed the notion that exercise is boring. If you find yourself saying these words you need to look behind this vague generality and identify exactly what it is about your fitness activity that leads you to feel this way. Is it possible that you have structured your exercise sessions so rigidly that there is no room for creativity, spontaneity, and play? If you find yourself doing the same exercise, on the same day, at the same time, year in and year out, maybe you need to vary

Making changes in your level of physical activity is not an easy process. You will probably find that you go through a series of steps, like those listed below, each time you try to make such healthy changes in your behavior. To receive the health promotion and physical fitness benefits of regular activity you may need to improve your current physical activity pattern. The following tips will help you as you progress through the stages of behavior change.*

Precontemplation → Contemplation

If you have never thought about making healthy changes in your level of physical activity or you do not intend to make any changes within the next six months you might want to consider:

- assessing your current aerobic fitness level (Activity for Wellness 5.1) to determine if you need to become more physically active.

Contemplation → Preparation

If you have been seriously considering making some changes in your level of physical activity, but have not yet attempted any changes, try to thoughtfully answer the following questions:

- How do I think or feel about striving for a more optimal level of body fat, aerobic capacity, muscular strength and endurance, and flexibility, that may help me to have more energy, attain my desired body weight and shape, and increase my level of well-being both now and in the future? Am I willing to change my lifestyle permanently to achieve this goal safely?

Preparation → Action

If you are ready to make some definite plans for becoming more physically active, such as walking or bicycling, during the next month, or if you have already made small changes in the past

but were not able to maintain those changes as a permanent part of your lifestyle, consider the following actions:

- Make a resolution to yourself to begin to improve your level of physical activity; for instance, make a commitment to yourself to begin to add thirty minutes of aerobic activity to your day.
- Set a specific date to begin your new behavior, for example, "starting Monday I will walk briskly with my friend Jill for fifteen minutes and bicycle alone for ten minutes, five days a week."

Action → Maintenance

If you have recently started to make some healthy changes in your activity level, the following tips will help you continue on this healthy path:

- Write a behavior change contract, such as found in chapter 1, and find a support person who will help you keep with your plan; have your support person sign your contract.
- Give yourself rewards *often* for meeting your goals and objectives; rewards should be things you really enjoy, but that you are willing to do without if you do not meet your goal.

Maintenance

You have made important changes in your exercise habits that you have practiced for six months or longer, now you need to focus on maintaining your healthy choices every day:

- Review the suggestions on page 191; these suggestions will help you learn how to deal with inevitable lapses in your exercise plan so that you maintain your active lifestyle for a lifetime.

* Based on Prochaska, Norcross and DiClemente's transtheoretical model. See Prochaska, J. O., Norcross, J. C. & DiClemente, C. C. (1994). *Changing for Good.* New York: William Morrow and Company.

your routine. Try a new aerobic activity now and then, or ask a friend to share your fitness activities and make it a social occasion. You could even combine the two suggestions and join a friend who is already involved in a different kind of activity. Let people show you the ropes of their favorite exercise. Remember, variety is the spice of life (see A Social Perspective 5.1).

The best way to assure yourself of leading an active physical lifestyle is to choose aerobic activities you enjoy. If jogging is not for you, try swimming, bicycling, aerobic dance, walking, or any of the other many

activities that offer aerobic benefits. Table 5.9 offers suggestions that will help you begin or continue a physically active lifestyle that will provide you with the health promotion benefits discussed in this chapter. It's up to you to try new fitness activities; choose an activity that sounds fun and investigate how to participate in that activity safely. The recommended readings at the end of this chapter should help you with your investigation. Seek out a support group; find friends or family members who would be interested in participating with you. And most of all, have fun.

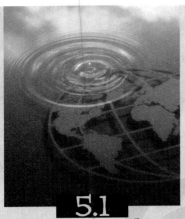

5.1

A Social Perspective

Meditation in Motion: Tai Chi

From karate and judo to aikido and tae kwon do, the martial arts are becoming increasingly popular among people in the U.S., many of whom practice them primarily as exercise or sport, rather than for self-defense. One of the most attractive of these is tai chi chuan, or simply tai chi (pronounced tie-jee), prominently featured in Bill Moyers's recent television series *Healing and the Mind.* Though it originated as a self-defense technique, tai chi has been practiced in China for centuries as an art form, religious ritual, relaxation technique, and exercise for people of all ages, even people in their eighties and nineties. Today, every morning in San Francisco's Washington Square park (as in public spaces across the U.S.) you can see hundreds of people—mostly Asian—performing the slow, balanced, low-impact movements of tai chi. As a means of strengthening muscles, improving balance, and reducing stress, tai chi has much to offer.

Tai chi involves dozens of fluid, graceful, dancelike postures, performed in sequences known as "forms," which at first glance resemble karate in slow motion or swimming in air. Unlike many martial arts, it does not call for punches or kicks. Instead, it is based on the concept of withstanding aggression without force—yielding to a punch and using an attacker's momentum against him. It calls for concentration, balanced shifting of body weight, and muscle relaxation—thus it is often called "moving meditation." Though tai chi movements are slow, they can provide a fairly intense workout. The benefits of tai chi include:

Strengthening. Tai chi helps tone muscles in the lower body, especially the thighs, buttocks, and calves.

Increases flexibility. The choreographed exercises gently take your joints through their full range of motion. One recent study found that the controlled movement of tai chi can be helpful for people with arthritis (but check with your doctor first). Other research has found that it can aid recovery from injuries.

Improves posture. Your head, neck, and spine are usually aligned, thus minimizing strain on the neck and lower back.

Enhances balance. Tai chi calls for smooth, slow movement that requires balance, coordination, and body awareness. That's why many college and professional sports teams include tai chi as part of their training.

Induces relaxation. For many people, tai chi has some of the same psychological benefits of yoga. The concentration on the body's fluid motion and on breathing helps them relax and relieve tension and anxiety.

May even provide a modest aerobic workout. An Australian study from 1989 as well as a Taiwanese study last year found that a regular program of tai chi works the heart as much as other types of moderate exercise.

Tai chi requires no special clothing or equipment and can be done anywhere—even in a small space. The best way to learn tai chi is in a class from an experienced instructor who can guide you through the positions. Tai chi classes are often available at the Y, health clubs, colleges, and adult education programs. Check the Yellow Pages under "martial arts instruction." Classes generally begin with meditation and warm-ups and end with a cooldown period. Books and videos may also be helpful, though these seldom can take the place of a qualified instructor. It takes years to truly master tai chi, but within a few weeks you can learn several movements and start to reap the physical and mental benefits.

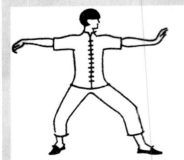 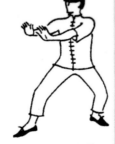

Postures from two common forms: the "single whip" (left) and "grasping the bird's tail" (right). The essence of tai chi is movement, however, not static poses.

What Do You Think?

1. Would you consider trying to learn Tai Chi as a way to increase your daily physical activity? Explain your rationale.
2. What factors might account for the growing popularity of Tai Chi as a form of exercise and stress management?

Reprinted by permission from the *University of California at Berkeley Wellness Letter,* © Health Letter Associates, 1994.

Summary

1. The key to leading a physically active lifestyle is to find aerobic activities that you consider play.

2. There are many benefits of physical activity, including psychological, cardiovascular, weight control, and disease prevention.

3. Fitness can be described as the ability to function efficiently. The American College of Sports Medicine has delineated four major components of fitness; cardiorespiratory endurance, muscular fitness, flexibility, and body composition.

4. There are four generally accepted principles of fitness: overload, specificity, individual differences, and reversibility.

5. Aerobic exercise causes a sustained increase in heart rate and uses the large muscles of the body for an extended period of time. Long-distance running, bicycling, brisk walking, and swimming are considered good aerobic activities.

6. Aerobic exercise has two major goals: to increase the total amount of blood and oxygen circulated throughout the body during exercise and to improve the ability of the large skeletal muscles to utilize the oxygen circulated.

7. Anaerobic exercise requires an intense, maximum burst of energy and is of short duration. A tennis serve and a 100-yard dash are examples of anaerobic exercise.

8. There are many ways to measure physical fitness. A stress test and Cooper's one-mile walking test are two good ways to measure aerobic fitness levels.

9. When designing an aerobic exercise program it is important to consider frequency, intensity, and time (F.I.T.).

10. The American College of Sports Medicine and the Centers for Disease Control and Prevention recommend that all adults, in order to receive *health promotion benefits* of physical activity, should accumulate thirty minutes or more of moderate-intensity physical activity on most, preferably all, days of the week.

11. The American College of Sports Medicine recommends that healthy adults who want to receive the *physical fitness benefits* of physical activity should participate in vigorous aerobic exercise three to five days a week.

12. Target heart rate is the specific percentage of an individual's maximal heart rate; it is the rate that is the goal when exercising aerobically.

13. It is important to begin each exercise session with an appropriate warm-up period and end it with a cooldown period. Warm-ups and cooldowns help to prevent exercise injuries.

14. Stretching exercises are good activities to include in the warm-up and cooldown periods. Stretching also makes an important contribution to total fitness by increasing flexibility.

15. The American College of Sports Medicine suggests that aerobic exercise programs progress gradually from very low-level activities to more strenuous activities. Three stages of conditioning are recommended: the initial-conditioning stage; the improvement-conditioning stage; and the maintenance stage.

16. People don't *find* the time to exercise. They must *make* time. Choosing activities that are enjoyable and playful helps, as will building a support network for play. Experiment with physical activity as one avenue to wellness.

Recommended Readings

American College of Sports Medicine. (1992) *ACSM Fitness Book.* (Champaign, Illinois: Leisure Press).

The ACSM Fitness Book provides an easy-to-follow overview of beginning a fitness program to improve cardiovascular endurance, muscular fitness, flexibility, and body composition. Measures are included for testing yourself on all four measures of physical fitness. Tips are also provided on how to select appropriate exercise equipment and fitness books or videos.

Institute for Aerobics Research. (1990) *The Strength Connection: How to Build Strength and Improve the Quality of Your Life.* (Dallas, Tex.: Institute for Aerobics Research).

This well-written book focuses on the health and fitness benefits of a balanced fitness program. While aerobic activity is covered, this book focuses on the contributions of strength and flexibility to total fitness. Assessment tests and suggested strength and flexibility programs are offered.

White, Timothy P., and the editors of the University of California at Berkeley Wellness Letter. (1993) *The Wellness Guide to Lifelong Fitness.* (New York: REBUS).

This practical and beautifully illustrated book offers valuable guidance on how to participate in a wide variety of physical activities. Walking, running, swimming, cycling, aerobic movement, stretching, and strength training are all discussed in some detail.

References

1. Centers for Disease Control. (1993) *Health, United States, 1992 and Healthy People 2000 Review* (Washington, D.C.: U.S. Government Printing Office).

2. U.S. Department of Health and Human Services. (1991) *Healthy People 2000: National Health Promotion and Disease Prevention Objectives* (Washington, D.C.: U.S. Government Printing Office), 610.

3. "Prevalence of sedentary lifestyle—behavioral risk factor surveillance system, United States, 1991." (1993) MMWR 42 (29): 576–579.

4. Magnus, Marcia H. (1991) "Cardiovascular health among African-Americans: A review of the health status, risk reduction, and

intervention strategies." *American Journal of Health Promotion* 5 (4): 284.

5. Lewis, Cora E., James M. Raczynski, Greg W. Heath, Richard Levinson, and Gary R. Cutter. (1993) "Physical activity of public housing residents in Birmingham, Alabama." *American Journal of Public Health* 83 (7): 1016–1020.

6. Cheadle, Allen, David Pearson, Edward Wagner, Bruce M. Psaty, Paula Diehr, and Thomas Koepsell. (1994) "Relationship between socioeconomic status, health status, and lifestyle practices of American Indians: Evidence from a Plains reservation population." *Public Health Reports* 109 (3): 405–413.

7. "Prevalence of Sedentary Lifestyle," 576–577.

8. Sheehan, George. (1988) "Pursuing happiness." *The Physician and Sportsmedicine* 16 (1): 45.

9. "Which exercise is best for you?" (1994) *Consumer Reports on Health* 6 (4): 40.

10. Girdano, Daniel A., George S. Everly, Jr., and Dorothy E. Dusek. (1990) *Controlling Stress and Tension: A Holistic Approach,* 3d ed. (Englewood Cliffs, N.J.), 263.

11. Powers, Scott K., and Edward T. Howley. (1994) *Exercise Physiology: Theory and Application to Fitness and Performance,* 2d ed. (Dubuque, Iowa: Brown & Benchmark Publishers), 83.

12. "A lifelong program to build strong bones." (1993) *UC Berkeley Wellness Letter* 9 (10): 4–5.

13. "Which exercise is best for you?" 37.

14. Smith, E. L. and C. Gilligan. (1987) "Effects of inactivity and exercise on bone." *The Physician and Sportsmedicine* 15 (11): 91–92, 95–96, 98–99, 102.

15. Paffenbarger, Ralph S., Jr., Robert T. Hyde, Alvin L. Wing, I-Min Lee, Dexter L. Jung, and James B. Kapert. (1993) "The association of changes in physical-activity level and other lifestyle characteristics with mortality among men." *The New England Journal of Medicine* 328 (8): 538–545.

16. Girdano, Daniel A., George S. Everly, Jr., and Dorothy E. Dusek, *Controlling Stress and Tension,* 270.

17. "Women on the walk." (1992) *Nutrition Action Healthletter* 19 (2): 4.

18. "Research notes: Exercise." (1993) *Nutrition Week* XXIII (47): 7–8.

19. Seer, Beth. (1993) "Actively avoiding diabetes." *American Health* XII (5): 88.

20. Schardt, David. (1993) "These feet were made for walking." *Nutrition Action Healthletter* 20 (10): 6.

21. "New guidelines offer exercise standards." (1991) *The Physician and Sportsmedicine* 19 (4): 38–39.

22. Herbert, William G., Victor F. Froelicher, and John D. Cantwell. (1991) "Exercise tests for coronary and asymptomatic patients: Risk factors and methods." *The Physician and Sportsmedicine* 19 (2): 56.

23. "Pulsepoints: More than half (54%) of Americans." (1993) *American Health* XII (8): 10.

24. Haskell, William L. (1994) "Health consequences of physical activity: Understanding the challenges regarding dose-response." *Medicine and Science in Sports and Exercise* 26 (6): 649–660.

25. Pate, R. R., Pratt, M., Blair, S. N., Haskell, W. L., Macera, C. A., Bouchard, C., Buchner, D., Ettinger, W., Heath, G. W., King, A. C., Kriska, A., Leon, A. S., Marcus, B. H., Morris, J., Paffenbarger, R. S., Patrick, K., Pollock, M. L., Rippe, J. M., Sallis, J., & Wilmore, J. H. (1985) "Physical activity and public health: A recommendation from the Centers for Disease Control and Prevention and the American College of Sports Medicine." *JAMA* 273: 402–407.

26. American College of Sports Medicine. (1991) *Guidelines for Exercise Testing and Prescription,* 4th ed. (Philadelphia: Lea & Febiger).

27. "Exercise without injury." (March, 1990) *U.C. Berkeley Wellness Letter:* 4–5.

28. American College of Sports Medicine. (1986) *Guidelines for Exercise Testing and Prescription,* 3rd ed. (Philadelphia: Lea & Febiger).

29. "Racquetball players." (1982) *Independence Health Plan Newsletter* 2 (3).

30. Bennion, L. J., E. L. Bierman, and J. M. Ferguson. (1991) *Straight Talk About Weight Control: Taking Pounds Off and Keeping Them Off.* (Mount Vernon, N.Y.: Consumers Union), 242.

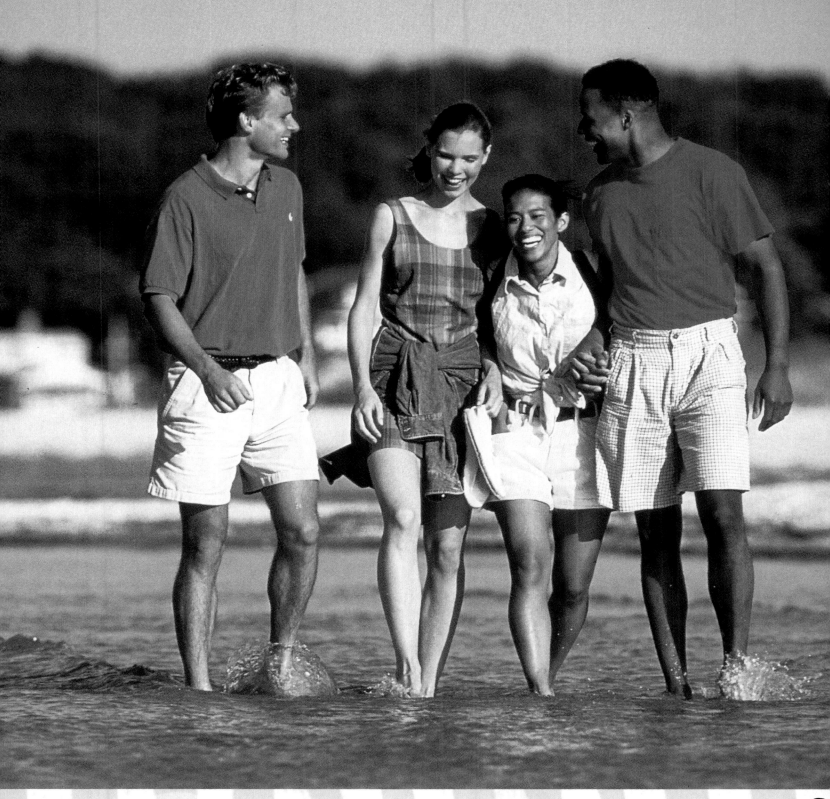

Relationships, Social Support, and Well-Being

UNIT II

Unit I concentrated on your wellness level as an individual. Our relationships with others are also an essential part of wellness. In Unit II we will consider intimate relationships and their impact on health and well-being.

Sexual relationships serve as a beginning point for examining intimate relationships. In chapter 6, you will learn about sexuality and lifestyle choices, as well as the factors that influence those choices. Decisions about sexual behaviors and lifestyle options, and the relationships that develop as a result of those decisions, can have a profound effect on your level of well-being.

When sexual intimacy leads to pregnancy, new family relationships are born. In chapter 7, the structure and function of the female and male reproductive systems are presented as a foundation for discussions about pregnancy and parenting, as well as about family planning, which is discussed in chapter 8. The decision to become a parent, and the timing of starting or adding to your family, will have many and varying effects on your health and well-being and that of significant others in your life.

Human Sexuality: Behavior and Relationship Options

Chapter 6

Student Learning Objectives

Upon completion of this chapter, you should be able to:

1. define human sexuality;
2. differentiate between gender identity and gender roles giving an example of each;
3. classify influences on gender identity and gender roles as biological or social;
4. explain the concept of androgyny and assess whether you are currently adopting an androgynous gender role;
5. list and describe the phases of human sexual response for both the female and male;
6. describe the concept of a sexual orientation continuum;
7. identify and briefly describe the types of theory that attempt to explain the development of sexual orientation;
8. differentiate among Sternberg's three components of a love relationship;
9. analyze Sternberg's ten rules of love in terms of enhancing communication between people who love each other;
10. assess your current love relationships for intimacy, passion, and commitment;
11. analyze the characteristics you seek in a romantic partner;
12. identify common research limitations regarding the study of human sexual behavior;
13. explain the strengths of the National Health and Social Life Survey in terms of describing sexual behavior in the U.S.;
14. describe common sexual behaviors and their prevalence in the U.S.;
15. briefly describe four common sexual performance problems;

16. list four sources of referral that could help you locate a certified sex therapist, and five questions you should ask a therapist before you start treatment;
17. describe common sexual relationship lifestyle options and their demographic profiles;
18. analyze whether or not U.S. society privileges some people's differences at the expense of others;
19. evaluate five social and technological developments that have affected sexual relationships in the U.S.

Chromosome: a threadlike structure containing genes, found in the nucleus of every cell.

Zygote: the term for a human egg (ovum) that has been fertilized by a sperm cell (spermatozoon) before the process of cell division begins.

Testes: the primary male reproductive organs, also known as testicles, that produce sperm and testosterone.

Testosterone: the primary male sex hormone. Testosterone stimulates the development of a male physique and reproductive organs. It also maintains the viability of the adult reproductive organs.

Penis: the external male reproductive organ that contains the urethra through which both sperm and urine are discharged.

Epididymis: a structure in the male reproductive system located over the testes whose major function is the temporary storage of sperm.

Vas deferens: a structure of the male reproductive system that originates in the scrotum, circles the bladder, and eventually joins with the urethra. Its function is to transport sperm from the epididymis to the urethra.

Our relationships with others, which offer us opportunities to fulfill our need to love and be loved, are an essential aspect of wellness. In this chapter we will look at sexual relationships as a beginning point for examining intimate, loving relationships.

The college years are often a time of exploration in terms of finding and maintaining intimate love relationships. In this chapter you will learn about sexual behavior and lifestyle choices, as well as the factors that influence those choices. You will be afforded an opportunity to explore sexual lifestyle options, and the relationships that develop as a result of such decisions. There is no doubt that intimate relationship decisions will have a profound effect on your level of well-being, now and throughout your life.

Defining Human Sexuality

Much has been written about human sexuality, but there is not one widely accepted definition. In looking at sexuality from a wellness perspective, **sexuality** refers to our need for love and personal fulfillment, the pursuit of sexual pleasure, as well as the desire to reproduce. Sexuality also includes our awareness of and reaction to our sense of femaleness and maleness, and that of everyone with whom we interact.[1] The term sexuality encompasses femininity, masculinity, desire, satisfaction, love, loss, intimacy, loneliness, caring, sharing, touching, jealousy, rejection, self-esteem, and joy.

Gender Identity and Gender Roles

One important component of sexuality is **gender,** or the sociocultural expression of one's masculinity or femininity. When discussing the influences that are thought to be related to how children acquire behaviors that are gender appropriate, according to a particular culture, researchers differentiate between **gender identity** and **gender role.** Gender identity refers to an *individual's sense* of being female or male. Most children identify themselves as either male or female by the time they are three years old. Gender

role, on the other hand, refers to *society's expectations* of what are appropriate female and male feelings, thoughts, and actions. Over the years, research studies addressing the determinants of gender have identified numerous influences. These influences on gender are commonly grouped as biological and social.

Biological Influences on Gender

Biological factors influence sexuality in several important ways. First, there are chromosomal variations, but virtually everyone is either a genetic male or a genetic female (see figure 6.1). Genetic blueprints, established at the moment of fertilization, cause the fetus to develop either female or male internal and external reproductive organs. At conception, an X-shaped **chromosome** from the egg and either an X- or Y-shaped chromosome from the sperm are paired, and are referred to as the 23rd chromosome pair. If a **zygote** has two X chromosomes for the 23rd chromosome pair, the sex of the developing embryo will be female. If the 23rd pair of chromosomes is XY, the developing embryo will be a male.

For the first six weeks of gestation female and male embryos look the same. It is believed that the general blueprint for human development is female. However, during the seventh week of development, the Y chromosome, if present, stimulates the male **testes** to begin to develop. Soon the testes begin to produce **androgens,** or male sex hormones, the most potent of which is **testosterone.** The variety of male sex hormones stimulate the embryo to develop male reproductive organs, such as a **penis, epididymis, vas deferens,** and **seminal vesicles.** If sufficient amounts of androgens are *not* present, the embryo will continue to develop as a female. **Ovaries** will begin to form during the eleventh or twelfth weeks of gestation.

A second biological influence on gender involves the prenatal sexual differentiation of the brain. Researchers have begun to investigate the possibility that female and male brains are structurally and functionally different. Much of the research to date has focused on an area of the brain called the **hypothalamus,** and the changes that occur to it, probably during the second trimester of

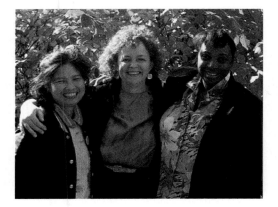

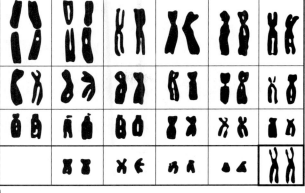

Figure 6.1: This illustration depicts the genetic differences between women and men.
In (a) you see the chromosome structure of a female and in (b) the chromosome structure of a male. You should note that the *only* difference appears in the 23rd chromosome pair, located in the lower right corner of each illustration. The female 23rd chromosome pair contains two X-shaped chromosomes while the male 23rd pair consists of one X-shaped and one Y-shaped chromosome.

a.

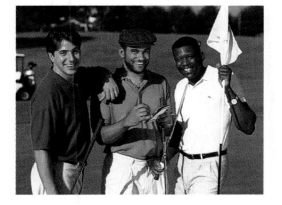

b.

fetal development.[2] It is believed that once the Y-shaped sex chromosome triggers sufficient production of testosterone in a male fetus, the testosterone is carried in the blood to the hypothalamus where it causes an *insensitivity* to **estrogen,** the female sex hormone. In a female fetus, where there is little androgens present, a *sensitivity* to estrogen develops. This sensitivity to estrogen is believed to be important in regulating a woman's menstrual cycle, beginning in puberty. The research into prenatal sexual differentiation of the brain is still in its infancy. Areas of the brain other than the hypothalamus may also be affected by sex hormones, influencing gender in presently unknown ways.

In any event, these genetic and hormonal influences on gender form the basis of the *nature* perspective in the nature versus nurture debate. The nature perspective argues that a person is born to be either a man or a woman. It suggests that a person's physical gender, male or female, and several respective characteristics such as aggressiveness, mathematical skills, verbal skills, and nurturing behavior are determined at the

moment of fertilization. Furthermore, this view of gender identity and gender roles proposes that such genetic gender traits have been passed down through the human race because they have been traits that helped the human species survive and reproduce. This view of gender determination is controversial, however. Opponents of the nature perspective contend that biology is *not* destiny, and that social influences (the nurture perspective) play an important role in both gender identity and gender roles.

Social Influences on Gender

Social influences are believed to affect gender identity and gender roles through the process of social expectations and imitation. These influences operate through social rewards and punishments as molders of an individual's gender-related behavior.

Social learning theory suggests that society directs a child's development of either male or female characteristics through rewards and punishment, as well as through the process of role modeling and imitation. Both the role modeling and reinforcement of stereotypic gender roles is pervasive in the

Seminal vesicles: two small glands found in the male reproductive tract at the end of the vas deferens. These glands produce fluid that contains a simple sugar which provides nutrients for the sperm. Additionally, they produce prostaglandins that help in stimulating sperm locomotion as well as contractions of the female's reproductive tract, both of which aid in the transport of sperm through the female reproductive tract.

Ovaries: the primary female reproductive organs that produce mature eggs and estrogen, the female sex hormone.

Hypothalamus: a small part of the forebrain, located below the cerebrum, that is linked to both the thalamus and the pituitary gland.

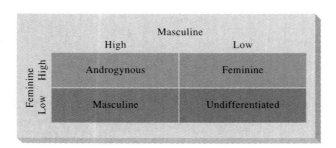

	Masculine	
	High	Low
Feminine High	Androgynous	Feminine
Feminine Low	Masculine	Undifferentiated

through example and social reinforcement, encourage people to think and act within gender-role stereotypes.

Most human-sexuality researchers believe that gender identity and gender roles are influenced by both biological and social factors. Although biology dictates genetic gender and may influence brain development in unknown ways, society strongly influences how women and men think and act in terms of gender identity and gender roles. This middle-of-the-road perspective embraces the notion that you are a product of *nature* (your biological self) and *nurture* (your social environment).

Gender-Role Classification

In the U.S. today gender role is not solely a choice between female or male roles. Many individuals choose to behave in ways that allow them to exhibit both male and female characteristics. This gender role is labeled **androgyny,** and has become more socially acceptable in the U.S. over the past twenty years.

The concept of androgyny asks us to think of gender roles as consisting of a mixture of masculine and feminine traits. Individuals who exhibit mostly masculine traits would be accepting the traditional masculine role while people who exhibit a high level of traditionally female traits would be taking a feminine gender role (see figure 6.2). Individuals who have high levels of both masculine and feminine traits would be considered to be following an androgynous gender role. And finally, some individuals may exhibit low levels of both traditional male and female traits and are considered to be undifferentiated in terms of gender-role classification. What gender role have you adopted at this point in your life? Activity for Wellness 6.1, the Bem Sex-Role Inventory, will help you determine your gender-role classification.

Another important aspect of human sexuality involves the physiological response to sexual arousal. Sexual arousal and orgasm satisfy the desire for sexual pleasure and biologically reinforce a behavior that often leads to the reproduction of the human species.

Human Sexual Response

Until 1966 relatively little was known about the physiological events involved in human sexual arousal. William Masters and Virginia Johnson

U.S. and can be found in educational, courting, marital, and occupational settings.

In the U.S., infant boys may be treated more roughly than infant girls. Traditionally, boys are expected to be more aggressive, athletic, ambitious, and unemotional than girls. Girls, on the other hand, are traditionally expected to be more affectionate, tender, maternal, and outwardly emotional than boys. Such traditional gender roles are often modeled for children by their parents, other adults, and television. For instance, if women are always responsible for the cooking and cleaning at home, they are modeling these behaviors as appropriate gender roles for women. If men are always responsible for doing the yard work, such as mowing the lawn, they are modeling gender-role behavior as well. Children observe and imitate the gender behaviors of the adults in their lives.

Parents and other adults also reward or punish certain gender-role behaviors. For example, when a parent praises (rewards) their son for playing with trucks or their daughter for playing with dolls, they are teaching gender roles. When young children take on behaviors associated with the opposite **gender-role stereotype** they may be told that this is not appropriate behavior for a girl or boy. Children may even be labeled as a "sissy" or "tomboy." These responses serve as negative reinforcement or punishment for behaviors that are viewed as inappropriate. Adults too receive positive reinforcements for following gender-role stereotypes and negative feedback for straying from socially accepted gender roles.

The social influence (nurture) perspective suggests that society guides people into a male or female role with every phase of a person's life carrying a masculine or feminine expectation, behavior, or attitude. Social learning theory suggests that cultures,

Gender-role stereotype: an oversimplified and often greatly distorted idea of how each gender should think, feel, and behave. Gender-role stereotypes are often sanctioned and rewarded by the dominant culture.

Androgyny: the adoption of behaviors that exhibit high levels of both male and female characteristics.

The Bem Sex-Role Inventory: Are You Androgynous?

The following items are from the Bem Sex-Role Inventory. To find out whether you score as androgynous, first rate yourself on each item, on a scale from 1 (never or almost never true) to 7 (always or almost always true).

Item	*Your Rating*
1. self-reliant	_____
2. yielding	_____
3. helpful	_____
4. defends own beliefs	_____
5. cheerful	_____
6. moody	_____
7. independent	_____
8. shy	_____
9. conscientious	_____
10. athletic	_____
11. affectionate	_____
12. theatrical	_____
13. assertive	_____
14. flatterable	_____
15. happy	_____
16. strong personality	_____
17. loyal	_____
18. unpredictable	_____
19. forceful	_____
20. feminine	_____
21. reliable	_____
22. analytical	_____
23. sympathetic	_____
24. jealous	_____
25. has leadership abilities	_____
26. sensitive to the needs of others	_____
27. truthful	_____
28. willing to take risks	_____
29. understanding	_____
30. secretive	_____
31. makes decisions easily	_____
32. compassionate	_____
33. sincere	_____
34. self-sufficient	_____
35. eager to soothe hurt feelings	_____
36. conceited	_____
37. dominant	_____
38. soft-spoken	_____
39. likable	_____
40. masculine	_____
41. warm	_____
42. solemn	_____
43. willing to take a stand	_____
44. tender	_____
45. friendly	_____
46. aggressive	_____
47. gullible	_____
48. inefficient	_____
49. acts as a leader	_____
50. childlike	_____
51. adaptable	_____
52. individualistic	_____
53. does not use harsh language	_____
54. unsystematic	_____
55. competitive	_____
56. loves children	_____
57. tactful	_____

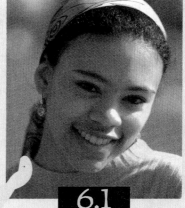

6.1

Activity for Wellness

58. ambitious	_____
59. gentle	_____
60. conventional	_____

Scoring

a) Add up your ratings for items 1, 4, 7, 10, 13, 16, 19, 22, 25, 28, 31, 34, 37, 40, 43, 46, 49, 55, and 58. Divide the total by 20. That is your masculinity score.

b) Add up your ratings for items 2, 5, 8, 11, 14, 17, 20, 23, 26, 29, 32, 35, 38, 41, 44, 47, 50, 53, 56, and 59. Divide the total by 20. That is your femininity score.

c) If your masculinity score is above 4.9 (the approximate median for the masculinity scale) and your femininity score is above 4.9 (the approximate femininity median) then you would be classified as androgynous on Bem's scale.

From: Janet S. Hyde, *Half the Human Experience: The Psychology of Women,* 3d ed. Copyright © 1985 D.C. Heath and Company, Lexington, MA. Reprinted by permission.

---

opened the door to this kind of research by publishing their observations of humans during sexual arousal.[3]

Masters and Johnson described two major physiological events that occur during sexual response: vasocongestion and myotonia. **Vasocongestion** occurs when blood fills the sexual organs such as the penis or **vulva.** **Myotonia** refers to the muscles becoming tight and rigid. Masters and Johnson also separated the human sexual response cycle into four consecutive phases: excitement, plateau, orgasmic, and resolution.

Excitement Phase

The first phase of sexual response is termed the **excitement phase.** During this phase the female begins to secrete vaginal fluids. These

Vulva: the anatomical name for the female external genitalia. The vulva consists of two paired folds of skin that surround the female's vaginal and urethral openings and extend to the clitoris.

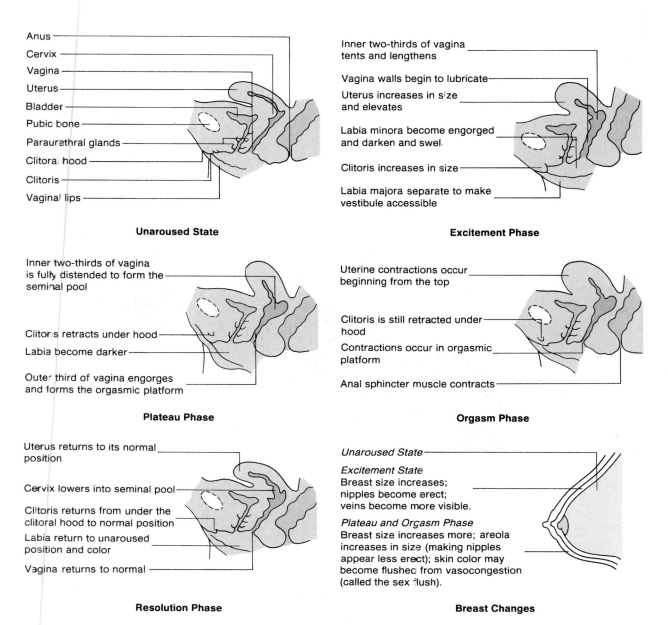

Unaroused State

- Anus
- Cervix
- Vagina
- Uterus
- Bladder
- Pubic bone
- Paraurethral glands
- Clitoral hood
- Clitoris
- Vaginal lips

Excitement Phase

- Inner two-thirds of vagina tents and lengthens
- Vagina walls begin to lubricate
- Uterus increases in size and elevates
- Labia minora become engorged and darken and swell
- Clitoris increases in size
- Labia majora separate to make vestibule accessible

Plateau Phase

- Inner two-thirds of vagina is fully distended to form the seminal pool
- Clitoris retracts under hood
- Labia become darker
- Outer third of vagina engorges and forms the orgasmic platform

Orgasm Phase

- Uterine contractions occur beginning from the top
- Clitoris is still retracted under hood
- Contractions occur in orgasmic platform
- Anal sphincter muscle contracts

Resolution Phase

- Uterus returns to its normal position
- Cervix lowers into seminal pool
- Clitoris returns from under the clitoral hood to normal position
- Labia return to unaroused position and color
- Vagina returns to normal

Breast Changes

Unaroused State

Excitement State
Breast size increases; nipples become erect; veins become more visible.

Plateau and Orgasm Phase
Breast size increases more; areola increases in size (making nipples appear less erect); skin color may become flushed from vasocongestion (called the sex flush).

Figure 6.3: Physical changes in the female during the sexual response cycle

Cervix: the opening of the uterus which connects with the vagina.

Scrotal skin: skin that forms a sac that is suspended in the groin of males and houses the two testes.

Clitoris: a small erectile organ located in the female at the top of the labia. Like the male penis, the clitoris becomes erect and sensitive when sexually stimulated.

Orgasm: the climax of sexual excitement, consisting of sudden muscle contractions followed by a distinct release of sexual tension.

fluids make the vagina more supple and less sensitive to friction. The vagina, **cervix,** and vulva expand due to vasocongestion, and the nipples become erect (see figure 6.3).

The male excitement phase begins with the penis becoming erect due to vasocongestion. The **scrotal skin** becomes smooth and the testes are drawn closer to the body (see figure 6.4).

Plateau Phase

The **plateau phase** follows the excitement phase. During the plateau phase the female's vagina continues to swell until it reaches the

"orgasmic platform," which causes the opening of the vagina to narrow by 30 percent or more. Additionally, the **clitoris** withdraws into its hood. The inner vaginal lips display color changes indicating that **orgasm** is imminent. Changes in skin color may occur in other parts of the female body as well. There may also be an increase in breast size.

For the male during the plateau stage the head of the penis and the testes increase in size. A male may also experience a skin color change around his penis. A small amount of **seminal fluid,** which may contain viable sperm, may drip from the penis.

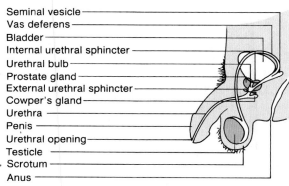

- Seminal vesicle
- Vas deferens
- Bladder
- Internal urethral sphincter
- Urethral bulb
- Prostate gland
- External urethral sphincter
- Cowper's gland
- Urethra
- Penis
- Urethral opening
- Testicle
- Scrotum
- Anus

Unaroused State

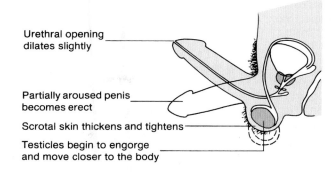

- Urethral opening dilates slightly
- Partially aroused penis becomes erect
- Scrotal skin thickens and tightens
- Testicles begin to engorge and move closer to the body

Excitement Phase

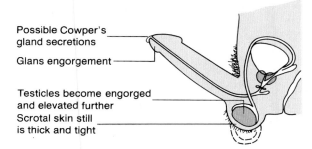

- Possible Cowper's gland secretions
- Glans engorgement
- Testicles become engorged and elevated further
- Scrotal skin still is thick and tight

Plateau Phase

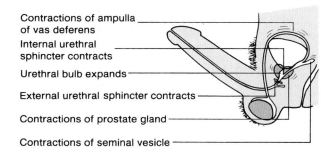

- Contractions of ampulla of vas deferens
- Internal urethral sphincter contracts
- Urethral bulb expands
- External urethral sphincter contracts
- Contractions of prostate gland
- Contractions of seminal vesicle

Orgasm Phase: Emission Stage

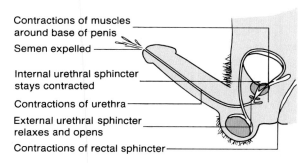

- Contractions of muscles around base of penis
- Semen expelled
- Internal urethral sphincter stays contracted
- Contractions of urethra
- External urethral sphincter relaxes and opens
- Contractions of rectal sphincter

Orgasm Phase: Expulsion Stage

- Rapid partial decrease in size of penis; then slow return to unaroused state and size
- Testicles become smaller and move down from the body
- Scrotal skin thins and becomes more loose

Resolution

Figure 6.4: Physical changes in the male during the sexual response cycle

Orgasmic Phase

The **orgasmic phase** is the third phase of sexual response. Orgasm for humans is the sudden release of sexual tension resulting in pleasurable feelings. Orgasm is a feeling of physical satisfaction unlike any other moment of the sexual response cycle.

Female orgasm involves anywhere from three to fifteen quick rhythmic muscular contractions of the uterus and vagina. Other muscle groups of the female's body may contract during orgasm as well. Females are capable of multiple orgasms, which is a rapid return to orgasm after an orgasmic experience (see figure 6.3).

Orgasm for the male begins with the pooling of semen into the **urethra.** Two sphincter muscles close off the urethra to the

bladder during this stage. One sphincter muscle opens to the penis allowing semen to exit, propelled by several short muscular contractions. The release of semen (**ejaculation**) does not necessarily occur simultaneously with orgasm. Males can release semen without experiencing an orgasm or experience the pleasurable sensations of orgasm without releasing average quantities of semen.

Resolution Phase

The final stage of sexual response is the **resolution phase.** During this phase both males and females return to their pre-excited state. Blood is pumped away from the sexual organs and muscles begin to relax. Heartbeat, respiration, and brain-wave patterns also

Seminal fluid: the fluid component discharged from the male reproductive tract at ejaculation. This fluid contains sperm, fructose to supply the sperm with an energy source, and prostaglandins that are thought to help move sperm to the fallopian tubes for possible fertilization of an egg.

Male urethra: a tube that conducts urine from the bladder, through the penis, to the exterior of the body. This tube also conducts semen from the male reproductive system to the exterior of the body.

Ejaculation: the expulsion of semen from the urethra, usually accompanied by orgasm.

Figure 6.5: Continuum of sexual orientation. This continuum ranges from exclusive heterosexuality, which Kinsey and associates (1948) rated as 0, to exclusive homosexuality (rated 6). People who are about equally attracted to both sexes (ratings 2 to 4) are bisexual.

From Alfred C. Kinsey, et al. *Sexual Behavior in the Human Male*, 1948. Reprinted by permission of The Kinsey Institute for Research in Sex, Gender, and Reproduction, Inc.

Exclusively heterosexual behavior	0
Largely heterosexual, but incidental homosexual behavior	1
Largely heterosexual, but more than incidental homosexual behavior	2
Equal amounts of heterosexual and homosexual behavior	3
Largely homosexual, but more than incidental heterosexual behavior	4
Largely homosexual, but incidental heterosexual behavior	5
Exclusively homosexual behavior	6

return to their pre-excited state. In males, a recovery period, often referred to as a **refractory period,** often takes place before a second orgasm can be experienced (see figure 6.4). The length of time needed for recovery varies with different men and increases as men grow older.

Many factors can affect the sexual response cycle, including the circumstances of sexual arousal (erotic literature, fantasies), drugs (legal and illegal), health, and age. The brain is an integral part of this cycle. Keep in mind that individuals go through the sexual response cycle in different ways. Even the same individual may experience sexual arousal in many ways, under different circumstances.

Another important aspect of human sexuality involves **sexual orientation.** Sexual orientation can be defined as the direction of an individual's sexual interest, either toward individuals of the opposite sex, the same sex, or both.

Sexual Orientation

Sexual orientation is often thought of as a continuum ranging from **heterosexual orientation** at one end to **homosexual orientation** at the other. An orientation somewhere between heterosexual and homosexual is labeled as **bisexual,** indicating that an individual is sexually attracted to both men and women. As early as 1948, Kinsey and his colleagues proposed a seven-point continuum depicting the range of sexual *behavior* seen in humans (see figure 6.5). One of the most important contributions of Kinsey's continuum was the acknowledgment that there is a range of

sexual behavior between exclusively heterosexual and exclusively homosexual behavior. In fact, it is this range of behavior that makes defining a person's sexual orientation so difficult. For instance, would you consider a man to be homosexually oriented if, as an adolescent boy, he had one sexual encounter with someone of his own sex, but throughout the rest of his life desired sexual relationships with women? Would a female prisoner be considered homosexually oriented if she had a sexual relationship with another female while she was in prison and denied access to relationships with men, even though her preference would be to have sexual relationships with men? Or would you consider a man to be heterosexual because he has never engaged in sexual behavior with another man, even though he finds men more sexually attractive than women?

A recent survey of sexual behavior in the United States[4] has shed some light on the issue of sexual orientation. Researchers at the University of Chicago asked a random sample of 3,432 people in the U.S. between the ages of eighteen and fifty-nine questions about a variety of aspects concerning their sexual behavior. In terms of sexual orientation, the researchers point out that at least three different measures relate to understanding sexual orientation, including having a *sexual attraction* to one sex or both, engaging in *sexual behavior* with individuals of one sex or both, and one's *perceptions of* his or her *identity* as either heterosexual, homosexual, or bisexual. Each of these measures produced a different view of sexual orientation and sexual behavior in the United States. For instance, while 5.5 percent

Heterosexual orientation: a form of sexual orientation where individuals are sexually attracted to and often engage in sexual activities with opposite-sex partners.

Homosexual orientation: a form of sexual orientation where individuals are sexually attracted to and often engage in sexual activities with same-sex partners.

Development of Sexual Orientation

Despite considerable research on sexual orientation, the development of heterosexuality, bisexuality, or homosexuality is still uncertain. Over the years, many theories on sexual orientation have been proposed. Some have been conclusively disproven, but none has been conclusively proven. Such theories can be categorized as biological, psychological, or cultural. Each of these categories influences the others, and all seem to influence our choice of sexual partners.

Biological Theories

During the 1990s the likelihood that biological factors contribute to the development of sexual orientation has received increasing emphasis. Evidence that biology plays at least some role has come from preliminary studies linking measurable differences in the size of several parts of the brain to sexual orientation. Further, evidence for a biological influence comes from studies showing that identical twins, who are genetically alike, have a greater rate of concordance (similarity) in their sexual orientation than do fraternal twins, who are not genetically alike.

One of the first biological factors to be examined for a relationship to sexual orientation was the sex chromosomes. No visible differences in the sex chromosomes or other chromosomes of heterosexual, bisexual, and homosexual people was evident. Gay or straight males are XY while lesbian or straight females are XX. Whether there are specific genes for sexual orientation, which might be present on any of the chromosomes, is unknown at this time. If genes do influence sexual orientation, they probably act by affecting the prenatal hormonal conditioning of the brain, which may (many authorities would say probably) influence our sexual orientation.

The role of sex hormones in influencing sexual orientation has been researched, but much conflicting information has been published. Hormones can have organizing or activating effects. Little, if any, activating effect of hormones on sexual orientation during adolescent or adult life is apparent. Hormones may very well, however, exert an organizing influence on sexual orientation early in fetal development. Many researchers now believe that prenatal hormone-influenced sexual differentiation of the brain does contribute to our sexual orientation.

Psychological Theories

Even if sexual orientation is conclusively proven to have biological roots or influences, psychological factors will still almost certainly be recognized as influencing how we express our sexuality. To expect that any single mechanism could account for so complex a phenomenon as human sexual orientation seems unrealistic.

Many psychological theories on sexual orientation have been proposed, but none has gained universal acceptance. Psychological theories on sexual orientation often presume that the normal pattern of development is toward a heterosexual orientation and that a homosexual orientation is the result of something going astray in that development. This frame of mind, however, can build a bias into research, making it difficult to formulate and test a theory that adequately explains the development of heterosexual, bisexual, and homosexual orientations.

The American Psychiatric Association, in its official *Diagnostic and Statistical Manual of Mental Disorders,* third edition, revised (DSM-IIIR) does not list homosexuality as a disorder. The closest applicable diagnosis is "persistent and marked distress about one's sexual orientation" in which the distress rather than the orientation is viewed as a disorder.

Cultural Theories

Different expectations for females and males exist in every known society. Although the behavioral boundaries between the sexes vary considerably from culture to culture, there is a general expectation in every society that most adult men and women will cohabit (live together) and produce the next generation. Social pressure is thus applied for members to engage in heterosexual behavior. The general rule is that one should have a mate of the other sex and produce children.

Those behaviors that are considered to be homosexual vary from culture to culture. What is considered homosexuality in one culture may be considered appropriate behavior within gender roles in another culture. For example, in the U.S., fellatio and anal intercourse between two males is generally (unless

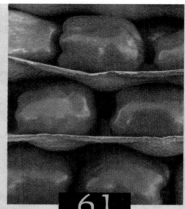

6.1
Of Special Interest

force is involved) considered homosexual behavior for both parties. However, in some cultures, such as Mexico, Brazil, Greece, Turkey, and Morocco, only the passive recipient (insertee) is considered homosexual while the active insertor is not.[1] Further, some societies, such as those in the highlands of New Guinea, have incorporated what in many cultures are considered homosexual acts into their male rituals. For example, the swallowing of semen through fellatio by young males is considered essential for proper growth, strength, and masculinity.

Regardless of whatever biological and/or psychological factors may eventually be proved to influence sexual orientation, culture provides another dimension that cannot be ignored.

---

[1]Carrier, J. M. "Homosexual behavior in cross-cultural perspective." In *Homosexual Behavior,* Ed. by Judd Marmor, New York: Basic Books, 1980.

Source: Adapted from Byer, Curtis O., and Louis W. Shainberg. (1994). *Dimensions of Human Sexuality.* Fourth Ed., Madison, WI: Brown & Benchmark Publishers, p. 373–374.

What Do You Think?

1. Which theories discussed here make the most sense to you in terms of influencing sexual orientation? What factors did you consider when answering this question?
2. How important do you think research into the development of sexual orientation is?

of the women respondents reported that they found the thought of having sex with someone of the same sex very appealing or appealing, and 4 percent of the women reported being sexually attracted to other women, fewer than 2 percent reported that they had actually engaged in sexual behavior with another woman during the past year. Additionally, about 4 percent of the women stated that they have had sex with another woman at some time during their lives. However, when asked about their perception of themselves in terms of sexual orientation, only 1.4 percent of the women respondents stated that they considered themselves to be homosexual or bisexual. The same pattern was seen with the adult male respondents. While approximately 6 percent of the male respondents reported being sexually attracted to other men, only 2 percent reported engaging in sexual behavior with other men during the past year, and 9 percent reported previous sexual behavior with another man at some point during their lives. However, only 2.8 percent of the male respondents identified their perceived sexual orientation as homosexual or bisexual.

Research on sexual orientation has identified several important conclusions. First, the range of desires, behaviors, and perceptions that define various aspects of heterosexual, bisexual, and homosexual orientation are complex. Second, sexual orientation does not appear to be a static state. People's behaviors, desires, and perceptions about their sexual orientation may change throughout their lives. Third, individuals with homosexual and bisexual orientations, measured in terms of sexual attraction, sexual behavior, and self-identity, are clearly a minority group in the United States.[5]

Another aspect of sexuality affecting both men and women, regardless of sexual orientation, is the need for loving relationships. As Maslow's hierarchy of human needs points out, once survival and safety needs are met humans seek to fulfill their need for love, affection, and belongingness.

Love Relationships

From the first written word to today's most elegant research, people have given advice to each other about love relationships. Today,

with the large number of love relationships that do not stand the test of time, psychologists, sociologists, and other scientists have begun major studies of loving relationships. Important questions have been asked, including What is love? and What ingredients go into a successful loving relationship?

Two terms that are often associated with human sexuality are love and sex. Although often related, love and sex are different human experiences. We will explore both of these experiences and their relationship to each other.

What is Love?

Researchers have conducted investigations into the common components of love and have subsequently developed theories to explain this phenomenon. Robert J. Sternberg, professor of psychology and education at Yale University, has identified three core components of love that he envisions as sides of a triangle[6] (see figure 6.6). These components include commitment, intimacy, and passion.

Commitment is described by Sternberg as the cognitive component of love. He defines commitment as a short-term decision to love someone and a long-term decision to maintain that loving relationship. Levels of commitment vary from one loving relationship to another. Sternberg points out, for instance, that often the love of a parent for a child is distinguished by a high level of unconditional commitment. Parent-child relationships also tend to be high in **intimacy,** the second component of Sternberg's model.

Sternberg defines intimacy as the emotional aspect of love. Intimacy includes closeness, sharing, communication, and support. Communication may be the heart of intimacy. Honest communication with our loved ones can help us to understand them and ourselves better. It also helps to build trust and caring. Of Special Interest 6.2 presents ten suggestions for successful loving relationships, many of which hinge on honest communication.

The final component of Sternberg's love triangle is **passion.** Sternberg perceives passion as the motivational aspect of love and the component that leads to physiological arousal. Social psychologist

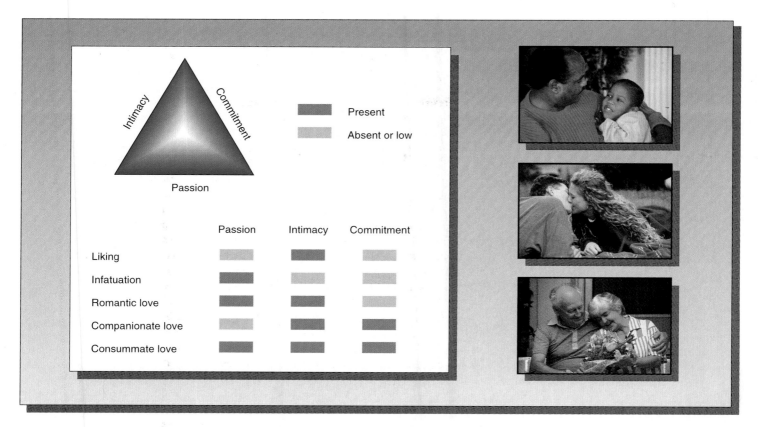

Figure 6.6: Sternberg's triangle of love

David Myers adds that passionate love is usually expressed physically.[7] Additionally he notes that, in passionate love relationships, partners often have expectations of exclusivity and an intense fascination with their romantic partners.

In loving relationships, the depth of love experienced (which corresponds to the size of the total triangle in Sternberg's model) and the strength of the individual components of love (represented by the length of the individual sides of the triangle) are known to vary. The depth and components of love may vary among the different people in our lives. For instance, the type of love we feel for our lover is different from the love we might share with a friend, parent, or child. Additionally, love often changes dimensions during the course of a relationship. A romantic love relationship in which passion played an important role may, over time, develop into a strong friendship that is without much

passion but is stronger in commitment and intimacy. Sternberg calls this companionate love. Myers notes that the emphasis on passion in romantic love relationships often fades, usually several months to several years into a romantic relationship. He notes that lasting romantic relationships evolve into companionate love.

Consummate, or complete, love—love with equal amounts of passion, intimacy, and commitment—is something that many of us strive for, especially in romantic relationships. It is important to remember, however, that there are important benefits that can be attained from a variety of loving relationships. In fact, as was discussed in chapter 1, a variety of loving relationships that include family, friends, and an intimate partner can be especially important to helping us achieve our wellness goals. Activity for Wellness 6.2 will help you assess love relationships in your life based on Sternberg's model of love.

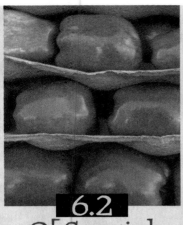

6.2

Of Special Interest

Ten Rules of Love

Sternberg* spells out ten rules that people who seek a satisfying love relationship should find helpful:

1. *Successful partners do not take their relationship for granted.* The seeds of a relationship's destruction are planted when partners take one another for granted. When we are dating, we often make a special effort to impress each other by paying attention to the way we look, act, and set priorities. In dating, we are usually aware of the possibility of losing each other, so we put forth an extra effort to keep the relationship stimulating. Dating is like an agreement written in paper and pencil, whereas marriage is like an agreement etched in stone, says Sternberg, but stone is not indestructible and, under certain conditions, crumbles.

2. *Successful partners make their relationships a priority.* In dating, we often put the relationship first because we want something—the love and possibly the marital commitment of the other individual. As time passes, the press of careers, family, and other matters tempt us to give less attention to the relationship. The relationship can share first place with other priorities, but, once it drops below them, its life is jeopardized.

3. *Successful partners actively seek to meet each other's needs.* Active, self-initiated meeting of your partner's needs shows you care and understand your partner. Don't wait for your partner to request something; anticipate his or her wants and desires. Do whatever it is that satisfies your partner's needs before you are asked, and the value of what you do will be much greater.

4. *Successful partners know when, and when not, to change in response to the other.* Successful partners in a love relationship are flexible and adaptive, willing to change to satisfy a partner's needs. Only by being flexible can partners meet the challenge to grow that each change in the nature of the relationship demands. Successful partners not only know when to give in as the situation demands, but also when not to give in. They are aware of what they can be and what they cannot be; they do not strive to meet requests they know are impossible or compromise in being true to themselves.

5. *Successful partners value themselves.* Abraham Maslow distinguished between deficiency love and being love. In deficiency love, you seek out another individual to attain something you lack in yourself; in being love, you seek out another individual to enhance an already competent self. Most loves are probably a combination of deficiency and being loves, a blend that varies over time. If you seek self-worth in another individual that you cannot find in yourself, you probably will be disappointed.

6. *Successful partners love each other, not their idealization of each other.* It is much easier to fall in love with an ideal person than a real person. An ideal person is flawless, does not make unreasonable demands, has all the characteristics we want in a true love, and does not talk back. The problem with an ideal love is that such a person exists only in one's mind. You can be in love with an idealized person rather than a real person, and the relationship can go on for some time; you tend to see only what you want to see and ignore or make excuses about your lover's flaws. Sooner or later, though, the bubble bursts as you eventually get to know your partner. You become disappointed because your partner is not the ideal love you initially thought. In a successful relationship, partners love each other for who they are, not for what they want each other to be.

7. *Successful partners tolerate what they cannot change.* We can change some things in our partner; other things we cannot change. A key ingredient of a successful love relationship is the wisdom to recognize which is which. If your partner is short and you want someone tall, you are not going to be able to change that characteristic. You must either accept your partner's short stature or give up the relationship. If your partner is moody and has been that way for a long time, he or she will probably continue to be moody. If you want to make the relationship work, you may have to cope with your partner's moody tendencies.

8. *Successful partners are open with each other.* We all have faults, but most of us are not very willing to admit them. Sometimes the easy way out is to lie or hold back the truth instead of divulging errors and shortcomings. The problem is that omissions, distortions, and flat-out lies can be damaging to a relationship. Once they start, they tend to spread and can ultimately destroy the relationship. Once you see you can get by with a small lie, you may tell a bigger one next time. Eventually the relationship becomes only a shell. When the partners talk, they say empty things because the relationship has lost its depth and trust.

9. *Successful partners make good times together and grow through the bad ones.* They participate in joint activities that are enjoyable and provide companionship. Instead of waiting for good times to happen, they create them. At the same time, they recognize that life is not always perfect. Successful partners, though, use the bad times as opportunities to grow. You can be truly honest with each other and still not prevent problems from developing in a relationship; however, by using problems as an opportunity to cope and grow mutually, you can come out stronger.

10. *Successful partners do unto the other as they would have the other do unto them.* It is easy to want to give less than we get. If you really want a relationship to work, see things from your partner's point of view and treat your partner the way you want to be treated. This helps you develop the empathy and understanding that are important in a successful love relationship.

What Do You Think?

1. Do you see components of communication, both verbal and nonverbal, as essential to Sternberg's ten rules of love? Explain your answer using specific examples.

2. How many of Sternberg's ten rules of love do you currently practice in a romantic love relationship? Do you think these ten rules apply equally well to love relationships that are of a nonromantic nature?

Successful Loving Relationships

Loving relationships that contribute to high-level wellness are a goal of most people. But what factors influence successful loving relationships? This was a question researched by Robert Sternberg and Michael Barnes of Yale University. To aid in our understanding of successful relationships, Sternberg and Barnes studied twenty-four couples involved in romantic relationships.[8] Each couple was given a love scale to complete in four different ways, indicating (1) their feelings toward their current romantic partner, (2) how they thought their current romantic partner felt about them, (3) their feelings toward an ideal, yet realistic, other member of a couple, and (4) how they thought an ideal, yet realistic, other member of a couple would feel toward them. Results from these love scales were then compared with the subjects' perceptions of satisfaction and happiness in their current romantic love relationships. Several important factors were identified by this study.

1. The higher a person's score on the love scale, the greater his or her satisfaction with the relationship. In other words, those who personally felt more loving toward their partners were happier with that relationship.

2. The level of discrepancy between an individual's real feelings for his or her partner and expectations for how he or she should ideally feel greatly influenced the reported satisfaction with the current relationship. Thus, for those who perceived their current relationships as being close to their ideal love relationships, there was more satisfaction and happiness. In fact, it appears that the amount of love felt for a significant other, and the comparison of the real to an ideal, seem to carry equal weight as factors that predict successful loving relationships.

3. For many of the couples measured in this study, the love scale scores were not highly correlated. Often, one member loved more intensely than the other. As a factor in predicting successful loving relationships, however, it was found that a person's *perception* of how a lover felt about him or her was more important than how the lover *really* felt.

4. Finally, the most important predictor of a successful love relationship was the difference between the way a person would ideally *like* his or her partner to feel and the way the person *thinks* the partner *really* feels about him or her. Thus, if a person felt that his or her partner was either under involved or over involved in the love relationship, as compared with the ideal image, the person was much less satisfied with the relationship.

5. As a last note to the study, Sternberg and Barnes noted that a "liking" scale developed by Zick Rubin of Brandeis University was a better predictor of successful relationships than Rubin's "love" scale that was used in this study. Sternberg points out that "no matter how much a person loves his partner, the relationship is not likely to work out unless he likes her as well."[9]

It seems clear, from this research, that our *own perceptions* of our love for another and of that person's love for us are at the heart of satisfaction and happiness in loving relationships. Equally important are our expectations of how relationships *should* be.

Serious research in the area of love and love relationships is still in its infancy. As more research results become available we will have a more complete picture of the components of successful love relationships. As often occurs in research, studies of love relationships have answered some questions while generating many more. If our perception of another person's love for us is critical to a satisfying relationship, how are these perceptions formed? Additionally, what factors shape the development of our "ideal" notions of loving relationships? Research into partner selection has shed some light on our notions of an "ideal" partner.

Partner Selection

What characteristics do men and women look for in a potential romantic partner? According to the research of psychologist David Buss, men and women often look for similar characteristics, most importantly kindness, understanding, and intelligence.[10] Men and women do differ, however, on the value they place on certain characteristics. Men place a higher value on physical attractiveness than do women. On the other hand, women appear to place more value on

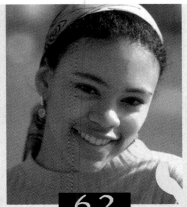

Activity for Wellness

Sternberg's Triangular Love Scale

What are the components of your love relationship? Intimacy? Passion? Decision/commitment? All three components? Two of them?

To complete the following scale, fill in the blank spaces with the name of one person you love or care about deeply. Then rate your agreement with each of the items by using a nine-point scale in which 1 = "not at all," 5 = "moderately," and 9 = "extremely." Use points in between to indicate intermediate levels of agreement between these values. Then consult the scoring key at the end of the scale.

Intimacy Component

_____ 1. I am actively supportive of _____'s well-being.

_____ 2. I have a warm relationship with _____.

_____ 3. I am able to count on _____ in times of need.

_____ 4. _____ is able to count on me in times of need.

_____ 5. I am willing to share myself and my possessions with _____.

_____ 6. I receive considerable emotional support from _____.

_____ 7. I give considerable emotional support to _____.

_____ 8. I communicate well with _____.

_____ 9. I value _____ greatly in my life.

_____ 10. I feel close to _____.

_____ 11. I have a comfortable relationship with _____.

_____ 12. I feel that I really understand _____.

_____ 13. I feel that _____ really understands me.

_____ 14. I feel that I can really trust _____.

_____ 15. I share deeply personal information about myself with _____.

Passion Component

_____ 16. Just seeing _____ excites me.

_____ 17. I find myself thinking about _____ frequently during the day.

_____ 18. My relationship with _____ is very romantic.

_____ 19. I find _____ to be very personally attractive.

_____ 20. I idealize _____.

_____ 21. I cannot imagine another person making me as happy as _____ does.

_____ 22. I would rather be with _____ than with anyone else.

_____ 23. There is nothing more important to me than my relationship with _____.

_____ 24. I especially like physical contact with _____.

_____ 25. There is something almost "magical" about my relationship with _____.

good earning capacity. What do you look for in a potential romantic partner? Activity for Wellness 6.3 will help you assess the value that you place on a variety of partner characteristics.

We have all heard the old saying "opposites attract." This, however, does not appear to be the case when it comes to selecting a romantic partner for a long-term committed relationship. Buss has studied similarities and differences between spouses and found that the similarities are indeed striking.[11] Couples in Buss's study were similar in age, race, religion, ethnic background, and socioeconomic status. They often grew up within driving distance of each other. Additionally, Buss found that

attitudes, opinions, and worldviews were also very much alike among the couples. As couples live together, over time certain compatibilities become more important.[12] Sharing values, a willingness to tolerate flaws and to make changes in response to each other, communicating effectively, and sharing religious beliefs seem to be especially important in the long run.

The results of a nationally representative study of sexual practices in the U.S., reported in 1994, has confirmed Buss's findings. Robert Michael and his colleagues state that "on every measure except religion, [including race/ethnicity, age, and educational level] people who are in any stage of a sexual relationship are remarkably similar to each

_____ 26. I adore _____.

_____ 27. I cannot imagine life without _____.

_____ 28. My relationship with _____ is passionate.

_____ 29. When I see romantic movies and read romantic books I think of _____.

_____ 30. I fantasize about _____.

Decision/Commitment Component

_____ 31. I know that I care about _____.

_____ 32. I am committed to maintaining my relationship with _____.

_____ 33. Because of my commitment to _____, I would not let other people come between us.

_____ 34. I have confidence in the stability of my relationship with _____.

_____ 35. I could not let anything get in the way of my commitment to _____.

_____ 36. I expect my love for _____ to last for the rest of my life.

_____ 37. I will always feel a strong responsibility for _____.

_____ 38. I view my commitment to _____ as a solid one.

_____ 39. I cannot imagine ending my relationship with _____.

_____ 40. I am certain of my love for _____.

_____ 41. I view my relationship with _____ as permanent.

_____ 42. I view my relationship with _____ as a good decision.

_____ 43. I feel a sense of responsibility toward _____.

_____ 44. I plan to continue my relationship with _____.

_____ 45. Even when _____ is hard to deal with, I remain committed to our relationship.

Scoring Key

Add your ratings for each of the three sections—intimacy, passion, and commitment/decision—and write the totals in the blanks below. Divide each subscore by 15 to get an average subscale score.

_____ ÷ **15** = _____
intimacy   intimacy average
subscore   rating

_____ ÷ **15** = _____
passion   passion average
subscore   rating

_____ ÷ **15** = _____
decision/   decision/
commitment   commitment
subscore   average rating

An average rating of 5 on a particular subscale indicates a moderate level of the component represented by the subscale; for example, an average rating of 5 on the intimacy subscale indicates a moderate amount of intimacy in the relationship you chose to measure. Following this example further, a higher average rating would indicate a higher level of intimacy, and a lower average rating would indicate a lesser amount of intimacy. Examining your ratings for each of the three subscales will give you an idea of how you perceive your love relationship to be composed of various amounts of intimacy, passion, and decision/commitment.

Sternberg's Triangular Love Scale (adapted) from _The Triangle of Love_ by Robert J. Sternberg. Copyright © 1988 by BasicBooks, Inc. Reprinted by permission of BasicBooks, a division of HarperCollins Publishers, Inc.

other. And married people are even very likely to have the same religion."[13] Michael and his colleagues point out that some individuals do have successful romantic relationships with people who are very different from themselves, but this is an exception—not the rule. Additionally, Michael and his colleagues believe the pattern of "like attracts like" holds true for homosexuals as well as heterosexuals.

Michael and his colleagues propose that it is easier for individuals in a romantic relationship to share their lives with each other when they have similar backgrounds and interests. Additionally, they believe that social networks, consisting of family, friends, and business associates, exert subtle and not so subtle influences on individuals to select a romantic partner that will fit into these social groups. The case of Tom and Kathy illustrates how like attracts like. Tom and Kathy met in their junior year of college. Tom, a communications major, met Kathy, an English major, in a required professional writing course. They "hit it off" right away. As Tom and Kathy began to get to know each other they quickly found that they had much in common, including a love of scuba diving, tennis, writing, and country music, as well as having grown up in small communities nearby. Tom and Kathy's friends approved of the relationship: they were glad that Tom and Kathy were happy, and they enjoyed having another friend who

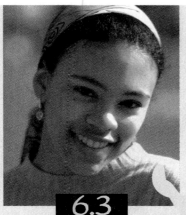

6.3

Activity for Wellness

What Do You Look for in a Romantic Partner?

Some of the most common characteristics people look for in a romantic partner are listed below. Rank order these characteristics in terms of their importance to *you* in looking for a romantic partner. The most important characteristic would be ranked #1, while the characteristic least important to you would be ranked #13.

Characteristic	Your Rank
A. adaptability	_____
B. kindness and understanding	_____
C. religious orientation	_____
D. creativity	_____
E. physical attractiveness	_____
F. good health	_____
G. desire for children	_____
H. good housekeeper	_____
I. college graduate	_____
J. exciting personality	_____
K. intelligence	_____
L. good heredity	_____
M. good earning capacity	_____

David Buss, a psychologist at the University of Michigan, has studied the characteristics that men and women look for in a romantic partner.* He found that men and women ranked the characteristics listed above in the following order, from most to least important:

Men: B,K,E,J,F,A,D,G,I,L,M,H,C

Women: B,K,J,F,A,E,D,M,I,G,L,H,C

1. How do you compare with the gender norms from Dr. Buss's study?

2. Comparing the male and female rankings of important characteristics of a romantic partner, what do you see as the most important similarities and differences?

3. Are there important characteristics that *you* look for in a romantic partner that are not listed above?

*Buss, David M. (1985) "Human Mate Selection," *American Scientist, 73:* 47–51.

shared similar interests. Tom's and Kathy's parents also approved of the relationship and were especially pleased that their children had found romantic partners who were educated and yet wanted to stay near home after graduation. Tom's parents were especially relieved, as Tom's last girlfriend Elizabeth came from an extremely wealthy New York City family, and expected to return to the city after graduation to pursue a career in fashion design. While Tom's parents regarded Elizabeth as caring and intelligent, they felt uncomfortable about her wealth and didn't want their son to move away once he finished school. Their messages to Tom about the relationship were subtle, yet unmistakable. These subtle pressures from Tom's family

likely played a role in his decisions to both end his romantic relationship with Elizabeth and continue his relationship with Kathy.

Most romantic love relationships have some element of physical and emotional passion. Such passion is often displayed through a variety of sexual behaviors.

Sexual Behavior and Pleasuring

There are many ways that individuals communicate their sexual thoughts and feelings. Some of the more common sexual behaviors include kissing and touching, masturbation, oral-genital stimulation, and sexual intercourse. Before we examine these sexual behaviors, however, it is important to recognize the limitations of sexuality research.

Sexuality Research

It is a difficult task to describe the sexual behavioral profile of a particular society. Questionnaires, telephone surveys, mail surveys, and personal interviews make up the majority of data-collection techniques used in sexuality research. These techniques are prone to error. For example, some people do not respond to sexuality surveys, so the results of many studies reflect only the sexual attitudes and behaviors of those people who did respond. It is quite possible that people who respond to sexuality surveys are different from nonresponders, especially regarding sexual behavior. Because of this nonresponse factor, it is difficult for researchers to construct a sample of people who are representative of all persons in the U.S. or even smaller groups such as Southerners or Washingtonians.

Another problem with sexuality research involves time. Sexuality studies tend to represent attitudes and behaviors for a certain time frame. Ten years, ten months, or even ten days later, a person's attitudes may have changed.

Certain groups of people, such as the very rich, the very poor, and the young, are generally inaccessible to researchers. Additionally, social institutions often erect barriers to sexuality research. For instance, public schools have traditionally discouraged research examining the sexual behaviors of students.

Another major limitation of sexuality research involves the need to rely on the memories of subjects. People who respond to surveys may be unable to recall the details of their sexual behavior, especially five, ten, or twenty years after the fact. Others may feel that their answers are too personal to share with strangers. Collectively, these factors render our knowledge of sexual behavior, like many other types of human behavior, incomplete.

The lack of scientifically valid studies of human sexual behavior has, in the past, limited our understanding of the types of sexual behavior people in the U.S. typically engage in, how often they participate, and with whom. In 1992, however, social scientists at the University of Chicago undertook a scientifically accurate study of the sexual behaviors of a random sample of 4,369 U.S. English-speaking adults between the ages of eighteen and fifty-nine.[14] This study, called the National Health and Social Life Survey (NHSLS), was statistically designed to provide a representative sample of adults in the U.S. Special consideration was given to sampling a large enough number of Blacks and Hispanics that the data for these minority groups could be statistically analyzed separately. Unfortunately, the NHSLS sample did not include large enough numbers of homosexuals to be able to analyze that data separately. This was largely due to the difficulty in identifying gay men and lesbians during the sampling phase of the study.

In order to ensure a nationally representative sample, the NHSLS randomly selected geographical areas of the country. For each selected geographical area, cities, towns, rural areas, neighborhoods, and finally households were also randomly selected. Once households were randomly identified, a person who met the study criteria (age eighteen to fifty-nine, and English-speaking) was randomly selected from eligible household members. Once subjects were identified, they were interviewed in person by a trained interviewer. Interviewers in the NHSLS were able to interview over 72 percent of the individuals randomly chosen for this study—an exceptionally high response rate for any study. The NHSLS results, based on the responses of 3,159 adults, have given us our first scientifically valid picture of the typical sexual behaviors of people in the U.S. As we discuss a variety of sexual behaviors in this chapter, results from the NHSLS will be highlighted.

Kissing and Touching

Sexual stimulation can be communicated through all sensory receptors in the body. Two common avenues for communicating sexual stimulation are kissing and touching. These behaviors, however, are not always intended as sexual behaviors. Many people use a kiss or a touch to communicate love. A mother kissing her child or one friend hugging and kissing another friend after a long absence are examples of nonsexual intentions.

Sexual activity with another person often begins with kissing and touching. Many parts of the human body are receptive to stimulation from both kissing and touch. Areas of the body that are especially receptive to sexual stimulation are known as erogenous zones and commonly include the mouth, ears, inner surfaces of the thighs, the breasts, and the genitals.

Masturbation

Usually a person's sexual experience begins with self-discovery of his or her own body and the pleasures of being sexually aroused. Self-stimulation of the body for the purpose of sexual pleasure is defined as **masturbation.**

According to the National Health and Social Life Survey scientists, masturbation is a common sexual practice in the U.S. today.[15] Among adults age eighteen to fifty-nine, about 60 percent of the men and 40 percent of the women reported that they had masturbated during the past year. Additionally, approximately 25 percent of the men and 10 percent of the women told interviewers that they masturbated at least once a week. Among the participants of this nationally representative sample, individuals who masturbated were also more likely to have sex with partners as well. The NHSLS scientists conclude that "masturbation is not a substitute for those who are sexually deprived, but rather it is an activity that stimulates and is stimulated by other sexual behavior."[16]

Over the years, social and cultural forces in the U.S. have attempted to discourage people from masturbating. For instance, masturbation has been condemned as sinful by both the Christian and Jewish faiths. Additionally, scores of myths have been invented to discourage people from masturbating. Masturbation, however, remains a common sexual practice, and is considered by sexuality experts to be a normal and natural way of expressing sexuality.

Oral-Genital Stimulation

A sexual behavior that has become more popular among certain groups of people in the U.S. is oral-genital stimulation. **Cunnilingus** is the term used to describe oral stimulation of the female genitals. **Fellatio** is the term used to describe oral stimulation of the male genitals.

According to the National Health and Social Life Survey findings, 68 percent of women and 77 percent of men in the U.S. have performed oral sex on a partner at some point in their lifetime, while 73 percent of women and 79 percent of men have had oral sex performed on them at least once during

their lifetime (see figure 6.7).[17] Rates of oral sex, however, are markedly different for people of various social groups, especially groups defined by race/ethnicity and education level. Oral sex appears to be more popular among young Whites and people who have higher levels of education. Oral sex is reported to be less common among Blacks, those with a high school education or less, and members of conservative Protestant religious groups.

Respondents of the National Health and Social Life Survey were asked to rate the appeal of a variety of sexual behaviors, using a rating scale of "very appealing" to "not at all appealing." Only three sexual behaviors—vaginal intercourse, watching a partner undress, and oral sex—were reported to be appealing by a significant number of respondents. However, in the case of oral sex, responses ranged from high appeal to low appeal, indicating that while some people find oral sex very appealing others feel equally strong that it is not a sexual activity they wish to engage in.

Vaginal Intercourse

Vaginal intercourse, sometimes referred to as **coitus,** is defined as sexual activity in which there is insertion of the penis into the vagina. What do we know about contemporary sexual behavior in the U.S. as it relates to vaginal intercourse? Today the majority of people experience vaginal intercourse for the first time at a young age and outside of marriage. Results from the 1991 Youth Risk Behavior Survey,[18] conducted by the Centers for Disease Control and Prevention, indicated that 36 percent of fifteen-year-old females, and 44 percent of fifteen-year-old males reported that they had engaged in vaginal intercourse. Additionally, 66 percent of seventeen-year-old females, and 68 percent of seventeen-year-old males had participated in vaginal intercourse.

There are serious health concerns associated with teenage vaginal intercourse. The high rate of teen pregnancy and the effects of a pregnancy on both the teen parents and the child are of primary concern to public health professionals. Additionally, exposure to a variety of sexually transmitted diseases is an ongoing concern. The U.S. Department of Health and Human Services recognized teen sexual intercourse as a

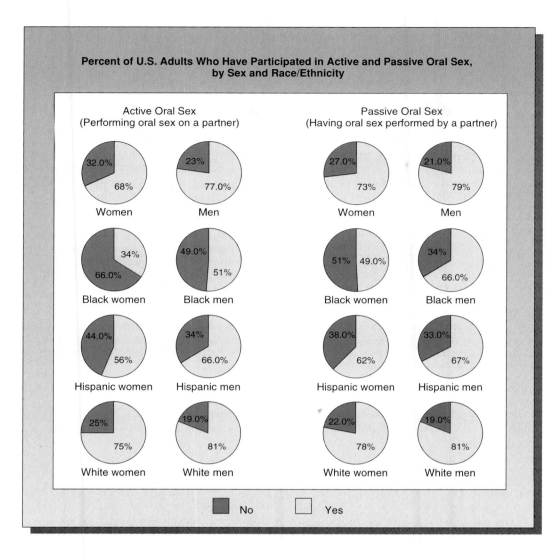

Percent of U.S. Adults Who Have Participated in Active and Passive Oral Sex, by Sex and Race/Ethnicity

Active Oral Sex (Performing oral sex on a partner)

- Women: 32.0% No, 68% Yes
- Men: 23% No, 77.0% Yes
- Black women: 34% No, 66.0% Yes
- Black men: 49.0% No, 51% Yes
- Hispanic women: 44.0% No, 56% Yes
- Hispanic men: 34% No, 66.0% Yes
- White women: 25% No, 75% Yes
- White men: 19.0% No, 81% Yes

Passive Oral Sex (Having oral sex performed by a partner)

- Women: 27.0% No, 73% Yes
- Men: 21.0% No, 79% Yes
- Black women: 51% No, 49.0% Yes
- Black men: 34% No, 66.0% Yes
- Hispanic women: 38.0% No, 62% Yes
- Hispanic men: 33.0% No, 67% Yes
- White women: 22.0% No, 78% Yes
- White men: 19.0% No, 81% Yes

■ No   □ Yes

Figure 6.7: What Do You Think?

1. What similarities and differences does this data depict between men and women in terms of having participated in oral sex actively as opposed to passively?
2. What similarities and differences does this data depict between Blacks, Hispanics, and Whites in terms of having participated in oral sex actively as opposed to passively?

priority in its *Healthy People 2000* objectives for the nation (see table 6.1). To date, some progress has been achieved in influencing sexually active teens to return to **sexual abstinence** after experiencing vaginal intercourse. Between 1988 and 1991 there was a 4 percent increase in the percent of girls fifteen to seventeen years of age who returned to sexual abstinence following a period of being sexually active. For boys of the same age the increase in abstinence among those who were previously sexually active was 9 percent between 1988 and 1991. However, we are still far from the year 2000 goal of having 40 percent of *ever* sexually active girls and boys abstaining from sexual intercourse (see table 6.1).

Another area of concern is the increasing number of teens reporting that they have engaged in sexual intercourse. The number of fifteen-year-old females and males who have *ever* engaged in vaginal intercourse increased 33 percent between 1988 and 1991. The increases for seventeen-year-old males and females during that same time were 3 percent and 32 percent respectively.

In adult sexual relationships, vaginal intercourse can be an important means of expressing both intimacy and passion. The National Health and Social Life Survey has provided us with a snapshot of the current status of vaginal intercourse among U.S. English-speaking adults between the ages of eighteen and fifty-nine. According to the NHSLS, only vaginal sex was found to have universal appeal (see figure 6.8).[19] For all other sexual behaviors studied, including oral-genital stimulation, anal intercourse, and

Sexual abstinence: a premeditated decision not to have sexual intercourse for a specific period of time.

1. **Reduce the proportion of adolescents who have engaged in sexual intercourse to no more than 15 percent by age 15 and no more than 40 percent by age 17.** (Update: adolescents 15 years, 36 percent of females and 44 percent of males in 1991, up from 27 percent and 33 percent respectively in 1988; adolescents 17 years, 66 percent of females and 68 percent of males in 1991, up from 50 percent and 66 percent respectively in 1988.)

2. **Increase to at least 40 percent the proportion of ever sexually active adolescents aged 17 and younger who have abstained from sexual activity for the previous 3 months.**

(Update: 25 percent of ever sexually active females 15–17 years, and 36 percent of ever sexually active males 15–17 years in 1991, up from 23.6 percent and 33 percent respectively in 1988.)

3. **Increase to at least 85 percent the proportion of people aged 10–18 who have discussed human sexuality, including values surrounding sexuality, with their parents and/or have received information through another parentally endorsed source, such as youth, school, or religious programs.** (Baseline: 66 percent of people 13–18 years had discussed sexuality with parents in 1986.)

Source: *Healthy People 2000 National Health Promotion and Disease Prevention Objectives.* Department of Health and Human Services, Washington, D.C., 1991; *Healthy People 2000 Review 1993.* Department of Health and Human Services, Washington, D.C., 1994.

---

having a same-gender sex partner, significant numbers of men and women reported a lack of appeal. Additionally, 95 percent of the 3,159 respondents reported that they had participated in vaginal sex the last time they had sex. Eighty percent of respondents reported that they had vaginal sex every time they had participated in sexual activity during the past year. It is important to note that both heterosexual and homosexual respondents are included in this data; however, the number of homosexual respondents was low.

The National Health and Social Life Survey also asked respondents how often they had sex each month. The results indicated that adults in the U.S. can be divided into three groups in terms of frequency of sex.[20] Approximately one-third of adults have sex with a partner two or more times a week. An additional one-third have sex with a partner several times a month. The remaining one-third have partnered sex only a few times a year, or not at all. Sex frequency rates for various racial/ethnic groups, religious groups, and educational levels were remarkably similar. Only three factors were associated with frequency of sex, including age, marital/**cohabiting** status, and the length of time partners have been a couple. Generally, those individuals in marriages or cohabiting

report having the most sex. However, the frequency of sex is highest for those ages twenty-five to twenty-nine, and decreases as people age. The NHSLS researchers were surprised at the generally low frequency of sex reported in the U.S., but they point out that their data indicates that most U.S. adults say that they are satisfied with their sex lives. This may confirm the often stated belief that couples who communicate their sexual needs to each other and reach a consensus on the frequency of sexual intercourse in their relationships seem to be satisfied with their relationships regardless of the actual frequency of sex.

Anal Intercourse

Anal intercourse, sometimes referred to as **sodomy,** is defined as the insertion of the penis into the **anus.** Anal intercourse is a sexual behavior that is practiced by both heterosexual and homosexual couples as a part of sexual pleasuring. While some people find anal intercourse to be an appealing aspect of sexual behavior, many others report that it is not appealing to them at all (see figure 6.8). Yet there appears to be some discrepancy between what people find appealing and what they actually do sexually. For instance, according to the National Health and Social Life Survey results,[21] only

Cohabiting: a living arrangement in which two people who are not married to each other share both bed and board.

Sodomy: a term often used legally to define "unnatural sex acts" that may be determined by a state to be illegal. Anal intercourse, as well as oral-genital stimulation and sex with animals, is usually listed as a sexual behavior prohibited as sodomy.

Anus: a small opening at the lower end of the intestines, below the rectum, through which feces is discharged.

The Appeal of Selected Sexual Practices

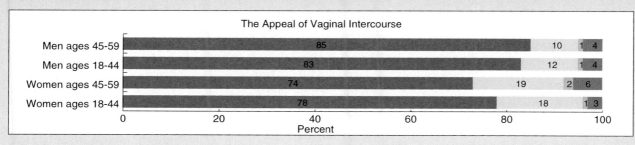

The Appeal of Vaginal Intercourse

Men ages 45-59	85 / 10 / 1 / 4
Men ages 18-44	83 / 12 / 1 / 4
Women ages 45-59	74 / 19 / 2 / 6
Women ages 18-44	78 / 18 / 1 / 3

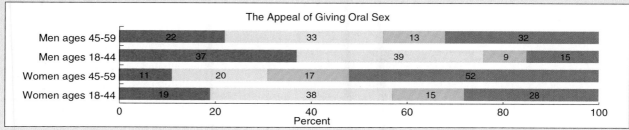

The Appeal of Giving Oral Sex

Men ages 45-59	22 / 33 / 13 / 32
Men ages 18-44	37 / 39 / 9 / 15
Women ages 45-59	11 / 20 / 17 / 52
Women ages 18-44	19 / 38 / 15 / 28

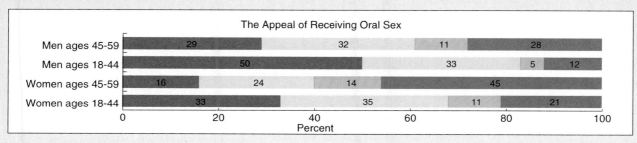

The Appeal of Receiving Oral Sex

Men ages 45-59	29 / 32 / 11 / 28
Men ages 18-44	50 / 33 / 5 / 12
Women ages 45-59	16 / 24 / 14 / 45
Women ages 18-44	33 / 35 / 11 / 21

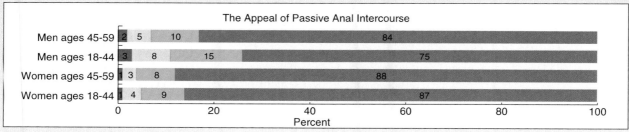

The Appeal of Passive Anal Intercourse

Men ages 45-59	2 / 5 / 10 / 84
Men ages 18-44	3 / 8 / 15 / 75
Women ages 45-59	1 / 3 / 8 / 88
Women ages 18-44	1 / 4 / 9 / 87

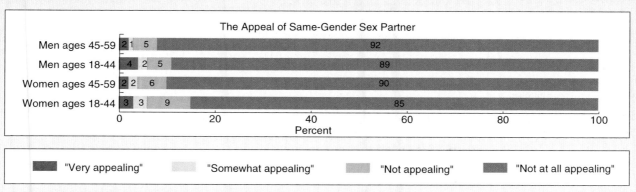

The Appeal of Same-Gender Sex Partner

Men ages 45-59	2 / 1 / 5 / 92
Men ages 18-44	4 / 2 / 5 / 89
Women ages 45-59	2 / 2 / 6 / 90
Women ages 18-44	3 / 3 / 9 / 85

■ "Very appealing" ■ "Somewhat appealing" ■ "Not appealing" ■ "Not at all appealing"

Figure 6.8: What Do You Think?

1. Men and women in the Health and Social Life Survey rated a number of sexual behaviors in terms of how personally appealing they were. Some of the results are depicted here in graphic form. Rank order the sexual behaviors in terms of their ratings for being "very appealing." Do these rankings vary by sex or age? Did any of the appeal ratings surprise you?

2. What social and biological factors do you think may account for the similarities and differences noted in your answer to question 1? What source of evidence did you use to answer this question?

5 percent of women age eighteen to forty-four and 4 percent of women age forty-five to fifty-nine reported that they found **passive anal sex** to be very or somewhat appealing. Yet 20 percent of the female respondents reported engaging in passive anal sex during their lifetime, and 9 percent of female respondents reported having anal sex with an opposite-gender partner within the past twelve months. The percents were similar for men: eleven percent of men age eighteen to forty-four and 7 percent of men age forty-five to fifty-nine reported that they found passive anal sex to be very or somewhat appealing. The NHSLS also studied **active anal sex** in males and found that 14 percent of men age eighteen to forty-four and 8 percent of men age forty-five to fifty-nine reported active anal sex to be very or somewhat appealing. Yet 26 percent of men reported participating in anal sex during their lifetime, and 10 percent of the male respondents reported participating in anal sex with an opposite-gender partner within the past year.

Anal intercourse is considered to be a high-risk sexual behavior in terms of disease transmission for several reasons. First, bacteria and other **pathogens** are commonly found in and around the anus. If the pathogens come into contact with the urethra or vagina, infection can result. Secondly, there is special danger for the passive recipient of anal intercourse. The tissue of the anus and **rectum** is easily torn during anal intercourse, and these tears provide easy access for pathogens, such as **HIV,** to enter the blood stream of the passive or receptive partner. Public health authorities recommend that a lubricated latex condom *always* be used if people engage in anal sex. Yet even with condom use, anal sex remains a high-risk sexual behavior.

Sexual Attitudes and Beliefs

It has been a long-held belief that a person's general attitudes, values, and beliefs dictate the sexual behaviors in which he or she participates. For instance, if an individual has a conservative, traditional Judeo-Christian belief system, he or she would be less likely to engage in premarital sex because it is not sanctioned by his or her religion. The National Health and Social Life researchers decided to study this phenomenon as part of their national study of sexual behavior in the

U.S.[22] Interviewers asked subjects questions such as "If a man and a woman have sex relations before marriage, do you think it is always wrong, almost always wrong, wrong only sometimes, or not wrong at all?" Considering responses to nine such questions covering issues like abortion, same-gender sex, premarital sex, and extramarital sex, the researchers were able to cluster responses into three broad attitudinal categories. The *traditional* category describes individuals whose religious beliefs always serve as a guide for sexual behavior. These respondents—about one-third of the sample—did not condone homosexuality, abortion, premarital sex, or extramarital sex. The second category was labeled *relational* and describes individuals who believe that love should always be present before a relationship proceeds to sex. For these respondents—not quite half of the sample—marriage is not a necessary prerequisite for sex. Most individuals in this category, however, did not condone extramarital sex. The final category, *recreational*, describes individuals who view sex as an acceptable activity for pleasure regardless of whether two people love each other. These respondents—approximately one-quarter of the sample—were more likely to be opposed to laws that would restrict the sale of pornography to adults.

As you can see in figure 6.9, women tend to have more traditional attitudes than men, while men have a greater tendency to have recreational attitudes toward sex. This is especially true of Black men and women. Of the Black male respondents in the NHSLS, 42.3 percent were categorized as having *recreational* attitudes toward sex, while only 8.9 percent of the Black female respondents were so categorized. This data tends to support the belief that many more men than women are looking for sexual pleasure, while more women than men tend to be looking for love and marriage. This is especially true for nonmarried men and women. The NHSLS researchers conclude that their findings

> seem to confirm the notion that people's beliefs about sexual morality are part of a much broader social and religious outlook that helps define who they are. . . . Membership in a particular attitudinal group is closely associated with what their sexual practices are. It is even correlated with

Passive anal sex: during an act of anal sex, having a penis inserted into one's anus.

Active anal sex: during an act of anal sex, inserting one's penis into another person's anus.

Pathogens: organisms that can produce disease in a host.

Rectum: the end segment of the large intestine that connects to the anal canal and stores feces prior to defecation.

HIV: Human immunodeficiency virus; the virus that is believed to cause the symptoms associated with AIDS (acquired immune deficiency syndrome).

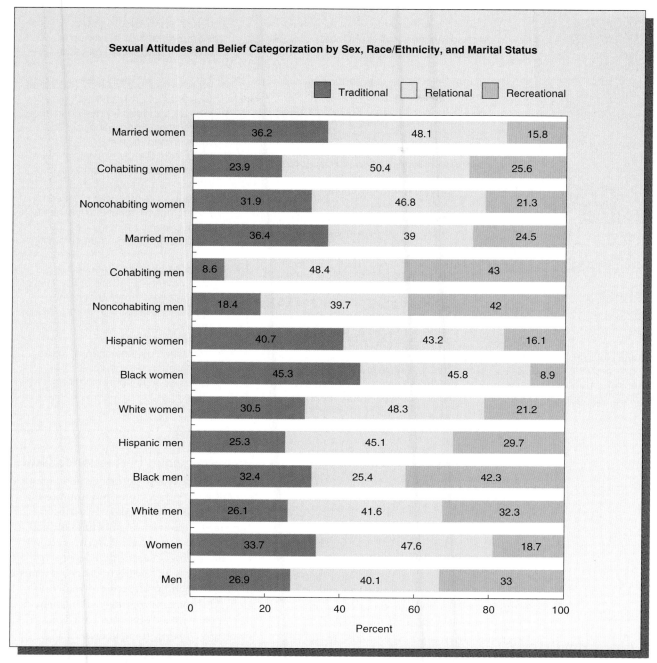

Sexual Attitudes and Belief Categorization by Sex, Race/Ethnicity, and Marital Status

Legend: ■ Traditional □ Relational ▨ Recreational

Group	Traditional	Relational	Recreational
Married women	36.2	48.1	15.8
Cohabiting women	23.9	50.4	25.6
Noncohabiting women	31.9	46.8	21.3
Married men	36.4	39	24.5
Cohabiting men	8.6	48.4	43
Noncohabiting men	18.4	39.7	42
Hispanic women	40.7	43.2	16.1
Black women	45.3	45.8	8.9
White women	30.5	48.3	21.2
Hispanic men	25.3	45.1	29.7
Black men	32.4	25.4	42.3
White men	26.1	41.6	32.3
Women	33.7	47.6	18.7
Men	26.9	40.1	33

Percent (x-axis: 0 to 100)

Figure 6.9: What Do You Think?

1. The National Health and Social Life Survey results categorized respondents according to their attitudes and beliefs about life in general and sexual behaviors in particular. The traditional category describes individuals whose religious beliefs always guide decisions about sexual behavior. The relational category describes individuals who believe you should be in love before engaging in sexual behavior, and the recreational category describes individuals who believe that sex and love do not necessarily have to go together. Looking at the data presented here, what groups are most likely to hold traditional beliefs about sexual behavior? What groups are most likely to hold relational beliefs about sexual behavior? What groups are most likely to hold recreational beliefs about sexual behavior?

2. How might this data help to explain conflicts between young men and women as they attempt to negotiate sexual relationships? (Hint: compare the data for men and women on each variable presented.)

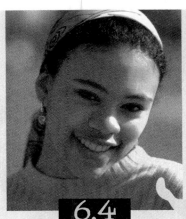

6.4
Activity for Wellness

How to Find a Certified Sex Therapist

If sometime during your life you have a sexual performance problem that is persistent and troubling, you should seek help from a *certified* sex therapist. Most states do *not* have legal requirements for individuals who call themselves sex therapists. Therefore, the old saying "buyer beware" applies to the search for professional help for sexual performance problems. The following checklist will help you locate a trained, certified sex therapist.

❑ Ask your family physician, college health center counselors, or a state or county mental health department for a referral to a *certified* sex therapist practicing in your area.

❑ Contact the American Association of Sex Educators, Counselors, and Therapists (AASECT). This organization certifies sex therapists and is willing to provide the names of certified sex therapists who practice in your geographical area. AASECT is located in Washington, D.C. and can be contacted by telephone at (202) 462–1171.

❑ Once you have located the *certified* sex therapists in your area, you should interview each therapist before you begin treatment. Ethical therapists should be willing to answer the following questions:

1. What is their profession? (Common examples of professions that provide appropriate training include psychology, counseling, social work, and medicine.)
2. Where did the therapist earn his or her professional graduate degree? (Check to make certain the therapist's degree was granted by an accredited college or university.)
3. What specific training does the therapist have in human sexuality and sex therapy?
4. What types of treatment do they recommend? (Beware of therapists who suggest that you become sexually involved with them. This is unethical and not accepted practice for sex therapists.)
5. What fees do they charge? (Many therapists are expensive; however, prices do vary from one therapist to another.)

---

how often people think about sex and how often they have sex. . . . Overall, people's sexual opinions and their behavior mesh quite closely. We cannot tell whether the opinions prompted the behavior or whether the behavior prompted the opinions, or both, but the relationship is clear.[23]

What are your personal beliefs and attitudes about sexual intercourse and other forms of sexual behavior? How do you determine when sexual intercourse would be an appropriate expression of intimacy and passion? Are your personal attitudes and beliefs more traditional, relational, or recreational? If you have a romantic partner, do you understand his or her attitudes and beliefs about sexual behavior? Take some time to think about your beliefs and the impact they have on your sexuality and general well-being.

Sexual behavior with a partner often brings intimacy and pleasure to couples. However, it can also be a source of frustration or distress if a couple experiences one of the many types of sexual dysfunctions.

Common Sexual Performance Issues

People view sexual performance and orgasm from different perspectives and in terms of their definitions of sexuality. In addition, each culture has its own guidelines for how males and females should perform sexually.

During the last several decades people in the U.S. have been learning more about human **sexual dysfunction.** The term "dysfunction" implies that something is not working right or to its full potential. When the word dysfunction is used with "sexual" it implies something is not working right sexually. But how do we define "right?" For example, Phil and Mary are in their twenties and Phil reaches orgasm soon after penetration of Mary. Neither Phil nor Mary view their sex lives together as a problem. On the other hand, John and Donna, also in their twenties, are experiencing the same sexual response pattern as Phil and Mary. Neither John nor Donna, however, is satisfied with their sexual relationship due to what they term premature ejaculation. When a couple perceives that there is a problem with their sexual relationship, especially if the problem is persistent, it should be addressed. Activity for Wellness 6.4 provides tips for locating an ethical, certified sex therapist who is trained to provide assistance in overcoming sexual performance problems.

One of the first steps in addressing a sexual performance problem is to determine whether the cause is physiological, psychological, or both. There are many physiological factors that can affect how people perform sexually. Diseases such as **diabetes,** drugs such as alcohol and cocaine, and injuries, especially to the central nervous system, can result in a female or male having difficulty or being unable to become sexually aroused or responsive. More commonly, a variety of psychological factors can also affect sexual performance. Factors such as lack of sexual knowledge, fear of sexual failure, guilt, and insecurity are commonly associated with sexual performance problems.

There are several common behaviors that are often considered to be sexual dysfunctions. All of these dysfunctions can be situational. They can occur with certain sexual partners or only under certain conditions. For example, a male may be unable to gain an erection with one sexual partner, yet experience no erectile difficulties with another.

Anorgasmia

Anorgasmia is the inability to reach orgasm. This is often situational. There are adult males and females who have never experienced orgasm in their lifetimes. Anorgasmia is usually associated with females, but males can also experience situational anorgasmia. In most cases of anorgasmia, males and females are sexually responsive. They simply do not reach orgasm.

Erectile Dysfunction

The term **erectile dysfunction** has begun to replace the term impotence. Erectile dysfunction describes the male's inability to have an erection of sufficient strength and duration to perform intercourse. There are few adult males who have not experienced, at one time or another, the inability to have or maintain an erection. Often the problem is situational.

Premature Ejaculation

This dysfunction concerns the duration of intercourse. One way of defining **premature ejaculation** is in terms of the couple's satisfaction. Premature ejaculation implies that one or both partners are not satisfied with the duration of their episodes of sexual intercourse due to the male's loss of erection following orgasm.

Dyspareunia

Dyspareunia is the term for painful intercourse, which may occur in any of the four sexual response phases. Both males and females can experience dyspareunia. **Antihistamines** and vaginal infections can cause dyspareunia in females. Sexually transmitted diseases in both males and females can cause dyspareunia. People who experience dyspareunia should seek medical advice.

Most people will probably experience one or more of these dysfunctions in their lifetimes. Any time sexual performance is perceived as a problem it is prudent for the individual or couple to seek expert advice.

Sexuality and Lifestyle Options

There are a variety of lifestyle options that influence how we express our sexuality at any given point in time. Being single, married, or living with a sexual partner outside of marriage are all relationship options common in the U.S. today.

Single Lifestyle

Everyone is single at some point during his or her lifetime. The traditional goal of single people was to find a partner and marry. Today, however, a greater proportion of people are choosing to remain single for longer periods of time as compared to a few decades ago. The number of never-married single people age twenty to twenty-nine has increased significantly since 1970. Currently, 37.5 percent of the total U.S. adult population (age eighteen and older) is single. The percent of never-married single adults varies by race/ethnicity, with 37.4 percent of Blacks, 27.9 percent of Hispanics, and 20.5 percent of Whites fitting this description.[24] Previously married singles, either separated, divorced, or widowed, comprise 15.8 percent of the U.S. population.

For some individuals, being single is a stepping-stone to marriage. For others being single is a lifestyle option chosen for the benefits it carries. For instance, many single individuals believe that their careers are a greater priority than marriage, at least during

Diabetes: a metabolic disorder caused by lack of insulin or resistance to insulin, resulting in the body not being able to metabolize sugar for energy. Uncontrolled diabetes can result in life-threatening complications.

Antihistamines: drugs used to treat symptoms of allergy.

certain periods of their lives. Still others remain single because of the difficulty in finding a suitable marriage or cohabiting partner. Most people want to marry someone who is close to them in age. Yet after age thirty, there are fewer males than females for every age group.[25] This is due, in large part, to the fact that by their forties men die at a higher rate than women. When other "suitability" factors such as marital status and education level are considered, the numbers of suitable men are dramatically reduced.[26] This is especially true for older women and women with more education.

Many single individuals expend considerable resources and energy locating potential romantic partners. A large number of people select intimate partners from their school or work settings. In the National Health and Social Life Survey, 38 percent of married respondents, 28 percent of cohabiting respondents, and 39 percent of respondents in a noncohabiting partnership that lasted more than one month reported that they met their partners at work or school.[27] Many single people also rely on family, friends, or coworkers and classmates to introduce them to potential romantic partners. In the National Health and Social Life Survey,[28] 35 percent of married respondents, 40 percent of cohabiting respondents, and 36 percent of respondents in a noncohabiting partnership that lasted more than one month reported that they were introduced to their partners by mutual friends. Family members also played an important role in partner selection, with 15 percent of married respondents, 12 percent of cohabiting respondents, and 8 percent of respondents in a noncohabiting partnership that lasted more than one month stating that they were introduced to their partners by a family member.

Dating

A common method of getting to know a potential romantic partner is dating. People use dating to find partners for relationships that range from nonsexual companionship to recreational sexual intimacy to a lifelong committed relationship. Even after a potential romantic partner has been located, it can be difficult for men and women to feel confident about asking another person to go on a date. Table 6.2 provides some suggestions for improving date-seeking skills.

Dating can be both exciting and frustrating because each person brings unique attitudes, values, beliefs, experiences, and expectations to a relationship. During the course of any relationship there may be differences in the expectations and goals each partner has for that relationship. When dating, it is important that each partner communicate his or her present goals for the relationship and strive to reach mutually acceptable goals and expectations. Both early on and periodically in a relationship individuals should discuss their views on being in a loving relationship. Sternberg's model of love, which sees love relationships as composed of various levels of passion, intimacy, and commitment, can serve as a guide for discussion.

Passion is described as the physical aspect of a love relationship, and is typically expressed through a variety of sexual behaviors. In a dating relationship it is important for each partner to assess his or her individual expectations of acceptable sex behaviors and communicate these expectations verbally. This includes the relationship as it currently exists, as well as expectations for the future should the relationship continue. Couples may agree to, or rule out, an array of sexual behaviors. For instance, Drucilla and Malcolm are college sophomores who have been dating for several weeks. After discussing their sexual expectations, they mutually decide that they will limit their current sexual contact to kissing and hugging. Malcolm, however, has expressed his desire for the relationship to progress to vaginal intercourse once he and Drucilla have dated for several months. Drucilla, on the other hand, has *relational* beliefs that direct her to wait until she is sure that she and Malcolm love each other before engaging in such intimate sexual contact. While Malcolm and Drucilla have reached an agreement on their current sexual relationship, they will have to reassess their individual expectations in the near future if they continue to date.

Being able to sincerely and honestly communicate with a romantic partner about sexual behaviors and other important aspects of the relationship and each partner's life is a sign of intimacy in a relationship. As a relationship progresses over time, communication and trust become more

The college years are a time for meeting people and making new friends. For many college students this involves dating new acquaintances, a process that can be uncomfortable. This is especially true of initiating the first date. The following tips will help you improve your date-seeking skills.

Precontemplation → Contemplation

If you have never thought about making changes in how you seek out dates, or you do not intend to make any changes within the next six months, you might want to consider:

- assessing your current dating patterns. When was the last time you asked someone new out on a date? Do you want to date someone new? If so, do you feel comfortable approaching that person and asking for a date?

Contemplation → Preparation

If you have been seriously considering improving your date-seeking skills, but have not yet attempted any changes, try:

- making a list of topics that you are interested in and know something about. Keep this list in mind when you are trying to make friendly small talk, one of the preliminary ways we get to know someone enough to feel comfortable asking them for a date.
- getting to know someone of the gender you wish to date, but for now choose someone that you have no desire to date. This will allow you to practice making small talk under less threatening circumstances.
- practicing your greeting skills. As you pass individuals you might be interested in dating on campus, say hello.

Preparation → Action

If you are ready to make some definite plans for improving your dating skills during the next month, or if you have already made small changes in the past but were not able to maintain those changes as a continuing part of your lifestyle, consider the following actions:

- set a specific date to begin your new date-seeking behaviors.

- choose a person in one of your classes that you might like to date. Sit down next to him or her and say hello.
- choose an appropriate topic from your small talk list and begin a conversation with the person. Be sure to introduce yourself by name, and give some other personal information such as your major, or where you are from, or why you are taking the class.
- decide on where you would like to go before you ask the person out. Group settings, such as movies or restaurants, are often less threatening for a first date. Practice asking the person out in front of a mirror or a friend.

Action → Maintenance

If you have recently made some changes in date-seeking, the following tips will help you continue:

- ask the person for a date just the way you rehearsed it. If the person has other plans, be ready to respond in a friendly manner such as "maybe another time." If this person is interested in dating you, he or she will let you know through friendly eye contact, body language, and conversation. If these signs are there, ask again soon for a date.

Maintenance

You have made important changes in your date-seeking behavior. Keep up your momentum by:

- actively being friendly to people you may not know. Greet them and talk with them. You may be introducing yourself to someone who will become an important part of your life.
- do not interpret a rejection for a date as a catastrophe. You may meet people who, for any number of reasons, are not ready or able to date you. Keep yourself open to new opportunities for friendship and dating.

Based on Prochaska, Norcross and DiClemente's transtheoretical model. For more information see Prochaska, J. O., Norcross, J. C. & DiClemente, C. C. (1994). *Changing for Good.* New York: William Morrow and Company, Inc.

important. Honestly talking about each partner's strengths and weaknesses, hopes and dreams, and past and present life experiences helps to build intimacy in a loving relationship.

Commitment expectations often differ among people in romantic relationships. Again, communicating expectations early on in the relationship, as well as periodically, is especially important. Some individuals want to date but do not want to progress to any exclusive commitment such as going steady or becoming engaged. Others would be willing to live with a romantic partner, but do not wish to make the legal or spiritual long-term commitment that defines marriage. For example, a person may not want marriage until after college graduation, and not want children until after age thirty. This factor may play a role in the direction and form of the relationships he or she seeks. Discussing commitment expectations with a partner adds a great deal to understanding individual goals and overall direction in life. It also helps both partners understand and judge for compatibility the purpose, motives, and commitment level each partner brings to a developing relationship. Honest communication also decreases the risk of experiencing disappointment and hurt, and can ease the pain of rejection when one accepts that the relationship failed, and not the person.

In practice, the more each partner defines the passion, intimacy, and commitment expectations they bring to a relationship the more likely it is that a relationship will meet their expectations. Paying attention to the components of love helps to build a satisfying loving relationship.

Cohabitation

Cohabitation describes a living arrangement in which two people who are not married to each other share both bed and board. Cohabiting couples in essence live as married couples without being legally married.

Rates of cohabitation have increased dramatically over the past twenty-five years, tripling in the 1970s and almost doubling in the 1980s.[29] Overall, nearly half of the single population in the U.S. less than age thirty-five have cohabited for some period of time. In addition, more than one out of four separated or divorced persons under age thirty are cohabiting.[30] In a given year, more than

2.5 million heterosexual couples are cohabiting, which is nearly 5 percent of all married and unmarried couples in the U.S.[31]

Couples who cohabit usually do so for one of three reasons.[32] First, some couples participate in what is often termed part-time or limited cohabitation. In this form of cohabitation, a couple who is dating start to spend more time at one of the partner's residence. They may begin to spend the night and leave some of their belongings there. Gradually, the couple finds that they are, for all practical purposes, living together.

For others, however, cohabiting *is* a step that they believe will lead them to marriage. Living together prior to marriage is a conscious choice that is often viewed as a "trial marriage." A recent study conducted by the American Council on Education found that 51 percent of almost 300,000 U.S. college freshmen believed that couples should live together before marriage. It appears that this belief often translates into action, as half of all *first* cohabitations do result in marriage. These marriages seem to face a greater risk of ending in divorce.[33] A number of studies have found an increased rate of divorce among couples who cohabited prior to marriage, with results ranging from a 33 percent to an 80 percent greater risk of divorce.[34] Many explanations have been offered for this higher risk of divorce. It has been suggested that people who have cohabited may (1) have more extramarital affairs that could disrupt a marriage, (2) have less of a commitment to the institution of marriage, or (3) have less impulse control and patience, qualities that may be important to successful long-term relationships.[35] It is important to note that the studies on cohabitation and divorce do not prove that the act of cohabitation prior to marriage *causes* divorce. Rather, it it likely that individuals who choose to cohabit prior to marriage have different attitudes and values compared to people who do not cohabit prior to marriage, and it may be these attitudes and values that predispose them to also choose divorce.

A third reason couples choose to cohabit is to have a substitute marriage. In this instance, a couple does make a long-term commitment to each other similar to marriage, but for any number of reasons they do not formally marry. This form of cohabitation may be the only available choice for homosexual couples who are prevented from legally marrying a same-sex partner.

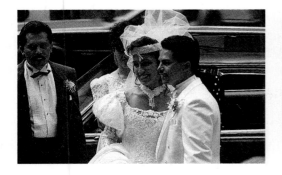
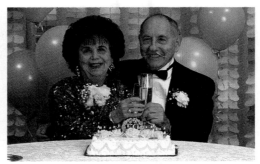

Figure 6.10: What Do You Think?

1. It is estimated that approximately 70 percent of males and females will marry at some point during their lives. Yet relatively few marriages make it to the 50th anniversary. What factors do you think contribute to this phenomenon?

2. How important do you think lasting marriages are for society? for families? for individuals involved in a marriage? What evidence did you use to reach your conclusion?

Marriage

Marriage is the personal commitment of two people to share forever their feelings, thoughts, failings, and triumphs. The marriage bond is a legal bond and is often practiced as a spiritual bond. The marriage ceremony is the formal act of two people announcing to the world; and possibly their God, that they have joined their lives forever.

In the traditional view, marriage creates a foundation for the family that serves as the workshop for human emotional, spiritual, physical, intellectual, and social development. The husband and wife form a human bond of purpose, which unites them to their ancestors. Each spouse becomes responsible for the other and for any children they might bear.

In the U.S. today, people overwhelmingly seek out this traditional form of marriage (see figure 6.10). People tend to marry partners who are similar to themselves in terms of economic, racial, and religious backgrounds. Additionally, we tend to marry spouses who have lived or are living close to our homes. First-time marrieds tend to marry spouses close to their own ages. The median marital age at first marriage for U.S. males is 26.2 years, and for females 23.8 years. Less than 2 percent of married couples comprise interracial marriages in the U.S. Table 6.3 illustrates the distribution of single and married people for various age groups. Keep in mind that the married column includes people who are remarried. For men, by age twenty-five just over 80 percent are single and by age thirty-five over 70 percent are married. By age twenty-five 65 percent of the women are single and by age thirty-five 70 percent are married.[36]

There are two basic mores of marriage. The first is that the husband's and wife's sexual activity is limited to each other. The second is that the husband and wife are personally and socially responsible for each other and their children. The spouses are the family providers, protectors, teachers, and counselors.

Why are so many people attracted to marriage as a lifestyle? Marriage offers people the chance to experience intense human compassion and support for a lifetime. Married people can build their relationship over time until love and friendship become one. They can be molders and givers of life and love. They can share their compassion with children. Additionally, marriage offers economic benefits and support, as well as providing a heritage of ancestors and the possibility of heirs. On the average, married people are happier, healthier, and live longer than never-married people.

Divorce

During the last quarter-of-a-century the U.S. divorce rate increased markedly, almost doubling between 1965 and 1995.[37] Presently, the divorce rate has stabilized with the median age at divorce for men in the U.S. at 35.6 years and women, 33.2 years. The median duration of *first* marriage is eight years.[38] Based on the high rate of divorce one may conclude that the institution of marriage is failing; however, the majority of divorced people remarry. Forty-five percent of all marriages are remarriages. However, remarriages tend to be less stable than first marriages. Based on marriage's popularity, it is reasonable to assume that people in the U.S. are more likely divorcing their spouses, rather than divorcing themselves from marriage.

Divorced people are faced with the task of reassembling their lives and lifestyles. They must deal not only with legal matters of divorce but also with the emotional and social aspects. In some cases divorced persons must sever ties with family, friends, and neighbors. Most divorced people seek out

TABLE 6.3 — Marital Status of the Population, by Sex and Age:1992

Sex and Age	Total	Single	Married	Widowed	Divorced
Male	100.0	26.2	63.3	2.9	7.6
18 to 19 years old	100.0	97.7	2.3	*	*
20 to 24 years old	100.0	80.3	18.3	*	1.4
25 to 29 years old	100.0	48.7	46.3	0.1	4.8
30 to 34 years old	100.0	29.4	63.0	0.1	7.5
35 to 39 years old	100.0	18.4	70.8	0.5	10.3
40 to 44 years old	100.0	9.2	77.8	0.6	12.4
45 to 54 years old	100.0	7.3	79.5	1.0	12.2
55 to 64 years old	100.0	5.6	82.2	3.5	8.7
65 to 74 years old	100.0	4.6	79.1	10.2	6.1
75 years old and over	100.0	3.5	70.2	23.7	2.6
Female	100.0	19.2	59.1	11.7	9.9
18 to 19 years old	100.0	90.0	9.3	—	0.6
20 to 24 years old	100.0	65.7	32.0	0.1	2.2
25 to 29 years old	100.0	33.2	58.5	0.3	8.0
30 to 34 years old	100.0	18.8	69.8	0.7	10.7
35 to 39 years old	100.0	12.6	73.7	1.1	12.6
40 to 44 years old	100.0	8.4	74.3	2.0	15.4
45 to 54 years old	100.0	5.3	73.6	4.6	16.4
55 to 64 years old	100.0	4.0	69.6	14.9	11.4
65 to 74 years old	100.0	4.4	53.0	35.9	6.7
75 years old and over	100.0	5.4	25.6	65.0	4.0

Percent Distribution

What Do You Think?

1. Looking at the column of data on single men, what trend do you see as men age? Does the same trend exist for single women?

2. What trends exist by age for married men and married women? What factors may explain the differences in trends seen in the percent of married men compared to married women for ages eighteen to thirty-nine and for ages forty to seventy-five and older?

*Represents or rounds to zero.

Source: Data from the U.S. Bureau Of The Census, *Statistical Abstract Of The United States: 1993*, 113th Edition, Table #61, Washington DC. 1993

---

another mate. That task requires they reenter the dating arena and learn new dating rules that apply to divorced people. In most cases divorced people will be anxious about this new lifestyle and possibly apprehensive over their ability to readjust.

On the positive side, most divorced people do adjust and find a new sense of independence and self-worth. Sometimes the feeling of being freed from a failed marriage is a personal relief.

Divorce and Children

One-parent families have increased dramatically since 1960. There are over one million children involved in divorce each year. Twenty-three percent of families in the U.S. with children under the age of eighteen report only one parent as the head of household.[39] Eighty-five percent of the single-parent households are headed by females. The markedly low proportion of single-parent fathers across all racial groups is remarkably similar, and most likely this is a function of family courts' propensity to award child custody to the mother.

Understandably, there is concern as to whether divorce has any ill effects on children. Several researchers have concluded

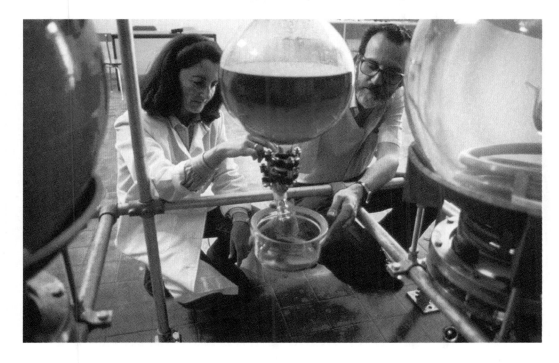

Figure 6.11: What Do You Think?

1. What type of gender roles do you see portrayed in this photograph? Explain your perspective.
2. Do you think that certain professions or jobs *should* be done by *only* females? or *only* males? What scientific evidence can you cite to support your opinion?

divorce adversely affects adolescent girls regarding their self-esteem and sexual relationships.[40] There is growing concern that nonremarried mother households have long-term negative effects on boys.[41] There is additional research that indicates children living with the same sex divorced parent are happier, more socially competent, and have a higher self-esteem than those children living with the opposite sex divorced parent.[42] One should not conclude that all children from divorced homes will suffer permanent ill effects. However, most researchers and professionals in the field agree that divorce is a stressful and emotionally upsetting experience for children. It is for this reason that parents, and people interacting with children from divorced homes, be perceptive to these children's needs, fears, misguided guilt, and confusion regarding the disruption of their family and lives.

Personal and Social Influences on Sexuality

The social environment influences both how we perceive ourselves and others and the ways we choose to express our sexuality. Some of the more important interactions between personal and social influences affect our choice of gender roles and the relationship options we select.

Gender Roles and Society

A personal association with either a masculine, feminine, or androgynous role is a person's gender identity. One's personal sense of being masculine or feminine may follow traditional gender roles or may include behaviors, attitudes, and characteristics that are not part of the stereotypic gender role (see figure 6.11).

Each society has historically devised a variety of gender-role guidelines for males and females. Despite the many variations between societies, within each society there is a minimum of duplication between gender roles. Historically gender roles within a society were often compatible and specialized. For example, the male was the provider and the female the preparer, the male the model of strength and the female the model of compassion, and so on.

Over the centuries such specialized roles developed from social idiosyncrasies and from the belief that males and females were biologically and intellectually different and therefore best suited for different life tasks and roles. On the other hand the case has been made that males and females are human beings first and neither gender has a monopoly on a given emotion, ability, or intellectual vocation. Furthermore, stereotypic gender roles have been perceived to stifle human development and serve only to limit the range of emotional and personal options in life (see A Social Perspective 6.1).

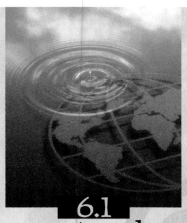

6.1

A Social Perspective

In a Male-Centered World, Female Differences Are Transformed into Female Disadvantages

The search for fundamental biological differences between men and women is misguided. We already know the truly potent differences between the sexes—women can become pregnant and can breast-feed their infants, while men, on average, are bigger and stronger. Even if we were to discover differences with more power than these have to shape our lives or to limit our chances for equality, the fact remains that biological differences are given real meaning by the ways in which a culture interprets and uses them.

Put somewhat differently, social change—what I like to call cultural invention—can so radically transform the context in which human beings live their lives that people can often be liberated from what in earlier times were thought to be intrinsic biological limitations. This, of course, is why human beings can fly today even though they have no wings.

The problem for women thus is not simply that they are different from men, whether biologically or in some other way. The problem for women—and what limits their chances for equality—is that they are different from men in a social world that disguises what are really just male standards or norms as gender-neutral principles. In other words, the difficulties women face stem from the fact that they are different from men in an "androcentric" or male-centered world, one in which almost all policies and practices are so completely organized around male experience that they fit men better than they do women—and hence automatically transform any and all male/female differences into female disadvantages.

This privileging of male experience frequently involves the male body. Consider, for example, that the Centers for Disease Control included in their early diagnostic criteria for HIV infection only those medical conditions that showed up in men, thereby denying women access both to the appropriate diagnosis for their medical conditions and to emerging experimental treatments.

Consider as well that the U.S. Supreme Court ruled in the 1970s that pregnancy could be excluded from an employer's disability-insurance package, even if it covered every medical condition that could conceivably occur in a man—including those, like diseases of the prostate, that are unique to men. Why? Because, the Court argued, pregnancy is "unique to women" and thus deviates from what, in an androcentric society, are seen as "normal," thus gender-neutral, medical conditions.

If we want to understand gender inequality, it is much more important to shift from an analysis of difference *per se* to an analysis of the ways in which the social structure privileges some people's differences at the expense of others'.

Adapted from: Sandra Lipsitz Bem. (August 17, 1994) "In a Male-Centered World, Female Differences are Transformed into Female Disadvantages." *The Chronicle of Higher Education*, B–1 - B–2.

What Do You Think?

1. Do you agree with Dr. Bem's premise that, in the U.S. social structure, male differences receive privilege at the expense of female differences? Provide several examples that support your position.

In our society, there are always certain individuals and organizations trying to influence others to adopt particular sets of gender-role behaviors. Because gender-role behaviors are not necessarily right or wrong, each of us can create our own individual sexual identity. Your expression of your sexuality is a part of your personality, personal interactions, and social experience. That is why it is so important that you are satisfied with your sexual identity. It is a key to your overall wellness.

Prolonged Adolescence

Four hundred years ago people married in their early teens, about the time they reached puberty. Seventy years ago people in the U.S. married in their late teens, just a few years after they reached puberty. Today people in the U.S. marry in their mid-twenties, about one decade after they reach puberty. There is now a ten-year time lag from when most young people seek out sexual relationships to when they get married.

Prolonged adolescence has been necessitated by society's ever-increasing need to have trained and educated workers. More and more young people today wait to complete college before starting a career and marriage. Although society has extended the youth's occupational training period, it is not able to postpone the youth's desire for human intimacy and sexual relationships.

Prolonged adolescence encourages young people to enter into sexual relationships of convenience that do not hinder or jeopardize their future education or career goals. This pattern of partner selection encourages relationships in which the participants place personal goals before relationship needs. The pressure to marry when "you are ready," or when the "timing is right" is brought to bear by both friends and family. In turn young people learn to place their needs first in such relationships of convenience. These same individuals when they marry may have little or no experience in placing their partner's needs first, nor have experience in the gesture and art of compromise.

Increased Life Span

An increased life span has also influenced sexual relationships in the U.S. During colonial times the average life span in the U.S. was about thirty-five years. If you married and had children at age sixteen you would probably not live to see your grandchildren or your twenty-fifth anniversary. Today if you marry at age eighteen it could be a sixty-year commitment! This has caused some people to question the wisdom of marriage without the option of divorce. On the other hand, it has caused others who oppose divorce to be even more committed to the view that marriage and family are the foundation of society and binds it together.

Fertility Technology

Another factor challenging sexual relationships is fertility technology. Today people have the option to postpone procreation or to procreate artificially through the use of **artificial insemination, surrogate mothers,** or **sperm banks.** Unwanted pregnancies can be prevented and people can choose to be sexually active and not procreate before they believe they are socially ready. This makes sexual intimacy during prolonged adolescence less a threat to an individual's future marital and career goals. Young people can continue to pursue their educational, occupational, and sexual goals without having a pregnancy jeopardize their plans. The number of females having their first child between the ages of thirty and thirty-nine has increased markedly.

Single people can become parents. Married couples can remain childless.

Remarried people can remain childless or decide to procreate and start a second family. Fertility technology has added several new options to the sexual lifestyle in the U.S.

Leisure Time

As the number of average working hours decreases people gain more free time. This increased leisure time grants people additional opportunities to locate sexual partners. In turn, people have more time to invest in one or more ongoing sexual relationships. Leisure time has contributed to the number of relationships and social options open to single and married people.

Occupational Opportunities Available to Women

Improved occupational opportunities provide women with the independence and freedom to maintain their single lifestyles indefinitely. Occupational opportunities give married and single females the economic independence to move from one relationship to another. Occupational opportunities also increase partner selection opportunities. The more people someone is able to meet, the greater the chance for a relationship to develop. Working acquaintances and friendships have the possibility of developing into loving relationships for married as well as single people.

Human Sexuality and Well-Being

Sexuality is a vital component of being human. Each of us has sexual needs, desires, and hopes that we attempt to fulfill in life. As we grow and mature, we become more acquainted with our sexual selves—our gender identity, our sexual orientation, and our physiological and emotional responses to sexual stimulation. We also learn about the sexual needs and desires of significant others in our lives, and we make decisions about love relationships, sexual relationship options, and the types of sexual behaviors we will experience. Gaining a greater understanding of sexuality and intimate relationship decisions will help you navigate toward higher levels of well-being.

Artificial insemination: using means other than vaginal intercourse to introduce semen into the female vaginal tract.

Surrogate mothers: paid or unpaid female volunteers who make their reproductive organs available for procreation and pregnancy through artificial insemination. Surrogate mothers agree to give the child to the prospective parents following childbirth.

Sperm banks: Organizations that solicit and store sperm donations for use in artificial insemination.

Summary

1. Sexuality not only refers to the pursuit of sexual pleasure and reproduction, but also to our need for love and personal fulfillment. Sexuality includes our awareness of and reaction to our own characteristics of maleness and femaleness and to that of everyone with whom we interact.

2. Gender role is a group or societal view of what is masculine and feminine. Gender identity is an individual's sense of being either male or female.

3. A person's gender is believed to be influenced by both biological and social influences.

4. Androgynous people exhibit and utilize both masculine and feminine behaviors and thoughts and, thus, do not limit themselves to a stereotypic gender role.

5. Masters and Johnson separated the human sexual response cycle into four consecutive phases: excitement, plateau, orgasm, and resolution. They also described two major physiological events that occur during sexual response: vasocongestion and myotonia.

6. Sexual orientation is often thought of as a continuum ranging from a heterosexual orientation at one end to homosexual orientation at the other. Heterosexual orientation describes individuals who are attracted to people of the opposite sex, while homosexual orientation describes people who are attracted to others of the same sex. Bisexuals, individuals who are sexually attracted to both men and women, would be located in the middle of the continuum.

7. Sexual orientation can be defined by one or all of the following: sexual attraction, sexual behavior, and personal identification of a particular orientation. It is currently unknown why individuals have a particular sexual orientation. Biological, psychological, and social theories all attempt to explain the cause of sexual orientation.

8. Many researchers have studied love relationships in order to define love and successful love relationships. Sternberg describes love as consisting of various amounts of intimacy, passion, and commitment.

9. Sternberg makes ten suggestions for successful love relationships: do not take a relationship for granted; make the relationship a priority; actively seek to meet each other's needs; know when and when not to change in response to each other; value yourself; love each other, not an idealization of each other; tolerate what you cannot change; be open with each other; make good times together and grow through the bad ones; and do unto the other as you would have them do unto you. Most of these suggestions hinge on honest communication.

10. Men and women often look for similar characteristics in a romantic partner, most notably kindness, understanding, and intelligence. Women, however, typically place a higher value on a potential partner's earning capacity while men typically place a higher value on a potential partner's physical attractiveness.

11. The difficulty of using random selection techniques and a generally high nonresponse rate in sexuality research make it difficult for researchers to construct a sample of people who are representative of all people in the U.S. Additionally, sexuality studies tend to represent attitudes and behaviors for a certain time frame.

12. In 1992, the National Health and Social Life Survey (NHSLS) was administered to a random sample of English-speaking adults in the U.S. Over 72 percent of the sample participated in the face-to-face interview process that gave us our first scientifically valid snapshot of sexual behavior in the U.S.

13. Masturbation is defined as self-stimulation of the body for the purpose of sexual pleasure. Masturbation is a common sexual practice in the U.S. today, and is considered by sexuality experts to be a normal and natural way of expressing sexuality.

14. Cunnilingus is defined as oral stimulation of the female genitals. Fellatio is defined as oral stimulation of the male genitals. Some people find oral sex to be very appealing while others feel strongly that it is not a sexual behavior they wish to engage in. The NHSLS found oral sex to be most popular among young Whites and people who have higher levels of education.

15. Vaginal intercourse is defined as sexual activity in which there is insertion of the penis into the vagina. Today, the majority of people in the U.S. experience vaginal intercourse for the first time at a young age and outside of marriage. According to the NHSLS, vaginal intercourse appears to have universal appeal with 95 percent of respondents reporting that they had vaginal intercourse the last time they had sex.

16. Anal intercourse, commonly defined as the insertion of the penis into the anus, is a sexual behavior practiced by both heterosexual and homosexual couples for sexual pleasuring. According to the NHSLS, a small percent of people in the U.S. find anal intercourse appealing. Anal intercourse is considered a high-risk behavior for infectious disease transmission.

17. The NHSLS has categorized people into three groups based upon their sexual attitudes, values, and beliefs. The *traditional* category describes individuals whose religious beliefs always guide their sexual behaviors. The *relational* category describes individuals who believe that love should always be present before sex occurs. The *recreational* category

describes individuals who view sex as an acceptable activity for pleasure regardless of whether or not love is present.

18. There are several common sexual performance behaviors that are often considered to be sexual dysfunctions, including anorgasmia, erectile dysfunction, premature ejaculation, and dyspareunia. Certified sex therapists can often help individuals and couples achieve a satisfying sexual relationship.

19. There are several lifestyle options commonly found in the U.S. today, including a single lifestyle, cohabitation, marriage, and divorce. Marriage is the most common adult lifestyle option, with an estimated 70 percent of adults marrying at some time during their lives.

20. Many social factors influence an individual's expression of sexuality, including gender roles; prolonged adolescence; increased life span; improved fertility technology; more leisure time; and greater occupational opportunities for women.

Recommended Readings

Robert T. Michael, John H. Gagnon, Edward O. Laumann, and Gina Kolata. (1994). *Sex in America: A Definitive Survey*. Boston: Little, Brown and Company.

Michael and colleagues present results of their nationally representative study of adult sexual behavior in the U.S. This well-written book examines common sexual myths by comparing them to the results of the National Health and Social Life Survey. Explanations of the social influences on sexuality are insightful.

Michael et al. give us our first scientifically valid snapshot of sexual behavior in the U.S.

David G. Myers. (1992). *The Pursuit of Happiness*. New York: William Morrow and Company, Inc.

Social psychologist David Myers has written a book that describes what is currently known about the components of well-being and happiness. Two chapters—"The Friendship Factor," and "Love and Marriage"—describe the contribution of loving relationships to happiness and well-being.

Robert Pool. (1994). *Eve's Rib: The Biological Roots of Sex Differences*. New York: Crown Publishers.

This well-written book describes recent advances in our understanding of sex and gender differences. Pool writes about technical research developments in an engaging manner that reads like a mystery.

References

1. Byer, C. O. & L. W. Shainberg. (1994). *Dimensions of Human Sexuality*. Madison, WI: Brown & Benchmark Publishers, p. 4.
2. Rathus, Spencer A., Jeffrey S. Nevid, and Lois Fichner-Rathus. (1993). *Human Sexuality in a World of Diversity*. Boston: Allyn and Bacon, p. 157.
3. W. H. Masters & V. E. Johnson. (1966). *Human Sexual Response*. Boston: Little, Brown and Company.
4. Michael, Robert T., John H. Gagnon, Edward O. Laumann, and Gina Kolata. (1994). *Sex in America: A Definitive Survey*. Boston: Little, Brown and Company.
5. Michael et al., *Sex in America*, p. 171, 177.
6. Sternberg, R. J. (1988). *The Triangle of Love*. New York: Basic Books.
7. Myers, David G. (1992). *The Pursuit of Happiness*. New York: William Morrow and Company, Inc., 166–168.
8. Sternberg, R. J. (April, 1985). "The measure of love," *Science Digest: 60*, 78–79.
9. Sternberg, "The measure of love."
10. Buss, David M. (1985). "Human mate selection," *American Scientist, 73*: 47–51.
11. Buss, "Human mate selection."
12. Segall, Michael. (November, 1987). "Your mental love map," *American Health*: 52–57.
13. Michael et al., *Sex in America*, p. 45.
14. Michael et al., *Sex in America*, p. 15–41.
15. Michael et al., *Sex in America*, p. 155–168.
16. Michael et al., *Sex in America*, p. 165.
17. Michael et al., *Sex in America*, p. 139–142.
18. National Center for Health Statistics. (1994). *Healthy People 2000 Review 1993*. DHHS Publication No. (PHS) 94–1232–1. Washington, D.C.: U.S. Government Printing Office.
19. Michael et al., *Sex in America*, pp. 135, 145.
20. Michael et al., *Sex in America*, pp. 114–115.
21. Michael et al., *Sex in America*, pp. 140, 146–147.
22. Michael et al., *Sex in America*, pp. 230–246, 286.
23. Michael et al., *Sex in America*, pp. 240, 244.
24. U.S. Bureau of the Census. (1993). *Statistical Abstract of the U.S.: 1993*. Washington, D.C.: U.S. Government Printing Office.
25. U.S. Bureau of the Census. (1992). *Statistical Abstract of the United States: 1992*. Washington, D.C.: U.S. Government Printing Office.
26. Michael et al., *Sex in America*, pp. 82–83.
27. Michael et al., *Sex in America*, p. 72.
28. Michael et al., *Sex in America*, p. 71.
29. Myers, David G., *The Pursuit of Happiness*, p. 161.
30. Landers, R. (1990). "Are Americans still in love with marriage?," *Editorial Research Reports, 1* (25): 382–95.

31. U.S. Bureau of the Census. (1990). *Statistical Abstract of the United States: 1990*. Washington, D.C.: U.S. Government Printing Office.

32. Kammeyer, K. C. W. (1990). *Marriage and Family: A Foundation for Personal Decisions* (2nd ed.) Boston: Allyn & Bacon, Inc.

33. Demaris, A., & K. V. Rao. (1992). "Premarital cohabitation and subsequent marital stability in the United States: A reassessment," *Journal of Marriage and the Family*, 54: 178–190.

34. Myers, David G., *The Pursuit of Happiness*, p. 162.

35. Myers, David G., *The Pursuit of Happiness*, p. 163.

36. U.S. Bureau of the Census. (1993). *Statistical Abstract of the U.S.: 1993*. Washington, D.C.: U.S. Government Printing Office.

37. National Center for Health Statistics. (1995). "Advance report of final divorce statistics, 1989 and 1990," *Monthly Vital Statistics Report*, 43 (9): 16, 19.

38. National Center for Health Statistics, "Advance report of final divorce statistics, 1989 and 1990," p. 9.

39. U.S. Bureau of the Census. (1993). *Statistical Abstract of the U.S.: 1993*. Washington, D.C.: U.S. Government Printing Office.

40. Hetherington, E. M. (1991). "The role of individual differences and family relationships in coping with divorce and remarriage," In P. A. Cowan & E. M. Hetherington (Eds.), *Family Transitions*. Hillsdale, New Jersey: Erlbaum.

41. Hetherington, "The role of individual differences and family relationships in coping with divorce and remarriage."

42. Furstenberg, F. F. (1988). "Childcare after divorce and remarriage," In E. M. Hetherington & J. D. Arasteh (Eds.), *Impact of Divorce, Single-Parenting, and Stepparenting on Children*. Hillsdale, New Jersey: Erlbaum.

Parenthood: Pregnancy and Child Care

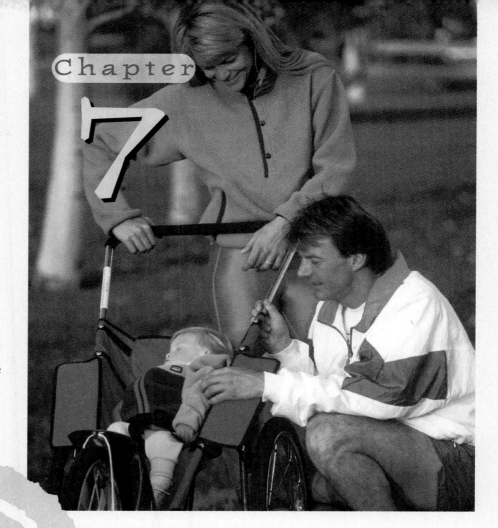

Student Learning Objectives

Upon completion of this chapter you should be able to:

1. list the functions of key hormones that regulate the human reproductive system;

2. identify and describe the functions of the male external and internal reproductive organs;

3. describe the controversy surrounding male circumcision;

4. identify and describe the functions of the female external and internal reproductive organs;

5. explain the ovarian cycle;

6. trace the paths of an ovum and sperm through the female reproductive tract to the point of implantation;

7. describe the female reproductive cycle;

8. evaluate the evidence currently available regarding the effects of nonparental primary caregivers on the well-being of children;

9. evaluate personal motives, expectations, and other factors that play a role in the decision of whether or not to become a parent;

10. describe the role of love in a parent-child relationship;

11. describe prenatal health behaviors that increase the chances for a healthy pregnancy and baby;

12. describe the social advantages and disadvantages of fetal rights legislation;

13. identify the stages and events in prenatal development for both the mother and her fetus;

14. list several common prenatal tests and evaluate their advantages and disadvantages;

15. describe the stages and events in childbirth;

16. list several advantages and disadvantages of breast-feeding;

17. identify the five main categories of childbirth options available to parents in the U.S., describing at least two examples for each category;

18. define infertility and explain the most common causes of male and female infertility;

19. describe three currently available male and female infertility options, identifying the ethical concerns of each option;

20. describe three prominent social influences on pregnancy and parenting.

A clear understanding of the human reproductive system is essential knowledge for you as a college student and as an adult in the midst of making some critical life decisions. Decisions about becoming a parent and raising children are ones that affect lifestyle and personal well-being for many years to come. Health behavior choices you make now have implications for a healthy pregnancy and childbirth experience, a healthy newborn, and your adaptation to parenthood. Whether you are female or male, your personal health decisions are important. Table 7.1 illustrates many of the national health objectives for the year 2000 that are related to pregnancy and child care.

Most people contemplate what it would be like for them to be parents. In doing so it is common to underestimate the demands of parenthood and taking responsibility for a new life. It is difficult to appreciate fully the devotion that is required to take care of that life through infancy, early childhood, and adolescence. Likewise, until one has been a parent, it is equally as difficult to explain the joys of creating and nurturing a life. People who choose to be parents hope to create and nurture a healthy baby. Most people who make this choice are able to conceive and create a healthy baby. For persons who want to be parents but have been unable to conceive their own child, new technology is available to increase their chances of becoming parents in this way. Moreover, the possibility of adopting children permits responsible individuals and couples a clear option of selecting parenthood. Parenthood is perhaps the most complex and challenging task that people will ever undertake. After considering the pros and cons of parenthood, some people choose not to be parents. This chapter explores the intricacies of the human reproductive system, the features of pregnancy and development during pregnancy, and the possibilities and potential of parenthood.

The Reproductive System

The human species is **dimorphic** because it has two unique reproductive forms, a male and a female. Together the male and the female form the human reproductive system. Not all living creatures are dimorphic. There are species of animals that are asexual and consequently have no male or female form. Dimorphic species have more variation and adaptability because two individual members contribute genes to their offspring. In the case of humans the contributed genes from the male and the female combine to form a single cell, called a **zygote.** The zygote develops into a new member of the human race.

The Primary Reproductive Organs

The primary human reproductive organs are the **testes** in males and **ovaries** in females. The testes and ovaries have several important functions. First, the sperm produced by the testes and the eggs produced by the ovaries carry genetic information. Each sperm carries either an X or Y sex **chromosome.** Each egg carries only an X chromosome. If a zygote is formed by an X-carrying sperm the offspring will be female, because the new pair of sex chromosomes will both be X chromosomes. If the zygote is formed by a Y-carrying sperm the offspring will be male, because the new pair of sex chromosomes will be one X and one Y. The second function of the testes and ovaries is to produce hormones—testosterone and estrogen respectively—that cause **secondary sex characteristics,** the physical changes that lead to sexual maturity. The testes' and ovaries' third function is to produce hormones that maintain the viability of the reproductive organs.

Gonadotropins

The brain is responsible for the regulation of the human reproductive system. The part of the brain that monitors and regulates the reproductive system is the **hypothalamus** (see figure 7.1). The hypothalamus communicates its directions with **hormones,** chemicals that stimulate organs of the body into performing certain tasks. The hormone used by the hypothalamus to stimulate the testes and ovaries is called the **gonadotropin-releasing hormone,** or GnRH. The purpose of GnRH is to set off a chain of chemical events that cause the testes to produce sperm and the

Zygote: the term for a human egg (ovum) that has been fertilized by a sperm cell (spermatozoon) before the process of cell division begins.

Chromosome: a threadlike structure containing genes, found in the nucleus of every cell.

Hypothalamus: a small part of the forebrain, located below the cerebrum, that is linked to both the thalamus and the pituitary gland.

1. **Increase to at least 75 percent the proportion of mothers who breast-feed their babies in the early postpartum period and to at least 50 percent the proportion who continue breast-feeding until their babies are 5 to 6 months old.** (Update: 54 percent during early postpartum period, and 19 percent at age 5–6 months, in 1992.) (Special Target Populations: Low-income mothers, Black mothers, Hispanic mothers, American Indian/Alaska Native mothers.)

2. **Increase smoking cessation during pregnancy so that at least 60 percent of women who are cigarette smokers at the time they become pregnant quit smoking early in pregnancy and maintain abstinence for the remainder of their pregnancy.** (Update: 31 percent quit smoking during pregnancy in 1991, down from 39 percent in 1986.) (Special Target Population: Females with less than a high school education.)

3. **Increase to at least 60 percent the proportion of primary caregivers who provide age-appropriate preconception care and counseling.** (Baseline: the following percent of primary caregivers routinely inquired about family planning with 81–100 percent of female patients of childbearing age in 1992: pediatricians 18 percent, nurse practitioners 53 percent, obstetrician/gynecologists 48 percent, internists 24 percent, and family physicians 28 percent; the following percent of primary caregivers routinely counsel about family planning with 81–100 percent of patients in 1992: pediatricians 36 percent, nurse practitioners 53 percent, obstetrician/gynecologists 65 percent; internists 26 percent, and family practitioners 36 percent.)

4. **Reduce the incidence of fetal alcohol syndrome to no more than 0.12 per 1,000 live births.** (Update: 0.39 in 1992, up from 0.22 in 1987.) (Special Target Populations: American Indians/Alaska Natives, and Blacks.)

5. **Reduce low birth weight to an incidence of no more than 5 percent of live births and very low birth weight to no more than 1 percent of live births.** (Update: 7.1 percent of live births were low birth weight in 1991, up from 6.9 percent in 1987; 1.3 percent of births were very low birth weight in 1991, up from 1.2 percent in 1987.) (Special Target Population: Blacks.)

6. **Increase to at least 85 percent the proportion of mothers who achieve the minimum recommended weight gain during their pregnancies.** (Update: 75 percent in 1988, up from 67 percent in 1980.)

7. **Reduce the cesarean delivery rate to no more than 15 per 100 deliveries.** (Update: 23.6 in 1992, down from 24.4 in 1987.)

8. **Increase abstinence from alcohol, cocaine, and marijuana by pregnant women by at least 20 percent.** (Baseline: 79 percent of pregnant women abstained from alcohol, 99 percent from cocaine, and 98 percent from marijuana in 1988.)

9. **Increase to at least 90 percent the proportion of all pregnant women who receive prenatal care in the first trimester of pregnancy.** (Update: 76.2 percent of live births were to women who received prenatal care in the first trimester in 1991, up from 76 percent in 1987.) (Special Target Populations: Blacks, American Indians/Alaska Natives, and Hispanics.)

10. **Increase to at least 90 percent the proportion of women enrolled in prenatal care who are offered screening and counseling on prenatal detection of fetal abnormalities.** (Note: this objective will be measured by tracking use of maternal serum alpha-feto protein screening tests.) (Baseline: 29 percent in 1988.)

11. **Reduce the prevalence of infertility to no more than 6.5 percent.** (Baseline: 7.9 percent of married couples with wives aged 15 through 44 in 1988.) (Special Target Populations: Black couples and Hispanic couples.)

From *Healthy People 2000 National Health Promotion and Disease Prevention Objectives,* 1991, and *Healthy People 2000 Review 1993,* 1994. Department of Health and Human Services, Washington, D.C.

---

ovaries to produce eggs, as well as producing additional hormones to maintain the reproductive organs.

Luteinizing Hormone

When GnRH is secreted by the hypothalamus it causes the **pituitary** to secrete **luteinizing hormones (LH)** into the bloodstream. In males, LH stimulates the testes into producing **testosterone,** the primary male sex hormone. Although the physiological process is not completely understood, testosterone prevents atrophy (wasting away) of the male reproductive organs. Testosterone is the biological stimulant for males' socially and sexually

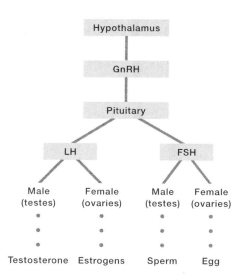

Figure 7.1: Hormonal direction of the human reproductive system

Pituitary gland: an endocrine gland the size of a pea, located beneath and attached to the hypothalamus in the brain. The pituitary secretes various hormones when it receives hormone releasing factors from the hypothalamus.

Figure 7.2: Male reproductive organs

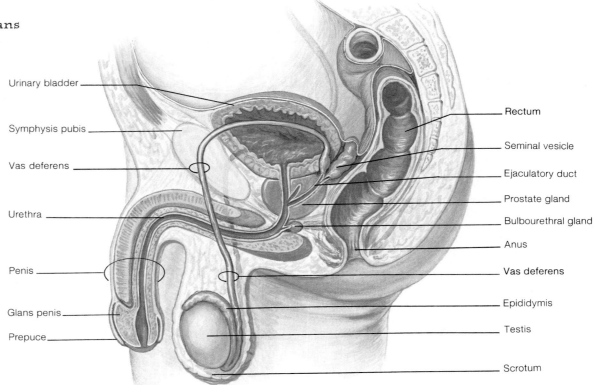

Urinary bladder

Symphysis pubis

Vas deferens

Urethra

Penis

Glans penis

Prepuce

Rectum

Seminal vesicle

Ejaculatory duct

Prostate gland

Bulbourethral gland

Anus

Vas deferens

Epididymis

Testis

Scrotum

aggressive behaviors. Additionally, testosterone causes the adolescent male to develop the adult male physique, including broad shoulders, pubic hair, enlargement of the penis and scrotum, enlargement of the larynx and vocal chords, and thickening of the skin.

In females, LH stimulates the ovaries to produce the primary female hormone **estrogen,** which has several functions. In preadolescent females estrogens cause the development of the breasts. Estrogens also cause the female to develop the feminine physique by adding fat deposits in the abdomen, buttocks, and hips. Estrogens are also responsible for the enlargement of reproductive organs. In post pubertal females, estrogens stimulate and maintain the female reproductive organs. Estrogens also cause eggs to mature and prepare the uterus for pregnancy.

Follicle-Stimulating Hormone

The pituitary, when stimulated by GnRH, also secretes **follicle-stimulating hormone (FSH).** In females FSH stimulates the ovaries to produce eggs. In males FSH stimulates the testes to produce sperm.

The Male Reproductive System

The male reproductive system is composed of the primary reproductive organs, the testes, and the secondary reproductive organs, the seminal vesicles, prostate gland, and bulbourethral glands (see figure 7.2).

Scrotum

The **scrotum,** a skin sac suspended in the groin area at the base of the penis, houses two testes. The scrotum is suspended from the body in order to maintain the temperature of the testes at approximately 3.6 degrees (Fahrenheit) cooler than normal body temperature. This lower temperature is necessary for the production of sperm. Muscle fibers in the scrotum contract and relax in response to external temperature. In cold weather, the muscle fibers contract and move the testes closer to the body for warmth, whereas in warm weather the muscles relax and move them farther away from the body.

The testes are the primary male reproductive organs. The testes produce sperm and testosterone. Inside the testes are numerous highly coiled tubes known as the **seminiferous tubules.** It is inside these seminiferous tubules that sperm are produced.

In the spaces between the seminiferous tubules lie the **Leydig cells,** which produce testosterone (see figure 7.3).

Epididymis

As sperm mature, they migrate from the seminiferous tubules into the **epididymis.** The literal meaning of the word epididymis is "over the testes," which accurately describes their location. The epididymis also provides a fluid for storing sperm.

It takes approximately seventy-four days to manufacture sperm. The male manufactures approximately 200 million sperm per day. Viable sperm remain stored in the epididymis for approximately two to four weeks. After such time they are reabsorbed by the body.

Vas Deferens

Each epididymis empties into a **vas deferens.** The vas deferens are approximately eighteen inches long and are partially housed inside the scrotum. The vas deferens circle the bladder and ultimately join with the urethra. The walls of the vas deferens are lined with **cilia.** Contraction of the vas deferens, coupled with the action of the cilia, combine to transport sperm through the vas deferens.

Semen

When exiting the body, sperm reside in a fluid called **semen.** Seminal fluid is produced by the epididymis and the secondary male reproductive organs, which include the seminal vesicles, prostate gland, and bulbourethral glands.

Seminal Vesicles

The **seminal vesicles** are two small glands found at the end of each vas deferens, just before the vas deferens enter the prostate gland. The seminal vesicles produce a fluid containing a simple sugar that provides nutrition for sperm. About 60 percent of the total volume of semen is made up of the fluid produced by the seminal vesicles. The seminal vesicles also secrete prostaglandins, which stimulate the sperm into undulating their tails for locomotion. Prostaglandins also stimulate the female's reproductive tract into contractions. These combined actions help to transport sperm through the female reproductive tract.

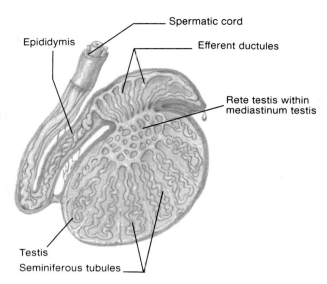

Figure 7.3: Cross section of scrotum

From Kent M. Van De Graaff, *Human Anatomy*, 3rd edition. Copyright © 1992 Wm. C. Brown Communications, Inc. Reprinted by permission of Times Mirror Higher Education Group, Inc., Dubuque, Iowa. All Rights Reserved.

Labels: Epididymis, Spermatic cord, Efferent ductules, Rete testis within mediastinum testis, Testis, Seminiferous tubules

Prostate Gland

The **prostate gland** is a small walnut-shaped gland located at the base of the bladder. The ejaculatory duct and the urethra pass through the prostate gland. The prostate secretion, which makes up about 15 to 30 percent of the semen, is alkaline, opalescent in color, and possesses the characteristic seminal odor. The prostate secretions neutralize: (1) the waste products of sperm; (2) the acid found in the **male urethra;** and (3) the acidic environment of the female reproductive tract. Without the neutralizing action of the prostate fluid many sperm would die, making fertilization of the egg impossible.

Urethra

The urethra has two functions. It is the tract that urine passes through from the bladder to the penis, and the tract that semen passes through.

Bulbourethral Glands

Two **bulbourethral glands** (also referred to as Cowper's Glands) are connected to the urethra as it enters the penis. They are about the shape and size of a pea. These glands create an alkaline secretion that sometimes appears as a droplet prior to ejaculation. Occasionally this droplet may contain viable sperm. The exact purpose of the bulbourethral glands' secretion is not known. Its secretions may provide a neutralizing effect on any urine left in the urethra prior to ejaculation.

Cilia: tiny hairlike projections that line certain parts of the body, whose constant motion helps to move particles away from that part of the body.

Semen: the fluid component discharged from the male reproductive tract at ejaculation. This fluid contains sperm, fructose to supply the sperm with an energy source, and prostaglandins that are thought to help move sperm to the fallopian tubes for possible fertilization of an egg.

Male urethra: a tube that conducts urine from the bladder, through the penis, to the exterior of the body. This tube also conducts semen from the male reproductive system to the exterior of the body.

Penis

The reproductive function of the penis is to deposit semen in the female reproductive tract. The approximate length of the adult male penis when flaccid (not stimulated) is between two and one-half, and four and one-half inches. This increases to approximately six inches when erect.

Internally, there are three spongelike chambers that run the length of the penis. When the male is sexually stimulated these chambers fill with blood causing the penis to become erect.

The head of the penis, called the **glans,** is an especially sensitive area of the penis, containing many nerve endings. The glans is covered by loosely fitting skin called the **prepuce** or **foreskin.** It has been a common practice in the U.S. to remove the foreskin at birth or soon after. This operation is called **circumcision.**

During the last twenty years the American Academy of Pediatrics has reversed its recommendation on routine neonatal male circumcision on several occasions. Presently the American Academy of Pediatrics recommends routine neonatal male circumcision. The lack of consensus regarding the health and medical benefits for routine male circumcision is a result of the divided published research on the issue. Some research indicates that uncircumcised infant males are more likely to experience urinary tract infections than circumcised males.[1] Authors have suggested that by circumcising the male, his female sexual partners may have a lower risk of cervical cancer. In addition some authors argue that male circumcision provides some protection against penile cancer and HIV infection.[2] However there is just as compelling evidence that uncircumcised males do not have a higher incidence of urinary tract infections, that there is no relationship between cervical cancer and uncircumcised men, and that the foreskin does not provide additional protection against penile cancer and infection from HIV or other sexually transmitted diseases.[3] Since there is not a consensus regarding the need for routine circumcisions, and given that male circumcision is the second most common surgical operation in the U.S., it is prudent that the risks, benefits, and procedures (e.g., use of local anesthesia) be discussed with a physician to determine whether circumcision is necessary. The parents requesting

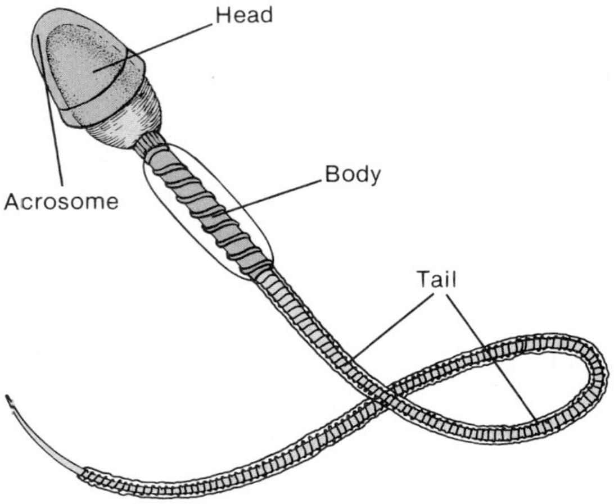

Figure 7.4: A sperm cell is highly adapted for reaching and penetrating a female egg

From John W. Hole, Jr., *Human Anatomy and Physiology*, 4th edition. Copyright © 1987 Wm. C. Brown Communications, Inc. Reprinted by permission of Times Mirror Higher Education Group, Inc., Dubuque, Iowa. All Rights Reserved.

circumcision of their male newborn should take into consideration that it is a medical procedure, and like all medical procedures errors can be made resulting in damage, permanent incapacitation of the male's penis as a sexual organ, and life-threatening surgical complications.

Sperm

The sperm cell is truly unique. The sperm has three basic parts, including the head, middle piece, and the tail. Atop the head is the **acrosome,** a structure that contains an **enzyme** that breaks down the coating of cells that surround the egg, enabling a sperm to penetrate. The middle piece, or body of the sperm, is partially responsible for generating energy. The tail is responsible for the sperm's mobility (see figure 7.4).

Sperm can swim about one inch an hour. However, on the average, sperm reach the **fallopian tubes** sixty to ninety minutes after being deposited into the female reproductive tract. The female tract is much longer than two inches and this suggests that the sperm's journey is aided by the contractions of the female reproductive tract.

Ejaculation

Sperm leave the body via ejaculation. **Ejaculation** is the expulsion of semen from the urethra and is usually associated with **orgasm.** Ejaculation and orgasm, however, can occur independently. Semen and sperm

Enzyme: a protein substance that speeds up biochemical reactions.

Fallopian tubes: two tubes found in the internal female reproductive tract that lie between the uterus and the right and left ovaries. With rare exceptions, these tubes are the site of fertilization.

Orgasm: the climax of sexual excitement, consisting of sudden muscle contractions followed by a distinct release of sexual tension.

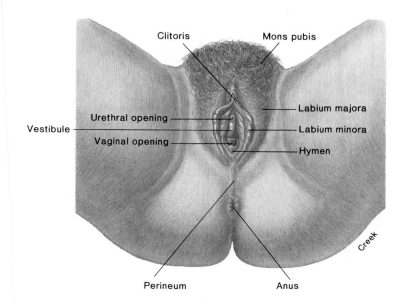

Figure 7.5: The external female genitals

From Kent M. Van De Graaff, *Human Anatomy*, 3rd edition. Copyright © 1992 Wm. C. Brown Communications, Inc. Reprinted by permission of Times Mirror Higher Education Group, Inc., Dubuque, Iowa. All Rights Reserved.

leave the urethra in the following order: first the fluid from the bulbourethral glands is expelled, then the prostatic fluid, followed by sperm. Finally the seminal fluid is released.

There are several factors that can reduce the male's **sperm count,** or the number of sperm found in one ejaculation. These factors range from fever to tight underwear. Altitude (either living in elevations well above sea level or traveling frequently in airplanes) can also reduce sperm count. Stress, whether caused by the battlefield or emotional distress, can also reduce the male's sperm count. Drugs, poor nutrition, and several diseases, such as **mumps, diabetes mellitus,** and **gonorrhea,** can also affect a male's sperm count.

The average ejaculation contains three milliliters of semen with an average range of 10 to 100 million sperm per milliliter. There are reports of males fathering children with only two to four million sperm in their entire ejaculate. As a benchmark, however, it seems that when the male's sperm count drops below 20 million per milliliter, fertilization of the egg becomes difficult.[4]

External Female Reproductive System

The external female reproductive structures are the vulva and the breasts. The breasts are secondary reproductive organs.

Vulva

The external female genitals (see figure 7.5) are all referred to as the **vulva.** The **labia majora** (Latin for "major lips") are paired folds of skin that surround the clitoris, urethral opening, and vaginal opening. The **labia minora** (Latin for "small lips") are paired folds of skin that extend along the vestibule. The labia minora and labia majora merge to form a clitoral hood. The **clitoris** is similar to the penis in structure and function. It is composed of erectile tissue that swells with blood and becomes erect when stimulated. The shaft of the clitoris is referred to as the glans. All of the external female genitals are sensitive to touch, especially the clitoris.

The **vestibule** is the area enclosed by the labia minora. The **introitus** is the opening of the vagina. An imaginary line from the introitus to the anus is the area called the **perineum.** This area is sometimes surgically cut during childbirth in an operation called an **episiotomy.** The episiotomy is done to prevent tearing of the perineum during childbirth.

The **hymen** partially covers the introitus. The hymen often remains intact until the female's first experience of sexual intercourse. Although the intact hymen has been used as proof of virginity over the centuries, there are several problems with such an assumption. Some females are born with partially torn hymens, while others may tear their hymens prior to first intercourse (e.g., by the insertion of tampons).

The **Bartholin's glands** lie inside the labia minora, one on each horizontal side of

Mumps: a viral infection typically occurring in young children. The most distinct symptom of mumps is the presence of swollen salivary glands on the sides of the face. If the infection spreads to the testicles it can cause sterility.

Diabetes mellitus: a metabolic disorder caused by lack of insulin or resistance to insulin, resulting in the body not being able to metabolize sugar for energy. Diabetes can be controlled through diet, exercise, and medication. Uncontrolled diabetes can result in life-threatening complications.

Gonorrhea: a bacterial sexually transmitted disease that if left untreated, can result in sterility.

Hymen: a membrane that partially covers the vaginal opening.

Figure 7.6: Cross section of the female reproductive organs

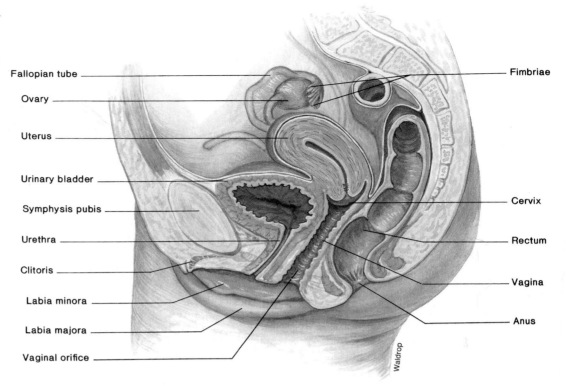

Fallopian tube — Ovary — Uterus — Urinary bladder — Symphysis pubis — Urethra — Clitoris — Labia minora — Labia majora — Vaginal orifice — Fimbriae — Cervix — Rectum — Vagina — Anus

Waldrop

Progesterone: a steroid hormone responsible for preparing the inner lining of the uterus for pregnancy, and, if pregnancy occurs, maintaining the uterus throughout the pregnancy while preventing ovulation during that period.

Menopause: the cessation of the female's menstrual or reproductive cycles.

Graafian follicle: a small, estrogen secreting gland in the ovary, containing a maturing egg. When the egg is fully matured, the graafian follicle ruptures, releasing the egg, a process known as ovulation.

the introitus. They secrete a mucus that appears prior to female orgasm. The exact function of the Bartholin's glands and their secretions is unknown.

Breasts

The breasts are secondary reproductive glands that are responsible for nurturing the product of reproduction, the infant. Each **breast** contains fifteen to twenty milk ducts, all of which open to the external nipple. The nipple is highly sensitive to stimulation. The action of hormones (prolactin, progesterone, and estrogens) causes a female to produce milk after childbirth. Breast size has no relation to the quantity or quality of milk produced by lactating females. An overwhelming majority of females are capable of breast-feeding following childbirth.

Internal Female Reproductive System

The internal female reproductive system contains a number of important structures (see figure 7.6). These include the ovaries, fallopian tubes, uterus, and vagina.

Ovaries

The ovaries are the primary female reproductive organs and have two main functions: to produce eggs and to produce estrogen and **progesterone.** Females have two ovaries that measure a little over an inch across. The female is born with all the potential eggs she will use throughout her reproductive lifetime. In fact, a peak of some seven million immature eggs are produced while the female fetus is developing. From that peak throughout her lifetime the quantity of immature eggs decline to where she has approximately two million or so at birth, one million at puberty, and less than 200,000 at **menopause.**

During the female's reproductive cycle several immature eggs begin to mature. Usually just one of these eggs fully matures and the remaining eggs are dissolved in the ovaries. An egg that fully matures is contained in a **Graafian follicle.** When the Graafian follicle ruptures it releases the egg from the ovary into the fallopian tube. This event is called **ovulation.** Some women experience discomfort, pressure, or pain around the time of ovulation. The phenomena is called **mittelschmerz,** meaning middle pain. Mittelschmerz may occur on either side of the abdomen, depending on which ovary is ovulating (see figure 7.7).

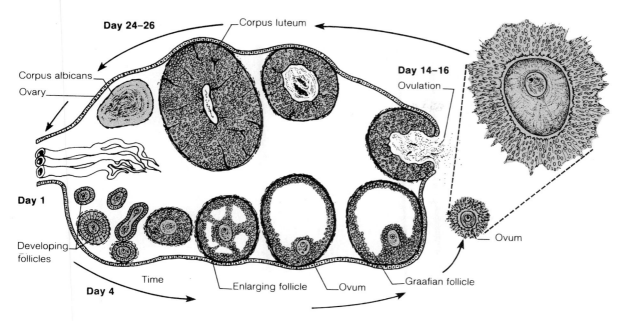

Figure 7.7: The ovarian cycle

At no one time are all the structures illustrated present. At the beginning of the ovarial cycle, several follicles start to develop. One of these becomes a mature Graafian follicle, while the others regress. The mature Graafian follicle releases its egg (ovulation). If there is no fertilization, the corpus luteum starts to regress in about ten days. If fertilization occurs, the corpus luteum secretes hormones to maintain the pregnancy.

From John W. Hole, Jr., *Human Anatomy and Physiology*, 4th edition. Copyright © 1987 Wm. C. Brown Communications, Inc. Reprinted by permission of Times Mirror Higher Education Group, Inc., Dubuque, Iowa. All Rights Reserved.

Fallopian Tubes

Once the egg is released by the ovary, it enters a fallopian tube. Each fallopian tube is approximately four inches long and is connected at one end to the uterus. The other end of the fallopian tube consists of fingerlike projections called **fimbriae** that lie close to the ovaries. Because the fimbriae are not directly connected to the ovary, there is some speculation about the process by which an egg leaves the ovary and is subsequently "picked up" by the fallopian tube.

The fallopian tube's contractions and the action of the cilia push the egg through the tube, where the egg awaits fertilization. The egg travels at the rate of about one inch per day. With rare exceptions, fertilization will take place in the fallopian tubes (see figure 7.8).

The estimated time an egg can be fertilized after ovulation ranges from as short as two hours to as long as three days. There have been viable sperm found in the fallopian tubes seventy-two hours or more after being deposited in the vagina. This enhances the likelihood of fertilization. Thus it is possible for a female to have intercourse one day, ovulate the next day, and become pregnant the following day. If an egg is not fertilized it soon begins to degenerate. If an egg is fertilized it becomes a zygote and quickly begins to divide into a mass of vibrant cells as it completes its trek through the fallopian tube, on its way to the uterus.

Uterus

The **uterus** is a hollow, muscular, pear-shaped organ that is approximately three inches long and two inches wide in its nonpregnant state. The opening of the uterus into the vagina is called the **cervix.** The uterus has three layers: the perimetrium; myometrium; and endometrium. The **perimetrium** is the outermost layer. The **myometrium** is the muscular layer (*myo* means muscle), which is essential for birthing and menstruation. The **endometrium** is the innermost layer and is responsible for secreting fluids and nutrients for the developing fetus. The endometrium is where the fertilized egg will usually implant. During pregnancy the uterus will increase in size by 200 times.

The uterus has several important functions. It is the preferred site for **implantation,** or the attachment of the zygote to the uterus. In addition the uterus has the necessary vascular arrangements for nurturing a fetus. The uterus also assists in transporting

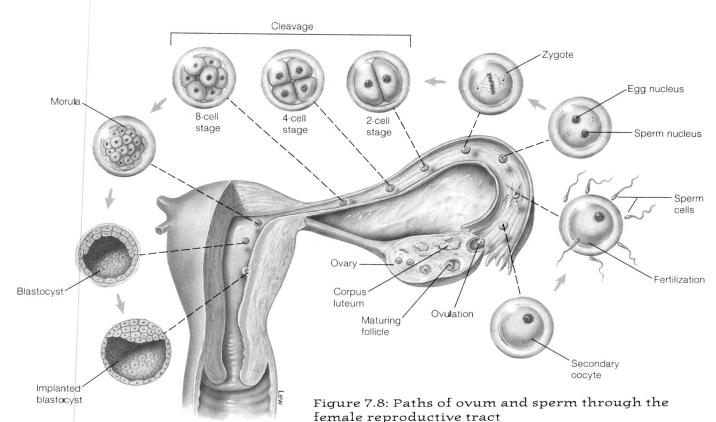

Figure 7.8: Paths of ovum and sperm through the female reproductive tract

From Kent M. Van De Graaff and Stuart Ira Fox, *Concepts of Human Anatomy and Physiology*, 3rd edition. Copyright © 1992 Wm. C. Brown Communications, Inc. Reprinted by permission of Times Mirror Higher Education Group, Inc., Dubuque, Iowa. All Rights Reserved.

sperm up to the fallopian tubes and moving the fetus through the reproductive tract during childbirth. Finally, the uterus contains the necessary muscular contractions for **menstruation.** Menstruation is the cyclical bleeding that signals the beginning of the next reproductive cycle.

The uterus undergoes a series of changes in preparation for a zygote. In the beginning of the reproductive cycle estrogens cause the endometrium to thicken about one-eighth of an inch. This layer of tissue and fluids is necessary for the preservation and development of an embryo. Estrogens cause the mucus around the cervix to change in its consistency and become less acidic. The mucus becomes clear and elastic. This change in the cervical mucus enhances the probability of sperm penetrating the cervix and continuing on to the fallopian tubes. There is also growing evidence that the cervical mucus prevents defective sperm from passing on through the fallopian tubes.[5]

If the egg is not fertilized, the **corpus luteum** of menstruation disintegrates causing a marked decrease of hormones in the bloodstream. About twenty-four hours after

this decrease in hormonal blood levels menstruation commences. The myometrium begins to contract and the layer of blood, mucus, and membranes attached to the endometrium is sloughed off through the cervix and vagina. The menstrual phase usually takes from two to five days. During menstruation the hypothalamus will detect the reduced levels of hormones in the bloodstream and release GnRH to start the next reproductive cycle.

Vagina

In its unstimulated state the **vagina** is approximately three to five inches long, and connects the cervix to the external genitals. The cervix actually protrudes into the vagina. The vagina functions to transport sperm to the uterus and to transport the products of menstruation to the external genitals. It is also the passageway for childbirth.

Female Reproductive Cycle

The female reproductive cycle is plotted from the first day of menstruation to the day before the onset of the next menstruation. Average female reproductive cycles range from twenty

Corpus luteum: the temporary endocrine gland in the ovary that secretes hormones. Its purpose is to prevent menstruation during pregnancy.

to forty-five days. The part of the female reproductive cycle that causes the greatest time variation is the follicular phase, which is the time from menstruation up until ovulation. For most females, however, the time from ovulation to menstruation is about the same, approximately fourteen days.

A female's first menstruation is called **menarche.** Menarche usually occurs between the ages of eleven and fifteen for U.S. females. The cessation of menstruation is called menopause, which usually occurs between the ages of forty-five and fifty for U.S. females. During menopause the menstrual cycle becomes irregular and less frequent. In a period of usually one to two years the menstrual cycle will eventually cease.

There are scores of factors that may alter a female's reproductive cycle. These factors include the most obvious, pregnancy, to the more subtle such as diet and stress. Seemingly unrelated factors may affect the healthy functioning of the female reproductive organs. Many such factors have been suggested including tight-fitting clothing, fabric softener, brands of toilet paper, laundry detergent, bubble bath, and deodorant tampons.[6]

Discomfort, pain, unusual bleeding, foul odor, or discharge are indicators of potential reproductive health problems. Females should be aware of what is normal for them regarding their reproductive cycles. Females experiencing unusual cycles should contact their physicians. Together they can decide what course of action, if any, is necessary.

Dysmenorrhea

Dysmenorrhea is painful menstruation. The majority of females, at one time or another, experience dysmenorrhea. Dysmenorrhea can be caused by high levels of prostaglandins in the bloodstream, which cause the uterus to contract. There are prescription and over-the-counter medications available, such as ibuprofen, that inhibit natural prostaglandin secretions, thus relieving pain. However, the diagnosis and treatment of amenorrhea should be performed by a qualified physician.

Amenorrhea

Primary amenorrhea is the absence of menstruation by age sixteen. **Secondary amenorrhea** is the absence of menstruation for six months or longer in a female who has previously established a pattern of normal reproductive cycles. The prevalence of secondary amenorrhea is approximately 3 percent of the female population. Some complications of amenorrhea include **infertility,** and possibly **osteoporosis** and endometrial cancer. Primary amenorrhea may also contribute to psychosexual problems. The causes of amenorrhea range from extreme emotional or physical stress, to hormonal or nutritional deficiencies. The diagnosis and treatment of amenorrhea should also be performed by a qualified physician.

Premenstrual Syndrome

Premenstrual syndrome (PMS), a chronic disorder that encompasses emotional, behavioral, and physical symptoms, has received a great deal of attention and publicity. Yet despite such attention, the causes and effective treatment for PMS are unknown. PMS signs and symptoms may include: violence towards others, crying spells, binge eating, hostility, paranoia, depression, irritability, fatigue, and **edema.** These changes occur a week prior to the onset of menstruation and end with menstruation.[7] This is a key criterion of PMS.

Many treatments have been suggested as potential remedies for PMS including sleep, exercise, lifestyle alterations, caffeine, **mild tranquilizers,** and **diuretics.** One of the more controversial treatments is the use of progesterone. Although some researchers have recommended progesterone therapy in the second half of the menstrual cycle, positive results have not been confirmed in double-blind studies, and additional studies report that drug therapy is not indicated for a considerable proportion of patients.[8]

Toxic-Shock Syndrome

Toxic-shock syndrome (TSS) is an infection caused by a common staphylococcus bacterium. The signs and symptoms of TSS are fever, headaches, sore throats, diarrhea, rash, vomiting, hypertension, dizziness, and disorientation.

In 1980 a commercial superabsorbent tampon was linked to TSS. In 1990 the FDA standardized absorbency labeling. In addition, manufacturers are marketing tampons with lower absorbency rates. The result has been a substantial lowering of the TSS death rate. Women who choose to use tampons should select products with a low absorbency rate (6–15g).[9]

Infertility: the inability to conceive.

Osteoporosis: a disease condition of the bone resulting from a decline in bone mineral content and predisposing it to injury and fracture.

Edema: the swelling of body tissue due to fluid retention.

Mild tranquilizers: drugs which relax the muscles and reduce anxiety; sometimes called minor tranquilizers.

Diuretics: drugs that increase the amount of urine produced and excreted. Diuretics are often used to treat edema.

Premenstrual syndrome (PMS): a condition ranging in severity that some women experience several days before the onset of menstruation that is characterized by some of the following symptoms: tension, anxiety, mood change, depression, headache, breast tenderness, water retention, and other symptoms. Severity usually diminishes close to onset of the menstrual period. Exact causes of PMS are unknown but may relate to changes in estrogen and progesterone during the menstrual cycle.

1. Small children require continuous
   adult supervision and nurturing.
   How might this affect the lives of
   the parents of young children?
2. What safety hazards would
   unsupervised young children be
   exposed to on a typical day in their
   own home?

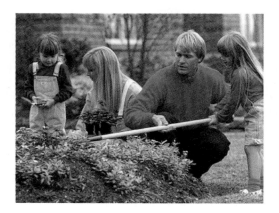

Parenthood

There are a variety of ways to become a
parent: natural procreation, artificial
procreation, adoption, and by marrying into a
family with children. Parents can be either
married or single. Single parenthood can
result from divorce, death, long separations
due to occupational commitments, or from
choosing parenthood without marriage.

Most people, at some point in their
lifetimes, will contemplate their desire to
become a parent. The choice to become a
parent is a momentous decision. People who
become parents acquire the ultimate
responsibility—the responsibility for another
human being.

First-time parents are often amazed how
a child can dramatically and sometimes
radically change their lifestyles. For the first
few years of a child's life, continuous adult
supervision and nurturing are required.
Parents find themselves adjusting their daily
schedules in order to accommodate this new
life. Children can make demands on their
parents' occupational as well as recreational
commitments. Parenting requires a great deal
of time (see figure 7.9).

Many parents spend large amounts of
energy and resources to locate apartments that
allow children, neighbors with playmates for
their children, and schools that meet their
standards. In addition good day care for infants
and other preschool-age children is a major
concern in the U.S. In general, parents labor at
establishing a social and physical environment
that supports and enhances their children's
wellness (see Of Special Interest 7.1).

Although a child is an added expense to
a family's budget, economics alone rarely
decide the question of having children.
Nevertheless, some people do decide to
postpone parenthood until they obtain a
well-paying job, buy a house, or save up
enough money. Whatever a couple's financial
circumstances, it is reasonable for them to
discuss the financial implications of
parenthood. There is no magic figure under
which a child should not be brought into the
world, but future parents should work out a
family budget. Estimates range from $4,100 to
$10,000 per year to raise a child in a two-
parent, two-child household. By a child's
eighteenth birthday the inclusive costs of
raising that child may range from $80,000 to
$160,000 and will increase considerably if the
child goes on to college.[10]

Making the Decision to Parent

The essential question to prospective parents
is: Why do you want to become a parent? Do
you need an excuse to go to Disney World, or
attend little league games? Do you want to
carry on the family name, or provide
grandchildren for your parents to spoil? Do
you want to relive your childhood through
your child? Do you want to have your child
do and be what you could not accomplish or
become? Or, do you truly want to be part of
some other person's life, joys, sorrows, and
hopes? Do you want to be the first person a
child loves and trusts? Do you want to
experience the depths of your compassion
and personal self-worth?

Discovering the reasons why you want to
become a parent will reveal some clues as to
what kind of relationship will develop
between you and your child. No one can
predict who will be a good parent. You may
explore your motives for wanting to be a
parent by yourself and with your mate.
Activity for Wellness 7.1 can help you in
this exploration.

As you ponder the parenthood decision
you will inevitably discover or rediscover your
own motives and goals in life. Contemplating
parenthood will cause you to review your
priorities in life. Parenthood is one of the
most important decisions any human being
will make.

Working Moms

Today's typical U.S. family has changed dramatically, moving away from the traditional role of mothers staying home to raise the children. In fact, over half of all mothers with children less than one year of age work outside the home. Many parents and child-development specialists alike worry about the effects of nonparental caregivers raising the next generation.

A great deal of research has been directed at gaining a better understanding of the effects of nonparental day care on young children. Results to date indicate that the emotional and cognitive development of children who begin day care *after age one* is not significantly different from developmental patterns seen in children who are cared for by a parent.[1] However, this may not be true for children who begin routine day care before age one.

Many psychologists believe that it is very important for children to bond with their mothers during the first year of life. They fear that children who spend a large portion of time in the care of nonparental caregivers during their first year of life may have a less secure bond with their mothers. This insecurity may, in turn, affect them throughout their lives in ways as diverse as problem solving and the ability to form caring relationships. This fear, however, is not universally held by psychologists and child-development specialists. Some professionals propose that if children are placed in *high quality* day care with nurturing adults, it may have a positive benefit of helping them to learn to develop a number of caring relationships at an early age.

Dr. Michael Lamb, a researcher at the National Institute of Child Health and Human Development (NICHD) recently completed a study designed to shed light on these issues. Lamb looked at the results of thirteen previous studies to determine trends in the data. He found that infants (defined as children in the first year of life) who were cared for by someone other than their mothers for more than five hours per week, were somewhat more likely to be insecure. This was especially true of infants enrolled in day care centers. Research into the effects of day care on child development, however, is still in its infancy and scientists caution that more research must be completed before we have an adequate picture of the positive and negative effects of nonparental child care. Studies that measure the *quality* of day care received are especially important.

Most studies conducted to date have been retrospective, meaning that they examined the cognitive and emotional development of older children and then looked back to see which children had been cared for by mothers and which by another caregiver. Prospective studies are a more powerful and expensive way to answer research questions. Currently, the NICHD is sponsoring a national prospective study that is following the development of over 1,000 infants and young children, evaluating both the type and quality of child care received, and its relationship to cognitive, social and language skill development. It will be several years before the results of this study will be available to help us understand the child care conditions which best promote well-being.

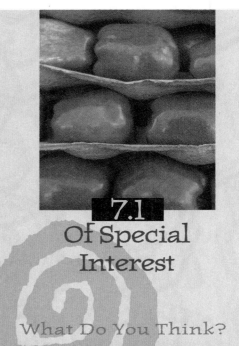

7.1 Of Special Interest

What Do You Think?

1. How important do you think it is for parents to be the primary caregivers for their children from birth to age one? What evidence have you used in developing this opinion?
2. If you have children, how did you decide upon who would participate in caring for them? What factors did you have to consider when making this decision?
3. If you do not have children yet, but are planning to have them in the future, what factors will you consider when making the decision about who will participate in caring for your children?

[1]Chellar, Susan. (July/August, 1993). "Working moms." *American Health*, p. 57.

Parenting

Since the 1950s people in the U.S. have been preoccupied with the art and science of parenting. The media attempts to tell parents the "best" way to nurture their child, from toilet training to detecting drug abuse. The subject of parenting has been both popular and profitable. Still, there is no magic parenting formula that reduces parenting to a science or guarantees the child will be all the parent hoped for.

Rather than discussing *how* to parent, it is more enlightening to explore what parenting is. The vocation of parenting requires that the parent love his or her child. Without this love, parenting is reduced to caretaking. Love is the foundation of the parenting relationship. The parent will be the

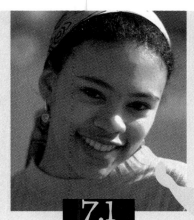

7.1

Activity for Wellness

Do I Want to Be a Parent?

Do I want to be a parent? The answer to this question is not obvious to everyone. The decision of whether or not to be a parent is one of the most important ones you will ever make. We have many pressures on us where deciding to be a parent is concerned. We have the influence of our own parents and grandparents who might expect us to help them to become grandparents and great-grandparents respectively. We have our siblings and our friends who are having children. They may provide a subtle influence on us to want to be like them, or cause us to feel that we are not equal in some way because they have children and we do not. We have the pressures of being sexually active and the possibility of being a parent by accident rather than by choice. We have religious influences that support the notion of creating more "sons and daughters" to advance the faith. We also have the ecologists from whom we hear about the overpopulated earth and the lack of a bright future for children being brought into the world now. Ultimately, the answer to the question posed is ours. Arriving at an answer should involve a careful and deliberate process. Some of the questions shown here will help you to think through matters. You may have different responses to these questions in the years ahead, but they are good questions to revisit from time to time as the issue of becoming a parent gets raised.

Have a friend answer the questions too, and talk about your responses together.

- Do I like spending time with children and doing the things they like to do?
- Will having a child make my life happier and richer?
- What will the impact of having a child be on me? on my partner? on our relationship with each other?
- What does it take financially to raise and support children?
- Is it my purpose in life to create or nurture another life?
- Childrearing is teaching—do I like teaching?
- Do I have the patience for a 24-hour-per-day job?
- Am I able to control my emotions as I must to care for children?
- What is my philosophy about child discipline?
- Could I accept the responsibility for the well-being of another individual and myself?
- Do I understand the parenting style around which I was raised? What did I learn from that experience?
- Is my partner able to accept shared responsibilities for childrearing and are my partner's views of childrearing similar to my own?
- What are the most important elements of raising a child from infancy to young adulthood, and how do these elements change through the years?
- Do my partner and I have any life goals that would be significantly compromised by having children?

first person this new being will place all of its trust and dependence upon. The child will discover and view the world and himself/herself through the sights, sounds, touches, and lives of the parent. The parent is the child's first, and no doubt most important, teacher.

Parental Expectations

All parents have expectations for their children. Some expectations are usually shared with the child, some are understood without verbal communication, and some are unknown to the child. These expectations include the values, lifestyles, accomplishments, mannerisms, and personality a parent envisions for his or her child. Parents might want their male child to be, among other things, honest, hardworking, and a professional athlete. Parents might want their female child to be, among other things, feminine, trustworthy, and successful in the business world. The virtues of such expectations are a matter of personal conviction. Such expectations will, however, affect the parent-child relationship and ultimately parenting.

Children who behave contrary to their parents' expectations may be unaware that their behavior is in conflict with their parents' expectations, unable to assume responsibility to fulfill their parents' expectations, or simply unwilling to fulfill these expectations. For example, a child may pursue playing the guitar as a possible occupation "unaware" that his parents would rather he become a gourmet chef. A parent may scold a child for talking during religious services, but the child may be "unable" to comprehend the request because of her young age. A young boy aware of his parents' expectations for him not to date may be "unwilling" to comply because of his personal attraction to a special friend.

Parenting becomes easier when children are aware of parental expectations. Parents who expect their child not to use profanity, not to talk to strangers, and to be respectful toward elders need to tell the child of these expectations. In cases where a child is unable or unwilling to fulfill such expectations, parents can either enforce their expectations, modify them to meet the abilities or desires of the child, or withdraw them totally.

The decision to enforce, modify, or withdraw an expectation is based on the parents' values and judgment. Children will inevitably not meet all of their parents' expectations. Parents need to assess the unique personality and feelings of their child when their expectations are not met. Is what they are requiring of or denying their child a self-serving indulgence on the part of the parent? One example might be a child who enjoys classical literature but whose parents believe he or she should take more business courses because the occupational outlook in classical literature is limited. In this case, a compromise is certainly possible. Another example might be a parent who denies his or her child permission to date because the parent believes this will increase the child's chances of an early marriage or an unwanted pregnancy. The child may find dating personally fulfilling and at the same time want to remain sexually abstinent and not marry until after college. In this case, the expectations of the parent and child may be identical, but this fact may be unknown to either of them.

In any case, as children mature they have more influence on their parents' expectations. Children seek personal independence as they mature. Ultimately, children either reject or accept some, or many, of their parents' expectations. This process will find both parent and child using a variety of techniques to debate the merits of an expectation, which may be the true purpose of parental expectations. Nonetheless, the child ultimately decides which expectations are reasonable and worthy of pursuit.

Enforcing Parental Expectations

Some parents believe that they have no control over their children. Such a view is an underestimation of their parental control. Parents possess the most powerful human intoxicant known: love. Parents may give their children love without question, they may make their love conditional, or they may deny their children love.

Parenting where parental love is in question can only be burdensome. The child soon learns that he or she is only lovable under certain conditions, or not lovable at all. Denying love to a child changes the kind of parenting experience that will develop. Children who are only shown love when they do chores or remain silent during adult conversation may, in turn, view love as a reward and punishment exercise. In practice these children may themselves use love as a behavior modification tool to control other persons. There are few if any virtues to this practice. Parental love is *the* essential ingredient in parenting. Love's omnipresence underlies all parent-child interactions. Children value their parents' love and this, in turn, makes them receptive to their parents' desires and needs. Most children accommodate their parents' expectations as best they can.

Pregnancy

There are numerous health concerns that affect wellness before and during a pregnancy. That is why **prenatal care,** which involves the combined efforts of health professionals and mother to create a healthy environment for the developing unborn child, is essential to the wellness of both mother and infant.

Prenatal Care

Ideally, a woman and man attempting to become pregnant should begin prenatal care *before* pregnancy. Several health considerations should be addressed, including physical health, family history of genetic disorders, drug use, nutrition, and sexual activity.

Physical Health Status

The first consideration is the physical health of prospective parents. The mother and father-to-be need to be at the most optimal level of health possible. This includes eating a nutritious diet, participating in regular physical activity, attaining or maintaining optimal weight, and practicing stress-management techniques. Pregnancy and parenting are rigorous experiences for both the mother and father. Starting the experience in good physical health will be of great help in managing both the physical and emotional aspects of becoming parents. Additionally, the mother-to-be should avoid becoming infected with German measles (**Rubella**) or a sexually transmitted disease (STD) just before or during pregnancy, as these conditions may lead to pregnancy complications and birth defects.

Prenatal care: actions taken by a future mother and her mate to increase the chances of birthing a healthy baby and reducing the health risks of pregnancy and childbirth for the future mother.

Rubella: a virus-induced infection that, if acquired by a woman during pregnancy, may result in fetal malformations.

Genetic Counseling

Prospective parents should determine whether there is a history of hereditary disease in their families. Couples may consider genetic counseling as a means of determining the likelihood of producing a child with a genetic disorder. Such counseling would educate the prospective parents on the nature of a particular disorder and the medical options available to them and their future child.

Avoiding Drug Use

Parents-to-be should consider their use of drugs *prior to* and *during* the pregnancy. For males, preliminary evidence indicates that alcohol use one month prior to conception *may* be related to low birth weight.[11] Cigarette smoking by prospective fathers may also affect a developing fetus, and after the birth will put the child at risk for a variety of respiratory problems. While the evidence for drug use in a father-to-be is not yet conclusive, the prudent course of action would be to abstain from drug use prior to conceiving and during pregnancy.

Drug use by women attempting to become pregnant is also problematic. It may be as long as four to five weeks after a missed period when a pregnancy is confirmed. For women not planning a pregnancy the lag may be greater. The day a woman is informed she is pregnant is not the day her pregnancy began. Confirming a pregnancy five weeks after a missed period is actually the seventh week of pregnancy. By the fifth week of pregnancy the artery that will become the heart is already beating.

The embryo/fetus is most vulnerable to chemicals during the first twelve weeks of pregnancy.[12] Potentially harmful chemicals can be introduced to the embryo/fetus via the mother's blood (see A Social Perspective 7.1). One such chemical is alcohol. Alcohol consumption during pregnancy has been linked to an increase in spontaneous abortions, as well as congenital heart defects, retardation, physical malformations, and other deformities.[13] Select congenital defects produced by the mother's consumption of alcohol are referred to as **Fetal Alcohol Syndrome (FAS).** Any congenital defect caused by the mother's alcohol consumption is referred to as **Fetal Alcohol Effect (FAE).**

Maternal alcohol abuse may be the most frequent environmentally known cause of mental retardation in the Western World.[14]

There are many other chemicals commonly used that may cause problems for the mother or embryo/fetus. The antibiotic tetracycline, if taken during pregnancy, can cause staining of the infant's teeth and stunt the growth of long bones.[15] Other antibiotics may cause congenital **cataracts.** Chemicals from tobacco smoke increase the risk of spontaneous abortion, **stillbirth,** low birth weight,[16] and **ectopic pregnancies.**[17]

Caffeine remains in the pregnant mother's body much longer than it would if she were not pregnant. There is a body of evidence that suggests caffeine intake (>300 mg per day) may result in low-birth-weight infants and fetal growth retardation.[18] However studies have also indicated that caffeine may not present a significant risk to the fetus.[19] The prudent course of action for pregnant women would simply be to avoid all caffeine in food, drink, and over-the-counter drug products.

Excessive amounts of vitamins such as A, D, and B_6 have also been associated with fetal defects. Additionally, although not drugs, pregnant females should avoid X-ray radiation and hot tubs.

Acknowledging the fact that there is no definitive evidence in all cases, the judicious course of action is for the female to avoid the use of all prescription, over-the-counter, and illegal drugs from the first day of the reproductive cycle she chooses to become pregnant until after childbirth (see table 7.2).

Mothers who breast-feed should check with their physicians before ingesting prescription or over-the-counter drugs, alcohol, nicotine, and caffeine since these substances pass into the breast milk in small amounts. However, many physicians prescribe multiphasic birth control pills for new mothers after breast-feeding is established. Even though the multiphasic birth control pills are safe and do not interfere with breast-feeding, they do tend to cause a reduction in the amount of breastmilk.

Regarding the pregnant woman's household and worksite, she should avoid airborne drugs via second-hand smoke such as tobacco and second-hand exposure to marijuana.

Fetal Alcohol Syndrome (FAS): a pattern of abnormalities found in the newborns of women who drank alcohol during pregnancy. This condition consists of a pattern of specific congenital and behavioral abnormalities. Current research suggests even low to moderate alcohol consumption may be problematic.

Cataracts: a common occurrence with aging in which the lens of the eye becomes increasingly opaque, resulting in obscured vision.

Stillbirth: the birth of a fetus at or later than 28 weeks gestation, that has no heart beat or respiration.

Ectopic pregnancies: pregnancies with implantation of the zygote occurring outside the uterus, most commonly implanting in one of the fallopian tubes.

Fetal Rights

The National Association for Perinatal Addiction Research and Education estimates that each year in the U.S. 375,000 infants are born with drugs in their body. There is a growing willingness of social welfare agencies and district attorneys to prosecute women who give birth to babies already addicted or suffering from drug poisoning including alcohol, cocaine, and heroin. On July 13, 1988 Jennifer Johnson, a cocaine addict, was convicted of delivering a controlled substance to a minor based on the fact she had delivered the drugs to her two children through their umbilical cords, after the babies were born, but before the cords were severed from their placentas. However most cases of women giving birth to infants addicted to drugs have not resulted in a conviction. The legal question is whether the fetus's life and health is protected under state and federal child protection laws. An example is Margaret Reyes who after being warned by medical personnel of the danger of narcotic use to her unborn child gave birth to twin boys both addicted to heroin and suffering from withdrawal. The California Court dismissed the case ruling child endangerment laws do not apply to the unborn child.[1]

In contrast state courts, such as Massachusetts, have ruled if a fetus is killed during a reckless vehicular crash, then the fetus is a person and the perpetrator is liable for homicide and civil penalties as a result of that loss of life. In addition if a man in the act of domestic violence causes a spontaneous abortion, then he is charged with homicide.

This legal double standard has prompted several new laws directed at protecting the rights of a fetus. Several state court decisions, including that of New York, have ruled in gross cases of neglect where there is imminent danger of impairment of physical condition, that an unborn child is a *person* under New York State's abuse and neglect statute.

Opponents to fetal rights legislation argue such laws and rulings are intrusive and coercive in that they would oppress women of childbearing age and deny their right to privacy. They warn that drug-addicted women may seek an abortion in order to avoid detection and subsequent prosecution. In addition they say racial minorities and the poor would be disproportionately affected by such policies.

What Do You Think?

1. Does a pregnant woman have a responsibility to protect the health and safety of a fetus she intends to carry to full term?
2. Should the death or injury of a fetus be considered that of a *person,* in criminal and civil laws, for all perpetrators except that of its fetal mother?

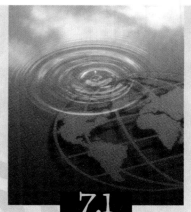

7.1
A Social Perspective

3. If a pregnant woman aborts her drug addicted fetus to avoid prosecution under state child abuse laws, is that punishable under state and federal laws regarding the intentional destruction of the physical evidence of a crime?
4. Could rulings defending the rights of a drug addicted fetus be applied to health-related behaviors of a pregnant woman in areas such as tobacco smoking, intentional dieting, or strenuous athletic activity?

---

[1] E. Viano, "Creating Fetal Rights and Protecting Pregnant Women's Constitutional Rights." In P. J. Venturelli, *Drug Use in America* (Boston: Jones & Bartlett, 1994).

Nutrition during Pregnancy

The nutritional needs of women increase significantly during pregnancy. The Recommended Dietary Allowances reflect this greater need (see table 7.3). The average pregnant woman needs to increase her intake of calories by about 15 percent so that her minimum daily count is about 2,400 calories. The National Academy of Sciences recommends that during pregnancy a woman gain twenty-five to thirty-five pounds.[20] This weight gain will vary somewhat during a pregnancy, with the greatest weight gain occurring during the last six months. A pregnant woman should average a gain of slightly less than one pound a week during the last six months.

Maternal weight gain during pregnancy is directly related to infant birthweight and by association to length of **gestation,** fetal growth, and infant mortality. Black mothers are less likely than White mothers to achieve the recommended weight gain during pregnancy. Another factor is age, where teenage mothers are less likely than women in their twenties to achieve the minimum recommended weight gain.

In addition to more calories, the need for protein, vitamins, and minerals also increases. Although many physicians prescribe a vitamin/mineral supplement for pregnant women, this does not negate the need for a well-balanced diet. Pregnant women need to pay special attention to their food intake

Gestation: the time from the formation of a zygote until childbirth. In humans, the average gestation is 266 days.

TABLE 7.2 — Partial List of Common Drugs Having Potentially Dangerous Effects on the Embryo/Fetus

Cold and Allergy Medications

- Actifed
- Alka-Seltzer Plus
- Chlor-Trimeton
- Contact
- Co-Tylenol
- Dristan
- Drixoral
- Sudafed-Plus
- Benadryl
- Nytol
- Sinutab Maximum Strength

Aspirin Preparations

- Alka-Seltzer
- Anacin
- Bayer
- Bufferin
- Excedrin
- Maximum Strength Midol
- Vanquish

Aspirin-substitute Preparations

- Anacin-3
- Comtrex
- Co-Tylenol
- Datril
- Vanquish

Cough Suppressants

- Benylin DM
- Naldecon DX
- Robitussin products
- St. Joseph Cough Syrup
- Sudafed Cough Syrup
- Vicks products

Source: Data from J. Sussman and B. B. Leavitt, *The Complete Pregnancy Guide*, 1989, Bantam Books, New York.

regarding protein, iron, calcium, sodium, and B-complex vitamins (see table 7.4).

Sexual Activity during Pregnancy

Most obstetrical physicians support the idea that intercourse during a normal pregnancy is quite safe for the fetus and the mother. Physical changes during pregnancy, however, may affect sexual behavior.[21] An expecting couple that understands these physiological changes may prepare for and cope with them. Many couples thus enjoy intercourse throughout the pregnancy.

Physiological changes will vary between the three trimesters. Table 7.5 presents the major alterations in sexual response during pregnancy. During the first trimester women may experience fatigue and **morning sickness,** both of which may decrease interest in sex. During that same time, however, congestion of blood vessels in the breasts and pelvic area may cause an enhanced erotic response. It is not uncommon for women to experience greater intensity of orgasm during the first two trimesters. In the third trimester the congestion of blood in the pelvic area is not well relieved during the **resolution stage** of sexual response and may be a cause of discomfort. Also during the third trimester abdominal size may preclude intercourse in the male superior position, but alternative positions may be used.[22]

Certain problems of pregnancy may contraindicate intercourse and orgasm during specific phases of the pregnancy. A physician's consultation is important in determining if such problems exist. If there are no contraindications, it is safe for a couple to continue intercourse throughout the pregnancy as they may desire.[23]

Benefits of Prenatal Care

Prenatal care increases the chances of a mother bearing a healthy, normal-weight baby. This is an important benefit, as birth weight is an important predictor of infant

Morning sickness: the nausea and vomiting a pregnant female may experience throughout the day or night, but commonly in the morning.

Resolution stage: the stage of human sexual response, following the orgasmic stage, characterized by the loss of sexual tension and a return to a preexcitement stage.

Dietary Allowance	Pregnant	Lactating	
		First 6 months	Second 6 months
Protein (gm)	60	65	62
Fat-Soluble Vitamins			
Vitamin A (µg RE)	800	1300	1200
Vitamin D (µg)	10	10	10
Vitamin E (mg ∝ TE)	10	12	11
Vitamin K (µg)	65	65	65
Water-Soluble Vitamins			
Vitamin C (mg)	70	95	90
Thiamine (mg)	1.5	1.6	1.6
Riboflavin (mg)	1.6	1.8	1.7
Niacin (mg NE)	17	20	20
Vitamin B_6 (mg)	2.2	2.1	2.1
Folate (µg)	400	280	260
Vitamin B_{12} (µg)	2.2	2.6	2.6
Minerals			
Calcium (mg)	1200	1200	1200
Phosphorous (mg)	1200	1200	1200
Magnesium (mg)	300	355	340
Iron (mg)	30	15	15
Zinc (mg)	15	19	16
Iodine (µg)	175	200	200
Selenium (µg)	65	75	75

TABLE 7.3 — *Recommended Dietary Allowances for Pregnant and Lactating Women Recommended by the Food and Nutrition Board*

RE = retinol equivalents

TE = tocopherol equivalents

NE = niacin equivalents

Reprinted with permission from *Recommended Dietary Allowances: 10th edition.* Copyright © 1989 by the National Academy of Sciences. Courtesy of the National Academy Press, Washington, D.C.

health status. Specifically, low birth weight (<2,500 grams) is strongly associated with infant mortality. A recent study has indicated that the earlier in the pregnancy prenatal care begins, the more likely the mother will bear a normal weight infant. This was true for all ethnic groups studied including Hispanics, Mexicans, Puerto Ricans, Cubans, Whites, and Blacks.[24]

Prenatal care will also allow for the detection of potential and actual pregnancy problems. For example, one tool in prenatal care is ultrasonic fetal examinations. **Ultrasound** machines can produce an image of the fetus using relatively harmless sound waves. These tests can provide data about how the fetus is developing and whether any medical attention is required to treat the fetus while in the womb or soon after birth. Prenatal care enables the parents to select options that will reduce the risk of pregnancy complications and congenital disorders. The physician becomes an important consultant during this time.

Prenatal Development

Pregnancy begins when an egg is fertilized (see figure 7.10) and ends with childbirth. It takes approximately 266 days (or thirty-eight weeks), about nine calendar months, for a baby to develop fully.

Ultrasound: high frequency sound waves, undetectable to the human ear, used to examine the inner structures of the body.

TABLE 7.4   *Daily Food Guide during Pregnancy*

The Five Food Groups	*How Much Each Day—Servings and Sources*
Fruits and Vegetables	
Fruits and vegetables contain vitamins, minerals, and fiber, a natural laxative. The dark-green leafy vegetables and deep yellow vegetables are rich in vitamin A. The dark-green leafy vegetables are also valuable for iron, vitamin C, magnesium, folacin, and riboflavin.	Eat *at least one* serving of a good source of vitamin A *every other day:* • Apricots • Pumpkin • Broccoli • Sweet potatoes • Cantaloupe • Winter squash • Carrots • Dark-green leafy vegetables— beet greens, chard, collards, kale, mustard greens, spinach, turnip greens Eat *at least one* serving of a good source of vitamin C *every day:* • Broccoli • Tomatoes • Brussels sprouts • Dark-green leafy • Cantaloupe vegetables—chard, collards, • Cauliflower kale, mustard greens, • Green or sweet red pepper spinach, turnip greens • Grapefruit or grapefruit juice • Cabbage • Orange or orange juice • Strawberries • Watermelon Select *two* servings of other vegetables and fruit *each day:* • Beets • Peas • Cherries • Corn • Potatoes • Grapes • Eggplant • Squash • Pears • Green and wax beans • Apples • Pineapple • Lettuce • Bananas • Plums
Meat, Fish, Poultry, Eggs, Dried Beans and Peas, Nuts	
Meat, fish, poultry, eggs, dried beans and peas, seeds, nuts, and peanut butter supply protein as well as vitamins and minerals. Protein is needed to help build new tissues for both mother and baby.	Eat *three* servings of protein food *daily:* These amounts equal one serving: • 2 or 3 ounces lean meat (remove the extra fat when possible). Some examples: 1 hamburger, 2 thin slices of beef, pork, lamb or veal, 1 lean pork chop, 2 slices luncheon meat, 2 hot dogs. • 2 or 3 ounces of fish. Some examples: 1 whole small fish, 1 small fish fillet, 1/3 of a 6 1/2 ounce can of tuna fish or salmon. • 2 or 3 ounces of chicken, turkey, or other poultry. Some examples: 2 slices light or dark meat turkey, 1 chicken leg, 1/2 chicken breast. These amounts equal one-half serving: • 1/2 to 3/4 cup cooked dried beans, peas, or lentils, garbanzos (chick-peas) • 2 to 3 tablespoons peanut butter • 1 or 2 slices cheese • 1 egg • 1 cup tofu • 4 to 6 tablespoons nuts or seeds

The Five Food Groups	How Much Each Day—Servings and Sources
Milk and Milk Products	

Four 8-ounce glasses of milk or milk products are needed daily to give mother and baby the calcium and other nutrients needed for strong bones and teeth. Choose milks that have vitamin D added. You may select whole milk, buttermilk, low-fat milk, or dry or fluid skim milk. Low-fat milk and skim milk have fewer calories than whole milk. Milk or cheese used in making soup, pudding, sauces, and other foods count toward the total amount of milk you use.

Drink *four* 8-ounce glasses of milk or eat the equivalent in milk products *daily:*

These amounts equal the calcium in one 8-ounce glass of milk:

- 1 cup liquid skim milk, low-fat milk, or buttermilk
- 1/2 cup evaporated milk (undiluted)
- 2 one-inch cubes or 2 slices of cheese
- 1/3 cup instant powdered milk
- 1 cup plain yogurt, custard, or milk pudding

These amounts equal the calcium in 1/3 cup of milk:

- 2/3 cup cottage cheese
- 1/2 cup ice cream

Whole-Grain or Enriched Breads and Cereals

Breads and cereal foods provide minerals and vitamins, particularly the B vitamins and iron, as well as protein. Whole-grain breads and cereals provide essential trace elements such as zinc, and also fiber, a natural laxative. Check the labels on breads and cereals to make sure that they are made with whole-wheat or whole-grain flour or are enriched with minerals and vitamins.

Eat *four or five* servings of whole-grain or enriched breads, cereals, and cereal products *every day:*

These amounts equal one serving:

- 1 slice of bread
- 1 muffin
- 1 roll or biscuit
- 1 tortilla or taco shell
- 1/2 to 3/4 cup cooked or ready-to-eat cereal, such as oatmeal, farina, grits, raisin bran, shredded wheat
- 1 cup popcorn (1 1/2 tablespoons, unpopped)
- 1/2 to 3/4 cup noodles, spaghetti, rice, bulgur, macaroni
- 2 small pancakes
- 1 section waffle
- 2 graham crackers or 4 to 6 small crackers

These amounts count as two servings:

- 1 hamburger bun or hotdog roll
- 1 English muffin

Fats and Sweets

This group of other foods includes margarine, butter, candy, jellies, sugars, syrups, desserts, soft drinks, snack foods, salad dressings, vegetable oils, and other fats used in cooking. Most of these foods are high in fat, sugar, or salt. Use them to meet additional caloric needs after basic nutritional needs have been met. Eating too much fat and too many sweets may crowd out other necessary nutrients.

No specific number or types of servings are recommended for fats and sweets.

Source: Adapted from *Prenatal Care,* Public Health Service Publication No. (HRSA) 83–5070, Washington, D.C., 1983.

Stage	Changes
Excitement and plateau	Breasts—tenderness, discomfort, enhanced erotic response; milk letdown after orgasm in late pregnancy
	Labia—feeling of fullness
	Vagina—increased secretions, feeling of fullness
	Cervix—may bleed more easily at coitus, may be more sensitive
Orgasm	Tonic uterine contractions, transient fetal bradycardia, greater intensity (or first orgasm)
Resolution	Often poor or inadequate in late pregnancy

From George W. Dameron, Jr., "Helping Couples Cope with Sexual Changes Pregnancy Brings," in *Ortho Forum*, 3(3): 8 (1983). Reprinted by permission of Ortho-McNeil Pharmaceutical, Inc.

Figure 7.10: What Do You Think?

1. Pregnancy begins when an egg is fertilized. Can you explain how the egg (ovum) and sperm each reach the fallopian tube where fertilization most commonly occurs?

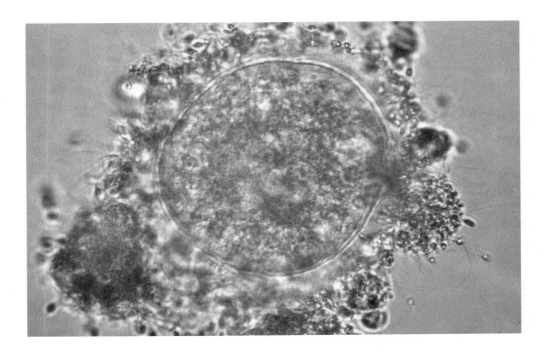

Pregnancy is divided into three phases called trimesters. The **first trimester** begins at the point of fertilization and continues to the end of the third month. The **second trimester** begins at the beginning of the fourth month and continues to the end of the sixth month. The **third trimester** begins at the beginning of the seventh month and continues until childbirth. Pregnancies that last until the ninth month are called **full-term pregnancies.**

Implantation

By the sixth or seventh day after fertilization the fertilized egg will have traveled through the fallopian tubes where fertilization occurred and implanted itself in the uterus. The female does not experience any physical sensation resulting from implantation. Sometimes implantation may cause "spotting," or bleeding, and this bleeding could be misdiagnosed as the onset of menstruation.

Embryonic Period

For the first eight weeks after fertilization the developing baby is called an **embryo.** By the end of the first month the embryo is two-tenths of an inch long. The brain, eyes, spinal cord, nose, limbs, liver, pancreas,

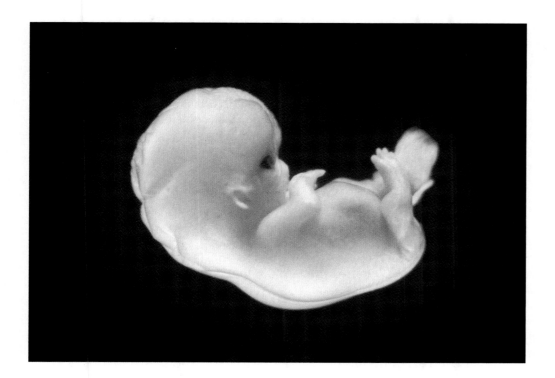

Figure 7.11: What Do You Think?

1. By the end of the second month, an embryo has fingers, toes, and many other human features. What signs and symptoms of pregnancy might the mother of this embryo be experiencing?

and gallbladder have begun to develop. The tube that will become the heart begins to pulsate.

By the end of the second month the embryo has fingers, toes, blood vessels, lips, ears, eyelids, and a nose (see figure 7.11). Testicular tissue appears in male embryos, but female embryos will not begin to develop their reproductive organs until the following month. The embryo is now 1.2 inches long and weighs 1 gram (0.04 ounces).

During the embryonic period, important membranes begin to form. The outer membrane, the chorion, and the inner membrane, the amnion, are tissue sacs that enclose the developing embryo, and later the fetus, until childbirth. These sacs hold **amniotic fluid** in which the embryo is submersed. The amniotic fluid acts as a barrier to physical shock and also serves to maintain the proper temperature.

The **placenta** also begins to form during the embryonic period. The placenta is a temporary organ that transfers nutrients and oxygen to the embryo and later to the fetus. The placenta secretes hormones in order to maintain the pregnancy. The placenta is expelled by uterine contractions after childbirth.

The embryo, and later the fetus, are connected to the placenta by an **umbilical cord.** The umbilical cord contains two arteries and one vein. The maternal blood is circulated through the uterine side of the placenta. Although the two circulatory systems never physically mix, the placenta allows nutrients and oxygen to pass from the maternal blood to the embryo/fetal blood. The placenta also allows the waste products of the embryo/fetal blood to pass through to the maternal blood.

Fetus

During the third month of pregnancy the embryo becomes a **fetus.** At the end of the third month the fetus has toenails, fingernails, fingerprints, and an excretory system. The fetus will demonstrate breathing motions by moving amniotic fluid in and out of its lungs. The fetus is able to move its fingers, arms, and neck. Additionally, the fetus will weigh two-thirds of an ounce and be four inches long.

By the end of the fourth month, the fetus weighs about six ounces and is about eight to ten inches long. During the fourth month **quickening** usually occurs. Quickening is the first fetal movement felt by the mother. The fetus will move its arms and legs and also demonstrate a swallowing reflex.

By the end of the fifth month the fetus weighs about one pound and will be about twelve inches long. The fetal heartbeat can now be heard with an ordinary stethoscope and beats approximately 150 times per

Fetus: the medical term for an embryo that has developed for at least eight weeks.

minute. The fetus will respond to lights and sounds and will spend part of its time awake and part asleep. The youngest fetus to survive outside its mother had an estimated gestation age of nineteen weeks.

By the end of the sixth month (second trimester) the fetus weighs about one-and-one-half pounds, is about fourteen inches long, and is very active. Mothers will regularly feel the movement of the fetus from then on. Ninety percent of the final fetal birth weight is yet to be gained.

By the end of the seventh month the fetus will usually turn upside down, head first into the birthing position. Babies not born in the head-first position are called breech. **Breech births** include buttocks first, legs first, or shoulder first presentations. Breech births can cause medical complications for both mother and infant. During the seventh month the fetus is covered with lanugo, a downy hair that will shed before birth. The eyelids, which fused closed in the third month, will reopen. The fetus may begin to suck its thumb during the seventh month. The brain and nervous system are completely developed. The chances are better than 50 percent that the fetus will survive childbirth if born in the seventh month. The fetus now weighs about four pounds.

By the end of the eighth month the fetus can taste sweet substances.[25] The fetus has a 95 percent chance of surviving childbirth. By the ninth month (full-term pregnancy) the survival rate in childbirth is better than 99 percent. The fetus is less active because of its cramped environment. All fetal eyes are blue and will change to another color (if genetically predetermined) when exposed to light following childbirth. The same is true of fetal skin color, which is pink or blue-pink. The genetically predetermined skin color will not fully appear until after its exposure to light. A full-term infant will weigh from six to nine pounds and measure about twenty inches.

Multiple Births
Identical twins, which come from the same fertilized egg, are formed sometime between fertilization and implantation, when the fertilized egg separates into two masses. Identical twins will be nearly exact duplicates of each other from their physical appearance to their blood type.

Fraternal twins are created from two eggs that were fertilized independently. Thus fraternal twins do not share identical chromosomes. Fraternal twins are not identical in appearance or physiology. Approximately 70 percent of all twin births are fraternal and the remainder identical. Multiple births of three or more can be fraternal, identical, or both.

Pregnancy Indicators
There are several bodily changes caused by the hormones produced during pregnancy. The first such signs include the absence of menstruation, tingling nipples, enlarged or sensitive breasts, increased pigmentation around the nipples, increased urination, fatigue, and morning sickness. Morning sickness refers to the nausea and vomiting a pregnant female may experience throughout the day or night. These signs and symptoms are said to be "presumptive indicators" of pregnancy.

When presumptive indicators of pregnancy appear most women choose to have a pregnancy test. Pregnancy tests are based on the detection of a hormone in the female's blood or urine. This hormone, produced by the implanted embryo, is called **human chorionic gonadotropin (HCG).**

Laboratory pregnancy tests that use urine as the medium to detect HCG can be administered as early as the first week after a missed menstrual period. The most sensitive pregnancy blood test is the radioimmunoassay, which can detect HCG as early as twenty-three days after the last menstrual period or one week "before" a missed menstrual period. This test is performed by a medical laboratory, takes about twenty-four hours, and is between 95 and 99 percent reliable.[26]

There are over-the-counter (OTC) pregnancy tests a woman can perform herself. In general, these tests are less accurate than the ones performed by laboratory technicians. OTC kits that test specifically for HCG are the most accurate.

Physiological Maternal Changes
During the first trimester the pregnant woman's breasts will swell and tingle. Her nipples may darken and broaden. She will urinate more frequently and her bowel movements may become irregular. She may experience nausea and be revolted by particular foods. During the second trimester the pregnant woman may experience **hemorrhoids,** nosebleeds, and edema.

Hemorrhoids: enlarged veins that may protrude from the wall of the anus.

Edema, coupled with additional conditions such as high blood pressure and protein in the urine, may indicate **pre-eclampsia,** also known as **toxemia.** If pre-eclampsia develops into **eclampsia** (seizures), then the life of the mother can be threatened. Eclampsia results in coma and convulsions. In order to save the life of the mother a physician can perform an abortion or preterm delivery of the fetus.

A pregnant woman usually experiences the first movements of the fetus in the second trimester. During the third trimester there is increased pressure on several organs including the uterus, stomach, bladder, and lungs. These conditions may result in shortness of breath and heartburn. Nulliparous women (those who have never given birth) may experience "dropping," which occurs when the head of the fetus drops into position within the pelvis.

Prenatal Testing

Amniocentesis is a test used to discover genetic disorders, chromosomal abnormalities, sex-linked disorders, sex and other information about the developing fetus. The physician performing amniocentesis obtains a sample of the amniotic fluid. This is accomplished by first using a noninvasive test (ultrasound) to map the position of the fetus inside the uterus. A local anesthetic is then used on the female's abdomen, after which a needle is inserted through the abdominal wall and a sample of amniotic fluid is withdrawn. The results of the test can take from two to four weeks to prepare. Because amniocentesis needs to be performed sometime between the fourteenth and sixteenth week of pregnancy, the option of abortion is available to parents who choose to terminate a pregnancy based on the results of the test.

The proportion of mothers and fetuses that suffer ill effects from amniocentesis is less than 1 percent.[27] It is possible that a healthy fetus may be spontaneously aborted as a result of amniocentesis. Candidates for amniocentesis are parents with a family history of genetic disorders (e.g., African-Americans with **sickle cell trait/disease**), women who have borne children with birth defects, and pregnant women over the age of thirty-five.

One of the major drawbacks to amniocentesis is that it has to be performed relatively late in the pregnancy. A procedure called **chorionic biopsy** involves the physician obtaining a sample of the **chorionic tissue** through the vagina. On the positive side the chorionic biopsy provides information about fetal genetic defects as early as the seventh week of pregnancy. On the negative side there is concern that this method carries a greater risk of spontaneous abortion than amniocentesis.

There are additional screening tools available to physicians and parents to determine the health of the fetus. With new high-resolution ultrasonography physicians can confirm certain fetal defects. There is a maternal blood test, the **Alpha Fetoprotein Blood Test,** which can detect birth defects of the brain and spinal cord such as **spina bifida.** This test involves only a sample of the mother's blood. **Percutaneous Umbilical Blood Sampling (PUBS)** is a method of prenatal testing. The physician, guided by a real-time ultrasonography, inserts a needle into one of the blood vessels in the umbilical cord to draw a sample of blood. This is a variation of a fetoscopy procedure in which the instrument, fetoscope, is inserted into the uterus allowing the physician to take blood and tissue samples as well as view the fetus. Additional diagnostic tools are available, and this fact underscores the value of supervised prenatal care by a qualified physician (see table 7.6).

What if amniocentesis revealed that a woman was pregnant with twins, one having **Down's syndrome** and the other perfectly healthy? Parents would be faced with a perplexing decision of whether to abort a healthy fetus along with its genetically deficient sibling or to raise a healthy child along with its Down's syndrome sibling. When such a situation arose in 1980, the parents decided to abort the Down's syndrome fetus immediately and continue the pregnancy for the healthy fetus. Both procedures were successful.[28]

The ethical issues, however, remain. Should a woman with a multiple pregnancy be allowed to eliminate one or more fetuses to reduce the number of her offspring and/or select the most desirable fetus?

The option of prenatal testing with subsequent abortion has led to an ethical debate as to whether there is a personal responsibility on the part of the parents to bear and raise children with congenital disorders. Is it morally irresponsible to abort a

Pre-eclampsia and true eclampsia: the accumulation of toxic substances in the blood that produces symptoms such as headache, hypertension, fluid retention in the lower trunk and limbs of the body, and other symptoms. If neglected or left untreated the condition may worsen and lead to coma, convulsive disorders (true eclampsia) or even death.

Sickle cell disease: a hereditary disease that affects primarily people of African descent. Defective hemoglobin causes the red blood cells to become sickle shaped, resulting in anemia and often severe complications such as kidney or heart failure.

Chorionic tissue: a membrane that completely surrounds an embryo once implantation occurs.

Spina bifida: a condition in which infants are born with a spinal column that does not close completely, leaving the spinal cord exposed.

Down's syndrome: a congenital disease caused by the presence of an extra number-21 chromosome, resulting in mental deficiency and a variety of physical defects.

TABLE 7.6 The Gene Screen: Looking in on Baby

The Problem	The Effects	Who's at Risk	Tests and Their Accuracy*	What Can Be Done?
Alpha$_1$ anti-trypsin deficiency	Enzyme deficiency that can lead to cirrhosis of the liver in early infancy and pulmonary emphysema and degenerative lung disease in middle age.	1 in 1,000 Caucasians	Amniocentesis, CVS Accuracy varies, but can sometimes predict severity	No treatment
Alpha thalassemia	Severe anemia that reduces ability of the blood to carry oxygen. Nearly all affected infants are stillborn or die soon after birth.	Primarily families of Malaysian, African, and Southeast Asian descent	Amniocentesis, CVS Accuracy varies; more accurate if other family members tested for gene	Frequent blood transfusions
Beta thalassemia (Cooley's anemia)	Severe anemia resulting in weakness, fatigue, and frequent illness. Usually fatal in adolescence or young adulthood.	Primarily families of Mediterranean descent	Amniocentesis, CVS 95 percent accurate	Frequent blood transfusions
Cystic fibrosis	Body makes too much mucus, which collects in the lungs and digestive tract. Children don't grow normally and usually don't live beyond age twenty.	1 in 2,000 Caucasians	Amniocentesis, CVS Accuracy varies; more accurate if other family members tested for gene	Daily physical therapy to loosen mucus
Down's syndrome	Minor to severe mental retardation caused by an extra twenty-first chromosome.	1 in 350 women over age thirty-five; 1 in 800, all women	Amniocentesis, CVS Nearly 100 percent accurate	No treatment
Duchenne's muscular dystrophy	Fatal disease found only in males, marked by muscle weakness. Minor mental retardation is common. Respiratory failure and death usually occur in young adulthood.	1 in 7,000 male births	Amniocentesis, CVS 95 percent accurate	No treatment
Fragile x syndrome	Minor to severe mental retardation. Symptoms, which are more severe in males, include delayed speech and motor development, speech impairments, and hyperactivity. Considered one of the main causes of autism.	1 in 1,200 male births; 1 in 2,000 female births	Amniocentesis, CVS 95 percent accurate	No treatment
Hemophilia	Excessive bleeding affecting only males. In its most severe form, can lead to crippling arthritis in adulthood.	1 in 10,000 families with a history of hemophilia	Amniocentesis, CVS 95 percent accurate	Frequent transfusions of blood with clotting factors

The Problem	The Effects	Who's at Risk	Tests and Their Accuracy*	What Can Be Done?
Neural tube defects				
Anencephaly	Absence of brain tissue. Infants are stillborn or die soon after birth.	1 in 1,000	Ultrasound, amniocentesis, 100 percent accurate	No treatment
Spina bifida	Incompletely closed spinal canal, resulting in muscle weakness or paralysis and loss of bladder and bowel control. Often accompanied by hydrocephalus, an accumulation of spinal fluid in the brain, which can lead to mental retardation.	1 in 1,000	Ultrasound, amniocentesis Test works only if the spinal cord is leaking fluid into the uterus or is exposed and visible during ultrasound	Surgery to close spinal canal prevents further injury; shunt placed in brain drains excess fluid and prevents mental retardation
Polycystic kidney disease	Infantile form: enlarged kidneys, leading to respiratory problems and congestive heart failure. Adult form: kidney pain, kidney stones, and hypertension resulting in chronic kidney failure. Symptoms usually begin around age thirty.	1 in 1,000	Infantile form: ultrasound 100 percent accurate Adult form: amniocentesis 95 percent accurate	Kidney transplants
Sex chromosome abnormality	Minor to severe developmental and learning disabilities, caused by missing X or extra X or Y chromosome.	1 in 500	Amniocentesis, CVS Nearly 100 percent accurate	Hormonal treatments to trigger puberty
Sickle-cell anemia	Deformed, fragile red blood cells that can clog the blood vessels, depriving the body of oxygen. Symptoms include severe pain, stunted growth, frequent infections, leg ulcers, gallstones, susceptibility to pneumonia, and stroke.	1 in 500 Blacks	Amniocentesis, CVS 95 percent accurate	Painkillers, transfusions for anemia, antibiotics for infections
Tay-Sachs disease	Degenerative disease of the brain and nerve cells, resulting in death before the age of five.	1 in 3,000 Eastern European Jews	Amniocentesis, CVS 100 percent accurate	No treatment
Trisomy 13 (Patau syndrome)	Severe mental retardation and heart, kidney, and other organ defects, caused by the presence of an extra thirteenth chromosome. Usually fatal soon after birth.	1 in 20,000; women over age thirty-five have increased risk	Amniocentesis, CVS, ultrasound Nearly 100 percent accurate	No treatment
Trisomy 18 (Edwards syndrome)	Severe mental retardation and heart defects, caused by presence of an extra eighteenth chromosome. Usually fatal soon after birth.	1 in 8,000; women over age thirty-five have increased risk	Amniocentesis, CVS, ultrasound Nearly 100 percent accurate	No treatment

*Cannot predict severity unless otherwise indicated.

Researched by Valerie Fahey, *Hippocrates,* May/June 1988. Excerpted from *Health,* © 1993. Reprinted by permission.

fetus who is marginally or minimally handicapped as a result of a genetic disorder? Should the government provide specialized health-care benefits to parents who choose to bear children with severe physical disorders? Is it possible for a pregnant woman to have a sample of her blood tested to reveal the sex of her fetus? Should a woman be allowed to abort a fetus because it is not a boy or a girl? Is it criminal for a pregnant woman to cause harm or death to her fetus as a result of her health behaviors? For example alcohol consumption, tobacco smoking, low calorie dieting, strenuous physical activity, or high-risk sexual activity. These are only some of the questions faced by parents-to-be and society.

Childbirth

The physiological changes responsible for bringing about childbirth are not fully understood. There is strong evidence that prostaglandins produced by the uterus and fetal membranes are responsible for initiating **labor.** The childbirth process causes the delivery of the infant, placenta, and fetal membrane. This is accomplished by regular rhythmic uterine contractions that push the fetus toward the vulva.

There are several early signs that childbirth is about to begin. One sign is the expelling of the mucus plug that had closed off the cervix during pregnancy. The mucus plug, formed early in the pregnancy, provides protection against fetal infection. Childbirth often begins a few hours or days after this sign.

Another early sign is the rupturing of the **amniotic sac** (sometimes called the bag). The sac will break before labor begins in one out of ten births. The expectant mother will feel the warm fluid exit the vagina. Childbirth will usually commence within twenty-four hours after the amniotic sac breaks.

The process of childbirth consists of three stages of labor. All three stages are usually longer for a woman's first baby. The entire childbirth process usually lasts from four to twenty-four hours or longer.

First Stage of Labor

The **first stage of labor** begins with the onset of uterine contractions and lasts until the cervix is completely dilated. During this stage of labor uterine contractions will become

progressively stronger and arrive in shorter time intervals. When the contractions are two minutes apart and last forty-five seconds or longer, the birth of the baby is imminent. This is when the amniotic sac usually ruptures. Just prior to this time a physician or licensed midwife can introduce optional medications to reduce discomfort or pain (see figure 7.12).

Second Stage of Labor

The **second stage of labor** begins when the cervix is fully dilated and ends with the birth of the infant. During this stage, the strong uterine contractions push the fetus through the birth canal (vagina).

Before crowning, which is when the infant's head is at the vulva, an **episiotomy** may be performed. An episiotomy is the surgical cutting of some of the tissue between the anal and vaginal openings to prevent this tissue from tearing during labor. This surgical incision widens the vaginal opening. The tissue is stitched together after childbirth. An episiotomy after crowning is a risky procedure because of the close proximity of the infant's head.

Episiotomies in the U.S. have been criticized as unnecessary procedures. The physician usually performs an episiotomy before crowning as a preventive measure, so it is difficult to determine whether the episiotomy was really needed. Critics of the procedure cite studies indicating that considerably fewer episiotomies are performed, or considered necessary, for European women. Since the episiotomy is usually a preventive measure, expectant parents should discuss with their childbirth supervisor the circumstances in which they would approve the procedure.

As soon as the infant's head is accessible, the oral and nasal openings are drained of fluids and mucus. The procedure is repeated until the infant draws its first breath of air. When the infant is stable and responsive, the umbilical cord is usually cut. The physician often places silver nitrate or an antibiotic into the infant's eyes to prevent infection.

Third Stage of Labor

Following the birth of the infant the uterus continues to contract in order to expel the placenta and the remains of the fetal membranes. The placenta and fetal

Labor: a series of contractions of the uterus and abdominal muscles that help to expel the fetus, placenta, and membranes during childbirth. The average length of labor ranges from 8–12 hours.

Amniotic sac: a clear, fluid-filled membrane that develops during the embryonic period and surrounds the embryo, and later the fetus, providing a protective and nurturing environment until birth.

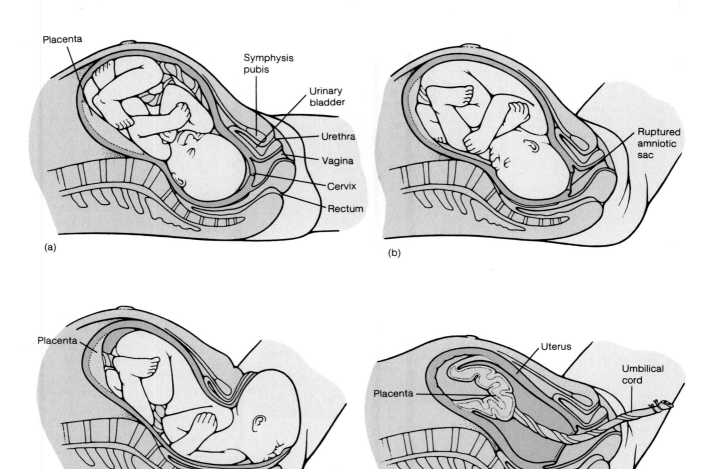

(a)

(b)

(c)

(d)

Placenta

Symphysis pubis

Urinary bladder

Urethra

Vagina

Cervix

Rectum

Ruptured amniotic sac

Placenta

Uterus

Umbilical cord

Placenta

Schenk

Figure 7.12: Birth
(*a*) Fetal position prior to birth;
(*b*) stage of dilation; (*c*) stage of
expulsion; (*d*) placental stage.

From Kent M. Van de Graaff, *Human Anatomy*, 3rd edition. Copyright © 1992 Wm. C. Brown Communications, Inc. Reprinted by permission of Times Mirror Higher Education Group, Inc., Dubuque, Iowa. All Rights Reserved.

membranes are referred to as the **afterbirth.** This process comprises the **third stage of labor.** It is essential that no remnants of the afterbirth remain in the uterus, since they could lead to increased bleeding or infection.

Breast-Feeding

After childbirth a yellowish fluid called **colostrum** will be secreted by the breasts. Colostrum contains several antibodies that can protect the newborn from illness, allergies, respiratory diseases, and diarrhea. Two to three days after childbirth the breasts will be able to secrete milk. Human milk contains sugar, protein, calcium, and water. Animal milks such as cow's milk, and products made from these animal milks (formulas), are not chemically or nutritionally equivalent to human milk. Human milk helps the newborn's digestion. There is some evidence that the milk from mothers of premature infants may be especially suited to

the premature infant.[29] The proportion of women choosing to breast-feed increased during the 1970s, reaching a peak in 1984. Currently slightly more than half of mothers initially breast-feed their newborns with only 18 percent continuing to the infant's sixth month of life. There are ethnic differences in mothers who breast-feed their children. Fifty-nine percent of White mothers breast-feed in comparison to 48 percent of Hispanic mothers and 23 percent of Black mothers.[30] Milk production subsides within a few days after the mother does not begin nursing, or stops nursing (see figure 7.13).

Breast-feeding has several advantages which are making it a practice that more women are turning to. Pediatricians and mothers alike seem to report that breast-fed babies are healthier babies and are less likely to contract allergies. If a mother breast-feeds, her uterus returns to its prepregnant state sooner. Moreover, the mother herself may regain her own prepregnancy size at a more

1. Most childbirth supervisors recommend that women breast-feed their infants. What do you think are the most important advantages and disadvantages of breast-feeding?
2. How could your local community encourage new mothers to breast-feed their infants? Are your suggestions realistic and feasible?

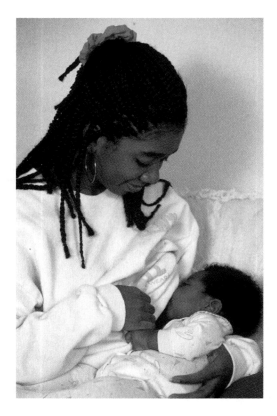

rapid rate. Many women report that their sexual responsiveness is restored faster if they breast-feed. Bonding between the mother and the infant may be enhanced if breast-feeding is performed. There may be some other practical reasons to breast-feed: it is less costly than buying formula, it is more convenient than preparing formula, and the milk is always at just the right temperature.

There are some drawbacks to breast-feeding. Breasts sometimes leak milk, and require special bras to protect clothing. Although some women report breast tenderness, the discomfort is usually of a short-term nature. While breast-feeding can be done practically anytime, it can also seem burdensome to a tired mother or make her feel like some of her own life has become restricted.

To assist women in breast-feeding, special bras have been created to permit it to be done discretely in public. For women who prefer more privacy and comfort while breast-feeding, an increasing number of public places, such as department stores and malls, have established special rooms that promote this practice. In addition, the use of breast pumps allow mother's milk to be obtained and stored for use at a later time. Thus, a

Nurse midwife: registered nurses who have received advanced training in assisting women through pregnancy and childbirth.

Obstetrician: a physician who specializes in pregnancy and childbirth.

father can take an active role in feeding the infant, and form a bond with his infant in a way similar to that which the mother is able to.

Childbirth Options

There are several childbirth options available to expectant parents. These options can be grouped into five categories: childbirth supervisors; childbirth facilities; childbirth courses; childbirth techniques; and childbirth witnesses. Parents may choose any combination from this array of options.

Some years ago, Manuel and Juanita were a bit overwhelmed with the thought of being expectant parents and deciding what doctors, hospitals, and techniques would be best for their child. Should they have a **nurse midwife** and a home birth instead of the customary hospital birth? They also wrestled with the fear that their child may be born with a physical deformity or that the birth may be complicated or even life-threatening for Juanita and the baby. The expense of a hospital birth worried them. The couple decided to buy a life insurance policy and they began thinking about providing for the child now and in the future. Even though the birth of the baby was still months away, the focus of their relationship, as well as the bonds of their relationship, changed dramatically. Reassurance was provided to them by Juanita's **obstetrician.** Her interactive style and desire to answer Manuel's and Juanita's questions made her a great comfort to them. Juanita later gave birth to Vilma. Many years later, Juanita was a great resource for Vilma as she had her own family and gave birth to twins—Christina and Maria.

Childbirth Supervisors

The person in charge of childbirth, the **childbirth supervisor,** may be a physician, a nurse midwife, a lay midwife, or a layperson. The childbirth supervisor is a key person during childbirth, but each of these supervisors has a different level of childbirth skill. Because every childbirth episode carries a degree of risk, it is prudent to consult a physician to assess the medical risks and health of both the mother and future child.

There are physicians who will refuse to take part in childbirth if the parents opt for a particular assistant, place, or technique. On the other hand there are physicians who will agree to be on call in case of a medical emergency during childbirth. Parents may opt for a **medicated childbirth,** in which case they may desire additional medical personnel who specialize in medicated deliveries. These matters should be clarified before, or soon after, pregnancy is confirmed.

Childbirth Facilities

It is important that future parents select a childbirth facility that meets both their birthing and emotional needs. Some facilities emphasize medical services while bypassing family needs in terms of togetherness and bonding. Some facilities do just the opposite. There are also facilities that combine both medical care and family care during childbirth.

Childbirth facilities include hospitals, birthing clinics, and home deliveries. Ninety-nine percent of all births are in hospitals. With few exceptions, comprehensive hospitals offer the emergency care and equipment needed when the mother or infant experiences medical complications during or soon after childbirth. Eighty to 90 percent of all births do not require extraordinary medical care or equipment. Birthing clinics specialize in childbirth and attempt to provide a home setting rather than a hospital setting. Birthing clinics are often physically or professionally attached to hospitals. They may have the same level of childbirth emergency care and equipment as a comprehensive hospital. Home births usually occur in the parents' residence, so it provides the most familiar and convenient setting for the family. Home births, however, increase the distance and time between emergency care and the mother and infant.

Childbirth Courses

In prepared childbirth courses, expectant family members, prior to delivery, learn about the process and skills of childbirth. This method usually involves familiarizing the parents with the childbirth process, facilities, personnel, and equipment that will be involved in their child's birth. Some courses prepare the entire family, including brothers and sisters, for the childbirth process. There are scores of childbirth courses, which use a variety of approaches. Most courses are helpful in preparing the family for the events of childbirth and the days that follow.

Childbirth Techniques

Currently, there are a variety of childbirth techniques used in the U.S. The traditional method of having the woman lying flat on her back is rarely used and most physicians employ the use of gravity by having the laboring woman recline in a semi-sitting position. Other common positions include the hands-and-knees, side-lying, and squatting positions. In addition to comfort, each position has physiological advantages for the mother and baby. Although childbirth education is not required, it is highly recommended, so that the woman and her labor partner may work as a team with the physician. Even if a woman is unable to attend classes, it is the physician's responsibility to inform the mother of the risks, benefits, and available alternatives for all the birthing options. One delivery option is the use of **electronic fetal monitoring (EFM)** devices. Some EFM devices are designed to be inserted in the vagina to monitor the fetus's vital signs prior to delivery. There is controversy over whether the risks of EFM devices outweigh their benefits.[31] In any event, such options should be explained and consent obtained prior to the birth.

There is also the birthing chair in which the mother sits upright and the law of gravity assists her in the delivery. Studies indicate that the birthing chair reduces the duration of the second stage of labor by one-half (see figure 7.14).

The Lamaze method of childbirth teaches the mother to relax and to control her breathing during labor. In Lamaze, the childbirth supervisor acts as the mother's coach during the birth (see figure 7.15).

Another method of birthing is the **cesarean section** (C-section), a surgical procedure in which an incision is made in the mother's lower abdomen and the uterus. The infant is then removed through the abdominal cavity. The rate of cesarean sections increased from a low of 4.5 percent in 1965 to a high of 24 percent in 1989. Since 1989 the rate has stabilized at 22.6 percent.[32] There is an ongoing debate as to what proportion of cesarean sections are unnecessary.[33]

The cesarean section is not the medically preferred method of delivery because of the increased risk of maternal mortality when

Medicated childbirth: childbirth in which one or more drugs are used by the mother during labor and delivery.

Figure 7.14: What Do You Think?

1. The birthing chair allows gravity to assist the mother during delivery. If you or your female partner were pregnant, how important would it be for you to find a birthing facility that provided a birthing chair or other contemporary childbirth options?

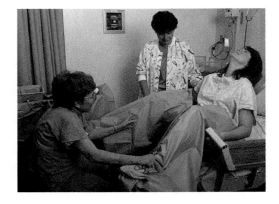

Figure 7.15: What Do You Think?

1. In the Lamaze birthing method each mother-to-be has a coach to aid in the childbirth process. Do you know anyone that has given birth using the Lamaze method? Were they pleased with the experience?

2. What childbirth education classes are available in your local community? What childbirth techniques do they advocate?

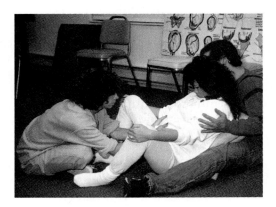

Epidural: an anesthetic administered to some women during labor and delivery to reduce pain associated with the birthing process.

compared to vaginal delivery (2:20,000 vs. 1:20,000). There are several instances in which a cesarean section is medically indicated to prevent maternal or infant injury or death. Some examples include: breech birth, prolonged labor, fetal distress, diabetes, hypertension, and preventing the fetus from contracting an infectious disease (e.g., herpes, hepatitis B, or gonorrhea) while passing through the vagina. The phrase "once a cesarean section, always a cesarean section" is not true for all women. A considerable proportion of women follow a cesarean birth with a normal vaginal birth.

Natural childbirth implies that the woman chooses to use relaxation and breathing techniques instead of pain-relieving medications while in labor. For women who choose the use of medication, the most common method of pain relief is the **epidural.** After an anesthesiologist inserts a thin, plastic catheter into the epidural space

surrounding the spinal column, the pain-relieving, nerve-blocking medication slowly drips through tubing for the duration of labor and birth. The other kinds of medications used during childbirth range from mild tranquilizers (Valium) to muscle relaxers (Demoral). However, since every medication has potential side effects, it is important for the pregnant woman to discuss all available medication options with her physician prior to the onset of labor. Parents should understand that most drugs administered during childbirth will cross the placental barrier. The risk of birth complications depends on the drug, the dose, and when and how it is administered.

Childbirth Witnesses

Witnesses to the birth of a child can include a husband, children, immediate family, or friends. Parents may want to use a camera to document the birth.

Parents need to decide how much time they and their loved ones will spend with the newborn. Some childbirth facilities place severe restrictions on who may visit with the newborn child and its mother and when. The parents also need to decide who will see, touch, and care for the infant right after birth. Hospital settings tend to place the most restrictions on the parents' access to their newborn child. Expectant parents should select a facility that will meet their physical as well as family needs.

Not all childbirth supervisors and facilities will accommodate all childbirth options. In addition, medical insurance companies are often very selective in the kinds of childbirth facilities and practitioners they will cover. All these options and details should be worked out prior to delivery. Mother, father, and other children can use this time to prepare to welcome the family's newest member.

Infertility

A couple is considered **infertile** when they are unable to conceive after one year of repeated sexual attempts without practicing birth control, or when the woman is incapable of carrying the fetus to a live birth. Estimates vary but approximately 14 percent of couples in the U.S. will experience infertility resulting in involuntarily childless, or fewer naturally conceived children than they desire.[34]

One option for both infertile males and females is adoption. Adoption may not be less expensive or less frustrating than medical attempts to bring about a successful live birth for an infertile couple. However adoption, like procreation, has the potential to fulfill both the parents' and child's lives.

A specific physiological cause can be diagnosed in approximately 85 percent of all infertile couples. A couple's infertility can be a result of male, female, or some combination of male and female factors (see figure 7.16). Two factors contributing to infertility are women delaying childbirth, and the rise in STDs.

Common causes of female infertility are blocked fallopian tubes, endometriosis, and failure to ovulate. **Endometriosis** is a condition in which a piece of the endometrium in the uterus tears off and grows in the pelvic cavity on adjacent reproductive organs, such as the fallopian tubes or ovaries. This tissue acts exactly as endometrial tissue in the uterus, thickening during certain stages of each reproductive cycle and then attempting to slough off excess tissue at the time of menstruation. Endometrial tissue in the pelvic cavity, however, cannot be expelled from the body. It therefore continues to increase with each cycle, causing severe abdominal pain in some women. "Hostile mucus" has been identified as another cause of female infertility. Hostile cervical mucus does not allow sperm to pass through the cervix into the vagina. This is due, in part, to the cervical mucus containing sperm antibodies that immobilize sperm.

Common causes of male infertility are low sperm counts and low mobility of sperm. Low mobility of sperm is a condition in which a considerable proportion of the total sperm in a male's ejaculate is not active enough to accomplish fertilization. The male may also develop an autoimmune response to his own sperm. In this case his body produces antibodies that destroy his sperm or prevent their development. Another cause of male infertility is erectile inhibition, or the inability to have and maintain an erection. Erectile inhibition is common among diabetic males, due to their circulatory difficulties.

A common combined cause of infertility is a woman's allergic reaction to sperm. In such cases she produces antibodies that attack and destroy sperm, in effect producing a natural spermicide.

Male Infertility Options

Infertile males can sometimes father children by using erectile enhancers or artificial insemination.

A penile implant is a surgical technique that has been somewhat successful in overcoming erectile inhibition. A surgeon can implant semirigid rods into the penis so that the male constantly has a partially rigid penis. Another device that can be implanted in the penis is an inflatable, cylinder-shaped balloon. The male, using a pump implanted in the scrotum, pumps up the device with fluid stored in a bag inside the abdomen. With this device the male can control his erection.

Artificial insemination occurs when some means other than the penis is used to introduce semen into the vaginal tract of the uterus. For example, a physician can use a syringe to squirt semen into the vaginal tract. The majority of artificial inseminations use semen from a paid or unpaid donor or *Artificial Insemination by Donor (AID)*. AIH is *Artificial Insemination by Husband*. Estimates vary, however, approximately 15,000 to 20,000 children a year are born in the U.S. as a result of artificial insemination. The inheritance and other legal rights of AID children, and the substantiation of who is the legal father and his liabilities as the paternal father, remain unresolved legal questions.

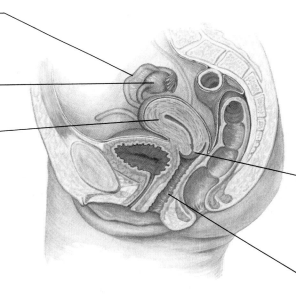

Vas deferens (the sperm duct) carries sperm out of the testicles. If it is blocked by scars from infection or surgery, the sperm are trapped.

Urethra (the urine and sperm passageway) may harbor infections that can spread and damage the sperm duct.

Penis may be unable to deliver sperm into the vagina if the erection is incomplete.

Seminal vesicle contributes nutrients and fluid for sperm transport. Too much or too little fluid can be detrimental to fertility.

Prostate gland can harbor infections that might affect sperm motility, or movement.

Epididymis is a single coiled tube in which the sperm mature after leaving the testicle. Infections here may prevent sperm from reaching the sperm duct.

Testicle may produce sperm that are too weak or too few in number to reach the egg in the fallopian tube. Hormonal signals from brain and pituitary gland may be weak.

Scrotum may contain a varicose vein, or varicocele, which allows for backward flow of warm blood. This heats up the testicle, interfering with sperm production.

a.

Male

Fallopian tube, which normally carries the egg to the uterus, may be blocked by scars from infection. If so, egg cannot move or sperm will be unable to reach egg.

Ovary can fail to produce eggs because it receives no hormone signal from the brain and pituitary gland.

Uterus, or womb, may not be hospitable to the egg. Most often, hormone imbalances affect the endometrium (the inner lining of the uterus) and prevent the egg from implanting.

Cervix (the opening to the uterus) may be hostile to sperm. Some women develop a plug of mucus within the passageway that blocks the sperm.

Vagina may harbor infections that destroy sperm or prevent cervix from accepting sperm. (Some vaginal infections also may spread to the fallopian tubes.)

b.

Female

Figure 7.16: Causes of infertility

Data from Earl Ubell, "Encouraging News for Childless Couples," in *Parade Magazine*, May 6, 1984, as appeared in John W. Hole, Jr., *Human Anatomy and Physiology*, 5th edition. Copyright © 1990 Wm. C. Brown Communications, Inc. Reprinted by permission of Times Mirror Higher Education Group, Inc., Dubuque, Iowa. All Rights Reserved.

Female Infertility Options

Infertile women can sometimes produce genetic offspring through ovum transfer, hormone therapy, surrogate mothers, and in vitro fertilization.

Blocked fallopian tubes can sometimes be repaired with microsurgery. A method called low tubal ovum transfer allows surgeons to capture a Graafian Follicle from the ovaries and insert it in the fallopian tube at the point beyond the blockage. In this way the egg bypasses the blocked portion of the tube and fertilization can take place naturally.

Females who do not ovulate can be prescribed clomiphene, an oral drug that stimulates the secretion of FSH and LH. If clomiphene proves unsuccessful, a series of injections using human menopausal gonadotropins (HMG) may be tried. This drug acts directly on the ovaries to induce ovulation. These drugs are not without side effects. A couple should discuss the health risks of hormonal therapy with their physician. If pregnancy occurs with the use of HMG there is one chance in five that it will be a multiple birth.

Surrogate Mothers

Some infertile couples have contracted with surrogate mothers to bear their babies. **Surrogate mothers** are paid or unpaid volunteers who make their reproductive organs available for procreation and pregnancy.

Surrogate mothers can be artificially inseminated by the male of an infertile couple, in which case the male becomes the baby's genetic father and the surrogate mother its genetic mother. The three "parents" agree, however, usually with the assistance of a lawyer, that the surrogate mother will lay no claim to parent the baby once it is born. This allows the infertile female to become the baby's familial mother.

Many events could occur that would place surrogate contracts in legal limbo. Surrogate mothers have refused to give up their babies. What happens if a surrogate mother is accused of consuming alcohol and thereby damages the baby? Who is legally and financially responsible for a child if any, or all, of the "parents" refuse custody?

In Vitro Fertilization

The technique that results in "test-tube babies" is called **in vitro fertilization (IVF).** IVF solves some fertility problems while creating other social issues. IVF involves removing the egg from the ovaries, fertilizing it artificially in a laboratory dish, incubating it for a short time, and then implanting it inside the uterus. This technique enables females with blocked fallopian tubes or no fallopian tubes to be the genetic parents of their children.

The first successful animal IVF took place in 1947, and the first successful human IVF was performed in 1972. There are now over 100 medical centers in the U.S. performing this service. In the U.S. there are over 2,300 live births a year as a result of IVF.[35]

IVF also makes it possible for a female without a uterus to become the genetic parent of her child by using the services of a surrogate mother. In such a case the egg is removed from the female without a uterus, artificially fertilized by her mate's sperm in a laboratory dish, incubated, and then implanted in a surrogate mother. An infant produced this way would be the genetic product of the infertile couple with the surrogate mother acting only as a human incubator. Here the surrogate or birth mother is not the genetic mother of the child she bore.

IVF raises numerous legal and ethical questions. For example, the woman receives hormones which cause her ovaries to produce several eggs. All of these eggs are retrieved from the ovaries and fertilized. Only those fertilized eggs that appear healthy and comprise only four cells will be placed into the uterus. Subsequently, there are leftover fertilized eggs. If they are sold to someone else, is that "baby selling," which is illegal? If they are destroyed, is that an abortion? How can a female have an abortion when she is not pregnant? Are IVF embryos orphans of the state?

Animal breeders have used a technique called twinning to produce identical offspring from a prize animal. Twinning involves a relatively simple technique of splitting one embryo into two or more masses. Each newly formed embryo could be an identical twin. By using IVF and twinning, it is possible for a couple to order identical twins, have them both immediately, or choose to freeze one or two for a later pregnancy five, ten, or twenty years later.

From a personal perspective the desire of an infertile couple/person to have a child impacts on every aspect of their emotional, social, physical, intellectual, and often spiritual health. It is common for an infertile couple's hopes and dreams to rest on producing a son or daughter. For this reason they are willing to endure surgery, invest large sums of money, and even submit to experimental reproductive techniques. Unfortunately the realities of reproductive technology demonstrate that they are more unsuccessful than successful cases. In some cases reproductive clinics may have success rates, where success is measured by live births, at or near 0 percent. Thus it is important that infertile people carefully select and research their infertility specialist and clinic.

Personal and Social Influences on Pregnancy and Parenting

Many social factors that occur during our lifetimes impact upon our sexuality. These factors range from parental and formal sex education to medical advancements, on through political and social agendas. The following are three social segments that can have a considerable affect on our sexuality and wellness.

Sexuality and Family Life Education

For centuries many people believed that "talking about sex" would increase the likelihood of promiscuous sexual behavior. So generations of schoolchildren grew up learning about the digestive system, respiratory system, and other systems, while parents and clergy supposedly taught children about the reproductive system. Unfortunately, most parents and clergy reneged on their duty to teach children and young adults about the human reproductive and sexual response systems. By default, friends, television, movies, and other media became the primary "sex teachers."

Ironically, many school "sex education" courses have contributed their share of misinformation. School sex education courses are under constant pressure from external influences such as PTAs, churches, health departments, and politically active groups to teach various points of view. In addition, many courses are taught by people not academically

or emotionally prepared for sound instruction. Rarely does a school employ a full-time teacher trained specifically in human sexuality. Only thirteen states require sex education in all schools.[36] It is not surprising that public schools in the U.S. have been repeatedly criticized for not providing effective and meaningful sex education to students.

Teenagers' lack of information regarding sexual conduct, coupled with their relatively high rate of sexual activity, combine to thwart society's efforts to prevent unintended pregnancies, teenage marriages, and the spread of sexually transmitted diseases. Should teenagers be required to complete a high school sex education course taught by a professionally prepared sex educator? Is one-half semester of sex education during a teenager's four year high school program enough time to prepare to make decisions regarding his or her sexuality, procreation, fertility, relationships, child-rearing, and sexual health-related problems?

Infertility Issues

IVF and reimplantation techniques offer reproductively healthy couples new procreation options. Some females might desire to be the genetic and familial parents of their children but also desire to forego pregnancy. Careers such as modeling, entertainment, or professional sports may be a factor in the prospective mother's desire to retain her figure. Pregnancy may be viewed as a handicap by females who choose to remain in their professions during and following pregnancy. Reimplantation using surrogate mothers is an option that would allow such individuals to be the genetic and familial mothers of their children, without experiencing the rigors of pregnancy or childbirth. It is possible today for a female to be the genetic mother of her child without ever having intercourse, going through pregnancy, or giving birth.

Fertility procedures such as artificial insemination, surrogate mothers, and reimplantation techniques have produced options for both fertile and infertile people. Should only married couples have access to these procedures? Should single persons, gay men, or lesbians have access to such techniques? Should the government subsidize these procedures for the economically disadvantaged?

As these procedures become more commonplace there will be an ever-increasing interest in, and medical necessity for, children

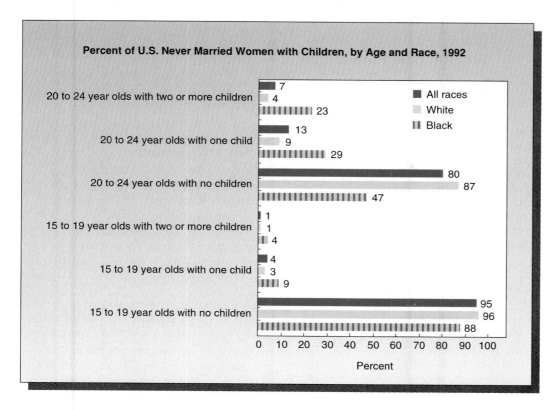

Percent of U.S. Never Married Women with Children, by Age and Race, 1992

Legend:
- All races
- White
- Black

20 to 24 year olds with two or more children
- 7
- 4
- 23

20 to 24 year olds with one child
- 13
- 9
- 29

20 to 24 year olds with no children
- 80
- 87
- 47

15 to 19 year olds with two or more children
- 1
- 1
- 4

15 to 19 year olds with one child
- 4
- 3
- 9

15 to 19 year olds with no children
- 95
- 96
- 88

Percent
0 10 20 30 40 50 60 70 80 90 100

Figure 7.17: What Do You Think?

1. What childbearing differences does this data illustrate comparing Black and White young, never married U.S. women?
2. What factors do you think might account for the differences in childbearing patterns illustrated here? What evidence did you rely on to identify such factors?

Source: Data from *Statistical Abstract of the United States*, 1993, U.S. Bureau of the Census, U.S. Government Printing Office.

to know the identity of their genetic parents and siblings. Inherently people want to know their genetic roots and ancestry. Also, in matters of illness, medical emergency, and procreation it may be imperative to obtain a genetic history. Currently, there is no national consensus on whether or not records of a child's genetic parents should be kept or destroyed, or whether a child has a right to those records. Is the donation of sperm, eggs, or embryos the equivalent of donating blood to another person? Does the contribution of genes, in the form of sperm, eggs, and embryos, constitute the creation of life and ancestry?

The next generation may consider pregnancy an optional form of procreation. In any event, artificial procreation procedures and artificially created embryos have become a legal quagmire. Legal issues include the responsibilities, liabilities, and rights of everyone involved, including physicians, donors, parents, children, and the artificially created products of human conception.

Social Support for Parenting

The "typical" U.S. family—that is, mom, dad, and two kids—is no longer typical. More than one-half of marriages end in divorce and in most instances, the mother assumes custody of the children. A growing number of never-married women are choosing to have one or more children without a husband. Indeed 52 percent of never-married Black females age twenty to twenty-four have one or more biological children[37] (see figure 7.17). Many of these women and children exist at the poverty level. Working outside the home is often not a choice but rather a necessity. The need for good day-care facilities to assist single mothers raising their children is becoming a significant part of the social safety net.

Women comprise a large share of the workforce. They spend a good part of the day at work and require social supports to help maintain their family's level of wellness. Employers are starting to see that there are economic payoffs to underwriting child care and health services for their female employees. Some businesses have created their own day-care centers at the workplace so that employees can be close to their children. Parents can visit their children on lunch or other breaks, and are available in case their child becomes ill or requires their presence. Prenatal programs at the worksite are beginning to multiply. The issues surrounding government's and private industry's financial support for childbearing and parenting in the workplace are being openly debated. No doubt this area of debate

TABLE 7.7 Tips for Preparing for Caregiving to Children

Adapting to being a parent can be difficult. What training does one get for the realities of parenting? Most of us were raised around adults who were our biological parents, adoptive parents, foster parents, or "acting parents," but seldom thought about the caregiving experience. You may be able to reduce the anxiety associated with parenting and make a wiser decision about becoming a parent at all by thinking through some of the tips provided below.

Precontemplation → Contemplation

If you have never thought about being a parent, consider:

- Using the phone book and other resources, develop a list of organizations that teach classes about pregnancy, childbirth, and parenting.
- Contact a "Big Brothers" or "Big Sisters" program in your area and find out what kind of services they need volunteers to provide.

Contemplation → Preparation

If you have thought about what it means to be a supportive parent but have not prepared yourself for the task, try:

- Developing a list of your own personal resources that might be valuable to pass on to a "next generation."
- Make a list of things you do as part of your daily routine, and note how each would change as a result of being a parent of an infant? of a toddler or preschooler? of a boy versus a girl?

Preparation → Action

Having taken inventory of your own abilities and strengths, advance your plan to examine your parenting potential by:

- Identifying time in the next thirty days to carry out a plan to supervise and provide caregiving for a child. Circle the date on your calendar.
- Telling others about your activity, and letting them know you are actually preparing for a future role as a parent.

Action → Maintenance

Having successfully demonstrated your parenting ability (or identified your limitations in caregiving), you can explore things further by:

- Celebrating your accomplishment or examining how to improve your experience.
- After completing a caregiving task involving a child, making a promise to repeat that task or perform another one.
- Making a firm appointment (e.g., next Friday at 3:00 P.M.) to engage yourself again in a child caregiving task.

Maintenance

You are well on your way to being a caregiver. Keep up your momentum by:

- Diversifying your repertoire of activities with children and youth of different ages.
- Identifying a person you know who has children with whom you can volunteer to partake in their care.
- Inviting a roommate, classmate, or other friend to help you with one of your activities or outings that involves children.

Based on Prochaska, Norcross, and DiClemente's transtheoretical model. See Prochaska, J. O., Norcross, J. C. and DiClemente, C. C. (1994), *Changing for Good*. New York: William Morrow and Company, Inc.

concerns an essential issue regarding the future well-being of people in the U.S. Should government provide tax incentives for businesses that provide on-site day-care centers for their employees?

Children are a valued resource of nearly every society. They represent the vitality and immortality of both the culture and the individual. Thus procreation is both a cultural and personal contribution. Our ancestors basically dealt with the question, How many children? You will be presented with much more complicated questions such as: Should you become a parent?, How and when will you procreate?, How will you raise your child?, and As a working parent who should pay for your prenatal care, childbirth, childbirth leave, and child care? Table 7.7 lists some considerations for caregiving to children.

Summary

1. Males and females contribute genes to their offspring. The genes combine and form a single cell called a zygote. The zygote will develop into a new member of the human race.

2. The testes and ovaries produce sperm and eggs, both of which carry chromosomes. They also produce hormones that are responsible for development of secondary sex characteristics and maintenance of the reproductive organs.

3. The formation of a zygote is called fertilization.

4. The hormone used by the hypothalamus to stimulate the testes and ovaries is called the gonadotropin-releasing hormone, or GnRH.

5. Luteinizing hormone (LH) stimulates the testes into producing testosterone, the primary male sex hormone. In the female, LH stimulates the ovaries into producing estrogen, the primary female hormone.

6. Follicle-stimulating hormone (FSH) stimulates the testes into producing sperm. In the female, FSH stimulates the ovaries into producing mature eggs.

7. The seminal vesicles produce a fluid containing a simple sugar that provides nutrition for sperm. The prostate gland secretions neutralize (1) the waste products of sperm, (2) the acid found in the male urethra, and (3) the acidic environment of the vagina.

8. Ovulation occurs when the Graafian follicle, which contains the mature egg, ruptures and the egg is released from the ovary into the fallopian tube.

9. Parents, because they are parents, inherit the ultimate responsibility of providing for their child's wellness.

10. Parental love is *the* essential human ingredient in parenting. Love's omnipresence underlies all parent-child interactions.

11. Prenatal care increases a mother's chance of bearing a healthy baby. Prenatal care also allows for the detection of potential and actual pregnancy problems.

12. Although there is no definitive evidence in all cases, it seems that the prudent course of action is for the pregnant female to avoid the use of all prescription, over-the-counter, and illegal drugs from the first day of the reproductive cycle she chooses to become pregnant until after childbirth. In cases where the mother chooses to breast-feed, this period of drug abstinence should continue until the child is weaned.

13. Pregnancy is divided into three phases called trimesters. The first trimester is from the point of fertilization to the end of the third month. The second trimester is from the beginning of the fourth month to the end of the sixth month. The third trimester is from the beginning of the seventh month until childbirth.

14. Amniocentesis, chorionic biopsy, and PUBS are prenatal tests used to discover genetic disorders, chromosomal abnormalities, and sex-linked diseases.

15. The first stage of labor begins with the onset of uterine contractions and lasts until the cervix is completely dilated. The second stage of labor begins when the cervix is fully dilated and ends with the birth of the infant. The third stage of labor expels the placenta and fetal membranes (afterbirth).

16. Expectant parents have several childbirth options. These options can be grouped into five categories: childbirth supervisors, childbirth facilities, childbirth courses, childbirth techniques, and childbirth witnesses.

17. It is important that future parents select a childbirth facility that meets both their birthing and emotional needs.

18. A couple's infertility can be a result of male, female, or a combination of male and female factors. Common causes of female infertility are blocked fallopian tubes, endometriosis, and failure to ovulate. Common causes of male infertility are low sperm counts and low mobility of sperm.

19. There are important social influences on our ability to procreate and parent, including the family life education received, technological innovations that help infertile couples conceive, and social supports for the task of parenting well.

Recommended Readings

J. Christen & J. Greger. *Nutrition for Living*. New York: Benjamin/Cummings, 1994.

Chapter 15 of this work details the elements for good nutrition during pregnancy and lactation. Included are essential requirements for infant nutrition and a comparison of infant commercial formulas. Chapter 16 explores children's nutritional requirements, eating behaviors, and social influences on their diet.

B. Martin, H. Hart, & S. Jenkins. *Child Development and Child Health*. Boston: Blachwell Scientific Publications, 1990.

The text, authored by British pediatricians, approaches child development in terms of physical, cognitive, and social growth, and in the context of child behavior. The book details a comprehensive profile of developmental norms and health concerns, and a prospective of British medicine as it relates to the topics.

D. Suggs & A. Miracle (Eds.) *Culture and Human Sexuality*. Pacific Grove, California: Brooks/Cole, 1993.

The editors examine the cultural influences on peoples' sexuality, sexual behavior, and sexual attitudes. The range of topics span from eating disorders to relationship expectations for men and women.

References

1. H. Snyder, "To Circumcise or Not," *Hospital Practice* 26.1 (1991): 201–207; T. E. Wiswell et al., "Declining Frequency of Circumcision: Implications for Changes in the Absolute Incidence and Male to Female Sex Ratio of Urinary Tract Infections in Early Infancy," *Pediatrics* 79.3 (1987):338.

2. N. Touchette, "HIV-1 Link Prompts Circumspection on Circumcision," *Journal of NIH Research* 3 (1991):44–46; M. S. Wilkes & S. Blum, "Current Trends in Routine Newborn Male Circumcision in New

York State," *New York State Journal of Medicine* 90 (1990):243–246.

3. R. L. Polland, "The Question of Routine Neonate Circumcision," *New England Journal of Medicine* 322 (1990):1312–1315; E. J. Schoen, "The Status of Circumcision of Newborns," *New England Journal of Medicine* 322 (1990):1308–1312.

4. P. M. Hanno and A. J. Weim, *A Clinical Manual of Urology* (Norwalk: Appleton-Century-Crofts, 1987).

5. Hanno and Weim, *A Clinical Manual of Urology*.

6. M. L. Pernoll and R. C. Benson, *Current Obstetric and Gynecologic Diagnosis and Treatment* (Norwalk: Appleton & Lange, 1987); David M. Neuman, "Causes of Genitourinary Symptoms in Women," *Journal of the American Medical Association* 252 (1984):13.

7. Pernoll and Benson, *Current Obstetric and Gynecologic Diagnosis and Treatment*.

8. E. Freeman et al., "Ineffectiveness of Progesterone Suppository Treatment for Premenstrual Syndrome," *Journal of the American Medical Association* 264 (1990):349–353; L. Gise, "Premenstrual Syndrome: Which Treatments Help?" *Medical Aspects of Human Sexuality* 25.2 (1991):62–68; Pernoll and Benson, *Current Obstetric and Gynecologic Diagnosis and Treatment*.

9. Centers for Disease Control, "Reduced Incidence of Menstrual Toxic-shock Syndrome United States, 1980–1990," *Morbidity and Mortality Weekly Report* 39.25 (1990):421–423.

10. M. Lino, "Expenditures on a Child by Husband-Wife Families," *Family Economics Review* 3 (1990):2–12.

11. "Fathering Healthy Babies," *UC Berkeley Wellness Letter*, 10 (7):1–2.

12. R. L. Brendt & D. A., "Teratology," in R. D. Eden, F. H. Boehm, & M. Hare (Eds.), *Assessment and Care of the Fetus: Physiological, Clinical, and Medicolegal Principles* (Norwalk, CT: Appleton & Lange, 1990); I. M. Beckman, M. D. Bobak, Jensen, and M. K. Zalar, *Maternity and Gynecologic Care* (St. Louis: C. V. Mosby Co., 1989).

13. J. J. Mulvihill, "Fetal Alcohol Syndrome," in *Teratogen Update:*

Environmentally Induced Birth Defects Risks, eds. J. L. Sever and R. L. Brent (New York: Alan R. Liss, 1986), 13–18.

14. O. S. Ray and C. Ksir, *Drugs, Society, & Human Behavior* (St. Louis: Mosby, 1993).

15. B. Strong and C. Devault, *Understanding Our Sexuality* (New York: West Publishing, 1988).

16. M. Werler, B. Pober, and L. Holmes, "Smoking and Pregnancy," in *Teratogen Update: Environmentally Induced Birth Defects Risks*, eds. J. L. Sever and R. L. Brent (New York: Alan R. Liss, 1986), 131–139.

17. J. Coste, N. Job-Spira, and H. Fernandez, "Increased Risk of Ectopic Pregnancy with Maternal Cigarette Smoking," *American Journal of Public Health* 81.2 (1991):199–201.

18. L. Fenster et al., "Caffeine Consumption during Pregnancy and Fetal Growth," *American Journal of Public Health* 81.4 (1991):458–461.

19. J. R. Niebyl, "Teratology and Drugs in Pregnancy and Lactation," in J. R. Scott et al., Danforth's *Obstetrics and Gynecology* (Philadelphia: Lippincott, 1990). Sixth edition.

20. National Center for Health Statistics, "Advance Report of Maternal and Infant Health Data from the Birth Certificate, 1991," *Monthly Vital Statistics Report* 42 (11) (1994):1–32.

21. J. S. Greenberg, C. E. Bruess, K. D. Mullen, and D. W. Sands, *Sexuality: Insights and Issues* (Dubuque, Iowa: Wm. C. Brown Publishers, 1989), 328.

22. G. W. Dameron, "Helping Couples Cope with Sexual Changes Pregnancy Brings," *Ortho Forum* 3.3 (1983):7.

23. Greenberg et al., *Sexuality: Insights and Issues*, 328.

24. J. Becerra et al., (1991) "Infant Mortality Among Hispanics," *Journal of the American Medical Association*, 265 (2):217–221.

25. Jensen, Bobak, and Zalar, *Maternity and Gynecologic Care*.

26. A. J. Ingalls and M. C. Salerno, *Maternal and Child Health Nursing* (St. Louis: C. V. Mosby Company, 1987), 63.

27. Jensen, Bobak, and Zalar, *Maternity and Gynecologic Care*.

28. T. Kerenyi and U. Chitkara, "Selective Birth in Twin Pregnancy with Discordancy for Down's Syndrome," *New England Journal of Medicine* 304.25 (1981):1525–1527.

29. S. A. Atkins, G. H. Anderson, and M. H. Bryan, "Human Milk: Comparison of the Nitrogen Composition in Milk from Mothers of Premature and Full-Term Infants," *American Journal of Clinical Nutrition* 33 (April 1980):811–815; R. Schanler and W. Oh, "Composition of Breast Milk Obtained from Mothers of Premature Infants as Compared to Breast Milk Obtained from Donors," *Journal of Pediatrics* 96 (1980):679–681.

30. A. A. Ryan et al., "Recent Declines in Breast-Feeding in the United States," *Pediatrics* 88 (1991):719–727.

31. K. K. Shy et al., "Effects of Electronic Fetal-Heart-Rate Monitoring, as Compared with Periodic Auscultation, on the Neurologic Development of Premature Infants," *New England Journal of Medicine* 322 (1990):588–593.

32. National Center for Health Statistics, "Advance Report of Maternal and Infant Health Data from the Birth Certificate, 1991," *Monthly Vital Statistics Report* 42 (11) (1994):1–32.

33. R. Stafford, "The Impact of Nonclinical Factors on Repeat Cesarean Section," *Journal of the American Medical Association* 265:1 (1991):59–63.

34. J. J. Sciarra, "Infertility: A Global Perspective on the Role of Infection," *Annals of the New York Academy of Sciences* 626 (1991):478–483.

35. American Fertility Society, "In-Vitro Fertilization—Embryo Transfer (IVF-ET) in the United States: 1990 Results from IVF-ET Registry," *Fertility and Sterility* 57 (1992):15–24.

36. D. Haffner, *Sex Education 2000: A Call to Action* (New York: Information and Education Council of the United States, 1990).

37. U.S. Bureau of the Census, *Statistical Abstract of the United States: 1993*, Washington, DC: 1993 (113th Edition).

Birth Control: Options for Preventing Unintended Pregnancy

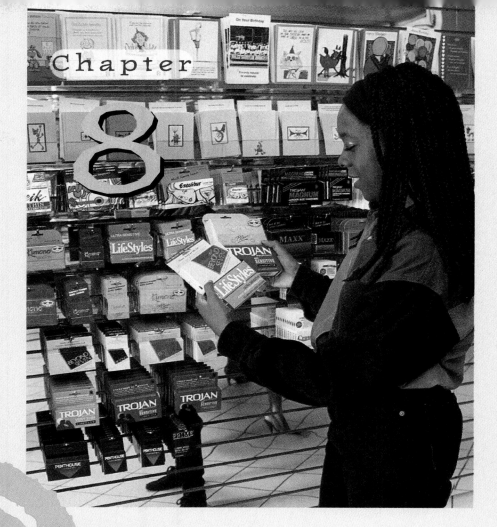

Chapter 8

Student Learning Objectives

Upon completion of this chapter you should be able to:

1. list the seven major objectives of family planning;
2. describe the four general categories of birth-control methods and give one example of each category;
3. describe common factors an individual can use to consider the acceptability of birth-control methods;
4. define and describe the theoretical and use effectiveness ratings for birth-control methods currently available in the United States;
5. assess both the health risks and health benefits associated with birth-control methods currently available in the United States;
6. compare the costs of the various birth-control methods currently available in the United States, both in terms of monetary costs and inconvenience;
7. describe the current reversibility estimates for birth-control methods available in the United States;
8. compare and contrast sexual abstinence and periodic abstinence as birth-control methods;
9. describe the similarities and differences of the diaphragm and cervical cap;
10. compare and contrast the male and female condom;
11. describe the correct way to use spermicides;
12. list the steps a woman would go through to become and remain an IUD user;
13. compare and contrast oral contraceptives, Norplant, and Depo-Provera as birth-control methods;
14. identify several birth-control methods being tested and developed for the U.S. market;
15. compare and contrast male and female sterilization as birth-control methods;
16. discuss the personal, social, and political concerns regarding current abortion rulings in terms of the mother, biological father, and fetus;
17. identify several consequences of world overpopulation.

Many college students face the important decision of whether or not to use birth control, and if so, which method may be best suited to their needs and circumstances. Decisions about sexual relationships and the options available regarding pregnancy, sexually transmitted diseases, and reproductive health can have a profound effect on well-being. Sound decision making requires a knowledge of medical technology, in some cases skills to effectively apply a technology, an understanding of the benefits, limitations and risks of the technology, and an awareness of your personal convictions and needs regarding sexual behavior. This chapter will help you to discover the available options for preventing unintended pregnancies and, in some cases, sexually transmitted diseases as well.

Preventing Unintended Pregnancy

Birth-control methods are an important tool of family planning. The goal of family planning is to help individuals control their fertility through preventive measures that ultimately enhance the health of the mother, her infant, and the entire family (see table 8.1). The goals of family planning center around preventing unintended pregnancies, as well as planning for the number and spacing of intended pregnancies.

It has been estimated that over 50 percent of women in the U.S. aged fifteen to forty-four use some method of birth control (see figure 8.1). However by eliminating the women who were not at risk for an unintended pregnancy such as women who were pregnant, **postpartum** women, women trying to become pregnant, women sterilized for health reasons and so on, then the estimate is upgraded to 90 percent of women at risk of an unintended pregnancy use some method of birth control.[1] According to the National Center for Health Statistics,[2] only 63 percent of young women 15 to 19 years old report using contraceptives during their first act of intercourse; 81 percent, however, report contraceptive use during recent intercourse.

The *Healthy People 2000* report recognizes the family planning service needs of young people in the U.S. (see table 8.2), and focuses specifically on encouraging young people to abstain from sexual intercourse, postpone sexual intercourse, and if sexually active, to increase the use of contraceptives to help prevent both pregnancy and sexually transmitted diseases. Some progress has been made toward the *Healthy People 2000* objectives for the nation.[3] The proportion of previously sexually active adolescent boys and girls reporting that they had not had sexual intercourse in the past three months increased slightly, from 23.6 percent in 1990 to 25 percent in 1991 for boys, and from 33 percent to 36 percent for girls during that same time. Additionally, there has been a slight increase in the number of sexually active adolescents (both male and female) who reported using contraception during recent sexual intercourse. Yet, the *Healthy People 2000* report also points out that an estimated 56 percent of pregnancies in the United States are unintended. If you are currently sexually active, or if you plan to become sexually active at some point in the future, the common birth-control methods profiled in this chapter should help you make informed decisions regarding birth-control choices.

Birth-Control Categories

There are four general ways birth-control methods can prevent a live birth. They can be categorized under the following headings: natural, mechanical, chemical, and invasive. It is possible for a single method of birth control to employ two means of preventing a live birth each from a different category, such as a spermicidal condom.

Natural

Natural birth-control methods involve techniques that do not use any devices, chemicals, or surgical procedures to directly prevent **fertilization.** People using natural birth-control methods attempt to predict the time of **ovulation,** and then practice sexual abstinence or another method of birth

Postpartum: the first few days following the birth of a child.

Fertilization: the creation of a single cell, formed when the genes from the female's egg and genes from the male's sperm unite.

Ovulation: the process by which the ovary releases a mature egg.

TABLE 8.1 — Objectives of Family Planning

- To avoid unwanted pregnancies
- To regulate intervals between pregnancies
- To decide the number of children in the family
- To control the time at which births occur in relation to the parents' age
- To facilitate wanted births for women with fertility problems
- To avoid pregnancy for women with serious disease whom an imposed pregnancy would place at additional risk

- To provide women who are carriers of genetic disease with the option of avoiding pregnancy

The overall goal of these objectives is to improve the health of the mother, the baby, and the family. Child spacing, limitation of family size, and timing of the first birth are recognized preventive health measures.

From Jean D. Neeson and Katharyn A. May, *Comprehensive Maternity Nursing: Nursing Process and the Childbearing Family.* © 1986 J. B. Lippincott Company, Philadelphia, PA. Reprinted by permission.

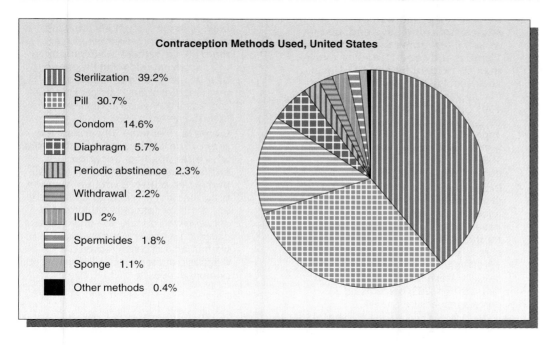

Contraception Methods Used, United States

- Sterilization 39.2%
- Pill 30.7%
- Condom 14.6%
- Diaphragm 5.7%
- Periodic abstinence 2.3%
- Withdrawal 2.2%
- IUD 2%
- Spermicides 1.8%
- Sponge 1.1%
- Other methods 0.4%

Figure 8.1: What Do You Think?

1. What factors account for the popularity of sterilization as a birth-control method?
2. Why do you think periodic abstinence, the IUD, spermicides, and the contraceptive sponge have such a low level of utilization in the United States?

Source: Data from *Facts in Brief Contraceptive Use,* 1993, the Alan Guttmacher Institute, New York, NY.

control during the time a mature egg could be fertilized. Some couples rely on **coitus interruptus** (withdrawal) during this time; however, failure rates for withdrawal are high. Because of this, we do not consider withdrawal to be a viable birth-control method, and do not recommend reliance on it to prevent pregnancy.

Mechanical

Mechanical birth-control methods prevent fertilization or end **implantation.** Some mechanical devices prevent fertilization by mechanically blocking sperm from entering the uterus during intercourse. Examples of such devices include the condom, diaphragm, and cervical cap. Other mechanical devices, such as the intrauterine device (IUD), end implantation.

Chemical

Chemical birth-control methods employ chemicals that either prevent fertilization or end implantation. Examples of chemical methods include spermicides, which kill sperm, and hormones, such as birth-control pills, which attempt to prevent ovulation or end implantation.

1. **Reduce pregnancies among girls aged 17 and younger to no more than 50 per 1,000 adolescents.** (Update: 3.3 per 1,000 females 10–14 years, and 74.3 per 1,000 females 15–17 years in 1990 down from 3.6 per 1,000 for females 10–14 years and up from 70.9 per 1,000 females in 1985.) (Special Target Populations: Black adolescent girls aged 15–19; Hispanic adolescent girls aged 15–19.)

2. **Reduce to no more than 30 percent the proportion of all pregnancies that are unintended.** (Baseline: 56 percent in 1988.) (Special Target Population: Black females.)

3. **Reduce the proportion of adolescents who have engaged in sexual intercourse to no more than 15 percent by age 15 and no more than 40 percent by age 17.** (Update: adolescents 15 years, 36 percent of females and 44 percent of males in 1991 up from 27 percent and 33 percent respectively in 1988; adolescents 17 years, 66 percent of females and 68 percent of males in 1991 up from 50 percent and 66 percent respectively in 1988.)

4. **Increase to at least 40 percent the proportion of ever sexually active adolescents aged 17 and younger who have abstained from sexual activity for the previous 3 months.** (Update: 25 percent of ever sexually active females 15–17 years, and 36 percent of ever sexually active males 15–17 years in 1991 up from 28.6 percent and 33 percent respectively in 1988.)

5. **Increase to at least 90 percent the proportion of sexually active, unmarried people aged 19 and younger who use contraception, especially combined method contraception that both effectively prevents pregnancy and provides barrier protection against disease.** (Update: 81 percent of females 15–19 years for recent intercourse in 1991 up from 78 percent in 1988; 83 percent of high school males for recent intercourse in 1991 up from 78 percent in 1990; 14 percent of males 17–19 years report condom and oral contraceptive use at last intercourse, 1990–91 down from 15 percent in 1988.)

6. **Increase the effectiveness with which family-planning methods are used, as measured by a decrease to no more than 5 percent in the proportion of couples experiencing pregnancy despite use of a contraceptive method.** (Baseline: 14 percent failure of contraceptive method in 1990–91 down from 15 percent in 1988.)

7. **Increase to at least 90 percent the proportion of pregnancy counselors who offer positive, accurate information about adoption to their unmarried patients with unintended pregnancies.** (Pregnancy counselors are any providers of health or social services who discuss the management or outcome of pregnancy with a woman after she has received a diagnosis of pregnancy.) (Baseline: 60 percent in 1984.)

From *Healthy People 2000 National Health Promotion and Disease Prevention Objectives.* Department of Health and Human Services, 1991; *Healthy People 2000 Review 1993,* Department of Health and Human Services, 1994, Washington, D.C.

Invasive

Invasive birth-control methods involve a physician entering the body in order to surgically alter the internal reproductive organs or to end a pregnancy. Examples of these methods include sterilization and abortion.

These four basic categories of birth control each consist of a variety of techniques. An individual or couple may use more than one method from different categories. For example, a woman may utilize a diaphragm and a spermicide simultaneously. A couple may practice rhythm and use a

condom. A spermicidal condom can also be a dual method selected by a couple.

Factors Influencing Birth-Control Choices

The decision about which birth-control method, if any, to use is complicated. In addition to understanding how each method prevents pregnancy, it is important to consider additional factors such as the effectiveness, safety, cost, and reversibility of each method. These factors should be judged in light of personal circumstances as well as

Am I Going to Like This Method of Birth Control?

It is important to choose a method of birth control that works well to prevent pregnancy. It is also important to choose a method you will like! Ask yourself these questions so you can judge carefully.

What type of birth control are you thinking about? _____

Have you ever used it before?

_____ yes _____ no If yes, how long did you use it? _____

_____

Circle Your Answer

Are you afraid of using this method?

yes   no   don't know

Would you rather not use this method?

yes   no   don't know

Will you have trouble remembering to use this method?

yes   no   don't know

Have you ever become pregnant while using this method?

yes   no   don't know

Will you have trouble using this method carefully?

yes   no   don't know

Do you have unanswered questions about this method?

yes   no   don't know

Does this method make menstrual periods longer or more painful?

yes   no   don't know

Does this method cost more than you can afford?

yes   no   don't know

Does this method ever cause serious health problems?

yes   no   don't know

Do you object to this method because of religious beliefs?

yes   no   don't know

Have you already had problems using this method?

yes   no   don't know

Is your partner opposed to this method?

yes   no   don't know

Are you using this method without your partner's knowledge?

yes   no   don't know

Will using this method embarrass you?

yes   no   don't know

Will using this method embarrass your partner?

yes   no   don't know

Will you enjoy intercourse less because of this method?

yes   no   don't know

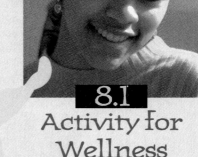

8.1
Activity for Wellness

Will this method interrupt lovemaking?

yes   no   don't know

Has a nurse or doctor ever told you not to use this method?

yes   no   don't know

- Do you have any "don't know" answers? Ask your instructor or physician to help you with more information.
- Do you have any "yes" answers? "Yes" answers mean you may not like this method. If you have several "yes" answers, chances go up that you might not like this method; you may need to think about another method.

From Robert A. Hatcher et al., *Contraceptive Technology,* 12th edition, 1984–1985. Copyright © 1984 Irvington Publishers. Reprinted by permission.

---

the social environment in which we interact (see Activity for Wellness 8.1).

Effectiveness

Effectiveness estimates calculate the chances of procreating if you use a particular method of birth control. Birth-control effectiveness measures can be divided into two categories, theoretical effectiveness and use effectiveness. **Theoretical effectiveness** is the maximum effectiveness of a method if there is no human error. For example, in theory some birth-control pills are 98 percent effective in preventing fertilization or ending implantation. This theoretical effectiveness assumes that the pills are of the right quality, the user follows directions, and the user has been prescribed the correct type and dose of hormone(s). In other words theoretical effectiveness rates reflect the method's effectiveness under ideal conditions.

Use effectiveness is derived from a sample of people who have used a particular birth-control method. Use effectiveness rates are often lower than theoretical effectiveness rates. Use effectiveness rates reflect the human error involved in using a particular birth-control method and are usually based on the experience of typical users during the first year of use.

Both theoretical and use effectiveness rates need to be considered when contemplating a particular birth-control method. The human error involved in a particular method may not always be within the control of the user. People may follow the

TABLE 8.3 — Contraceptive Failure Rates*

Method	Perfect Use	Average Use
No method (chance)	85.0	85.0
Spermicides	3.0	30.0
Sponge	8.0	24.0
Periodic abstinence	9.0	19.0
Cervical cap	6.0	18.0
Diaphragm	6.0	18.0
Condom	2.0	16.0
Pill	0.1	6.0
IUD	0.8	4.0
Tubal sterilization	0.2	0.5
Depo-Provera	0.3	0.4
Vasectomy	0.1	0.2
Norplant ®	0.04	0.05

What Do You Think?

1. If you were going to pick the most effective birth-control method based on perfect use, which method would you choose? Would your answer change if you used average use ratings?

2. Which methods have the greatest variation between perfect and average use? What factors might explain the differences?

3. What factors, other than effectiveness in preventing pregnancy, would you consider in selecting a birth-control method?

*Estimated percentage of women experiencing an unintended pregnancy in the first year of use. Perfect-use rates are given for the most commonly used type of contraceptive method (e.g., the calendar method of periodic abstinence, the copper IUD, and combined oral contraceptives).

Source: Data from *Facts in Brief, Contraceptive Use,* 1993. Alan Guttmacher Institute, New York, NY.

directions to the letter but may have purchased a faulty birth-control chemical or device, or one that is not compatible with their body chemistry or reproductive cycle. Generally, the correct use of a method and the motivation to use it conscientiously are the most important variables related to achieving a particular method's maximal effectiveness. Table 8.3 presents failure rates for common birth-control methods.

Safety

Assessing both the health risks and benefits of birth-control methods should be an important component of your birth-control decision-making process. Each birth-control method is accompanied by health risks ranging from minor nuisance side effects to more severe effects such as infection, hospitalization, or perhaps even death. Studies of various birth-control methods have identified select groups of people who may be at a higher risk of experiencing ill effects, or reduced effectiveness from a particular method.

Contraindications for a birth-control method indicate the conditions under which it should not be used. For example, women with a history of breast cancer or who are currently breast-feeding should not use **Norplant.**

Some birth-control methods also decrease the risk of certain health problems. It has long been recognized, for instance, that condoms reduce the risk of contracting several **sexually transmitted diseases** (STDs). It is important that you weigh the risks and benefits of each method, especially as they relate to your personal wellness and your susceptibility or exposure to certain health problems.

Cost

There are several costs to consider when selecting a birth-control method. The most obvious cost is monetary. Many of the most effective birth-control methods involve the purchase of materials, either over-the-counter (OTC) or by a physician's prescription. There may also be the expense of a physical

Norplant: a series of surgically implanted rods, placed just under the skin, that are designed to leak progesterone into the surrounding tissue to accomplish birth control.

Sexually transmitted diseases: any of a host of diseases that have the potential to be transmitted interpersonally through sexual or other intimate body contact.

examination. Monetary costs can be viewed as short term and long term. Some methods may cost more money in the short term due to the cost of seeing a physician and purchasing a major birth-control device. Norplant is a good example of a birth-control method with greater start-up costs. Current estimates indicate that it costs between $500 and $600 for a physical examination and the insertion of implants. There is an additional cost of $100–$200 for the removal of the implants when a woman no longer wants the Norplant in her arm. Other birth-control methods have their costs spread out over time, such as the regular purchase of **condoms** (at 25 cents or more a piece for male condoms and over $3 a piece for female condoms).

A second important cost to consider is that of inconvenience or dissatisfaction. If a birth-control method causes you or your partner great embarrassment, decreased pleasure, or increased health risks, this may be a high cost to your well-being.

Reversibility

Reversibility estimates refer to the ability of an individual to procreate after discontinuing the use of a particular birth-control method. Reversibility estimates are recorded in terms of percentages. A 100 percent reversibility estimate means that the individual's ability to procreate will be fully restored after discontinuing the use of a method. A 10 percent reversibility estimate indicates that only one out of ten individuals will be able to procreate after discontinuing the use of a method.

The reversibility of a birth-control method may encourage or discourage individuals from using that particular method. For example, a young married couple who presently do not want children but do want children in the future will reject birth-control methods that can or may reduce their future ability to have children. On the other hand, a married couple with two children may decide that a nonreversible birth-control method is acceptable.

There are circumstances in which an individual may regret selecting a method with little or no reversibility. For instance, a couple experiencing a tragedy in which their child dies in an accident, or a divorced person who remarries and then desires to procreate with his or her new

spouse, may regret their selection of a nonreversible birth-control method. Decisions regarding irreversible methods of birth control should therefore be made only after careful consideration of the alternatives. Indeed there is a growing number of people who regret their decision to be sterilized.[4] This is at a time when sterilization is the most popular birth-control method in the United States, and the developed world.[5]

In this chapter, we will review all of the birth-control methods currently available in the United States. As you learn about each method, evaluate them in terms of their effectiveness, safety, cost, and reversibility, as well as in terms of your own life circumstances and preferences.

Sexual Abstinence

Sexual abstinence, when used as a birth-control method, requires a premeditated decision not to have sexual intercourse for a specific period of time. For example, a couple may practice sexual abstinence until marriage or until they are engaged to be married. Sexual abstinence can be practiced by couples who have and have not been sexual partners. As a birth-control method, abstinence does not preclude sex play; however, it is possible, although rare, that sex play resulting in male ejaculation near the vagina can result in a pregnancy. Abstinence is a sophisticated birth-control method that requires self-confidence and emotional maturity.

Abstinence: Weighing the Benefits and Risks

As with any method of birth control, there are both benefits and risks associated with sexual abstinence that each couple must weigh. Some couples choose abstinence as a relief from other methods of birth control and their associated risks. Abstinence may also help highlight aspects of a couple's sex life other than intercourse. When strictly followed, sexual abstinence is an extremely effective method of birth control that also reduces the chances of contracting a sexually transmitted disease.

There are several potential disadvantages of abstinence as a birth-control method. Abstinence may stress a couple's relationship due to one or both partners' desire for sexual

Condoms: cylindrical sheaths made of rubber, animal skin, or polyurethane that are placed either over the male's penis (male condom) or in a woman's vagina (female condom) to prevent fertilization by trapping semen.

Sexual abstinence: a premeditated decision not to have sexual intercourse for a specific period of time.

TABLE 8.4 — How to Figure the "Safe" and "Unsafe" Days for the Calendar Method of Rhythm

If Your Shortest Cycle Has Been (# of Days)	Your First Unsafe Day Is	If Your Longest Cycle Has Been (# of Days)	Your Last Unsafe Day Is
21*	1st Day	21*	11th Day
22	2nd	22	12th
23	3rd	23	13th
24	4th	24	14th
25	5th	25	15th
26	6th	26	16th
27	7th	27	17th
28	8th	28	18th
29	9th	29	19th
30	10th	30	20th
31	11th	31	21st
32	12th	32	22nd
33	13th	33	23rd
34	14th	34	24th
35	15th	35	25th

*Day 1 = First day of menstrual bleeding.

From R. Hatcher, J. Trussell, G. Stewart, F. Stewart, D. Kowal, F. Guest. W. Cafes, and M. Policaret *Contraception Technology, 16th Revised Edition,* 1994. Contraceptive Technology New York: Irvington Publishing Co., Inc., 1994.

intercourse. Additionally, an impromptu decision to abandon abstinence without the replacement of another birth-control method leads to a high probability of pregnancy.

Periodic Abstinence

Periodic abstinence methods are designed to estimate when ovulation is occurring in the female. These birth-control methods prevent fertilization by requiring couples to refrain from intercourse or to practice another birth-control method for a specified time just before and after ovulation.

Calendar Method

The **calendar method,** sometimes called the rhythm method, is the simplest of the ovulation prediction methods. The calendar method requires the female to record her reproductive cycles using the first day of menstruation as day one and the day before her next menstruation as the last day. After accurately recording eight consecutive cycles, the shortest cycle and the longest cycle are used to determine the days in which the female is ovulating. Table 8.4 shows one way in which couples using the calendar

method can calculate the "unsafe" period during the female's reproductive cycle. For example, if the female's shortest cycle was twenty-six days and the longest cycle was thirty-three days, then the unsafe period is from day six to day twenty-three of her reproductive cycle.

There are several ways to calculate the unsafe period; this is just one example. Most formulas take into consideration: (1) that ovulation varies from cycle to cycle; (2) that viable sperm can be found in the reproductive tract seventy-two hours after being deposited; and (3) that the fertilized egg may be viable for as long as forty-eight hours.

Basal Body Temperature Method

Basal body temperature is defined as the lowest body temperature naturally reached by a healthy person. The **basal body temperature (BBT) method** calculates ovulation by plotting when the female's body temperature decreases slightly, followed by a sharp rise of 0.4 degrees F or more. The female is instructed to take her body temperature, orally or rectally, with a special thermometer for several cycles. A rise in temperature occurs between twenty-four and

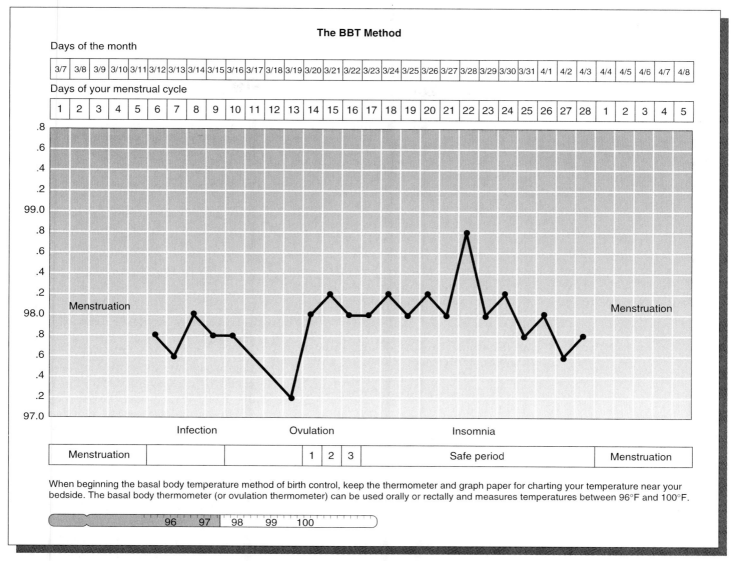

Figure 8.2: The BBT Method of Birth Control

- In the morning, just after waking and before any activity, take your temperature and record it as a dot on the chart like the one shown.
- Note on the chart any event other than ovulation that might make your temperature rise. Insomnia, infections, tension, even using an electric blanket may cause a daily rise in temperature.
- Note your menstruation period on the chart.

- Keep this chart for six months. Your safe days for intercourse will be from three days after the sudden drop in temperature until three or four days after your period is over. For some women, it is difficult to attend to the temperature-taking procedure first thing in the morning. It has been shown that if the temperature is taken regularly at 5:00 P.M., or at bedtime, these temperatures can be charted in the same way as the basal body temperature. Whenever you choose to measure your temperature, accuracy and consistency are of great importance.

seventy-two hours after ovulation (see figure 8.2). A woman using the BBT method should avoid sexual intercourse from day one of her cycle until her BBT has remained elevated for three consecutive days.[6]

Cervical Mucus Method

The **cervical mucus method** estimates ovulation by the change in consistency of the female's cervical mucus. During preovulation and postovulation times the mucus is thick and cloudy. During ovulation the cervical mucus is clear, slippery, and elastic. The mucus can be obtained by the female using one or two fingers to collect a sample from her **cervix.** The fourth full, consecutive day following peak slipperiness of the cervical mucus marks the end of the unsafe period.[7]

Cervix: the opening of the uterus which connects with the vagina.

Symptothermal Methods

The **Symptothermal method** combines the BBT and cervical mucus methods. This combination should logically yield improved use effectiveness rates.

Periodic Abstinence Methods: Weighing the Benefits and Risks

Periodic abstinence methods have several major benefits. First, there are limited major health risks for the user. Additionally, these methods do not rely on drugs or medical devices.

Men and women can easily share the responsibility for this method of birth control by jointly participating in the record keeping aspects of the method and by mutually avoiding intercourse during "unsafe" time periods. If another birth-control method is used during unsafe times, the couple can easily alternate between a male birth-control method such as the male condom, and a female method such as spermicides or a diaphragm.

Periodic abstinence methods require the user to obtain accurate measurements and to maintain diligent records for prolonged periods of time. Abstinence or additional birth-control measures must be instituted during unsafe times. Some females may have unsafe time periods for as long as twenty-one consecutive days, requiring prolonged abstinence. The BBT method estimates when ovulation has occurred, not when ovulation is about to occur. This contributes to potential failures of this method.

Periodic abstinence methods are contraindicated for women with a history of irregular reproductive cycles. Women with such a history have a reduced ability to predict ovulation accurately and should not rely on these methods as a form of birth control.

Diaphragm

The **diaphragm** consists of a shallow rubber dome two to four inches in diameter that is stretched over a flexible spring in its outer ring. The diaphragm is inserted over the cervix, preventing fertilization by trapping the sperm in the vaginal tract and not allowing it to enter the **uterus** and **fallopian tubes.** It is recommended that a spermicide always be used along with the diaphragm to increase effectiveness. A woman using a diaphragm, or her partner, puts a tablespoon of a spermicide on the inside of the diaphragm dome, as well as around the inside of the rim. The diaphragm is then inserted into the vagina with the inner side facing up (see figure 8.3). Diaphragms laced with a spermicide can be inserted up to thirty minutes prior to intercourse and must remain in place for six to eight hours after intercourse. If intercourse is repeated within that time, additional spermicide should be inserted into the vagina. Upon removal, the diaphragm should be washed with warm water and mild soap, rinsed, dried, and stored away from heat and light.

Women are fitted for diaphragms by a physician. The fitting is preceded by a consultation that includes a medical examination and directions on how to insert, remove, maintain, and use the diaphragm. The diaphragm should be checked for proper fit and quality by a physician once a year. If a woman has a weight gain or loss of ten pounds or more, an abortion, or a pregnancy, she should be reexamined before using her diaphragm. Women need to regularly check their diaphragm carefully inspecting for cracks and small holes. In addition, the diaphragm should be replaced every two to three years.

The Diaphragm: Weighing the Benefits and Risks

There are several important advantages associated with diaphragm use. The diaphragm does not pose serious health risks to the user; in fact, it may decrease the risk of cervical cancer.[8] The diaphragm does not alter a woman's hormonal functions, and is considered to be a safe and reliable birth-control method. When used with a spermicide, the diaphragm is almost as effective as the birth-control pill. Additionally, the diaphragm is 100 percent reversible.

One major drawback associated with diaphragm use is forgetfulness. Understandably, if the user forgets to insert the device it can not provide any protection against pregnancy. Some users have reported allergic reactions to the rubber in the diaphragm or to the spermicide. Diaphragm use may increase the incidence of urinary tract infections.[9] Finally, there is uncertainty

Uterus: a hollow, muscular, pear-shaped organ found in the internal female reproductive system.

Fallopian tubes: tubes found in the internal female reproductive tract that lie between the ovaries and the uterus. With rare exceptions, these tubes are the site of fertilization.

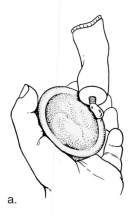

a.

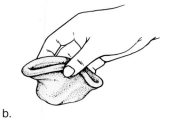

b.

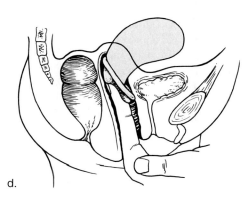

c.

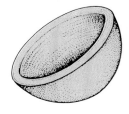

d.

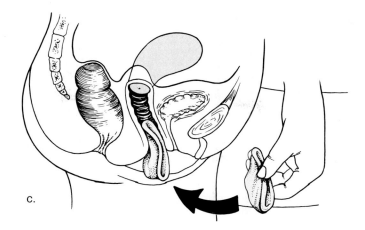

Figure 8.3: Insertion of the diaphragm:
(*a*) spermicide is applied around the rim and in the dome; (*b*) the diaphragm ready for insertion; (*c*) insertion before intercourse; (*d*) placement with dome covering cervix for correct positioning during and following intercourse.

From Kenneth L. Jones, *Dimensions of Human Sexuality*, Copyright © 1985 Wm. C. Brown Communications, Inc. Reprinted by permission of Times Mirror Higher Education Group, Inc., Dubuque, Iowa. All Rights Reserved.

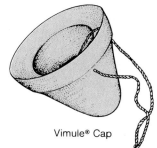

Dumas Cap   Vimule® Cap   Prentif® Cavity Rim Cervical Cap

Figure 8.4: Three types of cervical caps:
(*a*) Dumas Cap, (*b*) Vimule® Cap, (*c*) Prentif® Cavity Rim Cervical Cap.

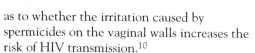

TABLE 8.5

Danger Signs of Toxic-Shock Syndrome

- Fever (temperature of 101 degrees Farenheit or more)
- Diarrhea
- Vomiting
- Muscle aches
- Rash (like sunburn)

vagina, a history of **toxic-shock syndrome** (see table 8.5), repeated urinary tract infections, or cervical, vaginal, or pelvic infections.[11]

Cervical Cap

The **cervical cap** is a thimble-sized and shaped device made of rubber or plastic (see figure 8.4). It is placed over the cervix and held in place by suction. Often used simultaneously with a spermicide, the cervical cap prevents fertilization by not

as to whether the irritation caused by spermicides on the vaginal walls increases the risk of HIV transmission.[10]

Some women should not use the diaphragm. The diaphragm is contraindicated for women with abnormalities of the uterus or

Toxic Shock Syndrome (TSS): a bacterial infection usually established in the vagina and associated with products and devices that block the vaginal tract. However, the causes of TSS are not entirely clear, and premenarchial girls and men have contracted the infection.

allowing sperm to enter the uterus. After a medical examination, which should include a **Pap test,** the female is fitted for a cervical cap.

The Cervical Cap: Weighing the Benefits and Risks

At the time of fitting, the female will be instructed on the insertion, removal, and care of the cap. The cap must remain inserted for six to eight hours after ejaculation. Although the cap has been left inserted by some women for weeks at a time, there is concern that prolonged insertion deteriorates its quality and leads to failure. For this reason, it is currently recommended that the cap be left in place for no longer than forty-eight hours.[12] Like the diaphragm, the cervical cap is most effective when used in combination with a spermicide. The spermicide should be placed inside the dome of the cervix before it is inserted by a woman or her partner.

As with many other mechanical methods of birth control the cervical cap usually presents no serious health risk to the user. The cervical cap does not need to be removed after each episode of intercourse, thus spontaneity is not compromised. Additionally, this method is 100 percent reversible.

There has been concern as to whether the cervical cap reduces the risk of cervical cancer as well as the diaphragm. Most cervical cap users do not use spermicides. Since the diaphragm is often used along with a spermicide, and spermicides may play a role in reducing cervical cancer, that fact may account for the difference. Other reasons for the difference may be that cervical caps are retained in the vagina for a longer duration, or the fact that cervical caps do not shield the same amount of the cervix and surrounding tissue as the diaphragm, or a combination of these factors.

Some women may have problems using the cervical cap. The skill required to insert the cap is greater than that involved in inserting the diaphragm, and some women may not be able to correctly insert it. Allergic reactions to the rubber

or plastic that is used to make the cervical cap may occur. It is possible for the cervical cap to become dislodged during sexual intercourse. After prolonged use irritation of the cervix is possible as well as a vaginal odor. Women using the cervical cap should have a Pap test three months after beginning its use to check for any cervical abnormalities. Additionally, because the cervical cap may remain in place for as long as forty-eight hours, it is advisable for the female to be alert for early signs of **pelvic inflammatory disease (PID)** (see table 8.6) and toxic-shock syndrome (TSS). The cervical cap is contraindicated for women experiencing the following conditions: cervical, vaginal, or pelvic infections; allergies to rubber or spermicide; abnormal Pap smears; abnormalities of the uterus or vagina; history of toxic-shock syndrome; or a full-term delivery within the past six weeks.[13]

Vaginal Contraceptive Sponge

Until recently, the vaginal sponge, a soft, polyurethane pad containing a spermicide, was available as an over-the-counter birth control method for women in the U.S. (see figure 8.5). In 1995, however, Whitehall-Robins Healthcare, the manufacturer of the vaginal sponge, discontinued production of this contraceptive device due to problems in the manufacturing processs. The company specifically cited an inability to meet FDA standards for preventing bacterial contamination of the vaginal sponge during production.

There are several potential disadvantages to the use of the contraceptive sponge, the most common of which are the possibility of a vaginal discharge or vaginal odor and itching. The contraceptive sponge may discourage **cunnilingus,** which some partners may view as a disadvantage. The sponge can be torn or shredded by unsuccessful attempts to remove it from the vagina. There have been a few cases of TSS among women using the contraceptive sponge. These cases, however, are rare. Risk

Pap test: a microscopic examination of cells taken from the cervix used as an early detection procedure for cancer of that site.

Pelvic Inflammatory Disease (PID): a general infection of the female reproductive tract, usually as a complication of an undiagnosed or untreated sexually transmitted disease, and having the potential to cause sterility.

Cunnilingus: the oral stimulation of the female's genitals.

TABLE 8.6

Signs and Symptoms of Pelvic Inflammatory Disease (PID)

Abdominal pain	Fever
Back pain	Chills
Leg pain	Vomiting
Pelvic pain	

Persons at Risk of Pelvic Inflammatory Disease

Multiple sexual partners
History of PID
Recent insertion of IUD

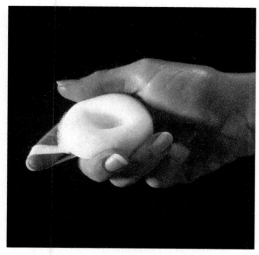

Figure 8.5: The vaginal sponge. What Do You Think?

1. The contraceptive sponge which is no longer available in the U.S., was one of the most popular over-the-counter contraceptives. How important do you think the loss of this over-the-counter birth control option is to the U.S. consumer?

2. What beliefs lead you to this conclusion?

of TSS can be decreased by leaving the sponge in place no longer than twenty-four hours, avoiding its use up to eight weeks after childbirth or an abortion, avoiding its use during menstruation, and avoiding its use if the female has a history of TSS.[14] Finally, the effectiveness of the contraceptive sponge is not as good as the diaphragm or other available methods of birth control. It is estimated that the contraceptive sponge has a use effectiveness of 72–82 percent.[15] Contraindications for use of the vaginal sponge include: allergic reaction to the spermicide or sponge, history of TSS, or abnormalities of the vagina.[16]

Male Condoms

The male condom is a cylindrical sheath made of rubber or animal skin that provides a barrier to the passage of sperm, as well as **pathogens,** to a partner. A male condom is used by unrolling the condom over the erect penis. A condom can be applied by the male user, or by his partner. The condom prevents fertilization by trapping semen in its tip or built-in reservoir. In order to prevent tearing of the condom and leakage of sperm, a one-half inch space (void of air) must be left at the tip of condoms without built-in reservoirs (see figure 8.6). **Spermicidal condoms** are standard condoms laced, both on the inside and the outside, with a spermicide.

Condoms are marketed in various shapes and colors and with or without lubrication. All condoms must be lubricated before use. Unlubricated condoms can be lubricated with K-Y jelly or another water-based lubricant before being inserted into the vaginal tract. Vaseline, and other oil-based lubricants, should not be used for lubrication as it weakens the rubber and may cause it to deteriorate.

One condom is used for each ejaculation and must be removed prior to loss of erection to prevent semen from leaking into the vagina. The condom should be held at the base of the penis as the penis is withdrawn from the vaginal tract.

Pathogens: organisms that can produce disease in a host.

Figure 8.6: What Do You Think?

1. Condoms provide protection against pregnancy and several sexually transmitted diseases. Do you think college students who select condoms as their birth-control method do so with disease prevention in mind? What is your source of evidence?

2. Condom vending machines are now available on many college campuses in student dormitories. Do you think that this is appropriate? Explain your rationale.

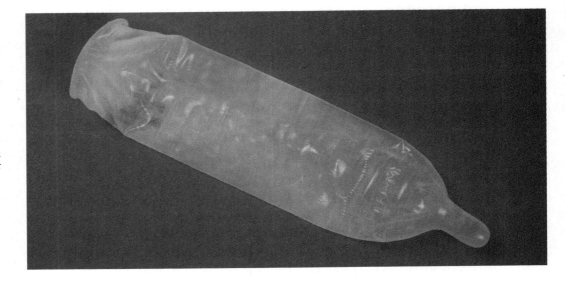

Amniotic fluid: fluid found in the amniotic sac surrounding a developing embryo/fetus, that acts as a barrier to physical shock and helps maintain proper temperature.

Miscarriage: a naturally occurring termination of pregnancy before the fetus is capable of extrauterine life.

Labia: two paired folds of skin that surround the female's vaginal and urethral openings and extend to the clitoris.

Male Condoms: Weighing the Benefits and Risks

Male condom use presents no serious health risk, and it is believed to decrease the risk of (both partners) contracting STDs, including HIV.[17] With a decreased risk of females contracting STDs there is a concurrent decrease in the chances of developing cervical cancer.[18]

Condoms used during pregnancy may decrease the chances of **amniotic fluid** infections and intrauterine infections that can lead to a **miscarriage.**[19] Additionally, the condom is currently the only available male birth-control method that is very effective and 100 percent reversible.

Some men believe that the condom reduces penis sensitivity. This may be viewed negatively by both males and females. Other couples may view the placement of the condom as an interruption of foreplay. This disadvantage can be overcome, as illustrated by couples who have incorporated the placement of the condom as part of their sex play. There is a possibility that either the male or female partner may be allergic to the rubber condom. Switching to a natural condom may alleviate this problem, however, natural condoms do not offer the same protection against STDs as the latex rubber condom. A new polyurethane male condom, that was approved for marketing by the FDA in 1993, may be a solution for individuals who are allergic to rubber condoms. Condoms sometimes slip off or tear, reducing the effectiveness of this method. Additionally,

condoms are especially sensitive to heat, and may become damaged if left in hot environments such as automobile glove compartments or hip wallets.

Female Condoms

One of the newest birth-control methods available is the vaginal pouch, more commonly known as the **female condom.** Approved by the FDA in 1993, the female condom was first made available to family planning clinics. It is now available to all women as an over-the-counter birth-control device, at a cost of about $3.00 each. The female condom is a disposable lubricated polyurethane cylindrical tube with flexible rings at each end (see figure 8.7). To insert the condom, the ring at the closed end is compressed and inserted into the vagina in a manner similar to a diaphragm (see figure 8.8). The ring helps anchor the condom around the cervix while the rest of the condom lines the vagina. The ring at the open end of the condom remains outside the body, surrounding the **labia.**

Female Condoms: Weighing the Benefits and Risks

One of the most important benefits of the female condom is that it is the only female birth-control method currently available that offers women good protection against sexually transmitted diseases, as well as preventing pregnancy. With the great increase in sexually transmitted HIV infections in

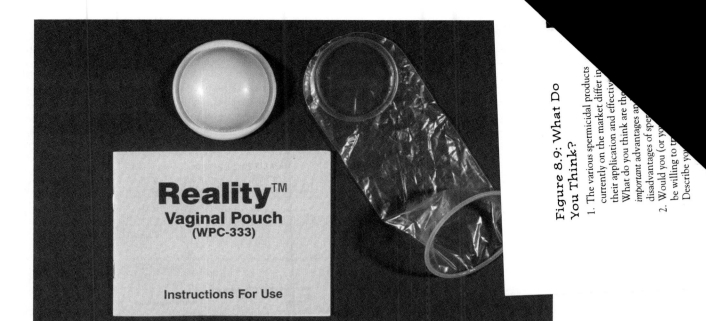

Figure 8.9: What Do You Think?

1. The various spermicidal products currently on the market differ in their application and effectiveness. What do you think are the important advantages and disadvantages of spe...

2. Would you (or you... be willing to t... Describe yo...

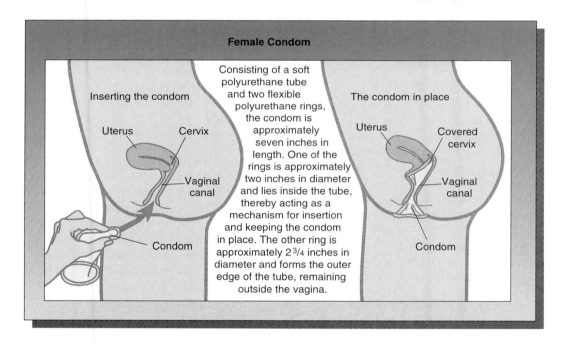

Figure 8.8: Female condom insertion

Female Condom

Inserting the condom

Uterus

Cervix

Vaginal canal

Condom

Consisting of a soft polyurethane tube and two flexible polyurethane rings, the condom is approximately seven inches in length. One of the rings is approximately two inches in diameter and lies inside the tube, thereby acting as a mechanism for insertion and keeping the condom in place. The other ring is approximately 2 3/4 inches in diameter and forms the outer edge of the tube, remaining outside the vagina.

The condom in place

Uterus

Covered cervix

Vaginal canal

Condom

women, the female condom is an important breakthrough. The female condom may be especially useful to women who cannot convince a male partner to use a male condom.

The female condom increases a woman's nonprescription birth-control choices and can be readily available when sexual intercourse is desired, as the condom can be applied immediately before intercourse. Current use effectiveness ratings estimate that the female condom is 88 percent effective in preventing

pregnancy under normal use, and can be increased to as much as 97 percent when the female condom is used correctly.[20]

The potential disadvantages of the female condom are similar to those of the male condom. Some individuals may believe that using a female condom will interrupt spontaneity. However, as with male condoms, the placement of the female condom can be a shared activity that becomes part of foreplay. In rare instances, irritation and allergic reactions have been noted.

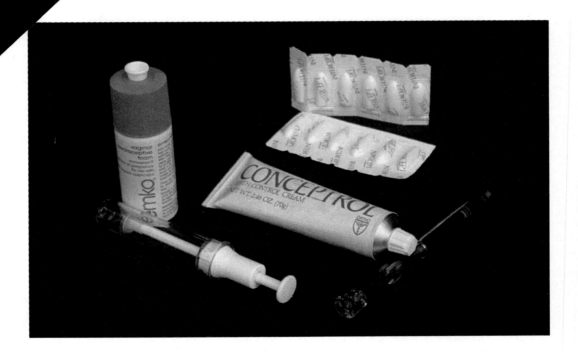

Spermicides (Foams, Creams, Jellies, Suppositories)

Spermicides are chemicals placed at the opening of the uterus prior to intercourse. They prevent fertilization by destroying sperm or blocking sperm from passing through the uterus. There are a variety of spermicidal products on the market, which differ in their application and effectiveness (see figure 8.9). Spermicides are available as foams, creams, jellies, and **suppositories.** Foam spermicides are the most effective and easy to use. For maximum effectiveness spermicides should be inserted no earlier than thirty minutes prior to intercourse. One chemical application is required for each ejaculation. The product should not be removed from the vaginal tract for six to eight hours following intercourse.

Spermicides: Weighing the Benefits and Risks

Spermicides are believed to pose no serious health risks for the user, and may provide some protection against other STDs and PID. Foams may also improve vaginal lubrication during intercourse. Additionally, spermicides can be purchased at virtually any drug store as a fairly inexpensive over-the-counter product. Spermicides are also 100 percent reversible.

There are a few potential disadvantages associated with the use of spermicides. Spermicidal tablets and suppositories require a minimum waiting period of ten to fifteen minutes after insertion to give them time to dissolve and offer birth-control protection. Individuals may not feel comfortable performing cunnilingus when spermicides are used, and some couples may view this as a disadvantage. Additionally, the use of spermicidal products usually results in a vaginal discharge after intercourse. After prolonged use of a spermicide, females may experience vaginal infections or irritation. Spermicides are contraindicated for men or women who experience an allergic reaction to the chemicals.[21]

Intrauterine Device (IUD)

The **IUD** is a plastic device approximately one, to one and one-half, inches long that is inserted into the uterus through the vaginal tract by a physician. There are two types of IUDs, nonmedicated and medicated (see figure 8.10). The nonmedicated IUD is made of plastic and works mechanically to prevent implantation. Medicated IUDs (e.g., Copper T, Progestasert T) leak chemicals, such as copper or hormones, to prevent implantation.

IUDs are not designed to prevent ovulation. Although it is not known exactly

Suppositories: a drug in solid form that is intended to be inserted into the vagina or rectum.

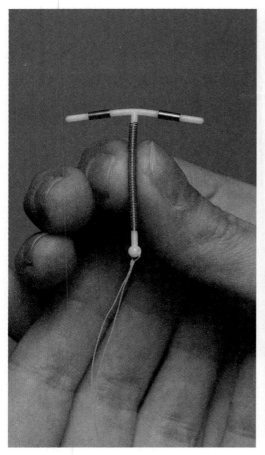

a.

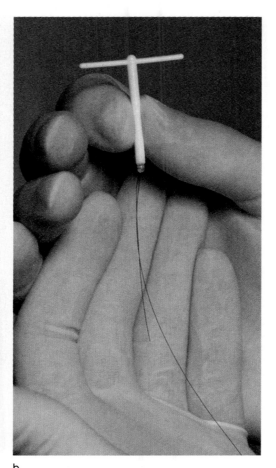

b.

Figure 8.10: What Do You Think?

1. There are currently two types of IUDs available in the U.S.: (a) the Copper T 380A, and (b) the Progestasert T. It is estimated that only two percent of women in the U.S. using a birth-control method select an IUD. What factors do you think account for this low level of use?
2. Would you (or your sexual partner) be willing to try an IUD? Describe your thinking.

how IUDs work, it is believed that they prevent or terminate the implantation of a fertilized egg in the lining of the uterus.

Currently the Progestasert T and the Copper T 380A (Paragard) are readily available in the U.S. through physicians. Both are medicated IUDs with the Copper T 380A designed to leak copper into the uterus for up to eight years, and the Progestasert T designed to leak a **progesterone** into the uterus for up to a year.

If a female and her physician decide the IUD is indicated, a series of preliminary exams are required before its insertion. These exams include a medical history and tests for sexually transmitted diseases and pregnancy. After the IUD is inserted the physician will teach the female how to check for the string (tail) that is attached to the IUD. Periodic checking is required to assure that the IUD has not been expelled.

Women with an IUD should have a medical examination three months after insertion and yearly pelvic examinations thereafter. Medicated IUDs need to be replaced at regular intervals. IUD users should immediately consult a physician if they suspect they are pregnant, have contracted a sexually transmitted disease, have developed a pelvic inflammatory disease, or experience unusual vaginal bleeding, abdominal discomfort, or pain.

IUDs: Weighing the Benefits and Risks

When deciding to use any form of birth control it is important to investigate both the method's advantages and disadvantages. This is especially important with the IUD. The major advantage of the IUD revolves around the fact that it is a highly effective birth-control method that requires no pre-intercourse planning.

There are many potential disadvantages to the use of an IUD. As many as 20 percent of IUD users will expel the IUD in the first year of use. The IUD can be expelled without the female's knowledge. Some IUD users

Progesterone: a steroid hormone responsible for the preparation of the inner lining of the uterus for possible pregnancy. If pregnancy occurs, it maintains the uterus and prevents ovulation.

1. There are a wide variety of birth-
control pills available on the market
today, and "the pill" is the second
most widely used method of birth
control in the U.S. What factors do
you think account for this high level
of use?
2. What do you think are the *most
important* advantages and
disadvantages of birth-control pills?

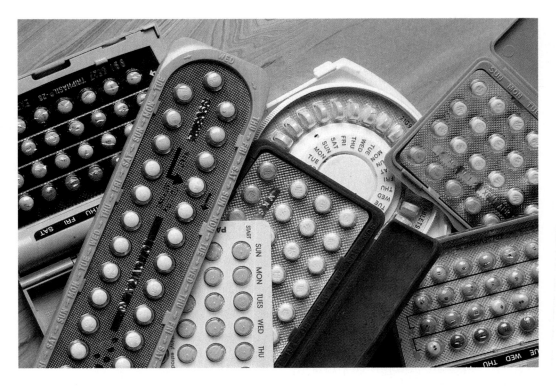

experience symptoms such as **anemia,**
cramping, spotting, and backaches. For the
first three cycles immediately following
insertion, the IUD user is required to use a
backup birth-control method. Additionally,
there is substantial evidence, although not
without its critics, that IUDs increase the risk
of Pelvic Inflammatory Disease (PID).[22] The
string of the IUD may act as a passageway for
bacteria to enter and infect the reproductive
tract. Studies have indicated that PID occurs
50 percent more often in women using IUDs
than in females using no birth-control
method. Just one or two episodes of PID can
cause **sterility** in a woman.

In 1 percent of all IUD insertions the
uterus is perforated. In rare cases the IUD can
pass through a tear in the uterus and fall into
the abdominal cavity, requiring surgical
removal. IUDs can also cause cervical
perforations. There is a 1 to 2 percent chance
that pregnancy will occur while the IUD is in
place and this can lead to medical
complications such as miscarriage, PID, and
maternal death. Furthermore there is an
increased risk of tubal pregnancy. One in
thirty IUD-user pregnancies is **ectopic** (the
fertilized egg implants outside the uterus).
Users with IUDs that release hormones have
an even greater risk of ectopic pregnancies
than regular IUD users.[23]

The IUD is contraindicated for the
following conditions: pregnancy, PID (recent
or chronic), women concerned for their
future fertility, severe **dysmenorrhea,**
abnormal Pap smears, abnormal uterine
bleeding, use of **anticoagulant drugs,** a
history of ectopic pregnancies, or multiple
sexual partners.[24]

Oral Contraceptives

There are three classifications of oral birth-
controlling hormones; **monophasic,
multiphasic,** and **minipills.** Monophasic
preparations release the same dose of an
estrogen and progestin each day. Multiphasic
preparations release varying doses of an
estrogen and/or progestin each day. Minipills
release low doses of only a progestin. There
are over fifty brand name oral birth-
controlling hormones using thirty-three
different formulations available in the U.S.
today. The prescribing trend has been
towards low-dose estrogen multiphasic
preparations.[25] Low-dose estrogen pills and
minipills either prevent fertilization or allow
fertilization but inhibit implantation
(see figure 8.11).

Women who take oral birth-control pills
usually take a monthly series of pills, one pill a
day for twenty-one days or twenty-eight days,

Anemia: a decreased ability of the
blood to carry oxygen, due to a decrease
in the amount of hemoglobin in the
blood.

Sterility: the inability to have children.

Dysmenorrhea: painful menstruation.

Anticoagulant drugs: drugs that
impede blood clot formation.

depending on the brand prescribed. Birth-control pills are most effective when taken at about the same time each day. In the case of minipills it is essential that the women ingest the pill at the same time each day. It is common for women on the birth-control pill to miss a period occasionally. If no pills have been forgotten during that month, the likelihood of pregnancy is small. If, however, a woman has forgotten to take one or more pills and misses a period, she should contact her physician and use another form of birth control until a pregnancy test can be completed.

Birth-Control Pills: Weighing the Benefits and Risks

There are several advantages associated with the use of birth-control pills. This method of birth control is one of the most effective and does not require interruption of the sexual act. The use of birth-control pills also regularizes the menstrual cycle and may eliminate **mittelschmerz** (the pain experienced during ovulation) as well as reducing menstrual duration, flow, and cramps.[26] Studies have also suggested that birth-control pills may provide protection against specific types of cancer, such as endometrial and ovarian cancer.[27] Generally, the effects of birth-control pills are reversible, with 90 percent of women beginning regular ovulation three months after discontinuing birth-control pill use.

There are some disadvantages to the use of birth-control pills. This method of birth control can produce pseudo-pregnancy signs and symptoms such as nausea, water retention, breast enlargement, breast tenderness, spotting between menstrual periods, and increased vaginal discharge. Many of these side effects are temporary and may subside by having a physician switch the brand of birth-control pills taken.

Birth-control pills have some serious risks, such as an increased risk of heart attack, stroke, blood clots, gallbladder disease, and liver tumors. In non-African American females there is an increased risk of **hypertension.** Birth-control pills have also been associated with an increase in female yeast infections, although this can be controlled by reducing the amount of estrogen. There is also a reported increased risk of chlamydial inflammation of the cervix.[28] Females who use progestin-only pills increase their risk of ectopic pregnancy.[29] Use of progestins may also cause hair loss, **jaundice,** rash, darkened skin, and depression. Additionally, it may increase the growth of existing cancers. A **false negative** reading for the **tuberculin skin test** is more likely to occur in women who use the birth-control pill. Also, the results of other medical laboratory tests, such as thyroid, vitamin, and sodium tests, can be altered for women taking birth-control pills. Because birth-control pills affect body metabolism, the use and excretion of vitamins and minerals can be altered, especially for vitamins A, B_2, B_6, B_{12}, C, folic acid, and the minerals iron and copper. Birth-control pills may cause contact lenses to fit snugly. Contact lenses should be removed immediately at the first sign of vision problems, such as blurred vision.

Birth-control pills have been demonstrated to be less effective when a woman takes certain drugs that may interfere with the absorption of the birth-controlling hormones (see table 8.7). When such drugs must be taken for a short duration, it is recommended that additional backup birth-control methods be used. If such drugs are needed for a long-term treatment program another nonhormonal method of birth control should be selected.

There are a number of conditions that, if present, should stop women from taking birth-control pills. These contraindications include: (1) a history of heart attacks, strokes, **angina,** blood clots, breast or uterine cancer, undiagnosed genital bleeding, **sickle-cell disorders,** or liver tumors; (2) a current pregnancy or while nursing an infant; or (3) being thirty-five years or older *and* smoking cigarettes.[30]

Most health professionals believe that it is safe for young, healthy women who do not have the contraindications just mentioned, to use birth-control pills. Most healthy, young birth-control pill users do not experience serious side effects. However, if you are using the birth-control pill it is wise to watch for certain danger signs, including severe abdominal or chest pain, shortness of breath, dizziness or weakness, severe headache, loss of or blurred vision, speech problems, numbness, or severe calf or thigh pain.[31] If you experience any of these symptoms, call your physician immediately.

Hypertension: abnormally high arterial blood pressure of a chronic nature.

Jaundice: a yellowing of the skin due to the presence of too much bile pigment in the blood.

False negative: an erroneous test outcome that implies a person does not have a disorder when in fact he or she may.

Tuberculin skin test: a test that determines whether a person has been in contact with the bacteria that causes tuberculosis.

Angina: severe chest pain resulting from restricted blood flow through the coronary arteries.

Sickle-cell disorders: a hereditary disorder that affects primarily people of African descent. Defective hemoglobin causes the red blood cells to become sickle shaped resulting in anemia, and often severe complications such as kidney or heart failure.

TABLE 8.7 — Medications That Affect Birth-Control Pill Effectiveness

Anticonvulsants	Antibiotics
(Decreased oral contraceptive activity) Phenobarbital Phenytoin Primidone	*(Decreased oral contraceptive activity)* Ampicillin Tetracycline Nitrofurantoin Penicillin

Antituberculous agents

(Decreased oral contraceptive activity)
Rifampin

What Do You Think?

1. How important is it for you to inform the physician treating you for a non-reproductive disease or disorder that you are currently using birth-controlling hormones?

2. How could you find out about additional OTC and prescription medications that may interfere with the action of birth-controlling hormones?

Source: Data from Donald L. Goode and Cynthia Ramadei, "Oral Contraceptive Agents, Part 2: Risks and Benefits" in *Family Practice Recertification,* 8:13, 1986.

Figure 8:12: What Do You Think?

1. Norplant capsules are 34 mm long and 2.4 mm wide. To insert these capsules, a health-care provider places a template against a woman's arm and marks the ends of the six slots on her skin with a ball-point pen or similar marker. When inserting the capsules, the provider lines up each capsule with one of the marks. Capsules should be inserted just under the skin. Do you think that Norplant will become a popular method of birth control? Explain your thinking.

2. Would you (or your sexual partner) be willing to try Norplant? What factors would influence such a decision?

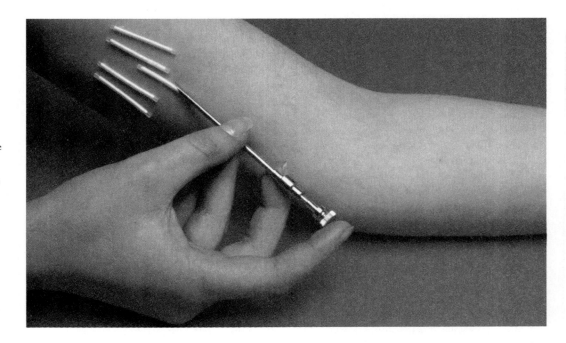

Norplant

Norplant, first approved for use in the United States in 1991, is a long-acting implant comprised of six small, soft rods that are surgically placed or injected under the skin (see figure 8.12). In the U.S., the implant site is usually the arm. However, international experience with the implantation site suggests that behind the knee may be more suitable for cosmetic reasons. The Norplant rods continuously release a low amount of a synthetic progestin called levonorgestrel, for as long as five years. Norplant is believed to work by keeping a woman's body from producing the hormones that are required for ovulation.

Norplant: Weighing the Benefits and Risks

Norplant has several important advantages. First, it is one of the most effective birth-control methods currently available to women in the U.S.; only 1 percent of five-year Norplant users become pregnant.[32] Because the implant releases progestin at a constant rate, less of the hormone is required to be effective. This also minimizes health risks for the user.[33] Once the implants are surgically placed, they can remain in place and effectively prevent pregnancy for up to five years. Other than routine checkups, a woman using Norplant does not have to remember to do anything for this method to be effective. Additionally, Norplant is reversible, with fertility promptly returned once the implants are removed.[34] A recent study[35] evaluated 115 women's satisfaction with Norplant, as compared with 148 women using birth-control pills, and found that 60 percent of the respondents who were using Norplant were satisfied with this method.

There are some important disadvantages to the use of Norplant. One of the most prominent problems reported in the news media is the concerns generated over the removal of Norplant implants. Because fibrous tissue will grow around the rods, it is expected that surgical removal of the rods will take at least fifteen minutes. In rare cases it may take as long as an hour and require significant amounts of local anesthetic. Some women have reported severe pain and scarring from the removal of Norplant. In 1994, 400 women initiated a class action suit against the pharmaceutical company that makes Norplant because of pain and suffering resulting from the removal process.[36] These women are seeking financial compensation for damages they sustained, as well as an injunction against the pharmaceutical company preventing them from selling Norplant to any physicians who have not received training on both the insertion and removal of the implants. Currently, there is no requirement that physicians be trained before inserting or removing Norplant, although 28,000 physicians have voluntarily been trained by the pharmaceutical company.

Women who weigh over 155 pounds have a higher probability of becoming pregnant in their second year of use of Norplant, as compared with lighter women.[37] In addition, they have a higher likelihood of having an ectopic pregnancy, in part because of the dose-to-body weight ratio, and also because Norplant is associated with producing enlarged **ovarian follicles.**

The proportion of women who decide to discontinue the use of Norplant ranges from 76–90 percent in the first year of use, and 33–78 percent by the fifth year of use. Because of the relatively high discontinuation rate, it is prudent for a female using birth-controlling hormones for the first time to use an oral progestin-only product (preferably levonorgestrel) to judge whether the effects are compatible with her body and lifestyle. Using Norplant to discover whether progestin-only hormones are acceptable to the user is a very costly procedure.

Norplant's most common side effect, experienced by half to nearly all users, is menstrual changes. Nearly 45 percent of Norplant users experience an abnormal bleeding pattern. Other popular reasons for women terminating the use of Norplant include pregnancy, frequent irregular bleeding, spotting, **amenorrhea,** dysmenorrhea, pelvic pain, headache, dizziness, nausea, depression, loss of appetite, hair loss, increase in facial or body hair, weight gain, pain at the implant site, infection at the implant site, acne, and other skin problems.[38]

Some women should not use Norplant. The contraindications are similar to those for the birth-control pill, and include a history of liver disease or tumors, unexplained vaginal bleeding, currently breast-feeding, or a history of breast cancer or blood clots.[39]

Depo-Provera

Depo-Provera is an injectable birth-control method that became available in the U.S. in 1992. Originally developed in 1969, FDA approval of Depo-Provera was delayed because of studies showing a relationship between Depo-Provera exposure and breast cancer in animals. The World Health Organization (WHO) has studied the use of Depo-Provera in over 11,000 women, mostly from New Zealand and Thailand.[40] Their results, published in the British Medical Journal *Lancet* in 1991, concluded that using Depo-Provera did not increase a woman's risk for breast cancer. This study was an important piece of evidence leading to FDA approval for Depo-Provera. However, not all consumer groups accept the conclusions of the FDA and WHO. The National Women's Health Network has pointed out that

Ovarian follicles: a cavity in the ovary where the ova or egg develops.

Amenorrhea: a lack of menstrual periods.

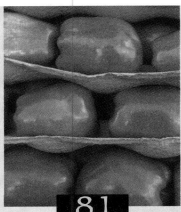

8.1
Of Special Interest

Contraceptives for Tomorrow—and the 21st Century

Barrier Methods

Lea's Shield: A one-size-fits-all diaphragm-type device that has been approved in Canada and several European countries. A large-scale U.S. clinical study was completed in 1993. But an official of Yama Inc., the Millburn, N.J., developer and manufacturer, says it can't predict when the product will be available because additional studies may be required by the FDA.

Femcap: A cervical caplike device that comes in three sizes. Approval expected by end of the decade.

Disposable Diaphragm: A diaphragm that would release the traditional spermicide nonoxynol-9. Not clear whether it would be available before the end of the century.

Polyurethane Male Condom: A new polyurethane condom, produced by London International Group, was cleared for marketing by the Food and Drug Administration (FDA) in 1993. It reportedly has improved feel and durability. Other types are being tested in volunteers.

Chemical Barriers

Researchers are looking at alternatives to current spermicides in an effort to find something that would be less irritating to vaginal tissue and would also protect against sexually transmitted diseases. Some versions are in early testing. These products could be as long as seven to ten years away from marketing.

Hormonal Methods

Rings: The most likely candidate in the hunt for new contraceptives in the next few years is a doughnut-shaped rubber ring inserted into the woman's vagina that releases low doses of synthetic hormones. The advantage is that a woman could insert or remove it whenever she wished but it could be effective for six months or longer. Expected by the year 2000.

Implants: An improved version of Norplant containing two rods instead of six—easing removal—could go on the U.S. market soon. A one-capsule implant that would last two years is currently being tested. Biodegradable implants, which would eliminate the need for removal, are at least three to five years away.

Skin Patches: This device would deliver hormones through the skin and could be easily removed and replaced by the user. The Population Council has tested it in women volunteers and is seeking a manufacturer.

Injectables: Studies are ongoing on injectables that would contain estrogen as well as progestin in order to minimize the abnormal bleeding patterns that often occur with Depo-Provera and Norplant. One product being introduced by the World Health Organization, known as Cyclofem, could be registered in the U.S. within the next two to three years.

Intrauterine Devices (IUDs): A frameless IUD that would eliminate pressure against the uterus, minimizing cramping, is undergoing clinical trials in Europe. An IUD that releases the hormone levonorgestrel and reduces excessive bleeding has been approved in Finland and Sweden.

Vaccines for Women: The most advanced testing is on vaccines that interrupt the action of a hormone necessary to maintain pregnancy—human chorionic gonadotrophin (HCG). However, because the vaccine acts after the egg is fertilized, companies may be unwilling to pursue them in the face of political anti-abortion opposition. Vaccines that prevent fertilization are too early in development to be available this century.

Male Hormonal Methods: A drug known as testosterone enanthate has been tested in men for several years and may reduce sperm counts low enough to protect against pregnancy. Major drawbacks are a weekly injection schedule and a long lag time before it becomes effective.

Vaccines for Men: A vaccine currently being tested in men would suppress a brain hormone—luteinizing hormone-releasing hormone—which indirectly controls production of sperm. The vaccine shuts down the testes to eliminate not only sperm production but testosterone as well. To avoid impotence and loss of libido, the user would need to supplement the vaccine with testosterone. In contrast, a vaccine using another hormone important to reproduction—follicle stimulating hormone—has eliminated sperm but maintained normal testosterone levels in monkeys. Male vaccines are not expected to be available this century.

From "Birth Control Choices" in *CQ Researcher,* 4:666, 1994. Congressional Quarterly, Washington, D.C. Reprinted by permission.

What Do You Think?

1. Do you think there is a need for new methods of birth control?
2. Would you (or your sexual partner) be interested in using any of the methods described here? Explain your rationale.
3. What are some of the safety, effectiveness, reversibility, and ethical problems with these new birth-control methods?

baseline breast cancer rates in New Zealand and Thailand are less than breast cancer rates in the U.S., and therefore cannot accurately represent the Depo-Provera related breast cancer risk of women in the U.S. This controversy is likely to continue until more prospective epidemiological evidence on large numbers of U.S. Depo-Provera users becomes available.

One injection of Depo-Provera, a synthetic progesterone, will prevent ovulation for twelve weeks. Additionally, Depo-Provera is believed to cause changes in the lining of the uterus that make pregnancy less likely.[41] It is recommended that a woman who wants to begin using Depo-Provera receive her first injection within five days following her menstrual period. Depo-Provera's birth-control effects are immediate, but the hormone loses its strength after twelve weeks, making the timing of future injections critical.

Depo-Provera: Weighing the Benefits and Risks

One of the most important benefits of Depo-Provera is its convenience. Following an injection, Depo-Provera is immediately effective and does not require a woman or her partner to take any other action to prevent pregnancy. It does, however, require that women faithfully keep appointments for injections every three months as long as they wish to continue using this method of birth control. Depo-Provera is also considered to be extremely effective in preventing pregnancy. Like Norplant, Depo-Provera has a 99 percent effectiveness rate. Depo-Provera is considered a reversible birth-control method; however, the median amount of time it takes to conceive following the last injection is ten months,[42] with a range between four and thirty-one months.

The use of Depo-Provera is not without side effects. The most common side effect is a disruption in a woman's normal menstrual cycle. When first using Depo-Provera, many women report irregular bleeding or spotting. These effects often disappear after a few injections. In approximately half of the women using Depo-Provera for a year, menstruation stops completely. For those women who continue to menstruate, the blood flow is often less and cramps are reduced. In fact, many women view this side effect as a benefit of Depo-Provera.

Other side effects of Depo-Provera use include weight gain, headaches, weakness, and fatigue, as well as dizziness, nervousness, and abdominal pain. **High density lipoproteins (HDL)** decrease significantly in Depo-Provera users.[43] Additionally, researchers have reported that bone density decreases in long-term users of Depo-Provera,[44] causing concern that this birth-control method may increase the risk of **osteoporosis.**

As with other methods of birth control that we have discussed in this chapter, not all women should use Depo-Provera. The contraindications are the same as those for Norplant: women with a history of liver disease or tumors, unexplained vaginal bleeding, a history of breast cancer or blood clots, or who are currently breast-feeding, should not select Depo-Provera as their birth-control method.[45] Additionally, if a woman intends to try to become pregnant within the next year or two she should select another temporary birth-control method.

Voluntary Sterilization

Sterilization is a surgical and permanent method of birth control. Voluntary sterilization is usually accomplished in men by closing off the tubes through which sperm passes (vas deferens) and in women by closing off the tubes through which the egg travels (fallopian tubes). The surgeon's skill is directly related to the success and medical complications associated with sterilization. You should select a physician that performs more than 100 procedures per year of the basic type of sterilization you will receive.[46] Voluntary sterilization is the most popular method of birth control in the U.S., and the developed world.[47] Presently, operations for reversing voluntary sterilization have low success rates. Therefore sterilization procedures should be considered as permanent. Studies have shown that the men and women most likely to regret their decision to use sterilization as a birth-control method are those who made their decision soon after a divorce, pregnancy, or abortion.

High density lipoproteins (HDL): a type of lipoprotein that carries cholesterol from the bloodstream to the liver, where it can be excreted from the body. High blood HDL levels may help protect individuals against coronary artery disease.

Osteoporosis: a condition affecting mostly the elderly, especially women, resulting from a decline in bone mineral content, making bones susceptible to fracture.

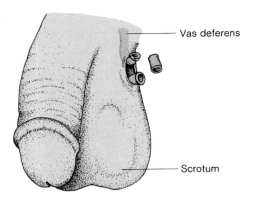

Vas deferens

Scrotum

Additionally, individuals who regretted a sterilization decision were more likely to have been sterilized at a relatively young age.[48]

Vasectomy

A **vasectomy** involves blocking the vas deferens, usually by cutting and tying (see figure 8.13). The first human vasectomy was performed in 1894 over 100 years ago.[49] A vasectomy prevents fertilization by blocking sperm from entering the upper portion of the vas deferens during ejaculation. The procedure takes about twenty minutes and is usually performed in a physician's office. Most males can return to normal sexual activity within a week. A backup birth-control method should be used for several months following the operation, because sperm may be present between the upper portion of the vas deferens and the urethra. A semen analysis will confirm if there are any sperm present in the male's **ejaculate.** If two consecutive semen analyses indicate sperm are not present then the male can engage in unprotected intercourse. Most vasectomized males cannot detect any change in the quantity or quality of their semen.

Vasectomy: Weighing the Benefits and Risks

There are two major advantages associated with vasectomy. It is a very effective long-term male birth-control method, and it seems to present no serious health risks to the male.

As with any method of birth control, there are potential risks. Following a vasectomy, most men will experience some postoperative discomfort for a day or two. Additionally, the male will be sexually incapacitated for approximately a week. Postoperative complications are rare (seen in

4–5 percent of cases) and most commonly include local swelling and inflammation.[50] Serious medical complications, such as infection of the **epididymis,** are very rare.[51] While vasectomies have a very high success rate, in one in 1000 vasectomies the vas deferens naturally repairs itself and allows sperm to pass through the urethra once again.

Approximately 10 percent of men who elect to have a vasectomy later request a reversal operation.[52] The effectiveness of reversal operations, measured by pregnancy following the reversal, ranges from 18 to 60 percent.[53]

The major contraindication for vasectomy relates to the permanence of this method of birth control. Unless a man and woman are *100 percent certain* that childbearing is no longer desired, it would be best to select a reversible birth-control method.

Female Sterilization

Sterilization in women prevents fertilization by stopping sperm from reaching an egg in the fallopian tube. There are several types of female sterilization procedures currently in use. **Tubal ligation** involves tying, or cutting and tying the female's fallopian tubes (see figure 8.14). **Electrocoagulation** uses electricity to seal a portion of each tube. Because of the increased chance of injury this method has become the least popular with U.S. physicians. **Thermocoagulation** uses heat to melt away a portion of each tube.

The most commonly performed surgical procedures are the **minilaparotomy** and the **laparoscopy.** For the minilaparotomy, a physician makes a tiny incision just above the pubic hairline. The physician then inserts an instrument to lift the fallopian tubes and bring them out of the abdominal cavity so that they can be cut and tied, clipped, or cauterized. The physician then lets the fallopian tubes slip back into place in the abdominal cavity.

During a laparoscopy, a physician makes a tiny incision just below the naval and inserts a lighted, tubular instrument into the abdominal cavity. This instrument helps the physician locate the fallopian tubes (see figure 8.14) so that they can be cut and tied, clipped, or cauterized.

Minilaparotomy and laparoscopy procedures are usually done on an outpatient basis under anesthesia and can be completed

Ejaculate: the fluid component discharged from the male reproductive tract at ejaculation that contains sperm cells; commonly known as semen.

Epididymis: a structure in the male reproductive system located over the testes whose major function is the temporary storage of sperm.

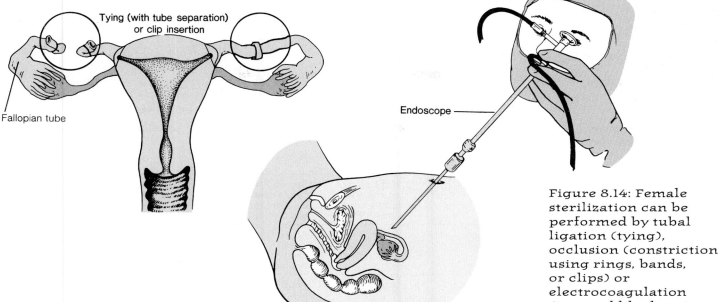

Tying (with tube separation)
or clip insertion

Fallopian tube

Endoscope

in about fifteen minutes. Within two days following the surgery, most women are able to resume their normal activity levels. Women can resume sexual activity as soon as they feel comfortable doing so.

Female Sterilization: Weighing the Benefits and Risks

Sterilization is a very effective long-term female birth-control method. It does not affect a woman's ability to enjoy sex. Additionally, sterilization has no long-term side effects.

There are some potential disadvantages to female sterilization. The most important may be that this method of birth control is considered to be irreversible. It is estimated that about 3 percent of women who undergo sterilization attempt to have the surgery reversed.[54] Most often, this request is motivated by remarriage and a desire to have children with the new spouse. The success of reversal operations appears to depend in large part on the amount of the fallopian tube that was destroyed.[55] The normal fallopian tube is between eight and thirteen centimeters long. Most sterilization procedures destroy between two and five centimeters of tube. Studies indicate that live birth rates following reversal surgery vary by the technique used to

occlude the fallopian tubes.[56] Live birth rates range on average from 41 percent following reversal of electrocoagulation to 84 percent after reversal of clips used to clamp the fallopian tubes closed. Not all women who have been sterilized, however, are candidates for reversal surgery. Age, health status, ovulation patterns and amount of damage to the fallopian tubes are common screening criteria used to determine a woman's eligibility for reversal surgery. Therefore, women who elect female sterilization as a birth-control method should consider it to be an irreversible method.

The major contraindication for female sterilization relates to the permanence of this method of birth control. Unless a woman and her partner are *100 percent certain* that childbearing is no longer desired, it would be best to select a reversible birth-control method.

Abortion

It is estimated that approximately one out of every four pregnancies in the United States is terminated by induced abortion.[57] The use of abortion as a birth-control method is an important and hotly debated issue that has been going on for some time (see Of Special Interest 8.2). In 1973, the United States Supreme Court (*Roe v. Wade*) established the

The effectiveness ratings for birth control methods in the following chart are based on several studies. Sometimes birth control fails because of the method itself, and sometimes due to human error, such as incorrect use or failure to use. Each method has possible risks and side effects, and some cannot be used by individuals with certain medical problems.

Type	Estimated Effectiveness	Risks/Side Effects	Sexually Transmitted Disease (STD) Protection	Convenience	Availability	Cost
Male Condom	About 85%	Rarely, irritation and allergic reactions	Helps protect against STD, including herpes and AIDS	Applied immediately before intercourse; used only once and discarded	Non-prescription	25¢ to $2.50 each
Female Condom	An estimated 74–79%	Rarely, irritation and allergic reactions	Same as male condom, only not as effective	Applied immediately before intercourse; used only once and discarded	Non-prescription	$2.50 each
Spermicides Used Alone	70–82%	Rarely, irritation and allergic reactions	Unknown	Applied no more than one hour before intercourse	Non-prescription	$8, with refills $2–$5
Sponge	72–82%	Rarely, irritation and allergic reactions;difficulty in removal; very rarely, toxic shock syndrome	None	Can be inserted hours before intercourse and left in place 24 hours; used once and discarded	No longer available	NA
Diaphragm	82–94%	Rarely, irritation and allergic reactions; difficulty in removal; very rarely, toxic shock syndrome	None	Inserted before intercourse; can remain 24 hours, but more spermicide needed if intercourse is repeated	Rx	$13–$25 plus medical exam fees & spermicides
Cervical Cap with Spermicide	At least 82%	Abnormal Pap test; vaginal or cervical infections; very rarely, toxic shock syndrome	None	Can remain in place for 48 hours; may be difficult to insert	Rx	$13–$25 plus medical exam fees & spermicides
Pills	97–99%	Blood clots, heart attacks, strokes, gallbladder disease, liver tumors, water retention, hypertension, mood changes, dizziness, nausea; not for smokers	None	Pill must be taken regularly, regardless of frequency of intercourse	Rx	$15–$35 per month plus medical exam fees
Implant (Norplant)	99%	Menstrual cycle irregularity; headaches, nervousness, depression, nausea, change of appetite, breast tenderness, weight gain, enlarged ovaries and/or fallopian tubes, excessive body and facial hair; may subside after first year	None	Effective 24 hours after implantation for approximately 5 years; can be removed by physician at any time	Rx; minor outpatient surgical procedure	$500–$800 for a five year implant
Injection (Depo-Provera)	99%	Side effects similar to those with Norplant	None	One injection every three months	Rx	$30–$75 for three months plus medical exam fees
IUD	95–96%	Cramps, bleeding, pelvic inflammatory disease, infertility; rarely, perforation of the uterus	None	After insertion, stays in place until physician removes it	Rx	$150–$500 to insert
Periodic Abstinence	Very variable, perhaps 53–86%	None	None	Requires frequent monitoring of body functions and periods of abstinence	Instruction from physician or clinic	physician or clinic fee
Surgical Sterilization	Over 99%	Pain, infection, and, for female tubal ligation, possible surgical complications	None	Vasectomy is usually performed in a doctor's office; tubal ligation is performed in an operating room	Surgery	$250–$500 for vasectomy, $1,000–$2,500 for tubal ligation

Source: Data from "Choosing a Contraceptive" in *FDA Consumer,* September 1993.

The Abortion Controversy

Whether or not a woman has the right to abort the embryo or fetus she is carrying is a highly controversial issue. Adding to the heat of the debate has been the use of emotionally loaded labels, such as pro-choice or pro-life.

The "Pro-Choice" Argument

Those who favor a woman retaining this right of choice are generally identified as **pro-choice**. Pro-choice individuals believe that abortion should be a strictly personal matter and that a pregnant woman has the right to decide for herself whether or not to have an abortion because she has an undeniable right to control her own body. They contend that this right entitles her to the support and advice of trusted friends and professionals. They also believe that the woman should not be subject to interference from the state, church, or any other self-appointed guardian of public morality. In addition, they argue that a pregnant woman has a right to easy access to a qualified physician who is an expert at performing abortion, regardless of the woman's ability to pay for the procedure.

The "Pro-Life" Argument

Pro-life, or right-to-life, proponents hold that from the moment a sperm cell fertilizes an egg, new life has been created. They contend that the developing embryo or fetus is a separate growing organism, and as such cannot be considered an integral part of the mother's body. They hold that this developing embryo is not only human but that it also has legal rights, including the right to life, at any stage of its development. Rejecting abortion-on-demand as a method of curtailing population increases, pro-life individuals argue that abortion not only poses physical and emotional hazards to a woman, but that it constitutes a denial of basic moral and religious principles. They view the "quality of life" ethic, in which a person decides that the quality of his or her life takes precedence over the quality of someone else's life, as discriminatory. Such an ethic, they contend, contrasts with the "absolute value of life" ethic as characterized by Hippocratic, Jewish, and Christian philosophy.

What Do You Think?

1. On a continuum of "pro-life" philosophy to "pro-choice" philosophy, where do you personally stand? Explain your position.
2. Do you know someone who has had an abortion? If so, do you know what considerations went into her decision

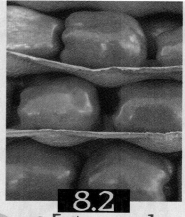

8.2
Of Special Interest

to have the abortion? How did it affect her emotionally? Physically? What about her partner? Did they have counseling? How does she feel about the abortion now?
3. What do you think you would do if you (or your partner) became unintentionally pregnant? How would your decision affect you and your partner's lives at this time? A year from now? Five years from now?

Source: Adapted from Curtis O. Byer & Louis W. Shainberg, *Dimensions of Human Sexuality,* 4th edition. Madison, WI: Brown & Benchmark Publishers, 1994, p. 557.

---

conditions under which an abortion on demand can be legally performed in the United States. In the **first trimester** of pregnancy, no state can outlaw a woman's right to an abortion. During the **second trimester** states can control the circumstances under which a woman may have an abortion. While in the **third trimester,** states can outlaw abortion except in cases where the life or health of the pregnant woman is at stake. Since 1973, all fifty states, under this ruling, have legislated a host of regulations for second-trimester abortions. Several of these laws have been challenged in the U.S. Supreme Court.

In 1989 the United States Supreme Court (*Webster v. Reproductive Health Services*) upheld a Missouri law that requires physicians to test the fetus for viability before performing abortions at twenty weeks or

greater gestation, and cut public funding for abortions in Missouri. This ruling also invited states to experiment with laws that limit access to abortion.

More recently, in 1992 the United States Supreme Court (*Planned Parenthood v. Casey*) ruled as constitutional a Pennsylvania law that required (1) a twenty-four hour waiting period prior to an abortion, (2) physicians to inform women seeking abortions of other options available to them, (3) parental notification for minors requesting abortions, and (4) physicians to provide statistical information about their abortion patients. This same ruling, however, stated that a woman did not have to notify her husband before having an abortion. Such a requirement was ruled an "undue burden" on the woman, as it could expose her to potential abuse. It seems that the states are

First trimester: that period of pregnancy beginning with fertilization and continuing to the end of the third month.

Second trimester: that period of pregnancy beginning with the fourth month and continuing to the end of the sixth month.

Third trimester: that period of pregnancy beginning with the seventh month and continuing until childbirth.

currently free to place restrictions on access to abortion as long as they do not place "undue burden" on women.[58]

It is estimated that, in the U.S., there are about thirty-three abortions for every 100 live births. According to the Alan Guttmacher Institute,[59] the most likely recipient of an abortion is a twenty to twenty-four year old, White, unmarried woman who has never had either a live birth or an abortion. Most abortions (90 percent) are performed during the first trimester of pregnancy, with 51 percent being performed before the ninth week.

When birth-control efforts fail the result is an unintended and possibly unwanted pregnancy. Abortion is considered by some people as a "backup" birth-control method to be used if the first method of choice fails. Abortion, however, is not the only choice available to individuals confronting an unintended pregnancy. Carrying the fetus to full term and then either keeping the baby or placing the baby up for adoption are options to be considered in the decision-making process.

Types of Abortion

The medical definition of **induced abortion** is the termination of a pregnancy before the embryo or fetus is capable of extrauterine life. Abortions that occur naturally are termed miscarriages, or spontaneous abortions. There are several types of induced abortions. How far along a woman is in her pregnancy will determine, in part, the abortion method used.

Vacuum Aspiration

Vacuum aspiration can be performed up until the fourteenth week of pregnancy. This technique requires the cervix to be **dilated** to allow access to the uterus. Once the cervix is dilated the physician uses a suction tube to remove the uterine lining.

Vacuum aspiration abortions can be performed under general or local anesthesia. If local anesthesia is used the procedure can be done on an outpatient basis. In the United States, vacuum aspiration is the method of choice, accounting for 97 percent of all abortions.[60]

RU-486

Mifepristone or **RU-486** is the French developed abortion pill. Its anti-progesterone effects thwart the proper development of the **endometrium** and **placenta,** resulting in a chemically induced abortion. RU-486 can be administered up until the forty-seventh day of pregnancy or approximately four weeks after the female's last menstrual period. The effectiveness of RU-486 alone is 80 percent, but as high as 96 percent when used in combination with prostaglandin injections or pills. Forty-eight hours after consuming RU-486 the female is given prostaglandin and the embryo is expelled within the following twenty-four hours. This is a critical time period when the female should be closely monitored for adverse reactions. Common side effects of the combined use of RU-486 and prostaglandin include heavy menstrual bleeding and considerable menstrual cramping lasting for up to two weeks. In 4 to 5 percent of the cases the female experiences hemorrhaging. Females who fail to abort are advised to schedule themselves for a surgical abortion. There remain unanswered questions regarding the side effects and risks of RU-486 on adolescent females, on women who use the drug for multiple abortions, and failures requiring women to undergo a surgical abortion.

RU-486 may not be the drug of choice when used soon after unprotected intercourse. For decades U.S. physicians and family planning clinics have prescribed standard high-dose progestin birth-control pills to be used as abortifacients or as *morning after pills*. Thus the common U.S. birth-control pill may be the drug of choice for women seeking chemical abortions soon after fertilization. RU-486 may be best slated for use from the third, through the sixth week of pregnancy.

In 1994 The Population Council of The United States began human testing of RU-486. As of the printing of this textbook, the FDA, upon completion of the human studies on RU-486, would then consider whether to approve RU-486. If RU-486 is approved, it is almost certain that it will be approved only in combination with another standard abortifacient, of which prostaglandin is the leading candidate.

Dilation and Evacuation

Dilation and evacuation is a second trimester abortion procedure that may be performed from the thirteenth to the twentieth week of pregnancy. This technique is very similar to

Dilated: enlarged or expanded.

Endometrium: the innermost layer of the uterus that secretes fluids and nutrients for the developing embryo.

Placenta: a temporary organ that transfers nutrients and oxygen from the mother to the developing embryo/fetus. This organ also secretes hormones that maintain the pregnancy.

Informed consent/abortion: an example.

Before you give your consent, be sure you understand both the pros and cons of having an abortion. This form outlines possible complications that can occur with an abortion and the danger signs you should watch for after an abortion. If you have any questions as you read, we will be happy to discuss them. Also, remember that your consent is entirely voluntary. You can change your mind any time before the abortion procedure is begun.

As you read, please check (✓) each section.

I am aware that my three alternatives regarding this pregnancy are parenthood, adoption, and abortion. ☐

I understand the medical procedure that will be used in the termination of my pregnancy. ☐

I authorize the administration of anesthetic and the disposal of any tissue removed during the abortion. ☐

If complications or problems occur during my abortion, I authorize my physician to perform any *other* procedure and to administer medications that are necessary for my well being, or to have me admitted to a hospital. ☐

I understand that possible complications of abortion include:

infection
bleeding
perforation of the uterus
incomplete abortion, which may require a repeat procedure
continuing pregnancy
damage to the uterus or nearby internal structures (bladder, rectum, intestines, blood vessels, and nerves)
loss of future fertility
death ☐

I understand that no medical procedure is 100 percent successful, and that an abortion procedure cannot guarantee successful results. ☐

I have freely chosen to have this abortion and understand that it is my responsibility to return for follow-up care as advised, or sooner if problems occur. ☐

Figure 8.15: An example of an informed-consent document

the vacuum aspiration abortion: both methods require dilation of the cervix and use suction to remove the uterine contents. Because the fetus is further along in its development, the dilation and evacuation procedure requires a greater dilation of the cervix, the use of forceps to remove fetal tissue, and the use of a special tool to scrape the uterine wall.

Chemical Abortions

In **chemical abortions** a toxic substance is introduced into the amniotic sac resulting in the premature delivery of a dead fetus. **Saline, urea,** and **prostaglandins** are the most common substances used to induce chemical abortions. These methods are used during the second trimester or up until the twenty-fourth week of gestation.

Hysterotomy

The **hysterotomy** is identical to a small **cesarean section.** An incision is made in the female's lower abdomen and then her uterus. The fetus is then removed. This procedure is usually done between twenty and twenty-four weeks of gestation. Hysterotomy is considered major intrauterine surgery and carries with it the inherent risks of such major surgery.

Complications of Abortion

Abortions are an expensive method of birth control; they also carry substantial health risks, both physical and emotional. Although rare, abortions may fail (0.1–0.3 percent) allowing the pregnancy to continue.[61] Before a woman decides to have an abortion she should be educated about the total range of options available for dealing with an unwanted pregnancy. Additionally, she should be aware of the potential complications resulting from abortion. Many clinics and hospitals that perform abortions require that a woman sign an informed-consent document such as the one shown in figure 8.15 as a method to ensure a woman has been fully educated regarding her options.

Saline: a solution used in chemical abortions that contains sodium chloride.

Urea: the chemical form of nitrogen that is excreted in urine.

Prostaglandins: a group of compounds produced by the human body that have powerful hormone like effects, and may result in pain.

Cesarean section: the surgical opening of the abdomen and uterus for childbirth.

Physical Health Risks

The physician's skill and abortion experience are factors in the effectiveness and subsequent health risk of the procedure. Some of the major physical health concerns of abortion include the following:

- The female may develop a secondary infection as a result of an abortion.
- Females having abortions may experience uterine blood clots, injury to the intestines, hemorrhage, perforation of the uterus, and laceration of the cervix.
- Females with past abortions have been reported to have a greater risk of future pregnancy failures and infant mortalities; however, some experts believe that the data reported regarding this issue are not conclusive.[62]

Emotional Health Risks

There are also important emotional health issues related to abortion. Guilt, anger, and sadness are only a few of the many emotions that may be experienced by a woman and her partner upon consideration of or use of an abortion. It is very important that women considering an abortion receive unbiased professional counseling.

Birth Control: Personal and Social Influences

There are many personal and social influences that impact on the decision to use, or not use, any particular birth-control method. These variables range from family and religious beliefs or traditions to an awareness of concerns with overpopulation.

Effective birth-control options have improved dramatically since the 1960s. With improved effectiveness came a greater opportunity for people to have real control over their fertility. Many individuals have taken advantage of the option to postpone pregnancy and childbearing until they have met other goals such as establishing a career. Additionally, some people are acutely aware of the economic and environmental threat that overpopulation poses for humanity. These individuals may view themselves as world citizens and take their personal role in family planning quite seriously (see A Social Perspective 8.1).

The ability to plan a family reliably should, theoretically, lead to fewer unintended pregnancies. Many individuals, however, do not practice effective birth control. Certain religious groups, such as the Roman Catholic church, exert a strong influence on their members to avoid chemical or mechanical birth-control options, which they view as immoral. Other individuals choose, often by default, to have unprotected sexual intercourse. This may result from a lack of knowledge regarding effective methods of birth control or from a real or perceived lack of access to such methods. This is especially prominent with sexually active teenagers.

Numerous studies have reported the lack of birth-control use among teenagers.[63] However, a recent study by the Alan Guttmacher Institute reported that 70 percent of fifteen to seventeen year-old women, and 80 percent of eighteen to nineteen year-old women regularly use birth control.[64] It has also been noted that 83 percent of high school males reported using birth control during recent intercourse.[65] While this data may look encouraging, it does not tell us whether the birth-control methods are being used correctly. One recent study looked at the difference between perceived and actual condom skills among patients at a sexually transmitted disease clinic.[66] Over 3,000 patients were asked to demonstrate their condom skills using a penile model. While 89 percent of these patients *believed* that they could correctly put on and take off a condom, the average correct skills test score was 60 percent, indicating only a moderate level of condom skills. Men were more likely than women to *believe* that they could correctly use condoms, however, their *actual* condom skills were not significantly different from the skills of the women studied.

Decisions regarding the use or nonuse of birth-control methods are complex. A detailed investigation of available birth-control options, including their effectiveness, cost, safety, and contraindications, is an important step in decision making for sexually active individuals. Personal beliefs and social influences should also be assessed for the role they might play in any particular situation. Table 8.9 provides some suggestions for making healthy changes in your lifestyle in order to prevent unintended pregnancy. Each sexually active individual and couple must take the responsibility for careful decision making about birth control and family planning. Such decisions have the potential to impact positively on your quest for higher levels of wellness.

Population's Insidious Impact on the Health of the Planet

Without a stable population, people become as endangered as other species. Achieving stability should be our goal.

The term "demographic transition" refers to the way birthrates and death rates have historically proceeded from high to low levels. Such studies of population trends can be useful but are not necessarily predictive. Transition appears to occur in three phases. At first, both birthrates and death rates are high or in balance, so little, if any, population growth occurs. In the second phase, death rates fall because of improved living conditions—better health care, increased food production, expanded social services—but birthrates remain high. In this stage, populations grow rapidly. Finally, in the third phase, economic and social gains combined with lower infant mortality rates reduce the desire for large families and birthrates decline. As the gap between birthrates and death rates narrows, population growth slows. When a population has reached the point of equilibrium between birthrates and death rates, and is able to maintain a state of zero population growth (i.e., there are no net gains in the number of people in a given population), then the population is said to have stabilized. Some countries have even advanced to a fourth stage in which death rates are higher than birthrates and population has declined.

The problem in the developing world is that most of these countries get stuck or "trapped" in the second phase of the demographic transition. Modern medical technology and improved diets reach these populations and decrease death rates before a modern economy has been able to develop and encourage lower birthrates. Populations continue to grow at a rapid pace, outstripping the ability of these countries to meet the needs of such a large number of people. This places undue stress on the land and natural resources as well as negating the modest economic gains of an incipient modern economy. Per capita income declines. If this trend is accompanied by declines in per capita food production (as in much of sub-Saharan Africa over the last decade), rising food imports will increase external debt, putting further stress on the economy. People lose all hope of attaining a better life for themselves, and political instability results. The population then has grown beyond the capacity of the immediate environment to peacefully sustain it.

What Do You Think?

1. It is predicted that the world's population will double in the next 100 years. What would be some of the more important problems that will

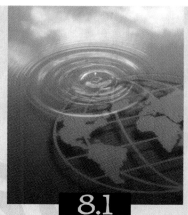

8.1
A Social Perspective

result if the predicted ten billion world population estimate is reached in that time period? What is your source of evidence?

2. How will these problems affect you personally, or potentially affect your children and grandchildren?

3. Do you feel any personal responsibility to plan your family and limit the number of children you will have? Explain your reasoning.

Reprinted by permission of The Putnam Publishing Group from *The National Audubon Society Almanac of the Environment* by Valerie Harms. Copyright © 1994 by The National Audubon Society, Inc.

Making changes in health-related behavior is not an easy process, especially when it comes to decisions about birth control—a decision that involves both the male and female sexual partner. The following tips will help you as you progress through the common stages of behavior change.*

Precontemplation → Contemplation

If you and your sexual partner have never thought about making healthy changes in how you attempt to prevent *unintended* pregnancy or you do not intend to make any changes within the next six months you might want to consider:

- assessing your current risk of *unintended* pregnancy. If you are sexually active, do you want to become pregnant? If not, are you correctly using a reliable method of birth control? (Information provided throughout this chapter can help you assess correct use and reliability of various birth-control methods.)

Contemplation → Preparation

If you and your sexual partner have been seriously considering making some changes in birth-control use, but have not yet attempted any changes, try to thoughtfully answer the following questions:

- How do my sexual partner and I think and feel about the possibility of becoming pregnant? Am I, and my sexual partner, willing to make birth-control changes to decrease the chance that we will experience an unintended pregnancy?

Preparation → Action

If you and your sexual partner are ready to make some definite plans for more effectively preventing an unintended pregnancy during the next month, or if you have already made small changes in the past but were not able to maintain those changes as a continuing part of your lifestyle, consider the following actions:

- Study the variety of birth-control options currently available. Discuss with your sexual partner the sharing of responsibility for birth control, and the risks and benefits of the various methods. Jointly make a decision on which birth-control method is best for your individual circumstances.
- Set a specific date to begin your new birth-control method. Some over-the-counter birth-control products can be used immediately. Other birth-control methods may involve making an appointment with a physician to gain access to the birth-control product.

Action → Maintenance

If you have recently made some healthy changes in birth-control use, the following tips will help you continue on this healthy path:

- Regularly discuss the birth-control method you have chosen with your sexual partner. Include issues of responsibility, correct use and side effects. If the method is satisfactory for both partners the discussion will reinforce your choice. If the method is not satisfactory, the discussion will help you make a change in methods that will help you maintain optimal birth-control protection.

Maintenance

You have made important changes in preventing an unintended pregnancy that you have practiced for six months or longer; now you need to focus on maintaining your healthy choices every day:

- Talk to your sexual partner about birth control; offer each other support for regularly and correctly using the birth-control method you have chosen.

*Based on Prochaska, Norcross and DiClemente's transtheoretical model. See Prochaska, J. O., Norcross, J. C. & DiClemente, C. C. (1994). *Changing for Good.* New York: William Morrow and Company, Inc.

Summary

1. The major goal of family planning is to enhance the health of families through planned births.

2. Birth-control methods can be grouped into four categories: natural, mechanical, chemical, and invasive.

3. When deciding on a method of birth control, it is important to consider the effectiveness, safety, cost, and reversibility of each available method.

4. Theoretical effectiveness ratings estimate the effectiveness of birth-control methods if used perfectly; use effectiveness ratings take into account the errors that occur with human use.

5. Each birth-control method has certain health risks associated with it, ranging from minor side effects like irritation and allergic reactions to more serious health problems such as perforation of the uterus or heart attacks. Many birth-control methods provide health benefits in addition to pregnancy prevention. For instance, condoms help protect against sexually transmitted diseases, and oral contraceptives may decrease the risk of endometrial and ovarian cancer. It is important for each individual to weigh both the risks and benefits before selecting a birth-control method.

6. Sexual abstinence involves a decision to refrain from sexual intercourse for a period of time, such as until marriage or engagement. Periodic abstinence is a birth-control method based on predicting when a woman ovulates and refraining from sexual intercourse during that time each month when pregnancy would be most likely to occur. Periodic abstinence requires frequent monitoring of body functions.

7. The diaphragm and cervical cap are mechanical methods of birth control that are used with chemical spermicides. These birth control methods are available by prescription. The cervical cap can remain in place for up to 48 hours, while it is recommended that the diaphragm be left in place no longer than 24 hours.

8. The condom is a mechanical method of birth control that prevents sperm from reaching the uterus. Both male and female condoms are available over-the-counter and are helpful in preventing sexually transmitted diseases as well as pregnancy. Spermicides are often used in conjunction with condoms.

9. Spermicides are chemicals that prevent fertilization by destroying sperm. Spermicides come in a variety of forms, including foams, creams and suppositories. They must be applied no longer than one hour prior to intercourse, and must be reapplied before each separate act of intercourse.

10. An IUD (intrauterine device) is a plastic device approximately one and one half inches long that is inserted by a physician into a woman's uterus through the vaginal tract. IUDs probably work by ending implantation of a fertilized egg. Before a woman is given an IUD, her physician should take a medical history and test for sexually transmitted diseases and pregnancy. A woman using an IUD will need to be checked by a physician three months after insertion, and each year thereafter.

11. Oral contraceptives, Norplant, and Depo-Provera are all prescription birth-control methods that use birth-controlling hormones to prevent pregnancy. Oral contraceptives are taken as pills, while Depo-Provera is given by injection. Norplant consists of six small rods that are surgically placed under the skin for as long as five years. All three forms of birth-controlling hormones are highly effective methods of birth control, however, each has side effects and risks that may be unacceptable to some women.

12. There are several contraceptives currently under review or development in the U.S., including barrier methods such as the polyurethane male condom and a disposable diaphragm, chemical barriers involving newly formulated spermicides, and hormonal methods such as improved implants and injectables.

13. Voluntary sterilization is a surgical, permanent, and highly effective method of birth control that is the most popular form of birth control in the U.S. Male sterilization blocks the vas deferens, while female sterilization blocks the fallopian tubes. Male sterilization is less expensive than female sterilization.

14. Several types of abortions are used to terminate pregnancies at different stages of fetal development. Vacuum aspiration is the most common method of abortion in the U.S. today. Another abortion method, RU-486, has received a great deal of attention, and is currently being tested by the FDA to determine whether or not it will be granted approval for use in the United States.

15. There are many personal and social influences that impact on an individual's decision to use, or not use, a particular birth-control method. Some of the more common influences include family and religious beliefs or traditions, career goals, lack of knowledge of or access to birth-control methods (especially for teenagers), as well as concerns about overpopulation. Each sexually active individual and couple should carefully and responsibly consider their decisions about birth control and family planning.

Recommended Readings

Byer, Curtis O., & Louis W. Shainberg. *Dimensions of Human Sexuality*, 4th ed. Madison, WI: Brown & Benchmark Publishers, 1994.

This human sexuality textbook contains an excellent and up-to-date chapter on birth-control methods (chapter 18

"Contraception"). Its coverage of contraception among teenagers and young adults is especially well done.

"Birth Control Choices." 1994. *CQ Researcher*, 4 (28):649–672.

This issue of *CQ Researcher* focuses on the question "Do American women need better birth-control products?" It highlights concerns about RU-486 availability and the question of whether oral contraceptives should be available as an over-the-counter birth-control method. The issue ends with an annotated bibliography that is exceptionally well done.

Hatcher, Robert, et al. *Contraceptive Technology*. 16th rev. ed. New York: Irvington Publishers, 1994.

This book is one of the classic sources for information on the range of available birth-control methods. It is revised every two years by experts in the field of birth control.

References

1. W. Mosher & W. Pratt. (1990). Contraceptive use in the United States, 1973–88. National Center for Health Statistics #182, 1–10.

2. Department of Health and Human Services. (1994). *Healthy People 2000 Review, 1993*. Washington, D.C.: U.S. Government Printing Office.

3. Department of Health and Human Services. *Healthy People 2000 Review, 1993*.

4. L. Wilcox et al., "Risk Factors for Regret After Tubal Sterilization: 5 Years of Follow-up in a Prospective Study," *Fertility & Sterility* 55:5 (1991):927–933; S. Henshaw and S. Singh, "Sterilization Regret Among U.S. Couples," *Family Planning Perspectives* 18 (1986):238–240.

5. United Nations Population Fund, *Population Policies and Programmes: Lessons Learned From Two Decades of Experience*, N. Sadik (Ed.) New York: New York University Press, 1991.

6. R. Hatcher et al., *Contraceptive Technology*, 16th Revised Edition. (New York: Irvington Publishers, 1994), 336.

7. R. Hatcher et al., *Contraceptive Technology*, 16th Revised Edition. (New York: Irvington Publishers, 1994), 337.

8. F. Parazzini et al., "Barrier Methods of Contraception and the Risk of Cervical Neoplasia," *Contraception* 40:5 (1989):519–530; "Barrier Contraceptives Lower Cervical CA Risk," *Medical Aspects of Human Sexuality* 21.12(1987):27.

9. B. Foxman, "Recurring Urinary Tract Infection: Incidence and Risk Factors," *American Journal of Public Health*, 80:3 (1990):331–333; "A Barrier That Can Bother the Bladder," *Emergency Medicine* 18.6 (1986):81–82.

10. M. Rekart, "The Toxicity and Local Effects of the Spermicide Nonoxynol-9," *Journal of Acquired Immune Deficiency Syndromes* 5:4(1992):425–426.

11. R. Hatcher et al., *Contraceptive Technology*, 16th Revised Edition. (New York: Irvington Publishers, 1994), 204.

12. R. Hatcher et al., *Contraceptive Technology*, 16th Revised Edition. (New York: Irvington Publishers, 1994), 197.

13. R. Hatcher et al., *Contraceptive Technology*, 16th Revised Edition. (New York: Irvington Publishers, 1994), 204–207.

14. D. A. Eschenbach, "Pelvic Infections and Sexually Transmitted Diseases," in J. R. Scott, *Danforth's Obstetrics and Gynecology* (Philadelphia: Lippincott, 1990) Sixth Edition; A. Reingold, "Toxic Shock Syndrome and the Contraceptive Sponge," *Journal of the American Medical Association* 255 (1986):242–243.

15. Choosing a contraceptive. (September, 1993) *FDA Consumer*, 18–20.

16. R. Hatcher et al., *Contraceptive Technology*, 16th Revised Edition. (New York: Irvington Publishers, 1994), 204–205.

17. W. Cates & K. Stone, "Family Planning, Sexually Transmitted Diseases and Contraceptive Choice: A Literature Update-Part 1," *Family Planning Perspectives* 24:2 (1992): 75–84.

18. M. Slattery et al., "Sexual Activity, Contraception, Genital Infections, and Cervical Cancer: Support for a Sexually Transmitted Disease Hypothesis," *American Journal of Epidemiology* 130.2 (1989):248–258.

19. W. Darrow, "Condom Use and Effectiveness in High-Risk Populations," *Sexually Transmitted Diseases* 16.3 (1989):157–160; Richard L. Naeye, "Coitus and Associated Amniotic-Fluid Infections," *New England Journal of Medicine* 301 (1979):1198–1200; R. Snowden, M. Williams, and D. Hawkins, *The IUD: A Practical Guide* (London: Croom Helm, 1977).

20. Female condom: Equal protection. (1994) *Consumer Reports on Health* 6:34.

21. R. Hatcher et al., *Contraceptive Technology*, 16th Revised Edition. (New York: Irvington Publishers, 1994), 206.

22. R. Burkman, N. Lee, H. Ory, and G. Rubin, "Response to The Intrauterine Device and Pelvic Inflammatory Disease: The Women's Health Study Reanalyzed," *Journal of Clinical Epidemiology* 44.2 (1991): 123–125; R. Kronmal, C. Whitney, and S. Mumford, "The Intrauterine Device and Pelvic Inflammatory Disease: The Women's Health Study Reanalyzed," *Journal of Clinical Epidemiology* 44.2 (1991):109–122.

23. M. Pernoll and R. Benson, *Current Obstetric and Gynecologic Diagnosis and Treatment*. (Norwalk, Conn.: Appleton and Lange, 1987.)

24. United Nations Population Fund, *Population Policies and Programmes: Lessons Learned From Two Decades of Experience*. N. Sadik (Ed.) (New York: New York University Press, 1991); R. Burkman, N. Lee, H. Ory, and G. Rubin, "Response to 'The Intrauterine Device and Pelvic Inflammatory Disease: The Women's Health Study Reanalyzed'," *Journal of Clinical Epidemiology* 44.2 (1991):123–125.

25. B. Gerstman et al., "Trends in the Content and Use of Oral Contraceptives in the United States, 1964–88," *American Journal of Public Health* 81(1991):90–96.

26. Neeson and May, *Comprehensive Maternity Nursing*, 184.

27. R. A. Hatcher et al. (1990). *Contraceptive Technology: 1990–91* (15th rev. ed.). New York: Irvington Publishers.

28. L. Speroff & P. Darney, *A Clinical Guide for Contraception* (Baltimore: Williams & Wilkins, 1992).

29. L. Speroff & P. Darney, *A Clinical Guide for Contraception* (Baltimore: Williams & Wilkins, 1992).

30. Rathus, S. A., Nevid, J. S. & Fichner-Rathus, L. (1993). *Human Sexuality in a World of Diversity*. Boston: Allyn and Bacon, 345.

31. Reinisch, J. M. (1990). *The Kinsey Institute New Report on Sex: What You Must Know to Be Sexually Literate*. New York: St. Martin's Press.

32. Darney, P. D. (1994). Hormonal implants: Contraception for a new century. *American Journal of Obstetrics and Gynecology* 170: 1536–1543.

33. Darney, Hormonal implants, 1536–1543.

34. Darney, Hormonal implants, 1536–1543.

35. Eilers, G. M., & Swanson, T. K. (1994). Women's satisfaction with Norplant as compared with oral contraceptives. *Journal of Family Practice* 38:596–600.

36. Birth control choices. (1994). *CQ Researcher* 4:649–672.

37. R. Hatcher et al., *Contraceptive Technology*, 16th Revised Edition. (New York: Irvington Publishers, 1994), 289.

38. A. P. McCauley & J. S. Geller, "Decisions For Norplant Programs," *Population Reports* Series K/Number 4 (1992):1–32.

39. Segal, Marian. (May, 1991). Norplant: Birth control at arm's reach. *FDA Consumer*; Anthony, Joseph. (1994). Contraceptive: What's best for you? *American Health* XIII(3):70.

40. Stehlin, Dori. (1993). Depo-Provera: The quarterly contraceptive. *FDA Consumer* 27(2):11–13.

41. Stehlin, Depo-Provera:, 11–13.

42. Stehlin, Depo-Provera:, 12.

43. D. R. Mishell et al. (Eds) *Infertility, Contraception, and Reproductive Endocrinology* (Cambridge, England: Blackwell Scientific Publications, 1991).

44. T. Cundy et al. "Bone Density in Women Receiving Depo Medroxyprogesterone Acetate for Contraception," *British Medical Journal* 303:6793 (1991):13–16.

45. Stehlin, Depo-Provera:, 12.

46. R. Hatcher et al., *Contraceptive Technology*, 16th Revised Edition. (New York: Irvington Publishers, 1994), 402.

47. W. D. Mosher, "Contraceptive Practice in the United States," *Family Planning Perspectives* 22 (1990):198–205.

48. I. Chi, D. Gates, & S. Thapa, "Performing Tubal Sterilizations During a Woman's Postpartum Hospitalization: A Review of the United States and International Experiences," *Obstetrical & Gynecological Survey* 47:2 (1992):71–79; L. Wilcox et al., "Risk Factors for Regret After Tubal Sterilization: 5 Years of Follow-up In A Prospective Study," *Fertility & Sterility* 55:5 (1991):927–933.

49. D. Wolfers and H. Wolfers, *Vasectomy and Vasectomania* (St. Albans, England: Mayflower, 1974).

50. Rathus et al., *Human Sexuality in a World of Diversity*, 363.

51. Reinisch, *The Kinsey Institute new report on sex: What you must know to be sexually literate.*

52. J. Jarow, "Quantitative Pathologic Changes in the Human Testis after Vasectomy," *New England Journal of Medicine* 20 (1985):1252–1256.

53. Reinisch, *The Kinsey Institute new report on sex: What you must know to be sexually literate.*

54. Ramos, Andreas, and Huggins, George. "Tubal sterilization: When is it the right choice?" *Medical Aspects of Human Sexuality* (December, 1991): 38–45.

55. "Voluntary Female Sterilization: Number One and Growing." (1990). *Population Reports*, Series C, Number 10, p. 18.

56. "Voluntary Female Sterilization," p. 18.

57. National Center for Health Statistics. (1991). "Induced terminations of pregnancy: Reporting states, 1988," ed. by Kenneth D. Kochanek. *Monthly Vital Statistics Report*, U.S. Department of Health and Human Services, Vol. 39, No. 12, Supplement, 30 April, 1991.

58. Salholz, E., Azar, V., Clifton, T., Chideya, F., Glick, D., Mason, M., and Miller, S. "Abortion angst." *Newsweek* (13 July, 1992):16–19.

59. Henshaw, S. K. and Van Vort, J. eds. *Abortion Factbook, 1992 Edition: Readings, Trends, and State and Local Data to 1988*. The Alan Guttmacher Institute, New York, NY, 1992.

60. L. Koonin et al., "Abortion Surveillance—United States, 1989," *Morbidity & Mortality Weekly Report* 44:SS–5 (1992):1–33.

61. R. Hatcher et al., *Contraceptive Technology*, 16th Revised Edition. (New York: Irvington Publishers, 1994), 483.

62. Pernoll and Benson, *Current Obstetric and Gynecologic Diagnosis and Treatment*, 609.

63. J. Forrest & S. Singh, "The Sexual and Reproductive Behavior of American Women," *Family Planning Perspectives* 22:5 (1990):206–214.

64. The Alan Guttmacher Institute, *Sex and America's Teenagers*, (New York: The Alan Guttmacher Institute, 1994).

65. Department of Health and Human Services. *Healthy People 2000 Review, 1993*.

66. Langer, L. M., Zimmerman, R. S., & Cabral, R. J. (1994). "Perceived versus actual condom skills among clients at sexually transmitted disease clinics." *Public Health Reports* 109 (5):683–687.

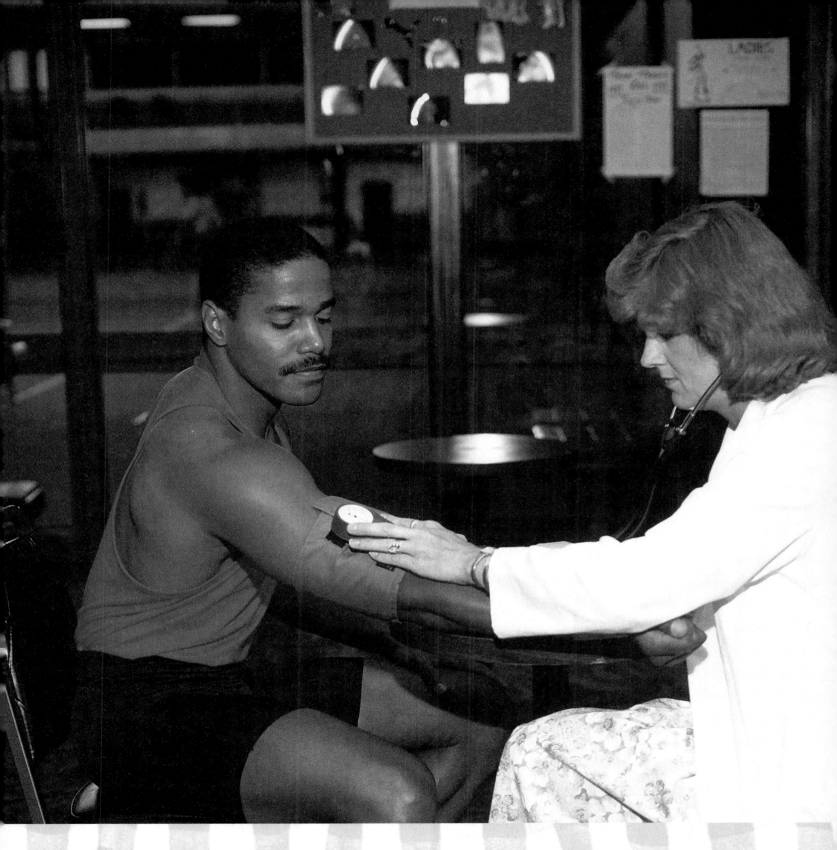

Preventing Major Threats to Well-Being

An important aspect of promoting health and well-being is understanding disease and injury risks that may compromise our ability to live life to the fullest. Unit III focuses on the leading causes of death and disability, examining both disease and injury causation and prevention strategies.

Chapter 9 focuses on preventing intentional and unintentional injuries—leading causes of death and disability in adolescents and young adults. In this age group, motor-vehicle crashes account for the majority of injury and death from unintentional injury. Recently, however, other forms of injury have been identified as significant public health problems. Violent and abusive behaviors, such as homicide, suicide, acquaintance rape, spouse abuse, and child abuse are receiving more attention as health problems affecting young people. For people of all ages, learning how to navigate more safely through our dangerous world is an important step in attaining well-being.

Unit III also presents the important communicable and noncommunicable diseases that may be roadblocks to high-level wellness. The common cold, sexually transmitted diseases, AIDS, cardiovascular disease, cancer, diabetes, emphysema, and other diseases pose significant threats to health and wellness. Chapter 10, 11, and 12 will help you learn a variety of ways to moderate the risk factors that contribute to the disease process.

While the major goal of Unit III is to help you reduce your risk of death and disability from disease and injury, it is also important to acknowledge that death is an eventuality for us all. Yet, the reality of death can lead us to appreciate life in a way no other event could. Chapter 13 will help you in your study of the phenomenon of death and dying and in understanding how to provide support to friends and loved ones when they experience death and dying. It may also help you to appreciate and live your life to the fullest.

Intentional and Unintentional Injury: Safer Living in a Dangerous World

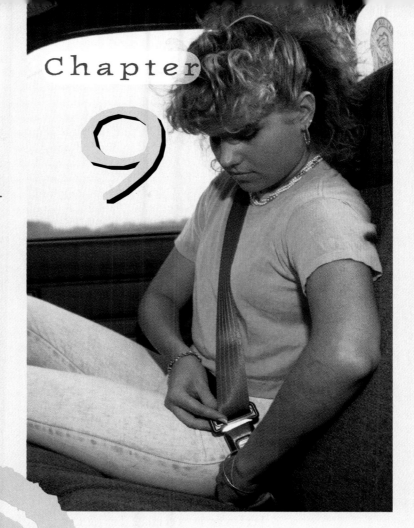

Chapter 9

Student Learning Objectives

Upon completion of this chapter, you should be able to:

1. describe the current social influences on intentional and unintentional injury;
2. analyze levels of violence depicted on current prime time and children's television shows;
3. list and identify two reasons why some individuals are willing to take risks that can be a threat to life and health;
4. define the term "accident," and explain why someone would argue that there are no "accidents";
5. list ten factors that contribute to unintentional injuries;
6. identify and describe the role played by the three Es in reducing risks associated with unintentional injury from motor-vehicle crashes;
7. assess your level of defensive driving skills;
8. describe suicide rate differences between minority and majority populations;
9. distinguish between "myths" and "realities" regarding suicidal behavior;
10. list five characteristics related to suicide behavioral profiles;
11. describe how to help someone who is suicidal;
12. analyze the relationship between homicide rates and socioeconomic status, race/ethnicity, and gender;
13. identify the two factors most often associated with occurrence of homicide;
14. list at least five recommendations for the prevention of homicide;
15. describe techniques to manage anger;
16. define acquaintance rape and list at least three safety precautions that may prevent its occurrence;
17. analyze the relationship between alcohol abuse and violence;
18. identify several ways in which violence is present in domestic settings;
19. explain the relationship between various social conditions and the occurrence of domestic violence;
20. assess your personal safety habits and determine where you need to improve your risk reduction habits.

S ince 1950, the death rate for adolescents and young adults in this country fell 20 percent, from 128.1 to 101.6 per 100,000 population.[1] In that time, deaths from cancer and heart disease have been reduced 40 and 65 percent respectively, but homicide rates have doubled, suicide rates have tripled, and death rates from unintentional injury have increased and remain the leading cause of death for this age group.

In this chapter we will examine a broad range of topics and issues, including a variety of both unintentional and intentional injuries. It is a primary objective of this chapter to demonstrate that the death, lost years of life, disability, and suffering from these events represent an important and complex public health threat (see figure 9.1). Individuals, communities, and the nation must work together to decrease injury rates and improve levels of well-being for all citizens.

Social Influences on Intentional and Unintentional Injury

As we move toward the end of the century to the year 2000 and toward the end of the second millennium, we have come to recognize change as an important part of our lives. Increases in the speed of communications and other improvements in technology have made our world smaller, but at the same time have forced us to be influenced by a greater number of events than ever before.

Few people in the U.S. living during the sixties have forgotten where they were during three political assassinations—John F. Kennedy, Martin Luther King, and Robert F. Kennedy. The seventies were dwarfed by the Vietnam war, the conspiracies surrounding the Watergate scandal, and the subsequent resignation of a U.S. president. It was also the decade of the emergence of the women's movement as a substantial force and the decade of *Roe vs. Wade*. Few of us old enough to understand will forget the results of a fundamentalist revolution in Iran and the violation of our sensibilities with the

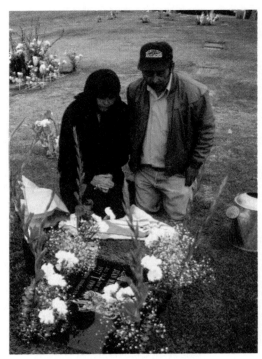

Figure 9.1: What Do You Think?

1. The anguish on these parents' faces is seen with increasing regularity across the U.S. as the incidence of violence increases. What factors do you believe are associated with the increasing homicide rate, especially among young Black men for whom it is the leading cause of death?

capture of fifty-six U.S. hostages in that country. In the early eighties our attention was riveted for 444 days to the fate of the remaining fifty-two Americans. The degradation of the U.S. spirit by this act of violence surely contributed greatly to the loss of Jimmy Carter's reelection to the presidency. This event seemed to mark a point at which we began to learn how violent our world can be.

The eighties brought to us some of our most important lessons in the politics of health. At a time when we know more about health than ever before, when we recognized as national policy that more than 70 percent of illness and death was preventable, when we believed that technology could help us treat or cure almost any disease, when supply-side economics fostered incredible growth in our economy, and when the civil rights

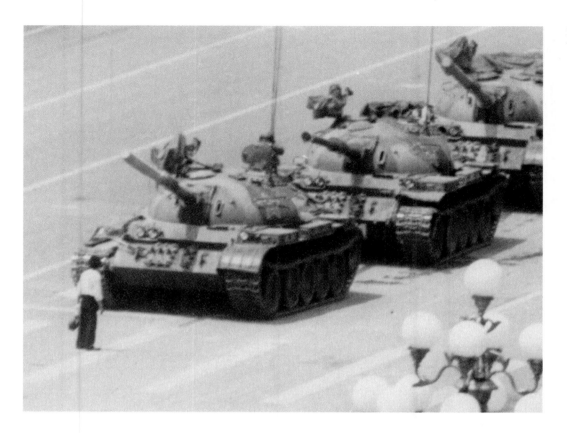

Figure 9.2: What Do You Think?

1. In spite of danger there are often those still willing to stand up for what they believe. Do you have beliefs that are so important to you that you would stand up for them like the college student from Tienanman Square did in this photo? Explain your thinking.

movements for minority populations and women had a substantive and recognizable history, we learned these lessons.

1. That the U.S. home is one of the most violent places on the planet as a result of accidental injury and death, and the physical and emotional trauma associated with child abuse, spouse abuse, elder abuse, sexual abuse across all social categories, other forms of domestic violence, and increased numbers of broken homes.

2. That intentional and unintentional injury and death could occur anywhere and at any time, as characterized in the following events: the attempted assassination and subsequent wounding by handgun of a U.S. president, his press secretary, and a secret service agent; the attempted assassination by handgun of the pope; the assassination by handgun of John Lennon; many media stories of serial killers; and the addition of new terms to the vocabulary—drive-by shootings and cluster suicides.

All of this happened in a decade when international violence once again riveted us to our televisions. Few among us will forget the many threats of terrorism in the 1980s, perhaps best illustrated by the succession of Americans and others taken hostage in the Middle East and the murder of more than 200 U.S. marines in Lebanon while they slept in their barracks; the U.S. responses to such violence as the bombing of Libya; the invasions of Grenada and Panama; and the crushing of the youthful attempt at democratization in Tienanman Square (see figure 9.2).

In the decade of the eighties we were treated to big box office violence in such films as *Texas Chain Saw Massacre*, the *Halloween* movie series making Freddie a famous name, *Rambo*, *Predator*, *Terminator*, *Young Guns*, and *Die Hard*. In the eighties we seem to have learned that if you have a problem you solve it with violence; that the person with the biggest gun is right; and that the way to end disagreement is with force. In *Power Shift*, Alvin Toffler[2] refers to three forms of power—violence, money, and knowledge. The first of these may be the hallmark of the eighties.

Now, midway through the nineties, where do we stand on these issues? Global

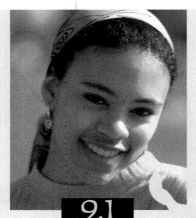

9.1
Activity for Wellness

Logging Television Violence

How common is television violence? Watch one primetime television show and one children's television show this week, and analyze them for violence.

Name of show:

_____

Type of show:

_____

Network or station:

_____

How many violent incidents were in the show?

_____

How many of these were committed by "bad guys"?

_____

What kind of incidents?

_____

How many violent incidents were committed by "good guys"?

_____

What kind of incidents?

_____

What weapons were used?

_____

Did the characters ever use nonviolent strategies to resolve conflicts?

_____

If so, how?

_____

_____

_____

Name of show:

_____

Type of show:

_____

Network or station:

_____

How many violent incidents were in the show?

_____

How many of these were committed by "bad guys"?

_____

What kind of incidents?

_____

How many violent incidents were committed by "good guys"?

_____

What kind of incidents?

_____

What weapons were used?

_____

Did the characters ever use nonviolent strategies to resolve conflicts?

_____

If so, how?

_____

_____

_____

Were you surprised with your results? Talk to classmates and share your results.

_____

communications continue to selectively show us the benefits of violence and power. Most will remember August 4, 1990 as the date that Saddam Hussein invaded Kuwait, which led subsequently to Desert Shield and Desert Storm. Beginning in March 1991, Americans were triumphantly welcomed home as victors following Desert Storm—yet thousands of Kurds and Shiites were still being slaughtered. The early 1990s also saw the terrorist bombing of the World Trade Center in New York City, the massive suicide and homicide associated with David Koresh and his followers in Waco, Texas, and the terrorist bombing of the Federal Building in Oklahoma City that killed hundreds of people, including children attending a day-care center housed in the building. Add to that the political violence

seen throughout the world in places such as Bosnia, Haiti, and Somalia, and it is easy to come to the conclusion that violence may well be the hallmark of the nineties as well. Even our entertainment for children has become more violent in the 1990s. Television shows such as the Power Rangers and Beavis and Butthead are extremely popular, and violent. (Activity for Wellness 9.1 will help you study television violence today.)

What is the legacy of "might makes right"? Examine the following statistics taken from *Healthy People 2000*[3]

- 2.2 million people are victims of violent injury each year
- the U.S. ranks first among industrialized nations in violent death rates

- the total number of deaths in the U.S. caused by violent and unintentional misuse of firearms is greater than the total of the next seventeen nations combined
- together, suicide and homicide constitute the fourth leading cause of years of potential life lost to people under sixty-five years of age in the U.S.
- unintentional injuries constitute the fifth leading cause of death in the U.S., with approximately 89,000 deaths annually

This chapter is designed to examine some of the issues related to the **years of potential life lost** and **disability days** suffered as a result of both unintentional and intentional injury and death. Basically, in the former category motor vehicle crashes account for the vast majority of deaths and injuries, with poisoning, drowning, and residential fires the next biggest contributors to the problem. The latter category includes **suicide, homicide** and other forms of violent and abusive behavior.

Why a Chapter on Injury and Violence in a Book about Wellness?

If you were to reexamine the definition of wellness and the models presented in chapter 1 describing its multidimensional nature, you would find that most of what will be presented in this chapter is consistent with these concepts. Moving towards wellness is one of the very ways most of the consequences of violence and injury can be prevented—resulting in continued years of optimal functioning and creative adapting. Recognition of the threats, consequences, and actions that can be taken to minimize the kinds of violence and injury discussed here can contribute to such adaptation.

Risk-Taking Behavior

Why are some individuals willing to take **risks** that can be such a threat to life and health? Let's examine some pertinent issues based on work by Dixon and Clearwater.[4]

Although risk may be real, individual perceptions of risk can vary from person to person, and from time to time in one person. Two different people may interpret a situation entirely different in terms of the potential for risk; with one concluding that there is very little risk and another that risk to health is dramatic. How many among us would walk a tightrope strung one thousand feet above the ground? How many of us would evaluate a risk the same at age forty as age twenty?

A second reason is that perceived reward can cloud the assessment of risk. Some people might be willing to work in vary hazardous environments (e.g., the clean-up following a nuclear accident in a reactor) for a high enough price, while others would not consider it at any price. Money, however, is only one form of reward that modifies our evaluation of risk. Taking risks in return for potential social admiration is another circumstance in which there is a potential for reward; and this is one that is particularly prevalent among young adults. Fighting is an example of the kind of behavior some engage in for this reason. Driving a car very fast may be the result of an attempt at social admiration or may be instigated by another type of reward—convenience.

In each case, a risk is evaluated by attempting to balance the rewards and the potential dangers. In the absence of a perception of threat, or when the potential rewards extend beyond the perceived risk, an individual will ordinarily fail to take the kinds of actions that reduce the threat of unintentional or intentional injury. Perhaps the most important thing that this chapter can do is to help you clarify your perception of risk so that you make daily behavioral choices that are appropriate to your continued optimal functioning.

Safety

The term **safety** refers to the minimization of risk while maximizing quality of life. To make safe choices in life, you must be able to accurately assess the risks of a given situation and be aware of the range of alternative choices that might decrease risk.

Safety experts often refer to the three Es in reducing risks associated with injury—engineering, education, and enforcement. The first—engineering—refers to all the measures that can be taken in the design and production of consumer products (e.g., clothing, motor vehicles) as well as measures designed to minimize risk from environmental exposure (e.g., unsafe roads,

Years of potential life lost: the difference between a person's life expectancy and that person's age at death. This is used as one measure of the consequences of early death.

Disability days: the number of days during a year when a person is not able to engage in his or her usual activities because of an injury or illness.

Risks: the probability or likelihood that injury, disease, damage, or other negative consequences will follow an action.

Safety: the application of knowledge, skills, and attitudes in any situation to minimize risks.

1. **Reduce deaths caused by unintentional injuries to no more than 29.3 per 100,000 people.** (Update: 29.2 per 100,000 in 1992, down from 34.7 per 100,000 in 1987.) (Special Target Populations: American Indians/Alaska Natives, Black males, White males.)

2. **Reduce deaths caused by motor-vehicle crashes to no more than 1.9 per 100 million vehicle miles traveled and 16.8 per 100,000 people.** (Update: 1.8 per 100 million vehicle miles traveled in 1992, down from 2.4 per 100 million vehicle miles traveled in 1987; 15.4 per 100,000 people in 1992, down from 18.8 per 100,000 in 1987.) (Special Target Populations: Children 14 years and under, People 15–24 years, People 70 years and over, American Indians/Alaska Natives, Motorcyclists, Pedestrians.)

3. **Reduce drowning deaths to no more than 1.3 per 100,000 people.** (Update: 1.9 per 100,000 people in 1991, down from 2.1 per 100,000 in 1987.) (Special Target Populations: Children aged 4 and under, Males 15–34 years, Black males.)

4. **Reduce residential fire deaths to no more than 1.2 per 100,000 people.** (Update: 1.5 per 100,000 people in 1991, down from 1.7 per 100,000 in 1987.) (Special Target Populations: Children 4 years and under, People 65 years and over, Black males, Black females, Residential fire deaths caused by smoking.)

5. **Increase use of occupant protection systems, such as safety belts, inflatable safety restraints, and child safety seats, to at least 85 percent of motor vehicle occupants.** (Update: 66 percent of motor vehicle occupants in 1993, up from 42 percent in 1988.) (Special Target Population: Children 4 years and under.)

6. **Increase use of helmets to at least 80 percent of motorcyclists and at least 50 percent of bicyclists.** (Update: 62 percent of motorcyclists in 1991, up from 60 percent in 1988; 5–10 percent of bicyclists in 1991, compared to 8 percent in 1988.)

Source: Data from *Healthy People 2000 National Health Promotion and Disease Prevention Objectives,* 1991; and from *Healthy People 2000 Review, 1993,* 1994. Department of Health and Human Services, Washington, D.C.

work hazards). Enforcement refers to adhering to the many regulations and laws that have been passed based on professional assessment of risk (e.g., traffic laws, use of child-proof product containers, and mandated waiting periods and background checks when purchasing firearms). Finally, education refers to the kinds of choices we make as individuals that can be affected by knowledge, attitudes, and skills which can modify the risks associated with injury (e.g., driving too fast, use of mood modifying substances while operating motor vehicles, and using violence to settle conflicts).

In this chapter you will be presented with an assessment of the risks related to unintentional injury, homicide, suicide, acquaintance rape, and domestic violence. Additionally, an array of safety recommendations will be offered that address engineering, education, and enforcement. It is our hope that you will gain insight into the importance of recognizing injury risks and making appropriate choices and adaptations.

Unintentional Injuries

Healthy People 2000 introduces its listing of year 2000 health objectives with the following points:[5]

1. Unintentional injury comprises a family of complex problems involving many different sectors of society. No single force working alone can accomplish everything needed to reduce the number of injuries.

2. Alcohol use is intimately associated with the causes and severity of many unintentional injuries. Efforts to reduce death and disability from unintentional injuries must be combined with efforts to reduce alcohol and other drug abuse.

Listed in table 9.1 are the primary objectives cited for college-age populations in the area of unintentional injuries.

The term that is most frequently used to describe unintentional injury has been the

Ten Leading Causes of Death by Age Group—1991

Rank	<1	1-4	5-9	10-14	15-24	25-34	35-44	45-54	55-64	65+	Total
1	Congenital Anomalies 7,685	Unintentional Injuries 2,665	Unintentional Injuries 1,739	Unintentional Injuries 1,921	Unintentional Injuries 15,278	Unintentional Injuries 14,774	Malignant Neoplasms 16,909	Malignant Neoplasms 39,922	Malignant Neoplasms 94,195	Heart Disease 597,267	Heart Disease 720,862
2	SIDS 5,349	Congenital Anomalies 871	Malignant Neoplasms 580	Malignant Neoplasms 526	Homicide 8,159	HIV 9,488	Heart Disease 12,397	Heart Disease 30,374	Heart Disease 74,985	Malignant Neoplasms 354,768	Malignant Neoplasms 514,657
3	Short Gestation 4,139	Malignant Neoplasms 526	Congenital Anomalies 279	Homicide 381	Suicide 4,751	Homicide 7,801	HIV 12,259	Unintentional Injuries 7,137	Bronchitis Emphysema Asthma 10,432	Cerebro-vascular 125,139	Cerebro-vascular 143,481
4	Respiratory Distress Synd. 2,569	Homicide 428	Homicide 138	Suicide 265	Malignant Neoplasms 1,814	Suicide 6,514	Unintentional Injuries 11,752	HIV 4,728	Cerebro-vascular 9,744	Bronchitis Emphysema Asthma 76,412	Bronchitis Emphysema Asthma 90,650
5	Maternal Complications 1,536	Heart Disease 332	Heart Disease 128	Congenital Anomalies 208	Heart Disease 990	Malignant Neoplasms 5,319	Suicide 5,767	Cerebro-vascular 4,720	Diabetes 7,011	Pneumonia & Influenza 68,962	Unintentional Injuries 89,347
6	Placenta Cord Membranes 962	Pneumonia & Influenza 207	HIV 69	Heart Disease 153	HIV 613	Heart Disease 3,425	Homicide 4,571	Liver Disease 4,450	Unintentional Injuries 6,556	Diabetes 36,528	Pneumonia & Influenza 77,860
7	Unintentional Injuries 961	HIV 155	Pneumonia & Influenza 68	Bronchitis Emphysema Asthma 78	Congenital Anomalies 449	Liver Disease 858	Liver Disease 3,591	Suicide 3,983	Liver Disease 6,047	Unintentional Injuries 26,444	Diabetes 48,951
8	Perinatal Infections 881	Perinatal Period 140	Bronchitis Emphysema Asthma 44	Pneumonia & Influenza 67	Pneumonia & Influenza 256	Cerebro-vascular 813	Cerebro-vascular 2,530	Diabetes 3,034	Pneumonia & Influenza 3,738	Nephritis 17,963	Suicide 30,810
9	Pneumonia & Influenza 607	Septicemia 91	Benign Neoplasms 39	Cerebro-vascular 52	Cerebro-vascular 219	Pneumonia & Influenza 759	Diabetes 1,553	Bronchitis Emphysema Asthma 2,337	Suicide 3,241	Athero-sclerosis 16,568	HIV 29,555
10	Intrauterine Hypoxia 599	Benign Neoplasms 76	Cerebro-vascular 34	HIV 35	Bronchitis Emphysema Asthma 209	Diabetes 658	Pneumonia & Influenza 1,444	Homicide 2,112	Nephritis 1,695	Septicemia 15,888	Homicide 26,513

Age Groups

Source: National Center for Injury Prevention and Control

CDC
CENTERS FOR DISEASE CONTROL AND PREVENTION

Figure 9.3: What Do You Think?

1. For which age group is injury (unintentional, homicide, and suicide) the biggest problem? How did you arrive at your answer?
2. For which age group is injury the least problem? Explain your rationale.
3. According to the data presented in this chart, which form of injury is the biggest health concern for people in the U.S. in general?

Source: Data from the National Center for Injury Prevention and Control, Centers for Disease Control and Prevention, Atlanta, GA.

word **"accident."** What is an accident? Is there really any such thing as an accident? The National Safety Council[6] defines accident as a "sequence of events which usually produces unintended injury, death, or property damage." There is, however, an important movement currently under way to help people recognize that there is no such thing as an "accident." What we call accidents are really the result of a series of events that could be prevented with appropriate attention to certain factors.

Unintentional injuries rank as the leading cause of death for every age group from one year to thirty-four years of age in the U.S. (see figure 9.3).[7] Motor-vehicle deaths account for more than 40 percent of all deaths for persons aged sixteen to nineteen.[8] Motor-vehicle deaths are the second leading cause of death for African-American males aged fifteen to forty-four (with only homicide exceeding this death rate). The death rate from all unintentional injuries among young people is almost double the death rate from the second leading cause of death for that group—homicide. Alcohol consumption is a major factor in motor-vehicle accidents resulting in serious injury and death. It is estimated that almost 25 percent of all fatally injured drivers have a blood alcohol concentration high enough to be considered legally intoxicated.[9]

Dixon and Clearwater[10] suggest that accidents are primarily social in nature— "that is, most factors that contribute to accidents are caused by people and thus can be eliminated." They further suggest that there is a mistaken belief among most that

TABLE 9.2   *Factors Contributing to Unintentional Injury*

Type	Contributing Factors
Traffic	Alcohol
	Speed
	Vehicle and road conditions
	Driver error
Fires	Smoking
	Cooking
	Heating defects
	Electricity defects
	Lightning
	Hazardous storage of products
	Inadequate or absent sprinklers
	Inadequate or absent smoke detectors
	Inadequate or absent fire extinguishers
Poisoning	Curiosity combined with inability to read
	Absence of child-proof caps
	Absence of Mr. Yuk warning stickers
	Mixing medications
Occupational hazards	Uneven surfaces
	Unguarded machinery
	Impeded means of egress
	Exposures to toxic chemicals

Source: Data from D. Leviton, *Horrendous Death, Health, and Well-Being*, 1991, Hemisphere Publishing Corporation, New York, NY.

accidents stem from only one cause; rather, each one is the result of many associated contributing factors. Table 9.2 contains a brief listing of some contributing factors, such as alcohol and road conditions.

Preventing Injury from Motor Vehicle Crashes

Strategies for preventing death and disability from motor vehicle crashes can be categorized using the three Es—engineering, education, and enforcement.

Engineering

In 1966 the National Traffic and Motor Vehicle Safety Act became law, creating and empowering the National Highway Traffic Safety Administration to set safety standards for new cars beginning with the 1968 model year. Since that time many safety improvements have been added to automobiles, including collapsible steering assemblies, dashboard padding, and dual braking systems.[11]

An important safety feature found in all new cars today are seat belts with shoulder straps. It is estimated that use of seat belts prevented 4,800 motor vehicle deaths and 120,000 serious injuries in 1990 alone.[12] If all automobile drivers and passengers correctly used the seat belts available in their vehicles, the decreases in death and disability would be even more dramatic. To be most effective, seat belts should be worn "over the shoulder, across the chest, and low on the lap."[13] Some automobiles are currently equipped with automatic seat belts, reducing the problem of motivating people to correctly "buckle up."

Air bags are another form of occupant protection that have been proven effective in preventing death and disability from motor vehicle crashes (see figure 9.4). Air bags are becoming a standard item on all cars; 90 percent of 1994 models came with driver-side air bags and 66 percent had front-seat passenger air bags as well.[14] Used in combination with seat belts, air bags offer important protection to car occupants. By

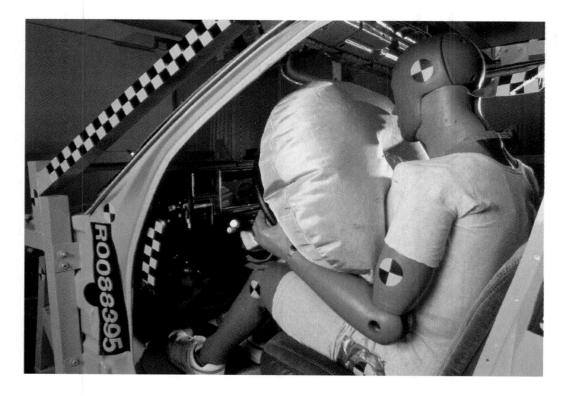

Figure 9.4: What Do You Think?

1. Continuing death and injury from automobile accidents have led to increased research, and now the availability of air bags in automobiles. Does the automobile you ride in most often have air bags?
2. Why do you think it took auto manufacturers so long to start putting air bags in all cars?

1999, air bags will be a requirement in all cars, pickup trucks, and vans sold in the U.S.

Education

Learning to drive defensively may be one of the most important skills you can acquire to prevent death and disability from motor-vehicle crashes. If you have not previously taken a driving course, it would be a good investment in your personal safety to consider it. Most communities have driving schools that teach **defensive driving skills.** To help you locate defensive driving schools in your area you can call the National Traffic Safety Institute at 800–732–2233 (west of the Mississippi River), or 800–334–1441 (elsewhere). Activity for Wellness 9.2 will help you determine how knowledgeable you are about defensive driving skills.

As discussed previously, driving while under the influence of alcohol dramatically increases the chances of becoming involved in a motor vehicle crash. Educational campaigns to prevent drunk driving, such as those sponsored by MADD (Mothers Against Drunk Driving), are important strategies for reducing drunk driving. Combining information dissemination with environmental changes, such as designated driver programs, as well as legislative strategies, appears to have the

greatest chance for reducing drunk driving. (Drinking and driving are discussed in more detail in chapter 15.)

Enforcement

Often, when safety hinges on human behavior, it is not enough to educate people about the safe alternatives. Sometimes mandatory measures are necessary to protect the health of the public. This is certainly the cases with motor vehicle crashes. The National Committee for Injury Prevention and Control recommends several mandatory measures aimed at reducing the death and disability associated with motor vehicle crashes. One strategy involves raising state and federal excise taxes on alcohol. This measure would have a great impact on alcohol-related death and disability in young people, who typically have less disposable income to spend on alcoholic beverages. It has been estimated that tax increases indexed to the rate of inflation could reduce deaths associated with alcohol-related motor vehicle crashes in young people eighteen to twenty years of age by 15 percent.[15]

The Third National Injury Control Conference[16] recommends that states adopt and enforce laws requiring the immediate surrender of a driver's license if a driver is found to have a **blood-alcohol concentration**

Defensive driving skills: specific skills necessary to reduce the likelihood of motor-vehicle crashes. These skills include specific acts taken with the assumption that other drivers or road and environmental conditions are likely to increase the risk (e.g., waiting to see if a car stops at a red light before proceeding through an intersection.)

Blood-alcohol concentration (BAC): a measure of the amount of alcohol found in the blood of an alcohol user.

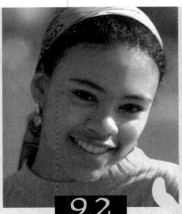

9.2

Activity for Wellness

Driving Like the Pros

Driving an automobile, or even riding in one, may be the most dangerous thing you do. At some time in their lives, according to the National Traffic Safety Institute, half of all Americans will be involved in a serious car crash, or will have an immediate family member involved in one. Seat belts, air bags, safer cars, and, of course, sobriety are prime elements in safety. Still, driving skills are an equally important element. You can learn to drive defensively: to avoid putting yourself in a dangerous situation, and to react intelligently in a crisis, should one develop.

Think of it this way: the safest driver of all may well be the professional racer. Though he's going 200 mph, he's wearing several seat belts, the chassis in his vehicle is a case of steel tubing, and most important, he's trained to react to danger up ahead. We can't all be racing drivers; yet we could be better drivers than we are. If you've never had a real driving course, and especially if your reaction time isn't as fast as it used to be,

defensive-driving training is worth considering. There are other potential benefits, too, besides being a safer driver: most localities will remove citations for moving violations, if any, from your permanent driving record when you complete a course. Most insurance companies offer graduates, particularly those over fifty-five, a break in premiums.

See how you fare on this quiz. (*Some questions have more than one correct answer.*)

1. The safest way to brake is
   a. as fast as possible.
   b. as far in advance as possible.
2. In moderate town traffic, with another car at a safe distance in front of you, you're being tailgated. What do you do?
   a. Tap the brakes and start to slow down—gradually, keeping an eye on the rearview mirror.
   b. Increase your speed to the allowable limit.
   c. Try to pass the car in front of you.
   d. Pull over to the right.
3. You're heading toward a green light at an intersection. A pedestrian (not in the crosswalk and walking against the light) steps off the curb and starts across without looking. Your first move is to
   a. sound the horn but don't give in. A little scare will do him good.
   b. change lanes to avoid him.
   c. begin braking, anticipating a full stop if necessary, and sound the horn.
4. Preparing to change lanes on a multilane highway, which of the following should you do?
   a. Check your rearview mirror.
   b. Check your side mirror.
   c. Take your eyes off the road momentarily and glance at the lane you're planning to move into.
   d. Turn on your directional signal.
   e. Be aware of what traffic in front of you is doing.

5. You've swerved to the right to avoid a collision on a two-way highway, and your right wheels drop off the pavement and are riding on the shoulder. To get back on the road you
   a. accelerate, cutting the wheel to the left.
   b. don't brake, but take your foot off the accelerator. Hold the wheel steady. When the car slows, check the traffic and steer back onto the pavement.
   c. brake sharply and try to pull off the road altogether. When you've got the car under control, pull onto the road again.
6. On a two-way highway, in what's clearly marked as a no-pass zone with limited visibility, a car pulls out to pass you, and you wonder if he's going to make it. Your best move is to
   a. speed up, hoping he'll duck behind you.
   b. ignore him—it's his problem.
   c. reduce your speed so he can get around you faster.
7. The *most* important factor in defensive driving is
   a. quick reflexes.
   b. anticipating trouble.
   c. skill at vehicle handling.
   d. strict observation of the law.
8. You're most likely to go into a skid
   a. in a steady downpour.
   b. in the first few minutes of a light rain.
9. Which of the following road conditions up ahead should tell you to reduce your speed?
   a. A deep pothole.
   b. Leaves on the pavement.
   c. Any bridge, when the temperature is just above freezing.
10. Your car is skidding (see diagram on p. 13). What's the safest reaction?
    a. Turn the wheel to the right.
    b. Turn the wheel to the left.
    c. Brake as hard as possible and avoid turning the wheel until you've stopped the car.

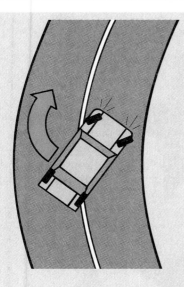

11. In two-way highway traffic, an oncoming car suddenly pulls into your lane. What action do you take?
    a. Brake hard and sound your horn.
    b. Move quickly into the left lane.
    c. Blow your horn, and head to the shoulder.
12. The best position for your hands on the steering wheel is
    a. at "10" and "2" o'clock position.
    b. at "8" and "4" o'clock.
    c. wherever you're most comfortable.
    d. at "9" and "3" o'clock.
13. True or false: Underinflated tires are safer, particularly in hot weather.
14. You realize you're heading into a curve too fast. Therefore you should
    a. brake sharply.
    b. brake gradually.
    c. avoid braking but take your foot off the accelerator.

Answers

1. (b) A basic principle of defensive driving is never to get into a situation that calls for slamming on the brakes. This can throw you into a skid and injure you and your passengers. Good braking technique: pump the brakes, reapplying as you come to a full stop. However, according to Professor Donald Smith, Highway Traffic Safety Program, Michigan State University, if you are forced to brake fast and have disc brakes, "threshold" braking is the best technique: push the brake just short of locking and hold it there.
2. (a) and (d), depending on circumstances. If the tailgater is daydreaming, tapping your brakes (and activating the brake lights) should wake him up. If he's being aggressive, you've politely signaled him to let up. If he doesn't stop tailgating, pull over as soon as you can and let him pass.
3. (c) Always yield the right of way to a pedestrian, even when he's in the wrong. Let him know you're there. A diversionary swerve could put you in the path of an oncoming car. Also, the pedestrian might dart into your pathway.
4. (all) All steps are essential, but some people forget (c). You always have a blind spot (about a car length behind you on either side) and may not be able to see an overtaking vehicle in either mirror. Always glance over your shoulder before making your move. The signal light (turned on several seconds in advance) will help protect you as well.
5. (b) Braking hard or jerking the wheel can cause you to skid into oncoming traffic. Don't brake but do reduce your speed and stay on a steady course. Then, after checking traffic, make a sharp quarter turn to the left to put yourself back on the road, then straighten out.
6. (c) Passing is always a cooperative venture. If this reckless driver has a head-on collision, you might be hurt, too.
7. (b) Obeying the law and vehicle-handling skills are all important. But anticipating trouble up ahead, and acting to prevent it, can make the speed of your reflexes far less important and thus may prevent many collisions.
8. (b) A little water plus the oil and dirt on the road form a slick film. A heavy rain will wash it clean. Be extra careful during the first half hour of a rainfall.
9. (all) The pothole may only jar you, but it could damage your car or even cause you to lose control. Leaves can send you into a skid. And even though there's no ice on the road, a bridge is about 6°F colder than a highway and may be hazardous when the road is not.
10. (b) Turn the wheel straight down your lane. That is, if your rear wheels are skidding left, as in the diagram, turn with the skid—that is, to the left. Don't brake, as this increases skidding.
11. (c) Don't move left, which could put you in someone else's pathway. Always more right when heading off the road.
12. (d) And some expert drivers recommend that you hook your thumbs lightly over the horizontal spokes. This gives you a feel for the front tires and is a good way to get a quick grip if you strike a pothole.
13. False. An underinflated tire is more likely to skid, whether in hot weather or on wet or icy pavement. Because underinflation allows a tire to "flap" slightly and thus to create more heat, it's also likelier to blow out. Even for desert driving, keep tires at the recommended maximum air pressure, and check them weekly. The number should be printed on the side of the tires; or check the instruction manual if the car still has its original tires.
14. (b) Take your foot off the accelerator, and brake before you get into the curve, but gradually release brakes as you get into it. Once you're rounding the curve, accelerate. This will help you steer safely around it and onto the straightaway.

Reprinted by permission from the *University of California at Berkeley Wellness Letter*, Health Letter Associates, 1989.

1. In many states, wearing a helmet
   while operating a motorcycle is
   required by law. These states have
   decided that safety education
   promoting helmet use is not
   enough—enforcement of the law is
   also required. Do you believe that
   motorcycle helmet laws are good?
   Explain your position.

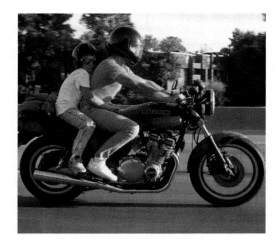

(BAC) of 0.08 percent or greater (0.00
percent for people under twenty-one years of
age). Additionally, the conference
recommends strict enforcement of minimum
legal drinking age laws, both for selling and
consuming alcohol. Also, the conference
supports mandatory seat belt, child safety
seat, and helmet laws as measures to reduce
death and disability due to motor vehicle
crashes (see figure 9.5).

We have focused so far on injuries that
are unintentional—what some people might
call *accidents*. Another category of injury,
however, merits our attention as a major
threat to health and well-being. Risk factors
for intentional injury, directed at oneself or
others, and strategies to decrease that risk will
be our final focus in this chapter.

Intentional Injury from Violent and Abusive Behavior

As stated earlier, violent and abusive
behavior includes suicide, homicide, sexual
abuse, elder abuse, spouse abuse, child abuse,
and many other forms of interpersonal
violence. Health professionals consider
violence and abusive behaviors to be
important public health problems. Table 9.3
provides an overview of some of the *Healthy
People 2000* objectives for the nation related
to this area. In this chapter, we focus on
several of these types of violence—suicide,
homicide, a form of sexual abuse known as
acquaintance rape, and domestic violence.

Suicide clusters: a group of suicides
that are related in some way (i.e.
occurring among a group of friends or
acquaintances, or in one geographic
location in a short period of time).

Suicide: Purposely Taking One's Own Life

Most attempts at suicide are unsuccessful, but
the actual number of suicides each day in the
U.S. may never be known with certainty. A
depressed and socially alienated person who
leaves a suicide note can be recorded as a
suicide statistic, but not all suicides are so
obvious. Is a drug-overdose an accident or a
suicide? Is a one-car accident on a clear day
and on dry pavement really an accident? One
cannot say for sure.

Why do different rates of suicide exist?
What causes one group of people to be so
much more prone to attempt suicide? Only
now are the answers to these questions
beginning to be explored. The explanation is
likely to be multifaceted and require
considerable investigation before causative
factors, rather than mere associated factors,
are clarified.

Typically, more suicides occur in the
month of April than in any other month,
possibly because of the sharp contrast
between a state of despair in the mind and
the awakening of spring. Because many
people are alone and lonely, the holiday
season around Christmas and New Year's Day
also has an elevated rate. Of all the major
religions in the U.S., the greatest proportion
of suicides is by Protestants, followed by
Catholics, then Jews. City dwellers are more
likely to attempt suicide than people residing
in rural settings. Military personnel are more
suicide prone than civilians, and persons who
have no children are at greater statistical risk
for suicide than people who do have children.
Suicide risk increases with age. Persons over
age sixty-five are the most likely to commit
suicide; however, youth constitutes a special
case. Suicides among youth are increasing
faster than for any other age group. Though
the eighth leading cause of death overall,
suicide is second in the fifteen- to nineteen-
year-old group. Although the suicide rate in
the general population has remained stable
for a decade, the rate among young people in
the U.S. is now 300 percent higher than the
rate forty years ago.[17] Relatively little is
known about the factors that contribute to
suicide in general and youth suicide in
particular, especially about **suicide clusters**
(see A Social Perspective 9.1). We do know,

1. **Reduce homicides to no more than 7.2 per 100,000 people.** (Update: 10.8 per 100,000 people in 1991, up from 8.5 per 100,000 in 1987.) (Special Target Populations: Children 3 years and under, Spouses 15–34 years, Black males, Hispanic males, Black females, American Indians/Alaska Natives.)

2. **Reduce suicides to no more than 10.5 per 100,000 people.** (Update: 10.9 per 100,000 people in 1992, down from 11.7 per 100,000 in 1987.)(Special Target Populations: Adolescents 15–19 years, Males 20–34 years, While males 65 years and over, American Indian/Alaska Native males.)

3. **Reduce weapon-related violent deaths to no more than 12.6 per 100,000 people from major causes.** (Update: 16.9 per 100,000 people in 1991, up from 14.8 per 100,000 in 1987.) (Special Target Populations: Firearm-related violent deaths, Knife-related violent deaths.)

4. **Reduce to less than 25.2 per 1,000 children the rising incidence of maltreatment of children younger than age 18.** (Baseline: 22.6 per 1,000 in 1987.) (Special Target Types of Maltreatment: Physical abuse, Sexual abuse, Emotional abuse, Neglect.)

5. **Reduce physical abuse directed at women by male partners to no more than 27 per 1,000 couples.** (Baseline: 30 per 1,000 couples in 1985.)

6. **Reduce assault injuries among people aged 12 and older to no more than 8.7 per 100,000.** (Update: 11.0 per 100,000 in 1991, down from 11.1 per 100,000 in 1986.)

7. **Reduce rape and attempted rape of women aged 12 and older to no more than 108 per 100,000 women.** (Update: 140 per 100,000 women in 1991, up from 120 per 100,000 women in 1986.) (Special Target Population: Women aged 12–34.)

8. **Reduce by 15 percent the incidence of injurious suicide attempts among adolescents aged 14 to 17 to a target of 1.8 percent.** (Update: 1.7 percent in 1991, down from 2.1 percent in 1990.)

9. **Reduce by 20 percent the incidence of physical fighting among adolescents aged 14–17, to a target of 110 incidents per 100 students per month.** (Baseline: 137 incidents per 100 students per month in 1991.)

10. **Reduce by 20 percent the incidence of weapon-carrying by adolescents aged 14–17, to a target of 86 incidents per 100 students per month.** (Baseline: 107 incidents per 100 students per month in 1991.)

11. **Reduce by 20 percent the proportion of weapons that are inappropriately stored and therefore dangerously available.** (No baseline data currently available.)

Source: Data from *Healthy People 2000 National Health Promotion and Disease Prevention Objectives,* 1991; and from *Healthy People 2000 Review, 1993,* 1994. Department of Health and Human Services, Washington, D.C.

however, that suicide is more prevalent in males, and in White males in particular (see figure 9.6).

Approximately eleven young adults in every 100,000 will succeed in committing suicide each year in this country. Looked at another way, more than 6,500 young people will take their own lives this year. Suicide attempts are about eight times more common than suicide completions. Whereas over 75 percent of those who commit suicide are

male, 60 to 70 percent of those who attempt suicide are female. Approximately 50 percent of those who attempt suicide are under thirty years of age, but 44 percent of those who commit suicide are over forty years of age.

Among minority groups, the rate of suicide is highest among Native American populations and the elderly female Asian populations. The age distribution patterns of suicides among American Indians and Alaska Natives is different than that of the general

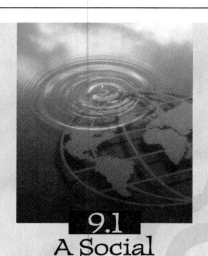

9.1
A Social Perspective

Is Suicide Contagious?

A relatively rare phenomenon, the youth suicide "cluster." has become a focus of research since the early 1980s. By one definition, a suicide cluster is "a group of suicides, suicide attempts, or both, that occur closer together than would normally be expected in a given community." Such clusters account for only about 1–2 percent of all suicides among adolescents and young adults. But the inherent drama of suicide claiming the lives of a locality's young people as if by contagion ensures that a cluster will receive wide coverage in the local—and sometimes the national—news media.

Charlotte Ross, executive director of the Youth Suicide National Center in San Mateo, Calif., cites a number of theories as to why a suicide cluster develops.* "[A]t any given time [there are] a number of people who are particularly vulnerable," she says. The triggering mechanism could be the sudden death of a friend or acquaintance, or even "a story in a newspaper, a film, a TV show, that either deliberately or inadvertently suggests that suicide is a solution to a problem."

Ross herself feels the forces setting a suicide cluster in motion are more complex than that. "One of the things that's not been sufficiently explored is the grief reaction of young people," she says. "It has certainly been underestimated how much young people grieve for their friends, how much they identify [with them]." Guilt also may play a pivotal role. "Many times, young people feel they should have done something" to prevent a friend's suicide, Ross says, "so they become depressed themselves."

While a suicide cluster is in progress, it can seem unstoppable as it seemingly feeds upon itself. But eventually it does end, prompting suicide-prevention experts to ask themselves, once again, "why?" Ross suggests the answer may be disarmingly simple: "You run out of highly vulnerable kids who are susceptible."

A 1989 study of two teenage suicide clusters that occurred in Texas earlier in the decade indicated how difficult it is to draw an all-purpose profile of at-risk young people. On the one hand, the 14 youngsters who committed suicide were more likely "to have had more than two different adults in the role of parents" than were the non-suicidal teenagers in a control group. This seemed to suggest a potential source of intra-family conflict. On the other hand, the "school performance, work performance [and] overall social relationships" of the suicides were similar to those of the control-group members. Some of the suicides were close friends, but others had had no direct contacts with the rest of their cluster. Further clouding the picture was a finding that the youths who committed suicide were less likely than control-group members to have watched television programs about suicide.

---

*Margaret O. Hyde and Elizabeth Held Forsyth, authors of *Suicide: The Hidden Epidemic,* theorized that the second and subsequent suicides in a cluster represent "a tragic plea for positive attention, an attempt to enjoy in death the same high status as the first suicide." They also suggested that some youngsters who are pulled into a suicide cluster "may harbor the 'magical' or juvenile belief that they are all powerful and can reverse death, can have death without dying." See Margaret O. Hyde and Elizabeth Held Forsyth, *Suicide: The Hidden Epidemic* (1986 edition), p. 32.

What Do You Think?

1. What do you think makes people so vulnerable that the suggestion of suicide can cause them to actually commit the act?
2. Describe what you think a rational approach to dealing with community education about suicide would consist of. How would the potential for inciting a "suicide cluster" be dealt with?

From "Teenage Suicide" in *CQ Researcher,* 1:374–375, 1991. Reprinted by permission of Congressional Quarterly, Inc., Washington, D.C.

---

population, with the greatest risk in the fifteen to twenty-four year age group. In the general population, the risk increases with age. The death rate for American Indian and Alaska Native youth has increased from 22.8 deaths per 100,000 in the years 1985–87, to a rate of 26.3 for the years 1989–91.[18] This rate is much greater than the general youth suicide rate of 13.1 per 100,000 in 1989–91.

Though there are many unanswered questions about causal relationships, the literature on Native American populations indicates that several factors appear significantly related to the high rates of suicide.[19] Cultural conflict or the difficulty all tribes have with relating to the dominant U.S. culture and the conflict created with their tribal customs, is one factor associated with Native American suicide rates. Rapid social change in U.S. culture has resulted in a breakdown and disorganization of tribal systems. This social disorganization is also associated with the high suicide rates. Additionally, unemployment and lack of meaningful work is an important factor. Native Americans have unemployment rates as high as 80 percent for some tribes.

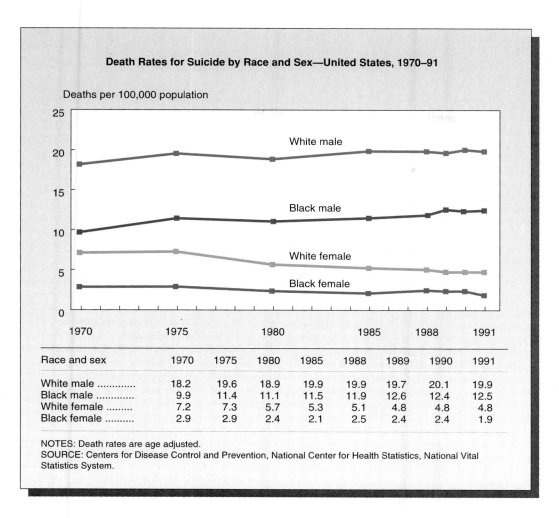

Death Rates for Suicide by Race and Sex—United States, 1970–91

Deaths per 100,000 population

Race and sex	1970	1975	1980	1985	1988	1989	1990	1991
White male	18.2	19.6	18.9	19.9	19.9	19.7	20.1	19.9
Black male	9.9	11.4	11.1	11.5	11.9	12.6	12.4	12.5
White female	7.2	7.3	5.7	5.3	5.1	4.8	4.8	4.8
Black female	2.9	2.9	2.4	2.1	2.5	2.4	2.4	1.9

NOTES: Death rates are age adjusted.
SOURCE: Centers for Disease Control and Prevention, National Center for Health Statistics, National Vital Statistics System.

Figure 9.6: What Do You Think?

1. Generally, what overall trend do you see for suicide rates in the United States from 1970 to 1991?
2. What trends do you see for women as opposed to men in terms of their suicide rates from 1970 to 1991?

Source: Data from National Center for Health Statistics, National Vital Statistics System (see related *Health, United States*, 1993, table 52). Centers for Disease Control and Prevention, Atlanta, GA.

Suicide Profiles

Who is likely to be a candidate for suicide? It is very difficult to tell since suicide is a complex behavioral pattern determined by biological, psychological, social, and environmental influences.[20] Our knowledge tends to be limited because of the difficulties associated with studying suicide behavior. But there are some things that we do know. Many teenagers who commit suicide do so following acute disciplinary crises, rejection, or humiliation.[21] Revenge or anger may also play a role. When young adults commit suicide, the target of their anger is often parents, a romantic partner, or someone else who may have rejected that person.[22] Some young people threaten suicide to manipulate the behavior of others, such as partners in a relationship, or to divert attention from family or marital conflicts.[23] Some suicide attempts occur in order for a young person to "atone for one's sins."[24] Another primary reason for suicide

attempts appears to deal with stress or loss of loved ones or when someone feels there is no other way out.[25]

Research suggests that the best indicator of the probability of suicide is behavior. Not a single behavior, but clusters of high-risk behaviors that are suggestive of suicidal tendencies. While all of the triggers of suicide remain somewhat in doubt, associated behavior changes and life crises, such as those just discussed, *may predispose some adolescents and young adults* to suicide.[26] Table 9.4 summarizes these potential triggers.

Suicide Prevention

How can you help a person who hints at suicide? First, all expression of suicide intent, talk of death, or threats about suicide must be taken seriously. If you know someone who has undergone noticeable behavior changes or has experienced a major life crisis or multiple crises you should be alert to warning signals. Friends should assume the role of

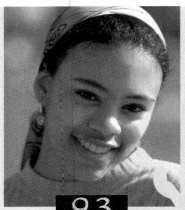

9.3
Activity for Wellness

Can You Tell Myth from Reality?

One way to minimize some of the problems we face is to recognize the potential for self-destructive behavior. Which of the following statements are true?

	True	False
1. Adolescents who talk about killing themselves rarely commit suicide.	___	___
2. The tendency toward suicide is inherited and passed from generation to generation.	___	___

	True	False
3. The suicidal person wants to die and feels that there is no turning back.	___	___
4. Suicidal people are mentally ill.	___	___
5. If someone attempts suicide, that person will always entertain thoughts of suicide.	___	___
6. If you ask an adolescent about suicidal intentions, you will encourage the young person to commit suicide.	___	___
7. Suicide is more prevalent among lower socioeconomic groups.	___	___
8. When a depression lifts, there is no longer any danger of suicide.	___	___
9. Suicide is a spontaneous activity that occurs without warning.	___	___

Answers
Each of these statements regarding suicide is a myth.

1. Many adolescents who commit suicide have indicated their intent; no threat should be ignored.
2. Suicide is a behavior, and is not inherited. Some disorders associated with the increased likelihood of acting on suicidal thoughts may be inherited.
3. Many people have sought help immediately following an attempted suicide.
4. There is a dramatic difference between being depressed or highly stressed and being diagnosed as mentally ill. Many who have attempted suicide could not have been diagnosed as mentally ill.
5. Most adolescents who have considered suicide do so for only brief periods in their lives. A young person who attempts suicide and survives, may never attempt it again with proper support and treatment.
6. Frequently asking a person about suicide will not only allow that person to unload built up anxiety and stress, but also reduce the likelihood of suicide.
7. Suicide does not discriminate by economic means.
8. Research suggests that the time of greatest risk of suicide is in the first three months after an adolescent begins recovery from severe depression.
9. Some youthful suicides may be spontaneous, but most are thought through in advance.

Revised and reprinted with permission, American Association of School Administrators, 1801 N. Moore St., Arlington, VA 22209–9988, (703) 875–0748.

responsive listeners rather than complain about the person's depression or distress. Help the person find sources of support through family members and other friends, churches or synagogues, suicide-prevention centers, campus counseling services, or community mental-health centers. A good friend should not operate alone in solving a problem or attempt to play therapist. Instead, help an individual inventory personal resources and urge him or her to seek assistance from an appropriate mental-health professional. A friend may need to be assertive enough to physically take a person to a place where professional help can be obtained. Table 9.5 summarizes the "Do's and Don'ts" of suicide prevention.

Homicide

Many people consider violence a societal disease. We may need to begin formulating our concept of violence as a public health problem and as a type of learned behavior. For more than a decade, there have been an average of more than 20,000 homicides in the U.S. per year—which is the highest rate of any industrialized nation in the world. Of these 20,000 deaths, more than

TABLE 9.4

Behavior Changes and Life Crises Associated with Youth Suicide

Behavior changes

Change in personal appearance
Insomnia or sleeplessness
Frequent somatic complaints
Decreased appetite or interest in food
Loss in concentration
Withdrawal from social situations
Expressions of hopelessness,
   worthlessness, depression, lack of caring
Mood swings
Increased use of alcohol or drugs
Academic failure
Frequent crying
Preoccupation with death or suicide
Giving away prized possessions or
   expensive items

Life crises

Death of a loved one
Separation/divorce of parents
Injury or illness of self or a loved one
Remarriage of a parent
Pregnancy
Moving
Romantic breakup
Severe disappointment
Severe physical or psychiatric illness
Failure at school or work

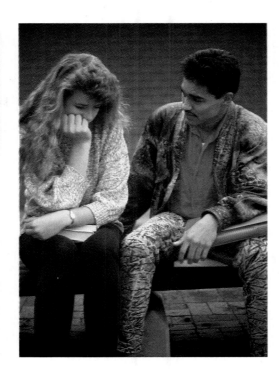

What Do You Think?

1. Suicide rates have risen dramatically for young people in the U.S. If you see signs of behavior change or life crisis in your friends or loved ones, do not ignore the possibility of suicide. What should the friend in this photo do if he suspects his friend is thinking about suicide?

African-American men and the lowest rates among White women. However, as Deborah Prothrow-Stith points out in her *Violence Prevention Curriculum for Adolescents,*

> when researchers have looked at the homicide rate in poor communities, it is always higher than in wealthier communities. And when poor communities in different parts of the country are compared, they often have about the same rate of homicide, regardless of the racial makeup of the community. A poor urban area that is largely White will have about the same homicide rate as a poor urban area that is largely Black.[29]

Among women, family members are most frequently the cause of the homicide; among men, acquaintances outside the immediate family are most frequently the cause. Table 9.6 contains a summary of some additional data on homicide that provides a clue to its nature. The most common known causes precipitating homicide, particularly among peers, are arguments, followed by homicide during the commission of another crime.[30] Contrary to most media accounts, gang violence and sexual assault appear to play a relatively small role in the overall picture of homicide in the U.S. today.

11,000 tend to occur between acquaintances (4,000 of these among family members) and the remainder (9,000) among strangers. It is worth examining some of the critical issues to help understand this phenomenon. For all races, homicide tends to be highest among twenty to thirty-four year olds; but for young adult African-American men, homicide is the leading cause of death.[27] There appear to be seasonal trends, with the highest rates of homicide occurring during the months of July and August,[28] which may be due to increased social contact during the summer months. Homicide rates are associated with race, with the highest rates among young

TABLE 9.5

Do's and Don'ts for Helping a Person Who Hints at Suicide

Do not ignore a suicide threat.

Do confront the individual if warning signs are present.

Do pay attention to signs of depression or isolation.

Do listen.

Do refrain from making judgments.

Do try to demonstrate that the negative feelings can pass with time.

Do allow the person to ventilate his or her feelings.

Do not leave the person alone.

Do express the loss you would feel if something happened.

Do let the person know that you care for him or her, no matter what has happened.

Do promise the person that you will not desert him or her.

Do mobilize the person's other friends and family members.

Do try to find out what has brought about the desperate feelings.

Do not react to suicide intent with horror or rejection.

Do not try "reverse psychology" by encouraging the act.

Do not try to argue the "merits" of suicide with the person.

Do not say that you "know how the person feels" if you have never been suicidal yourself.

Do not be fooled if the person says he or she felt really bad but suddenly feels "better."

Do not be afraid to get help, and get help immediately.

From Brent Q. Hafen and Kathryn J. Frandsen, *Youth Suicide,* Copyright © 1986 Cordillera Press, Evergreen, CO.

Preventing Homicide

The Prevention Workgroup on Assault and Homicide of the Surgeon General's Workshop on Violence and Public Health[31] made several important recommendations regarding the prevention of such violence. The Prevention Workshop believes that there should be a complete and universal federal ban on the manufacture, importation, sale and possession of handguns (except for authorized police and military personnel). Additionally, the manufacture, distribution, and sale of other lethal weapons such as martial arts items, knives, and bayonets should be regulated. Criminal penalties should be levied for possession of any weapon where alcohol is sold or served. The public should be made aware that alcohol consumption may also be hazardous to health because of its association with violence. A full employment policy should be developed and implemented for the nation, with immediate attention given to creating jobs for high-risk youths. Additionally there should be an aggressive policy to reduce racial discrimination and sexism. The cultural acceptance of violence should be decreased by discouraging corporal punishment at home, forbidding corporal punishment at school, and abolishing capital punishment by the state—all are models and sanctions of violence. Finally, the Prevention Workgroup recommends that there be a decrease in the portrayal of violence and violent role models on television and other media, and an increase in the presentation of positive, nonviolent role models.

Acquaintance Rape

Rape, the act of forcing someone to have sexual intercourse when he or she does not want to, is one of the most rapidly growing violent crimes in the U.S. One recent study estimated that 683,000 women age eighteen and older were raped in 1990.[32] Additionally, it is estimated that one out of every eight adult women will be raped sometime during their lifetime.[33] Women aged twelve to thirty-four appear to be particularly at risk for rape.[34]

There are many myths surrounding the crime of rape. Many people believe that most rapes are committed by strangers who attack victims when they are away from their homes. In fact, more than one-half of reported sexual assaults occur in the home—most often the victim's.[35] Additionally, most sexual assaults are committed by someone known to the victim. This is especially true of sexual assaults that occur on college campuses, where it is estimated that more than 80 percent of rapes are acts of **acquaintance rape.**[36]

Acquaintance rape is an important health problem on college campuses. Studies indicate that between 15 to 30 percent of

Acquaintance rape: an act of rape committed by someone known to the victim. The rapist may be a date, a friend, a family member, or casual acquaintance.

TABLE 9.6

Homicide Statistics and Characteristics

Homicide	Percentage
Involving handguns	50
Involving rifles	13
Involving knives or other sharp objects	19
Involving other weapons (e.g., fists)	18
Victims with alcohol in their blood	>50
Caused by arguments	47
Occurring during the commission of a crime	15
Related to youth gangs	1
With same race victim and assailant	90
With White victim	50
With Black victim	45
With victim and assailant in same family	20
With victim and assailant acquainted	55

(Involving handguns 50, Involving rifles 13, Involving knives or other sharp objects 19, Involving other weapons 18 bracketed = 100)

What Do You Think?

1. According to the data in this table, which activity will place you in the most danger of being a homicide victim?
2. Of the homicide factors listed in this table, which one does the media (television, newspapers, and magazines) present as the most dangerous threat to community well-being? Are there discrepancies between your answers to questions one and two? If so, please provide a rationale for the difference.

Source: Data from Deborah Prothrow-Stith, D.P., *Violence Prevention Curriculum for Adolescents,* 1987, Education Development Center, Boston, MA.

college women report having been a victim of forced sexual intercourse with someone they know.[37] Yet many college women do not label acts of forced sexual intercourse with someone they know as rape, and few victims tell anyone about what has happened to them. Many young acquaintance rape victims blame themselves, feeling that somehow it was their fault that they were sexually assaulted by a date or someone else they know. These victims may suffer severe psychological damage, including depression, anxiety, nightmares, sexual dysfunction, suicidal intentions, and fear in social situations.[38] Recent studies indicate that victims of acquaintance rape have higher levels of psychological distress than victims of stranger rape, and they tend to recover more slowly.[39]

Somehow society has not taught its young people that forced sex is *wrong* and that victims of sexual assault are *not* to blame. Several recent studies have investigated male and female attitudes toward acquaintance rape. These studies have found that some young men and women do not view acquaintance rape in the same manner as they do stranger rape. For instance, some students believe that acquaintance rape may be justified under certain circumstances and that the victim may be responsible. In a study of 400 Washington State University students, 19 percent of the men and 5 percent of the women believed that forced sexual activity might be acceptable "if the couple had been dating for a long time, if she had let him fondle her, if she wasn't a virgin or if she had 'led him on.' "[40] Such attitudes are formed early in life. A study of 1,700 students in Rhode Island, aged twelve to fifteen, revealed that one-fourth of the boys and one-sixth of the girls believed that if a man spent money on a woman on a date, he then had the right to force the woman to have sexual intercourse.[41] Attitudes such as these reflect a society that condones violence against women and has failed to teach its young people that forced sexual contact does not respect our fellow human beings and is *not* acceptable under any circumstances.

Preventing Acquaintance Rape

There are many safety precautions that both men and women can take to decrease the risk of being involved in an act of acquaintance rape. First, in dating situations know who you are going out with. If you do not know the person well, group dates and dates in public places with other people around are the safest. Do not let yourself be talked into going somewhere in private. This may increase the opportunity and pressure for sexual intimacy and decreases the chances that you could get help if you needed it.

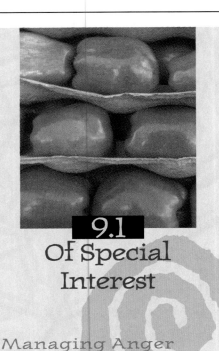

9.1
Of Special Interest

Managing Anger

Violence among young people is a complex problem with many causes and no simple solutions. It overlaps with other social problems whose victims are also disproportionately poor and African-American: racism, unemployment, inadequate schools and housing, alcohol and other drug abuse, teen pregnancy, and single-parent families. Until we can solve these problems, youth violence is unlikely to disappear. However, an innovative school program is teaching children and their parents to manage anger in more constructive ways.

Many children never learn how to deal with their anger nonviolently. Kids who grow up in families and societies where violence is the norm may not have the skills to resolve conflicts in other ways. Psychologists at Wright State University have developed a program called Positive Adolescent Choices Training (PACT) which is being incorporated into health education classes at nearby middle schools with primarily African-American students.* PACT's goal is to teach African-American children to avoid violence by talking instead of fighting. PACT participants use role play to learn how to peaceably handle disputes. For example, in one of the role plays a teenage boy confronts a friend who has insulted another friend. The students are directed to role play asking the friend to have a talk, during which the boy shares what he values about the friendship, states why he is angry, and proposes a possible solution to the problem. If the other boy doesn't like this solution, both boys talk until they negotiate a solution.

Preliminary studies show that PACT participants are better able to avoid violence and are less often suspended from school for fighting as compared to non-participants. But the students who show the most progress are those who have parents participating in a companion program known as Impact. Impact helps parents deal with their own anger towards their children in nonviolent ways. It stresses parental responsibility for disciplining children in positive, constructive, peaceable ways.

PACT and Impact are two promising school-based violence prevention programs. Long-term studies of their effectiveness, however, have yet to be conducted. Absence of social skills, such as anger management, is only one of many causes of youth violence. We must, as a community, begin to deal with the root causes of violence, such as unemployment and racism. However, until society is willing to commit resources to solve these complicated social problems, programs like PACT and Impact may help to minimize the death and disability due to violence.

What Do You Think?

1. Do you think that teaching children and youth how to manage their anger will decrease the homicide rate in the U.S.? Explain your thinking.
2. Why is it so difficult to address the other major causes of violence in the U.S.—poverty, unemployment, racism, drug abuse, and gun availability?

Source: From R. Henkoff, "Kids are Killing, Dying, Bleeding" in *Fortune,* August 10, 1992.

Communication of sexual desires and limits, by both men and women, is also important. When such desires and limits are not openly discussed, it is more difficult to communicate when the boundaries of one's personal space have been crossed. Patricia Rozée and her colleagues point out that women and girls may often be subtle and indirect in telling men when their sexual advances are unwelcome, and may therefore not be clearly communicating their message. For instance,[42]

standing or sitting uncomfortably when someone puts an arm around one's shoulders; changing the subject when a topic of conversation makes one feel uncomfortable; or answering questions vaguely that would have been better not asked.

It is important for women to immediately and clearly speak up and tell men when they do not like something that happens. Men should listen carefully and accept a woman's decision to refrain from sexual contact. Being turned down for sexual contact should not be viewed as a personal rejection. Accepting that when a woman says "no" to sexual contact it should be interpreted as "no," may help decrease the chances that acquaintance rape might occur.

stiffening the body and not returning an unwanted hug; crossing the legs and shifting position when someone's knee makes contact under a table or at the movies; turning the head so that a kiss headed for the lips lands on a cheek;

Avoiding the use of alcohol and other psychoactive drugs is another important strategy for preventing acquaintance rape. Several recent studies have found that the use of alcohol by the victim or the perpetrator of acquaintance rape is common. There are several important explanations for this finding.[43] First, many men expect to feel powerful and sexually aroused after drinking alcohol. Also, alcohol reduces people's capacity to analyze a situation and make sound decisions. Men may, for instance, easily misinterpret friendly cues from a woman as indicating a desire to have sex with him. Alcohol impairment can easily lead to misunderstandings about whether or not there was consent for sexual intimacy.

Alcohol impairment in the victim can also contribute to the risk of acquaintance rape. Women whose cognitive abilities are impaired from alcohol intoxication may miss important cues that her friendly behavior is being misinterpreted. An intoxicated woman may also be more likely to go to an isolated location where she will be less likely to be able to get help. Alcohol intoxication slows down a woman's cognitive and motor functions interfering with her physical ability to defend herself against rape. Clearly, all psychoactive drugs can interfere with the ability of both men and women to make sound judgments, and is best avoided.

What should a woman do if she has been raped? First, she should go to a safe place. Then she should call someone she trusts—a friend, family member, or rape crisis counselor—to be with her to help in dealing with the rape and its aftermath. It is important that both victims and trusted helpers remember that it is *not* the victim's fault that rape has occurred. The victim should be careful to preserve any evidence, including clothing she was wearing at the time of the rape. She should avoid showering, bathing, or douching, as this destroys evidence. The victim should go to a hospital emergency room for a medical examination and treatment as soon as possible. Counseling for the psychological effects is also important. Many cities have counselors who specialize in helping rape victims.

Acquaintance rape is a problem for both young men and women and for society in general. We need to begin to deliver the message—in our families, schools, and mass media—that forced sexual activity of any kind is wrong. Sexual assault, including rape, is an act of violence that should not be tolerated by society.

Domestic Violence: When Aggression Hits Home

Domestic violence is a serious and widespread problem that affects members of all social, economic, educational, racial, ethnic, and geographic groups. The American Public Health Association[44] defines domestic violence as:

> interpersonal abuse among family members who (1) have a structured social or familial relationship, which includes elder abuse, sibling abuse, child abuse, incest, and spouse abuse, or (2) have an intimate relationship.

Terms sometimes substituted for domestic violence include *family violence* and *intimate violence*. This type of injury-producing violence may consist of a single hostile act, or a series of aggressive episodes occurring over a long period of time, even years. It may produce physical injury, emotional injury, or other types of harm to the individual. Acts of violence may be overt, covert, or be represented simply as threat. Since acts of domestic violence encompass physical, emotional, and sexual abuse, as well as **incest** and neglect, and involve children, spouses, older people, and other groups, we will explore each of these in some detail.

Child Abuse and Neglect

In a little more than a decade, the number of reports of **child abuse** and **neglect** has risen by 50 percent. This increase results, in part, from better reporting and tracking methods, as well as more public awareness. The rise in cases also stems from more families living at or near the poverty level, abuse of alcohol or other substances, and diminishing resources available to families needing child protective services.[45] In a recent year there were nearly 3 million children reported as victims of abuse or neglect. There were about 1,300 child abuse and neglect related fatalities. About 86 percent of these deaths were to children under age five, and 46 percent of deaths were to children under one year of age.[46] Child abuse and neglect often reflects a *cycle of violence* in that the adult abuser was

Domestic violence: violence that is committed by and directed toward members of one's family or other individuals with whom there is an intimate relationship. Domestic violence includes partner abuse, rape, child abuse, elder abuse, and the like.

Incest: sexual relationships between close blood relatives, such as a father and daughter, or a brother and sister.

Child abuse: the maltreatment of children, which includes sexual maltreatment, as well as physical and emotional injury caused by improper care and discipline or neglect.

Child neglect: a type of child abuse that consists of failing to provide for the essential physical needs of a child, such as not providing adequate food or clothing.

1. What is the most common form of
child maltreatment (often called
child abuse) in the United States?
2. Did any of the data in this chart
surprise you? Explain your response.

Source: Data from the National Committee to
Prevent Child Abuse

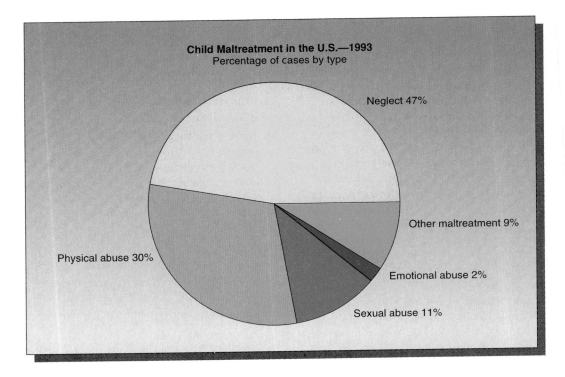

Child Maltreatment in the U.S.—1993
Percentage of cases by type

Neglect 47%

Other maltreatment 9%

Physical abuse 30%

Emotional abuse 2%

Sexual abuse 11%

himself or herself, abused as a child. A categorical breakdown of child abuse and neglect figures in the United States for a recent year is shown in figure 9.7.

Children are also the tragic victims of **sexual abuse.** Studies of adults suggest that anywhere from 6 percent to 63 percent of adult females were sexually abused as children.[47] Many child abuse experts agree that sexual abuse is the most underreported form of child maltreatment because of cultural taboos and historic laws against sexual activity with minors.[48] While females are more likely than males to be sexually abused, males are also victimized. Child sexual abuse perpetrators tend to be parents (77 percent) or other relatives (16 percent).[49] Frightening evidence is accruing that child sexual abuse even occurs at school, and like many other forms of sexual abuse, is underreported.[50]

Because of heavy media coverage, reports of child abuse in day-care centers or foster care centers have received national attention. It is important to bear in mind, however, that less than 1 percent of confirmed abuse cases occur in these facilities.[51]

Prevention and early intervention to reduce the level and consequences of child abuse and neglect are warranted. Among strategies for consideration are education programs for new parents (see chapter 7), including alternatives to corporal

punishment, special services programs for children with special needs (e.g., children with disabilities), more and better child day-care services for working parents, programs for abused children and young adults such as self-help and social support groups, and expanded family support care that includes crisis hot lines and counseling services.

Spouse and Partner Abuse

Relationship violence is a leading cause of injury for women.[52] A nationwide study revealed that 12 percent of wives had been assaulted by their husbands one or more times in the previous year.[53] The nature of partner abuse came to worldwide prominence during the 1995 murder trial of actor and former football star, O. J. Simpson, whose history of verbal and physical violence against his late ex-wife, Nicole Brown Simpson, was portrayed on television screens everywhere.

Annually within families, three to four million women are battered.[54] This figure is a conservative estimate of the actual total since surveys typically exclude non-English speakers, the very poor, people without telephones, and persons in hospitals or other institutions.

Partner abuse is the leading cause of injury among inner-city women between the ages of fifteen and forty-four years.[55] As many as one-third of women who go to hospital

Sexual abuse: any maltreatment of an individual that involves sexual coercion. This includes rape, incest, and any sexual activity between a child and an adult.

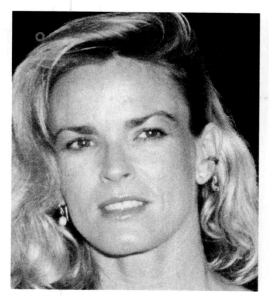

a.

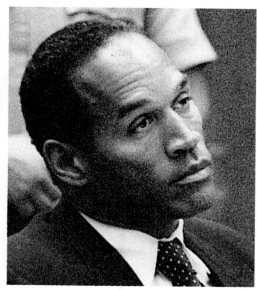

b.

What Do You Think?

1. Partner abuse may be more common than believed—crossing racial and socioeconomic lines. What effect do you believe the O. J. Simpson trial has had on domestic violence? What evidence has lead you to this belief?

emergency rooms do so because of symptoms stemming from ongoing abuse by a partner.[56] One estimate suggests that one-sixth of pregnant women in public health prenatal clinics have been abused in the past year.[57] Typically, victims of partner violence do not disclose their abuse.[58] As discussed earlier in this chapter women are the frequent recipients of sexual victimization and other forms of aggression by male acquaintances. A virtual epidemic of such sexual violence against women exists on many U.S. college and university campuses.

There are several important components to the successful intervention and prevention of partner abuse.[59] The provision of shelters and other safe environments for abuse victims, as well as comprehensive mental health and other health, legal, and social services for partner abuse victims, their children, and the abuser are essential. Treatments that take into account the diverse social, cultural, and economic needs of the abused and abusers are needed, as is better professional education of health-care practitioners for improved recognition and treatment of abuse. Finally, a justice system that holds abusers accountable for their violent behavior is essential to the prevention of death and disability related to partner abuse.

Elder Abuse

Of all forms of domestic violence and abuse, **elder abuse** may be the most difficult on which to obtain accurate figures.[60] Elderly victims are more likely to be unable or unwilling to report these episodes of maltreatment due to embarrassment, family loyalty, physical, emotional, or financial dependence on the perpetrators of abuse, fear of removal from the home, fear of social isolation, or fear of other negative repercussions.[61]

The factors that contribute to elder abuse are also not clearly delineated, but are presumed to be diverse. Caregiver burden and stress seem to place people at elevated risk of becoming an abuser. In addition, researchers have identified factors such as psychiatric illness and substance use as contributing to being a victimizer.[62]

Several elements are critical to protecting victimization of the elderly. First, **respite care** and older adult day-care services must become more plentiful and available to remove some of the burden from families that try to care for their older family members. Second, mechanisms that improve legal services, victim advocacy, and emergency and long-term shelter opportunities for older adults must be found. Case finding, case management, and crisis care for families and victims must become more systematic. Finally, better coordination of the justice system and other public agencies must occur.

Youth Violence

Violence and intentional injury have become predominant health problems among adolescent and young adult populations.[63] No prevention efforts have thus far demonstrated

Elder abuse: any maltreatment of elderly individuals, including sexual maltreatment, as well as physical and emotional injury caused by improper or violent care and neglect.

Respite care: temporary professional care provided for disabled individuals, with the intention of giving family caretakers a brief rest from caregiving responsibilities.

clear effectiveness.[64] In one study, violent behavior among African-American youth was associated with personal exposure to violence and victimization, hopelessness and depression, family conflict, corporal punishment, and self-assessed probability of still being alive at age twenty-five.[65] Violence among youth, however, is not uniquely a problem associated with race.[66]

According to a Centers for Disease Control and Prevention survey, 44.2 percent of high school youth reported having been in a physical fight during the preceding twelve months. When similar age youth not in school were assessed, the figure was 51.0 percent. Moreover, when weapon carrying was examined, 15.5 percent of school youth and 22.9 percent of nonschool youth indicated they had carried a gun, knife, club, or other weapon in the previous thirty days.[67] Initiatives to control youth violence are underway in many major U.S. cities, but presently, violence in schools, homes, and other settings is taking an upward course.

Addressing Domestic Violence Across Settings and Groups

Five sociological factors related to the cause of family violence have been identified. These elements include (1) high level conflict that goes hand-in-hand with family life; (2) male dominance in most family life, and society in general; (3) cultural norms that are tolerant of family violence and other forms of aggression; (4) the unintentional "training" that goes on in families that predisposes persons toward violence and aggression; and (5) the use of violence for socially-legitimate purposes.[68]

Many opinions exist as to how violence in general, and family violence in particular, should be treated. Possible interventions related to prevention and education, legal and judicial reform, and improved service diversity and delivery have been described. What may be most successful in the long run to curbing the trend of violence is the research that will shed more light on both the causes and the solutions.

Living Safer in a Dangerous World

Many dangers and risks exist in the complex world we live in. Some of the solutions to making this nation a safer place to live rely on governmental regulation and police protection. But you can do a great deal to decrease the risk that you will become an injury victim. Activity for Wellness 9.4 will help you assess your personal safety habits and help you determine where you need to improve your risk-reduction efforts.

As with other health-related behaviors, changes in your safety-related habits will not necessarily be easy. Table 9.7 will provide you with tips to guide you through the stages of behavior change.

It is clear that we live in a very dangerous world. While some threats are not within your personal control, there *are* many options available to you to decrease your risk of disability and death from intentional and unintentional injury (see figure 9.8). By taking responsibility for your safety and the safety of those around you, you are taking an important step toward wellness.

TABLE 9.7 — Tips for Making Changes in Your Safety Habits

Increasing safety precautions in your daily lifestyle is not an easy process. You will probably find that you go through a series of steps each time you try to make such changes. The following tips will help you as you progress through the stages of behavior change to enhance your chances for a safe and healthy life.

Precontemplation → Contemplation

If you have never thought about making safety changes or you do not intend to make any safety changes within the next six months you might want to consider:

- assessing your current safety-related behaviors to determine your strengths and weaknesses. Activity for Wellness 9.4 will help you determine how well you are protecting yourself against unintentional injury and violence.
- assessing your means of dealing with anger. The anger assessment located in the *Connections for Health Student Workbook* will help you determine if anger may be increasing your risk of injury.

Contemplation → Preparation

If you have been seriously considering making some safety changes but have not yet attempted any changes, try to thoughtfully answer the following questions:

- How do I think or feel about striving for a more optimal level of safety habits that help to decrease my chances of becoming an injury victim? Am I willing to change my lifestyle permanently to achieve this goal?

Preparation → Action

If you are ready to make some definite plans for improving your safety behaviors during the next month, or if you have already made small changes in the past but were not able to maintain those changes as a permanent part of your lifestyle, consider the following actions:

- Make a resolution to yourself to begin a certain safety change; for instance, make a commitment to yourself to stop becoming intoxicated by alcohol on dates to decrease your risk of being injured unintentionally or intentionally.
- Set a specific date to begin your new behavior, for example "starting Friday night, I will consume no more than one alcoholic beverage a day."

Action → Maintenance

If you have recently started to make some safety changes the following tips will help you continue on this healthy path:

- Write a behavior change contract, such as found in chapter 1, and find a support person who will help you keep with your plan; have your support person sign your contract.
- Give yourself rewards *often* for meeting your goals and objectives; rewards should be things you really enjoy, but that you are willing to do without if you do not meet your goal.

Maintenance

You have made important safety-related changes that you have practiced for six months or longer; now you need to focus on maintaining your healthy choices every day:

- Learn how to deal with inevitable lapses in your safety plan so that a lapse doesn't cause you to relapse permanently to a high risk lifestyle.

* Based on Prochaska, Norcross and DiClemente's transtheoretical model. See Prochaska, J. O., Norcross, J. C. & DiClemente, C. C. (1994). *Changing for Good.* New York: William Morrow and Company, Inc.

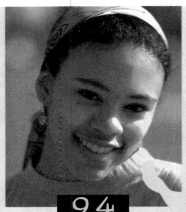

Activity for Wellness

How Safe Are You?

General Home Safety:
Answer each question with a YES or NO.

_____ 1. Should a child, teen, or woman alone answer a door to a stranger?

_____ 2. If you have a grease fire on the stove, should you stand back and throw water on it?

_____ 3. Is it appropriate to hide an extra key near your house or apartment door in case you lock yourself out?

_____ 4. When an electrical appliance smokes or sparks, should you unplug it immediately?

_____ 5. Are there any circumstances under which you could let another person use one of your prescription medicines?

_____ 6. For safety and violence prevention purposes, should you have locks on all of your bedroom doors?

_____ 7. Imagine you get a telephone call and the calling party says, "Sorry, I must have dialed the wrong number." Under this circumstance is it okay to give the person your phone number as long as you do not identify yourself?

_____ 8. Is 6 to 8 inches of bath water a safe level for a toddler?

_____ 9. If you have a swimming pool, is it acceptable to put a cover over the deep end when young children or nonswimmers are using the pool?

_____ 10. Is it acceptable to have candles to use in case of emergency blackouts?

Violence Prevention and Safety Practices for Those Home Alone:
Circle the letter(s) of the answer(s) that you believe to be the most correct response. (Some questions may have more than one correct response.)

11. If a child is home alone and a stranger calls and asks for a parent, the child should:
   a. hang up immediately.
   b. say "yes, they are home but busy; can I take a message?"
   c. say "no, but I can tell you how to get in touch with them."
   d. say "yes, but he or she is sick; can I take a message?"

12. You are home alone and a stranger knocks on the door and says through the door "hello, I have had an accident; can I use your telephone?" You should:
   a. get the number and make the call yourself.
   b. if your phone has a long cord, hand it out to the person.
   c. simply do not answer the door.
   d. tell the person to go to your neighbors.

13. Two children aged 8 and 10 are home alone. As the 10 year old is pouring juice, the glass bottle falls from his hands and breaks. He should:
   a. carefully pick up the glass—then wipe up the juice.
   b. use a broom and sweep it onto a dustpan and discard; wipe up the liquid.
   c. cover the mess and stay away from it—then show it to an adult as soon as possible.

14. You are home alone and fear someone is trying to break in. You should:
   a. immediately call 911.
   b. turn off all lights and hide.
   c. call 911 and sneak out another window or door.
   d. call 911 and yell that you have a weapon.

15. If you are at all concerned about being home alone, you should:
   a. tell someone about your fear and go over security procedures.
   b. turn on as many appropriate lights as possible.
   c. stay busy so you will not focus on fear.
   d. play the radio, stereo, or television.

16. If a child's babysitter breaks his parents' rules and drinks the parents' alcoholic beverages, the child should:
   a. tell the sitter that it is against the rules and he will have to tell his parents.
   b. hide all liquor or alcohol when the babysitter's attention is diverted.
   c. go to another room and ignore it.
   d. go to another room and then tell parents once they are home and the babysitter is gone.

Home Security Checklist
Answer YES or NO for any of the following questions that are relevant to your current living conditions.

Do You:

_____ 17. have and use automatic timers (at least 2) that go on and off at different but appropriate times?

_____ 18. have expensive or costly items (e.g., stereo equipment, computer hardware, quality art, silver, etc.) visible through any windows?

_____ 19. keep all doors locked even when you are there?

_____ 20. keep garage and utility doors locked at all times (except for time of immediate use) including when you are home?

_____ 21. have the outside of your dwelling well lit?

_____ 22. know your neighbors and have a communicative relationship with them?

_____ 23. always make sure your mail and paper are taken in at the appropriate times—even if you will be gone for a short time?

_____ 24. have an answering machine message that in no way implies you are "away" from your dwelling place?

_____ 25. have an answering machine that in no way implies that you live alone, or with another female (if you are female), or that you live alone with children?

_____ 26. appropriately store your valuables?

_____ 27. keep bushes, trees, and shrubs trimmed such that no one could hide without being seen?

_____ 28. have a visible (in large numbers) dwelling address?

_____ 29. have all security phone numbers (including police, fire, ambulance, and doctor) securely in place at all telephones in your house, apartment or dorm?

_____ 30. keep your car doors locked even when at your dwelling place?

_____ 31. (if you are a female) not list your first name in the telephone book?

_____ 32. keep your purse or wallet out of public viewing in your home?

_____ 33. have an in-place plan for what you would do if confronted with a potentially violent situation in your dwelling place?

_____ 34. know what you are supposed to do following a violent confrontation in your home?

_____ 35. keep anything that could be used as a lethal weapon out of sight?

_____ 36. if you have a gun, store your gun properly with both gun and ammunition hidden away in separate places?

Scoring

Explanations of correct answers follow. For each correct response to a question, give yourself one point. To determine your percentage of correct responses: (1) subtract the number of questions you omitted in Section III (Home Security Checklist) from 36, to determine your total number of questions; (2) divide the number of points you earned by the total number of questions you answered, and then multiply that number by 100.

95–100	Percent correct: **Excellent:** You have done a great deal to reduce the probability of injury in or near your home.
90–94	Percent correct: **Very Good:** You are well on your way to preventing injury in or near your home.
80–89	Percent correct: **Average:** Not bad, but a few extra steps can help secure your safety.
75–79	Percent correct: **Fair:** You are truly leaving too much to chance.
Below 75	Percent correct: **Poor:** You are endangering yourself, and possibly others.

Correct Answers:

Questions 1–10:

1. NO: Once you open the door, you would have little recourse to avoid confrontation or assault.

2. NO: This will just make the fire worse. You should respond by using a fire extinguisher which should be kept in the kitchen within easy reach of the stove. If the fire is out-of-control go to a neighbor's home and call 911 or your local fire department for help.

3. NO: Would-be thieves are accustomed to and knowledgeable about searching for hidden keys.

4. YES: This will help to prevent a fire.

5. NO: It is an unhealthy practice to share prescription medicine. A drug is prescribed with a particular disease and personal characteristics of the patient (height, weight, sex, previous health history, other medications, etc.) in mind. Additionally, there is always the possibility of an allergic reaction.

6. NO: There is too much of a chance that a small child could get locked in and not be able to get out by themselves. It may even be difficult for an adult to get in to rescue them. In addition, in case of a nighttime emergency, one's chances of safe escape are enhanced if they are not slowed down by having to unlock a door in a state of incomplete wakefulness.

7. NO: It is NEVER okay or appropriate to give an unknown person (by name _and_ voice recognition) your telephone number. This is true even for someone claiming to be a police officer, etc.

8. NO: No level of water in a bathtub for a toddler is safe _if_ that toddler is unattended for even the briefest time period.

9. NO: It is too easy for a person to get trapped under the pool cover.

10. NO: It is not acceptable to use candles, as they can get blown over or accidently knocked over, causing a fire.

Questions 11–16:

11. Answer = B
This response lets the caller believe adults are at home; thus, the child is less vulnerable.

12. Answer = C
Whenever you are home alone, never answer the door or let the person know that there's only one person at home. Even if the television and lights are on, do not answer the door. The "knocker" is likely to believe that the people inside are too involved to respond to the door. Do call 911 or the police and tell them a stranger came to your door reporting an accident had occurred.

13. Answer = C
Answer A is incorrect as there is too much chance of getting cut or slipping and getting injured. Answer B is incorrect as again, there is a chance of slipping on the damp floor or discarding the glass in a place that poses a hazard. The key is for adults to encourage children to perform the desirable behavior (Answer C) and to be honest. The adult should not punish the child who dropped the bottle, as this will encourage the children to lie or to try to clean up the mess, which puts the children at risk of injury.

14. Answer = A
If someone is trying to break into your home while you are there, you need to get help immediately! Answer B is incorrect as such behavior cues a would-be burglar that someone is, in fact, probably alone. Answer C is incorrect in terms of trying to sneak out. You may be caught by the intruder or an accomplice who are looking for other entry points to your home. Answer D is incorrect in terms of yelling that you have a weapon. Most people who are injured by an intruder's weapon have a weapon themselves. Not having a weapon decreases your chances of injury. Additionally, yelling that you have a weapon is likely to make an intruder believe that you are alone, and without a weapon.

15. Answer = All are correct and should be circled. Answer A is correct because having knowledge of security procedures and practicing them can increase your sense of security. Answer B is correct because lights may cause an intruder to believe that several people are in the house. Answer C is also correct. It is easy to create "self panic" if you dwell

Continued

unnecessarily on fears which are most often ungrounded. As the old saying goes, don't make mountains out of mole hills. Answer D is also correct, as the radio, music, or television will serve to distract you and will increase the chances that an intruder will believe more than one person is in the house.

16. Answer = D
Both answers A and B are incorrect, as they could inflame the babysitter causing him/her to do something that would put the child at risk. Answer C is also incorrect. If the child totally ignores this type of problem it could happen again, with potentially more dangerous outcomes such as a drunken fight. As answer D indicates, it is best to avoid the babysitter until the parents get home and the babysitter is gone. Yet, it is imperative that the child then inform the parents of the problem.

Questions 17–36:

17. YES: Automatic timers increase the chances that would-be intruders will believe that people are at home.

18. NO: Valuable items should not be easily visible through windows, as this invites trouble, even if people are obviously present.
19. YES: Many assaults and thefts occur because intruders simply "walk-up" and "enter" an unlocked door.
20. YES: Keeping garage and utility doors locked at all times prevents intruders from stealing, or from hiding and waiting for a better time to break into your home.
21. YES: Proper lighting decreases the probability of breakins, assaults, and "peeping Toms." A well-lighted area offers would-be criminals little or no security.
22. YES: Neighbors can better help each other in times of emergency if a cordial and trusting relationship exists.
23. YES: If you leave mail or newspapers to pile up, any number of people can and will know that your home is vacant. This increases the probability of theft.
24. YES: An answering machine that indicates you are away from home is an open invitation to theft.
25. YES: No one, male or female, adult or child, should let an unknown caller believe that they live alone or are

alone at home. Those who live alone are more often "targeted" for assault or theft.
26. YES: This will decrease the chances of having valuables stolen.
27. YES: Bushes etc. can be prime hiding places for intruders. Keeping them well trimmed will help to decrease the chances of assault, theft, or vandalism.
28. YES: Large and visible address numbers will help emergency personnel (police, fire, ambulances) more quickly and easily locate your home to offer their assistance.
29. YES: Valuable time can be lost searching for emergency phone numbers in a crisis. Keeping them posted by the telephone can save time, and maybe even a life.
30. YES: Keeping your car doors locked, even at home, can deter an intruder from breaking into the car to steal items or gain information about you or even "lay in wait" to assault you.

From the work of Karen King, Department of Public Health Education, University of North Carolina at Greensboro. Reprinted by permission.

Figure 9.8: What Do You Think?

1. How many of these risk reduction behaviors do you practice?
2. After reading this chapter, can you think of other risk reduction practices that should be added to this list?

Source: Data from *Closing the Gap: Homicide, Suicide, Unintentional Injuries, and Minorities,* Office of Minority Health Resource Center.

Risk Reduction Behaviors
Homicide, suicide, and unintentional injuries are health problems, and like other health problems, they have causes and risk factors. Although we still have a lot to learn, many public health researchers believe that individuals and families can reduce their risks in these ways:

Unintentional injuries
Wear safety belts and use child safety seats.
Discourage passengers from riding in open backs of pickup trucks.
Don't drink and drive.
Wear motorcycle helmets.
Use smoke detectors and check them monthly.
Install railings where falls may occur.
Swim only in designated areas and with other people.
Stop smoking (a primary cause of home fires).
Reduce tap water temperature to prevent burns.

Homicide
Choose television programs and other experiences for children that demonstrate appropriate and positive social behavior.
Obtain counseling for family conflicts.
Learn about effective, nonviolent child discipline methods.
Work to develop a community policy toward firearms.
Work to develop a community council on preventing violence.
Ask schools to institute violence prevention curricula.
Do not misuse alcohol and drugs.

Suicide
Obtain mental health counseling for depression.
Learn about community support groups, hotlines, and other mental health services.
Do not misuse alcohol and drugs.

Summary

1. More than two million people in the U.S. are victims of violent injury each year, with the U.S. ranking first among industrialized nations for such rates.

2. Unintentional and intentional injury are among the leading causes of death and disability in the U.S.

3. While the term *accident* is traditionally used to describe unintentional injury, it is perhaps not accurate enough when we recognize the series of events that must occur in order for such an outcome to take place.

4. Some individuals are more willing to take health risks than others. This may be due in part to the variety of ways that people interpret risk, as well as to the perceived rewards for taking a risk.

5. There are many factors that contribute to unintentional injury including variables such as alcohol use, human error, smoking, electrical defects, automobile and road conditions, and inadequate or absent safety devices such as smoke detectors.

6. The leading cause of death from unintentional injury is motor-vehicle crashes, over half of which are associated with the use of alcohol.

7. Death and disability from motor-vehicle crashes can be prevented by better engineering of the vehicles and roads, learning defensive driving skills, avoiding the use of alcohol when driving, and through enforcement of laws that mandate safety practices.

8. Suicide rates among young people in the U.S. have increased more than 300 percent over the past forty years. There are a number of behavioral clues that indicate someone is considering suicide.

9. If someone you know is showing signs of preparing to commit suicide it is important to listen to the person and help them find sources of support. Professional help should be sought; it may be helpful to offer to support the person by going with them to a health professional.

10. Homicide is now such a frequent cause of death and disability in young people that it is considered an important public health problem.

11. Homicides are most commonly precipitated by arguments among peers, or during the commission of another crime. Among women victims of homicide, the perpetrator is most often a family member; among male victims of homicide the perpetrator is most often an acquaintance outside the immediate family.

12. Recommended strategies for preventing homicide include gun control legislation and enforcement; a full-employment policy; reducing racial and sexual discrimination; discouraging corporal punishment; decreasing the portrayal of violence for entertainment; and teaching people how to cope with anger without violence.

13. Rape is one of the most rapidly growing violent crimes in the U.S. Acquaintance rape—being raped by someone you know—is especially troubling and a major form of sexual assault on college campuses.

14. Some strategies to help decrease the risk of acquaintance rape include avoiding the use of alcohol and other psychoactive drugs, communicating your desires and boundaries more clearly and assertively, and avoiding isolated environments where it is difficult to get help if needed.

15. An emerging type of violence is that in the home where children, spouses or partners, and older adults are the victims.

16. Violence among youth is one of the major health issues for persons under age twenty-five.

17. The world is a dangerous place; however, there are many factors that are within your control. Becoming more safety conscious will help decrease your risk of intentional and unintentional injury and may enhance your feeling of well-being.

Recommended Readings

Abbey, Antonia. "Acquaintance Rape and Alcohol Consumption on College Campuses: How Are They Linked?" *Journal of American College Health* 39 (1991): 165–69.

Acquaintance rape is an important health concern on college campuses today. Antonia Abbey discusses the prevalence of acquaintance rape on college campuses and then explores the link between acquaintance rape and alcohol consumption. Implications for preventing acquaintance rape are also discussed.

Leviton, D., ed. *Horrendous Death, Health, and Well-Being*. New York: Hemisphere Publishing Corporation, 1991.

This book examines the many causes of death that result from the actions of people, sometimes intentionally (e.g., homicide, war) and at other times unintentionally (accident, substance abuse). The authors of each chapter examine the economic, health, and well-being costs of these various causes of death at the national and global levels.

Warshaw, Robin. (1994). *I Never Called it Rape*. New York: HarperPerennial.

This easy-to-read book offers practical information on recognizing, fighting, and surviving date and acquaintance rape.

References

1. National Center for Health Statistics, *Prevention Profile, Health, U.S., 1989*. (DHHS Pub. No. [PHS] 90–1232. Hyattsville, Md.: USDHHS, 1990).

2. A. Toffler, *Power Shift* (New York: Bantam Books, 1990).

3. U.S. Department of Health and Human Services. *Healthy People 2000*. (Washington, D.C.: DHHS Publication No. [PHS] 91–50213, 1991).

4. M. I. Dixon and H. E. Clearwater. "Accidents," in *Horrendous Death, Health, and Well-Being*, ed. D. Leviton (New York: Hemisphere Publishing, 1991), 224.

5. USDHHS, *Healthy People 2000*, 270.

6. National Safety Council, *Accident Facts, 1986 Edition*. (Chicago: 1986).

7. DHHS. (1994). *Health, United States, 1993*. (Washington, D.C.: U.S. Government Printing Office).

8. *Injury Control in the 1990s: A National Plan for Action*. (May, 1993) (Association for the Advancement of Automotive Medicine).

9. Centers for Disease Control and Prevention. (1993). *MMWR Reprints*, pp. 15, 36, 50, 71.

10. Dixon and Clearwater, "Accidents," 222.

11. The National Committee for Injury Prevention and Control, *Injury Prevention: Meeting the Challenge* (Oxford: Oxford University Press, 1989):122.

12. Centers for Disease Control and Prevention. (1992). Increased safety belt use—United States, 1992. *MMWR* 41: 421–423.

13. The National Committee for Injury Prevention and Control, *Injury Prevention*, 130.

14. J. Poppy. (1994). The man who gave us the air bag. *Health* 8: 19.

15. The National Committee for Injury Prevention and Control, *Injury Prevention*, 126.

16. *Injury Control in the 1990s*, 33–35.

17. DHHS. (1992). *Youth Suicide Prevention Programs: A Resource Guide* (Washington, D.C.: U.S. Government Printing Office), 1.

18. DHHS, *Health, United States, 1993*, p. 107.

19. U.S. Department of Health and Human Services, *Report of the Secretary's Task Force on Black and Minority Health, vol. V: Homicide, Suicide, and Unintentional Injuries* (Washington, D.C.: U.S. Government Printing Office, 1985), 35–36.

20. T. C. Barrett, *Teens in Crisis: Preventing Suicide and Other Self-Destructive Behavior* (Arlington, VA: American Association of School Administrators, 9, 1989), 9.

21. Martti Heikkinen, Hilleve Aro, & Jouko Lonnqvist. (1993). "Life events and social supports in suicide." *Suicide and Life-Threatening Behavior* 23: 351.

22. Anthony G. Adcock, Stephen Nagy, & Janis A. Simpson. (1991). "Selected risk factors in adolescent suicide attempts." *Adolescence* 26: 818.

23. Barrett, *Teens in Crisis*, 9.

24. J. Landau-Stanton and D. M. Stanton, "Treating Suicidal Adolescents and Their Families," in *Handbook of Adolescents and Family Therapy*. (New York: Garner Press, 1985).

25. B. Q. Hafen and K. J. Frandsen, *Youth Suicide* (Evergreen, Colo.: Cordillera Press, 1986).

26. C. L. Tischler, P. C. McHenry, and K. C. Morgan, "Adolescent Suicide Attempts: Some Significant Factors," *Suicide and Life Threatening Behavior* 11.2(1981): 86–92.

27. DHHS. *Health, United States, 1993*.

28. Uniform Crime Report, *Crime in the United States* (Washington, D.C.: Department of Justice, Federal Bureau of Investigation, July 25, 1987).

29. Deborah Prothrow-Stith. (1987). *Violence Prevention Curriculum for Adolescents* (Boston: Education Development Center).

30. D. Prothrow-Stith, *Violence Prevention Curriculum for Adolescents* (Boston: Education Development Center, 1987), 24–25.

31. Foege, "Violence and Public Health," 53.

32. R. Hutcheson, "Study Says Rape Statistics Don't Paint True Picture," *Greensboro News and Record* (Friday, April 24, 1992) A1.

33. Hutcheson, "Study Says Rape Statistics Don't Paint True Picture."

34. DHHS, *Healthy People 2000*, 234.

35. North Carolina Crime Prevention Division, Department of Crime Control and Public Safety, "Sexual Assault and Prevention," undated brochure.

36. A. Abbey, "Acquaintance Rape and Alcohol Consumption on College Campuses: How Are They Linked?" *Journal of American College Health* 39 (1991): 165.

37. Abbey, "Acquaintance Rape and Alcohol Consumption on College Campuses: How Are They Linked?" 165.

38. D. G. Kilpatrick et al. "Rape in Marriage and in Dating Relationships: How Bad is it for Mental Health?" *Annals of the New York Academy of Sciences* Vol. 528 (August 1988): 335–344; C. A. Gidycz and M. P. Koss, "The Effects of Acquaintance Rape on the Female Victim," in *Acquaintance Rape: The Hidden Crime* ed. A. Parrot and L. Bechhofer (New York: John Wiley & Sons, Inc., 1991), 270–277; Hutcheson, "Study Says Rape Statistics Don't Paint True Picture."

39. B. L. Katz, "The Psychological Impact of Stranger versus Nonstranger Rape on Victims' Recovery," in *Acquaintance Rape: The Hidden Crime* ed. A. Parrot and L. Bechhofer (New York: John Wiley & Sons, Inc., 1991), 267.

40. J. Brothers, "Date Rape," *Parade Magazine* (September 27, 1987).

41. A. Rule, "Rape on Campus," *Good Housekeeping*, (September, 1989): 189, 240–242.

42. P. D. Rozée, P. Bateman, and T. Gilmore, "The Personal Perspective of Acquaintance Rape Prevention: A Three-Tier Approach," in *Acquaintance Rape: The Hidden Crime* ed. A. Parrot and L. Bechhofer (New York: John Wiley & Sons, Inc., 1991), 345.

43. Abbey, "Acquaintance Rape and Alcohol Consumption on College Campuses: How Are They Linked?" 166.

44. American Public Health Association, "9211 (PP): Domestic Violence," *American Journal of Public Health* 83.3 (1993): 458–463.

45. National Committee to Prevent Child Abuse, "Child Abuse Prevention," *National Association of Social Workers, Florida Chapter Newsletter* (March/April 1995): 16.

46. National Committee to Prevent Child Abuse, *National Association of Social Workers, Florida Chapter Newsletter*, 16.

47. National Committee to Prevent Child Abuse, *National Association of Social Workers, Florida Chapter Newsletter*, 16.

48. American Public Health Association, "9211 (PP): Domestic Violence," 459.

49. National Committee to Prevent Child Abuse, *National Association of Social Workers, Florida Chapter Newsletter*, 16.

50. Charol Shakeshaft and Audrey Cohan, "Sexual Abuse of Students by School Personnel," *Phi Delta Kappan* 76.7 (1995): 512–520.

51. National Committee to Prevent Child Abuse, *National Association of Social Workers, Florida Chapter Newsletter*, 16.

52. Centers for Disease Control, "Family and Other Intimate Assaults," *Morbidity and Mortality Weekly Report* 39.31 (1990): 525–529.

53. M. A. Straus and R. J. Gelles, *Physical Violence in American Families: Risk Factors and Adaptions to Violence in 8,145 Families*, (New Brunswick, NJ), 1990.

54. American Medical Association Council on Scientific Affairs, "Violence Against Women: Relevance for Medical Practitioners," *Journal of the American Medical Association* 267 (1992): 3184–3189.

55. American Public Health Association, "9211 (PP): Domestic Violence," 459.

56. Virginia P. Tilden, Terri A. Schmidt, Barbara J. Limandri, Gary T. Chiodo, Michael J. Garland and Peggy A. Loveless, "Factors that Influence Clinicians' Assessment and Management of Family Violence," *American Journal of Public Health* 84.4 (1994): 628–633.

57. J. McFarlane, B. Parker, K. Koeken and L. Bullock, "Assessing for Abuse During Pregnancy," *Journal of the American Medical Association* 267 (1992): 3176–3178.

58. Tilden et al., "Factors that Influence Clinicians' Assessment and Management of Family Violence," 628.

59. American Public Health Association, "9211 (PP): Domestic Violence," 461.

60. American Public Health Association, "9211 (PP): Domestic Violence," 459.

61. American Public Health Association, "9211 (PP): Domestic Violence," 459.

62. American Public Health Association, "9211 (PP): Domestic Violence," 459.

63. C. E. Koop and G. D. Lundberg, "Violence in America: A Public Health Emergency," *Journal of the American Medical Association* 267 (1992): 3076–3077.

64. M. L. Rosenberg, P. W. O'Carroll and K. E. Powell, "Let's Be Clear: Violence is A Public Health Problem," *Journal of the American Medical Association* 267 (1992): 3071–3072.

65. Robert H. DuRant, Chris Cadenhead, Robert A. Pendergrast, Greg Slavens and Charles W. Linder, "Factors Associated with the Use of Violence among Urban Black Adolescents," *American Journal of Public Health* 84.4 (1994): 612–617.

66. Durant, Cadenhead, Pendergrast et al., "Factors Associated with the Use of Violence among Urban Black Adolescents," 612.

67. Centers for Disease Control and Prevention, "Health Risk Behaviors Among Adolescents Who Attend and Do Not Attend School—United States, 1992," *Morbidity and Mortality Weekly Report* 43.8 (1994): 129–132.

68. American Public Health Association, "9211 (PP): Domestic Violence," 459.

Disorders of the Cardiovascular System: Influencing Your Odds

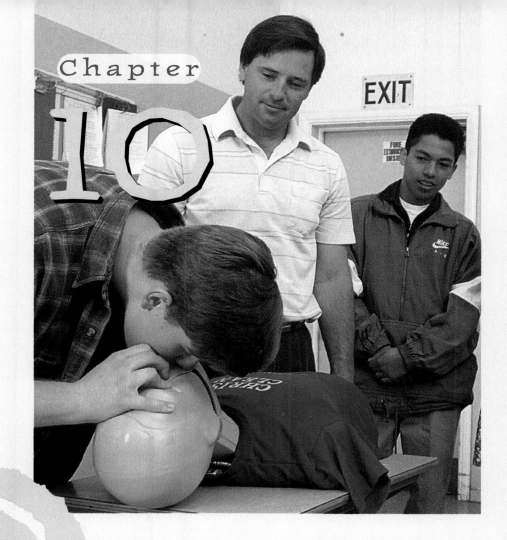

Chapter 10

Student Learning Objectives

Upon completion of this chapter you should be able to:

1. identify the health objectives of the nation for the year 2000 concerning cardiovascular disease;

2. describe the characteristics of normal heart function;

3. identify disorders affecting the cardiovascular system;

4. describe the symptoms of a heart attack and the appropriate emergency actions to follow;

5. explain how behavior patterns established or maintained during the college years influence risk of cardiovascular disease and premature death later in life;

6. list the major modifiable risk factors for cardiovascular disease;

7. identify potential barriers to cardiovascular disease risk reduction for you as a college student and for other adults;

8. identify several activities or behaviors that can lower your risk of premature cardiovascular disease onset and death;

9. estimate your risk of heart disease and stroke;

10. describe some of the major costs associated with failing to prevent premature cardiovascular disease;

11. compare and contrast cardiovascular disease morbidity and mortality for various special population groups.

Cardiovascular disease is responsible for more deaths in the U.S. than any other cause. Many of these deaths are premature deaths; that is, deaths occurring sooner than the typical life expectancy. Even if death is not an immediate consequence of cardiovascular disease, limitations on one's years of productive life can be imposed. The factors that influence development of diseases of the heart and circulatory system should be of particular interest to young adults in college and university settings since control of most of the relevant health compromising behaviors is still within their grasp.

In this chapter we will concentrate on wellness enhancement, delaying the onset of cardiovascular disease for as long as possible, and the implementation of practices that minimize the risk of cardiovascular disease formation altogether. We will not address the techniques of treating persons who have advanced levels of cardiovascular disease, except to illustrate the economic and medical futility of technological interventions when they are compared to prevention efforts.

In *Healthy People 2000* the health objectives for the nation that relate to cardiovascular disease prevention and control have been established. Some of these objectives are identified in table 10.1. As you examine the objectives that can be influenced by behavior change, ask yourself which activities are ones that you could improve in your own life. Notice too how some objectives have been specially targeted for African-Americans, Hispanics, Asian Americans, and Native Americans.

What Is Cardiovascular Disease?

The cardiovascular system consists of the heart, lungs, and a network of blood vessels that carry blood to the various parts of the body. Cardiovascular disease manifests itself in a variety of ways. All of the conditions listed below are examples of disorders related to the heart and the circulatory system:

- hardening of the arteries (arteriosclerosis)
- high blood pressure (hypertension)

- heart attack (myocardial infarction)
- chest pain (angina pectoris)
- irregular heartbeat (arrhythmia)
- stroke (cerebrovascular accident)
- congestive heart failure
- rheumatic heart disease
- congenital heart defects

Before we explore some of these disorders, however, it is useful to examine the function of the normal heart.

Normal Heart Function

The heart is a four-chambered muscular organ, a little larger than your fist, that continually pumps blood through the circulatory system. A heart contracts about 100,000 times per day and moves more than 4,300 gallons of blood through the body. If you can think of moving that same number of full gallon containers with great force, you can get some sense of the amount of work that the heart performs.

In humans and other mammals, the heart is divided into a left and a right side. Each side contains an **atrium,** a chamber in which blood collects, and a **ventricle,** a chamber that contracts to pump blood out of the heart. The right atrium receives **deoxygenated blood** concentrated with carbon dioxide from the body. This blood moves from the right atrium into the right ventricle, where it is pumped to the lungs to exchange its carbon dioxide for oxygen. Oxygen-rich blood moves from the lungs to the heart's left atrium and subsequently moves into the left ventricle. The left ventricle is the largest and most muscular of the heart's chambers. Its contractive force must be great enough to pump blood throughout the body (see figure 10.1).

The circulation of blood begins in the heart and lungs, moving oxygen and nutrients through **arteries, arterioles,** and **capillaries** to provide nourishment for the cells of the body, then through **venules** and **veins** back to the heart to repeat the process. You can think of the heart as a pump that "squeezes" blood through the body. The most vital part of the heart is the muscle itself, called the **myocardium.** Like all of the body's muscles, the myocardium must use oxygen and nutrients to do its work. The myocardium,

Arteries: blood vessels with elastic properties that carry blood away from the heart.

Arterioles: microscopic branches of the arterial system that connect arteries to capillaries.

Capillaries: the thinnest and most numerous type of blood vessel, and the site where gas and nutrient exchange occurs.

Venules: microscopic branches of the venus system that connect the capillaries to the veins.

Veins: blood vessels that receive blood from venules and return it to the heart.

TABLE 10.1

Selected Healthy People 2000 Objectives for the Nation Related to Cardiovascular Health and Disease

1. **Reduce coronary heart disease deaths to no more than 100 per 100,000 people.** (Update: 118 per 100,000 people in 1991, down from 135 per 100,000 in 1987.) (Special Target Population: Blacks.)

2. **Reduce stroke deaths to no more than 20 per 100,000 people.** (Update: 26.1 per 100,000 people in 1992, down from 30.4 per 100,000 in 1987.) (Special Target Population: Blacks.)

3. **Increase to at least 50 percent the proportion of people with high blood pressure whose blood pressure is under control.** (Update: 21 percent of people 18 and older for 1988–1991, up from 11 percent of people aged 20–74 for 1976–1980.) (Special Target Population: Males with high blood pressure.)

4. **Reduce the mean serum cholesterol level among adults to no more than 200 mg/dL.** (Update: 205 mg/dL in people 20–74 years for 1988–1991, down from 213 mg/dL for 1976–1980.)

5. **Reduce the prevalence of blood-cholesterol levels of 240 mg/dL or greater to no more than 20 percent among adults.** (Update: 20 percent of people aged 20–74 for 1988–1991, down from 27 percent for 1976–1980.)

6. **Reduce dietary fat intake to an average of 30 percent of calories or less and average saturated fat intake to less than 10 percent of calories among people aged two and older.** (Update: 34 percent of calories from total fat and 12 percent of calories from saturated fat for 1988–1991, down from 36 percent of calories from total fat and 13 percent of calories from saturated fat for 1976–1980.)

7. **Reduce overweight to a prevalence of no more than 20 percent among people aged twenty and older and no more than 15 percent among adolescents aged twelve–nineteen.** (Update: 33 percent for people aged 20 and older in 1988–1991, up from 26 percent of people aged 20–74 in 1976–1980; 21 percent for adolescents aged 12 through 19 in 1988–1991, up from 15 percent of adolescents in 1976–1980.) (Special Target Populations: Low-income women aged 20 and older; Black women aged 20 and older; Hispanic women— Mexican American, Cuban, and Puerto Rican—aged 20 and older; American Indians/Alaska natives; people with disabilities; Women with high blood pressure; and Men with high blood pressure.)

8. **Increase to at least 30 percent the proportion of people aged six and older who engage regularly, preferably daily, in light to moderate physical activity for at least thirty minutes per day.** (Update: In 1991, 17 to 24 percent of people aged 18–74 with number of days of exercise ranging from 5 to 7, up from 12 to 22 percent in 1985.) (Special Target Population: People 18–74 years.)

9. **Reduce cigarette smoking to a prevalence of no more than 15 percent among people aged twenty and older.** (Update: 27 percent in 1992, down from 29 percent in 1987.) (Special Target Populations: People with high school education or less 20 years and over; Blue-collar workers 20 years and over; Military personnel; Blacks 20 years and over; Hispanics 20 years and over; American Indians/Alaska natives; Southeast Asian males; Females of reproductive age [18–44 years]; Pregnant females; Females who use oral contraceptives.)

10. **Increase to at least 90 percent the proportion of adults who have had their blood pressure measured within the preceding two years and can state whether their blood pressure was normal or high.** (Update: 76 percent of people 18 years and over in 1990, up from 59 percent in 1985.)

11. **Increase to at least 75 percent the proportion of adults who have had their blood cholesterol checked within the preceding 5 years.** (Update: 63 percent of people aged 18 and over had their blood cholesterol checked in 1991, up from 59 percent in 1988; 50 percent of people age 18 and over reported they had had their blood cholesterol checked within the past 2 years as of 1991, down from 52 percent in 1988.)

Source: Data from *Healthy People 2000 National Health Promotion and Disease Prevention Objectives,* 1991; and from *Healthy People 2000 Review 1993,* 1994. Department of Health and Human Services, Washington, D.C.

Figure 10.1: Your heart and how it works

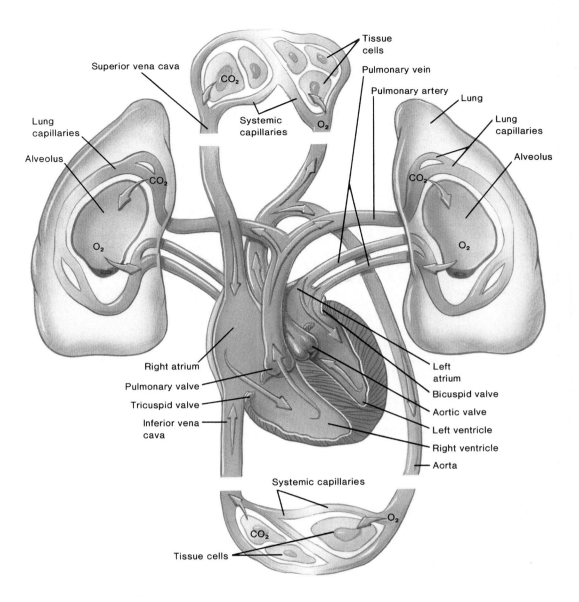

however, is unable to use the blood in the chambers directly. Instead, oxygen and other nutrients are supplied by **coronary arteries.** These arteries originate at the base of the **aorta,** the largest artery of the body, through which blood is pumped as it leaves the heart's left ventricle.

The pumping action or "beat" of the heart is regulated by a natural pacemaker consisting of specialized cells that generate electrical impulses. These tiny electrical impulses coordinate the contractions of the ventricles.

Each time the left ventricle contracts, blood flows into the heart because of the change of pressure. Valves between the atria and the ventricles open to permit blood to flow. When the ventricle receives the electrical impulse to contract, the valves between both atria and ventricles are closed by the pressure, and the blood is forced out of the heart to the lungs from the right ventricle, and to the rest of the body from the left ventricle.

Cardiovascular Disorders

As described above, the cardiovascular system is a network that delivers oxygen and nutrients throughout the body. Cardiovascular disease occurs when any one of a number of events takes place. Some of the things that can go wrong include a partial or complete block in the coronary arteries or elsewhere in the body, a loss in the pumping force of the heart muscle, a malfunction of the valves, or an alteration of the heart's electrical activity. Some cardiovascular diseases occur more commonly than others and are discussed in this chapter.

Arteriosclerosis

Arteriosclerosis, commonly called "hardening of the arteries," includes several conditions all of which produce a thickening of the walls of the arteries and a loss in elasticity. The most frequently seen form of this disorder is **atherosclerosis** (see figure 10.2).

Atherosclerosis is not something that happens only to middle-aged or old people. In reality, it is a lifelong process in which the walls of the arteries become thickened by deposits of fat, minerals, and other cellular debris. These deposits form what are called **plaques,** and actually injure the arterial walls. Some people seem to be especially sensitive or predisposed to the formation of plaques early in life. A diet that is high in fat, especially saturated fat, also may contribute to the early development of atherosclerosis (see chapter 3). As atherosclerosis progresses, arteries become less elastic, thereby prohibiting blood from moving smoothly and making blood more susceptible to forming clots. When a blood clot blocks or occludes one of the coronary arteries, the result is called a **coronary thrombosis,** one example of a heart attack.

Similarly, a clot in an artery of the brain may produce a **cerebral thrombosis,** a form of stroke.

High Blood Pressure

By definition, blood pressure is the force exerted against the walls of the arteries as the heart contracts and relaxes. The force is measured in millimeters of mercury (mm Hg), and a "typical" blood pressure is 120/80 (read 120 over 80). The "120" refers to the force exerted by the blood just as the heart contracts, and is called the **systolic** pressure. The "80" refers to the force exerted when the heart muscle is relaxed and is called the **diastolic** pressure.

When arteries are narrowed or become partially blocked, as in atherosclerosis, blood does not flow easily through them. As a result, the heart must pump harder to exert the same force to move the blood. This process increases blood pressure above normal levels. If this pressure elevation is maintained, the result is **hypertension,** or high blood pressure.

The conditions of hypertension and atherosclerosis are closely linked. As arteries narrow due to plaque formation, blood pressure increases. As blood pressure increases, arterial walls become increasingly damaged leading to the formation of still more plaques. Once underway, the process is hard to modify. High blood pressure can

Plaque: a yellowish swollen area in the arterial wall formed by deposits of lipids and other debris.

Figure 10.3: What Do
You Think?

1. Several blood pressure readings are
   necessary before hypertension can be
   diagnosed. Have you had your blood
   pressure measured recently?
2. What preventive activities could you
   begin now to decrease the risk that
   you will become hypertensive? If you
   already have high blood pressure,
   what activities will help you reduce
   your blood pressure?

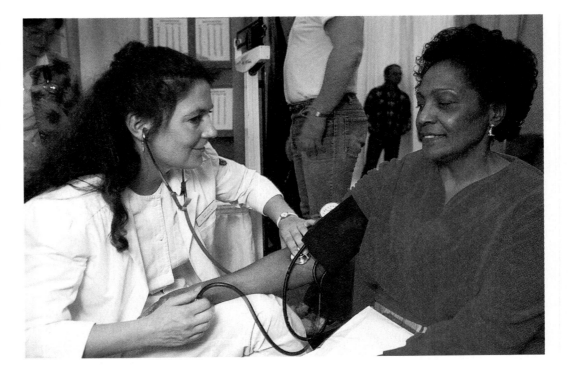

enhance the likelihood of an **aneurysm,** an
abnormal dilation or outpocketing of a major
artery, such as the aorta. An aneurysm can
burst. If it does, there is little chance for the
victim to survive since the internal bleeding
is so rapid and massive. Aneurysms may be
correctable by surgery, but not without
concurrent risk.

How "high" is high blood pressure? Health-
care providers disagree about the answer. A
person whose systolic pressure is consistently
above 160 mm Hg or whose diastolic pressure is
consistently above 95 mm Hg may have
hypertension. The American College of
Cardiology is more conservative in specifying its
upper limits of "normal," and suggests that
either a systolic pressure over 140 or a diastolic
pressure over 90 signals a problem.

One can never rely on a single blood
pressure measurement to diagnose
hypertension, as blood pressure can be
affected by a variety of circumstances. Stress,
exercise, and certain drugs may cause short-
term increases in blood pressure. Anxiety
over visiting a health-care provider, even
having one's blood pressure taken, can cause
a rise. A health-care professional ordinarily
will assess blood pressure on three or more
occasions before making a diagnosis of
hypertension (see figure 10.3).

Several steps can be taken to combat
hypertension if you are predisposed to
developing high blood pressure. First you can
avoid foods heavily concentrated in sodium.
Weight loss in obese persons also can help to
control high blood pressure. Most health
professionals attempt to control hypertension
through diet and exercise modifications
before introducing prescription drugs.
(Chapters 3, 4, and 5 provide many
suggestions for decreasing dietary sodium,
maintaining optimal body weight, and
participating in aerobic exercise.) People
should follow their health-care provider's
advice, for too often, people with
hypertension either fail to realize it, or fail to
take decisive action to control it.

Hypertension has been called the "silent
killer" because it often has no major signs or
symptoms. Many people never realize they
have high blood pressure until extensive,
even life-threatening damage has occurred.
Therefore, it may be useful to monitor your
blood pressure on a regular basis—several
times per year. The wide availability of home
blood pressure devices makes this practice a
realistic **secondary prevention** measure. If
you decide to purchase a home blood pressure
device, avoid cheap and unreliable
equipment (see chapter 18).

Secondary prevention: activities that
detect a disease condition early so that
the duration and severity of the disease
can be shortened.

Unfortunately, the mechanisms in the development of hypertension are not well understood. One estimate is that between 90 and 95 percent of all cases of hypertension are of unknown origin.[1]

Heart Attack

A heart attack is the result of any one of many cardiovascular disorders that can affect the heart muscle. The most common of these disorders is **coronary artery disease,** also known as **coronary heart disease (CHD)** or **ischemic heart disease.** It occurs when the coronary arteries are unable to supply the heart with an adequate supply of blood, as in the advanced stages of atherosclerosis. In this circumstance, known as **ischemia,** the person's health may be seriously threatened. A blood clot may form in a narrowed coronary artery, thus blocking the flow of blood to the heart muscle. When heart muscle cells are deprived of oxygen due to insufficient blood flow, those cells die. This type of heart attack is called a **myocardial infarction** or **MI.** If the blocked artery is a major blood supplier to the heart, the result may be sudden death or serious heart damage. This event is what some people describe as a massive coronary.

The heart appears able to develop a limited backup system for obtaining blood flow when an artery is blocked. This system is known as **collateral circulation.** Collaterals are tiny vascular channels that connect with major arteries. Normally, they carry little blood. However, if blood flow in a major artery becomes restricted, the small collaterals dilate and attempt to compensate for the impaired artery. How many collaterals the heart possesses, and to what extent they can compensate for a major arterial block are questions that continue to be researched.

Symptoms of a heart attack may vary but generally include one or more of the following events. The hallmark symptom of a heart attack is severe chest pain. Survivors have described the pain as "crushing" or "viselike" and compare it to what an elephant sitting on one's chest might feel like. The pain may radiate to other areas of the upper body, especially the jaw, shoulder, and arms. A person may experience dizziness, nausea, or even vomiting. The person may appear pale and cold but have beads of perspiration on the forehead. The pulse may be weak but rapid, and the person may begin to go into **shock.**

If you are with an individual experiencing severe chest pain, especially in combination with other symptoms, you should seek *immediate* emergency care. Many persons die unnecessarily each year because they fail to recognize symptoms and get help. You should know how to get in touch with the local emergency medical system. Such knowledge includes the telephone number of the fire-rescue service or having the number written in several prominent locations in your home. In most areas you can contact the emergency system by dialing 911, a central dispatch number for all emergency situations. Persons with a known heart condition should record emergency numbers when staying in hotels or other places away from home. This knowledge may be lifesaving in a variety of emergency situations.

A heart attack may be so severe that heartbeat and breathing cease. This situation is called **cardiac arrest,** and requires immediate action to maximize any hope of recovery. When such a crisis occurs, the well-prepared individual is in a position to perform **cardiopulmonary resuscitation (CPR).** CPR combines mouth-to-mouth resuscitation with closed heart massage in an effort to maintain breathing and circulation for the victim until help arrives. Physicians, nurses, and emergency medical and paramedical personnel have used CPR effectively for years. It is a skill that almost any layperson can and should learn. It is a *specialized* skill, however, that requires appropriate preparation and practice. Persons can find out more about CPR training by contacting local chapters of the American Red Cross or American Heart Association. Many hospitals and universities also offer citizen training and practice in CPR (see figure 10.4).

Angina

Another consequence of CHD is recurring chest pain known as **angina pectoris,** or simply, **angina.** Such pain occurs when restricted blood flow to the heart occurs. Angina may not be a constant source of discomfort for the person with CHD, but serious episodes can arise during periods of stress, emotional upset, physical exertion, or

Ischemia: a lack of sufficient blood flow to an organ resulting in an inadequate oxygen supply to that organ.

Shock: a situation in which blood flow is inadequate to return sufficient blood to the heart for normal function; associated with injury, trauma, heart attack, and other conditions; produces rapid but weak pulse, and shallow breathing; can be life-threatening if not addressed by proper first aid and advanced care.

Angina: chest pain, often characterized by heaviness and squeezing sensation as well as a numbness and tingling, caused by lack of oxygen (ischemia) to the heart muscle.

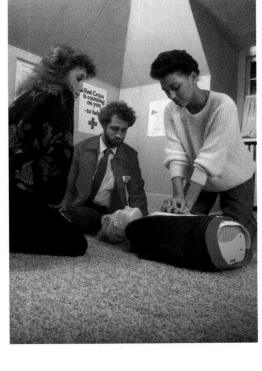

Congestive heart failure: inability of the heart to pump out all the blood that returns to it. Blood backs up in the veins that lead to the heart and fluid may accumulate in tissues, especially the lower extremities.

Edema: swelling due to an abnormal amount of fluid in body tissues. May be a side effect of congestive heart failure.

Cerebral arteries: arteries that carry blood, oxygen, and nutrients to the brain. Blockage in one of these arteries gives rise to a stroke.

Transient ischemic attack (TIA): a small stroke-like event that lasts only for a short time and is caused by a partially blocked blood vessel. A person having a TIA acts confused, dizzy, or loses short-term memory temporarily.

other circumstances when the blood supply demands of the heart are increased. Angina's discomfort often can be controlled by the self-administering of oral medication which dilates the constricted arteries. The absence of immediate relief following the introduction of the drug is a signal that a more serious heart-related event may be taking place, and requires immediate medical attention.

Arrhythmia

Arrhythmia means an irregular heartbeat. Normal heartbeat is regulated by electrical impulses originating in specialized bundles of cardiac cells. This system can malfunction, however. In extreme cases of electrical misfiring, the heart experiences a life-threatening situation known as **fibrillation.** During fibrillation, the pumping action of the ventricles is so irregular and insufficient that adequate circulation cannot be maintained. Minor problems in the heart's electrical conduction system are now controlled by drug therapy or by implantation of a small **pacemaker** device. The pacemaker is a battery operated unit that produces the electrical impulses that generate the appropriate heart rhythm.

Congestive Heart Failure

Congestive heart failure occurs when the heart muscle becomes damaged because of a heart attack, atherosclerosis, hypertension, rheumatic fever, or congenital heart defects. Damaged heart muscle lacks the contractive force to circulate blood properly. A failing heart may continue to work for years but does so less efficiently than a healthy heart. As the rate of blood flow decreases, blood returning to the heart "backs up," producing congestion or swelling in selective tissues. This accumulation of fluid in the tissues, called **edema,** occurs most often in the ankles and feet. However, fluid also may accumulate in the lungs (*pulmonary edema*) and result in labored breathing. Congestive heart failure reduces the kidneys' ability to excrete water and sodium, compounding the fluid retention and edema. A failing heart can lead to a heart attack.

Treatment for congestive heart failure requires multiple approaches. Some of these include rest, dietary changes, modification of daily activities, and drug therapy. Congestive heart failure can be a major confounding factor if an individual has other health compromising conditions under treatment. In the most advanced or extreme stages of congestive heart failure, treatment is limited to heart transplant surgery, and the long-term prognosis is poor.

Stroke

A **stroke** results from damage to arteries supplying blood to the brain. Blockage of **cerebral arteries** can produce death of the cells ordinarily nourished by these arteries. Such cell death is termed a stroke. If many brain cells are destroyed, the result may be partial paralysis, speech impairment, other psychomotor dysfunction, or death. Minor strokes occur if blood flow to the brain is reduced. A small stroke like this, called a **transient ischemic attack (TIA),** presents symptoms such as temporary dizziness, sensory loss, or confusion, and may be a forerunner of a more serious stroke.

In a recent year more than 500,000 people in the U.S. experienced a stroke and about 145,000 people died from one.[2] Men have a higher risk of stroke than women, but women who take oral contraceptives, and women who smoke increase their risk.[3]

African-Americans have a higher rate of death and disability due to stroke than do Whites, possibly because a high proportion of African-Americans have high blood pressure.[4] Sex and race factors cannot be controlled, but other factors that contribute to the risk of stroke can. Existing heart disease increases risk because an adequate supply of blood may not reach the brain, and because there is an increased likelihood of the formation of blood clots. Good management of existing heart disease, and prevention of it in the first place, are critical risk-reduction activities. Persons with **diabetes** (see chapter 11) have a higher risk of stroke than people without diabetes. Therefore, management of diabetes through diet, exercise, and proper medication are important measures.

Rheumatic Heart Disease

Rheumatic heart disease (RHD) usually results from bacterial infection of one or more layers of the heart, including the myocardium. RHD characteristically strikes children and youth four to eighteen years old about two weeks following a strep throat infection.[5] The myocardium can become inflamed and perform at a less than optimal level. An inner layer of the heart, the **endocardium,** also can be affected. When the endocardium is involved the heart valves, which regulate the flow of blood from chamber to chamber, may fail to open or close completely, producing a condition known as **stenosis.** The turbulence caused by blood rushing through a malfunctioning heart valve can be heard as a **heart murmur** with the help of a stethoscope. Even if the acute phase of this disease is treated successfully, the valves may become scarred, and thus, become sites where bacteria can accumulate and grow in the future to produce further damage. Replacement of defective heart valves may become necessary for normal life expectancy to occur.

Congenital Heart Disease

Congenital heart malformations occur in approximately 0.7 percent of live births and 2.7 percent of stillbirths.[6] A child born with a congenital heart malformation may suffer from inadequate oxygenation of the blood, and have a flesh tone that appears to be blue or dusky grey. Another congenital defect may be an incomplete formation of a septum, the partition between the heart chambers. Atrial and ventricular septal defects both can occur. Other malformations which affect heart performance also can occur. As one might guess, defects that are not treated surgically are likely to reduce life expectancy significantly.

Cardiovascular Disease: Personal and Social Influences

The best answer to the problem of cardiovascular disease is prevention. Although we cannot control all of the biological factors that contribute to cardiovascular disease, we can minimize many of the personal and social risks that play a role in CHD.

Scientists can identify several lifestyle factors that promote the development of cardiovascular disorders. Many people, however, have a difficult time following recommendations to decrease risk. Some people are "locked" into lifestyle patterns that are deeply rooted in tradition and habit. Others take on a fatalistic view of life, noting that "we all have to die sometime." Still other people ignore or reject any sense of susceptibility to cardiovascular disease, or engage in wishful thinking that whatever malady befalls them will be treatable by medical science. A growing number of people in the U.S. *are* recognizing that they can seize control of their lives, make conscious decisions concerning wellness lifestyles, and engage in practices that produce highly satisfying lives, while significantly reducing risk of premature illness. Some of these lifestyle options available to us are presented here.

Smoking

The more a person smokes, the greater is his or her likelihood of having a heart attack or stroke. Thus, someone who smokes a pack of cigarettes per day is at greater risk than someone who smokes just a few cigarettes. The most prudent choice is not to smoke at all. The death rate from heart attack is more than twice as high for smokers as for nonsmokers.[7] Smoking is the lifestyle factor that contributes most to cardiovascular diseases.

Diabetes: a chronic disease of the pancreas in which the body is unable to utilize sugars and other carbohydrates normally.

Rheumatic heart disease: damage done to the heart, particularly the heart valves, following one or more attacks of a strep bacterial-induced disease, rheumatic fever.

Endocardium: inner surface of the lining of the heart.

Stenosis: the constriction of a blood vessel or a heart valve.

Heart murmur: the abnormal sound made by the heart, particularly a heart valve, when blood passes through a damaged or constricted area as may occur following an episode of rheumatic fever.

Congenital heart malformations: defects in the heart that are present at birth.

Most smokers who have sustained the habit over time may have either a psychological or a physical dependence or both. The level of **nicotine** in tobacco is sufficient to cause physical addiction of the typical smoker.[8] Thus, many smokers find smoking cessation to be difficult. Moreover, newspaper and magazine advertisements, the inexpensive availability of tobacco products, and the presence of fellow smokers all undermine the best efforts. Chapter 15 provides more detail about tobacco and provides some tips for smoking cessation.

Hypertension

As noted earlier in this chapter, high blood pressure enhances the development of atherosclerosis and other disorders. Hypertension causes the heart to work harder. Persons who are aware of their hypertension should take medication as prescribed, eliminate excess sodium from their diet, and maintain an optimal body weight. However, many college students may not know that they have hypertension. A Purdue University study found elevated blood pressure in 9 percent of the males and 1.8 percent of the females screened.[9] Blood pressure monitoring provides regular feedback concerning the status of disease.

As with smoking many people have a hard time in changing their eating patterns, especially decreasing their sodium consumption. Practically every restaurant and home in the U.S. (unlike many other countries) has a salt shaker on the dinner table. Using the salt shaker liberally adds to the already high sodium content of many foods which were previously canned, frozen, or otherwise preserved. To assist health conscious people, sodium-free seasonings and spices can be substituted for salt without sacrificing flavor or taste. Chapter 3 provides many helpful suggestions for decreasing your sodium intake. Additionally, chapters 4 and 5 will help you in your goals of achieving optimal body weight and regular participation in aerobic exercise.

Dietary Fat

In chapter 3, we presented a detailed explanation of various types of fats. As many as 40 to 45 percent of the caloric intake of some persons in the U.S. is in the form of fat—about 10 to 20 percent more than what

is recommended.[10] Studies indicate that cardiovascular disease is lower in populations that consume less **trans-fatty acids** and **saturated fat.**[11] Consumption of these types of fat contributes to elevated levels of **blood cholesterol,** especially **LDL cholesterol** and **triglycerides.** It is also a factor in the development of obesity. Obesity itself does not affect the heart directly, but excess weight increases blood pressure, and inflates blood-cholesterol and blood-sugar. A person whose total blood-cholesterol exceeds 250 milligrams per deciliter (mg/dL) has three times the risk of premature heart attack as a person whose cholesterol is in the desired range (<200 mg/dL). With moderate dietary changes, exercise, and the maintenance of an optimal weight, cholesterol and triglycerides often can be maintained at levels that are health promoting.

While you have to be alert to your total blood-cholesterol (<200 mg/dL), you have to be aware of your relative levels of LDL and **HDL cholesterol.** According to the National Heart, Lung, and Blood Institute[12] (NHLBI) LDL levels below 130 mg/dL are desirable, while levels beyond 160 mg/dL are considered high. High LDL adversely affects risk of heart disease. Sustained HDL levels below 35 mg/dL are considered dangerously low. Generally, the higher the HDL the lower the risk of heart disease. Average HDL levels for men and women in the U.S. are 45 mg/dL and 55 mg/dL respectively. The mean total blood-cholesterol level for the U.S. population is 213 mg/dL, placing the population at risk of cardiovascular disease.

The NHLBI recommends that all adults over age twenty have their blood-cholesterol levels measured. While home cholesterol kits can estimate total cholesterol with reasonable accuracy, they do not partition it into LDL and HDL fractions. Therefore, having this test performed at a laboratory under the supervision of a health-care provider is recommended. People with undesirable HDL and LDL levels may be encouraged to make changes in their diet and physical activity, and may even be prescribed drugs to help manage their cholesterol.

Many U.S. college students and others are discovering that low fat, and even predominantly vegetarian meals are both less costly and deliciously refreshing when

Trans-fatty acids: a form of fatty acid derived from the process of hydrogenating food. These fatty acids, when consumed in foods, are believed to increase total and LDL cholesterol, and decrease HDL cholesterol, thus increasing a person's risk for coronary artery disease.

LDL cholesterol: low density lipoprotein; a type of lipoprotein that carries cholesterol from the digestive tract to other body cells. A high blood LDL level is associated with an increased risk of coronary artery disease.

Triglycerides: a fat compound that consists of three fatty acid molecules attached to a glycerol molecule. Triglycerides are stored in fat cells; elevated blood triglyceride levels are associated with an increased risk of cardiovascular disease.

HDL cholesterol: high density lipoprotein; a type of lipoprotein that carries cholesterol from the bloodstream to the liver, where it can be excreted from the body. High blood HDL levels may help protect individuals against coronary artery disease.

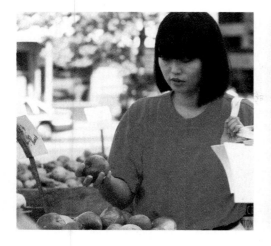
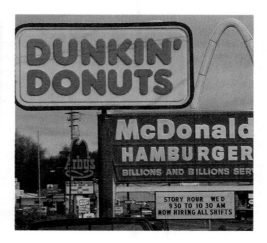

What Do You Think?

1. Food choices can have a great impact on several risk factors for coronary artery disease. What might help motivate college-age individuals to eat more low fat foods on a regular basis?

2. How does the availability of ready-to-eat high fat foods influence an individual's or a family's food choices?

compared to the high fat meals that are available at fast food eating establishments. Do we expect that you and your friends will call a complete moratorium on eating hamburgers, chicken wings, potato chips, and double cheese pizzas with pepperoni? No, of course not, but we hope that you will be more conscious of the food choices you do make, that you understand that these choices have consequences *now*, not just many years from now, and that you will be motivated to experiment with healthier alternatives (see Of Special Interest 10.1). Chapter 3 presents information on the fat content of many foods, and provides some easy-to-follow guidelines for implementing dietary changes that produce tasty meals and reduce your risk of coronary artery disease. In table 10.2, some tips for modifying your food choices are presented, attempting to take into account your particular stage of behavior change.

Stress and Personality

Some years ago it was widely accepted that development of cardiovascular disease was related, in part, to a behavior pattern referred to as the "type A" personality. The apparent relationship between heart disease and the type A individual was described in detail originally in the 1970s by Meyer Friedman and R. H. Rosenman in their classic book, *Type A Behavior and Your Heart*.[13] The type A person was seen as a highly competitive, hard-driving individual who felt a profound sense of urgency to complete tasks once they were started. As one looked around, most

type As were males, and it was hypothesized that this characteristic was more common to males because of society's tendency to rear males in an environment that fostered these traits. Although the role of the so-called type A behavior pattern in cardiovascular disease causation was never without some professional controversy, many educators and health-care practitioners cautioned people about controlling their temperament and minimizing the amount of unnecessary stress in their lives.

In the latter part of the 1980s, the type A connection to heart disease began to be diminished. Researchers began to notice that type A subjects who already had heart disease tended to show a greater ability to survive when a heart attack actually occurred.[14] Joel E. Dimsdale perhaps has put the controversy in the correct perspective for the 1990s when he writes:[15]

> This is a topsy-turvy career for a risk factor. In interpreting it, one should keep the following points in mind. First, there has been far too much fervor on both sides of the argument. Disappointed protagonists have been all too ready to dismiss summarily the findings of studies that contradict theirs, instead of asking what contradictory findings may mean. Dispassionate efforts to replicate findings are uncommon in this field. Second, one worries about whether the diagnostic criteria for type A behavior are sufficiently standardized. The

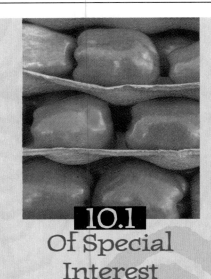

10.1
Of Special Interest

Fish Oil Capsules vs. Fish

A decade after fish oil capsules became widely available, they take up as much space as ever at drugstores and health-food stores. Scientists are still seriously studying the potential benefits of these supplements. Will these capsules prevent heart disease, and also help alleviate or prevent migraine headaches, arthritis, psoriasis, allergic asthma, and perhaps even some types of cancer, as claimed?

What's special about fish oil and pills made from it?

They contain relatively large amounts of polyunsaturated fatty acids popularly called omega-3s, which the fish get by eating plankton, particularly that growing in cold water. The major types of omega-3s in fish are called eicosapentenoic acid (EPA) and docosahexenoic acid (DHA). Fatty fish are the richest sources. When eaten by humans, these omega-3s, like aspirin, make platelets in the blood less likely to stick together and also reduce inflammatory processes in blood vessels. Thus they reduce blood clotting and plaque buildup in the arteries, lessening the chance of a heart attack due to a clot in coronary arteries. This may be one reason why Eskimos and the Japanese, whose diets include vast amounts of fatty fish, have such a low incidence of coronary artery disease.

Don't some plants contain omega-3s, too?

Yes. But leafy greens and some vegetable oils (such as walnut, linseed, or canola) contain only the short-chain omega-3 linolenic acid, not the longer-chain fatty acids found in fish oils. Fish are able to convert the linolenic acid in algae and other sea plants into EPA and DHA, and so can humans—but only to a very limited degree.

Can fish oil lower elevated cholesterol?

Yes, according to some studies; no, according to others. Still other studies have found that fish oil *raises* LDL ("bad") cholesterol, especially in diabetics and people with certain blood lipid disorders. However, substituting fish for meat (or other sources of saturated fat) should significantly lower blood cholesterol.

What about triglycerides?

Fish oil is known to reduce triglycerides, the major type of fat that circulates in the blood. While some scientists believe that elevated triglycerides may contribute to heart disease in some people, the connection remains unclear.

Does fish oil lower blood pressure?

Large doses of supplements *may* have a small effect in some people, but studies have had contradictory results. A recent review of thirty-one studies found that the most consistent (though still small) effect of fish oil on blood pressure was among people with both high blood pressure and high cholesterol.

Can fish oil help treat diabetes?

Not at this point. Some researchers hope that fish oil can help people with diabetes, who often have elevated cholesterol and triglyceride levels as well as clotting disorders, all of which may be ameliorated by fish oil. However, studies thus far have not shown that fish oil consistently benefits those with diabetes. In fact, some studies have shown that fish oil may actually cause a deterioration in blood sugar control and a rise in LDL cholesterol, especially in people with non-insulin-dependent diabetes.

---

behavior pattern is a heterogeneous hodgepodge, diagnosed by means of a semistructured interview or any of a series of self-administered questionnaires. The various scales agree with each other to a degree but are not tightly associated. As a result, it is possible that discrepant findings could be explained by different methods of diagnosing the type A behavior pattern.

It may be that certain degrees of type A behavior exist, and that only the most hard-driving, self-absorbed individual, whose personality actually is angry and hostile, is at risk of developing heart disease prematurely.[16] Furthermore, it is possible that factors associated with disease causation could in fact be beneficial to one's determination to overcome setbacks and promote recovery once disease already exists. Dimsdale concludes:[17]

> It is important to acknowledge that *something* is going on in terms of the relation between personality and heart disease. However, the nature of the influence is far more complex than is conveyed by the simple assertion that type A behavior is a risk factor for coronary artery disease.

What about arthritis and other inflammatory disorders?

This may be where fish oil holds the most promise, since little can be done to treat these disorders. Some scientists are hopeful that fish oil can help relieve inflammatory symptoms of some auto-immune diseases such as rheumatoid arthritis, but their research is only preliminary. Several studies have suggested that fish oil supplements, when taken with pain medication, can have at least modest effects in reducing joint swelling, easing morning stiffness, and lessening fatigue in people with rheumatoid arthritis. But other studies have not found a significant effect. There is also some preliminary evidence that fish oil may help reduce the itching and redness of psoriasis, another auto-immune disease.

Did people in the studies take fish oil pills or eat fish?

Nearly all the studies used pills—usually 8 to 20 capsules daily supplying 3 to 10 grams of omega-3s a day. You would have to eat nearly two pounds of salmon to get 10 grams of omega-3s.

Are there side effects of such high doses of omega-3s?

There are some serious concerns:

• The decreased ability of your blood to clot has a negative side. The same Eskimos who have a low incidence of heart disease have a high risk of hemorrhagic stroke, perhaps because of the decreased clotting ability of their blood. If you consume lots of fish oil, the anti-clotting effect may be dangerous in an accident or during surgery, though no studies have reported any bleeding problems. People with bleeding disorders, those taking anticoagulants, or those with uncontrolled hypertension (who are already at high risk for a stroke) should *not* take fish oil supplements.

• Large doses can cause nausea, diarrhea, belching, and a bad taste in the mouth.

• Like all fats, omega-3s are concentrated sources of calories—some recommended doses supply 200 calories a day.

• Fish oil in liquid or capsule form may contain pesticides or other contaminants, especially if it is made from fish livers, where these compounds tend to concentrate. These are usually removed in the manufacturing process, but there's no guarantee.

• Cod liver oil is overly rich in vitamins A and D, which can be toxic in high doses. There's no reason to take it.

• Prolonged consumption of fish oil may result in a vitamin E deficiency (polyunsaturated fats increase your need for E). Some manufacturers have thus added this vitamin to their supplements.

• Recent studies suggest that large doses of fish oil may suppress certain aspects of the immune system.

The bottom line

We still recommend fish, but not the routine use of fish oil supplements. If you have rheumatoid arthritis or psoriasis, fish oil supplements may be worth a try, but consult your doctor first. Many questions remain about their effectiveness and safety. None of the leading health or nutrition organizations recommends them. Should you take 3 to 6 capsules a day (providing as much omega-3s as 3.5 to 7 ounces of salmon), as some manufacturers recommend, or 20, the amount used in some studies? No one has any idea what the optimal dose is.

Moreover, it's unclear whether omega-3s supplements provide the same health benefits as the fish itself. These fatty acids may work with other elements in the fish not found in the supplements.

Fish itself is one of the best foods around: besides its oil, it is rich in protein, iron, B vitamins, and other nutrients, and it can take the place of meats that are high in saturated fat. Studies suggest that two or three servings of fish a week are enough to improve your cardiovascular health.

Reprinted by permission from the *University of California at Berkeley Wellness Letter*, Health Letter Associates, 1994.

What Do You Think?

1. What is an appropriate precaution to take prior to initiating the use of dietary supplements of any kind?
2. If one were to eat more fish in the diet, how would the preparation of the fish be an important factor in determining how good a substitute for red meat it actually is?

Chapter 2 presents a variety of stress-management techniques that *may* help decrease your risk of coronary artery disease, and that *will* increase your level of well-being if practiced regularly.

Physical Inactivity

A sedentary lifestyle or lack of exercise has been established as an independent risk factor for cardiovascular disease. In 1992, the American Heart Association upgraded "physical inactivity" from its list of cardiovascular disease *contributing* risk factors to the stronger category of *major risk factors*.[18] This upgrade places a sedentary lifestyle on a par with hypertension, smoking, and high LDL/low HDL cholesterol. A low activity level, when combined with consumption of large quantities of food, especially food high in fat, predisposes one further to obesity, which also is linked to cardiovascular disease.

Regular **aerobic exercise** strengthens the heart muscle, causing it to pump more highly oxygenated blood with each beat. Exercise may aid efforts to control cigarette smoking, hypertension, lipid abnormalities, diabetes, and emotional stress. Evidence suggests that regular, moderate, or vigorous occupational or leisure-time physical activity may protect

Aerobic exercise: activities that cause a sustained increase in heart rate and use the large muscles of the body continuously for an extended period of time.

TABLE 10.2 — Tips for Reducing Dietary Fat and Cardiovascular Disease Risk

In the U.S., where lifestyle revolves around eating foods high in fat, making changes in your diet can be challenging. You may make the transition to a reduced-fat diet however through following some of the tips provided below.

Precontemplation → Contemplation

If you have never thought about reducing your overall fat intake, try:

- Reading about the low-fat foods that are available to you, but that you rarely eat because of the self-imposed limitations on your diet.
- Keep a record of what you eat during a "typical" week.

Contemplation → Preparation

If you have thought about making dietary changes but have not yet done so, then:

- Read food labels in your cupboards and at the grocery store, noting calories, cholesterol, and percentage of calories from fat.
- Learn how food preparation contributes to fat and caloric intake.
- Ask your grocer about where low-fat foods are shelved.
- Plan what a main meal might consist of if it were 100 percent fat-free.

Preparation → Action

If you are ready to change your diet in the next month or have tried changing your diet in the past:

- Identify a date in the next thirty days when you will carry out your plan to modify your fat consumption. Mark the date on your calendar.

- Shop for snacks that are low in fat so that the next time you feel hungry or want to reward yourself with food, you will have a healthful snack available.
- Tell a friend that you are going to plan some health conscious meals, and invite him or her to assist. Make it a social experience.
- Invite a friend to a vegetarian restaurant.
- Plan meals for a whole day that are fat-free or are reduced fat.

Action → Maintenance

If you have recently started making dietary changes, the following tips may help you to continue this pattern.

- Avoid circumstances that "trigger" high fat and cholesterol foods.
- Diversify your repertoire of dining activities that limits your contact with fast-food chain restaurants and places where you are accustomed to having high-fat meals.
- Keep a diary of your food selections, estimating your caloric intake and the percentage of calories from fat.

Maintenance

You are making great progress in lowering your risk of cardiovascular disease.

- Become an advocate of healthier eating among your peers.
- Have your cholesterol and other lipids measured to monitor your progress toward a healthier heart.

against coronary heart disease and may improve the likelihood of survival from a heart attack.[19]

Fitness profiles and physical activity patterns of new college students show that neither men nor women exhibit high levels of cardiorespiratory fitness. Women may have slightly better conditioning than their male counterparts, however.[20]

Chapter 5 in this text provides valuable information about starting and maintaining

an aerobic exercise program that best meets your needs and interests. Research supports the belief that even low to moderate levels of physical activity can reduce cardiovascular disease risk.[21] This point should be of particular interest to persons who do not enjoy intense exercise, regardless of its nature, style, or mode, and to people whose motive for exercise is not necessarily to enhance endurance or cardiorespiratory function.

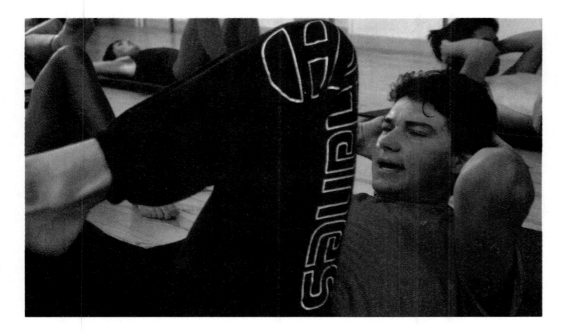

What Do You Think?

1. Regular participation in an aerobic exercise program can provide you with an enjoyable activity and decrease your risk for coronary artery disease. How many of your friends and family members participate at least three times a week, for at least twenty minutes a session, in an aerobic activity such as aerobic dance, walking, cycling, rowing, or stair climbing?
2. What might help motivate college-age people to regularly participate in aerobic exercise?

Aspirin: A Preventive Factor

The Steering Committee of the Physicians' Health Study Research Group showed in a study involving more than 22,000 subjects that individuals taking a 325 mg dose of aspirin every other day had a significantly lower occurrence of heart attack than persons in a control group who received an inert placebo.[22] Aspirin is an **anticoagulant,** a substance that inhibits the formation of blood clots. Thus, a person with atherosclerosis taking this dose of aspirin might be at less risk of heart attack since blood clots that can occlude narrowed arteries would be less likely to form. Although heart attack incidence was significantly less in the aspirin group, no comparable observation was made with respect to the incidence of stroke. Even when comparing both heart attack and stroke events, however, the aspirin group had a 23 percent lower occurrence of these types of episodes. While these findings are indeed encouraging for people predisposed to atherosclerosis, further research must be done. It is necessary for you to understand that taking aspirin does not alter the underlying disease process, only the probability of a sudden heart attack.[23] Since aspirin can be harsh on the digestive tract, cause blood loss, and even contribute to **anemia** in susceptible individuals, it must be determined whether its routine ingestion has more liability than benefit associated with it.[24]

Determining Your Cardiovascular Disease Risk and Developing A Plan for Wellness

As we have seen, several lifestyle factors are implicated in the development of the nation's number one killer, cardiovascular disease. By now you should have a clear idea of some of the factors which you can control regarding your personal risk. To assist you in determining your risk profile, Activity for Wellness 10.1 is presented. As you can see from the tables shown in Activity for Wellness 10.1, age begins to be a factor for heart attack as you enter your 30s, and for stroke as you enter your 50s. From what you have read in this chapter, however, it should be obvious that overall risk is cumulative over your life. Activity for Wellness 10.1 should be used primarily to illustrate how the modifiable risk factors are additive, although you can estimate a personal probability of experiencing a heart attack or stroke in the future.

The following example may help you. Suppose Adam, a twenty-year-old cigarette smoker, and his girlfriend, nineteen-year-old Elissa, are examining this wellness activity to compute Adam's risk of heart attack. Adam's recent cholesterol test showed a total cholesterol of 245 mg/dL but an HDL cholesterol of just 30. Repeated blood pressure readings have placed his systolic blood pressure consistently between 130 and

Anemia: a decreased ability of the blood to carry oxygen, due to a decrease in the amount of hemoglobin in the blood.

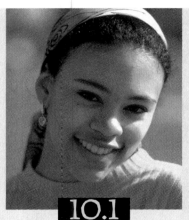

10.1

Activity for Wellness

Rating Your Risk

Okay, so you've had your cholesterol checked. You even know your HDL and LDL. You're eating less meat and cheese, exercising . . . doing all you can to cut your risk of heart disease.

But just what is your risk, anyway?

Using forty years of data from the Framingham Heart Study, the American Heart Association has created worksheets for health professionals to use to estimate their patients' risk of coronary heart disease and stroke. We've adapted them here so you can estimate your risk. If you have any questions about whether a risk factor applies to you, or if you want to discuss the results, see your doctor.

Key to Risk Factors

HDL-C—Your HDL ("good") cholesterol
Total-C—Your total cholesterol
SBP—Your systolic blood pressure (the higher of your two blood pressure numbers)
HYP RX—Do you take medication to lower your blood pressure? (Women will be adding more points for having a lower blood pressure. So far, researchers can't explain why.)
CVD—Have you had any of these:

- **heart attack?**
- **angina** (chest pain during physical activity)?

Heart Disease Risk Factor Prediction Chart

Men and Women

1. Find the Points that Correspond to Your Age

Men		Women	
Age	Pts.	Age	Pts.
30	−2	30	−12
31	−1	31	−11
32–33	0	32	−9
34	1	33	−8
35–36	2	34	−6
37–38	3	35	−5
39	4	36	−4
40–41	5	37	−3
42–43	6	38	−2
44–45	7	39	−1
46–47	8	40	0
48–49	9	41	1
50–51	10	42–43	2
52–54	11	44	3
55–56	12	45–46	4
57–59	13	47–48	5
60–61	14	49–50	6
62–64	15	51–52	7
65–67	16	53–55	8
68–70	17	56–60	9
71–73	18	61–67	10
74	19	68–74	11

2. Find the Points for Your Other Risk Factors

HDL Cholesterol		Total Cholesterol	
HDL-C	Pts.	Total-C	Pts.
25–26	7	139–151	−3
27–29	6	152–166	−2
30–32	5	167–182	−1
33–35	4	183–199	0
36–38	3	200–219	1
39–42	2	220–239	2
43–46	1	240–262	3
47–50	0	263–288	4
51–55	−1	289–315	5
56–60	−2	316–330	6
61–66	−3		
67–73	−4		
74–80	−5		
81–87	−6		
88–96	−7		

Systolic Blood Pressure

SBP	Pts.
98–104	−2
105–112	−1
113–120	0
121–129	1
130–139	2
140–149	3
150–160	4
161–172	5
173–185	6

Other Risk Factors

Factor	Pts.
Cigarette Smoker	4
Diabetic-Male	3
Diabetic-Female	6
LVH	9
0 points for each NO	

- **unstable angina,** or **coronary insufficiency** (the symptoms of a heart attack, but with no increase in the enzymes that signal heart muscle damage)?
- **intermittent claudication** (severe leg pain, usually upon exertion, that results from an inadequate blood supply)?
- **congestive heart failure** (symptoms like breathlessness and severely swollen ankles caused by the heart's failure to pump enough blood and oxygen)?

AF—Do you have a history of atrial fibrillation (irregular heart beats in the upper chambers of your heart)?
LVH—Has an electrocardiogram shown that you have left ventricular hypertrophy (an enlarged heart muscle)?

Example for Heart Disease Risk: A nonsmoking (0 points) 54-year-old woman (8 points) with total cholesterol of 227 (2 points), HDL ("good") cholesterol of 52 (−1 point), and systolic blood pressure of 131 (2 points), who doesn't have diabetes (0 points) or left ventricular hypertrophy (0 points), ends up with a total of 11 points.

According to the chart, she has a 3 percent chance of developing coronary heart disease within the next five years (compared to 8 percent for the average woman her age). Her risk over the next ten years is 6 percent (compared to 14 percent for the average woman her age).

Heart Disease Risk Factor Prediction Chart

Men and Women

3. Total the Points for All Your Risk Factors	
Age	_____
HDL-C	+ _____
Total-C	+ _____
SBP	+ _____
Cigarette Smoker	+ _____
Diabetes	+ _____
LVH	+ _____
Point Total =	_____

Note: Subtract minus points from total

4. Find Your Point Total and Corresponding Risk

Probability of Developing Heart Disease

Pts.	5 Yr.	10 Yr.	Pts.	5 Yr.	10 Yr.
1 or less	less than 1%	less than 2%	25	14%	27%
2	1%	2%	26	16%	29%
3	1%	2%	27	17%	31%
4	1%	2%	28	19%	33%
5	1%	3%	29	20%	36%
6	1%	3%	30	22%	38%
7	1%	4%	31	24%	40%
8	2%	4%	32	25%	42%
9	2%	5%			
10	2%	6%			
11	3%	6%			
12	3%	7%			
13	3%	8%			
14	4%	9%			
15	5%	10%			
16	5%	12%			
17	6%	13%			
18	7%	14%			
19	8%	16%			
20	8%	18%			
21	9%	19%			
22	11%	21%			
23	12%	23%			
24	13%	25%			

5. Compare Your Risk to the Average

Average 10-Year Risks

Age	Women	Men
30–34	less than 1%	3%
35–39	less than 1%	5%
40–44	2%	6%
45–49	5%	10%
50–54	8%	14%
55–59	12%	16%
60–64	13%	21%
65–69	9%	30%
70–74	12%	24%

Stroke Risk Factor Prediction Chart

Men

1. Find Your Age		2. Find the Points for Your Other Risk Factors			
Age	Pts.	SBP	Pts.	HYP RX	CVD
54–56	0	95–105	0	NO = 0	NO = 0
57–59	1	106–116	1	YES = 2	YES = 3
60–62	2	117–126	2		
63–65	3	127–137	3	Diabetes	AF
66–68	4	138–148	4	NO = 0	NO = 0
69–71	5	149–159	5	YES = 2	YES = 4
72–74	6	160–170	6		
75–77	7	171–181	7	Cigarette	LVH
78–80	8	182–191	8	Smoker	
81–83	9	192–202	9	NO = 0	NO = 0
84–86	10	203–213	10	YES = 3	YES = 6

Women

1. Find Your Age		2. Find the Points for Your Other Risk Factors			
Age	Pts.	SBP	Pts.	HYP RX	Cigarette Smoker
54–56	0	95–104	0	NO = 0	NO = 0
57–59	1	105–114	1	If Yes, add these points, depending on your SBP level:	YES = 3
60–62	2	115–124	2	SBP / Pts.	CVD
63–65	3	125–134	3	95–104 / 6	NO = 0
66–68	4	135–144	4	105–124 / 5	YES = 2
69–71	5	145–154	5	125–134 / 4	
72–74	6	155–164	6	135–154 / 3	AF
75–77	7	165–174	7	155–164 / 2	NO = 0
78–80	8	175–184	8	165–184 / 1	YES = 6
81–83	9	185–194	9	185–204 / 0	
84–86	10	196–204	10	Diabetes	LVH
				NO = 0	NO = 0
				YES = 3	YES = 4

Continued

Stroke Risk Factor Prediction Chart

Men and Women

3. Total the Points for All Your Risk Factors

Age		_____
SBP	+	_____
HYP RX	+	_____
Diabetes	+	_____
Cigarette Smoker	+	_____
CVD	+	_____
AF	+	_____
LVH	+	_____
Point Total	=	_____

5. Compare Your Risk to the Average

Average 10-Year Risks		
Age	Women	Men
55–59	3.0%	5.9%
60–64	4.7%	7.8%
65–69	7.2%	11.0%
70–74	10.9%	13.7%
75–79	15.5%	18.0%
80–84	23.9%	22.3%

Copyright © 1992, Center for Science in the Public Interest.

4. Find Your Point Total and Corresponding Risk

Men		Women	
Pts.	10-Yr. Risk	Pts.	10-Yr. Risk
1	2.6%	1	1.1%
2	3.0%	2	1.3%
3	3.5%	3	1.6%
4	4.0%	4	2.0%
5	4.7%	5	2.4%
6	5.4%	6	2.9%
7	6.3%	7	3.5%
8	7.3%	8	4.3%
9	8.4%	9	5.2%
10	9.7%	10	6.3%
11	11.2%	11	7.6%
12	12.9%	12	9.2%
13	14.8%	13	11.1%
14	17.0%	14	13.3%
15	19.5%	15	16.0%
16	22.4%	16	19.1%
17	25.5%	17	22.8%
18	29.0%	18	27.0%
19	32.9%	19	31.9%
20	37.1%	20	37.3%
21	41.7%	21	43.4%
22	46.6%	22	50.0%
23	51.8%	23	57.0%
24	57.3%	24	64.2%
25	62.8%	25	71.4%
26	68.4%	26	78.2%
27	73.8%	27	84.4%
28	79.0%		
29	83.7%		
30	87.9%		

139 mm Hg. Adam is not diabetic and has no history of an enlarged heart muscle. If Adam has a similar profile at age thirty, about what chance does he have of developing heart disease by age forty? What could he do to minimize his risk?

Elissa's father, James, is fifty-seven years old. Two recent cholesterol tests indicate James's total cholesterol to be 315 and 305 respectively. His HDL cholesterol is 30. James smokes less than half a pack of cigarettes per day, but he used to smoke two or more packs a day. His systolic blood pressure varies from 129 to 149. He has no medication which he takes currently. A few years back he was diagnosed with a sometimes irregular heartbeat, but has no other known illnesses or conditions. Should Elissa be concerned about her father's risk of heart attack? of stroke? Are there some things that James can do immediately to alter his risk profile?

The Cost of Inaction with Respect to Cardiovascular Disease Prevention

In the most recent year for which statistics are available, an estimated 407,000 **coronary**

Coronary artery bypass surgery: a surgical procedure that reroutes the blood supply in a coronary artery around a severe blockage.

Do Women and Minorities Get Equal Attention for Coronary Heart Disease?

It would appear that women and minorities do not get their fair share when it comes to diagnostic and intervention procedures for cardiovascular disease according to two independent reports. For example, one study indicated that women and African-Americans were much less likely than men and Whites to receive two specific types of interventions for advanced coronary artery disease: angioplasty and coronary artery bypass surgery. With angioplasty, narrowed coronary arteries are widened by the insertion of a deflated balloon on the tip of a catheter. Once inserted into the narrowed area, the balloon is inflated. With bypass surgery, the constricted coronary artery is "bypassed" through the surgical addition of a synthetic or actual blood vessel, after which, a more optimal blood flow to the heart muscle is restored. A

New York State Department of Health grant given to Dr. Michelle van Ryn of the State University of New York at Albany is expected to examine the reasons for the discrepancy in performance of these procedures on women and Black Americans. Researchers in St. Louis report that women are significantly less likely than men to have diagnostic tests and therapeutic interventions for coronary heart disease, even when their risks for heart attack are similar. Even after an abnormal exercise stress test, nearly two-thirds of the women had no further diagnostic testing, compared to about one-third of the men. Men were about twice as likely to undergo subsequent angioplasty or bypass surgery, or be given drug therapy. The cardiac death rate for the women whose medical records were examined was four times greater than for the men whose charts were reviewed.

Sources: Data from *The Public Health Memo* of the State University of New York at Albany School of Public Health 8.2 (1993):1; and *Consumer Reports on Health* 6.5 (1994):54.

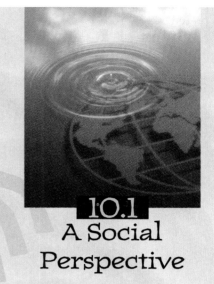

10.1 A Social Perspective

What Do You Think?

1. How would you explain the discrepancy found in these two independent reports? Is it sexism, racism, or are there other explanations?
2. To what extent do you think these examples are representative of discrepancies in care with respect to other disorders? Explain your reasoning.

---

artery bypass surgeries were performed on 265,000 patients.[25] Almost one out of two bypass procedures were performed on people under the age of sixty-five, and 73 percent of bypass procedures were performed on men (see A Social Perspective 10.1).[26]

Just under 1,900 heart transplant operations were performed in the U.S. in a recent year, a slight decrease in the number of such surgeries in the two previous years.[27] Approximately 6.9 percent of heart transplant recipients lived thirty days or less.[28] The five-year survival rate for transplant recipients on a **chemotherapy** program is 73 percent,[29] but the survival figure says nothing about quality of life and ability to perform the tasks of daily living.

In addition to the above surgeries, there were 58,000 operations performed on heart valves, 331,000 **angioplasty** procedures, over one million **cardiac catheterizations** for diagnostic purposes, 121,000 pacemaker implants, 518,000 open heart surgeries, and a total of more than 4.1 million

cardiovascular operations.[30] Statistics gathered by the National Center for Health Statistics and reported by the American Heart Association suggest that the annual frequencies of these procedures continue to increase.[31]

What do these procedures cost? American Heart Association estimates in 1994 extrapolated from 1984 data put the price tag of cardiovascular disease at over $128 million.[32] This figure includes the cost of physician and nursing services, hospital and nursing home services, the cost of medications, and the cost of lost productivity time resulting from disability.

As the mean age of the population in the U.S. continues to increase into the next century, cardiovascular disease will affect more and more people. Despite some important gains from research and an improved survival rate from heart attack and stroke, someone dies from cardiovascular disease in the U.S. every thirty-four seconds.[33] Prevention and wise selection of modifiable lifestyle options are the best alternatives to combat these astronomical costs.

Chemotherapy: the treatment of disease by the use of drugs.

Angioplasty: a procedure in which a balloon catheter is inserted into a blocked coronary artery. The balloon is then inflated in order to stretch the plaque and allow more blood to flow through the artery.

Cardiac catheterization: a procedure in which a small flexible tube (catheter) is inserted into an artery or vein in the arm or leg and fed through the vascular system to the heart.

Summary

1. Cardiovascular disease is responsible for more deaths in the U.S. than any other cause.

2. *Healthy People 2000* has established health objectives for the nation with respect to cardiovascular disease that are specific to age, sex, race, and ethnic group.

3. Cardiovascular disease includes many different disorders that affect the heart and the circulatory system.

4. The normal heart is a muscular organ that performs an enormous amount of work as it pumps blood throughout the body.

5. Oxygen and nutrients are supplied to the heart by coronary arteries. If these arteries become blocked or damaged, a heart attack may occur.

6. Atherosclerosis is a form of arteriosclerosis in which the walls of the arteries become thickened and lose their elasticity.

7. Hypertension is sometimes called a "silent killer" because symptoms may not be obvious, but it is a major risk factor for cardiovascular disease development.

8. A stroke occurs when a cerebral artery in the brain is blocked and the brain becomes deprived of blood and oxygen.

9. Several personal and social lifestyle factors contribute to the annual incidence of heart attack and stroke.

10. Smoking is the greatest single controllable risk factor in the causation of heart attack.

11. Dietary fat consumption beyond recommended levels can increase one's risk of developing heart disease.

12. Many American college students are physically less active than what is desired for prevention of heart disease.

13. The role of stress and personality in heart disease causation is complex, and not quite as clear as once believed.

14. Administration of aspirin may be a heart attack preventive action for some people, but the side effects and long-term effects of its use are controversial or unknown.

15. Mechanisms are available to assess one's risk of heart attack and stroke, and provide some guidance for lifestyle modification.

16. More than 4.1 million surgical procedures are performed annually in the U.S. to address cardiovascular disease.

17. The annual cost of cardiovascular disease in health care and lost productivity is estimated to be in excess of $128 million.

Recommended Readings

American Heart Association. *Heart and Stroke Facts*. Dallas, TX: 1995.

American Heart Association. *Heart and Stroke Facts: 1996 Statistical Supplement*. Dallas, TX: 1995.

These companion publications are updated annually, and include a review of normal heart function, major cardiovascular disorders, warning signals of heart disease and stroke, risk factors, and interventions. Facts and figures on cardiovascular disease are provided along with many fine illustrations. They are free upon request from your local affiliate of the American Heart Association.

Herbert Benson and Eileen M. Stuart, (eds). *The Wellness Book*. New York: Simon & Schuster, 1992.

This book provides many hints for lifestyle improvement, reiterating the importance of exercise, nutrition, and stress management. It contains a chapter on living with heart disease.

Editors of *Consumer Guide*. *Cholesterol: Your Guide for A Healthy Heart*. Lincolnwood, IL: Publications International, Ltd., 1994.

This guide puts cholesterol in perspective with other cardiovascular disease risk factors. It explores the role of nutrition, weight control, stress management, and exercise in an overall lifestyle program, and makes a case for cholesterol screening and cautions against fad dieting and other superficial wellness measures.

References

1. American Heart Association, *Heart and Stroke Facts* (Dallas, Tex.: 1993):7.

2. *University of California at Berkeley Wellness Letter* 10.4 (1994):7.

3. American Heart Association, *Heart and Stroke Facts*, 25.

4. *University of California at Berkeley Wellness Letter* 10.8 (1994):4.

5. David T. Purtilo and Ruth B. Purtilo, *A Survey of Human Diseases*, 2nd edition (Boston: Little, Brown and Company, 1989), 75.

6. Purtilo and Purtilo, *A Survey of Human Diseases*, 73.

7. *University of California at Berkeley Wellness Letter* 10.8 (1994):4.

8. Marlene Cimons, "Nicotine is Addictive, FDA Panel Says," *Los Angeles Times* (August 3, 1994):C1.

9. William K. Hahn, Jo A. Brooks, and Richard Hite, "Results of Blood Pressure Screening in White College Students," *Journal of American College Health* 38.5 (1990):235–237.

10. D. M. Hegsted, "Nutrition Standards for Today," *Nutrition Today* 28.2 (1993):34–36.

11. Walter C. Willett, M. J. Stampfer, J. E. Manson, et al., "Trans Fatty-Acid Intake in Relation to Risk of Coronary Heart Disease among Women," *Lancet* 341 (1993):581–585.

12. National Heart, Lung, and Blood Institute. *Report of the Expert Panel on Detection, Evaluation, and Treatment of High Blood Cholesterol Adults. National Cholesterol Education Program* (Washington, D.C.: U.S. Department of Health and Human Services, 1988).

13. Meyer Friedman and R. H. Rosenman, *Type A Behavior and Your Heart* (New York: Alfred A. Knopf, 1974).

14. David R. Ragland and Richard J. Braud, "Type A Behavior and Mortality from Coronary Heart Disease," *New England Journal of Medicine* 318 (1988):65–69.

15. Joel E. Dimsdale, "A Perspective on Type A Behavior and Coronary Disease," *New England Journal of Medicine* 318 (1988):110.

16. *University of California at Berkeley Wellness Letter* 10.8 (1994):5.

17. Dimsdale, "A Perspective on Type A Behavior and Coronary Disease," 112.

18. *University of California at Berkeley Wellness Letter* 8.11 (1992):1.

19. D. S. Siscovick, R. E. Laporte, and J. M. Newman, "The Disease-Specific Benefits and Risks of Physical Activity," *Public Health Reports* 100 (1985):180–189.

20. Edgar F. Pierce, Susan W. Butterworth, Tracey D. Lynn, et al., "Fitness Profiles and Activity Patterns of Entering College Students," *Journal of American College Health* 41.2 (1992):59–62.

21. James F. Sallis et al., "Moderate-Intensity Physical Activity and Cardiovascular Risk Factors: The Stanford Five-City Project," *Preventive Medicine* 15 (1986):561.

22. The Steering Committee of the Physicians' Health Study Research Group, "Preliminary Report: Findings from the Aspirin Component of the Ongoing Physicians' Health Study," *New England Journal of Medicine* 318 (1988):262–264.

23. John E. Willard, Richard A. Lange, and L. David Hillis, "The Use of Aspirin in Ischemic Heart Disease," *New England Journal of Medicine* 327.3 (1992):175–181.

24. Carlo Patrono, "Aspirin As An Antiplatelet Drug," *New England Journal of Medicine* 330.18 (1994):1287–1294.

25. American Heart Association, *Heart and Stroke Facts: 1994 Statistical Supplement* (Dallas, Tex.: 1993), 20.

26. American Heart Association, *Heart and Stroke Facts: 1994 Statistical Supplement*, 20.

27. American Heart Association, *Heart and Stroke Facts: 1994 Statistical Supplement*, 20.

28. American Heart Association, *Heart and Stroke Facts: 1994 Statistical Supplement*, 20.

29. American Heart Association, *Heart and Stroke Facts: 1994 Statistical Supplement*, 20.

30. American Heart Association, *Heart and Stroke Facts: 1994 Statistical Supplement*, 21.

31. American Heart Association, *Heart and Stroke Facts: 1994 Statistical Supplement*, 21.

32. American Heart Association, *Heart and Stroke Facts: 1994 Statistical Supplement*, 22.

33. American Heart Association, *Heart and Stroke Facts: 1994 Statistical Supplement*, 1.

Cancer and Other Noncommunicable Disease Threats to Wellness: The Body Under Siege

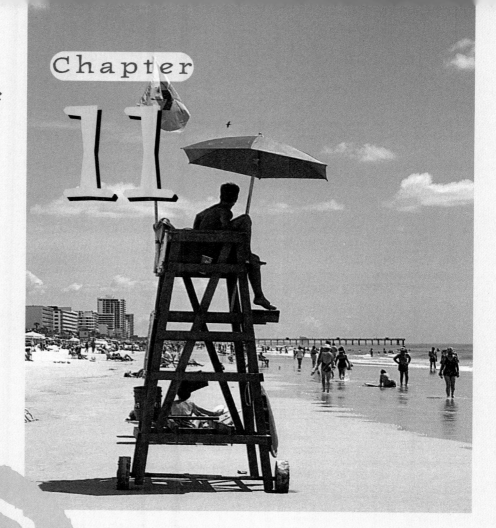

Chapter 11

Student Learning Objectives

Upon completion of this chapter you should be able to:

1. discuss the change in the pattern of illness seen in the U.S. over the past century;

2. distinguish between the traits of benign and malignant tumors;

3. list and discuss several personal and social influences that contribute to the development of human cancers;

4. compare selected U.S. statistics for cancer occurrence and cancer deaths among men and women;

5. compare and contrast the occurrence of chronic, noncommunicable diseases across the diverse groups of people in the U.S.;

6. explain why quackery in cancer treatment continues to thrive;

7. identify several things that a person can do to minimize the risk of developing some cancers;

8. describe some activities that people can undertake that will increase the chance that a cancer will be diagnosed early, when it is most treatable;

9. conduct a breast self-examination (women), a testicular self-examination (men), and a skin self-examination (men and women) explaining the rationale for the performance of each;

10. describe some of the consequences of having diabetes;

11. compare the threats to wellness posed by the respiratory ailments of asthma, emphysema, and chronic bronchitis;

12. identify the health objectives of the nation for the year 2000 as they relate to cancer and selected other noncommunicable diseases.

By the time you are in college it is likely that you will have known someone who has had **cancer.** Maybe you have had someone in your family develop cancer, or perhaps, even die from the disease. For many people cancer can arouse more fear than any other disease, including HIV/AIDS. While cancer can indeed be frightening, much has become known about its cause and treatment. Today, there is much that can be done to prevent cancer. Many kinds of cancer, that only a few years ago shortened life by many years, are now being treated successfully and cured.

The past century has seen enormous changes in the patterns of illness in the U.S., as well as changes in the causes of premature death. Deaths in the early 1900s could be characterized as due to communicable diseases, especially those affecting the respiratory system, such as pneumonia, influenza, and tuberculosis. From about the second half of the twentieth century up to the current time, communicable disease causes of death have been replaced largely by noncommunicable disease causes, many of them linked to lifestyle choices that we make. In this chapter we will examine a few of these diseases, concentrating particularly on the various forms of cancer.

Cancer

Cancer, which is probably as old as the oldest forms of life, is not a single disease. Instead, it is a collection of diseases that share certain traits. Scientists have identified more than 100 different types of human cancers, all of which arise ultimately from a single cell. The various forms of cancer account for about 1,252,000 new cases each year in the U.S., and about 547,000 deaths,[1] making cancer the second leading cause of death in the U.S.

In all living things known to get cancer, the disease process begins when something goes wrong within the cell's replication mechanism. Instead of an orderly and controlled pattern of growth and replacement, the abnormal cell follows a disorderly pattern of irregular and uncontrolled growth. How an error is introduced into the cell is poorly understood. Errors may result from many factors.

Chemicals from the environment, solar radiation, x rays or other radiation, foods, and food additives are all implicated to some extent in cancer causation. Some cancers may be caused by certain viruses. In addition, there simply may be random breakdowns in the cell giving rise to viable but abnormal new cells.

Few abnormal cells survive long enough to do much harm. They are seldom as virulent as normal, healthy cells. They may simply die or be eliminated by the body's immune system. But in the person with cancer, at least one abnormal cell survives and begins to engage in processes that may lead to the destruction of the host.

Some abnormal cells produce a lump or swelling called a **tumor** or **neoplasm.** Rarely do these swellings become a threat. The lump you get after bumping your head is, after all, only an accumulation of fluid and other cellular material underneath the skin. Even a tumor resulting from abnormal cell growth is usually not cancerous. Most lumps or tumors are classified as **benign** (noncancerous) and do not pose an immediate threat. **Malignant** tumors are cancerous though, and they almost always are life-threatening.

These two types of tumors differ in many ways. Benign tumors are almost always enclosed in a fibrous sheath or capsule. The cells that comprise benign tumors have the same physical characteristics of the normal surrounding tissue. Benign tumors grow by expansion only and seldom penetrate surrounding areas. They do not spread to distant parts of the body. Warts and moles are familiar benign tumors.

Malignant tumors do not confine themselves to the site of the body in which they arise. With rare exception, malignant tumors are not encapsulated and do not resemble surrounding cells. They fail to respond to normal growth-control mechanisms. They invade surrounding tissues and often spread to distant parts of the body, a process known as **metastasis.**

Though not cancerous, benign tumors can be dangerous. A benign tumor inside the skull may give rise to a fatal stroke if it inhibits blood from reaching the brain. Benign tumors as large as basketballs have been surgically removed from people after

Neoplasm or tumor: a new growth of tissue serving no physiological function.

Benign: usually in reference to a tumor, meaning noncancerous or nonmalignant; can be life-threatening if the tumor grows to a size where it interferes with function of surrounding tissue.

Metastasis: the spread of a previously localized cancer to new sites in the body, thereby increasing the life-threatening potential of the disease.

TABLE 11.1 A Comparison of Benign and Malignant Tumors

Trait	Benign Tumor	Malignant Tumor
Method of growth	Grows by expansion, displacing normal tissue	Invades, destroys, or incorporates adjacent structures
Metastasis	Does not metastasize	Most metastasize and develop distant colonies
Rate of growth	Usually slow; may be self-limiting	Grows slowly or rapidly
Architecture	Encapsulated	Not encapsulated
Potential for harm	Most without lethal potential but may grow to the point of compressing other cells or adjacent organs	Almost always has a lethal potential by killing the host by destroying essential cells; must be removed or destroyed

causing a deficiency in blood flow to vital organs, producing pain and interfering with digestion and other bodily functions.

While malignant tumors can produce the same kind of results, their principal threat arises from their ability to metastasize. Metastasis begins when a cell or cell mass breaks away from its primary site and is carried by the blood or lymph fluid elsewhere in the body. If even one cancerous cell exists, it has the potential of developing into billions of destructive cells (see table 11.1).

There are four major types of cancer, named according to the tissue from which they arise. **Carcinomas** are cancers of epithelial tissue such as the skin or the mucous membranes that line organs. **Sarcomas** are cancers originating in connective or supporting tissues such as bone, cartilage, fibrous tissue, and muscle. **Leukemias** are cancers of the blood-forming parts of the body, primarily the bone marrow and the spleen. **Lymphomas** arise in the lymphatic system.

Personal and Social Issues in Cancer Causation

While the exact mechanism that sparks abnormal cell growth is not understood completely, some conditions are so frequently associated with cancer's development that they are identified as predisposing factors. We might divide them into four categories:

occupational factors, medical factors, social factors, and biological factors.

Occupational Factors

A number of agents found in occupational settings may be related to specific types of cancer. In their classic review of avoidable cancer risks, Richard Doll and Richard Peto estimate that at least 4 percent of all cancer deaths result from occupational exposures.[2] Some of the agents encountered in various occupations are summarized in table 11.2.

Asbestos, one of the known occupational **carcinogens,** has received much attention. Because of its flame- and friction-retardant properties, asbestos is used in the automotive industry (brake linings), shipbuilding industry, and construction industry (insulation). It probably poses its greatest health threat, however, to workers involved in asbestos mining and milling. The tiny asbestos fibers lodge in the lung, producing a condition known as **chronic obstructive lung disease.** This condition may be a precursor to an otherwise rare form of lung cancer. Since asbestos has been used traditionally in the walls and ceilings of schools and other buildings, millions of people inadvertently may have received years of exposure to fibers. Other products now are substituted for asbestos where possible in construction projects. Because of the efforts of health personnel, scientists, labor-union personnel, and legislators, employers are now required by law to inform employees of known or suspected carcinogens in the

Chronic obstructive lung disease (COLD): a category of lung disease characterized by decreased ability of the lungs to perform gas exchanges. Emphysema and chronic bronchitis are common examples.

TABLE 11.2 Carcinogens and Occupations

Occupation	Suspected Carcinogen	Type of Cancer
Automobile mechanic	Petroleum products	Larynx, lung, nasal passages, scrotum, skin
Carpenter	Wood dusts	Nasal passages, sinus cavity
Dyer	Benzene and other aromatics	Bladder, leukemia
Farmer	Ultraviolet rays of the sun	Skin
Miner	Arsenic, asbestos, coal,	Liver, lung, skin; lung; bladder, larynx, lung, scrotum, skin;
	iron oxide, uranium	larynx, lung; bone, lung, skin
Painter	Benzene	Leukemia
Rubber worker	Vinyl chloride	Liver
Textile worker	Cadmium	Kidney, lung, prostate

What Do You Think?

1. Have you ever researched the careers you are personally considering in terms of your potential exposure to carcinogens?

2. How important is carcinogen exposure to you in terms of choosing your life's work? Explain your rationale.

work setting and to take precautionary measures to minimize risk.

Medical Factors

Medical exposure to carcinogens results from radiation, hormonal drugs, chemotherapeutic agents, and immunosuppressive drugs.

Exactly how much **radiation** exposure is safe is unknown. Several factors, though, are considered crucial. Radiation is known to have a cumulative effect. Small doses spread over years are not as harmful, however, as a single large dose. For years, the calibration of x ray equipment was inadequate, and doses were sometimes greater than intended. Radiation was also scattered rather than directed at a particular target site. With improvement in both diagnostic and therapeutic radiation techniques, it is probable that radiation-induced cancer will diminish.

Another celebrated example of cancer arising from medical exposure involves the substance diethylstilbestrol, or **DES.** DES was prescribed from the 1940s through the 1960s to women who experienced complications like bleeding or diabetes during pregnancy or who were believed to be at risk of a miscarriage.[3] Several million pregnant women were treated with DES.

In 1971, scientists found a link between DES and a cancer of the female reproductive organs. The cancer did not affect the women who actually took the drug; instead, it affected their daughters. DES and DES-type drugs are no longer prescribed for pregnant women. They do continue to be used for a number of other medical problems, however. For instance, DES-type drugs are useful in treating some of the undesirable symptoms of menopause and certain kinds of cancer of the breast and prostate. DES is also used as a "morning-after" birth-control pill in cases of rape and incest.

Social Factors

Without much doubt, the largest percentage of fatal cancers result from social exposures, especially involving the use of tobacco and alcohol. *Healthy People 2000* identifies several trends in smoking activity in the U.S. There appears to be an overall decline in the number of adults who smoke, particularly among males; however, an increasing number of smokers are smoking more heavily.[4] Mortality and morbidity rates are lower for smokers of low tar and nicotine cigarettes, the consumption of which now represents 40 percent of all cigarette sales. The gains made by changing to low tar and nicotine brands

Radiation: energy emitted or radiated in the form of waves or particles implicated in the cause of certain cancers, but also used in the treatment of some cancers.

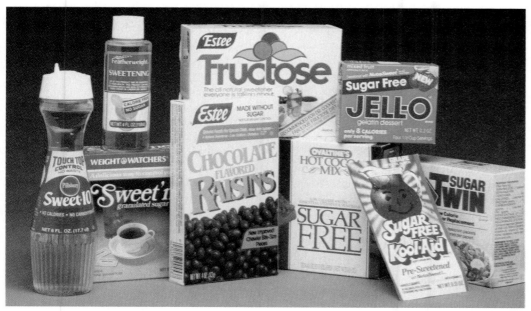

Figure 11.1: What Do You Think?

1. Efforts by the FDA to ban products containing saccharin resulted in great protest and the continued availability of saccharin in the U.S. Politicians and others say that the FDA has too much power. Do you think that the FDA should be able to place a ban on popular products that constitute a health hazard?

2. How do you think cancer-causing ingredients in the food supply compare in magnitude to other cancer-causing elements in our environment? What evidence did you use as the basis for your opinion?

may be negated, however, if smokers inhale more deeply or smoke more cigarettes to achieve the effect of higher tar and nicotine cigarettes.

While there is no evidence that alcohol is carcinogenic in itself, it does appear to act with other factors to cause cancers in the digestive tract. Because of its link to cirrhosis of the liver, alcohol may be at least indirectly responsible for the development of cancer of the liver as well.

There has been an increasing interest in the role of diet in both cancer causation and prevention. Dietary practices are closely related to tradition and culture, and certain cancers are linked to specific behaviors involving food preparation and consumption. In Japan, fish lovers enjoy such delicacies as salmon, salmon eggs, or codfish eggs, all heavily salted and seasoned. These large quantities of salt in the diet have been associated with the inflated rates of stomach cancer that exist worldwide, wherever salted fish is a staple.

Certain food additives are linked to some cancers. Most additives, though, serve useful purposes. Some provide protection from spoilage; some mask an otherwise unappetizing color; others enhance flavor. A wise consumer must weigh these benefits against the potential risks. The great American hot dog, for instance, contains *sodium nitrite*, which adds color and acts as a preservative. Sodium nitrite is converted, when ingested, into suspected carcinogenic substances known as **nitrosamines;** however, the untreated hot dog is pale gray, instead of the familiar red, and must be both fresh and carefully prepared to avoid growth of the bacteria that produce deadly botulism.

Other food additives have been associated with cancer. Artificial sweeteners, for example, have been the subject of much controversy. The first artificial sweeteners to come under suspicion and scrutiny were the **cyclamates.** Introduced in the 1950s and popularized in diet soft drinks during the 1960s, cyclamates were linked to bladder tumors. Because these substances had produced such tumors in laboratory rats, cyclamates were removed from the market in the U.S. in 1969.

Another popular artificial sweetener, **saccharin,** came under attack in 1977. Canadian studies involving both humans and laboratory animals provided evidence that saccharin intake substantially increased the risk of bladder cancer. The Canadian government banned the use of saccharin following publication of these studies. When the U.S. Food and Drug Administration announced its intent to carry out a similar ban, there was a loud protest from consumers. People raced to their grocers to buy up popular substances containing saccharin. Today, products containing saccharin are labeled with warning messages like those found on cigarette packages (see figure 11.1). New artificial sweeteners are likely to be scrutinized carefully for any cancer-causing potential.

Aspartame is another artificial sweetening product that appeared on the market during the 1980s in such name brands as Equal® and Nutrasweet®. Its use has become widespread in such merchandise as the leading selling diet soft drinks and other familiar items. No conclusive evidence supports concerns that aspartame poses a carcinogenic threat under circumstances of ordinary consumption.

Irish physician Denis Burkitt noted that cancer of the colon was second only to lung cancer as a cause of cancer death in Western Europe and North America, but it was virtually nonexistent in East Africa and some other parts of the world. Africans, he observed, ate about three times the amount of fiber (e.g., fruits, vegetables, whole grain cereals) consumed by westerners, who process most of the fiber out of their food. Burkitt reasoned that fiber's ability to absorb liquids and its general indigestibility made it pass rapidly through the digestive tract, presumably removing carcinogenic substances in the process before they could do damage.[5] Consumption of wheat bran appears to inhibit colon tumor development more than other dietary sources of fiber.[6]

Some investigators feel that it is the western diet of red meat and animal fats that is responsible for the high incidence of colon cancer. In many western countries, fats from beef, pork, lamb, fried foods, and cheese and other milk products account for 40 percent or more of the caloric intake. By contrast, in Japan, other Asian countries, and the East African countries studied by Burkitt where colon cancer is rare, fats constitute only 10 to 12 percent of the caloric intake.

Exact mechanisms may be unclear, but the presence of fat seems to enhance colon carcinogenesis through elevation of agents that act as promoters of tumor development. A high intake of dietary corn oil, beef fat, safflower oil, and lard increases colon carcinogenesis; however, diets high in olive oil, coconut oil, and fish oil do not appear to enhance one's susceptibility to colon cancer.[7] In summary, increased consumption of fiber-containing food and decreased dietary fat intake form the basis of a diet likely to do no harm and that may have the potential to reduce the likelihood of colon cancer development.

The pursuit of the golden tan is yet another sociocultural behavior that can have grave consequences. A tan provides various subtle messages in North America and elsewhere in the world. To some people, it represents affluence, indicating that the possessor can afford the Florida vacation, the Caribbean cruise, or the exotic "good life" described in travel brochures. To other people, a bronzed appearance is symbolic of health, of a rugged exterior, or of being in touch with nature. To still others, a tan is sensual or symbolic of sexual prowess. Tanning beds have become popular, and their radiation may be even more intense than that produced by the sun. They are not a safe alternative to suntanning.

For whatever reason a tan is pursued, sun worshipers are susceptible to the most common of all malignancies to attack humankind—skin cancer from the sun's ultraviolet rays (see figure 11.2). There are several varieties of skin cancer, and they form on or near the surface of exposed areas of skin. Fortunately, skin cancers grow slowly, usually remain localized, and seldom metastasize. These qualities make them treatable, usually on an outpatient basis.

More dangerous is a skin cancer known as **melanoma.** Melanomas are cancers of the cells that produce **melanin,** the pigment that gives skin its color. Melanomas are life threatening if they metastasize. Although they are more likely to occur on exposed areas of the body, they may also occur on covered areas. A change in the appearance of a mole may signal the development of melanoma, and it should promptly be examined by a physician.

Other sociocultural factors seemingly related to cancer incidence include having multiple sex partners (cancer of the cervix), obesity (cancers of the uterus and gallbladder), being beyond age thirty during one's first pregnancy (breast cancer), and never having borne children (ovarian cancer). Not all of these relationships can be explained readily; however, even if cause-and-effect relationships are eventually confirmed, it is unlikely that significant life-style changes would result without accompanying and profound cultural changes.

Biological Factors

Cancer research is a field that is rapidly changing, and one that has shed light on biological factors associated with cancer. One exciting research area is concerned with the

Melanoma: a serious type of skin cancer of the pigment-forming cells.

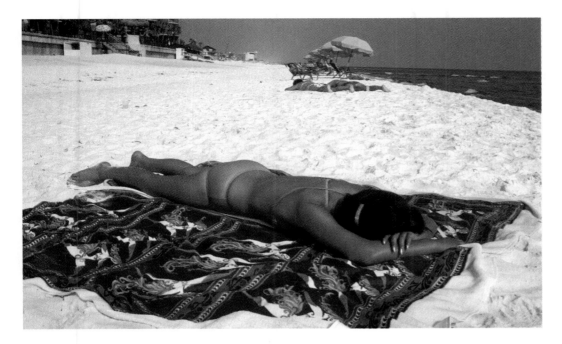

Figure 11.2: What Do
You Think?

1. Sunbathers are susceptible to skin
   cancer from the sun's ultraviolet
   rays. What cultural factors do you
   think encourage excessive sun
   exposure?
2. What factors do you think could be
   instrumental in getting people to
   decrease sun exposure?

study of genetics. Scientists have discovered **oncogenes** which may mutate and play an important role in the uncontrolled cell growth associated with cancer. Oncogenes now serve as "markers" that provide insight as to how cancers arise. The *ras oncogene* is associated with 50 percent of colon cancers and 90 percent of pancreatic cancers.

Cancer research also has identified **suppressor genes** which are part of the normal cell's protective mechanisms. If something goes awry in a suppressor gene, cancers may arise. For instance, a suppressor gene known as the "p53" gene is associated with both breast and lung cancer. With a particular type of cancer that seems to have a strong genetic component, as many as 90 percent of family members who inherit the p53 gene may develop cancer before age fifty. Screening for p53 is already being done, and in the future, having a means of altering the gene (genetic engineering) to reduce cancer risk is a real possibility.[9]

Obscuring the role of heredity in cancer causation is the fact that family members frequently follow similar lifestyles. They eat the same foods, share an environment, and are exposed to the same kinds of things. They may, therefore, have similar risks but no unique hereditary predisposition.

As cells and tissues grow older, they are less able to repair themselves and may be more susceptible to abnormal activity. By the age of twenty-five, risk begins to increase, with more cancers showing up in women until about age fifty-five, when cancer starts to occur more often in men. Some authorities believe that if other diseases, such as those of the cardiovascular system, did not claim so many lives prematurely, cancer would ultimately cause nearly everyone's death.

Sex appears to be a factor in the development of some cancers. While breast cancer can indeed occur in men, new cases in 1994 were 182 times more common in women.[10] The role of sex is a difficult one to assess because of the intervention of lifestyle variables.

About thirty years ago, when cigarette smoking was a male-dominated behavior, lung cancer was virtually unknown in females. Today, more women than ever are smoking cigarettes, and lung cancer has become the leading cause of cancer deaths for both men and women. This link between changing lifestyles and the resultant growth in lung cancer among women dispels some earlier views about the relation between sex and susceptibility to cancer.

Francis Peyton Rous demonstrated in 1911 that a virus infection could increase the incidence of cancer in chickens. Other studies similarly have shown a relationship between certain viruses and some kinds of cancer. Several viruses have been hypothesized as playing a role in the

Oncogene: a bit of genetic material or "gene" that plays a role in promoting the development of certain types of cancers.

Suppressor gene: a bit of genetic material or "gene" that plays a role in preventing abnormal cell growth of the type associated with cancer, and whose malfunction may contribute to the formation of some cancers.

Figure 11.3: Cancer
incidence and cancer
deaths by site and sex,
1995 U.S. estimates.

Source: Data from Phyllis Wingo, et al.,
"Cancer Statistics, 1995" in CA—A Cancer
Journal for Clinicians, 45.1 (1995):8–30,
American Cancer Society, Inc.

Cancer Incidence and Cancer Deaths by Site and Sex—1995 U.S. Estimates

Males

Cancer incidence*		Cancer deaths	
skin melanoma	3%	skin melanoma	2%
oral	3%	oral	2%
lung	14%	lung	33%
pancreas	2%	pancreas	5%
stomach	2%	stomach	3%
colo-rectal	10%	colo-rectal	9%
prostate	36%	prostate	14%
urinary	8%	urinary	5%
leukemia/lymphoma	7%	leukemia/lymphoma	8%
other sites	15%	other sites	19%
Total cases = 677,000		Total deaths = 289,000	

Females

Cancer incidence*		Cancer deaths	
skin melanoma	3%	skin melanoma	1%
oral	2%	oral	1%
breast	32%	breast	18%
lung	13%	lung	24%
pancreas	2%	pancreas	5%
colo-rectal	12%	colo-rectal	11%
ovary	5%	ovary	6%
cervix/uterus	8%	cervix/uterus	4%
urinary	4%	urinary	3%
leukemia/lymphoma	6%	leukemia/lymphoma	8%
other sites	13%	other sites	19%
Total cases = 575,000		Total deaths = 258,000	

*Does not include basal and squamous cell skin cancer, nor carcinoma in situ, except that of the bladder.

Free radical: unstable, naturally occurring substances which are believed to interfere with healthy cellular functioning, and contribute to the aging and disease processes.

Antioxidants: substances that prevent the formation of free radicals, or atoms in which there is an unpaired electron. Free radicals are natural byproducts of the body burning oxygen (oxidation). By inhibiting the formation of free radicals, antioxidants are thought to decrease the risk of developing a variety of chronic diseases, including heart disease and some cancers.

Folacin: a B vitamin, also known as folic acid, that aids in the formation of hemoglobin in the red blood cells and is necessary for the production of genetic material. Recently, daily consumption of 0–4 mg of folic acid by pregnant women has been associated with a reduction in neural tube defects in newborns.

development of human cancers as well. Among the most widely suspected viruses are Epstein-Barr virus (EBV), herpes simplex type II (HSV-II), and hepatitis virus type B. EBV, the causative agent in infectious mononucleosis, is linked to Burkitt's lymphoma, a cancer found mostly in China, and to a nasopharyngeal cancer found primarily in southern China and parts of Southeast Asia. HSV-II may play a role in development of some cervical cancers. Hepatitis B has been associated with liver cancers in some parts of Africa and Asia.

Another biological factor implicated in the development of some cancers are **free radicals,** naturally occurring substances believed to interfere with normal cell functioning through **oxidation** processes (see chapter 19).[11] It is theorized that **antioxidant** substances, particulary vitamins C and E and beta-carotene, may retard or eliminate the damaging effects of free radicals that give rise

to cancers of the oral cavity, esophagus, and reproductive tract. Although not an antioxidant, **folacin** has been associated with a decreased risk of cervical cancer.[12] Other factors may be involved in these prevention processes so the evidence about antioxidants and other vitamins remains controversial.[13]

Cancer Incidence and Mortality

While cancer can strike at virtually any part of the body, it occurs more commonly in certain areas (see figure 11.3). Some cancers of particular concern include lung cancer, colon and rectum cancer, breast cancer, uterine cancer, and testicular cancer.

Lung Cancer

Lung cancer is the leading cause of cancer deaths among both men and women. It is estimated that 87 percent of lung cancers

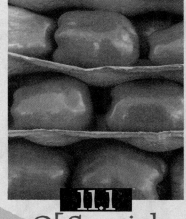
occur from people smoking cigarettes.[14] Lung cancer metastasizes easily and is one of the most virulent and difficult of all cancers to treat. It is seldom diagnosed in its early stages. Even with the most radical of therapeutic procedures, the five-year survival rate among lung cancer patients is only 13 percent.[15] Moreover, the survival rate with respect to lung cancer has improved only slightly during the past decade, and no significant change in this rate is on the horizon.

Colon and Rectum Cancer

Cancers of the colon and rectum are sometimes referred to as the "cancers no one talks about." As mentioned previously, dietary habits related to fat and fiber intake may be responsible, in part, for the relatively high incidence of these cancers in the U.S.

Because colorectal cancer tends to metastasize slowly, early detection can often result in complete cure through surgery and follow-up therapy. Delayed diagnosis, however, makes treatment more difficult. Changes in bowel habits and stool consistency or rectal bleeding not attributable to hemorrhoids are cause for a medical checkup. As with other cancers, survival rate is dependent on the actual site and stage of development.

Breast Cancer

Nationally, cancer of the breast is the number-two cancer killer of women. Early detection of breast cancer is essential for successful treatment. With early detection and treatment, breast cancer can show a five-year survival rate as high as 93 percent.[16] Delayed diagnosis can reduce the options for treatment and the probability of long-term survival. Under the age of thirty-five, the risk of breast cancer is minimal. Risk increases with age; about 75 percent of breast cancer patients are over the age of fifty. Women with a personal history of breast cancer are at high risk, as are women who have a history of breast cancer in their families (grandmother, mother, or sister). Women with breast lumps or thickenings, nipple discharges, or other abnormalities and women who are obese, childless, or had their first child after age thirty may also be at greater risk.

Besides a lump, thickening, swelling, puckering, or dimpling of the breast, any persistent skin irritation of the breast or nipple can signify breast cancer. Changes in the shape or appearance of the nipples or areolae should be reported to a physician, as should unusual pain or breast tenderness. **Breast self-examination (BSE)** should be practiced on a monthly basis as a means of early detection. Women should have their health-care provider check their BSE proficiency during office visits, request a breast physical examination if it is not provided routinely, and discuss the need for **mammography** (breast x ray) for early detection of breast cancer. More information about early detection is offered later in this chapter. Pamphlets that outline the steps of BSE are widely available as well. Women should ask their physicians for these pamphlets or inquire about them through local affiliates of the American Cancer Society (ACS).

Uterine and Cervical Cancer

Most uterine cancers arise in the cervix, the "neck" of the uterus that descends to the posterior end of the vagina, or in the lining of the uterus. For both of these sites, early symptoms include unusual bleeding or discharge. At its earliest stage a tumor can be confined to a single area, allowing for a relatively uncomplicated surgical removal. The lack of early detection and prompt treatment permits metastasis to occur.

The **Pap test,** named for its creator, George N. Papanicolaou, is an examination of cells taken from the cervix to detect abnormalities. The procedure takes minutes to administer, creates only minor discomfort, and can be performed in a physician's office. If the test reveals any abnormality, additional diagnostic techniques may be necessary.

While highly effective in detecting cervical cancer, the Pap test is less effective in detecting cancer of the uterine lining. Other diagnostic techniques are available, however.

Testicular Cancer

Although testicular cancer represents only 1 percent of all cancers in the male, it is the most frequently occurring type of solid tumor seen in late adolescence and early adulthood.[17] Unfortunately, many adolescent males are unaware of this potentially dangerous type of cancer. Because of the seriousness of testicular cancer and the importance of early detection to allow for effective treatment, **testicular self-examination (TSE)** is now being promoted.[18]

Other Cancers

Several other types of cancers can occur. Over 700,000 cases of skin cancer occur annually in the U.S.[19] Most of these skin cancers are of the basal or squamous cell variety and are almost 100 percent curable if diagnosed and treated early. Most skin cancers are related to experiencing excessive, unprotected exposure to sunlight and other forms of ultraviolet radiation, having a fair complexion, and having occupational exposure to such products as coal tar, pitch, creosote, radium, or compounds containing arsenic. As pointed out earlier in this chapter, the most serious type of skin cancer is malignant melanoma. Changes in skin color or in appearance of a wart or mole can be a sign of melanoma. A more thorough summary of the danger signs of malignant melanoma can be found in table 11.3

More than 28,000 new cases of leukemia (cancer of the blood-forming tissues) were diagnosed in 1994.[20] Leukemia has several varieties, a fact important in detection, treatment, and eventual survival. Leukemia is often thought of as a cancer of childhood, despite the fact that twelve times as many adults actually get the disease. Its cause has been linked to excessive exposure to radiation and occupational exposure to certain hydrocarbons, notably benzene. Treatment of many forms of leukemia has progressed markedly during the past thirty years, with chemotherapy the most common method of treatment.

Ovarian cancer accounted for about 24,000 new cases in 1994 and is the deadliest of all cancers of the female reproductive

Breast self-examination (BSE): the systematic exploration and palpation of the breasts with the hand to identify normal and abnormal or irregular features; a self-care early detection procedure for breast cancer.

Mammography: x ray examination of the breasts used in early detection of breast cancer.

Pap test: an examination of the cells of the cervix used as an early detection procedure for cancer at that site.

Testicular self-examination (TSE): the systematic exploration and palpation of the testicles with the hand to identify normal and abnormal or irregular features; a self-care early detection procedure for testicular cancer.

TABLE 11.3   *Warning Signs of Malignant Melanoma of the Skin*

Changes of a mole or other skin tissue in:

Size	sudden or gradual enlargement
Color	especially from edge of lesion to surrounding skin
Elevation	any area that becomes raised is suspicious
Surface	such as becoming scaly, crusty, ulcerating, bleeding, or oozing
Shape	particularly if irregular margins develop
Sensation	such as itching or soreness
Consistency	skin that becomes abnormally soft or brittle for instance
Surrounding Skin	redness, swelling, changes in flesh tones

system.[21] It mostly strikes women between the ages of sixty-five and eighty-four. While there are few risk factors for ovarian cancer that women can themselves control, early detection is important. The ACS recommends that women over forty have an annual cancer-related checkup.

Oral cancer accounts for about 29,600 new cases each year.[22] It occurs more than twice as often among men than among women. Risk factors are clear. People who smoke cigarettes, cigars, or pipes or who dip snuff or chew tobacco, as well as people who use alcohol frequently and to excess, are candidates for oral cancer.

Persons who dip snuff or chew tobacco may be at exceptional risk for oral cancer.[23] A regular observation made by dental health professionals in patients who use smokeless tobacco is the presence of white, patchy lesions, a condition known as **leukoplakia.**[24] This results from irritation of the tissue in the mouth and almost always is associated with the specific area of the mouth where tobacco is placed. Some of these lesions have the potential to become oral cancers. Tobacco contains cancer-causing nitrosamines. Their concentration in products such as snuff is 500 to 14,000 times higher than that allowed in food.[25] In one study, smokeless tobacco users had eleven times the risk of developing cancers of the mouth and gum as nonusers of any tobacco product.[26] A more in-depth discussion of this cancer and other health risks associated with tobacco products can be found in chapter 15.

Prostate cancer is the second leading form of cancer death in men.[27] About 80 percent of the cases of prostate cancer are diagnosed in men over age sixty-five. The number of new cases of prostate cancer is increasing (due largely to improved detection and diagnosis). The occurrence of prostate cancer is 30 percent higher in African-American men than in White men.[28] For reasons that are not known, African-American men have the highest incidence of this disease in the world.[29] The ACS recommends that men over the age of forty should have an examination of the prostate performed annually. This test requires the physician to insert a finger in the patient's rectum to locate and palpate the prostate gland. After age fifty, men should have a blood test as well that can help in early diagnosis of prostate cancer. Many middle-aged men experience a non-malignant enlargement of the prostate known as *benign prostatic hypertrophy* or BPH. BPH can arise from urinary tract infection or from unknown causes. Early symptoms of both prostate cancer and BPH can create difficulty in urinating, and pain in the lower back and thighs. Such symptoms need to be reported as soon as possible to a physician.

About 51,800 new cases of bladder cancer occurred in 1994.[30] This type of cancer presents more often in men than in women, Whites than in African-Americans, urban residents than in rural dwellers, and in dye, rubber, and leather workers than in other occupational groups. Smoking, however, is the greatest risk factor for bladder cancer. Smokers have a relative risk twice that of nonsmokers.

Pancreatic cancer is one of the most insidious forms of cancer because it has few symptoms until disease processes are firmly

Leukoplakia: white, patchy lesions of the mouth or the tongue considered sometimes to be a precursor of oral cancer.

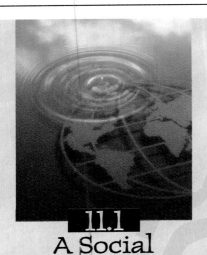

11.1

A Social Perspective

Cancers as They Affect Minorities in the U.S.

In estimating 1995 cancer incidence on behalf of the American Cancer Society, Phyllis Wingo, Tony Tong, and Sherry Bolden projected 1,252,000 new cancer cases in the United States. Among these new cases were approximately 120,000 among African-Americans and about 35,000 among other minorities (see table 11.4). Cancer incidence and mortality rates are often higher among African-Americans than among Caucasians. For instance, in 1991 cancer incidence rates were 439 per 100,000 population for Blacks, but 406 per 100,000 for Whites. For the same year, cancer deaths were 228 per 100,000 for Blacks and 170 per 100,000 for Whites.

African-Americans have both a higher occurrence of, and a higher death rate from cancers of the esophagus, cervix, stomach, liver, prostate, and larynx. The rate of esophageal cancer is more than three times that in Blacks as compared to Whites. African-Americans also experience more multiple myeloma (cancer of the bone and bone marrow).

A customary way of measuring cancer survival is in terms of five-year survival rate, the number of persons still alive five years after the diagnosis of disease. When all cancers are taken into consideration, African-Americans have a poorer five-year survival rate than Caucasians, 39 percent versus 55 percent. Much of this difference is due to the later seeking of treatment and later diagnosis among Blacks, in part, a consequence of access to care and economics. Ironically, many of these cancers are ones for which there are screening procedures.

Cancer incidence and mortality for other minorities varies. Cancer rates among Hispanics often are lower than those for Black or Whites. Since many cancers are linked to lifestyle, cultural differences in tobacco use, alcohol use, dietary patterns, sexual behaviors, and other factors provide insight about causes of disease. Cultural traditions, independent of socioeconomic factors, also may play a role in screening, diagnosis, and treatment.

What Do You Think?

1. What implications for prevention and early detection programs can you identify based on the information above and in table 11.4?
2. If cultural values and belief systems affect seeking out screening and follow-up care, how does this point apply to African-Americans? to Hispanic Americas? to Asian Americans? to Native Americans? How does it apply to you?

Sources: Data from Phyllis Wingo, et al., "Cancer statistics, 1994" in *CA—A Cancer Journal for Physicians*, 45.1 (1995) 8–30; and American Cancer Society, *Cancer Facts & Figures—1994*, (Atlanta: American Cancer Society, 1994), 18.

established. Little is known of its cause or prevention. Only 4 percent of pancreatic cancer victims are alive five years following their diagnosis.[31]

Lymphoma is a collection of cancers involving the body's lymph glands. Risk factors are poorly defined although persons with reduced immune system function, such as persons affected by the AIDS virus, and persons who have had organ transplants may be more susceptible. About 52,900 new cases and 22,750 deaths occurred in 1994.[32]

Cancer Treatment

Four particular treatments are presently used, separately and in combination, depending on the stage of the disease at the time of diagnosis and the aggressiveness of the individual cancer. These treatments include surgery, radiotherapy, chemotherapy, and immunotherapy. A fifth treatment, psychotherapy, is as yet unproven in its effectiveness.

Surgery

The development of successful cancer surgery was dependent on the development of modern medical technology, including blood transfusions, antibiotics, improved surgical techniques, and new anesthetics. Surgery is now the most common weapon against cancer. If tumors are confined to their sites of origin, surgery alone often can accomplish a complete cure. Surgery in combination with additional therapy can frequently achieve positive results, even after metastasis.

Radiotherapy

About one-half of all cancer patients receive radiation treatment, either alone or combined with surgery or chemotherapy. **Radiotherapy** is based on the fact that x rays stop cell growth and do so somewhat selectively. That is, x rays are more effective in destroying abnormal cells than in destroying healthy cells. It is effective as long as cancer cells are confined locally.

TABLE 11.4   *Cancer Deaths among Selected Groups of Minorities*

Cancer Site	African-Americans	Hispanic* Americans	Native Americans	Asian** Americans
Oral	1,274	204	31	78
Esophageal	1,987	233	532	48
Stomach	2,338	824	53	212
Colo-rectal	6,030	1,399	143	340
Liver and other biliary	1,405	860	81	273
Pancreas	2,933	810	77	173
Lung	15,201	2,727	371	646
Skin melanoma	119	89	8	5
Breast (female)	4,809	1,264	84	184
Cervical	983	292	42	27
Other uterine	921	207	14	29
Ovarian	1,067	369	34	70
Prostate	5,299	833	71	79
Bladder	841	221	22	29
Kidney	977	399	61	36
Brain & nervous system	681	429	26	38
Lymphatic	1,444	750	41	105
Leukemia	1,609	714	41	81
Multiple myeloma	1,680	314	26	27

*Persons classified as Hispanic origin on death certificates may be of any race. Incomplete data on death certificates may account for some inaccuracy. These data account for 90 percent of cancer deaths.

**Includes Japanese and Chinese Americans only.

Source: Data from the National Center for Health Statistics, *Vital Statistics of the United States, 1991.* Public Health Service, Washington, D.C., 1994.

What Do You Think?

1. What are the three leading causes of cancer deaths for African-Americans? Hispanic Americans? Native Americans? Asian Americans? Do the types of cancer deaths vary by racial/ethnic minority group?

2. What factors might account for the different types of cancer deaths noted for these minority groups? You may want to consider factors presented in tables 11.5 and 11.6.

Surgery and radiotherapy share some similar limitations. Both are local forms of treatment and therefore do not affect tumor cells that have been shed into the blood. Both forms of treatment, by necessity, must do some damage to healthy tissue. Radiotherapy, while a useful tool, has drawbacks that require considerable research and continued technological improvement.

Chemotherapy

More than fifty different cancer drugs are now used in the U.S. **Chemotherapy,** or drug therapy, has a major advantage over surgery and radiotherapy in that it is useful for treatment of diffuse tumors, such as leukemias, and malignancies that have

metastasized. Chemotherapy has produced astounding results for some forms of cancer.

A case in point is Hodgkin's disease. Precision x ray treatments combined with chemotherapy have increased five-year survival rates to 70 percent for advanced disease patients and 90 percent for patients whose disease is detected early. Significant improvements in survival have also been accomplished for cancers at several other sites.

Cancer chemotherapy has many side effects. Some side effects, such as nausea and vomiting, may be immediate and of short duration but intense. Though time passes and the patient begins to feel better, the prospect of another treatment day and the return of the unpleasantness must be faced. Side effects such as hair loss, weight loss, and fatigue are both less immediate and more cumulative in nature. Their presence, however, may be damaging to the patient's self-image and act as a constant reminder of the disease.

Many experimental drugs are presently undergoing clinical study to determine their effectiveness and safety. For the time being, existing drugs are saving many lives of cancer patients who only a few years ago would have been without hope.

Immunotherapy

Immunotherapy, the newest approach to cancer management, is based on a search for ways to stimulate the body's defenses to fight cancer cells. The goal is to accomplish the type of immune system mobilization that occurs when the body fights off chicken pox, an infected cut, or the common cold.

A problem is that since cancerous cells come from within the body, the body does not recognize them as hostile or alien. Thus, the immune system is not stimulated. Another problem relates to the fact that cancer is a collection of diseases rather than a single disease. There is, therefore, little chance of a single "immunization" being able to build up the body's resistance to all forms of cancer. Promising results are now coming from the world's laboratories, though.

Scientists hope that an antiviral protein produced in the body, called **interferon,** which helps to combat colds and influenza, may be useful for cancer treatment as well; however, theories that attempt to explain interferon's actual role in cancer management still greatly outnumber facts. In addition, interferon is expensive to produce and retrieve in pure form. While early experiments hint that interferon may be useful in cancer management, it is likely to be many years before sufficient research evidence substantiates these claims.

Scientists are excited about the potential of **monoclonal antibodies** for treating cancer.[33] These special disease-fighting antibodies are created by the genetic fusing of cancer cells with normal, healthy cells. They may have the potential to seek out and destroy specific cancer cells. Their use in cancer diagnosis and treatment is under study at the present time, and shows promise as a means of carrying cancer cell-destroying drugs and radiation to precise locations in the body which are affected by disease.

Cancer Quackery

Cancer quackery is a multimillion-dollar industry in the U.S. alone each year. When cancer strikes, many people do foolish, irresponsible, or dangerous things. One of the things they do is turn to "quacks." These practitioners offer the cancer patient friendly attentiveness, hope, or "secret" cures. The person with cancer may be desperate, so the practitioner who can make these offers has appeal. Quacks may be professionally educated physicians; however, many times they have no degree and no medical education whatsoever.

Responsible physicians do not offer secret cures or make guarantees about treatment interventions. Quack treatments can be especially dangerous to the patient who has cancer in its early stages. Trying useless gadgets or therapeutically worthless drugs is costly and wastes valuable time. Quacks may have no conscience about telling patients that they have cancer when in fact they do not. After a series of worthless but expensive "treatments," the patient is declared "cured." The practitioner takes the credit, which opens the door for the testimonial and exploitation of more people. Quacks cannot be recognized by their appearance alone. They are smart, friendly, and impressively attired. They provide warmth, act concerned, and give reassurance to patients who are filled with anxiety.

Cancer Prevention and Early Detection

The technology needed to prevent cancer or detect it early (when therapy is most beneficial) is evolving. As a result of new knowledge, the American Cancer Society provides the recommendations for prevention and early detection contained in this section. Important cancer risk factors are summarized in table 11.5. Specific behaviors that are believed to reduce cancer risk are described in table 11.6.

Lung cancer and nonmelanoma skin cancer are the best examples of malignancies largely preventable through prudent lifestyle

Interferon: an antiviral protein produced by the body that assists in immune response, and is thought to play a future role in the successful treatment of various diseases, including cancer.

Monoclonal antibodies: special factors which bolster the body's response to disease, especially by carrying targeted drugs and radiation to specific disease sites.

TABLE 11.5 — Summary of Cancer's Risk Factors

Colorectal

- History of rectal polyps
- Rectal polyps run in family
- History of ulcerative colitis
- Blood in stool
- Over age forty

Lung

- Heavy cigarette smoking over age fifty
- Started smoking before age fifteen
- Smoker working with/near asbestos

Uterine—Endometrial

- Unusual bleeding or discharge
- Late menopause (after age fifty-five)
- Diabetes, high blood pressure, and overweight
- Over age fifty

Uterine—Cervical

- Unusual bleeding or discharge
- Frequent sex in early teens or with many partners
- Low socioeconomic background
- Poor care during or following pregnancy

Breast

- Lump or nipple discharge
- History of breast cancer
- Close relative with history of breast cancer
- Over age thirty-five; especially over age fifty
- Never had children; first child after age thirty

Skin

- Excessive exposure to sun
- Fair complexion
- Work with coal tar, pitch, or creosote

Oral

- Heavy smoker and drinker
- Poor oral hygiene
- Snuff dipper or tobacco chewer

Ovary

- History of ovarian cancer among close relatives
- Over age fifty
- Never had children

Prostate

- Over age sixty
- Difficulty in urinating

Stomach

- History of stomach cancer among close relatives
- Diet heavy in smoked, pickled, or salted foods

---

choice. Since lung cancer is related to cigarette smoking, the best prevention against it is never to start smoking, to quit or reduce smoking if you already smoke, or to change to a lower tar brand. Smoking-cessation programs have helped many smokers overcome dependency on cigarettes.

If you must pursue the golden tan, or if prolonged exposure to the sun is unavoidable, you can still reduce the risks. Special caution should be exercised when in the mountains, where thin air transmits more of the sun's ultraviolet rays, or near water, where they are multiplied. When you are in the sun, be cautious.

1. Wear light clothing and a hat to protect exposed areas.

2. Use lotions that block the sun's rays and apply them often, especially after swimming. Sunscreen products are those that contain a **sun protection factor** or **SPF.** They are graded from two to forty, with the higher numbers providing greater screening protection.

3. Avoid using baby, mineral, olive, or vegetable oils during exposure. Although these products may moisturize the skin, they also enhance the burning power of the sun.

4. Avoid exposure during the midday hours when the sun's rays are particularly damaging. During the summer months, these hours are approximately 10:00 A.M. to 2:00 P.M.

Sun protection factor (SPF): a rating assigned to tanning and sunscreen products indicating the relative level of protection from solar radiation, where a higher-numbered rating is indicative of more protection.

TABLE 11.6 Behaviors Associated with Cancer Risk

Smoking

Cigarette smoking accounts for 90 percent of male lung cancers and 79 percent of female lung cancers, and about 30 percent of *all* cancer deaths. Persons who smoke two or more packs of cigarettes a day have death rates from lung cancer that are 12 to 25 times that of nonsmokers.

Sunlight

Virtually all of the cases of nonmelanoma skin cancer (>700,000 each year) in the U.S. are due to exposure to ultraviolet radiation. Sun exposure is also a major factor in the occurrence of melanoma.

Alcohol

Oral cancer and cancer of the larynx, throat, esophagus and liver occur more frequently among heavy drinkers. The risk is compounded in those individuals who smoke cigarettes or use chewing tobacco.

Spit Tobacco

Use of chewing tobacco and snuff, both forms of smokeless or "spit" tobacco have more oral cancer, and cancer of the larynx, throat, and esophagus.

Estrogen

The exact role of estrogen in cancer causation is controversial. Estrogen treatment for menopausal symptoms has been linked to endometrial cancer. Including progesterone as part of this therapy appears to reduce this risk.

Occupational Risks

Exposure to different chemicals and industrial products can increase risk of certain cancers (see also table 11.2). The best documented risk is exposure to asbestos and development of lung cancer, especially if accompanied by cigarette smoking.

Ionizing Radiation

Excessive exposure to radiation (x rays, radon in homes) may increase risks of certain cancers, especially if compounded by other risk factors and behaviors.

Diet

Maintain a desirable weight. Individuals 40 percent or more overweight increase their risk of cancers of the colon, breast, prostate, gallbladder, ovary, and uterus. *Eat a variety of fruits and vegetables.* These products are associated with decreased risk of cancers of the lung, prostate, bladder, esophagus, colon, and stomach. *Increase fiber as found in whole grain cereals, breads, pasta, vegetables, and fruits.* Evidence suggests a decreased risk of colon cancer. *Reduce overall fat intake.* High fat diets are associated with cancers of the breast, colon, and prostate. *Limit alcohol consumption* (see above). *Limit consumption of salt-cured, smoked, and nitrite-cured food products.* These products are associated with an elevated risk of esophageal and stomach cancer.

Source: Data from American Cancer Society, *Cancer Facts & Figures—1994,* (Atlanta: American Cancer Society, 1994).

---

5. Be aware of hazy or partially overcast days. Ultraviolet radiation can penetrate haze or clouds.
6. Avoid use of artificial tanning devices.

Methods exist for early detection of many cancers (see table 11.7). Most of these procedures require a visit to a physician's office. One test that can be self-administered by women is monthly breast self-examination (BSE) (see Activity for Wellness 11.1). Although a woman's risk of breast cancer remains low until she is in her forties, BSE is encouraged among women in their twenties and thirties, as well as among older women. BSE allows the woman to become familiar with the feel and texture of normal breast tissue. Unfamiliar lumps or changes can then be identified more easily.

The American Cancer Society recommends that women have a baseline mammogram by age forty.[34] Women between forty and forty-nine should have a mammogram every 1 to 2 years. After age fifty, women with no symptoms of breast disease should have a mammogram every year.

Despite the importance of mammography in breast cancer early detection, some women are reluctant to seek getting one. What determines whether or not a woman gets a mammogram? Researchers Suzanne M. Fuller, Robert J. McDermott, Richard G. Roetzheim, and Phillip J. Marty found that a woman's decision to have a mammogram was related both to her perceptions of breast cancer and to the screening process itself.[35] They also found that women of color were less likely than their White counterparts to pursue

TABLE 11.7 — General Guidelines for Your Cancer Early Detection Checkup

Ages twenty to forty years:

Your cancer-related checkup should be performed every three years, and include examination for cancers of the thyroid, testicles, prostate, oral cavity, ovaries, skin, and lymph nodes. Oral exams can be performed during regular preventive dental checkups that occur at the typically recommended six-month intervals. A physical breast exam by a qualified health provider should be performed at least once every three years. A baseline x ray of the breast (mammogram) should be obtained by age forty. Breast self-examination should be performed monthly. An annual pelvic examination and Pap test is recommended for women after age eighteen to check for cervical cancer and other abnormal conditions of the cervix and uterus. Persons with known health conditions, family histories of certain cancers, and other special health needs may require more frequent cancer detection examinations. Your physician or other qualified health-care provider can provide more specific personal guidance on the frequency for such examinations.

After age forty:

Your cancer-related checkup should be performed every year and include examination for cancers of the thyroid, testicles, prostate, oral cavity, ovaries, skin, and lymph nodes. A physical breast exam should be obtained annually. A mammogram should be obtained each year after age fifty. Between the ages of forty and fifty, guidance on the frequency of mammograms should be sought from your health-care provider. Breast self-examination should be performed monthly. An annual pelvic exam can assist in the early detection of cancer of the uterus. A Pap test, as part of a pelvic examination, should occur every one to three years depending on personal history, personal risk factors, and the advice of your health-care provider. An endometrial tissue sample at the time of menopause should be obtained if you are known to be at elevated risk of endometrial cancer (history of infertility, obesity, failure of ovulation, abnormal uterine bleeding, estrogen therapy). To detect colon and rectal cancers at an early stage, an annual digital rectal examination is recommended. In addition, after age fifty, a Guaiac slide test is recommended. Finally, a proctoscopic examination is recommended based upon personal history, personal risk factors, and the advice of your health care provider. Thorough consultation with your health-care provider includes your input so that care can be tailored optimally to meet your health-care needs.

---

breast cancer screening, a point which may relate to minority women's poorer prognosis when disease is discovered. The failure of some physicians to recommend a mammogram is less of a problem now than it was some years ago, but health-care provider reluctance still occurs. A woman between age thirty-five and forty would be well advised to address the subject of mammography with her primary health care provider. Mammography is underutilized as an early detection procedure.[36]

An early-detection test for testicular cancer in men can also be self-administered. The procedure for testicular self-examination is easy to perform (see Activity for Wellness 11.2).

The ACS recommends that adults should practice skin self-examination on a monthly basis to detect changes in the appearance of the skin that may signal skin cancers (see Activity for Wellness 11.3).

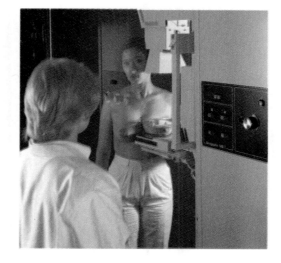

What Do You Think?

1. Mammography is an important screening test for the early detection of breast cancer. What do you think are some of the most important barriers that stop women from having a mammogram?
2. What incentives can you think of that, if offered, would increase the utilization of mammography? How realistic are your suggestions?

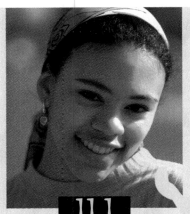

11.1
Activity for Wellness

Breast Self-Examination (BSE)

1. Stand before a mirror. Inspect both breasts for anything unusual, such as any discharge from the nipples, puckering, dimpling, or scaling of the skin.

   The next two steps are designed to emphasize any change in the shape or contour of your breasts. As you do them you should be able to feel your chest muscles tighten.

2. Watching closely in the mirror, clasp hands behind your head and press hands forward.

   Breast self-examination should be done once a month so you become familiar with the usual appearance and feel of your breasts. Familiarity makes it easier to notice any changes in the breast from one month to another. Early discovery of a change from what is "normal" is the main idea behind BSE.

3. Next, press hands firmly on hips and bow slightly toward your mirror as you pull your shoulders and elbows forward.

   Some women do the next part of the exam in the shower. Fingers glide over soapy skin, making it easy to concentrate on the texture underneath.

4. Raise your left arm. Use three or four fingers of your right hand to explore your left breast firmly, carefully, and thoroughly. Beginning at the outer edge, press the flat part of your fingers in small circles, moving the circles slowly around the breast. Gradually work toward the nipple. Be sure to cover the entire breast. Pay special attention to the area between the breast and the armpit, including the armpit itself. Feel for any unusual lump or mass under the skin.

   If you menstruate, the best time to do BSE is two or three days after your period ends, when your breasts are least likely to be tender or swollen. If you no longer menstruate, pick a day, such as the first day of the month, to remind yourself it is time to do BSE.

5. Gently squeeze the nipple and look for a discharge. Repeat the exam on your right breast.

6. Steps 4 and 5 should be repeated lying down. Lie flat on your back, left arm over your head and a pillow or folded towel under your left shoulder. This position flattens the breast and makes it easier to examine. Use the same circular motion described earlier. Repeat on your right breast.

Source: Data from the National Cancer Institute.

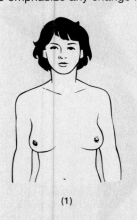

(1)

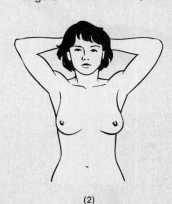

(2)

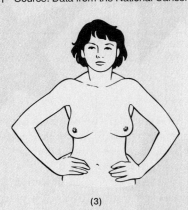

(3)

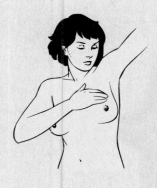

(4)

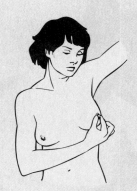

(5)

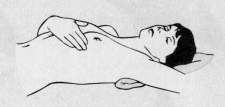

(6)

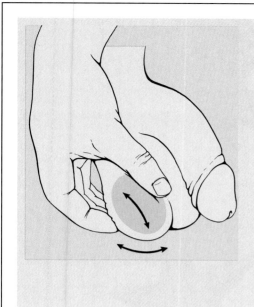

Testicular Self-Examination

1. Examine each testis separately with your fingers.
2. Your index finger, middle fingers, and thumb should be positioned as shown in the sketch.
3. Your testis should be gently rolled between your thumb and fingers; feel for small lumps or other abnormalities.
4. This examination ought to be conducted on a monthly basis; the best time is after a shower or hot bath when the scrotum is relaxed, and your testes are easily felt.
5. If you identify an abnormality, bring it to the attention of your physician.

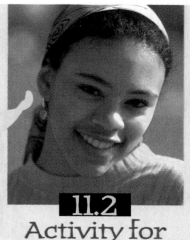

11.2
Activity for Wellness

This procedure may be especially valuable for persons with fair skin, persons who have a history of prolonged sun exposure, and persons whose occupation necessitates work outside. If you are unsure about your present commitment to self-examination or other cancer early-detection procedures, you may get some assistance by referring to table 11.8.

Also, become acquainted with cancer's seven warning signals (see table 11.9). Although these signs of cancer are not comprehensive, they do provide a clue to the most common cancers.

Other Noncommunicable Disease Threats

In addition to cancer, there are a number of other noncommunicable diseases that threaten a person in quest of high-level wellness. Some of these diseases include diabetes, emphysema, asthma, and chronic bronchitis.

Diabetes

Diabetes is a disease of the pancreas in which the body cannot make use of sugars and other carbohydrates in a normal way. The sixth leading cause of death in the U.S., diabetes is also a contributing cause of death due to other conditions, such as cardiovascular disease.

Normally, complex carbohydrates, when consumed, are broken down into a simple sugar called **glucose. Insulin,** a hormone produced by the pancreas, then acts on the glucose to facilitate its use by the body for energy. The diabetic either does not produce sufficient insulin or is unable to mobilize the insulin. Thus, excess glucose accumulates in the blood and may appear in the urine.

Diabetes arises from two distinct routes.[37] **Type I diabetes** is the result of destruction by the immune system of pancreatic beta cells. It is these beta cells that normally produce insulin. Type I diabetics require insulin-replacement therapy. **Type II diabetes** results from a combination of changes in insulin sensitivity and insulin secretion. It can be treated with diet therapy, oral medications, and occasionally, with administered insulin.

There are an estimated ten million diabetics in the U.S. Perhaps four million are unaware of their disease. It is a serious disease in itself but even more so because of the complications that can arise. High levels of glucose in the blood can have many harmful effects. Diabetes leads to damaged or narrowed coronary arteries. It precipitates hemorrhages in the capillaries of the retina of the eye, a condition that now ranks as the leading cause of blindness in the U.S. Diabetes contributes to kidney failure, when the body's waste-and-disposal system is no longer able to maintain the body's delicate chemical balance. Furthermore, diabetes gives rise to peripheral vascular disease, in which the extremities of the body do not receive an

Insulin: a hormone secretion of the pancreas necessary to convert carbohydrates into energy and sometimes used therapeutically to control diabetes.

Type I diabetes: diabetes arising from destruction of the beta cells of the pancreas that produce insulin.

Type II diabetes: diabetes arising from changes in insulin secretion or sensitivity of the body to insulin.

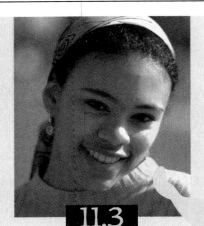

11.3
Activity for Wellness

Skin Self-Examination

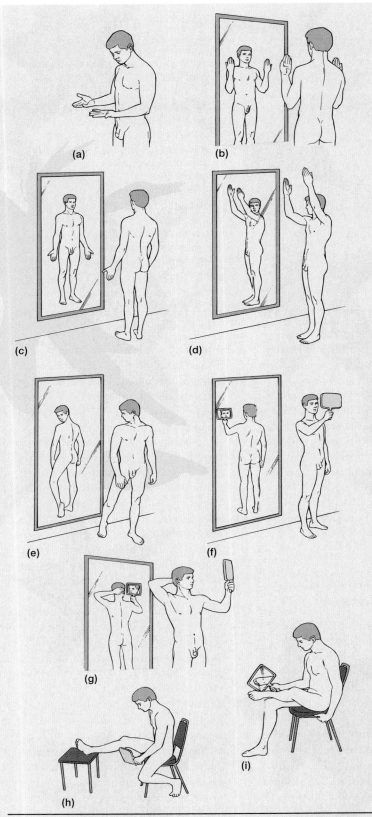

(a)

(b)

(c)

(d)

(e)

(f)

(g)

(h)

(i)

Source: Robert J. Friedman, et al., "Early Detection of Malignant Melanoma: The Role of Physician Examination and Self-Examination of the Skin," in *CA—A Cancer Journal for Clinicians*, 35(3):146–149, 1985, 1985, American Cancer Society, Inc.

TABLE 11.8 — Tips for Initiating Self-Examination for Cancer Early Detection

Self-examination may seem difficult at first if you have no history of performing these activities, or feel that the effort is a waste of time. The following tips may help you to adopt these important self-care procedures.

Precontemplation → Contemplation

If you have never thought about cancer early detection you may find the suggestion below to be helpful in giving the idea some consideration.

- Using the phone book, locate the local division of the American Cancer Society. Contact the office by phone, or better yet, stop in to obtain publications about self-examination and other early detection procedures.

Contemplation → Preparation

If you have given serious consideration to employing early detection practices, but have not yet done so, some of these steps may be of assistance.

- Ask your health-care provider about self-examinations appropriate for you. Go over the procedures together. Get questions answered.
- Make the decision to take action.

Preparation → Action

When you have made the decision to take action, the following activities may help you establish the practice.

- Identify a date in the next 30 days when you will carry out your plan. Circle the date on your calendar.
- Review the steps of the particular procedure you will employ. Remind yourself that the best outcome of self-examination is reassurance that everything is normal.

Action → Maintenance

If you are performing self-examination or participating in other early detection practices, these steps will help you to maintain your activity.

- After completing your first self-examination, pledge that you will repeat the procedure at the next scheduled interval (usually the next month).
- Make a firm appointment with yourself (e.g., the first of every month, every pay day, every fourth Sunday, etc.) to repeat the procedure. Tie the procedure to some other activity that is part of your normal routine.
- Tell a close friend or relative whom you trust about your practice of self-examination (breast, testicular, skin—whatever applies to you). Let people know that you are not "just thinking about" taking an active role in your own health care—but actually doing something about it.

Maintenance

Congratulations! You are doing some important steps to help yourself and those about whom you care. Additional things you can do include:

- Becoming a proponent and advocate of self-examination among relatives, friends, and peers.
- Diversifying your repertoire of self-care activities outside the realm of self-examination. Having many self-care activities shows you (and others) that you care about yourself.

TABLE 11.9

Cancer's Seven Warning Signals

Change in bowel or bladder habits
A sore that does not heal
Unusual bleeding or discharge
Thickening or lump in breast or elsewhere
Indigestion or difficulty in swallowing
Obvious change in wart or mole
Nagging cough or hoarseness
If *you* have a warning signal, see your doctor!

adequate supply of blood and thus leads to tissue death. In some cases, amputation of the affected body part may be necessary.

Symptoms of diabetes include frequent urination and thirst, extreme hunger, rapid weight loss, blurred vision or a sudden change in visual acuity, easy tiring, drowsiness, or general weakness after completion of relatively simple physical tasks. If these symptoms recur or persist, consult your physician.

Simple, relatively painless tests can detect the presence of diabetes. A physician may prescribe some combination of the following therapies for diabetes: diet modification, structured exercise, insulin

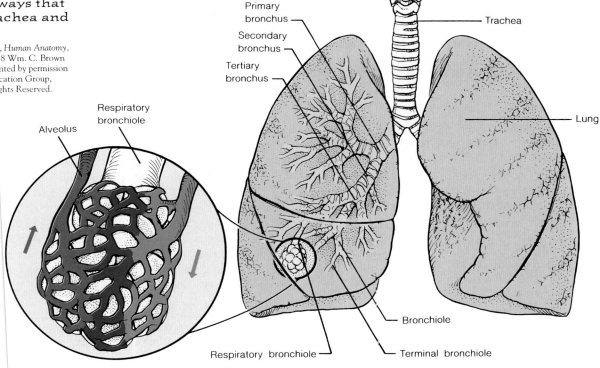

Respiratory bronchiole

Alveolus

Primary bronchus

Secondary bronchus

Tertiary bronchus

Larynx

Trachea

Lung

Bronchiole

Respiratory bronchiole

Terminal bronchiole

injections as needed, and oral medication. Diabetes cannot currently be cured, but it can be managed, especially with early detection.

Emphysema

Emphysema is a severe destructive lung disease that is presently incurable. Its development is gradual rather than sudden. Although it is most common in men between the ages of fifty and seventy, women are also affected. A high percentage of emphysema patients have a history of cigarette smoking. As with some other smoking-related disorders (e.g., heart disease and lung cancer) emphysema may show important increases in occurrence among women in the coming years.

Air pollution is also associated with the incidence of emphysema. It has been suggested, too, that people who lack a substance called *alpha one antitrypsin* may be particularly susceptible to emphysema and at an earlier age than normal.

Emphysema develops when the **bronchi,** passageways leading from the trachea (windpipe) to the lungs, become irritated and obstructed. Air becomes "trapped" in the lung beyond the obstruction. The bronchi are like the branches of a tree, branching smaller and

smaller until they terminate in clusters of air spaces in the lung, known as **alveoli** (see figure 11.4). Oxygen enters the blood from the alveoli and is exchanged for carbon dioxide. Emphysema damages the alveolar walls causing them to lose their elasticity. The capillaries that carry the blood for gas exchange also may be damaged. With less oxygen exchange possible, the person with emphysema experiences shortness of breath, making even simple physical tasks difficult. Even normal breathing is laborious for people who have advanced emphysema. Since emphysema also interferes with blood flow through the lung, the heart works harder in an effort to compensate. Under such strain, the heart may enlarge, leading to congestive heart failure.

The exact cause of emphysema is unknown, but the strong evidence of a relationship among cigarette smoking, air pollution, and emphysema suggests the wisdom of avoiding these agents.

If emphysema is diagnosed early, progressive disease may be halted. Breathing retraining, light exercises, and careful effort to minimize respiratory congestion can help people with emphysema to make the best use of their breathing capacity and lead ordinary lives.

Emphysema: a progressive loss of function or rupture of the alveoli of the lung resulting in an increased amount of difficulty in breathing.

Asthma

Asthma is an abnormal response of the air passageways to various environmental agents or events. Among asthmatics, airways can constrict suddenly, triggering shortness of breath and wheezing. Episodes may be mild, lasting only a few minutes, or severe to the point where airways are closed off resulting in unconsciousness and death. Severe asthma may produce panic and fear in the victim, especially if help is not immediately accessible. Such an emotional state can make the attack even worse.

According to the American Lung Association, "Psychological and inherited factors play a part in the disease. What may be inherited is the tendency to react to external and internal stresses in a particular way. However, environmental factors such as dusts and chemicals are often related to the first onset of symptoms.[38]

For many asthma suffers, episodes are triggered by substances such as pollen, spores, dust, molds, or animal dander. Food allergies are additional possibilities that lead to asthma attacks. The chemicals present in cigarette smoke present yet other potential sources of concern for some asthmatics. Asthma may be seasonal or year-round depending on the major contributing factors. It is a disease about which much remains unknown and for which individual variation in onset, periodicity, and responsiveness to treatment is considerable.

Recent advances in treatment and control have led to use of medicines such as aminophylline, epinephrine, isoproterenol, and cromolyn sodium for relief of symptoms.[39] Asthma is a disease whose threat to life should not be underestimated. Severe attacks constitute medical emergencies; therefore, persons who have had asthma diagnosed should follow the advice of their physicians carefully, take medication as prescribed, and have the telephone number of emergency assistance personnel readily available for themselves and their family members.

Chronic Bronchitis

Bronchitis is an inflammation of the lining of the bronchi. Accompanying this inflammation, typically, is an impaired air flow. Acute bronchitis, with its characteristic coughing and spitting, is often associated with the common cold or with influenza. Chronic bronchitis includes all the symptoms of the acute state, except that they are almost always present.

Bronchitis is caused by the irritation brought on by disease or infection and contact with air pollutants. A major pollutant is cigarette smoke. The person with chronic bronchitis experiences occasional acute episodes. If the source of the acute bronchitis is bacterial infection, antibiotic therapy can provide relief; however, permanent relief of the symptoms of chronic bronchitis requires elimination of the sources of irritation to the nose, throat, mouth, sinuses, and bronchi. Cigarette smoking should be eliminated, as should exposure to secondary smoke. If a person is exposed to dust and irritating fumes at work, a change of employment is recommended. That is, of course, more easily said than done. The following recommendations are for persons who experience chronic bronchial distress:

1. See your physician at the beginning of any cold or respiratory infection. Do not neglect even a slight cold.
2. Do not smoke.
3. Follow a nutritious diet and avoid obesity.
4. Participate in mild, but daily exercise, taking care not to tire yourself.
5. Ask your physician about being immunized against pneumococcal pneumonia and influenza.
6. Avoid exposure to colds and influenza at home or in public.

Healthy People 2000

Goals and objectives to reduce the prevalence of, and disability resulting from chronic diseases such as those discussed in this chapter comprise a major portion of *Healthy People 2000*. The implementation of relevant behavioral lifestyle changes for primary and secondary prevention would result in improvement in quality of life, while saving billions in health-care costs. Some of the objectives that relate to material examined in chapter 11 are shown in table 11.10.

TABLE 11.10

Selected Healthy People 2000 Objectives for the Nation Related to Cancer and Other Selected Chronic Diseases

1. **Reverse the rise in cancer deaths to achieve a rate of no more than 130 per 100,000 people.** (Age Adjusted Update: 133 per 100,000 people in 1992, down from 134 per 100,000 in 1987.)

2. **Reduce cigarette smoking to a prevalence of no more than 15 percent among people aged 20 and older.** (Update: 27 percent in 1992, down from 29 percent in 1987.) (Special target populations: People with high school education or less 20 years and over; Blue-collar workers 20 years and over; Military personnel; Blacks 20 years and over; Hispanics 20 years and over; American Indians/Alaska natives; Southeast Asian males; Females of reproductive age [18–44 years]; Pregnant females; Females who use oral contraceptives.)

3. **Reduce dietary fat intake to an average of 30 percent of calories or less and average saturated fat intake to less than 10 percent of calories among people aged 2 and older.** (Update: 34 percent of calories from total fat and 12 percent of calories from saturated fat for 1988–1991, down from 36 percent of calories from total fat and 13 percent of calories from saturated fat for 1976–1980.)

4. **Increase complex carbohydrates and fiber-containing foods in the diets of adults to five or more daily servings for vegetables (including legumes) and fruits, and to six or more daily servings for grain products.** (Baseline: 4.0 servings of vegetables and fruits for adults in 1989; 3.0 servings of grain products for females 19–50 years in 1985.)

5. **Increase to at least 60 percent the proportion of people of all ages who limit sun exposure, use sunscreens and protective clothing when exposed to sunlight, and avoid artificial sources of ultraviolet light (e.g., sun lamps, tanning booths).** (Baseline: 31 percent limit sun exposure, 28 percent use sunscreen, and 28 percent wear protective clothing according to 1992 data.)

6. **Increase to at least 80 percent the proportion of women aged 40 and older who have ever received a clinical breast examination and a mammogram, and to at least 60 percent those aged 50 and older who have received them within the preceding 1 to 2 years.** (Update: 66 percent of females age 40 and over ever received exams, and 51 percent of females 50 years and over received exams in preceding 1–2 years as of 1992, up from 36 percent and 25 percent respectively in 1987.) (Special Target Populations: Hispanic females 40 years and over; Low-income females 40 years and over; Females 40 years and over with less than a high school education; Females 70 years and over; Black females 40 years and over.)

7. **Increase to at least 95 percent the proportion of women aged 18 and older with uterine cervix who have ever received a Pap test, and to at least 85 percent those who received a Pap test within the preceding 1 to 3 years.** (Update: 91 percent of women with uterine cervix ever received Pap test, and 74 percent within the preceding 3 years in 1992, up from 88 percent of all women ever received Pap test, and 75 percent within the preceding 3 years in 1987.) (Special Target Populations: Hispanic females age 18 and older; Females 70 years and over; Females 18 years and over with less than a high school education; Low-income females 18 years and over.)

8. **Increase to at least 50 percent the proportion of people aged 50 and older who have received fecal occult blood testing within the preceding 1 to 2 years, and to at least 40 percent those who have ever received a proctosigmoidoscopy.** (Update: 30 percent received fecal occult blood testing within preceding 2 years, and 33 percent ever had proctosigmoidoscopy in 1992, up from 27 percent and 25 percent respectively in 1987.)

9. **Reduce diabetes to an incidence of no more than 2.5 per 1,000 people and a prevalence of no more than 25 per 1,000 people.** (Update: Incidence of 2.6 per 1,000 for 1989–1991, down from 2.9 for 1986–1988; prevalence of 28 per 1,000 for 1990–1992, with no change from the 1986–1988 baseline.) (Special Target Populations: American Indians/Alaska Natives; Puerto Ricans; Mexican Americans; Cuban Americans; Blacks.)

10. **Reduce diabetes-related deaths to no more than 34 per 100,000 people.** (Age Adjusted Update: 38 per 100,000 in 1991, with no change from the 1986 baseline.) (Special Target Populations: Blacks; American Indians/Alaska Natives.)

11. **Reduce to no more than 10 percent the proportion of people with asthma who experience activity limitation.** (Update: 21.8 percent in 1990–1992, up from 19.4 percent in 1986–1988.)

Source:*Healthy People 2000 National Health Promotion and Disease Prevention Objectives.* Department of Health and Human Services, Washington, D.C., 1991 *Healthy People 2000 Review 1993.* Department of Health and Human Services, Washington, D.C., 1994; Prevalence of Overweight Among Adolescents—United States, 1988–91. (1994) *MMWR,43*:818–821.

Summary

1. In the last century, the pattern of serious disease has shifted in the U.S. from being mostly communicable to being chronic and noncommunicable.

2. Cancer is often referred to as the most feared of all diseases, and ranks second to cardiovascular disease as a killer of people in the U.S.

3. Cancer is a collection of diseases that share the trait of abnormal cell growth.

4. Benign tumors are not cancerous and pose no immediate threat to health in most cases. Malignant tumors are cancerous and are usually life-threatening if not diagnosed and treated early in the disease process.

5. Cancer is spread through the body by metastasis.

6. The causes of cancer can be grouped by occupational, medical, social, and biological factors.

7. Oncogenes and suppressor genes are bits of genetic material that may play a role in cancer prevention and causation.

8. Free radicals and antioxidants are other biological factors that have received recent attention for the role they may play in cancer prevention and causation.

9. Cancer is largely a preventable disease. For example, smoking is directly related to 90 percent or more of all lung cancers. Most skin cancers could be eliminated if people took better precautions to avoid excessive sun exposure. Other examples of cancer-preventive practices can be identified.

10. Cancers may be treated by chemotherapy, radiation therapy, immunotherapy, surgery, and combinations of these procedures.

11. Monoclonal antibodies are being used to help the body fight cancer cells.

12. Cancer quackery is a multimillion-dollar a year business because people fall prey to "quacks" out of fear and desperation.

13. Not all cancers have early detection procedures but many do. All men and women should practice self-examination procedures as illustrated in this chapter, participate in other screening activities, and consult the advice of a qualified health-care provider concerning their personal cancer screening needs.

14. Diabetes is a major disease that can complicate other health conditions, including cardiovascular disease, as well as be life-threatening in and of itself.

15. Emphysema, asthma, and chronic bronchitis are all serious and potentially life-threatening disorders of the respiratory system. Appropriate responses to illness and lifestyle modifications still permit one to have a normal and productive life.

Recommended Readings

American Cancer Society. *Cancer Facts and Figures—1996*. Atlanta: American Cancer Society, 1996.

A publication updated annually with the latest in cancer facts and figures, including advances in prevention, early detection, and treatment.

Biermann, June, and Toohey, Barbara. *The Diabetic's Book*. New York: G. P. Putnam's Sons, 1994.

The Diabetic's Book is designed to help the person with diabetes to establish control of life, including control of personal emotions, diet, and meeting the needs of daily living.

Lorig, Kate, Laurent, Diana, Holman, Halsted, Gonzalez, Virginia, Sobel, David, and Minor, Marian. *Living A Healthy Life with Chronic Conditions*. Palo Alto, Calif: Bull Publishing, 1994.

This book offers many helpful hints for self-management for the person who lives with arthritis, asthma, diabetes, bronchitis, emphysema, or heart disease.

References

1. Phyllis Wingo, Tony Tong and Sherry Bolden, "Cancer Statistics, 1995," CA—A Cancer Journal for Physicians 45.1 (1995):8–30.

2. Richard Doll and Richard Peto, "The Causes of Cancer: Quantitative Estimates of Avoidable Risks of Cancer in the United States Today," *Journal of National Cancer Institute* 66 (1981):1193–1308.

3. U.S. Department of Health, Education and Welfare, *Questions and Answers about DES Exposure before Birth* (Washington, D.C.: NIH Publication No. 77-1118, 1977).

4. *Healthy People 2000, National Health Promotion and Disease Prevention Objectives* (Washington, D.C.: U.S. Department of Health and Human Services, 1991).

5. Bandaru, S. Reddy, "Dietary Fiber and Colon Cancer: Animal Model Studies," *Preventive Medicine* 16 (1987):559–565.

6. Bandaru, S. Reddy, "Dietary Fat and Colon Cancer: Animal Models," *Preventive Medicine* 16 (1987): 460–467.

7. Reddy, "Dietary Fat and Colon Cancer," 460–467.

8. American Cancer Society, *Cancer Facts & Figures—1994* (Atlanta: American Cancer Society, 1994), 2.

9. American Cancer Society, *Cancer Facts & Figures—1994*, 2.

10. American Cancer Society, *Cancer Facts & Figures—1994*, 10.

11. C. A. Rice-Evans and R. H. Burdon, *Free Radical Damage and Its Control*, (London: Elsevier, 1994).

12. University of California at Berkeley Wellness Letter, "Our Vitamin Prescription: The Big Four," *University of California at Berkeley Wellness Letter* 10.4 (1994):1.

13. American Medical Association Council of Scientific Affairs, "Diet and Cancer: Where Do Matters Stand?" *Archives of Internal Medicine* 153 (1993):5056.

14. American Cancer Society, *Cancer Facts & Figures—1994*, 22.

15. American Cancer Society, *Cancer Facts & Figures—1994*, 9.

16. American Cancer Society, *Cancer Facts & Figures—1994*, 10.

17. Vincent T. DeVita, *Cancer Treatment* (Washington, D.C.: U.S. Department of Health and Human Services, NIH Publication No. 80-1807, 1980).

18. Nancy Neef et al., "Testicular Self-Examination by Young Men: An Analysis of Characteristics Associated with Practice," *Journal of American College Health* 39 (1991):187–190.

19. American Cancer Society, *Cancer Facts & Figures—1994*, 15.

20. American Cancer Society, *Cancer Facts & Figures—1994*, 14.

21. American Cancer Society, *Cancer Facts & Figures—1994*, 15.

22. American Cancer Society, *Cancer Facts & Figures—1994*, 16.

23. U.S. Department of Health and Human Services, Public Health Service, *The Health Consequences of Smokeless Tobacco* (Washington, D.C.: U.S. Government Printing Office, Publication No. 36-2874, 1986).

24. Robert J. McDermott, Barbara J. Clark, and Kelli R. McCormack, "The Reemergence of Smokeless Tobacco: Implications for Dental Hygiene Practice," *Dental Hygiene* 61 (1987):348–353.

25. Gregory N. Connolly et al., "The Reemergence of Smokeless Tobacco," *New England Journal of Medicine* 314 (1986):1020–1027.

26. Heather G. Stockwell and Gary H. Lyman, "Impact of Smoking and Smokeless Tobacco on the Risk of Cancer of the Head and Neck," *Head and Neck Surgery* 9 (1986):104.

27. American Cancer Society, *Cancer Facts & Figures—1994*, 10.

28. American Cancer Society, *Cancer Facts & Figures—1994*, 10.

29. American Cancer Society, *Cancer Facts & Figures—1994*, 11.

30. American Cancer Society, *Cancer Facts & Figures—1994*, 16.

31. American Cancer Society, *Cancer Facts & Figures—1994*, 12.

32. American Cancer Society, *Cancer Facts & Figures—1994*, 14.

33. David M. Goldenberg, "New Developments in Monoclonal Antibodies for Cancer Detection and Therapy," *CA—A Cancer Journal for Clinicians* 44.1 (1994): 43–64.

34. American Cancer Society, *Cancer Facts & Figures—1994*, 10.

35. Suzanne M. Fuller, Robert J. McDermott, Richard G. Roetzheim and Phillip J. Marty, "Breast Cancer Beliefs of Women Participating in a Television-Promoted Mammography Screening Project," *Public Health Reports* 107.6 (1992):682–690.

36. Judith Sobel, Ann Curtin, and Deborah Fell, "The Oregon Breast Cancer Detection and Awareness Project: The Legacy of a Mammogram Screening Campaign," *Health Values* 15.1 (1991):3–8.

37. Andrew S. Krolewski et al., "Epidemiologic Approaches to the Etiology of Type I Diabetes Mellitus and Its Complications," *New England Journal of Medicine* 317 (1987):1390.

38. American Lung Association, *Facts in Brief about Lung Disease* (New York: American Lung Association, 1986), 11.

39. U.S. Department of Health and Human Services, "*What You Need to Know about Asthma*," (Washington D.C.: National Institute of Allergy and Infectious Diseases, 1990).

Communicable Diseases: Threats to Wellness Old and New

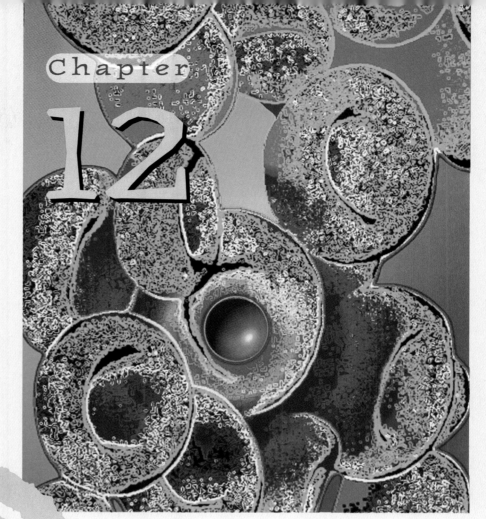

Student Learning Objectives

Upon completion of this chapter, you should be able to:

1. identify the public health agencies responsible for communicable disease control at the local, state, national, and international levels;

2. give examples of the health objectives of the nation for the year 2000 that target communicable disease control;

3. list several agents that can cause infection in a human being;

4. explain the body's defense mechanisms to infection;

5. explain the concept of immunity, and identify several ways of attaining immune status with respect to a disease;

6. describe the characteristics of the most common communicable diseases affecting people in the U.S.;

7. cite the recommended standards for immunization of selected communicable "diseases of childhood";

8. evaluate the status of HIV-related disease and other sexually transmissible diseases (STDs) in the U.S., including the methods for prevention, diagnosis, and treatment;

9. discuss why certain minority groups and women may require special consideration during the HIV/AIDS epidemic;

10. discuss several personal and social issues about STD control;

11. identify the factors that contribute to the practice of safer sex by you and by other college students;

12. estimate your comfort level with respect to negotiating "safer sex" with a partner;

13. identify resources for getting help on your campus and in your community should you think you might be infected by HIV or another STD;

14. apply disease prevention and health promotion measures for individual control of communicable diseases.

The reduction in incidence of communicable diseases is the most significant public health achievement of the past 100 years.[1] Their control is a fundamental aspect of most public health programs. While chronic diseases (e.g., cardiovascular disease, cancer, diabetes) have gained more prominence in developed countries during the twentieth century, and achievements have been made in the war against communicable diseases, prevention and control of infection has become more important than ever with the advent of threats to wellness such as Acquired Immune Deficiency Syndrome (AIDS).

Effective control of diseases requires that people have detailed knowledge of disease **epidemiology,** that is, surveillance of the person, place, and time factors that influence their development and spread. For infectious diseases that can give rise to large-scale outbreaks called **epidemics,** surveillance is performed by municipal, county, and state health departments at the local level, and the **Centers for Disease Control and Prevention (CDC)** at the national level. On a global scale, international control of infectious diseases is under the auspices of the **World Health Organization (WHO)** and other international agencies.

As a college student you should be aware of the communicable diseases that you are most likely to encounter. It is true that the stress of college life can decrease your resistance to some diseases such as flu, the common cold, and other disorders. Risky sexual practices can expose you to more serious diseases, including ones that can be both infectious and chronic, and in some instances, even life-threatening. A little common sense, a few easy self-care practices, and knowledge about your college or university health service can, however, minimize the adverse effects of most communicable diseases during the college years.

The health objectives of the nation for the year 2000, as reported in *Healthy People 2000,* highlight numerous issues related to the control of infectious diseases. A sample of these objectives is illustrated in table 12.1.

The Infectious Disease Cycle

Each communicable disease has a unique cycle of progression that may aid in its transmission and spread (see figure 12.1). The first trait or condition in a disease cycle is the presence of disease-causing organisms. Such organisms are called "germs," as everyone knows, or more precisely, **pathogens.** Pathogenic organisms, then, are disease causing, and each kind of pathogen is usually responsible for a specific disease or set of symptoms. Pathogens may be viruses, bacteria, fungi, spirochetes, protozoa, tiny worm-like creatures, insects, and other plant and animal organisms. What they have in common is that they are all small, often invisible to the naked eye.

A **reservoir** where pathogenic organisms can thrive and reproduce until they can infect people is a second condition that needs to be present for disease transmission. Some common reservoirs are animals (including people), soil, air, water, food, and inanimate objects. Some pathogens, such as those that cause **sexually transmissible diseases (STDs),** require special environments. For most STD-producing species, the warm, moist mucous membranes of the oral, genital, or anal regions of the body provide the receptive reservoir.

Pathogens require a **place of exit** from their reservoir to get to another person. For instance, germs from the common cold exit through the mouth and nose in the form of droplets when the infected person sneezes. Most STD-causing organisms, however, leave the body by means of the genitals, though they may also leave by way of the mouth, anus, or, in some cases, open sores or wounds in the skin.

Communicable diseases must have a **mode of transmission** from reservoir to person or from person to person. A mode of transmission is the means by which germs leave one person and enter another. **Direct contact,** or the direct spread of a pathogen from one person to another, is often a vehicle for transmission in diseases such as flu, chicken pox, measles, and the common cold. Sexual intercourse and other intimate physical contact are one form of direct contact and are the usual mechanisms for transmitting the STDs, hence the name.

Epidemiology: the study of the distribution and causes of disease.

Pathogen: an organism that can produce disease in a host.

Reservoir: an environment conducive to the maintenance of pathogenic organisms.

1. **Reduce indigenous cases (per 100,000) of vaccine-preventable diseases as follows: diphtheria among people aged 25 and younger to 0 cases** (Update: 3 in 1992, up from 1 in 1988); **tetanus among people aged 25 and younger to 0 cases** (Update: 7 in 1992, up from 3 in 1988); **polio (wild-type virus) to 0 cases** (Update: 0 in 1992, unchanged from 1988); **measles to 0 cases** (Update 2,237 in 1992, down from 3,058 in 1988 and 9,411 in 1991); **rubella to 0 cases** (Update: 160 cases in 1992, down from 225 in 1988 and 1,401 in 1991); **congenital rubella syndrome to 0 cases** (Update: 11 in 1992, up from 6 in 1988, but down from 47 in 1991); **mumps to 500 cases** (Update: 2,572 in 1992, down from 4,866 in 1988); **pertussis (whooping cough) to 1,000 cases** (Update: 4,083 in 1992, up from 3,450 in 1988 and 2,719 in 1991).

2. **Reduce epidemic-related pneumonia and influenza deaths among people aged 65 and older to no more than 7.3 per 100,000.** (Update: Average of 23.1 during 1987–1990, up from 9.1 for the influenza seasons of 1979–1980 and 1986–87.)

3. **Reduce pneumonia-related days of restricted activity as follows: 38 days per 100 people aged 65 and older** (Update: 63.5 days in 1992, up from 19.1 days in 1987); **24 days per 100 children aged 4 and younger** (Update: 19.4 days in 1992, down from 29.4 in 1987).

4. **Increase to at least 90 percent the proportion of primary care providers who provide information and counseling about immunizations and offer immunizations as appropriate for their patients.** (1992 Baseline: *DTP vaccination*—pediatricians 86 percent, nurse practitioners 76 percent, family physicians 89 percent; *Oral polio vaccination*—pediatricians 87 percent, nurse practitioners 76 percent, family physicians 89 percent; *Tetanus-diphtheria booster under age 18*—pediatricians 79 percent, nurse practitioners 71 percent, family physicians 70 percent; *Tetanus-diphtheria booster 18 years and over*—nurse practitioners 38 percent, obstetricians/gynecologists 4 percent, internists 29 percent, family physicians 74 percent; *Influenza vaccination 65 years and over*—nurse practitioners 42 percent, obstetricians/gynecologists 6 percent, internists 49 percent, family physicians 31 percent; *Pneumococcal vaccination 65 years and over*—nurse practitioners 33 percent, obstetricians/gynecologists 5 percent, internists 40 percent, family physicians 25 percent.)

5. **Confine annual incidence of diagnosed AIDS cases to no more than 98,000 cases.** (Baseline: 87,000 diagnosed cases in 1992, up from 49,000 in 1989.) (Special Population Targets: Gay and Bisexual Men, Blacks, Hispanics.)

6. **Confine the prevalence of HIV infection to no more than 800 per 100,000 people.** (Baseline: An estimated 400 per 100,000 people in 1989.) (Special Population Targets: homosexual men, intravenous drug abusers, women giving birth to live-born infants.)

7. **Increase to at least 50 percent the proportion of sexually active, unmarried people who used a condom at last sexual intercourse.** (Baseline: 19 percent of sexually active, unmarried women aged 15 through 44 reported that their partners used a condom at last sexual intercourse in 1988.) (Special Population Targets: sexually active young women aged 15–19 [by their partners], sexually active young men aged 15–19, intravenous drug abusers.)

8. **Reduce gonorrhea to an incidence of no more than 225 cases per 100,000 people.** (Update: 202 per 100,000 in 1992, down from 300 in 1989.) (Special Population Targets: Blacks, adolescents aged 15–19, women aged 15–44.)

9. **Reduce primary and secondary syphilis to an incidence of no more than 10 cases per 100,000 people.** (Update: 13.7 per 100,000 in 1992, down from 18.1 in 1989.) (Special Population Target: Blacks.)

10. **Reduce *Chlamydia trachomatis* infections, as measured by a decrease in the incidence of nongonococcal urethritis to no more than 170 cases per 100,000 people.** (Update: 210 per 100,000 in 1992, down from 215 in 1988 but up from 170 in 1990.)

11. **Reduce genital herpes and genital warts, as measured by a reduction to 142,000 and 385,000, respectively, in the annual number of first-time consultations with a physician for the conditions.** (Update: 139,000 and 218,000 respectively in 1992, down from 163,000 and 290,000 in 1988.)

Source: Data from *Healthy People 2000 National Health Promotion and Disease Prevention Objectives,* 1991; and from *Healthy People 2000 Review 1993,* 1994. Department of Health and Human Services, Washington, D.C.

Pathogens require a **portal of entry,** or place where they can get into the body. For the more familiar communicable diseases (such as the common cold, influenza, chicken pox) this place is the nose or the mouth. The portal of entry for the STDs is usually the genitals, though it may also be the mouth or the anus depending on individual sexual practices. Rarely, but occasionally, the portal of entry for some STDs may be an opening in the skin, such as a sore located on a part of the body quite distant from the genitals.

Communicable diseases have various **incubation periods.** The incubation period of a disease is the time lapse between exposure to, or introduction of the pathogen, and the actual onset of symptoms. Incubation periods are disease specific, which is another way of saying that they vary from disease to disease.

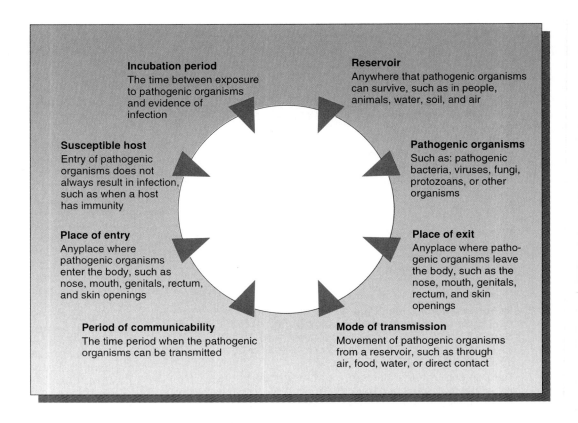

For example, the common cold has an incubation period of one to three days before symptoms occur. In the dreaded disease AIDS, the incubation period may be three years or more.

A disease may have a stage in which it is more easily transmitted than during other stages. This time is called its **period of communicability.** For example, a cold is most easily transmitted during its early stages. Genital herpes, an STD whose symptoms can be recurrent, is most easily transmitted during an outbreak in the infected individual; at other times, the risk of transmission may be relatively low. Syphilis, another important STD, may be easily transmitted during its primary or secondary stages but rarely transmitted at other times. Some STDs, however, are readily communicable virtually all of the time.

Pathogens may never make a person sick unless that person is what is called a **susceptible host.** That is, exposure to infection does not automatically result in disease. The body's arsenal of natural defenses includes the **immune system,** whose principal functions are the detection of and protection against diseases. Good overall health that results from proper nutrition and water

consumption, rest, and exercise may help to fight potential disease-causing invaders but can never guarantee absolute protection.

The Body's Response to Infection

An **infection** is the invasion of the body by pathogens that produce tissue injury or disease.[2] Usually, these infectious agents are microorganisms such as viruses, bacteria, fungi, protozoans, or other parasitic forms of life. Not all microorganisms cause disease in humans, however. Sometimes, too, the location of a particular microorganism determines whether it is "friendly" or "unfriendly." For example, the bacterium *Escherichia coli,* normally found in the lower part of the digestive tract, produces no symptoms of disease when maintained in that environment. However, when introduced to the body through the mouth by means of contaminated food or water, *E. coli* can cause severe diarrhea, vomiting, fever, and abdominal cramping.

What can happen when the body encounters a microorganism? According to Paul D. Ellner and Harold C. Neu, one of five possible events is likely.[3] First, the encounter

Susceptible host: An individual whose ability to fight off disease is compromised for some reason.

TABLE 12.2   *Types of Nonspecific Resistance*

Type	Description
Species resistance	A species of organism is resistant to certain diseases to which other species are susceptible
Mechanical barriers	Unbroken skin and mucous membranes prevent the entrance of some infectious agents
Enzymatic actions	Enzymes present in various body fluids act against pathogens
Interferon	A group of proteins (produced by cells in response to the presence of viruses) that interferes with the reproduction of the viruses in other cells
Inflammation	A tissue response to injury that helps to prevent the spread of infectious agents into nearby tissues
Phagocytosis	Neutrophils and macrophages engulf and destroy foreign particles and cells

From John W. Hole, Jr., *Human Anatomy and Physiology,* 6th edition. Copyright © 1993 Wm. C. Brown Communications, Inc. Reprinted by permission of Times Mirror Higher Education Group, Inc., Dubuque, Iowa. All Rights Reserved.

can result in no infection. The invading agent may not be virulent enough to produce infection. Second, the organism can "colonize" the body, but still not produce disease. Third, there can be an "inapparent infection." That is, the host develops no symptoms of illness, or develops an immunity to the invading agent. However, the host may become a carrier of the agent and be capable of passing it along to new hosts. These new hosts may in fact become infected and show disease symptoms. Fourth, the original host may show clinical symptoms of disease, later to develop either immunity or susceptibility to reinfection. And finally, the invading agent may be so virulent as to produce host death directly, or contribute to death because of other underlying illness.

To protect itself from foreign material, such as germs, your body has developed a sophisticated system for fighting off would-be invaders and eliminating pathogens that have penetrated the system. Part of your body's disease-fighting mechanism acts in general, nonspecific ways to protect you from a variety of pathogenic organisms. These mechanisms include species-specific resistance, epithelial barriers, enzymatic action, interferon, inflammation, and phagocytosis (see table 12.2). Another part of the disease-fighting system against infection is quite specific in that it protects against particular pathogenic agents. This part of the system provides a protection from disease known as **immunity.**

Species-specific resistance simply refers to the fact that human beings are resistant to certain diseases that may be lethal to birds, reptiles, or even other mammals. Similarly, diseases that can prove quite harmful to humans (e.g., gonorrhea) may be of no consequence to other animal species.

Skin, the mucous membranes that line organ systems, and other **epithelial structures** act as mechanical barriers to potential infections. Furthermore, **cilia,** tiny hairlike projections such as those of the respiratory tract, sweep out invading organisms and help to prevent the introduction of germs to the lungs and bronchial tubes.

Pathogenic organisms are susceptible to the action of certain **enzymes** contained in body fluid. Pepsin, an enzyme released in the stomach, neutralizes the effect of some pathogens that reach that part of the digestive tract. Similarly, an enzyme found in tears, called lysozyme, reduces the potentially harmful effects of many bacterial substances that find their way to the surface of the eye.

A protein-containing substance produced by infected cells, called **interferon,** has excited scientists recently for its apparent role in fighting diseases, especially those caused by viruses. Interferon can be taken in by noninfected cells, which subsequently become protected against the spread of disease. If interferon can be extracted from cells or manufactured efficiently, it has the potential to be a major weapon against many diseases.

Immunity: the state of being able to resist a particular disease by counteracting the potential effects of a foreign substance or pathogen

Epithelial structures: components of the body with epithelial tissue. Epithelial tissue is a type of tissue that lines all body surfaces, such as the outer layer of skin, and the inside lining of the digestive tract.

Enzyme: a protein substance that speeds up biochemical reactions.

Figure 12.2: Bone marrow releases undifferentiated lymphocytes that, after processing, become T-lymphocytes and B-lymphocytes.

From John W. Hole, Jr., *Human Anatomy and Physiology*, 7th edition. Copyright © 1996 Times Mirror Higher Education Group, Inc., Dubuque, Iowa. All Rights Reserved. Reprinted by permission.

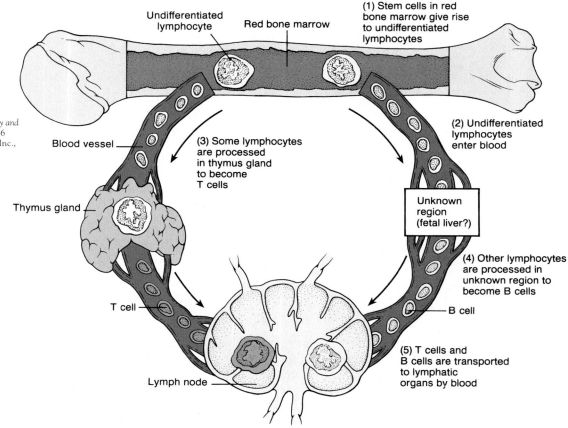

Undifferentiated lymphocyte — Red bone marrow

(1) Stem cells in red bone marrow give rise to undifferentiated lymphocytes

(2) Undifferentiated lymphocytes enter blood

Blood vessel

(3) Some lymphocytes are processed in thymus gland to become T cells

Unknown region (fetal liver?)

Thymus gland

(4) Other lymphocytes are processed in unknown region to become B cells

T cell

B cell

Lymph node

(5) T cells and B cells are transported to lymphatic organs by blood

White blood cells: A component of blood, also called leukocytes, capable of leaving the capillaries of the circulatory system in order to reach an infection site where they play a variety of roles in attacking the pathogen.

Phagocytosis: The process whereby white blood cells "eat" bacteria or other pathogens, by engulfing them and digesting them.

Lymph nodes: small, encapsulated oval bodies occurring in clusters in various parts of the body. Their primary functions are to filter lymph fluid and produce lymphocytes, playing an important role in the body's immune system.

Spleen: an organ of the lymph system located on the left side of the abdominal cavity. The primary functions of the spleen are to assist in the production of lymphocytes, filtering of blood, and destroying old red blood cells. In infants, it is also an important producer of red blood cells.

Inflammation is yet another response of the body to infection, although it can occur from other things as well, such as mechanical injury to the body. Four things characterize the inflammatory response; redness, swelling, heat, and pain. **White blood cells** generally accumulate at the site of inflammation and may form a thick fluid called **pus.** Once an infection has been brought under control, **phagocytosis,** or the removal of dead cells and other debris from the inflamed area by specialized cells, takes place. These special phagocytic cells are of two types: **neutrophils** and **monocytes.** Neutrophils handle small debris, while monocytes engulf and digest larger particles. Monocytes also give rise to **macrophages,** phagocytic cells concentrated in the lymph nodes, spleen, liver, and lungs.

As was stated, immunity is resistance to specific invading pathogens and the toxic substances they may release. Immunity involves several mechanisms in which selected cells identify the presence of foreign organisms and act to deactivate or remove them. Playing an important role in the immune response are special cells called **lymphocytes,** which originate in the bone marrow. Before reaching maturity, these undifferentiated cells are released from the marrow and are circulated through the body. About half of them reach the thymus gland, where they continue to mature and undergo additional changes. They become known as T-lymphocytes or **T cells** (for thymus-derived lymphocytes). Subsequent to this process, they are released to the blood where they comprise 70 to 80 percent of the circulating lymphocytes.[4] Lymphocytes accumulate at certain sites in the body more so than at others, such as the **lymph nodes** and the **spleen.**

Other undifferentiated lymphocytes released from bone marrow that do not travel to the thymus gland become B-lymphocytes or **B cells** (for bone marrow-derived lymphocytes). They comprise the remaining circulating lymphocytes, but like their T-cell counterparts, they also collect in the lymph nodes, spleen, bone marrow, and other locations (see figure 12.2).

Both T cells and B cells have receptors on their surfaces that can recognize foreign substances, known as **antigens.** Antigens are the proteins, polysaccharides, and other substances comprising or produced by attacking pathogens. When antigens are identified by the lymphocytes, immune response against them can be activated. T cells and B cells do not respond to antigens in identical ways, however. Some T cells attach themselves to antigens associated with certain types of bacteria, interacting directly with the invaders. This T cell response is known as **cell-mediated immunity.** With some kinds of viruses, T cells destroy the antigens produced on the membranes of infected cells, interfering with the virus-induced disease process.

There is more than one variety of T cell. **T-helper cells** stimulate the development of B cells or other T cells. **T-suppressor cells** inhibit growth of certain cell types. **Killer T cells** are able to destroy some kinds of cancer cells. This observation has led scientists to hypothesize that it is a disruption of normal T cell functions that contributes to at least some cancers in humans. This hypothesis is supported by the apparent relationship among declining T cell function, advancing age, and increased incidence of many types of cancer.

To combat antigens, B-lymphocytes produce and secrete substances called **immunoglobulins,** which are responsible for the production of **antibodies.** There are five major types of immunoglobulins, three of which are responsible for 80 percent of the production of antibodies. Immunoglobulins comprise the **gamma globulin** fraction of blood plasma. Antibodies produced are carried by body fluids to react with, and eliminate, specific antigens or antigen-bearing particles. This B cell response is known as **antibody-mediated immunity.** Occasionally, people lack the ability to form immunoglobulins and cannot produce the necessary antibodies for the B cell response. As a result of this deficiency, such individuals are highly susceptible to developing infectious diseases.

Types of Immunity

Immunity can occur via several pathways. Immunity may be a **naturally acquired active immunity** if a person is exposed to a living pathogen, subsequently develops disease, and then becomes resistant to that disease as a result of having produced T cells that serve as **memory cells.** That is, if the lymphocytes meet up with the same antigen again, they can respond appropriately, already having been sensitized to the antigen from the first encounter.

An **artificially acquired active immunity** can be produced in response to a **vaccine.** A vaccine may present antigen that stimulates an immune response against the disease-causing agent without actually producing symptoms of disease. Vaccines may contain viruses or bacteria that have been killed or weakened so that the severe symptoms of disease cannot be produced. They also may contain toxins of an infectious organism that have been modified in such a way so as to eliminate any toxic reaction. In each case, the antigen retains enough characteristics to stimulate the necessary immune response. Examples of such vaccines include those for **diphtheria, pertussis** (whooping cough), **tetanus, polio, rubella, measles, mumps, cholera,** and **typhoid fever.**

On some occasions, a person requires protection against pathogenic organisms but lacks the time necessary for active immunity. Under such circumstances, injections of gamma globulin fraction from the blood of persons already having immunity are given. This action provides the recipient with a temporary immunity usually lasting no more than a few weeks. Immunity received in this way is known as **artificially acquired passive immunity.** It is said to be passive because no antibodies are actually produced by the recipient. Since the lymphocytes of this individual have not been activated, that person remains susceptible to the pathogen involved after the passive immunity expires.

Yet another type of immunity is possible. During pregnancy, it is possible for selected antibodies to pass from the maternal bloodstream to the fetal bloodstream. The fetus thus acquires a temporary immunity to the pathogens for which the mother has developed active immunity. The fetus can be described as having **naturally acquired passive immunity,** protecting it from the diseases affected in some cases for up to a year (see table 12.3).

Autoimmune Disease: The Body Turned Against Itself

Under normal circumstances, the body's immune response is directed toward foreign proteins and other invading substances. The

Antibodies: immunoglobulin proteins that have been changed into plasma cells, or cells that make up the fluid portion of blood. The transformation from immunoglobulin to antibody occurs in order to counteract a specific antigen of an invading pathogen.

Diphtheria: a highly communicable infectious disease caused by the bacteria *Corynebacterium diphtheriae*. Common symptoms include a sore throat, weakness and mild fever, followed by a constriction of the air passage causing difficulty in breathing. Toxin produced by the bacteria can cause death from heart failure if not treated promptly.

Rubella: commonly known as German measles, this highly contagious infection is caused by a virus and is transmitted through respiratory secretions. Most commonly infecting children, its symptoms include enlarged lymph nodes in the neck, and a widespread pink rash. When the virus infects a pregnant woman, however, it can result in birth defects.

Cholera: a communicable infectious disease caused by the bacteria *Vibrio cholerae* transmitted through food or water contaminated with infected feces. Common symptoms include severe diarrhea and vomiting, often resulting in dehydration and circulatory collapse. If treated promptly and properly, the fatality rate is low. Without such care the fatality rate may exceed 50 percent.

Typhoid fever: a communicable infectious disease caused by the bacteria *Salmonella typhi*, transmitted through food or water contaminated with infected feces or urine. Common symptoms include fever, headache, weakness, red rash on the chest and abdomen, and a nonproductive cough.

TABLE 12.3   *Types of Immunity*

Type	Stimulus	Result
Naturally acquired active immunity	Exposure to live pathogens	Symptoms of a disease and stimulation of an immune response
Artificially acquired active immunity	Exposure to a vaccine containing weakened or dead pathogens	Stimulation of an immune response without the severe symptoms of disease
Artificially acquired passive immunity	Injection of gamma globulin containing antibodies	Immunity for a short time without stimulating an immune response
Naturally acquired passive immunity	Antibodies passed to fetus from mother with active immunity	Short-term immunity for infant, without stimulating an immune response

From John W. Hole, Jr., *Human Anatomy and Physiology,* 6th edition. Copyright © 1993 Wm. C. Brown Communications, Inc. Reprinted by permission of Times Mirror Higher Education Group, Inc., Dubuque, Iowa. All Rights Reserved.

Myasthenia gravis: a chronic disease characterized by excessive fatigue and weakness in certain muscles, often so severe the muscles are temporarily paralyzed.

Rheumatoid arthritis: a form of arthritis, or inflammation of the joints, most commonly affecting the joints of the fingers, wrists, feet, ankles, hips, or shoulder.

Multiple sclerosis: a chronic disease of the nervous system characterized by a variety of nervous system abnormalities such as shaky limbs, being unsteady or stumbling when walking, or having problems pronouncing words.

Smallpox: this now extinct contagious infection was caused by a virus and was transmitted through respiratory secretions or direct contact with skin sores. Its symptoms included high fever and a rash that left patients with scars.

body's own components are protected and preserved. For reasons that are not well understood, this protective mechanism can go awry, resulting in T cell and B cell mediated immune responses against the body's own tissues. Quite literally, the immune system attacks itself. Such an event is known as an **autoimmune reaction,** the consequences of which can be severe or even lethal.

Autoimmune disorders seem to occur more frequently in older individuals, suggesting that the aging process may precipitate unusual changes in the immune system. These disorders may come on the heels of severe viral or bacterial infections, they may stem from the presence of antigens in large quantity, or they may occur from the unsuppressed production of antibodies. Several diseases believed to have autoimmune origins have been identified. One of these disorders is **systemic lupus erythematosus (SLE),** where B-cell production of antibodies results in assaults on red blood cells, platelets, and lymphocytes. Some other autoimmune diseases you may have heard or read about include **myasthenia gravis, rheumatoid arthritis, insulin-dependent** (type I) **diabetes mellitus,** and **multiple sclerosis,** just to name a few.

Infectious Diseases of Interest in the U.S.

To address all possible infectious diseases that occur in the U.S., much less in the world, is

well beyond the scope of this chapter. We will examine some of the common infectious diseases found in the U.S. that are important to persons of college age. A number of these diseases are identified in table 12.4. If you were to travel to other parts of the world, the diseases encountered might be quite a bit different than these. Several of these disorders are known popularly as diseases of childhood, even though one's first personal contact with them may occur later in life. Examples of these diseases are **chicken pox,** diphtheria, measles, mumps, pertussis, poliomyelitis, and rubella. Diseases for which effective and safe immunizations exist and are typically provided are shown in table 12.5, along with the recommended timing of administration for infants and children. As a result of widespread immunization practices, the occurrences of many diseases have been reduced significantly. **Smallpox,** a disease formerly having worldwide importance, is believed to have been eliminated completely as a result of effective immunization programs. A little more than a generation ago, polio aroused fears not terribly unlike those associated today with AIDS. Thanks to the development of two different types of vaccines to prevent the disease, and the implementation of immunization programs for infants and children, polio is seen only rarely in the U.S. today. It is common practice for measles, mumps, and rubella immunizations to be given simultaneously.

TABLE 12.4   *Characteristics of Selected Human Infectious Diseases*

Disease	Type of Infectious Agent	Usual Routes of Transmission	Practical Treatment	Practical Prevention
Chicken pox	Virus	Person-to-person direct contact; airborne droplet	Selected antiviral drugs if started early after infection; isolation	Avoidance of contact and immunization
Diphtheria	Bacterium	Person-to-person direct contact	Isolation	Immunization
Acute gastroenteritis	Virus	Fecal-oral; fecal-respiratory	Fluid and electrolyte replacement	Personal hygiene and handwashing
Common cold	200+ viruses	Direct contact; airborne droplets; contact with freshly soiled articles	No specific treatment other than rest; avoid unnecessary use of antibiotics	Avoidance of direct contact with infected individuals
Hepatitis A	Virus	Fecal-oral; contaminated water, milk, food	Isolation	Personal hygiene and handwashing
Influenza	Virus	Direct contact; droplet infection	Fluid and electrolyte replacement; rest	Immunization when disease would complicate existing condition
Legionellosis (Legionnaires' Disease)	Bacterium	Airborne transmission	Selected antibiotic chemotherapy	Unknown
Lyme disease	Spirochete	Bites from infected ticks	Selected antibiotic chemotherapy	Avoidance of tick-infested areas
Measles	Virus	Droplet spread or direct contact	Isolation; rest	Immunization
Mononucleosis	Virus	Person-to-person via saliva; kissing	Rest	Unknown
Mumps	Virus	Droplet spread or contact with saliva	No specific treatment	Immunization
Pertussis (whooping cough)	Bacterium	Droplet spread or direct contact	Isolation; selected antibiotic chemotherapy	Immunization
Pneumonia	Bacteria; virus; other agents	Droplet spread or direct contact; contact with freshly soiled articles	Depends on specific causative organism	Depends on type; avoidance of crowded living conditions
Poliomyelitis	Virus	Fecal-oral contamination by direct or indirect means	None other than the protection of others	Immunization
Rubella	Virus	Direct contact or droplet spread	Isolation	Immunization
Strep throat	Bacterium	Direct contact or droplet spread	Selected antibiotic chemotherapy	Personal hygiene by self and others
Tetanus	Bacterium	Introduction of soil-borne organisms by means of a puncture wound	Administer tetanus immunoglobulin; tetanus antitoxin	Immunization
Toxic shock syndrome	Bacterium	Infected with *Staphylococcus aureus* associated with tampon use during menstrual period	Selected antibiotic chemotherapy	Elimination of or reduced tampon use
Tuberculosis	Bacterium	Airborne droplet spread or prolonged direct contact with infected individual	Selected antimicrobial chemotherapy	Improve social conditions that affect occurrence; immunization of contacts

Source: Data from *Control of Communicable Diseases in Man,* 15th edition, 1990, the American Public Health Association.

TABLE 12.5 Recommended Schedule for Active Immunization of Normal Infants and Children

Recommended Age*	Vaccine(s)†	Comments
2 months	DTP-1‡, OPV-1§	Can be given earlier in areas where diseases occur frequently.
4 months	DTP-2, OPV-2	6-week to 2-month interval desired between OPV doses to avoid interference.
6 months	DTP-3	An additional dose of OPV at this time is optional for use in areas with a high risk of polio exposure.
15 months″	MMR,# DTP-4, OPV-3	Completion of primary series of DTP and OPV.
24 months	HbPV**	Can be given at 18–23 months for children in groups who are thought to be at increased risk of disease, e.g., day-care-center attendees.
4–6 years††	DTP-5, OPV-4	Preferably at or before school entry.
14–16 years	Td‡‡	Repeat every 10 years throughout life.

*These recommended ages should not be construed as absolute, i.e., two months can be six to ten weeks, etc.

†For all products used, consult manufacturer's package enclosure for instructions for storage, handling and administration. Immunobiologics prepared by different manufacturers may vary, and those of the same manufacturer may change from time to time. The package insert should be followed for a specific product.

‡DTP-Diphtheria and Tetanus Toxoids and Pertussis Vaccine Adsorbed.

§OPV-Poliovirus Vaccine Live Oral; contains poliovirus strains types 1, 2 and 3.

″Provided at least six months have elapsed since DTP-3 or, if fewer than three DTPs have been received, at least six weeks since last previous dose of DTP or OPV. MMR vaccine should not be delayed just to allow simultaneous administration with DTP and OPV. Administering MMR at fifteen months and DTP-4 and OPV-3 at eighteen months continues to be an acceptable alternative.

#MMR Measles, Mumps, and Rubella Virus Vaccine, Live.

**Hemophilus b Polysaccharide Vaccine.

††Up to the seventh birthday.

‡‡Td-Tetanus and Diphtheria Toxoids Adsorbed (for adult use)—contains the same dose of tetanus toxoid as DTP or DT and a reduced dose of diphtheria toxoid.

Source: Data from *Morbidity and Mortality Weekly Report*, Vol. 35, No. 37:578, September 19, 1986, The Centers for Disease Control and Prevention, Atlanta, GA.

Similarly, diphtheria, pertussis, and tetanus immunizations are administered together.

An irony of the development of successful immunizations has been the parallel development of the mistaken belief that diseases like measles, polio, and other communicable disorders no longer pose a threat to people. Consequently, some individuals have become lax in getting themselves and their children properly immunized, thus setting the stage for a possible epidemic in the future. For control of these diseases, it is important that immunization practices be continued.

Influenza

Three types of **influenza** (flu) are recognized types A, B, and C. Typical influenza is recognized by the abrupt onset of fever, chills, muscle ache, sore throat, headache, and a nonproductive cough. Unlike some other respiratory ailments, flu can produce malaise that persists for several days. Influenza type A and influenza type B have presented themselves as epidemics in the U.S. almost annually.[5]

Thus far, influenza type C has occurred only rarely, usually as a minor, localized outbreak. Influenza viruses have the ability to modify their physical structure and properties, resulting in new strains, thus impeding the development of a permanent vaccine. Immunization for influenza variants may decrease the risk of disease or minimize its severity. Generally speaking, influenza immunization is recommended for older adults, and for persons with chronic diseases whose health would be severely compromised if they developed influenza.[6]

The Common Cold

If the common cold is not the most written about disease of all time, surely it must be the most talked about. There are some important facts to be noted about colds. Colds are caused by more than 200 different viruses.[7] One is likely to encounter and fall victim to two or three of these viruses annually, each lasting from seven to ten days. How does one "catch" a cold? If you are not sure, ask your friends, parents, and grandparents to see what they believe about catching a cold. Myths about cause, prevention, and treatment of colds abound. You may have heard that colds come from becoming chilled, from getting your feet wet, from sleeping in a draft, or from not wearing a hat on cold rainy, or windy days. Sound familiar? In fact, these so-called mechanisms do not explain the acquisition of colds whatsoever. It is true that the common cold is more "common" in the winter than in the summer. The explanation of this phenomenon is rather simple, though. It has little or nothing to do with the weather or nature's elements. Actually, people spend more time inside during the winter and come into close and prolonged contact with others in a restricted environment. Thus, the opportunity for passing along cold viruses through direct contact, droplet spread from coughing and sneezing, and handling freshly contaminated articles, is more prevalent. If you live or work in buildings where heat is supplied by large, forced air systems, the mucous membranes in nasal and respiratory passages that act as an early line of defense against infection may dry up and be rendered less effective against pathogenic organisms. The main reservoir of cold organisms is young children.[8] Hand-washing at regular intervals throughout "cold and flu season" may reduce exposure to some extent.

People spend large sums of money on cold prevention and treatment remedies. While taking large quantities of water soluble vitamin C may deplete the pocketbook, "enrich" the urine, and provide "psychological" defense against colds, it appears unlikely that this practice gives satisfactory protection for most people against the rhinoviruses that cause colds. If you take vitamin C either through supplements purchased at the pharmacy or through consumption of large volumes of orange juice and get fewer or milder colds, the result can be attributed primarily to good luck. The numerous medications purchased over the counter may help the symptoms (runny nose, burning, itchy eyes, sore throat, mild fever, and headache) associated with colds, but they will not help the cold go away any faster. Symptom relief should be managed carefully (see table 12.6).

There is no known cure for the common cold, and **antibiotics** are no exception. Antibiotics are not effective against the viruses that cause colds. They should be used only when secondary infections that are not viral in nature (**bacterial pneumonia, bronchitis, sinusitis, otitis media,** or **tonsillitis**) occur and are severe, and only under physician supervision. For decades, however, physicians have been hounded by their cold-suffering patients for prescriptions containing antibiotics. Physicians eventually may give in to their patients' pressure merely to avoid further badgering. Such practice is ill-advised for both patient and practitioner. Antibiotics used to "treat" colds can disrupt the normal population and distribution of nonpathogenic microorganisms in the body. Such disruption can produce symptoms and problems much more serious and unpleasant than the original cold.

Rubella

Many diseases are worthy of special consideration. For instance, rubella is a mild disease involving fever and rash. It seldom has serious complications for the person infected; however, it can have devastating consequences for more than 25 percent of the infants whose mothers acquire it during the first trimester of pregnancy.[9] Infants may experience congenital deafness, **cataracts,** mental retardation, heart defects, and a host of other functional or life-threatening disorders. Fortunately, most women have had the disease by the time they are of childbearing age, or have been immunized against it.

Lyme Disease

Lyme disease is a tick-borne infection caused by the spirochete *Borrelia burgdorferi*. Symptoms may not appear for several weeks

Antibiotics: a class of drugs commonly used to treat infections caused by bacteria or fungi. Antibiotics work by inhibiting the growth of these microorganisms.

Bacterial pneumonia: also known as pneumococcal pneumonia this infectious disease is caused by the bacteria *Streptococcus pneumoniae*, and is transmitted through respiratory secretions.

Otitis media: an inflammation of the middle ear that can be caused by either bacteria or virus. Common symptoms include severe pain and a high fever.

Cataracts: a common occurrence with aging in which the lens of the eye becomes increasingly opaque, resulting in obscured vision.

TABLE 12.6

Keeping Your Cold Under Control

Drink large quantities of fluids.

Fluids, especially if hot, soothe the throat and help to relieve congestion. Alcoholic beverages should be avoided because they tend to dehydrate the body.

Gargle with salt water.

One teaspoon of salt in warm water every four hours is recommended. This practice helps to reduce swelling in the throat.

Get plenty of rest.

Rest helps heal and restore.

Use disposable tissues instead of handkerchiefs.

Handkerchiefs can harbor germs for up to several hours.

Inhale warm moist air (steam).

A vaporizer, humidifier, or pan of water on a radiator can be used. Moderately warm to hot showers can be substituted. These practices soothe inflamed mucous membranes.

Take aspirin or acetaminophen according to label directions.

These products provide some relief to headache, muscle pain, and fever. Consult a physician if cold symptoms persist beyond a week.

Source: Data from *Managing the Common Cold*, 1988, American College Health Association.

---

after being bitten by a tick that carries *B. burgdorferi*, but may include skin lesions, malaise, muscle ache, fever, and other manifestations.[10] The disease came into national prominence in the late 1980s after some individuals who contracted the disease subsequently died from it. Although cases of Lyme disease have been seen in forty-six states, most outbreaks have been concentrated in Minnesota and Wisconsin, along the Atlantic coast from Massachusetts to Georgia, and in California and Oregon.

The reservoir for the tick which transmits infectious spirochete includes deer (especially the white-tail deer), wild rodents, and other small mammals. Although selected antibiotics can treat Lyme disease in its early stages, prevention through avoidance of tick-infested areas and the use of tick repellents is recommended.

Viral Hepatitis

Hepatitis is a disease whose primary symptom is the inflammation of the liver. It may be caused by reactions to drugs, toxic agents, excess alcohol intake, bacteria, or viruses. Most hepatitis results from one of five viruses labeled respectively, hepatitis A (HAV), hepatitis B (HBV), hepatitis C (HCV), hepatitis D (HDV), and hepatitis E (HEV). Of these different viral agents, HAV and HBV are the most important ones for your consideration.

HAV, also known as infectious hepatitis, is transmitted primarily by the fecal-oral route. Public health officials attribute outbreaks to contaminated water and food (often milk, meat, shellfish, and salads). Infection also is seen in persons in contact with children in day-care settings, persons who inject drugs, and men who have sex with other men.[11]

The incubation period for HAV is fifteen to forty-five days and is dose-related. A shorter incubation period is seen when a large infectious dose occurs. Overall, the incubation period averages about twenty-eight days. When symptoms occur, their onset may be abrupt and consist of fever, malaise, nausea, abdominal pain, and possibly diarrhea. The definitive symptom is **jaundice,** the yellowish appearance in skin tone that suggests liver impairment. Symptoms persist one to three weeks, but overall recovery may be much longer.[12]

Hepatitis B (HBV) is also known as serum hepatitis. Infection occurs from exposure to infective body fluids (blood, serum, saliva, semen, vaginal fluids), unscreened blood or blood products, accidental needle stick, contact with infected needles used in intravenous drug abuse, or by sexual contact.[13] As a result, HBV is sometimes classified as a sexually transmissible disease, a category of diseases that we will look at a little later in this chapter. The incubation period is forty-five to 180 days, but averages sixty to ninety days. Symptoms (fatigue, malaise, anorexia) may last one to four weeks, but persist for as long as six months. Approximately 20 percent of symptomatic patients develop jaundice. Recovery is slow, and some patients may progress to cirrhosis of the liver, cancer of the liver, and complete destruction of the liver cells, producing liver failure and death.[14]

Sexually Transmissible Diseases

Another important group of infectious diseases that commonly occur in the U.S. are the sexually transmissible diseases (STDs). Because of the high incidence of STDs in the college-age population an entire section of this chapter is devoted to understanding their causative agents, transmission, and prevention. Although authorities now recognize more than twenty disorders as being transmitted primarily by sexual means, there are a few STDs that are most likely to be problematic for sexually active persons, especially for persons who have casual or multiple sexual partners and do not use latex condoms for some measure of protection (see figure 12.3). Many of these STDs may already be familiar to you. The more familiar STDs discussed in this section are HIV/AIDS, gonorrhea, syphilis, chlamydia-related infections, genital herpes, genital warts, candidiasis, nonspecific vaginitis, trichomoniasis, pediculosis, scabies, and urinary tract infections.

HIV/AIDS

AIDS stands for **acquired immune deficiency syndrome,** a disorder first documented in the U.S. in 1981, through which the body's immune system is impaired to varying degrees. "Acquired" refers to the fact that AIDS is not inherited and is not explained by an underlying illness. "Immune deficiency" is the common trait that persons with confirmed cases of AIDS demonstrate. This trait refers to the body's inability to defend itself against a host of what are called **opportunistic diseases,** diseases that include certain infections and otherwise rare tumors. "Syndrome" refers to the variety of specific diseases that can occur. Persons with AIDS, therefore, are predisposed to diseases that immunologically healthy individuals would not normally encounter. Presently, there is no known cure for AIDS and no vaccine to prevent it. Furthermore, no major breakthroughs are expected for years to come. The best hope for persons with AIDS has

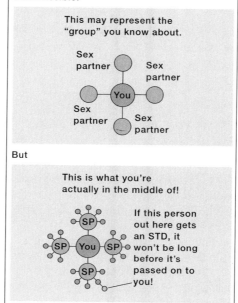

By sexually active, we don't mean simply having a lot of sex. Instead we are using the term to mean having sex with different people.

In general, the fact of life is that sooner or later, sexually active people will either be exposed to an STD, or get one.

By STD, of course, we mean sexually transmitted disease—that group of infections spread from person to person by sexual contact. The term STD includes syphilis, gonorrhea, nongonococcal urethritis, genital herpes, trichomoniasis, and more than ten other diseases, all of which are sexually transmissible.

This may represent the "group" you know about.

Sex partner / Sex partner / You / Sex partner / Sex partner

But

This is what you're actually in the middle of!

If this person out here gets an STD, it won't be long before it's passed on to you!

Figure 12.3: STDs: a fact of life for the sexually active

From *The Sexually Active and VD,* 1979 by the American Social Health Association, Research Triangle Park, NC. Reprinted by permission.

been the approval of a drug called **zidovudine,** formerly called **AZT,** which reduces some of the symptoms of disease and retards the disease progress. As we move through the 1990s, other drugs for the treatment of AIDS are expected to be developed, tested, and introduced for patients.

The cause of AIDS is a virus known as **human immunodeficiency virus,** or **HIV.** Previously, the virus was known as human T-lymphotrophic virus type III (HTLV-III) and lymphadenopathy virus (LAV). When reading literature about AIDS written before 1987 you are likely to see these terms. In common discourse, HIV is simply referred to as the "AIDS virus." This virus is able to compromise the infected person's immune system by attacking the body's T cells and reducing their ability to defend against certain opportunistic diseases (see figure 12.4). Recent data suggest that variants of the HIV virus, such as HIV-2, may be implicated in some cases of AIDS as well.[15]

Opportunistic disease: any otherwise rare disease that attacks a person whose immune system has been severely compromised, as during AIDS.

Figure 12.4: AIDS virus infection and replication in a human cell

The virus enters the cell and releases ribonucleic acid (RNA), its genetic material. Using the enzyme reverse transcriptase (RT), the virus converts its RNA into deoxyribonucleic acid (DNA), which enters the cell nucleus and combines with the cell DNA. The cell's altered genetic material then produces messenger RNA (mRNA), which codes for new virus.

Source: From *FDA Consumer,* 21(8), October 1987.

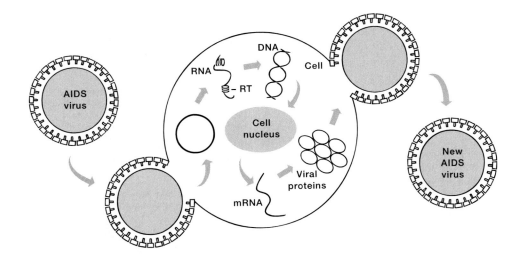

Cytomegalovirus: a salivary gland inhibiting virus that can affect numerous sites in the body.

Toxoplasma gondii: the causative agent in toxoplasmosis, a disease with mild to severe symptoms that can include fatigue, muscle pain, and swollen lymph glands.

TABLE 12.7

The Centers for Disease Control and Prevention's (CDC) Revised Definition of AIDS as of January 1993

- All HIV-infected adolescents and adults with fewer than 200 CD4+ T-lymphocytes
- Or HIV positive and one or more of the following:

  cryptosporidiosis
  cytomegalovirus
  isosporiasis
  Kaposi's sarcoma
  lymphoma
  lymphoid pneumonia (hyperplasia)
  Pneumocystis carinii pneumonia
  progressive multifocal leukoencephalopathy
  toxoplasmosis
  candidiasis
  coccidioidomycosis
  cryptococcosis
  herpes simplex virus
  histoplasmosis
  extrapulmonary tuberculosis
  other mycobacteriosis
  salmonellosis
  other bacterial infections
  HIV encephalopathy (dementia)
  HIV wasting syndrome
  pulmonary tuberculosis
  recurrent pneumonia
  invasive cervical cancer

Source: Data from The Centers for Disease Control and Prevention, Atlanta, GA.

It is estimated that in the U.S. alone, between 1.0 and 1.5 million people may be carriers of HIV.[16] On a global basis (see Of Special Interest 12.1) it is estimated that around 13 million people live with HIV and AIDS.[17]

Despite being infected with HIV, some people appear healthy and well, with no manifested symptoms of illness. Others develop minor symptoms three to six weeks after exposure to HIV. This illness typically lasts seven to twenty-one days, and consists of swollen lymph glands, a sore throat, fever, muscle aches, headache, and sometimes a rash. Following HIV infection, months or years may pass before an individual experiences the suppressed immune function and opportunistic diseases that define AIDS (see table 12.7). Current *estimates* indicate that it may take as long as twelve years for some individuals to progress from HIV infection to AIDS.

What are the so-called opportunistic diseases associated with AIDS? The most common diseases stemming from infection with HIV include an unusual cancer affecting the lining of blood vessels known as **Kaposi's sarcoma,** causing pink to purple flat or raised blotches on or under the skin or inside the mouth, nose, eyelids, or rectum; a severe infection, ***Pneumocystis carinii* pneumonia,** an otherwise rare but frequently lethal form of pneumonia that produces a dry cough, fever, and shortness of breath, **cytomegalovirus,** which infects the brain, eyes, lungs, and intestines, **Toxoplasma gondii,** a protozoan that can cause abscesses in the brain, and chronic yeast infections associated with **Candida albicans** showing up in the mouth, throat, esophagus, and elsewhere.

Ten Things You Need to Know about HIV/AIDS

1. **AIDS is a worldwide problem.**
   The AIDS pandemic has left no continent untouched. By mid-1994, WHO estimated that 17 million men, women, and children worldwide had been infected with HIV and about 4 million people had developed AIDS.

2. **HIV causes AIDS.**
   AIDS (acquired immunodeficiency syndrome) is the late state of infection with the human immunodeficiency virus, HIV. In some adults, AIDS can take more than 10 years to develop. Thus, a person infected with HIV may look and feel healthy for many years, but he or she can still transmit the virus to someone else.

3. **HIV is transmitted through intimate contact.**
   We know that HIV infection is transmitted primarily through unprotected sexual intercourse. Like other sexually transmitted diseases, it can also spread through infected blood or blood products and from an infected mother to her baby before, during, or shortly after birth (perinatal transmission).

4. **Sexual transmission of HIV can be prevented.**
   Sexual intercourse, whether heterosexual or homosexual, is the major route of transmission of HIV. The most effective way to prevent the sexual transmission of the virus is to abstain from sexual intercourse, or for two uninfected partners to remain mutually faithful. The risk of spreading HIV through sexual intercourse can be significantly reduced by the proper and consistent use of condoms. Safer sex practices that involve no penetration are also an effective way to prevent the sexual transmission of HIV.

5. **Infection through blood can be stopped.**
   Blood for transfusion can be tested for HIV infection and discarded if contaminated. Needles, syringes, and other skin-piercing instruments should be sterilized or discarded after each use and should never be shared.

6. **It is important to know how HIV is NOT transmitted.**
   HIV is a virus which does not survive easily outside the body. It is NOT spread by casual contact at work or school, by shaking hands, touching, or hugging. It is NOT spread through food or water, by sharing cups or glasses, by coughing or sneezing, in swimming pools or on toilets. It is NOT spread by mosquitoes or other insects. This means there is no danger of becoming infected through ordinary social contact.

7. **Isolating people with HIV infection or AIDS is not the answer.**
   Besides being a violation of their human rights, discrimination against people with HIV infection or AIDS—or those thought to be at risk of infection—also endangers public health:
   - It gives people outside the stigmatized group a sense that the threat of infection, and thus the need for personal precautions, has been removed
   - It drives the AIDS problem underground, making all efforts at prevention and care much more difficult

8. **Information and education are vital.**
   Until medical research finds a cure for AIDS or a vaccine to prevent infection, we must rely on changes in personal behavior to stop the spread of HIV. Therefore, information and education are vital in the fight against HIV/AIDS.

9. **AIDS and Families: Protect and Care for the Ones We Love!**
   Families can become more effective in both HIV/AIDS prevention and care. The concept of a family is not limited to relationships of blood, marriage, sexual partnership, or adoption but extends to a broad range of groups who share trust, mutual support, or have a common destiny. Families whose bonds are based on love, trust, nurture, and openness are best able to protect their members from infection and to give compassionate care and support to those affected by HIV/AIDS.

10. **There are things YOU can do to stop the spread of HIV/AIDS.**
    YOU can contribute to this global fight by making sure that you understand the facts about HIV/AIDS and by helping others to do the same. World AIDS Day is a special opportunity every year to focus attention on this urgent challenge that affects us all. It is marked around the world by thousands of different events designed to increase awareness, and to express solidarity and compassion. This World AIDS Day—and everyday—join the worldwide effort to stop the spread of HIV/AIDS.

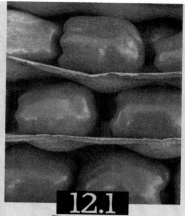

12.1 Of Special Interest

Source: Data from American Association for World Health, Washington, D.C.

What Do You Think?

1. How could you become more active in promoting AIDS prevention?
2. What resources exist on your campus and in your community to support AIDS prevention efforts?

What Do You Think?

1. It has taken the direct involvement of celebrities with HIV infection to arouse public attention, but even that might not be enough. Magic Johnson's HIV+ status was reported in 1991 and Olympic gold medalist Greg Louganis's HIV+ status was made public in 1995. Do you think that their admissions have affected people's sexual practices? Explain your rationale.
2. How can the misfortune of well-known celebrities be capitalized on to curb further growth of HIV infection?

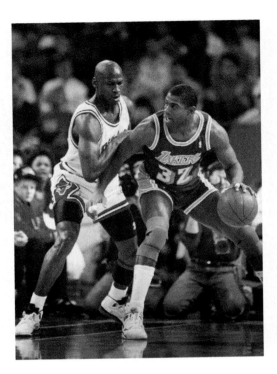

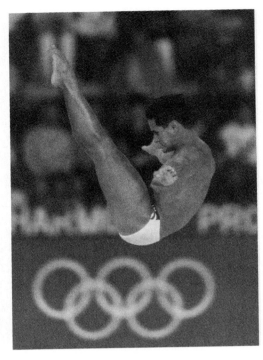

Tuberculosis or **TB** is an infectious disease of historic significance in that it was once a major killer. It is spread through airborne droplets and typically affects the lungs, although other parts of the body such as the spine and the brain can be affected. Although TB occurs less frequently in the U.S. than it once did, it has become a major opportunistic disease among people with HIV. In addition to these diseases, other disorders also are seen. Neurological involvement from the disease can result in a condition called **AIDS dementia complex,** which manifests itself through memory loss, difficulty in moving or speaking, or demonstration of erratic behaviors. Moreover, some persons with AIDS develop a **"wasting syndrome,"** which proves to be lethal. For the person living with AIDS, it is the opportunistic diseases and the body's inability to combat infection that actually causes death.

HIV/AIDS Prevention

How is the AIDS virus spread? There are two important things to bear in mind: (1) HIV has to be present in a person before it can be transmitted. *It is not a behavior alone that produces infection—one of the persons participating in the activity must be infected.* (2) HIV has to be transmitted to a place in the body where it can survive and multiply.

HIV resides within white blood cells called T-lymphocytes. It cannot live where there are no such cells. The virus will not infect a person by landing on their clothes or their unbroken skin. To give rise to infection, HIV must come into contact with body fluids, including, but not limited to, blood and semen.

Sexual Transmission of HIV.
Unprotected sex with a person infected by HIV can allow for contact with body fluids to occur. Next to blood, semen contains the highest concentration of the virus in men who are infected by HIV. This sexual fluid can be transmitted to a partner by means of vaginal intercourse, anal intercourse, oral sex, or artificial insemination. HIV can enter the bloodstream through tears in the vagina or anus and possibly through mucous membranes of the oral cavity. Sexual fluids from women can also transmit the virus. Although the concentration of HIV may be less in vaginal and cervical fluids, it is apparently high enough for transmission to occur. It is important to remember that menstrual blood also may harbor the virus, and along with sexual fluids, it can facilitate movement of the virus from person to person during vaginal intercourse or oral sex. Urine and feces contain lower concentrations of

Tuberculosis (TB): an infectious bacterial disease characterized by inflammations, abscesses, calcification of tissue, and other symptoms, affecting the respiratory system and other sites.

Wasting syndrome sometimes called "Slim Disease," this syndrome consists of severe weight loss, chronic diarrhea and weakness, and a persistent cough.

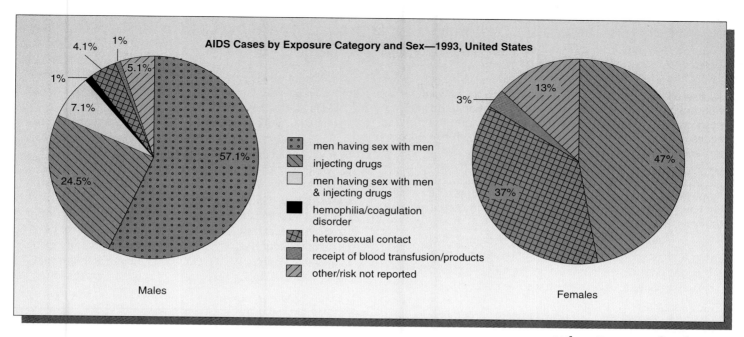

AIDS Cases by Exposure Category and Sex—1993, United States

Males:
- 57.1%
- 24.5%
- 7.1%
- 1%
- 4.1%
- 1%
- 5.1%
- 1%

Legend:
- men having sex with men
- injecting drugs
- men having sex with men & injecting drugs
- hemophilia/coagulation disorder
- heterosexual contact
- receipt of blood transfusion/products
- other/risk not reported

Females:
- 47%
- 37%
- 13%
- 3%

HIV than either blood or semen, but may be vehicles for transmitting the virus during sexual activity or if they come into contact with breaks in the skin.

It should be clear that having sex with multiple partners increases the risk of exposure to HIV. You must remember that when you engage in sex with a person, you are potentially coming into contact with the entire sexual history of that individual—meaning exposure to every sexual partner he or she has ever had. For example, if you have had five sexual partners in the past, and each of them had five sexual partners, and each one of those individuals had five sexual contacts, and so on, you can see that the possibility of being exposed not only to HIV but other sexually transmissible diseases becomes increasingly more likely. The only protection from sexual transmission of HIV infection is sexual abstinence. Since abstinence is neither a satisfactory nor a realistic expectation for many people, other steps of self-protection must be taken. A person must: (1) establish a sexual relationship that is mutually faithful with an uninfected partner; (2) avoid having sex with persons (such as prostitutes) known to have had multiple sex partners; and (3) use a latex condom during all sexually intimate contact with a partner whose sexual health status or sexual history is unknown to you or who is known to have engaged in practices

and behaviors that put him or her at risk of being infected, such as injecting drug use. Better yet, do not have sexually intimate contact with such persons. Table 12.8 provides some helpful tips for individuals attempting to establish safer sex practices as part of their personal plan for wellness and risk reduction.

What about the use of latex condoms that are lubricated with **nonoxynol-9,** the spermicide with HIV-inhibiting power that was being touted a few years ago? Recent evidence suggests that nonoxynol-9 lubricated condoms may not be as protective against HIV as once believed. Condoms that are prelubricated with nonoxynol-9 may have an insufficient quantity of the substance to provide adequate protection. Moreover, in some users, nonoxynol-9 has produced an inflammatory response in the mucous lining of organs such as the vagina or anus, possibly making these sites *more susceptible* to infection by HIV and other STDs.[18] A properly used latex condom provides reasonable disease protection.[19] Since nonoxynol-9 provides protection against some other STDs, use of a vaginal spermicide that contains nonoxynol-9 may give added disease and contraception protection when used with a latex condom, unless one of the partners has an allergic or other unfavorable physiological response to the nonoxynol-9.[20]

What Do You Think?

1. What are the top two HIV exposure categories for male AIDS cases in the United States?
2. How do the top two HIV exposure categories for males compare with the top HIV exposure categories for females?
3. How would these variations in exposure category impact on AIDS prevention messages?

Source: Data from HIV/AIDS Surveillance, Centers for Disease Control and Prevention, 1994.

As this chapter points out, throwing caution to the wind today with sexual relationships can have health compromising, or even deadly results. Still, many college students and other adults neglect common sense practices. The tips below encourage safer sex practices.

Precontemplation → Contemplation

If you are sexually active or about to become sexually active, but have never thought about your risk of contracting a sexually transmissible disease, consider:

- Seeing if there are any HIV awareness or support groups in your area or on your campus. Find out about their activities.
- Trying to imagine what it would be like for you to negotiate a sexual encounter, using safer sex guidelines.

Contemplation → Preparation

You may have read about abstinence, safer sex, or explored the use of condoms, but at this point you have not formulated a wellness plan. You might try:

- Having a dialogue with yourself or with a friend about negotiating safer sex. Practice what you would say and what a partner might say in return.
- Reading about available safer sex activities, but ones you do not participate in because of the limited concept of "sex" that you have allowed to have imposed upon yourself.
- Imagining a sexual encounter that consists only of non-genital touching. Focus on the sensation of just being touched by someone who cares about you.
- Reading condom labels, noticing what varieties there are in color, design, and packaging.

Preparation → Action

If you are ready to make some plans to protect yourself in the next thirty days and beyond, or have made efforts in the past without being able to sustain those lifestyle changes, try:

- Telling a close friend whom you trust about your decision to engage only in safer sex.
- Buying and carrying latex condoms.
- With a close friend whom you trust, practicing asking questions about sexual history so you will feel more confident and comfortable asking them to a potential sex partner.
- Opening a condom package and getting accustomed to the feel of a condom. If you are male, try putting it on correctly over your erect penis. If you are female, try putting it on correctly over an object that resembles an erect penis. Rehearse using a condom so you will not be ignorant or feel awkward if the circumstance to use one occurs.
- Seeing if your institution, its student health service, or a local radio station will sponsor a safer sex awareness day or week on campus, especially if you live in a residence hall or belong to a Greek organization. Organize appropriate activities that are fun but emphasize awareness of safer sex practices.

Action → Maintenance

The following tips may help you to sustain safer sex practices over time.

- Avoid situations and circumstances where heavy consumption of alcohol may occur, and poor judgments concerning safer sex may be more likely to occur.
- Do not consent to having sex with someone unless you believe you and this partner can have a mutually faithful, long-term, monogamous sexual relationship.
- Become an advocate of safer sex. Share your ideas with friends, other peers, and relatives.
- Develop a series of responses (polite and direct refusals) should someone attempt to convince you of the merit of having sexual intercourse without a latex condom.

Maintenance

You are taking steps that protect your health and that of someone you care about. Also try:

- Joining a campus group that promotes awareness of HIV and other STDs.
- Volunteering to be a peer educator, and give talks to new students at dormitories or at other settings about abstinence from or postponement of sexual intercourse, using latex condoms, and the merits of other safer sex practices.

Nonsexual Transmission of HIV. The primary mode of nonsexual transmission of the AIDS virus is by sharing contaminated needles used for injecting drugs. Blood containing the virus from one user is injected into the next person who uses the needle, and so on. There is no more efficient way of transmitting HIV than by this procedure.

Although it is now rare to be infected by receiving a blood transfusion, prior to 1985, before donated blood was screened, this mechanism of acquiring HIV was quite viable. Before screening procedures were implemented, infected blood—possibly several pints—might have been transfused directly into a patient's bloodstream, thus facilitating easy infection. Other blood products, such as Factor VIII (a clotting factor given to hemophiliacs), plasma, platelets, and red blood cells have transmitted

HIV as well. Careful screening of blood products and heat treating of Factor VIII virtually insures that no new infections develop. In addition to blood, organs that are donated for transplantation, and semen donated for artificial insemination, are tested for the presence of HIV.

A third mechanism for HIV to be passed in a nonsexual way is for an infected mother to infect her baby. Transmission of the virus in this way may occur in the uterus before delivery, by exposure to blood during delivery, or after birth through contaminated breast milk. Children who have HIV usually get it from their mothers through one of these modes. Some children, of course, have been infected as a result of receiving contaminated transfused blood or blood products prior to the adoption of screening procedures.

Finally, nonsexual transmission can occur through contact with urine and feces that are contaminated with HIV. It is important that individuals such as health-care workers who care for incontinent HIV-infected persons follow special sanitary procedures. Generally speaking, this means cleaning up body fluid spills with a household bleach solution consisting of one part bleach to ten parts water and wearing rubber gloves that are impenetrable to the virus.

Uncertain Modes of HIV Transmission. There are a few activities whose role in the transmission of HIV is unclear at the present time and that require additional research. Ear piercing equipment, toothbrushes, and razors can play host to infected blood *in theory*. Although no one is known to have acquired the AIDS virus from these tools, caution should be exercised in sharing them.

There is uncertainty about HIV transmission through saliva and across mucous membranes. HIV has been isolated in small quantities in the saliva of some infected individuals. Heavy kissing (i.e., tongue kissing, French kissing) does not appear to be an effective mode of transmitting HIV, but *in theory*, it could be. So-called dry kissing on the lips seems to be an implausible mechanism for virus transfer. To facilitate transfer of HIV by kissing, it would have to enter the bloodstream through a wound (e.g., a bleeding gum) or through the mucous membranes of the mouth, eyelid, and other sites. The only way to establish this would be to place live viruses at these locations and

follow up to see if infection occurred. Obviously, such an experiment cannot be performed. It is most difficult to isolate kissing as an independent risk factor for HIV transmission, since people who kiss one another deeply and passionately are likely to engage in other sexual activities that would place them at higher risk anyway.

Nonmethods of Transmission. How communicable is HIV? The high occurrence in homosexual men and injected drug users is consistent with the hypothesis that AIDS results from an agent transmitted sexually or through exposure to contaminated needles or blood. According to the Centers for Disease Control and Prevention, person-to-person transmission through ordinary social or occupational contact has not been shown. Thus, mechanisms such as sharing a glass, sharing hot tubs or swimming pools, and handling food are not viable. Also, there is no evidence of airborne or food-borne transmission. Furthermore, handshaking, hugging, and giving or getting messages are activities that do not transmit the virus since no exchange of blood, sexual fluid, or other body fluids take place. If casual contact with infected persons could facilitate transfer of HIV, members of households who care for, interact with, or have prolonged exposure to AIDS patients would be getting the virus. To date, none of these individuals have gotten infected through such a casual mechanism.

Biting insects (such as mosquitoes) do not transmit HIV. If they did, there would be a cross section (roughly equivalent proportions of old and young, male and female, African-American, and White, etc.) of the population infected, since insects do not discriminate among those they bite. Moreover, places in the world where mosquitoes are **endemic** would be more heavily affected by AIDS. Such is not the case. HIV is specific in attacking people; therefore, one does not get the virus from contact with dogs, cats, or other household pets.[21]

HIV Antibody Testing

If a person suspects that he or she has been exposed to the AIDS virus, it is important to have a blood test. Local health departments and university health services usually can provide specific information about where persons can be tested confidentially or anonymously. A **confidential test** means no

Endemic: diseases that occur frequently or commonly in a particular location or population.

one except the person tested and the health-care worker will know the test result. **Anonymous testing** means that the name of the person tested is never recorded. Each person tested is assigned a number, and the results of the test are recorded on a lab slip with a corresponding number.

There are two types of tests that may be performed—a relatively inexpensive screening test and a more expensive confirmatory test. These tests cannot tell if a person has AIDS or will develop AIDS. What they do is indicate whether the person has been infected by HIV. In infected persons, the virus stimulates the body to produce antibodies. It is the presence of antibodies that the tests actually detect. Following exposure to the virus, it may take from six weeks to six months for antibodies to appear; therefore, the testing procedure at this time cannot identify newly infected individuals. Thus, it may be necessary for an individual who suspects exposure to the virus to be tested more than once.

The "typical" pattern of testing may go something like this: A person is given the screening test, an **enzyme immunoassay,** or **EIA** test (also known as an **enzyme-linked immune sorbant assay** or **ELISA.** If the test is negative (i.e., no antibodies detected) and the exposure was not recent, the individual can be relatively certain of freedom from infection. If the test is positive, the individual will probably be asked to submit to another screening test. The reason for this is that sometimes **false positive results** occur due to the presence in the blood of things that can stimulate the presence of antibodies to HIV. If the second EIA test is negative, and exposure to HIV was not recent, once again the person can be relatively sure of being disease free. If the second test is also positive, the individual will be asked to take a confirmatory test, such as the one known as the **Western Blot Test.** If the result of the confirmatory test is negative, the individual can be reasonably certain of not being infected, since few **false negative results** are achieved. A person who tests HIV+ on the confirmatory test does carry the virus, may transmit it, and may go on in time to develop symptoms of AIDS.

There is much controversy about testing. Does an employer have a right to know if an employee carries the virus? What is the impact of a worker who is HIV+ on coworkers? Who has the responsibility of protecting the individual's right to privacy? What if a test result that is inaccurate becomes known? How will it affect the individual's life? Learning that one carries HIV can be emotionally traumatizing. How does one counsel such an individual? Suppose a false positive result is reported, and upon learning of this apparent outcome, the individual commits suicide. There are many questions to be answered and issues to be resolved where testing is concerned. Until other simple, precise, accurate, and inexpensive tests are developed, or until a cure or safe vaccine is discovered, everyone will struggle with the problems created by HIV/AIDS.

HIV/AIDS Update

Information about HIV/AIDS is constantly being updated. It is critical that people have access to accurate and reliable information about HIV/AIDS to protect themselves and others. Many cities have established telephone hot lines to address questions about the disorder. The U.S. Public Health Service operates a hot line (1–800–342–AIDS) from which referrals can be made, if necessary. Some state health departments also offer telephone services for persons with questions about HIV/AIDS. Telephone numbers can be obtained from local directories in most instances.

HIV/AIDS and Special Populations

HIV infection and AIDS have had a disproportionate impact on people of color and other minority groups in the U.S. since the disease was first recognized and described in 1981.[22] Although most HIV-related deaths have occurred among Whites, death *rates* (number of deaths/100,000 people) have been highest for African-Americans and Hispanics.[23] According to Stephen B. Thomas, Aisha Gilliam, and Carolyn G. Iwrey:[24]

> Major differences can be found in the high-risk behaviors leading to HIV infection practiced by whites and minorities who contract AIDS. Whereas 13 percent of white men with AIDS are IV drug abusers or had sex partners who were IV drug abusers, fully 41 percent of black and Hispanic men with AIDS fall into that category. Among women with AIDS, 50 percent of white women were

False positive result: an error in the outcome of a test that implies a person has a disorder when in fact he or she may not.

False negative result: an error in the outcome of a test that implies a person does not have a disorder when in fact he or she may.

IV drug abusers or had sex with partners who were IV drug abusers, in contrast to 72 percent of blacks and 80 percent of Hispanics who are in that category.

Deborah A. McLean writes:

Some common themes that unite African-American college students, increasing their vulnerability to HIV infection, include inaccurate and missing information about HIV transmission, beliefs about invulnerability that have both cultural and developmental origins, and behaviors that result from perceived expectations specific to African-American relationships between men and women. Because many students of color on predominantly white college campuses often feel marginalized and disempowered, attempts to reach them may be further complicated.[25]

In a San Francisco-based study of STD clinic patients, African-American men and women respectively were 1.6 and 3.7 times as likely as their White counterparts to have not used condoms during sexual intercourse.[26] In a Texas study of a low-income minority population, Hispanics were less knowledgeable than either Whites or African-Americans about AIDS, and just 58 percent of Hispanics knew that using a condom during sexual intercourse lowered the risk of contracting AIDS.[27]

The disparity in occurrence of sexually transmissible diseases is by no means limited to HIV infection. Syphilis, which we will discuss later in this chapter, experienced a startling increase in the late 1980s and early 1990s among inner-city ethnic groups of low socioeconomic status. Between 1985 and 1989, the incidence rose 132 percent among African-Americans.[28]

The contrast in AIDS knowledge among some Hispanics and other racial and ethnic groups may be explained, in part, by language barriers and subtle prejudicial attitudes toward people of color, individuals with less education, and persons who are poor. Knowledge deficiencies about HIV/AIDS, increases in frequency of risk behavior, and increases in new HIV cases also are reported with respect to Asian Americans.[29] There continues to be a need for culturally sensitive programs and publications that are salient to many minority groups (see figure 12.5).

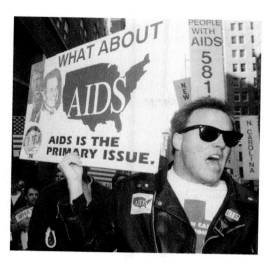

Figure 12.5: What Do You Think?

1. Why has HIV been a politically polarizing disease? Explain your thinking.
2. To what extent is a public outcry to find a cure or prevention for HIV-related conditions still lacking? What evidence do you have to base your answer on?

Women: Another Special Population

Any discussion of HIV/AIDS necessitates a close-up look at how HIV infection has affected women and how it could affect them in the future. It is a common myth that the "typical" person with HIV/AIDS is a male who has sex with other males or an injecting drug user. However, the number of women becoming infected with HIV is increasing faster than any other population.[30] Moreover, the World Health Organization estimates that over 13 million women worldwide will be infected with HIV by the year 2000.[31] Among women diagnosed with AIDS, 53 percent are African-American, 25 percent are Caucasian, and 21 percent are Hispanic.[32] Thus, women who also are members of some ethnic or racial minority groups may be especially susceptible to disease exposure.

While women who were infected a few years ago were likely to have become so as a result of injecting drugs, there has been a great rise in new infections among women receiving the virus through heterosexual contact. In heterosexual vaginal intercourse, it is easier to transmit HIV from a man to a woman than from a woman to a man. Semen has more contact with the vagina and other parts of the reproductive tract than vaginal secretions have with a man's genital tract. This greater exposure leads to a greater susceptibility to acquiring the AIDS virus.

Transmission of HIV from one woman to another through lesbian sex has not been well studied. More research concerning how risk of HIV among lesbians may differ is needed. Nevertheless, women having sex with other women should avoid taking a partner's vaginal secretions or blood (including menstrual blood) into the mouth, vagina, or anus.

How can women become less vulnerable to HIV infection? The main ingredient needed may be to address the issue of how women can negotiate safer sex with a partner. Achieving this end requires greater empowerment among women and better self-esteem for situations where negotiation is critical. In some societies, including the U.S., the subtle or blatant subordination of women often has brought about a powerlessness that leaves them vulnerable to sexual exploitation. To be effective, programs to change that status need to be sensitive to the diverse ethnic and cultural backgrounds of women at risk for HIV infection and other STDs (see Activity for Wellness 12.1).

Gonorrhea

Gonorrhea is one of the most frequently encountered communicable diseases in the U.S. Known by such street names as "clap," "drip," "dose," "strain," "gleet," and "jack," gonorrhea is caused by the bacterium *Neisseria gonorrhoeae*, which is common all over the world today. There is evidence that perhaps only 20 percent of the actual cases of gonorrhea get reported.[33]

Susceptibility to gonorrhea is considered to be general—that is, there appear to be no factors that predispose one to acquiring gonorrhea, other than being sexually active. Human beings are the only known reservoirs for *N. gonorrhoeae*. The highest attack rate is in young, sexually active adults in the twenty to twenty-four-year-old age group.[34] There is no way to acquire immunity to the disease, either by vaccine or by actually contracting gonorrhea.

Gonorrhea is transmitted via direct contact with the secretions of mucous membranes such as those of the urethra, cervix, vagina, anus, eyes, and throat. The contact involved in transmitting gonorrhea is almost always sexual in nature; however, an infant may acquire a gonorrhea infection of the eyes during passage from the birth canal of an infected mother. Because of this risk, the eyes of newborn infants may be treated with a 1 percent silver nitrate solution or erythromycin to minimize the possibility of infection developing. Use of this procedure, along with screening and treatment of pregnant women, has greatly reduced the occurrence of neonatal disease in developed countries.[35]

It is possible that contaminated fingers can also transfer infection from one region of the body to another; however, nonsexual infection (such as touching inanimate objects) is highly unlikely because *N. gonorrhoeae* dies rapidly when denied the warmth and moisture of mucous membranes.

Symptoms of infection usually appear within two to seven days after exposure but may take up to thirty days in some cases. These symptoms can vary for males and females.

In males, gonorrhea usually strikes first at the urethra, the tube-like structure that extends from the bladder to the tip of the penis. Urine is eliminated through the urethra and semen passes through it during sexual intercourse. Males may experience a burning sensation during urination due to the irritation of the urethra's mucosal lining. Many males may also notice an abnormal discharge from the penis. The penis itself may be red or swollen at the tip. Urination may become more frequent or become difficult. Occasionally, no symptoms are immediately evident.

In the female, gonorrhea seems to strike selectively at the cervix (the entrance of the uterus), but it also can appear elsewhere. As many as 80 percent of the females with gonorrhea have no immediate signs or symptoms to signal that something is wrong. In women with symptoms, there may be a foul smelling vaginal discharge. Since vaginal discharges are not uncommon, women should be alert to any change in the color, odor, or other appearances of discharges. If gonorrhea has affected the urethra, a woman may experience a burning sensation upon urination.

Gonorrhea can also infect the anal region, the oral cavity, and the eyes. Symptoms for males and females are identical. Gonorrhea that has affected the anus produces severe burning or itching. There may be a mucous discharge or blood and pus present in the stool. A throat infection acquired through oral-genital contact is likely to be only mild; it could easily be mistaken for a cold or other ailment. Eye involvement usually produces acute **conjunctivitis,** often severe and accompanied by pain and discharge.

Gonorrhea: a sexually-transmitted disease caused by a type of bacteria called *Neisseria gonorrhoeae*. Common symptoms include painful urination and a discharge of pus from the penis or vagina. If untreated, severe chronic diseases such as arthritis and inflammation of the heart valves may result.

Conjunctivitis: inflammation of the thin membrane covering the front of the eyeball and the lining of the eyelids.

AIDS Is Preventable!

At this time, AIDS cannot be cured, but it can be prevented! Education, knowledge, and practicing safe behaviors are the keys to prevention.

What Can I Do?

- **Get rid of the "This can't happen to me" attitude.** This sense of invincibility exists among most people, especially adolescents. You need to be aware of the trends of the disease and the behaviors that could put you at risk. HIV/AIDS affects people of all geographic locations, ages, races, ethnicities, social classes, and sexual orientations.
- **Practice abstinence or practice mutual monogamy with an uninfected partner—having sex only with one uninfected partner who has sex only with you.** These are the only foolproof ways to prevent sexual transmission of HIV. Although abstinence and mutual monogamy are the only foolproof methods, practicing SAFER SEX by adopting modifications in your sexual behavior can reduce your risk significantly.

Practice Safer Sex

Use latex CONDOMS. Condoms act as barriers to keep blood, semen, or vaginal secretions from passing from one person to another during sexual intercourse. When used consistently and correctly, latex condoms are highly effective in preventing HIV infection and other sexually transmitted diseases (STDs).

- **Consistent use** means using a condom from start to finish with each act of intercourse.
- **Correct use** should include the following steps:

  1. Use a new condom for each act of intercourse
  2. Put on the condom after the penis is erect and before any sexual contact (vaginal, anal, or oral)
  3. Hold the tip of the condom and unroll it onto the erect penis, leaving space at the tip of the condom, yet ensuring that no air is trapped in the condom
  4. Withdraw from your partner immediately after ejaculation, holding the condom firmly to keep it from slipping off

- **When buying condoms make sure they are latex.** Lamb-skin and natural membrane condoms are not an effective form of disease prevention because the pores in the material have been shown to allow the leakage of viruses.
- **If you use a lubricant during sex, be sure it is water-based,** such as glycerin or lubricating jelly. Never use an oil-based lubricant, such as petroleum jelly, cold cream, hand lotion, or baby oil.
- **Store condoms properly in a cool, dry place out of direct sunlight.** If you want to keep one with you, put it in a loose pocket, wallet, or purse for no more than a few hours at a time.
- **Do not use outdated condoms.** Check manufacturer's expiration date on the package.

Learn these facts so that you can protect yourself and others from infection. If your sexual behavior places you at risk, latex condoms used correctly every time you have sex can reduce, but not eliminate your risk. Aside from preventing HIV infection directly, widespread condom use could have a substantial indirect impact on the HIV/AIDS epidemic by preventing other STDs, some of which facilitate the transmission of HIV.

For additional information about condoms contact the CDC National AIDS Clearinghouse, P.O. Box 6003, Rockville, MD 20849–6003; 1–800–458–5231.

Avoid Drug Use

- **Non-injection drugs can kill too!** Drug abuse can cloud your judgment and cause you to forget what's important. When you get high you may mistakenly believe that nothing bad can happen to you. Drugs often decrease your decision-making abilities, lower your inhibitions, and may cause you to disregard safer sex precautions.

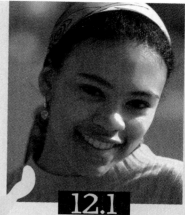

12.1
Activity for Wellness

- **Don't share needles!** Sharing needles is a very easy way to become infected with HIV. When people inject drugs into their bodies, some of their blood remains on the needle or syringe. When other people use the same needle, they could be shooting HIV directly into their bloodstream.
- **If you cannot stop injecting drugs, never share, rent, or borrow dirty injection equipment!** Use only sterile needles and syringes. Equipment must be cleaned before each use. First flush needles and syringes with water until the equipment is at least visibly clear of blood and debris. Then completely fill the equipment several times with full-strength household bleach. Make sure the "works" are also rinsed thoroughly with these disinfectants. After each bleach filling, rinse the equipment by filling with clean water several times.
- **Remember that ALCOHOL is a DRUG TOO!** The dangers and implications of drug abuse described above also apply to alcohol use because alcohol is a drug. Since its use is so widespread, especially among adolescents, alcohol is perhaps AIDS' greatest advocate!

Source: Data from American Association for World Health, Washington, D.C.

Figure 12.6: Gonorrhea infectious disease cycle

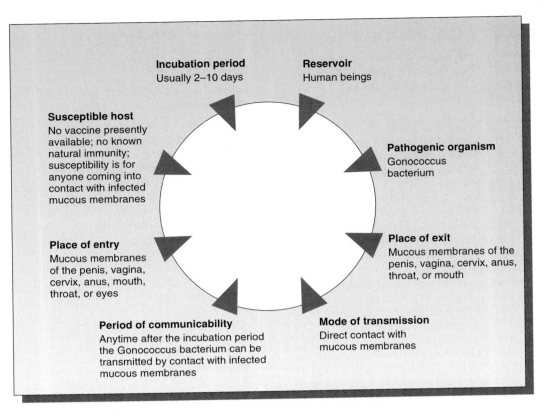

Incubation period
Usually 2–10 days

Reservoir
Human beings

Susceptible host
No vaccine presently available; no known natural immunity; susceptibility is for anyone coming into contact with infected mucous membranes

Pathogenic organism
Gonococcus bacterium

Place of entry
Mucous membranes of the penis, vagina, cervix, anus, mouth, throat, or eyes

Place of exit
Mucous membranes of the penis, vagina, cervix, anus, throat, or mouth

Period of communicability
Anytime after the incubation period the Gonococcus bacterium can be transmitted by contact with infected mucous membranes

Mode of transmission
Direct contact with mucous membranes

Nonspecific urethritis: an infection of the urethra whose cause cannot be tied to a single microorganism but is linked to many; considered to be a sexually transmitted disease.

Nonspecific vaginitis: an infection of the vagina whose cause cannot be tied to a single microorganism but is linked to many; may be sexually transmitted.

Pelvic inflammatory disease (PID): a general infection of the female reproductive tract, usually as a complication of an undiagnosed or untreated STD, and having the potential to cause permanent sterility.

Ectopic pregnancy: pregnancy with implantation of the zygote occurring outside the uterus, most commonly implanting in one of the fallopian tubes.

The period of communicability for gonorrhea is uncertain but probably lasts as long as discharges continue. This may be anywhere from three to six months. It is possible for gonorrhea to be transmitted even after clinical symptoms of the disease have subsided (see figure 12.6).

Diagnosis of gonorrhea is complicated by other STDs, **nonspecific urethritis** and **vaginitis** in particular, which are caused by a host of pathogens and mimic many of gonorrhea's symptoms. Precise diagnosis, therefore, requires cultures of discharge specimens. Repeated cervical cultures in females may be necessary to detect any residual infection. Under most circumstances gonorrhea is easily treated. It is now clear, however, that larger and larger doses of penicillin may be necessary to kill some resistant strains. Moreover, there are some strains that can even render the penicillin useless; these resistant strains are now responsible for 10 to 40 percent of the gonorrhea cases in the U.S.[36] One strain, PPNG, is responsive to nonpenicillin antibiotics, but should be treated rapidly for maximum effectiveness and reduced possibility of complications.

Untreated gonorrhea may result in irreversible complications. In the male,

infection may spread throughout the urinary and reproductive tracts. The channels through which sperm must pass may constrict or become blocked completely, thus decreasing fertility. In females, similar results may produce **pelvic inflammatory disease (PID).** PID can constrict the fallopian tubes, or even cause a complete blockage. If blockage is complete, sterility results. If it is partial, there is an increased risk of a tubal **(ectopic)** pregnancy, a medical emergency that can cause rupture, hemorrhage, or even death. Untreated gonorrhea in either sex may produce gonococcal arthritis in major joints and a generalized infection that irreversibly damages the brain, heart, liver, and other key organs.

To minimize the risk of contracting gonorrhea, sexually active people who have casual or multiple partners should use latex condoms during sexual episodes. This is their most reliable form of protection. The sexually active individual should also be selective about sexual partners and stay alert to obvious signs and symptoms of disease.

Syphilis

Nicknamed "syph," "pox," or "bad blood," **syphilis** is perhaps the best known of all the STDs. Once confined to certain parts of the world, syphilis now occurs universally. Its

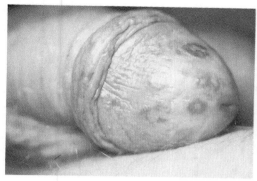

a.

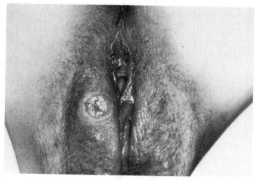

b.

Figure 12.7: What Do You Think?

1. Infectious sores, called chancres, characterize the primary stage of syphilis and often appear on the genitalia. What has contributed to the reemergence of syphilis as a serious disease in this country?
2. What public health measures are necessary to keep syphilis from rising beyond current levels?

causative agent, *Treponema pallidum,* belongs to a group of organisms that resemble bacteria, called **spirochetes.** Humans provide the only known reservoir for *T. pallidum.* There is no vaccine or other acquired immunity for syphilis. Although the potential for exposure to *T. pallidum* can be found worldwide, only about 30 percent of exposures result in infection.[37] The occurrence of syphilis, once declining and under control, rose in the 1980s and 1990s to reach its highest rate since 1950.[38] At least three reasons are thought to account for the reemergence of this disease: (1) the use of cocaine and other drugs has promoted high-risk sexual activity; (2) individuals with the highest risk practices have not had access to health care, have not sought health care, or have not given health a priority; and (3) persons most at risk often have been jobless, poorly educated, from dysfunctional families, and have had sex with multiple partners.[39]

Syphilis is transmitted by direct contact with infectious sores, called **chancres** (see figure 12.7), syphilitic skin rashes, or mucous patches on the tongue and mouth during kissing, necking, petting, or sexual intercourse. The disease also is transmissible between a pregnant woman and her fetus after the fourth month of pregnancy.[40] (Such transmission occurs when spirochetes in the mother's blood enter the circulatory system of the fetus.) Syphilis is not generally transmitted by inanimate objects such as drinking glasses or toilet seats, since spirochetes die rapidly when away from warmth and moisture. The incubation period for syphilis is from ten to ninety days, with twenty-one days being common (see figure 12.8). The blood test that is used in the diagnosis of this STD is likely to be negative during the incubation period.

Syphilis proceeds through several stages (see figure 12.9). In its **primary stage,** this STD is characterized by the appearance of a chancre at the primary site of infection. A chancre resembles a blister, pimple, or raised open sore. It is infectious and contains a large number of spirochetes. Despite their appearance, chancres are often painless and may be hidden in the mouth, throat, vagina, cervix, or anus, making detection difficult. Chancres are said to be self-limiting, that is, they heal themselves in from two to six weeks. After healing, however, a population of infectious spirochetes is left behind. Occasionally, primary syphilis also may be accompanied by swollen glands near the site of primary infection.

The primary stage ends with the disappearance of the chancre. The **secondary stage** then begins. Secondary stage symptoms may occur from six weeks to six months after the primary infection "disappears." These new symptoms usually include a rash or raised lesions anywhere on the skin. The rash is neither painful nor itchy, but it is infectious. White patches may appear in the mouth, nose, or rectum. These mucous patches also transmit disease. Additional symptoms at this stage may include patchy hair loss, mild fever and body aches, swollen glands, and some flu-like symptoms. Secondary symptoms disappear in two to six weeks but may recur for up to two years.

If still untreated, syphilis enters what is called the **latent stage.** At this point, symptoms are absent and the person is probably no longer infectious to others. The exception is the pregnant woman, who is still able to transmit disease to her fetus. The length of the latent stage is variable but can last at least five years, and perhaps as many as twenty years.[41]

Figure 12.8: Syphilis infectious disease cycle

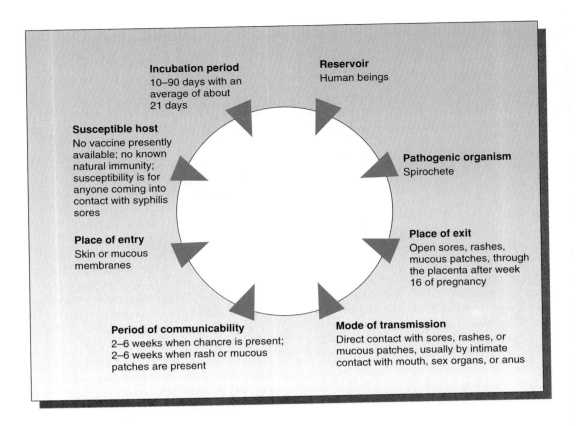

Incubation period
10–90 days with an average of about 21 days

Reservoir
Human beings

Susceptible host
No vaccine presently available; no known natural immunity; susceptibility is for anyone coming into contact with syphilis sores

Pathogenic organism
Spirochete

Place of entry
Skin or mucous membranes

Place of exit
Open sores, rashes, mucous patches, through the placenta after week 16 of pregnancy

Period of communicability
2–6 weeks when chancre is present; 2–6 weeks when rash or mucous patches are present

Mode of transmission
Direct contact with sores, rashes, or mucous patches, usually by intimate contact with mouth, sex organs, or anus

Figure 12.9: Stages of syphilis

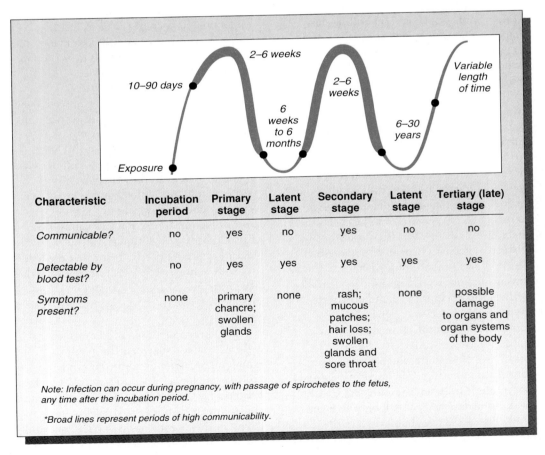

Characteristic	Incubation period	Primary stage	Latent stage	Secondary stage	Latent stage	Tertiary (late) stage
Communicable?	no	yes	no	yes	no	no
Detectable by blood test?	no	yes	yes	yes	yes	yes
Symptoms present?	none	primary chancre; swollen glands	none	rash; mucous patches; hair loss; swollen glands and sore throat	none	possible damage to organs and organ systems of the body

Note: Infection can occur during pregnancy, with passage of spirochetes to the fetus, any time after the incubation period.

*Broad lines represent periods of high communicability.

Tertiary or **late-stage syphilis** usually occurs between five and twenty years following initial infection. This condition leads to permanent disabilities and even death. Neurosyphilis, in which the brain and the spinal cord are affected, produces paralysis, insanity, and blindness. Cardiovascular syphilis includes major damage to the heart and the **aorta,** possibly resulting in death. A condition called late benign syphilis is characterized by the appearance of large destructive lesions virtually at any internal or external site.

Congenital syphilis can result from the infection of the unborn child. Spirochetes travel readily across the placenta from the woman to the fetus. Prior to the end of the fourth month of pregnancy the fetus is protected by a membrane known as Langhans' layer, but this membrane is temporary. Fetal infection can produce stillbirth, mild to severe damage of many body systems, or destruction not apparent until many years after birth.[42]

The period of communicability for syphilis is variable. It is clearly infectious in its primary and secondary stages. Active spirochetes are rendered harmless in twenty-four to forty-eight hours by adequate treatment with long-acting penicillin. For penicillin-sensitive individuals, antibiotics such as erythromycin or tetracycline are also effective. Infected individuals must be followed closely after treatment, and repeated blood tests must be performed to assure the complete absence of disease.

People hoping to avoid syphilis must avoid contact with syphilitic lesions. The use of a condom during sexual intercourse is beneficial, but a condom will not protect other exposed surfaces that may come into contact with lesions. Sexually active people who have multiple sex partners should undergo periodic screening for syphilis and other STDs. Early prenatal tests for this STD and periodic testing during pregnancy can assure that both mother and infant are disease-free. Many states continue to require blood tests for syphilis for people who are to be married. While this is one of the few control measures for syphilis, many states have undertaken initiatives to repeal the requirement for the premarital blood test, charging that it is not cost-effective.

Chlamydia-Related Infections

Infections caused by *Chlamydia trachomatis* may be the most common STDs in the U.S. today,[43] especially on the college campus.[44] This organism, an intracellular parasite, is responsible for more than one disease condition. Among these conditions are nonspecific urethritis (NSU), or **nongonococcal urethritis (NGU),** and **lymphogranuloma venereum (LGV).**

In the U.S., cases of NSU caused by the intracellular parasite *C. trachomatis* outnumber those of gonorrhea three-fold.[45] NSU involves an inflammation of the urethra, though no symptoms may be readily evident. If symptoms are present, they may resemble those of gonorrhea. NSU is said to be nonspecific because it appears to have a host of causative agents, including *C. trachomatis*, organisms known as T-mycoplasmas, and unidentified bacteria and protozoans. Transmission of NSU is probable during sexual intercourse, and transfer from mother to infant at birth is also possible. Infected newborns may experience conjunctivitis, pneumonia, and infections of the middle ear from these agents. Chlamydial eye infection in newborns may be prevented by the use of erythromycin or tetracycline ointment placed in the eyes immediately after birth. The use of silver nitrate solution may have some preventive capability as well.

To differentiate NSU from gonorrhea, cultures of smears or discharges must be examined in laboratory settings. The very organisms that are implicated in NSU may actually be present in healthy individuals too, colonizing their urogenital tracts, but without producing symptoms. Thus, when symptoms occur, pinning down the exact causative agent may be difficult. Ordinarily, the treatment of choice for NSU is tetracycline. Both partners should be treated in order to avoid the so-called Ping-Pong effect. Untreated acute NSU can produce multiple complications including inflammations of the **prostate, epididymis,** and rectum in the male and inflammations of the vagina, cervix, and rectum in the female. The most severe complication of NSU in females is PID, a condition that may contribute to infertility. NSU can be controlled by using condoms during sexual intercourse, and contacting sex partners when infection presents itself.

Spirochetes: a type of bacteria that has a spiral shape.

Aorta: the largest artery in the body that carries blood from the heart to the arterial and capillary network of the body.

Nongonococcal urethritis (NGU): an STD with symptoms like those produced in gonorrhea, but of different microorganism origin.

Lymphogranuloma venereum (LGV): a sexually transmitted disease caused by a type of bacteria called *Chlamydia trachomatis*. Symptoms include a small, painless sore on the penis or vulva, inflammation of surrounding lymph nodes and tissue, fever, chills, headache and joint pain.

Prostate: a small gland found in the male reproductive system at the base of the bladder. This gland secretes a fluid with a neutralizing action that protects sperm as they travel through the male and female reproductive tracts.

Epididymis: a structure in the male reproductive system whose main function is the temporary storage of sperm.

1. Blisters on the male and female genitals are a symptom of herpes. What precautions should one take prior to sex when one has a history of herpes infection?
2. Why is herpes so insidious a disease, especially for women?

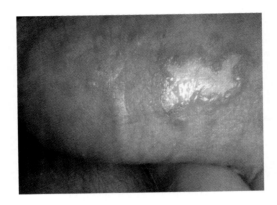

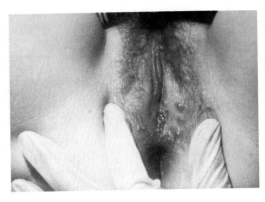

C. trachomatis also is responsible for the STD called lymphogranuloma venereum (LGV).[46] Symptoms include sores in the genital area that resemble pimples. LGV is most commonly seen among gay men and persons having multiple sex partners. Transmission occurs through direct contact with lesions, usually during sexual intercourse. Complications from LGV are rare, though inflammation of the urethra, cervix, and rectum are possible. Tetracycline provides reliable therapy for this STD.

C. trachomatis may be asymptomatic in up to 30 percent of males, including 7 percent of students at one university that was studied.[47] Unprotected sexual activity involving infected men can transmit the parasite easily.

Genital Herpes

Most people are familiar with **herpes simplex virus type I.** It is the cause of cold sores that occasionally affect many children and some adults. Cold sores generally appear on or around the mouth, and their symptoms are usually mild. Genital herpes, produced by **herpes simplex virus type II (HSV-II),** presents a different story. The sores caused by HSV-II form on the genitals and are transmitted during sexual intercourse. An infected pregnant woman may also pass on the virus to her infant during childbirth. The result for the newborn infant can be blindness, severe mental retardation, neurological damage, or even death.

Genital herpes is rapidly gaining attention as an STD. One reason is that thousands of new cases are being identified each year. Another reason for the recent concern is the lack of any known cure. The fact that herpes is a virus makes antibiotic drugs useless in treating the symptoms and eliminating infection from the body. In most

instances, herpes sores—the blisters and crusts they later form on the genitals—heal and disappear on their own in a few days or weeks. The virus itself, however, stays in a dormant stage; the absence of symptoms does not necessarily mean the absence of active virus. Herpes may reassert itself from time to time, causing the sores to reappear. The sores are usually visible and painful in both sexes; however, signs of herpes in women can be internal and painless. As with some of the other STDs, it is therefore possible for women to be unaware of the virus's presence (see figure 12.10).

What triggers recurrences of herpes is not well understood. Lowered resistance, other infections, chafing or irritation of the affected area, emotional upset, and even certain foods are factors implicated to some extent. In women, the onset of menstruation may occasionally produce a flare-up of this STD.

Though herpes has an effect on all of its victims, it need not "paralyze" them emotionally. If a few sensible points are observed, and some lifestyle alterations made, life can continue to be full and enjoyable. First, people with herpes infection are advised to be specifically conscientious about controlling the stressors that may aggravate the dormant HSV-II organism. Stress-management programs and routine relaxation, valuable assets for anyone's level of wellness, are particularly helpful for the person with herpes. During recurrence, sexual contact ought to be avoided. Even at other times, if procreation is not an objective, it is advised that a latex condom be used during intercourse to provide protection for the uninfected partner. Herpes blisters can appear in places not ordinarily protected from contact by a latex condom, though, thus limiting the effectiveness of condom use. The herpes infected person who eats a well-balanced diet, receives adequate rest, and practices the routines identified should experience only minimal life disruptions resulting from herpes.

The woman who has herpes needs to take a couple of additional precautions. There is a statistical association between HSV-II infection and the development of cancer of the cervix. Thus, a woman with herpes may be advised to have Pap tests slightly more often than other women her age. She should also be more conscientious about noticing any unusual vaginal bleeding. A physician is probably best able to determine the optimal frequency for periodic examinations.

Because of the danger of infecting the newborn infant, women who know they have herpes need to share this information with their physicians. **Cesarean deliveries** are generally advised when herpes is actively present.

Although no cure for genital herpes has been identified, some progress toward the relief of symptoms has occurred. Most traditional medical remedies are ointments applied topically to the affected areas. Most promising among these remedies is **acyclovir,** an antiviral drug that has demonstrated remarkable effects in recently infected individuals. Acyclovir as a topical ointment has not proven effective for persons experiencing a recurrent episode of herpes. An orally administered preparation of acyclovir has shown some success in preventing recurrences, however. Individuals who have been infected with the herpes virus should discuss treatment options with their personal physician.

Genital Warts (HPV)

Condyloma acuminata, also known as **genital warts** or **venereal warts,** are caused by a DNA virus of the papova virus group, called **human papilloma virus (HPV).** Although this disease occurs worldwide, it is only known to occur in sexually active individuals, and primarily by direct contact. These warts are really benign tumors, varying in size and shape, but frequently clustering in the genital and anal areas. Sometimes they are hidden from view. As long as they are present they can transmit infection. About fifty distinct HPV types have been identified.[48] At least two of these varieties (HPV types 16 and 18) have been associated with the subsequent development of cervical cancer in women.[49] There is some concern that the incidence of HPV infection is rising, especially among sexually active college women, placing them in a double jeopardy situation (STD infection and cervical cancer).[50] Males may also have long-term consequences from HPV infection, although exact linkages are still under study. Concern that this disease could be epidemic among college students even now is probably justified based on studies that demonstrate how commonly HPV shows up on routine Pap smears taken on college-aged women,[51] how unfamiliar college-aged women are with HPV,[52] and the generally well accepted level of sexual activity that occurs in college settings.

Candidiasis (Monilia)

Candidiasis, also known as monilia vulvovaginitis or just monilia, is a common yeast-fungus infection caused by *Candida albicans.* It produces clinical symptoms more frequently in women than in men. Candidiasis frequently may be acquired by other than sexual means. In fact, *Candida albicans* is a normal part of the human flora, such as those that reside inside the vagina. If this is so, why does it flare up? Why is candidiasis labeled an STD?

Acute episodes of candidiasis seem to occur when certain other predisposing factors are present. It is known to be more common in people with diabetes, individuals with certain immune deficiencies, women taking birth-control pills, and patients under broad-spectrum-antibiotic therapy.[53] Such circumstances may alter the normal acidity of the vagina, thus promoting an outbreak of the yeast organisms. Acute infections are accompanied by intense itching at the infected site, along with redness and perhaps swelling. In women, candidiasis may also produce vaginal discharges of a white, curd-like quality.

Complications from candidiasis are more aggravating than they are medically serious. The principal complication is recurrence, resulting when the infection is passed back and forth (Ping-Pong style) between partners. Consequently, when flare-ups occur, both partners are often treated. The most common and reliable treatment is topical application of nystatin for both partners.[54] Some women achieve relief from mild cases by douching with a solution of water and vinegar. The yeast organisms do not do well in acidic environments. Because candidiasis is so common, especially in women, some

Cesarean delivery: the surgical opening of the abdomen and uterus for childbirth.

physicians may prescribe topical nystatin over the telephone without examination or microscopic evidence. If your physician does this, special notice should be made of the progress of symptoms. If they persist beyond a week, examination by a physician is recommended. Acute episodes of candidiasis can generally be avoided or minimized by using condoms during intercourse, wearing clothes that are not tight fitting (to reduce perspiration), and keeping the genital area dry. An over-the-counter preparation that contains miconazole, and is sold in products such as Monostat, also can treat candidiasis intravaginally. It should, however, be used under the advice of a physician.

Nonspecific Vaginitis

Nonspecific vaginitis (NSV) is probably caused by the bacterium *Gardnerella vaginalis,* known to some scientists as *Haemophilus vaginalis,* whenever other organisms identified in the cause of NSV cannot be implicated. Symptoms of NSV are almost always restricted to females, though a male may experience itchy, burning symptoms of disease in his penis, similar to the vaginal symptoms that females report.

Symptoms in the female include a foul-smelling vaginal discharge, vaginal itching, and burning upon urination; however, the complete absence of symptoms is not uncommon. Treatment is accomplished with oral metronidazole, and transfer is prevented by the use of condoms.

Trichomoniasis

Trichomoniasis is caused by the presence of *Trichomonas vaginalis,* a protozoan, which may exist without symptoms in the vaginal flora of 50 percent of females in the U.S. between the ages of sixteen and twenty-five.[55] Susceptibility to "trich" is general, though clinical disease is usually restricted to females. Though the organisms can be acquired during sexual intercourse, they may also be picked up by nonsexual means from freshly soiled bedclothes, towels, and other items.

The female with trichomoniasis is most likely to notice acute disease during or shortly after menstruation. Symptoms may include a foul-smelling discharge, localized itching, redness, and burning during urination. Or, there may be no symptoms. Treatment of choice is oral metronidazole, usually given to both partners, since "trich" is another of the so-called Ping-Pong STDs. Males seldom experience any demonstrable symptoms. Females who suspect trichomoniasis should not douche before an examination, as this could make diagnosis difficult.

Pediculosis and Scabies

Pediculosis and **scabies** are two disorders more accurately labeled infestations than infections. Both are caused by parasites, pediculosis by the crab louse and scabies by the itch mite. These organisms may be found anywhere on the body but show a selective preference for the pubic hair. They lay their eggs at the base of the hair, just underneath the skin. The presence of these organisms is highly irritating. Crabs and mites can produce an agonizing itch after their eggs hatch. Transfer of these organisms can occur from person to person in a variety of ways. Direct body contact, particularly during physical intimacy, is a common mode. Contact with personal items such as clothes and bedsheets can often accomplish transfer. Other means are also possible.

Complications are rare, though secondary infections can result from breaks in the skin due to intense itching and irritation. Tight clothing and perspiration can aggravate the condition further. Treatment is provided by application of medicated shampoos. Reinfestation is prevented by good personal hygiene and careful laundering and ironing of clothes and bedding items.

Urinary Tract Infections

Urinary tract infections (UTIs) are often classified as bladder infections or cystitis and occur when pathogenic organisms enter the urethra and migrate to the bladder. Although they ordinarily are confined to the host, they can be sexually transmitted. Bacteria and other organisms may produce a UTI. Intestinal bacteria can produce infection when they are present in fecal matter that comes into contact with the urethra. This might occur when wiping the anal area following a bowel movement. Contact between the hands and the urethra or between the urethra and inanimate objects may also lead to infections. Women, perhaps because of their shorter urethras, are much more susceptible to UTIs than men. UTIs may be chronic in some women. Pathogens can sometimes be "flushed" from the system by having the individual drink eight to ten glasses of water per day. Because of the acidity of cranberry juice, physicians often prescribed it to prevent UTIs, believing that the acid killed the microbes implicated in causing the infection. Recent evidence suggests that cranberry juice is less effective at preventing UTIs than in limiting their complications.[56] It may be that compounds contained in cranberry juice prevent microorganisms from clinging to the walls of the urinary tract, and thus, produce the protective effect, rather than the actual acidity of the juice. It is important to know that cranberry juice may not be effective all by itself, and should not be seen as a replacement for proper treatment and follow-up. If you should have persistent symptoms of a UTI, be sure to consult a physician.

Personal and Social Issues Related to STD Control

Part of the reason why STDs pose a problem of such magnitude is that treatment of the infected individual solves only half the STD problem. Adequate treatment of sex partners through **contact investigation** is also necessary, although both laborious and expensive. There is even some disagreement as to who has the responsibility for contact investigation. Is it with the patient, the physician, or public health officials? Moreover, diagnosis of some STDs is occasionally difficult because most physicians do not screen for them on a routine basis, and some individuals, particularly women, may be infected but not notice any symptoms. The lack of early symptoms in women is characteristic of more than one of the STDs.

Also contributing to the proliferation of STDs is the fact that exact diagnosis of some STDs is extremely difficult without the availability of laboratory facilities. This is especially true of such STDs as gonorrhea, nonspecific urethritis, and nonspecific vaginitis, all of which have similar symptoms early in their development. Laboratories are expensive to build, staff, and supply, and therefore they are luxuries not found in all communities. Samples often must be sent great distances for accurate diagnoses, resulting in delays of several days.

Adding to this problem is the fact that some physicians fail to report cases of STDs to public-health agencies. Reporting is not required by law for all STDs, but for certain ones (syphilis, gonorrhea, and AIDS) reporting is mandatory. Support for physician training in the areas of STD diagnosis, treatment, and reporting may not be as strong as in many other areas of medical education.

Perhaps the most prevalent myth about STDs is that once symptoms disappear or treatment occurs, reinfection cannot take place. In fact, there are no vaccines and no acquired immunities for STDs. People can be infected over and over, and the reservoir for such disorders can be maintained indefinitely. Reinfection often occurs in the individual who is careless or reckless about sexual activity.

Due to the easing of sexual mores, there may also be greater opportunity than ever before for the transmission and spread of STDs. Improved fertility-control measures may enhance the frequency of sexual participation, or the number of sexual partners, thus increasing the chances of infection. Fertility-control measures such as birth-control pills may actually promote the proliferation of a natural yeast organism of the vaginal flora, *Candida albicans*. The pill creates an environment in some women that permits periodic growth of this yeast, leading to irritation of the genital area and other symptoms. Although a woman may not have contracted the organism by sexual activity, she can certainly transmit it to her partner by that means. Thus the "technology" of birth control has been somewhat of a mixed blessing. Moreover, through the early 1990s, the condom, the only contraceptive measure (other than abstinence) that provides a measure of protection against many STDs, may be unpopular. A study of women fifteen to forty-four years of age found that just 12 percent who were exposed to the risk of pregnancy used a condom.[57]

Despite their promotion by health educators and other health professionals, condoms continue to be underutilized, especially by persons whose risk of STDs may be high—persons with multiple sex partners and persons who have been treated previously for an STD infection. According to Mildred Z. Solomon and William DeJong:[58]

Historically, condom use in the U.S. has been associated with extramarital

Contact investigation: a mechanism for reducing the likelihood of an epidemic by asking persons treated for STDs to identify sexual partners who can be traced, examined, and successfully treated, if necessary.

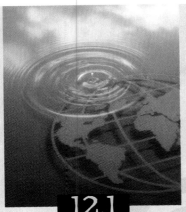

12.1

A Social Perspective

Are There Factors That Predict Safer Sex Among College Students?

With HIV+ status estimated to be approaching a figure as high as 1 percent on some campuses,* the time to understand what motivates safer sex practices is now. In a study at four New Jersey colleges, Ann O'Leary and her colleagues identified factors that predicted safer sex activity.** They examined knowledge about HIV, perceived risk of acquiring HIV, perceived social norms pertaining to safer sex on campus, negative expectations about condoms, perceived ability to discuss sexual history with a partner, and perceived ability to practice safer sex behaviors.

Knowledge about HIV was not a good predictor of safer sex practices, nor were perceptions about one's HIV susceptibility. According to O'Leary, et al.: "Students practicing riskier behavior, however, reported more negative expected outcomes from condom use, lower perceived self-efficacy to perform safer sex, more frequent sex under the influence [of alcohol or other drugs], and, surprisingly, *higher* perceived self-efficacy to discuss sexual history. Perceived social norms contributed with marginal significance to behavioral safety." Negative outcomes from condom use included beliefs that using a condom takes the fun out of having sex, that using a condom might make a partner angry or upset, or make the person suggesting its use feel silly, or actually scare a partner into thinking that the person suggesting condom use was infected with HIV or another STD. There is evidence that educational interventions that target behavioral change can favorably influence practice of safer sex,§ including greater self-efficacy with respect to discussing condom use,§§ and actually using condoms.§§§ As we approach the year 2000, it is critical that health officials and students in collegiate settings work together to help create an environment that minimizes the spread of sexually transmissible diseases.

Sources:
*H. D. Gayle, R. P. Keeling, M. Garcia-Tunon, et al., "Prevalence of HIV among College and University Students," *New England Journal of Medicine* 323 (1990): 1538–1541.
**A. O'Leary, F. Goodhart, L. S. Jemmott, and D. Boccher-Lattimore, "Predictors of Safer Sex on the College Campus: A Social Cognitive Theory Analysis," *Journal of American College Health* 40 (1992): 254–263.
§J. C. Turner, E. Korpita, L. A. Mohn, and W. B. Hill, "Reduction in Sexual Risk Behaviors among College Students Following Comprehensive Health Education Intervention," *Journal of American College Health* 41 (1993): 187–193.
§§N. D. Richie and A. Getty, "Did an AIDS Peer Education Program Change First-Year College Students' Behaviors?" *Journal of American College Health* 42 (1994): 163–165.
§§§T. M. Brien, D. L. Thombs, C. A. Mahoney, and L. Wallnau, "Dimensions of Self-Efficacy among Three Distinct Groups of Condom Users," *Journal of American College Health* 42 (1994): 167–174.

What Do You Think?

1. How easy is it for you to buy condoms? discuss condom use with a potential partner before engaging in sexual activity? use a condom from start to finish of a sexual episode? refuse sex if a condom is not available? find an alternative activity if a condom is unavailable? stop sexual activity if a condom is not available?

2. Do males and females differ with respect to their ability to apply the above skills or take the identified actions? What accounts for this difference? In the study by O'Leary, et al., how do you account for the finding that students who perceived their ability to discuss sexual history with a partner as high actually reported more risky sexual behavior?

sex, prostitution, and promiscuity. In addition, condoms are perceived by both men and women to impair the pleasure of sexual intercourse. Furthermore, introducing condom use can entail a difficult interpersonal negotiation that can result in distrust and embarrassment.

Other factors may negatively influence both men and women about condom use: fear of condom failure; interruption of lovemaking; lack of ready access; failure to plan for sexual intercourse; use of alcohol or drugs prior to sex; and the belief that insisting on using a condom will be offensive,

unnatural, or immoral where a partner is concerned.[59] Prior to the AIDS problem, condom use was not promoted much in the U.S. There was little effort devoted to social marketing of condoms—that is, promoting positive images associated with their use. Recent social marketing measures might be producing important attitudinal change. While some people continue to harbor many negative connotations about condoms, they also report that condoms provide peace of mind (about infection), no side effects, and convenience (see A Social Perspective 12.1). Interestingly, some condom users find that the reduced stimulation associated with

TABLE 12.9

Symptoms of STDs in Males

1. Burning during urination.
2. Any abnormal drip or discharge from the penis.
3. Any unusual or abnormal coloring in the urine.
4. Obvious presence of blood in the urine.
5. Sores, pimples, warts, or other unusual lesions on or near the genital area.
6. Soreness or redness on the penis or anus.

Symptoms of STDs in Females

1. Burning during urination.
2. Pain, itching, soreness, or redness on or around the vaginal or rectal areas.
3. Sores, pimples, warts, or other unusual lesions on or near the genital area.
4. Any unusual or abnormal discharge from the vagina.

condom use prolongs sex and that putting on a condom can in fact be sexually arousing—two highly desirable elements!

The present STD crisis can be attributed, in part, to public apathy about the subject, or public fears that taking measures to address the problem will make matters even worse or alienate people who take a strong moral stand on sexual activity outside of marriage. Administrators on university and college campuses debate whether or not to make inexpensive condoms available in vending machines in dormitories and other buildings. On the other hand, administrators wonder if by increasing availability to condoms, they also are condoning casual sexual activity and promoting moral turpitude. In some communities, the subject of STDs is ignored or tightly controlled in the public schools. Even when the STD is as serious as AIDS, teachers might be permitted to address only the epidemiology and historical significance of the problem—not how it is passed from person to person or how it could be prevented.

What to Do and Where to Go for Help

After being in a mutually monogamous sexual relationship for all of his nearly three years at college, Dennis had a one night stand with Trish, a woman he met at a friend's party. Since both Dennis and Trish had consumed quite a bit of alcohol, neither of them stopped to get a condom. Two days later the inside of Dennis's penis was sore, and when he tried to urinate, he did so with difficulty. When urine passed through his urethra, it created a painful burning sensation. Even when he was not trying to urinate, Dennis' penis felt as if it had a nest of bees buzzing around in it, and he felt as if he needed to urinate all the time. Efforts to do so produced no results, though. Five days later Dennis could feel swelling in his groin area and a dull but steady, painful ache in and around one of his testicles. While Dennis was pretty sure he had acquired an STD, he was too embarrassed to have it checked out and treated. A few days later his mind started working overtime and he began to worry that he might have gotten HIV. His symptoms caused him both physical and mental anguish. After nearly three weeks of discomfort, sleeplessness, anxiety, and making up excuses to his long-time girlfriend, Dennis finally went to the student health service on campus for an examination. What Dennis discovered was that he had a nonspecific infection, and one that required going through a series of antibiotics until one finally provided some relief many weeks later. His STD turned out to be one that did not result in chronic symptoms, or worse, one that was lethal, but Dennis discovered that casual sex could disrupt his life in a very profound and hurtful way.

The symptoms of STDs vary, though some STDs show symptoms that are remarkably similar to one another. A summary of common STD signs and symptoms, not unlike those that Dennis experienced, is presented in table 12.9.

If you have one or more symptoms that arouse suspicion of an STD, you should seek medical help *immediately*. Consultation with a physician also may be advisable if you suspect that you have been exposed to an infected person, whether or not signs of infection have appeared. Although the family physician is an appropriate person to contact, many people are reluctant to consult someone they know because of guilt or embarrassment. Other physicians certainly should be considered. Many communities have clinics exclusively for people with STDs. College campus health services can usually direct people to an appropriate source for STD tests.

Remember that not all physicians or clinics provide STD diagnostic and treatment services. If you are making an appointment to be examined for a suspected STD, be sure to ask if such services are available. Health centers and hospitals provide services with variable costs. Investigate these services and costs, and also look into the availability of free or low-cost clinics.

What is likely to happen during a trip to a clinic for an STD examination? In the waiting room you are likely to be instructed to "take a number." This ensures that names are not used in public and each person's confidentiality is protected. You will be requested to complete forms that ask for information about your purpose for coming in and your medical history. By law, all information you provide must be held in strict confidence.

Regardless of the exact STD symptoms, you are likely to be given a specific test for syphilis and possibly for gonorrhea as well. These tests are precautionary and routine. In the syphilis test, a blood sample is drawn from the arm. If any sores are present, fluid samples may be taken for examination.

If test results indicate the presence of one or more STDs, medications may be prescribed immediately. With women whose symptoms are vague or even absent, a complete pelvic examination may be required. Some tests take several days to a week for interpretation. If such tests are performed, the patient is usually asked to avoid any sexual contact until results are available and a diagnosis is made.

Next, you are likely to talk to a health counselor. This person may be a physician, nurse, health educator, or other specifically designated member of the health-care team. Part of the counseling process includes discussion of how you can help sexual partners. You may be requested to name sexual contacts. Providing the names of contacts will assist, however, in case control of STDs. If you are too embarrassed or uneasy about informing a partner, designated personnel from the clinic are likely to be available for such purposes. Dennis took

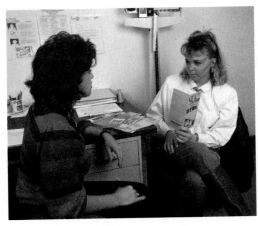

Figure 12.11: What Do You Think?

1. Health counselors provide guidance for individuals with STDs and help them control the spread of their diseases. How can more persons who think they have been exposed to an STD be persuaded to have a checkup?
2. Should persons with whom an infected person has had sex be contacted by health authorities? Should an infected person be required by law to name contacts, or merely encouraged to do so?

advantage of this option while at the student health service; he gave Trish's name to the physician, who asked professionals from the local health department to contact Trish. When they spoke to Trish they informed her that a previous sexual partner had been treated for a sexually transmitted disease and she should come in to be checked. Dennis' name was not mentioned, as this information is considered confidential. Trish had her checkup, and found out that she too had a nonspecific infection, NSV. Trish did not have any warning symptoms of this infection, and if Dennis had not let health professionals contact her, she may have experienced complications from the infection, as well as continuing to infect other sexual partners.

The counseling process concludes with a discussion of ways to prevent contracting STDs and usually a request to return to the clinic at least once for a follow-up examination. This return trip is to assure a complete cure; it is a vital part of disease control. You can usually rely on clinic personnel to be sensitive to your needs (see figure 12.11).

Minimizing the Risks of STDs

The best way of dealing with STDs is to prevent their occurrence in the first place. Most of the recommended precautions are

TABLE 12.10   *Personal STD Prevention Methods*

There is no fool proof way to prevent sexually transmitted diseases (STDs); however, practicing the known prevention methods listed here will significantly reduce your chances of becoming infected.

Sexual Abstinence
Refraining from sexual contact with others is an effective way to avoid STD infection through sexual transmission. (Some STDs, such as HIV-related disease, can be transmitted in other ways, such as through needle sharing during injecting drug use.)

Monogamy
Limiting your sexual contact to one uninfected partner will decrease your chance of becoming infected with a sexually transmitted disease.

Condom Use
Correctly using latex condoms during all genital sexual contact is an effective way to greatly decrease the chances that you will become infected with a sexually transmitted disease.

Selectivity
Avoid sexual contact with people who are sexually active with multiple partners. Additionally, limit your number of sexual partners as well. The more sexual partners someone has, the greater the likelihood that a STD will be transmitted.

Observation
Before becoming sexually active with someone, discreetly look for signs and symptoms of a STD. Blisters, sores, rashes, or discharges may indicate that a STD is present. Remember that signs and symptoms of STDs are *not* confined to the genital region of the body.

Urination
Urinate immediately following sexual activity, especially after sexual intercourse. It is believed that urination may wash STD pathogens out of the urethra, thus preventing infection.

Regular STD Checkups and Treatment
If you are sexually active, you should *request* that your physician or clinic give you a STD checkup *at least* once a year. Many STDs produce few or no signs or symptoms. Without special testing, you may have a hidden STD that could cause permanent damage if not treated promptly. Effective treatments or cures exist for many of the prevalent STDs. Additionally, regular checkups and treatment, if an STD is diagnosed, will help you prevent the possibility that you may infect your sexual partner with a STD.

Source: Data from the American Council on Healthful Living, Orange, NJ.

simple enough for everyone to follow (see table 12.10). Do not forget that with many STDs, it is what you cannot see that can hurt you. When symptoms do appear, have them checked out. If you are sexually active with more than one partner, periodic routine STD checkups may be a responsible precautionary measure on behalf of partners, as well as advisable for personal peace of mind. Embarrassment and guilt should not be barriers to informing a partner if you have an STD. Wouldn't you want to be informed if a partner just had an STD diagnosed? Having an STD is not likely to be looked upon as the highlight of your life, but it need not be the end of the world either.

A Final Word on Communicable Diseases

Like wars and natural disasters, new problems from communicable diseases seem to arise all the time. Before 1981, HIV was unknown. Now it is, perhaps, the most feared of communicable diseases. In 1994, an outbreak of a new disease from *hantavirus* claimed the lives of people in the southwestern United States, but also affected people in Florida, Rhode Island, and Indiana.[60] Old nemesis diseases, like syphilis, make comebacks because of changes in population, culture, and other conditions. As recently as 1995, tuberculosis was mounting a comeback, and not just in conjunction with persons of HIV+ status.[61] Although communicable diseases seem less threatening today than a hundred years ago, events remind us that they are not to be ignored. Moreover, diseases of other parts of the world could soon be having an impact on us here.

Summary

1. Control of infectious diseases by the year 2000 is a major health objective of the nation.
2. The body has several mechanisms for fighting off infection effectively.
3. Although brought under control to a large extent by sanitation procedures, antibiotic chemotherapy, and immunization, infectious diseases still pose threats to wellness.
4. While colds and the flu often can be troublesome, some common sense practices can help to control their symptoms and their communicability.
5. Like most infectious diseases, the STDs go through the infectious disease cycle.
6. AIDS is the newest of the STDs and one of the most dangerous. It may constitute the most important public-health challenge ever.
7. HIV/AIDS constitutes an even greater challenge for certain minority groups and women because of the generally low political clout they wield.
8. Some STDs are treated easily and effectively, but for others, there is no cure. Some STDs, such as herpes, may recur in the infected person. The absence of STD symptoms does not always mean the absence of disease.
9. The highest attack rate for gonorrhea, one of the classic STDs, is in the twenty- to twenty-four-year-old population.
10. Syphilis, once brought under control, has reemerged to become once again an important and dangerous STD.
11. *Chlamydia trachomatis* may be the most common STD on the college campus, and often produces no noticeable symptoms.
12. The presence of genital warts, also known as HPV, can be a significant STD problem on the college campus, and can lead to later, even more dangerous health problems, especially for women.
13. Numerous cultural, behavioral, and other factors act as barriers to adequate disease control. Appropriate contact investigation is a particularly vital STD control measure that often is not practiced.
14. For people who have an STD, there is help available through many channels. The best STD protection, however, is reliable prevention.

Recommended Readings

Ellner, Paul D., and Neu, Harold C. *Understanding Infectious Disease*. St. Louis: Mosby, 1992.

Ellner and Neu present methodical and clear explanations of the dynamics of disease infection and transmission, including present day diseases and ones of historic significance.

Hamann, Barbara. *Disease: Identification, Prevention, and Control*. St. Louis: Mosby, 1994.

This book covers communicable and noncommunicable diseases, and includes a historical perspective on humankind's treatment of disease through the ages.

Jackson, James K. *AIDS, STD, & Other Communicable Diseases*. Guilford, CT: Dushkin Publishing Group, 1992.

This easy-to-read and understand practical guide to prevention and control of communicable diseases, emphasizes those disorders most commonly affecting college-aged individuals.

References

1. *Healthy People 2000*, National Health Promotion and Disease Prevention Objectives, (Washington, D.C.: U.S. Department of Health and Human Services, 1991).
2. Paul D. Ellner and Harold C. Neu, *Understanding Infectious Disease*, (St. Louis: Mosby Year Book, Inc., 1992), 15.
3. Ellner and Neu, *Understanding Infectious Disease*, 22.
4. John W. Hole, Jr., *Human Anatomy and Physiology*, 5th ed. (Dubuque, Iowa: Wm. C. Brown Publishers, 1990), 741.
5. Abram S. Benenson, ed., *Control of Communicable Diseases in Man*, 15th ed. (Washington, D.C.: American Public Health Association, 1990), 225.
6. Centers for Disease Control, "Prevention and Control of Influenza," *Morbidity and Mortality Weekly Report* 39 (1990): 1–15.
7. Ellner & Neu, *Understanding Infectious Disease*, 27.
8. Ellner and Neu, *Understanding Infectious Disease*, 27.
9. Benenson, *Control of Communicable Diseases in Man*, 337.
10. Ellner & Neu, *Understanding Infectious Disease*, 259.
11. Ellner and Neu, *Understanding Infectious Disease*, 188.
12. Ellner and Neu, *Understanding Infectious Disease*, 188.
13. Ellner and Neu, *Understanding Infectious Disease*, 188.
14. Ellner and Neu, *Understanding Infectious Disease*, 189.
15. Centers for Disease Control, "Surveillance for HIV-2 Infection in Blood Donors—United States, 1987–1989," *Morbidity and Mortality Weekly Report* 39 (1990): 829–831.
16. Centers for Disease Control, "HIV Prevalence Estimates and AIDS Case Projections for the United States: Report Based upon a Workshop," *Morbidity and Mortality Weekly Report* 39 (1990): 12.
17. American Association for World Health, *AIDS and Families*, (Washington, D.C.: American Association for World Health, 1994), 6.
18. Robert Hatcher, James Trussell, Felicia Stewart, et al., *Contraceptive Technology*, 16th ed. (New York: Irvington Publishers, Inc., 1994), 155–156.
19. Hatcher et al., *Contraceptive Technology*, 155–156.

20. University of California at Berkeley Wellness Letter, "How Effective Are Condoms?" *University of California at Berkeley Wellness Letter* 9.3 (1992): 6.

21. U.S. Department of Health and Human Services, *The Surgeon General's Report to the American Public on HIV Infection and AIDS*, (Washington, D.C.: U.S. Government Printing Office, 1993), 8.

22. Deborah A. McLean, "A Model for HIV Risk Reduction and Prevention among African American College Students," *Journal of American College Health* 42 (1994): 220–223.

23. Centers for Disease Control, "Mortality Attributable to HIV Infections/AIDS—United States, 1981–1990," *Morbidity and Mortality Weekly Report* 40 (1991): 41–44.

24. Stephen B. Thomas, Aisha G. Gilliam, and Carolyn G. Iwrey, "Knowledge about AIDS and Reported Risk Behaviors among Black College Students," *Journal of American College Health* 38 (1989): 61–66.

25. McLean, "A Model for HIV Risk Reduction and Prevention among African-American College Students," 220.

26. Centers for Disease Control, "Heterosexual Behaviors and Factors that Influence Condom Use among Patients Attending a Sexually Transmitted Disease Clinic—San Francisco," *Morbidity and Mortality Weekly Report* 39 (1990): 685–689.

27. John F. Aruffo, John H. Coverdale, and Carlos Vallbona, "AIDS Knowledge in Low-Income and Minority Populations," *Public Health Reports* 106 (1991): 115–119.

28. Jane R. Schwebke, "Syphilis in the '90s," *Medical Aspects of Human Sexuality* 25.4 (1991): 44–49.

29. Gust A. Yep, "HIV Prevention among Asian-American College Students: Does the Health Belief Model Work?" *Journal of American College Health* 41 (1993): 199–205.

30. American Association for World Health, *AIDS and Families*, 22.

31. American Association for World Health, *AIDS and Families*, 22.

32. American Association for World Health, *AIDS and Families*, 22.

33. Ellner & Neu, *Understanding Infectious Disease*, 197.

34. Ellner and Neu, *Understanding Infectious Disease*, 197.

35. Ellner and Neu, *Understanding Infectious Disease*, 198.

36. Ellner and Neu, *Understanding Infectious Disease*, 201.

37. Benenson, *Control of Communicable Diseases in Man*, 422.

38. Barbara Hamann, *Disease: Identification, Prevention, and Control*, (St. Louis: Mosby Year-Book, Inc., 1994), 147.

39. Centers for Disease Control and Prevention, *Morbidity and Mortality Weekly Report* 40.19 (1991): 314.

40. Ellner & Neu, *Understanding Infectious Disease*, 254.

41. Benenson, *Control of Communicable Diseases in Man*, 421.

42. Ellner & Neu, *Understanding Infectious Disease*, 254.

43. Ellner and Neu, *Understanding Infectious Disease*, 203.

44. Robin G. Sawyer and Donald J. Moss, "Sexually Transmitted Diseases in College Men: A Preliminary Clinical Investigation," *Journal of American College Health* 42 (1993): 111–115.

45. Ellner & Neu, *Understanding Infectious Disease*, 203.

46. Ellner and Neu, *Understanding Infectious Disease*, 203.

47. Joshua E. Kaplan, Miriam Meyer, and Joanne Navin, "Chlamydia Trachomatis Infection in a Male College Student Population," *Journal of American College Health* 37 (1989): 159–161.

48. Ellner & Neu, *Understanding Infectious Disease*, 142.

49. American Social Health Association, *HPV and Genital Warts*, (Research Triangle Park, N.C.: American Social Health Association, 1991), pamphlet.

50. Arlene Loucks, "Human Papillomavirus Screening in College Women," *Journal of American College Health* 39 (1991): 291–293.

51. Loucks, "Human Papillomavirus Screening in College Women," 291.

52. Karen Vail-Smith and David M. White, "Risk Level, Knowledge, and Preventive Behavior for Human Papillomaviruses among Sexually Active College Women," *Journal of American College Health* 40 (1992): 227–230.

53. Ellner & Neu, *Understanding Infectious Disease*, 211.

54. Benenson, *Control of Communicable Diseases in Man*, 74.

55. Benenson, *Control of Communicable Diseases in Man*, 449.

56. Winifred Conkling, "The Cranberry Cure," *American Health* 13.5 (1994): 10.

57. Daniel R. Mishell, Jr., "Contraception," *New England Journal of Medicine* 320 (1989): 777–787.

58. Mildred Z. Solomon and William DeJong, "Preventing AIDS and other STDs through Condom Promotion: A Patient Education Intervention," *American Journal of Public Health* 79 (1989): 453–458.

59. Ann O'Leary, Fern Goodhart, L. S. Jemmott, and D. Boccher-Lattimore, "Predictors of Safer Sex on the College Campus: A Social Cognitive Theory Analysis," *Journal of American College Health* 40 (1992): 254–263.

60. Richard P. Wenzel, "A New Hantavirus Infection in North America," *New England Journal of Medicine* 330.14 (1994): 1004–1005.

61. Dick Menzies, Anne Fanning, Lilian Yuan, and Mark Fitzgerald, "Tuberculosis among Health Care Workers," *New England Journal of Medicine* 332.2 (1995): 92–98.

Coming to Terms with Death and Loss: A Wellness Perspective

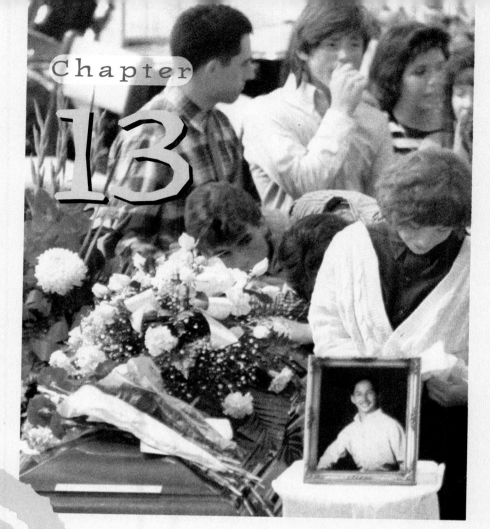

Chapter 13

Student Learning Objectives

Upon completion of this chapter you should be able to:

1. compare life expectancy among major racial and ethnic groups in the United States;
2. discuss the relationship of the study of death and dying to wellness;
3. describe historical and current ways people in the U.S. deal with the subject of death;
4. identify how technology has influenced the definition of death and raised moral and ethical questions concerning death;
5. describe the physiological reactions that occur when a body dies;
6. give the characteristics of ecological, humanistic, religious, reincarnation, and life-after-life perspectives about death;
7. describe the needs of the dying person as explained by Dr. Elisabeth Kübler-Ross;
8. explain the concept of hospice and its role in comforting the dying person and that individual's loved ones;
9. explain the body's reaction to grief, and the adjustment to the loss of a loved one;
10. describe the elements of a condolence call;
11. compare and contrast children's responses to death with that of adults;
12. review the elements of funerals that are shared among cultures and unique to some cultures;
13. provide advice on how to be a good consumer when the need to prepare a funeral arises;
14. explain the meaning of a living will, its enactment, and its legal application;
15. explain how one becomes identified as a uniform organ donor;
16. define euthanasia and mercy killing and explain their relevance to contemporary society;
17. give examples of different kinds of wills.

According to *Healthy People 2000*, the primary health goal of the nation by the 21st century is to increase the span of healthy life for people in the U.S.[1] Life expectancy at birth for Americans is approximately seventy-five years, an increase of twenty-eight years since 1900. This life expectancy is not, however, equal among racial and ethnic groups in the U.S. When years of *healthy life* are assessed, differences are especially apparent. African-Americans can expect the lowest life expectancy at sixty-eight years, with just fifty-six years unthreatened by disabling diseases or other conditions. More than 11 percent of African-Americans experience limitations of activity. This rate is not as high for Native Americans, among whom more than 13 percent have such limitations.[2] The greatest disparity in terms of healthy years is among low-income persons, regardless of race or ethnicity. The wellness strategy for the future must be to increase the span of unrestricted and productive life for all, to improve quality of life, and not merely to extend life expectancy.

The Growing Interest in Death Studies

Why does an examination of death appear in a text that purports to be about health and wellness? Since you might argue that "death" is the antithesis of "health," such a chapter might seem out of place. Is this an "antiwellness" chapter? To the contrary, this chapter is here because developing a philosophy about death may be an important step in appreciating the richness of life. No matter how well we insulate ourselves from the reality of death, we eventually must face events like the death of grandparents, parents, and siblings. Sometimes we must face the tragic and premature deaths of friends, peers, and siblings. These drastic changes in our lives require adaptation, a necessary element for wellness.

Sooner or later, we must face our own death, for to be born and experience life necessitates an eventual confrontation with death. For many people, the subject of death is an unpleasant one, but ultimately, one that is unavoidable. Everyone thinks about death at some point. We cannot feel, touch, see,

taste, or hear death. Therefore, we create a representation of it in the mind. Of all human experiences, none is more overwhelming in its implications than death; yet, it is perhaps the area of human experience about which we know the least.

So inquisitive about death are human beings that an entire field of study is now devoted to it. The field is called **thanatology,** and those who study the subject are called thanatologists. Questions about death and the fragile nature of life always have been central to human existence. In this last decade of the twentieth century, however, there seems to be an increased interest in this unfamiliar, yet intricate part of growth and development. What has spawned this interest? No one can say for sure. As Lynne Ann DeSpelder and Albert Lee Strickland write: "Life styles influence death styles."[3] To understand this concept more fully, it is necessary to consider some of the changing patterns of death in the U.S.

Personal and Social Issues Related to Death and Dying

Examine for a moment how the subject of death is addressed today. For many people, even the language of death is shrouded with euphemisms. It is apparent from the following examples that the way death is talked about is understood better by considering how it is *not* talked about. To say that one has "passed away," "perished," or "passed on" seems less harsh or blunt than to say that one has "died." The reality of death also may be softened if it is placed in a religious context. Thus, such phrases as "met his maker," "asleep in Christ," "in the arms of the Father," or "crossed over Jordan" are popular among Christians. Death may be dealt with in purposefully aggressive, even militaristic tones through remarks like "wasted," "greased," "annihilated," "liquidated," "terminated," "deep sixed," and "rubbed out," perhaps to lessen the reality of the meaning of "killed." Vague expressions of the concept of death are seen with terms like "succumbed," "expired," "checked out," or "departed." Perhaps to minimize anxiety about death more thoroughly, comedic

Thanatology: the formal study of death and dying.

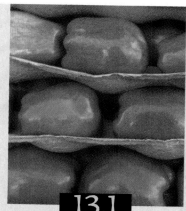
remarks such as "croaked," "kicked the bucket," "pushed up daises," "bit the dust," "bought the farm," "bit the big one," "went to Boot Hill," "cashed in," or, simply, "planted" are not uncommon. There are many illustrations of how death is *not* talked about (see Activity for Wellness 13.1).

Frequent and direct contact with death was a regular occurrence in the U.S. of yesteryear that was more rural and less mobile. Death was most likely to occur in the home, usually in the presence of family members of perhaps two or more generations. Today, death has become more institutionalized. An individual who lives to old age is more likely to die in a hospital or a long-term care facility such as a nursing home than in the family dwelling. Rather than having several generations of family members present, the dying person may be surrounded instead by professional staff members for whom death is a "job" and a "routine."[4]

In an era gone by, family and friends might have crafted a coffin from available wood, prepared the deceased individual for burial, held a wake or vigil in the home, and even prepared the grave and eventual burial right on the family's property or in a nearby church graveyard. Care for the dying person and disposition of the body after death were largely family tasks. Local "undertakers" and members of the clergy might have assisted in these activities, but their roles were not on the order they are in most familiar rituals today.

Nowadays, an entire industry attends to the needs of the deceased and surviving

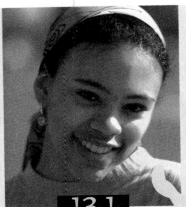

13.1
Activity for Wellness

Attitudes toward Death

The following items are not intended to test your knowledge, but rather, to help you assess some attitudes that you may have about death. Read each item carefully. Place a check mark next to the items with which you agree. Be as honest about your attitudes as possible. Mark nothing next to those items with which you disagree.

49 _____ The thought of death is a glorious thought.

47 _____ When I think of death I am most satisfied.

45 _____ Thoughts of death are wonderful thoughts.

43 _____ The thought of death is very pleasant.

41 _____ The thought of death is comforting.

39 _____ I find it fairly easy to think of death.

37 _____ The thought of death isn't so bad.

35 _____ I do not mind thinking of death.

33 _____ I can accept the thought of death.

31 _____ To think of death is common.

29 _____ I don't fear thoughts of death, but I don't like them either.

27 _____ Thinking of death is overvalued by many.

25 _____ Thinking of death is not fundamental to me.

23 _____ I find it difficult to think of death.

21 _____ I regret the thought of death.

19 _____ The thought of death is an awful thought.

17 _____ The thought of death is dreadful.

15 _____ The thought of death is traumatic.

13 _____ I hate the sound of the word death.

11 _____ The thought of death is outrageous.

To score this attitude scale, add up all the two-digit numbers to the left of each statement that you checked. Divide this sum by the total number of statements checked. Compare this number to those on the scale and the statements in the vicinity of your number. It will give you at least a rough idea of whether death is a subject that is a somewhat positive, somewhat negative, or rather neutral construct for you to consider in an intellectual sense. Compare your score to those of acquaintances. What experiences in your life do you think account for your present attitudes toward death?

From Dale V. Hardt, "Development of an Investigatory Instrument to Measure Attitudes toward Death," in *Journal of School Health*, Vol. 45, No. 2, February 1975, pp. 96–99. Copyright © 1975, American School Health Association, P.O. Box 708, Kent, Ohio 44240. Reprinted by permission.

What Do You Think?

1. Throughout the early part of the twentieth century, it was common for funeral rituals to be held in the home of the deceased, with family members and friends paying their last respects. What benefits might modern families be missing by moving funeral rituals to funeral "homes"?

Funeral director: a person whose educational background and professional preparation qualifies him or her to preserve and disinfect deceased human bodies in accordance with funeral custom for burial, cremation or other disposition, to provide grief counseling, and to carry out other related services when a person dies.

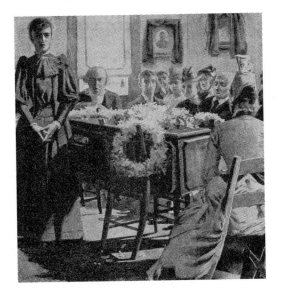

family members. A manufactured casket of various styles, designs, and quality is selected by family members from a **funeral director's** stock, in a manner not terribly unlike how a person shops for new shoes or a new car. Visitations at specialized funeral homes or chapels represent the new norm. The deceased is prepared for "viewing" by one or more professionals with embalming, mortuary science, and cosmetology skills. The deceased is disinfected, preserved, and restored to a "natural" lifelike appearance. To some people, this process diminishes the sad reality of death in a most tasteful way. To others, it conceals for as long as possible the fact that a loved one has died.

To a large extent, social and technological changes, along with increased life expectancies, have altered customs concerning death and burial in the U.S. For instance, the U.S. Department of Commerce reports that more than half of the deaths in 1900 involved persons of age fifteen or less.[5] In contrast, less than 5 percent of deaths occurred in this age group some eight decades later. In the past it was common for a mother to die in childbirth or for a parent or sibling to die as a consequence of acute infectious disease. A typical U.S. family today may go twenty years without losing one of its members to death. Thus, the probability of children and youth being confronted directly with death is less today than in 1900.

A social change that has modified our experiences with death is increased geographic mobility. Instead of having the ties of a multigenerational household, family members are likely to be scattered throughout the country. The decline in multigenerational households results in intermittent rather than daily contact of children, parents, and grandparents. The diversification in geography is likely to make the impact of a death less immediate, and the involvement of some family members in decisions following the death of a loved one less pronounced. With this change in mobility, coupled with other factors such as an increasing proportion of older Americans in the population, a growing prominence of the nuclear family, and fewer deaths among children and youth, fewer people are present when a death occurs.

Advances in medicine and related technologies have influenced the way we view death. To some people, the use of artificial organs, organ transplants, and other life-sustaining technologies has been nothing short of a miracle. To others, this technology has only served to confuse the issue of death by raising a series of controversial and volatile questions. Who shall have access to life-sustaining services? Are high-cost technologies affordable? When shall they be used? Who shall make the decisions about initiation, continuation, and cessation of use? What is the role of "quality of life" in their use? Indeed, there are no simple answers to these questions. Moreover, in the future, as now, each new technology will give rise to a whole new set of moral and ethical issues whose resolution will transcend the fields of medicine, law, religion, and philosophy.

In present times, people experience the deaths of older and younger persons differently.[6] We seem disposed to feel more remorse for the death of a small child. We view such a death as a greater injustice than the death of an older adult. We feel correspondingly greater sorrow, anger, regret, or bitterness when a young person dies. Are there any ethical justifications or implications resulting from these feelings? Should there be greater heroic medical efforts made to preserve a young life over that of an older person? These issues cause us to think about the meaning of life and our personal philosophy about living and dying.

What Does It Mean to Die?

Death is the cessation of physical life processes, the end of growth and development, and the termination of all responses to environmental stimuli. The process of dying, which culminates in death, takes place in stages, however. These stages include clinical death, brain death, and biological/cellular death.

In **clinical death,** heartbeat and respiration cease. Life-sustaining oxygen carried by the blood no longer circulates to the various sites in the body. The brain can maintain functioning for only a short time before its cells begin to die. Clinical death sometimes can be reversed through **cardiopulmonary resuscitation (CPR)** and other emergency life support procedures. To avoid irreversible brain damage or brain death, such restorative procedures must be initiated within approximately four minutes.

If the flow of oxygen is shut off from the brain, cells begin to die. A normal, functioning brain generates electrical activity that can be measured using an **electroencephalograph,** or **EEG.** Brain waves produced from electrical activity vary when a person is awake and asleep, but in either state, they show a series of peaks and valleys. In **brain death,** the EEG output is a flat line, indicating no electrical activity. Deprivation of oxygen for a period extending beyond about four minutes may produce brain damage, affecting physical or mental abilities even if oxygen flow subsequently is restored. In the absence of oxygen, it takes the brain about fifteen minutes to die completely.

Clinical death: the cessation of heart beat and respiration which will result in brain death if not reversed in a matter of a few minutes or less.

Cardiopulmonary resuscitation (CPR): Mouth-to-mouth resuscitation (often called rescue breathing) combined with external chest compressions, in order to maintain the circulation and breathing of an individual whose heart is not pumping blood on its own.

1. (a) This EEG printout shows a normal pattern of electrical activity generated by the brain. (b) When the brain dies, it ceases to generate electrical activity. Brain death is documented by an EEG when the output shows a straight line. How has our ability to measure the electrical activity of the brain with EEGs changed our personal and our medical-care system's view of the question "What is Death?"

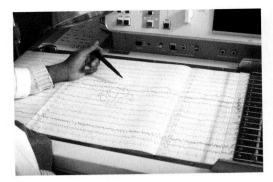

a.

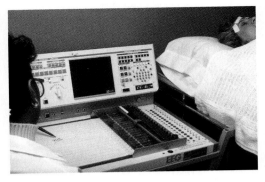

b.

Following brain death, the death of cells and the biological systems they comprise soon follows. At this point, the reversal of the symptoms of death is no longer possible. Not all parts of the body die at the same time, however. Muscle tissue may be responsive to artificially induced stimuli for a few hours. Hair and nails may continue to grow for days. It is possible to maintain flow of oxygen artificially to certain organs to keep them temporarily perfused, thus allowing for their use in transplantation.

Death brings with it several alterations in the body. After a few hours, the body may begin to take on a bloated appearance due to the accumulation of gases in the system that can no longer be dispersed. Changes in the chemistry of muscle tissue produce the familiar stiffness of the face, neck, trunk, and limbs that is associated with death. This condition, known as **rigor mortis,** begins to subside after a day or so. Since blood is no longer circulated throughout the body, the face and extremities take on a pale or bluish tint, even in darkskinned individuals. Blood clots and blood collect at the low points in the body, making those parts seem bruised. The surface temperature of the body approaches room temperature, and the elasticity of the skin becomes less apparent. Decomposition of the body begins shortly after death, a process whose speed depends on the nature of the physical environment where the body exists and the actual physical condition of the body just prior to death. Over time, decomposition breaks down soft tissues, leaving behind only the hardest tissues, the teeth and skeleton.

American Perspectives on Death

Like most people, you probably have given some thought to the subject of death. Maybe you have asked yourself what happens after death. Is there an afterlife? Is there a spirit that lives on when the body no longer contains life? Is there a consciousness in death? Is death merely the final stage of growth and development, after which there is nothing? If there is such a thing as "nothingness," what is it like? If you have considered such questions, you are not alone. These points have been argued by philosophers, theologians, and others almost since the beginning of time. If you have experienced the death of a friend or loved one, or had your own near-death encounter, perhaps you have succeeded in putting death in perspective or developed a certain philosophy concerning death.

Robert D. Russell discusses five distinct philosophies on life and death that have emerged in the U.S.[7] One of these points of view, the **ecological perspective,** sees all forms of life as equal in value and importance. Human existence is but one of these forms of life. Humans have both advantages and disadvantages where other species are concerned but no clear superiority. In the ecological view, life is a series of events through which individuals adapt to survive. Those members of a species that adapt best survive the longest; however, death is an inevitable consequence of having come into being. Death is a necessity, in part, because new life is based on the demise of old life. Decomposition is the basis for the formation of the earth. Plants grow and provide food for small animals, which in turn provide food for other animals, which in turn die and decompose to provide the earth with new life, and so on. The process of life and death, thus, is a continuous cycle. The ecological view assumes life to be a natural event, unguided by supernatural beings or any deity. Furthermore, it assumes there is no afterlife. In short, in the ecological perspective, species

Rigor mortis: a temporary condition following death in which the muscle tissue of the body undergoes chemical change resulting in stiffness.

come into being, grow and develop, die, and through their physical demise, give rise to new life.

The **humanistic perspective** shares some ideas with the ecological perspective but differs in that it sees human life and human relationships as more valuable and important than other forms of existence. Like the ecological perspective, the humanistic perspective sees death as the end of life and the end of all consciousness. Because humankind is seen as superior to other forms of life, it should be enriched and nurtured, sometimes even at the expense of other species. While a great value is placed on human life, when death comes, it should be met with dignity. In the humanistic perspective, a sense of immortality is achieved to the extent that a memory of the deceased, through his or her contributions and accomplishments, is left among those who survive. Consistent with this perspective is the belief that part of life's goal and opportunity is to create immortality in this way.

In the **religious perspective,** all forms of life are created by a supreme being, and human life is the highest form of life. This perspective is well illustrated in the Christian tradition. As such, the purpose of life is to obey God, to do God's will, and to seek eternal salvation in God's kingdom. If salvation is achieved, you gain eternal life in heaven, a reward for having lived a good life. If, on the other hand, you reject God and lead a life of sin and evil, the result instead shall be alienation from God in "hell." If you live a good life, and your mission for God is accomplished, for example, death may be seen only as the end of life on earth. If you subscribe to this perspective, death might very well be viewed as a celebration of the welcoming into the kingdom of God.

Somewhat foreign to Western tradition, but widely accepted on a global basis, is the **reincarnation perspective.** Although most Western scholars dismiss reincarnation, Ian Stevenson identified some twenty plausible instances where it could have accounted for observations that were made.[8] This philosophy sees existence as a continuous stream of experience, spanning many lifetimes. Death simply consists of leaving the earth plane and reentering the astral plane. In this examination of life and death, each life has a purpose; and this purpose is to reach the highest state of enlightenment possible. Furthermore, the purpose of life is the pursuit of selflessness. The quality of one's life and the nature of one's death may be determined by the experiences of previous lives. If life has been lived selflessly, then death is nothing to be feared. Death is but another opportunity to be selfish or selfless.

Finally, the **life-after-life perspective** is based on reports by persons who were clinically dead but who eventually were revived. People with near-death encounters give similar accounts of their experiences, prompting such individuals as physician Raymond A. Moody, Jr. to describe these reports in the books *Life after Life* and *Reflections on Life after Life.*[9] Recollections of these close encounters with death often include such events as hearing the pronouncement of death followed by a loud noise or ringing, the perception of moving through a long, dark tunnel, being "outside" of one's physical body, being in "spirit" form and perhaps looking down on one's lifeless body, recognizing previously deceased friends and relatives, seeing a bright light, having flashbacks of one's life, standing before a barrier, having a sense of being "judged," and returning to one's physical body, sometimes with a feeling of reluctance. Accounts of these events typically describe them as "good" and "peaceful" experiences. Of interest is the fact that such experiences are reported both by those who do not believe in an afterlife as well as by those who do. Moody's work and that of others have stirred much controversy; however, even thanatologists who accept these descriptions of near-death experiences reluctantly are baffled by the extraordinary similarity of detail given by people.[10] Apparitions of the dead, accounts of spiritualists, near-death experiences, out-of-body descriptions, deathbed observations, and spirit images appearing in photographs all contribute to the credibility of the life-after-life perspective.[11]

Needs of the Dying Person

Sometimes death is sudden, as in traumatic deaths from automobile accidents, falls, poisonings, and gunshots or as with certain natural causes of death such as stroke, heart attack, or **cardiac arrest.** When death occurs unpredictably or without warning, there is

Humanistic perspective: a philosophical view of life and death that sees human life as more significant than other life forms, and which identifies no after life experience.

Religious perspective: a philosophical view of life and death that values human existence, but which sees the union with a supreme being following death as giving birth to a much more valued eternal life.

Reincarnation perspective: a philosophical view of life and death that suggests that the spirit may occupy the bodies of different persons over many eras, and thus, have a continuous stream of experiences.

Life-after-life perspective: a philosophical view of life and death based on testimony from persons with near-death experiences that suggests the existence of a consciousness after the end of one's life on earth.

little or no time for the person to adjust to the notion of death. At other times, there is notification of impending death, such as following the diagnosis of a terminal illness. When an individual knows that death will occur at some "predictable" time, what goes through that individual's mind? How does one adjust? What does a person think about and do? What can be done to help a person come to terms with death?

A pioneer in the study of death and dying, psychiatrist Elisabeth Kübler-Ross, has provided thanatologists with a good deal of what is known about the psychology of the dying process. As a result of her interviews and discussions with hundreds of persons who were terminally ill, Dr. Kübler-Ross has suggested the existence of five psychological stages through which people may pass in adjusting to their own death.[12]

The first stage is one of *denial and isolation*. Upon learning of impending death, a person's first reaction may be, "No, not me!" "You must be mistaken, doctor!" "You must have someone else's records confused with mine!" The tendency is for the individual to seek a second, "more competent" opinion. By denying the truth, a person "buys" time to adjust to the bad news. Upon hearing confirmation that death is a certainty, the person may withdraw, isolate himself or herself socially, and for a short time at least, not want to talk about the diagnosis with anyone.

The second stage is one of *anger*. If the person's first reaction to the diagnosis of a terminal illness is "Not me," then a subsequent reaction may be the question, "Why me?" The feeling of anger arises when it is no longer possible to deny the probability of death. The response of "Why me, why now?" is not an unusual one when a person feels the unfairness of dying when others will go on living. Anger may be vented outwardly toward a physician or toward close friends and family members. Anger may consist of verbal abuse, frequent complaints, or episodes of impatience. Further questions like "What did I do to deserve this?" or "Why not someone else?" may be directed at God rather than at persons around the dying person.

In the third stage, the individual begins a process of *bargaining*. People learn early in life that they often can achieve a desired objective through bargaining. A frequent reaction following the stages of denial and anger is to "bargain" for more time and more life. Bargaining may be with God, such as, "Take me if you must, but let me live until my grandchild is born." Bargaining may also be displayed to a physician: "Doctor, just give me six months—there are some things I have to do." Sometimes bargaining arouses a person's will and energy to fight the disease. It provides the opportunity to put one's life in order, to take care of unfinished business, to overcome possible guilt stemming from feelings that one's life may not have been well spent, and to "mend fences" before death occurs. Bargaining is viewed as an important step in ultimately coming to terms with death.

The fourth stage is one of *depression*. When denial of death is no longer possible, anger is spent, and it is clear that bargains are only temporary departures from reality, depression may occur. The person thinks: "What will happen to my family after I am gone?" The person may worry and ask: "How will they get by without me?" The depression felt from such things as loss of job, radical change in lifestyle, and inability to care for one's family is known as **reactive depression.** The dying person also may become obsessed with the thought of a future that he or she will not be a part of and of a final separation from the family, friends, and world he or she has always known. This obsession is called **preparatory depression.** Depression may lead to at least a temporary repeat of alienation and social isolation.

The fifth stage of the dying process is *acceptance*. Given time and an opportunity to work through the grief of one's own loss of life, an individual eventually may come to terms with death. Depending on your perspective on death (ecological, humanistic, religious, reincarnation, life after life) death may be viewed as a new beginning. Most prominent religions have the notion of an afterlife as part of their doctrine. The opportunity to start over, or to be accepted into heaven, may prove comforting and help a person accept death. A person who is dissatisfied with the way life has been lived or who fears that death will not produce a positive reward may have a difficult time reaching acceptance. The stage of depression may recur or be prolonged. Alternatively, the urge to bargain for more time or to make up for past misdeeds and turn over a new leaf may take place.

Cardiac arrest: a condition characterized by the complete stopping of the heart beat.

Reactive depression: a depression that is triggered by, or can be linked to a specific event, such as a terminal diagnosis.

Preparatory depression: a depression that is triggered by an impending negative event, such as death.

Kübler-Ross observed that not all people experience each of the five stages, and those who do experience them do not necessarily do so in the same order. Moreover, some people find themselves in intermediate stages, regress in their acceptance of death, and repeat stages. Not everyone eventually comes to terms with death. For many, there is hope throughout the dying process that recovery may still occur.

Joan Retsinas points out that Kübler-Ross's work was done primarily with middle-aged cancer patients who may view death differently, than say, elderly patients.[13] Elderly people suffering from painful, chronic, debilitating illnesses may not be as likely to deny the deterioration of their bodies. Similarly, the older person, especially if experiencing pain, may be less apt to express anger. Since extended time may not offer an older individual joy, tranquility, or a chance to repair troubled relationships, "bargaining" may not occur. What may be viewed as depression in the elderly may be a withdrawn state more characteristic of "regression" than depression. While many of Kübler-Ross's patients never reached acceptance of their fate, such acceptance may be more forthcoming from someone whose life has spanned a large number of years.

How can knowledge of these stages help us to address the needs of the dying person? A person in the first stage can be supported by family and friends who recognize that time is necessary for the individual to prepare to meet the physical and psychological demands of impending death. Persons around the dying individual should try to accept and support the individual's attempts to seek help and hope.

The person in the second stage may seem openly hostile toward others. Individuals around the dying person should understand that this hostility, no matter how pronounced, is unrelated to them. Being cognizant of the anger felt by the dying person should help others be patient and supportive and allow the person to express any anger and despair. Kübler-Ross learned that most people who are dying want to talk about death.[14] While you should not force a person to talk about death, you should always be an attentive listener if or when the person does wish to talk. It is important that the dying person is not "killed off" socially long before actual death occurs, either because of others taking the anger personally or because avoiding the person is a means of coping with the discomfort of acknowledging a terminal condition. Expressions of love and acceptance may be especially important for the person in stage two.

Family members, friends, clergy, and health professionals may be unaware of a person in stage three if bargaining is done privately and in silence. If individuals close to the dying person are made aware of bargains, however, they can be as understanding and supportive as possible.

A person in the fourth stage of adjusting to death may need reassurance that significant others are managing and that, above all, they still love him or her. Encouragement for expressing feelings may be especially helpful to the person in this stage. At this time, the dying person may desire to have fewer visits, from fewer people, or visits of shorter duration. The person may talk less. It is helpful if visitors follow the person's lead in and out of conversation. This pattern is also characteristic of the person in stage five. The dying person may not seem to express much emotion. The mere physical presence of family members and friends, if desired by the dying person, may be all that is necessary to provide support at this stage.

In summary, while we have learned much about the needs of the terminally ill or dying person, there is much that is yet unknown. No two situations are alike because of individual differences in beliefs and philosophies about the meaning of life and the meaning of death. Acceptance of a person's impending death by those whose lives will continue, including caregivers, the emotional support provided by such individuals, and the dying person's self-efficacy and quality of relationships with others are variables whose impact on the dying process are not understood completely. It is possible, however, that caring, acceptance, patience, and understanding can be exchanged between the dying person and friends and family and that both can gain from the experience. If you are able to help another person come to terms with death you may gain important insight, not only about your own mortality but about the value of life in general.

Hospice: A Concept of Care for the Dying

A type of institutional care for the terminally ill growing in popularity is **hospice.** Hospice care seeks to permit death with dignity.

What Do You Think?

1. Hospice is a concept of care for the terminally ill. It may include special care in one's own home. What impact do you think the concept of hospice has had on the experience of dying in the United States?
2. Would you ever consider becoming a hospice volunteer?

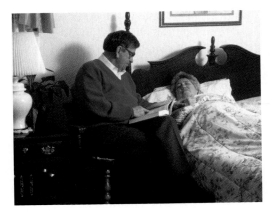

According to Charles A. Carr,[15] the specific tasks confronting individuals coping with dying include: (1) satisfying bodily needs and minimizing physical distress in a manner consistent with other values; (2) maximizing psychological security, autonomy, and richness in living; (3) sustaining and enhancing those interpersonal attachments of significance to the person; (4) addressing the social implications of dying; and (5) identifying, developing, or reaffirming sources of special energy, and in doing so, fostering hope. Hospice care is set up to work toward these goals better than traditional medical care for the terminally ill.

The concept of hospice developed in the 1950s and 1960s. Perhaps the most exemplary model of hospice care is that provided by St. Christopher's Hospice near London, England. At St. Christopher's, terminally ill patients are able to seek support from staff, family members, and friends, as well as from each other. Features such as social gatherings, extended visiting hours, encouraged visits by children, and even the welcoming of pets describe St. Christopher's Hospice. In short, a personal approach toward care not feasible in a typical hospital, nursing home, or other long-term care facility is possible.

Hospice is a concept in care and does not necessarily require a special facility for the terminally ill. In addition to the St. Christopher model, at least three other models of hospice care have evolved in the U.S. One of these approaches sets aside a section of a hospital to meet the special needs of the dying patient. Opponents of this approach argue that it is difficult to manage administratively and that once a patient is assigned to the hospice ward, a stigma of death is placed upon him or her. Such a stigma may be dysfunctional for the person who has not yet come to terms with dying.

A second hospital-based approach is more integrated with regular hospital services and does not include isolation of terminally ill patients. Staff members show greater sensitivity to the needs of the dying person and family members, counseling services are expanded, and the skills of specially prepared volunteers and professionals are employed to comfort persons who are dying.

A third model of service delivery is seen in home hospice care. This kind of care is likely to be provided by a private, but nonprofit community-based organization comprised largely of volunteers. These volunteers undergo training to make home visits, perform tasks such as grocery shopping and meal preparation, and provide social contact and care for persons who are dying.

Regardless of the hospice model employed, hospice workers, who often are volunteers, need to be exceptional communicators.[16] They must be good listeners, be able to interact easily with the terminally ill patient, and be able to talk freely about death and dying. Barbara Lafer[17] points out that the special demands placed on hospice workers create attrition among volunteers.

Understanding Grief

Grief is an intense emotion or feeling we experience when we are confronted with the loss of someone who has been part of our life. Grief, bereavement, and mourning are terms sometimes used synonymously to describe an individual's reaction to a death. The fine shades of difference in the meanings of these words are explained by Edgar N. Jackson.[18]

> Grief is always more than sorrow. Bereavement is the event in personal history that triggers the emotion of grief. Mourning is the process by which the powerful emotion is slowly and painfully brought under control. But when doctors speak of grief they are focusing on the raw feelings that are at the center of a whole process that engages the person in adjusting to changed circumstances. They are speaking of the deep fears of the mourner, of his prospects of loneliness, and of the obstacles he must face as he finds a new way of living.

Bereavement and grief bring about bodily responses that are both physiological and

Hospice: a special concept in the care of the terminally ill that accommodates the psychological, physical, and spiritual needs of the dying individual in a homelike environment.

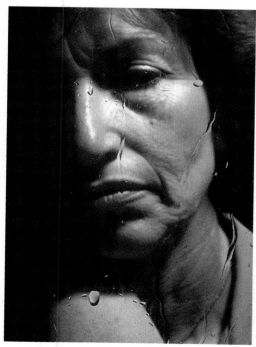

What Do You Think?

1. Grief is an intense emotional reaction resulting from important losses. What losses, other than the death of a loved one, might produce an intense grief response?

psychological in nature. For example, the death of a spouse, family member, or close friend are among the most traumatic life-change events that can be experienced by a college student.[19] People who experience such loss seem unable to function or act confused or are slow to respond. Behavior may be mechanical or robotlike. Life seems temporarily out of control, and biological processes appear to be retarded. There is a feeling of being emotionally drained, and eating and sleeping habits are disrupted.

Why do we grieve? Reason tells us that the person who has died is free of pain and suffering and is out of a troubled world. Moreover, most religions assure us that death releases the spirit to a richer and fuller existence. Among some older persons, death may even be anticipated with hope. Why then do we grieve? Grief is a shattering emotion stemming from the loss of love, the loss of emotional security, and the loss of a sustenance formerly provided by another's presence. Thus, we grieve for ourselves. We are sorrowful because we have been deprived. We ache because of separation from one whom we love and need.

We also grieve out of fear. Death changes our world as we know it. We are uncertain about what lies ahead. The fear of an unknown future is present for us throughout life, but for the most part, we can deny this fear or avoid thinking about it. Death is a reminder of the unrevealed future through which we must pass.

One's grief response may be tied to the purpose one feels she or he has in life. Having a high purpose seems to buffer the negative aspects of bereavement.[20] Having a strong internal locus of control and no significant downward slide in standard of living following the death of a loved one are factors also associated with adjustment to loss.[21]

We grieve, too, because of insecurity. The loss of a loved one sometimes makes us feel as if the solid ground beneath our feet has crumbled. Furthermore, we look at the reactions of people around us who comprise our "sphere of security" and see them crying, shattered, and acting in unpredictable ways. Such disorder adds to an already confused state and to our apprehensiveness about the future. In addition, some research has suggested that persons who have low purpose in life may experience more anger and grief following the loss of a loved one.[22]

Adjusting to the Death of a Loved One

Tasks that are central to processing grief and integrating loss after the death of a loved one include: (1) coming to an understanding that the person is no longer there, (2) addressing the feelings that accompany loss, and (3) reinvesting in your own life.[23] We must face the full reality of what has happened, and resist any detours to the truth. The sooner we can accept the fact of loss, the sooner the healing process can get underway. It is a necessary task to break the bonds that tie us to the person who has died. Doing so does not mean that we remove the person from our memory. Instead, it means we must declare our independence from the individual, adjust to life without the person, and let go of the past. Finally, we must facilitate the discovery of new interests, satisfactions, and creative endeavors. It may require giving ourselves permission to form new relationships and planting our seeds of energy where they will be the most fruitful. Perhaps we can find some consolation and reassurance in knowing that grief is relieved by the passage of time, the understanding and acceptance of the people around us, and the ongoing pursuit of creative activities (see table 13.1).

TABLE 13.1

What to Avoid Doing in a Grief Situation

- Being overly critical of your actions or engaging in self-condemnation
- Medicating yourself to relieve the pain of loss
- Engaging in self-pity
- Running away from the situation or taking a trip to sort things out (adjustment will have to take place at home, eventually)
- Becoming socially reclusive, or withdrawing from situations that put you in touch with other people
- Rejecting concern expressed by others
- Making decisions that can be put off to a later time
- Underestimating the human spirit's ability to rebound

How can you tell if grief is getting out of hand? When is mourning prolonged? These questions are difficult to answer. Therese A. Rando[24] identifies the six "R" processes of mourning necessary for the healthy reconciliation or accommodation of any loss. These processes include *recognizing the loss*, where one acknowledges and tries to understand what has happened; *reacting to the separation*, where one experiences the pain of loss and grief; *recollecting and reexperiencing the relationship*, where one reviews and remembers the person who has died; *relinquishing old attachments*, where one lets go of the past and begins to look toward the future; *readjusting but not forgetting*, where one moves forward but ties the life that is gone to what lies ahead; and finally, *reinvesting*, where one cultivates new relationships and new experiences.

While the grief people experience has many shared traits, responses to grief and mourning also can be highly individual. Extremes of emotion may sometimes signal difficulty in coping with loss. Elation, anger, suspicion, or depression at times when such feelings seem inappropriate can provide clues to friends. If grief appears to be out of control, it is important that the problem is identified and corrective steps are taken. Many personal resources are available and should be utilized as needed. Family members and friends, clergy, funeral directors, specialized grief counselors, and medical personnel all may be able to contribute to healing the person who is overcome with grief.

Maria and Marta are two sisters in their early twenties, and both are college students who lost their mother to breast cancer three months ago. Maria has worked through her grief and mourning by bearing the pain of the loss of her mother over time. She has tried to readapt to her environment and to reinvest in other personal relationships. Maria went through a period of time where she was unable to find a sense of meaning in life. This confusion has gradually subsided and she no longer thinks about the big questions of life and death. She avoids thinking about these issues because they remind her of the loss and the pain that continues. Marta went through a similar process of "letting go" of her mother. However, rather than a brief period of questioning life's meaning, she finds herself overwhelmed by life's lack of permanence, and of the suffering that is inherent in being alive. Marta still questions what life is really all about, and why people must die. In what ways is Maria's response a better adjustment than Marta's? In what ways has Marta made the better adjustment?

While it is impossible to insulate yourself from death and the grief that follows; it *is* possible to prepare for this aspect of life.[25] Through education and experience with loss, you can gain insight about the emotions of such a crisis. An honest study of thanatology can help you come to terms with death and dying, and many universities and community colleges now offer courses. Preparation for death can be done by developing a philosophy about life. Death is a threatening thought for people who have never explored the meaning that life has for them. Finally, providing support for others in their time of grief acquaints us with the resources available to assist us in our own time of grief and sorrow.

Expressing Condolence

When the relative of a friend dies, whether or not to visit the residence or funeral home to pay one's respects is an important concern. How long should I stay? What should I say or not say? Many people who feel awkward about making such calls have these questions on their minds.

An expression of condolence or sympathy serves several purposes, says Regina Flesch.[26] First and foremost, it offers help to friends and loved ones during turbulent times. It conveys a message to those who are mourning a loss that they are not alone and that their grief is shared. It tells an individual that despite the loss, friends will maintain ties now and in the future. It is a way of reminding the survivors that they are still bound to the living.

A visit need be only a few minutes but may be longer if it is evident that your presence is highly desired. If you are not able to stay longer at that time, it is useful to reassure people that you are available for help and that you will return as soon as possible. If you do not know what to say, perhaps it is comforting to realize that your presence and reaffirmation of friendship rather than your verbal expressions of sympathy are more important. Phrases such as "It's better this way" or "It was God's will," while said with good intentions, probably should be avoided. A simple, "I'm sorry about what has happened," or "I feel your loss" may be all that is necessary. Knowing that a condolence call can be simple without being trite or shallow should provide the confidence and sense of responsibility needed to overcome any reluctance about making it.

Lillian M. Range[27] and her colleagues had college students rate thirty potentially comforting remarks that might be made following a death. The three comments assessed as most comforting included: "If there is anything I can do, please let me know," "I'm here if you need someone to talk to," and "Put your faith in God." The three comments rated as least helpful were: "Didn't the funeral home do a good job!" "Did you know this was going to happen?" and "Was she or he in much pain?"

Children and Death

Just as adults are unable to shield themselves from the inevitability of death, so too are they helpless in defending their children from this reality of life. As with adults, a child's mental health is preserved through the frank acknowledgement of death rather than through its denial.

The abstract nature of death, combined with the mixed messages about death children receive, leads to ambiguity, misunderstanding, and fear. Many children are taught the bedtime prayer that begins "Now I lay me down to sleep." Subsequently they recite: "If I should die before I wake." While no transmission of fear is intended by this simple prayer, children may be afraid if they learn to equate going to sleep with the possibility of dying before they wake. This fear is enhanced when children are told by well-meaning adults that a deceased person is "just sleeping."

Children learn confusing messages from television and movies. They see a western hero or bad guy "die" on one channel, only to see him come alive again when the channel is changed. They see violence in cartoons such as those featuring Roadrunner and his coyote nemesis, in which the coyote is blown up, disintegrated, crushed, or knocked off a cliff, only to reappear in the next scene untarnished and ready for more action.

Terms such as "dead" and "die" are common to the vocabulary of childhood; however, the meaning of these terms, especially with respect to the finality of the construct they represent, may not be clear. Maria Nagy made one of the earliest but most important studies of children's views about death.[28] Nagy's investigation demonstrated recurrent questions that children have about death. What is death? What makes people die? What happens to people when they die? Where do people go? According to Nagy, children go through three phases in their awareness of mortality.

In phase one from ages three to five, a child may deny death as a regular and final process. Death is, indeed, like sleep—you are "dead" and then you are "alive" again. Death also may be equated with going on a journey. To this child, what is considered "death" occurs many times, such as when a parent goes to work or to the store, separates from sight, and then returns.

In phase two, from about ages five to nine, children can accept the idea that a person has died but may not yet comprehend the fact that death happens eventually to everyone, including themselves. Around the age of ten, children enter phase three and begin to recognize that death will happen even to them.

Psychologists point out that some adolescents and adults hold rather childlike views of death. They "know" that death is inevitable and final, but they carry out their daily activities more consistent with the conviction that personal death is really an unfounded rumor. They express this "denial" through the "personal fable" of adolescence, where high-risk behaviors are exhibited without apparent fear or alarm.

If possible, a child should discuss death with the family before a crisis occurs. Talking in a quiet, honest, and straightforward way encourages further dialogue. The learning process about death should be gradual and in stages that are consistent with a child's emotional and intellectual capacities. The attitudes that adults express about death in the presence of children are likely to be more important than the words through which these attitudes are conveyed. Involving the children in the sorrow that a family feels upon the death of a loved one can be a source of maturation. Children should be allowed to vent their emotions of grief. Adults need not feel that they must provide answers for all of a child's questions. Some questions have no clear-cut answers. Reassurance and support can help in those areas where answers are not possible. A child may assume responsibility for the death of a family member, believing his or her misbehavior is being punished. Adults should be on the lookout for children carrying such a guilt burden.

Children who are old enough to behave in a nondisruptive manner should be allowed to attend a funeral-home visitation or a funeral.[29] Parents should explain the process in advance so it will not be a source of anxiety. While a child's participation in a funeral can be encouraged, it should never be mandatory, no matter how therapeutic an adult thinks it might be. Keeping a sensitive child at home may be a prudent thing for adults to do. The child can share in the grief and mourning that the family experiences. A visit to the cemetery later on can reaffirm the death.

An unpleasant reality of life is that some children become terminally ill. Some research supports the notion that children over the age of four who have fatal illnesses generally anticipate their death.[30] Dialogue between mother and the dying child, and between mother and the child's siblings appears to be helpful for everyone. Other important factors may be the presence of the child at home, the specificity of the parent-led discussion, and the presence of religious faith as a source of emotional and spiritual support.

Cremation: the burning of a dead body to a state of ashes.

Universal Attributes of the Funeral Ritual

Each country, culture, or religion may have slightly different variations of the funeral custom. Hindu custom in India identifies death as being only one of a thousand such events that a person experiences. At death, male relatives may bear the body to a river, where it is immersed for purification. **Cremation** liberates the soul for reincarnation. If the heat of the fire is not sufficient to burst the skull, then the eldest son of the deceased must crush the skull to release the soul. In Ethiopia, mourning is a violent expression of emotion that includes wailing. In Mali, it is customary to hold a second funeral a year or more after an individual's death. Among Moslems in Egypt, cremation is prohibited, and burial is required to allow for the body to decompose to the original four elements of earth, air, water, and fire. People of Tibet hold what is called the "passing ceremony," where a single hair is plucked from the deceased to allow the spirit to pass out through the opening.

According to Paul E. Irion,[31] some anthropologists believe the origin of the funeral ritual grew out of a fear of offending the dead. The funerary right was for the appeasement of the dead, without which the deceased might be resentful and take revenge on the living. Respectful burial guaranteed peace.

Religious denomination may be a factor in directing the funeral custom. Traditional Roman Catholic funerals include a wake, a funeral Mass, and a liturgy at the graveside. Jewish funerals may vary but typically incorporate prayer and a period of mourning. Orthodox Jews may participate in preparing the deceased person's body for burial, and remain with it continuously until the actual burial occurs. Cremation as a means of disposal of a dead body is growing in popularity in the U.S., especially in Florida and California. How popular is cremation elsewhere in the world? In Japan, 98 percent opt for cremation compared to 70 percent in Great Britain, 68 percent in Denmark, 59 percent in Switzerland, but only 1 percent in Italy.[32]

While specific customs vary, certain attributes of the funeral ritual are shared from culture to culture. For instance, most cultures have a visual confrontation with the body of the deceased. This event is believed to affirm

TABLE 13.2

Criteria by Which Persons Select a Funeral Director

Personal acquaintance with the funeral director

Funeral director's reputation; previous use of services and satisfaction

Counseling and guidance abilities of the funeral director

Funeral director's sensitivity to the stress on the family

Funeral director's willingness to discuss prices in straightforward terms in person or over the telephone

Religious affiliation (if any) of the funeral home

Convenience of the funeral home's location

Recommendations by others

Funeral director's knowledge of community resources for the bereaved family

---

the reality of death psychologically and mark the beginning of the recovery and readjustment process for the survivors. Funerals, wherever they are held, have a specific intent. Funerals provide an opportunity for the survivors to receive the psychological and social support that will contribute to healing from their loss. The funeral also is meant to honor the dead, and a typical feature of the ceremony is the presentation of a eulogy about the person's life. The funeral often contains a religious ceremony, since most religions advocate the existence of an afterlife. Most funerals are marked by a procession and culminate in the disposition of the body.

The American Funeral Industry and the Consumer

At the time of the death of a close relative, we may be vulnerable consumers. When selecting funeral services, family members of the deceased can be financially victimized as a result of their emotional states. This point is not meant to imply that funeral directors as professionals are exploitive or unscrupulous. Quite the contrary, reputable funeral directors conscientiously uphold their ethics and standards as do persons in other

professions. Problems arise, however, when consumers are unaware of their decision options prior to planning a funeral. To assist consumers, the Federal Trade Commission has sponsored legislation to regulate the funeral industry. The following information outlines aspects of this important legislation.

Choosing a Funeral Director

Selection of a funeral director is a vitally important consumer task and one that should take place prior to the death of a loved one. Just as it is wise to select a physician or dentist prior to requiring medical or dental services, it is advantageous to identify a funeral director prior to requiring services. The elements to look for in a funeral director are summarized in table 13.2. These criteria will be more important to some people than others. Perhaps the best way to evaluate a funeral director is by visiting the establishment and seeing how funeral services are carried out there. Many proprietors of funeral homes view themselves as public servants and are willing to make themselves available for persons who desire to have the "mystery" of the industry clarified for them. Although it may seem peculiar to people not familiar with the funeral industry, directors take pride in their work and in their establishment. Time permitting, many will permit, and even encourage, public tours of their facilities. Such tours are commonplace during formal collegiate courses in thanatology.

Health and Safety Concerns of Funeral Directors

Directors by and large are on call twenty-four hours a day, 365 days a year. The pressure under which they must work as public servants can be stressful. In the 1990s, funeral directors, **embalmers,** and others who work with dead bodies must be especially safety conscious. They may encounter persons whose deaths were brought about by hepatitis, HIV-related infection, and other contagious diseases. While the immediate or official cause of death may appear on a death certificate, other unknown diseases may be present at the time of death that can be potential hazards to persons working around bodies. Precautions against accidental needle sticks, inadvertent contact with blood and other body fluids, and careful sanitation to protect themselves and the public are very real concerns of today's funeral director.

Embalmers: people who preserve dead bodies with chemicals.

Range of Services Provided

The death of a loved one requires a consultation with a funeral director in most cases. The funeral director is able to handle a variety of tasks in a competent manner that most people have limited or no experience with. The following items are likely to be discussed:

1. Personal information about the deceased.
2. Time, place, and type of funeral service.
3. Casket selection, perhaps even if cremation is to be performed.
4. Burial vault selection, if desired unless cremation is to be performed.
5. Cemetery arrangements.
6. Floral arrangements.
7. Preparation of the death notice for the local newspaper.

There are variations to this list, but these items are the ones most frequently discussed.

Pricing

In the past, many funeral directors offered families funeral "packages" in which prices were included in the cost of the casket selected. The package may have included unnecessary services or services not desired by the deceased person's family. The 1981 FTC legislation discourages this practice and promotes itemized price lists so that consumers can see exactly what they are purchasing. Funeral directors themselves are split over the merit of this legislation. There is evidence to suggest that it will lower the cost of a funeral, as well as evidence to suggest it will have the opposite effect. What to consider in selecting and pricing funeral goods and services are as follows:

1. *Newspaper notices.* A simple death notice is often done at no cost. A formal obituary is provided for the newspaper at a cost. It may be done by a family member or the funeral director, but it may be somewhat more expensive if handled by the director.
2. *Flowers.* They are customary but not required. Flowers may be ordered by either a family member or the funeral director, and prices may vary.
3. *Cemetery fees.* There is a charge for opening and closing a grave. Naturally, if a cemetery plot must be purchased, there is a substantial additional cost.

4. *Embalming.* Most states do not require this practice unless a person died of a highly contagious communicable disease; however, if there is to be funeral home visitation with a showing of the body, it is almost always strongly advised.
5. *Minimum service charge.* Most funeral homes charge a fee for the performance of such services as pickup and delivery of the body of the deceased, filing a death notice, and other services.
6. *Use of facilities.* If a visitation is to be held, there is a fee for use, setup, and arrangement of the funeral parlor or chapel. Visitations are, of course, optional.
7. *Hearse.* A fee is charged for the hearse, which may vary according to how far the body of the deceased is transported for burial or cremation.
8. *Limousine.* As with the hearse, a fee is charged to transport family members from the funeral home to the church or to the cemetery. This service is optional.
9. *Casket.* A casket is required for burial but not for cremation (see figure 13.1). If visitation is to be held prior to cremation, a casket may be rented. Caskets vary in cost from about $600 to $8,000 depending on their quality. Caskets are categorized as sealers and nonsealers, with the former being higher priced. It is seldom necessary to buy a sealer casket. Some funeral directors may try to suggest it as a "final gesture of love for the deceased." Try to ignore such suggestions unless having a sealed casket is of great importance to you.
10. *Alternative containers.* Most crematoriums require the body to be in a container. This container does not have to be a casket. Cremation containers can be purchased for as little as $50.
11. *Burial garments.* Most families provide burial clothes for the deceased. If they have no appropriate clothes, funeral directors can supply them at a cost.
12. *Burial vault.* State laws do not customarily require the use of grave liners or burial vaults. They are also not required if a body is to be interred in a **mausoleum.** Many cemeteries require vaults for burial to avoid the collapse of the grave and the need for maintenance, however. Local requirements can be

Mausoleum: a large vault or tomb for the dead.

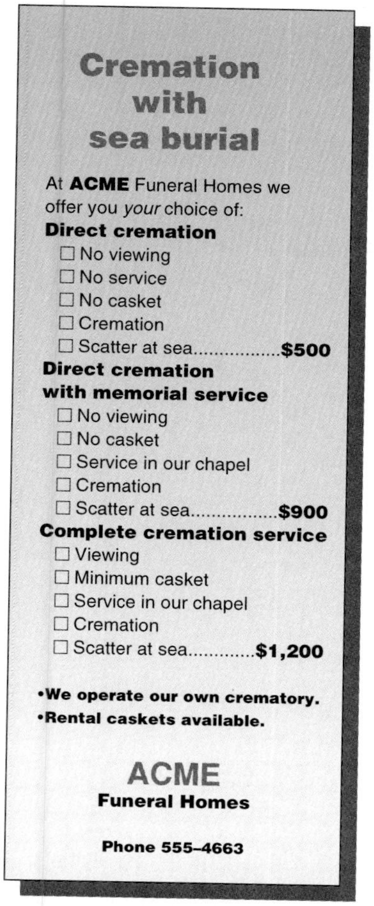

Cremation with sea burial

At **ACME** Funeral Homes we offer you *your* choice of:

Direct cremation
- ☐ No viewing
- ☐ No service
- ☐ No casket
- ☐ Cremation
- ☐ Scatter at sea..................$500

Direct cremation with memorial service
- ☐ No viewing
- ☐ No casket
- ☐ Service in our chapel
- ☐ Cremation
- ☐ Scatter at sea..................$900

Complete cremation service
- ☐ Viewing
- ☐ Minimum casket
- ☐ Service in our chapel
- ☐ Cremation
- ☐ Scatter at sea.............$1,200

- •We operate our own crematory.
- •Rental caskets available.

ACME
Funeral Homes

Phone 555–4663

Figure 13.1: Exceptions to burial are becoming more common in the U.S.

checked out. Vaults, like caskets, vary in price from $400 to $5,000 according to material.

Each family will arrange a funeral according to its own needs and preferences, making it as simple or as elaborate as desired. There are some good rules of thumb to keep in mind when planning a funeral. First, remember that funerals are for the living. Once a person has died, he or she cannot know or appreciate the funeral arrangements; therefore, the funeral should reflect the needs of the living. Also remember that life has to go on for those left behind, and there is no advantage to placing yourself in a burdensome economic position because of having to pay for an elaborate funeral. Finally, when in doubt about how elaborate a funeral ought to be, it may be helpful to be consistent with the person's financial means during his or her life.

Planning Your Own Funeral

We seldom think seriously about our own funeral, since most of us deny or reject the notion of personal mortality. A person who has had to make funeral arrangements for a loved one knows of the difficult decisions involved. By planning ahead, you can conscientiously avoid burdening those left behind with decisions when they may already be deeply burdened with feelings of loss, sorrow, and grief.

It is frequently difficult to obtain all the necessary information required for a death certificate. A person can assist in this task by having a document available and in a location where it is easily found that contains the following information: full name; social security number; city and state of official residence; birthdate and place; U.S. armed forces serial number if applicable; occupation; father's name and birthdate and place; mother's maiden name and birthdate and place.

It is also of enormous practical value to identify the locations of papers and important documents. These items might include wills, cemetery deeds, insurance policies, bank accounts, real estate deeds, birth and marriage certificates, stocks and bonds, negotiable papers, mortgages, contractual agreements, promissory notes, trust fund information, and any other pertinent materials.

Lastly, it is advantageous for those making funeral arrangements to know what kind of funeral you prefer. A person may identify such things as funeral home, clergy, type of funeral, pallbearers, music, readings, flowers, special requests, type of casket, type of vault, type of burial, name of cemetery, and cemetery plot numbers if owned.

The Living Will, Organ Donation, Euthanasia, and Mercy Killing

If all of this information seems excessive, it has tremendous practical value. There is one aspect of dying where a person can provide particular guidance for family members. Innovations in medical technology now make it possible for machines to provide limited heartbeat and breathing actions for persons unable to do these things for themselves. Such advances pose certain dilemmas for physicians, lawyers, patients, and members of a patient's family. If an individual's body is hopelessly ill or if the

FLORIDA LIVING WILL

INSTRUCTIONS

PRINT THE DATE

Declaration made this _____ day of _____, 19_____.

PRINT YOUR NAME

I, _____, willfully and voluntarily make known my desire that my dying not be artificially prolonged under the circumstances set forth below, and I do hereby declare:

If at any time I have a terminal condition and if my attending or treating physician and another consulting physician have determined that there is no medical probability of my recovery from such condition, I direct that life-prolonging procedures be withheld or withdrawn when the application of such procedures would serve only to prolong artificially the process of dying, and that I be permitted to die naturally with only the administration of medication or the performance of any medical procedure deemed necessary to provide me with comfort care or to alleviate pain.

It is my intention that this declaration be honored by my family and physician as the final expression of my legal right to refuse medical or surgical treatment and to accept the consequences for such refusal.

In the event that I have been determined to be unable to provide express and informed consent regarding the withholding, withdrawal, or continuation of life-prolonging procedures, I wish to designate, as my surrogate to carry out the provisions of this declaration:

PRINT THE NAME, HOME ADDRESS AND TELEPHONE NUMBER OF YOUR SURROGATE

Name: _____

Address: _____

_____ Zip Code: _____

Phone: _____

© 1993 CHOICE IN DYING, INC.

I wish to designate the following person as my alternate surrogate, to carry out the provisions of this declaration should my surrogate be unwilling or unable to act on my behalf:

PRINT NAME, HOME ADDRESS AND TELEPHONE NUMBER OF YOUR ALTERNATE SURROGATE

Name: _____

Address: _____

_____ Zip Code: _____

Phone: _____

ADD PERSONAL INSTRUCTIONS (IF ANY)

Additional instructions (optional):

I understand the full import of this declaration, and I am emotionally and mentally competent to make this declaration.

SIGN THE DOCUMENT

Signed: _____

WITNESSING PROCEDURE

Witness 1:

Signed: _____

Address: _____

TWO WITNESSES MUST SIGN AND PRINT THEIR ADDRESSES

Witness 2:

Signed: _____

Address: _____

© 1993 CHOICE IN DYING, INC.

Courtesy of Choice In Dying 11/93
200 Varick Street, New York, NY 10014 1-800-989-WILL

PAGE 2

Figure 13.2: Sample of a living will

Reprinted by permission of Choice In Dying, 200 Varick Street, New York, NY 10014. 212–366–5540.

---

brain is irreparably damaged, should that individual be kept alive by artificial means? If so, for how long? It is on this individual's family that the burden of reckoning with such a decision often falls. It is an agonizing decision to make because it necessitates a judgment about the quality of life.

A partial response to this issue has emerged with the advent of the "living will," a document available from Concern for Dying, an educational and service council that promotes death with dignity and patient involvement in decisions that affect the future quality of their lives (see figure 13.2). The living will is gaining validity as a legal document in many states. Its legal validity aside, it is still an important consideration for people, because it can provide guidance for physicians, family members, and others who may find themselves in a situation where a life versus death decision has to be made.

Concern over the legal and practical interpretation of living wills has prompted

some individuals to recommend **durable power of attorney** or **DPA** instead.[33] Where health care is concerned, a DPA allows people to appoint an agent to make medical decisions in the event they are no longer competent to make the decisions for themselves. A DPA is thought to be more powerful than a living will for three reasons: (1) the appointed person can assertively represent the patient's wishes better than a living will that might not be taken seriously, if even known about, (2) it can apply to terminal as well as nonterminal conditions, and (3) it permits decision making to be performed by a person who can apply what is known about the patient's wishes to the particular nuances of the present situation.

Another issue to which you can give consideration is the decision to become a uniform organ donor. More than 20,000 people receive an organ transplant each year in the U.S., and the demand for body parts is increasing. A major obstacle is the shortage

Durable power of attorney (DPA): a legal term which refers to one person being able to act on behalf of another individual whose competence to act on his or her own behalf may be compromised by coma, dementia, or other cause.

Where to Get Help with Your Funeral-Related Questions

- **American Association of Retired Persons**
  Provides free pamphlets about funerals and prepaid funeral planning.
  (202) 434–2277

- **Cemetery Consumer Service Council**
  Answers general consumer questions about funerals and cemetery related costs. (703) 379–6426

- **Continental Association of Funeral and Memorial Societies**
  Directs callers to local memorial societies, consumer groups that contract with funeral homes to provide low-cost funerals, cremations, burials, and related services. (800) 458–5563

- **National Funeral Directors Association**
  Offers free brochures for people wanting to acquaint themselves with services and costs associated with funerals.
  (414) 541–2500

- **U.S. Federal Trade Commission**
  Provides copies of public documents concerning funeral costs.
  (202) 326–2222

- **Cremation Association of North America**
  Provides free pamphlets upon request.
  (312) 644–6610

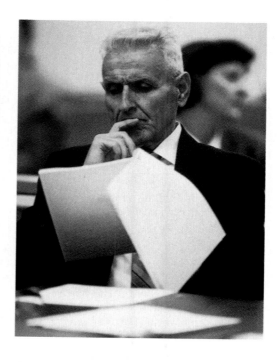

Figure 13.3: What Do You Think?

1. Jack Kevorkian has fueled the debate about the right to die. Do you agree with Kevorkian when he asserts that it is an acceptable activity for physicians to assist their patients in committing suicide if the patient wishes to end his or her life due to conditions such as intolerable pain or impending dementia?

of donors. The most common organs to be transplanted are corneas, hearts, kidneys, livers, bone marrow, and skin. Organs must be removed as soon as possible after death for their usefulness to be assured. If you are still in the decision process concerning obtaining a uniform donor card, the information in table 13.4 may be of assistance.

Euthanasia is the withholding of treatment or the removal of equipment that would prolong life through employment of heroic measures. The term euthanasia is derived from the Greek *eu*, meaning good, and *thanatos*, meaning death. Euthanasia allows for a person to select death with

dignity if he or she believes that heroic measures only postpone the inevitable while subjecting both the individual and family members to indignity.

Euthanasia is sometimes confused with **mercy killing,** a deliberate act performed either voluntarily or involuntarily to hasten death. This procedure is much more controversial than euthanasia. While people are inclined to equate voluntary mercy killing with suicide, they may see involuntary mercy killing to be synonymous with murder. This involvement of health-care providers has become prominent in the past few years because of the highly publicized role of a Michigan physician, Dr. Jack Kevorkian (see figure 13.3), in helping terminally ill patients and persons in extreme pain end their own lives. The concept of *assisted suicide,* is viewed by Kevorkian and his followers to be an ethical part of medical practice. Other authorities believe that "death by prescription" places both the patient and the practitioner in precarious legal, ethical, and moral positions. The issue presents legal philosophers much to debate in the coming years (see A Social Perspective 13.1).

Preparing a Will and Settling an Estate

A valid will is the basic document of almost every estate plan and is an essential measure

Euthanasia: an option in medical care whereby treatment is withheld in cases where such treatment would be judged as heroic or only temporarily delay impending death.

Mercy killing: an option in medical care whereby an action is taken to hasten death.

TABLE 13.4 Tips for Making the Decision to Complete A Uniform Organ Donor Card

Deciding to become an organ donor can be difficult for some people. The following tips may help you to work through the decision making process.

Precontemplation → Contemplation

If you have never thought about obtaining a uniform organ donor card, you might consider the following activities:

- Using the phone book and other resources, develop a list of places where you can obtain a Uniform Donor Card. Some of these places include the American Medical Association, the National Kidney Foundation, organ procurement centers, health departments, hospitals, and medical schools.
- Read about organ donation. Become informed of the legal aspects of signing an organ donor card and what to do should you wish to revoke the decision. Call the national hot line number (800) 24–DONOR.

Contemplation → Preparation

If you already have thought about becoming an organ donor and have familiarized yourself with what is involved, try:

- Reminding yourself of the peace of mind provided for loved ones when you die by their knowing that someone else's life may be saved or enhanced as a result of your generosity.
- Making the decision to take action to obtain a Uniform Donor Card.

Preparation → Action

Once you have prepared for the task of becoming an organ donor, take things to the next level. Try:

- Identifying a date in the next thirty days when you will carry out your plan. Circle the date on your calendar.
- Telling others about your decision to become an organ donor. Let people know that you are not "just thinking about" becoming an organ donor—but actually doing it.
- Making a firm appointment (e.g., next Monday at 1:00 P.M.) to obtain and sign your card.

Action → Maintenance

If you have gotten and signed your card, reaffirm the decision as the right decision by:

- Finding out how to have this new status of yours identified on your driver's license. Obtain a bracelet that further indicates your organ donor status.
- Regularly reaffirming your personal decision to be an organ donor. Look at your card and remind others of this status.

Maintenance

You have made a valuable decision for yourself, your family, and for the lives you might someday save. Maintain your confidence in your decision by:

- Encouraging an acquaintance to sign an organ donor card.
- Inviting a roommate, classmate, or other friend to participate in a health fair or related activity that acquaints the general public about the benefits of being an organ donor.

for the orderly distribution of property. A will contains the instructions of the **testator** (the will maker) for the disposition of his or her estate. What does an estate consist of? It consists of houses and land, businesses and business interests, stocks, bonds, mortgages, rights of various kinds including royalties and patents, life insurance policies, annuities, cash on hand, cash on deposit, and possessions known as personal property. The distribution of many of these estate components can be determined by will.

Because a will is a highly personal document that should be responsive to its maker's objectives, care must be exercised to assure the testator's intent is expressed clearly and that all reasonably anticipated contingencies are considered. A will remains inoperative until death because it may be modified or cancelled at the option of its maker. It is a wise decision to review a will periodically, perhaps every two to five years depending on a person's needs and wishes and changes in the law. Some important reasons

Testator: a person who makes or has a valid will that will become operable in the event of his or her death.

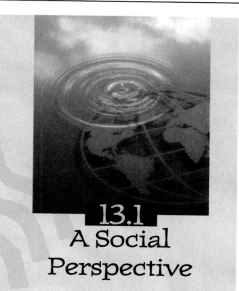
for making a will are listed in table 13.5. These reasons by no means apply only to older people or individuals who are married and have children. A will allows anyone, old or young, married or unmarried, to specify precisely how his or her property should be distributed in the event of death. Although so-called will kits can be purchased for a nominal fee and allow one to write a will alone, it may be just as easy, if somewhat more costly, to seek legal advice in preparing a will. The various types of wills are identified in table 13.6.

An individual who dies without a valid will is said to die **intestate.** Under this condition, each state's laws, rather than an individual's wishes govern the distribution of property. State laws vary too much to allow for generalizations about intestacy death. Dying intestate gives no discretion to the disposition of an estate beyond what the law allows. Thus, absolute control over the administration and disposition of an estate is achieved only by having a valid, up-to-date will.

A Final Word about the Study of Death

Much about death is, and may always remain, a mystery to us. The thought of death is something about which not all people will ever be comfortable. Although a brief study of death and dying cannot unlock all of the mystery or tear down all of the psychological barriers that people build to insulate themselves from death, it may help you come to terms with this aspect of life. From a wellness perspective, understanding what we can about death may help us in the enjoyment of life, in the seeking and appreciation of fulfilling experiences, and in relating in positive, caring ways to other people who have suffered the loss of a loved

TABLE 13.5

Reasons You Should Prepare a Will

You can arrange to give what you want to whom you want.

You may reduce the number or intensity of disputes over your property among relatives and friends.

You may reveal certain aspects of your financial affairs (e.g., a special savings account or trust fund) that are unknown to your survivors.

You can select a guardian for children who survive you.

You will minimize certain estate handling costs.

You can establish conditions (within limits) with which your beneficiaries must comply in order to obtain your bequests.

You can establish trusts for children, grandchildren, or others.

You can nominate a personal representative for administering your estate in accordance with its terms.

one. The acceptance of death may be an important achievement toward the development of a philosophy about the meaning of your life.[34] A careful examination of "death education" may, in fact, be better described as an exercise in "life education," thus enabling persons to progress in a positive direction on the wellness continuum. Is formal death education helpful to people? Results are mixed, but experiential programs that focus on personal feelings seem most likely to influence affective outcomes. Modest changes toward improved acceptance of death may be the best result that can be expected.[35]

TABLE 13.6 Kinds of Wills

Nuncupative (Oral) Will

Not legally binding in most states, it may be accepted in emergency situations. Even when considered legally binding it must have at least two witnesses. The facts surrounding nuncupative wills generally make them undesirable.

Holographic Will

Defined as a will totally in the handwriting of the testator. It does not require attestation by witnesses; however, it also is not legally binding in most states.

Attested Wills

A *joint* will is a combined effort of two or more people. Unless there is a special provision written into it, it legally binds the makers together. If one dies first, the surviving will makers may not change or revoke the will.

A *mutual* will is like a joint will but has what is called a "reciprocal provision." Each person signing the will leaves everything to the other person(s) or partner(s).

A *conditioned* will usually describes an event that must occur after the testator's death before the will becomes valid. These wills may originally have been developed to minimize the likelihood of a person being killed by heirs.

A *conventional* will, as is typically the case with attested wills, is overseen in preparation by legal counsel. It describes the distribution of property and administration of the testator's estate.

Summary

1. Not all groups of people in the U.S. enjoy the same life expectancy or the same number of "healthy years."

2. Thanatology, the study of death and dying, has become a topic of much study in recent years, and many colleges have entire courses devoted to it.

3. Many people avoid frank discussions about death. Death has become an institutional phenomenon involving professional funeral directors, and involves the family less directly than in earlier eras.

4. Technology has changed people's views of death and raised many questions for medicine, law, and philosophy about who makes decisions concerning life and death.

5. Death is the culmination of a series of physiological events that produce changes in the body. After one dies the body continues to change biochemically.

6. Typical perspectives on death come from ecological, humanistic, religious, life-after-life, and reincarnation points of view.

7. People who know they are dying tend to move among different psychological stages.

8. Hospice is a concept only about thirty years old whose various models of service delivery comfort dying persons and their families.

9. Grief is a complex emotion with psychological and biological components. People's responses to grief can vary.

10. Adjusting to the death of a loved one can be a difficult experience that interferes with normal activities of living.

11. Expressing condolence and sorrow when someone dies is a way of helping those who are left behind, and shows friendship and caring.

12. Children may have reactions to death that differ from those of adults.

13. In virtually all cultures, the funeral is an important final ritual, though its specific elements may vary considerably among cultures and regions.

14. The funeral industry can be complex to understand. It is wise to educate oneself prior to the time of having to make important decisions when a loved one dies.

15. To assist decision making of loved ones, the creation and enactment of living wills is being advocated.

16. Euthanasia, mercy killing, and assisted suicide are subjects receiving much attention by politicians, physicians and other health-care providers, and lawyers.

17. Everyone should consider having a legal will, and reviewing the consequences of dying intestate.

18. The study of death and dying can help one, in part, to prepare for the inevitable death of a loved one and for one's own death. An understanding about death may help one to live life more fully and completely.

Recommended Readings

DiGiulio, Robert. *After Loss.* Waco, TX: WRS Publishing, 1993. *After Loss* gives a personal account of the author's recovery after the tragic loss of his wife and child in an auto accident.

Moody, Raymond A., Jr. *Coming Back.* New York: Bantam Books, 1992. This well-written book explains the use of "regression hypnosis" to explore people's past lives, and provides research on detailed episodes of persons under hypnosis revealing past historic events.

Rando, Therese A. *Treatment of Complicated Mourning.* Champaign, IL: Research Press, 1993. Rando discusses people's responses to grief and bereavement, and examines the necessary steps for processing losses of any kind.

References

1. *Healthy People 2000, National Health Promotion and Disease Prevention Objectives* (Washington, D.C.: U.S. Department of Health and Human Services, 1991), 45.

2. *Healthy People 2000,* 50.

3. Lynne Ann DeSpelder and Albert Lee Strickland, *The Last Dance: Encountering Death and Dying,* 3rd ed. (Mountain View, Calif.: Mayfield, 1992), 5.

4. Robert Fulton and Greg Owen, "Death and Society in Twentieth Century America," *Omega* 18 (1987–88):379–395.

5. United States Department of Commerce, Bureau of the Census, *Social Indicators III* (Washington, D.C.: U.S. Government Printing Office, 1978), 71.

6. Nancy S. Jecker and Lawrence J. Schneiderman, "Is Dying Young Worse than Dying Old," *The Gerontologist* 34.1 (1994):66–72.

7. Robert D. Russell, "Some Perspectives on Death," unpublished paper (Carbondale, Ill.: Southern Illinois University, Department of Health Education).

8. Ian Stevenson, *Twenty Cases Suggestive of Reincarnation,* 2d ed. (Charlottesville, Va.: University of Virginia Press, 1974).

9. Raymond A. Moody, Jr., *Life after Life: The Investigation of a Phenomenon, Survival of Bodily Death* (Harrisburg, Pa.: Stackpole Books, 1976); Raymond A. Moody, Jr., *Reflections on Life after Life* (New York: Bantam Books, 1977).

10. Erlendur Haraldsson, "Survey of Claimed Encounters with the Dead," *Omega* 19 (1988–89):103–113.

11. V. Quinton Wacks, Jr., "Educating for Eschatological Concerns of the Older Adult: A Brief Report," *Death Studies* 12 (1988):329–335.

12. Elisabeth Kübler-Ross, *On Death and Dying* (New York: MacMillan, 1969).

13. Joan Retsinas, "A Theoretical Reassessment of the Applicability of Kübler-Ross's Stages of Dying," *Death Studies* 12 (1988):207–216.

14. Kübler-Ross, *On Death and Dying.*

15. Charles A. Carr, "A Task-Based Approach to Coping with Dying," *Omega* 24.2 (1992):81–94.

16. Stephen L. Coffman and Victoria T. Coffman, "Communication Training for Hospice Volunteers," *Omega* 27.2 (1993):155–163.

17. Barbara, Lafer, "The Attrition of Hospice Volunteers," *Omega* 23.3 (1991):161–168.

18. Edgar N. Jackson, Grief, in Earl A. Grollman, ed., *Concerning Death: A Practical Guide for the Living* (Boston: Beacon Press. 1974), 5.

19. Martin B. Mark, Thomas F. Garrity, and Frank R. Bowers, "The Influence of Recent Life Experiences on the Health of College Freshmen," *Journal of Psychometric Research* 19 (1975):87–98.

20. Ann Ulmer, Lillian M. Range, and Peggy C. Smith, "Purpose in Life: A Moderator of Recovery from Bereavement," *Omega* 23.4 (1991): 279–289.

21. Areila Lowenstein, Ruth Landau, and Aron Rosen, "Adjustment to Loss of Spouse as a Multivariate Construct," *Omega* 28.3 (1994): 229–245.

22. Karen S. Pfost, Michael J. Stevens, and Anne B. Wessels, "Relationship of Purpose in Life to Grief Experiences in Response to the Death of a Significant Other," *Death Studies* 13 (1989):371–378.

23. Izetta Smith, "Preschool Children 'Play' out their Grief," *Death Studies* 15 (1991):169–176.

24. Therese A. Rando, *Treatment of Complicated Mourning* (Champaign, Il.: Research Press, 1994).

25. Harriet Sarnoff Schiff, *Living Through Mourning* (New York: Viking Penguin, 1986), 105.

26. Regina Flesch, "The Condolence or Sympathy Call," in Earl A. Grollman, ed., *Concerning Death: A Practical Guide for the Living* (Boston: Beacon Press, 1974), 265–280.

27. Lillian M. Range, Andrea Wallston, and Pamela M. Pollard, "Helpful and Unhelpful Comments after Suicide, Homicide, Accident, or Natural Death," *Omega* 25.1 (1992):25–31.

28. Maria Nagy, "The Child's Theories Concerning Death," *Journal of Genetic Psychology* 73 (1948):3–27.

29. Schiff, *Living Through Mourning,* 43–53.

30. John Graham-Pole et al., "Communicating with Dying Children and Their Siblings: A Retrospective Analysis," *Death Studies* 13 (1989):465–483.

31. Paul E. Irion, "Changing Patterns of Ritual Response to Death," *Omega* 22.3 (1991):159–172.

32. Jennifer Barrs, "Funeral Business Passes on a Few Funny Facts," *Tampa Tribune* (April 28, 1994):B6.

33. Charles M. Culver and Bernard Gert, "Beyond the Living Will: Making Advance Directives More Useful," *Omega* 21 (1990):253–258.

34. Ross E. Gray, "Meaning of Death: Implications for Bereavement Theory," *Death Studies* 12 (1988): 309–317.

35. Joseph A. Durlak and Lee Ann Riesenberg, "The Impact of Death Education," *Death Studies* 15 (1991):39–58.

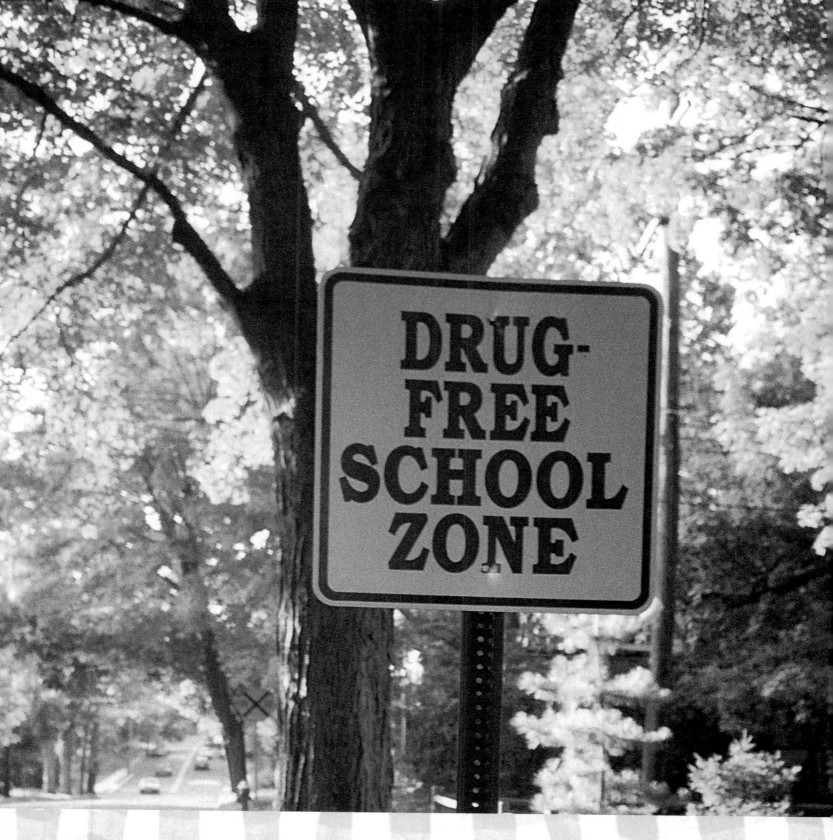

Minimizing Negative Health-Related Behaviors

As we have seen in earlier units, you can choose to live a wellness lifestyle. Taking responsibility for achieving wellness involves minimizing negative health-related behaviors.

Virtually everyone uses drugs of some kind, but many of the drugs we ingest are not typically called drugs. Chapter 14 will introduce you to five categories of drugs—herbal, over-the-counter, prescription, unrecognized, and illicit drugs. For many drugs, responsible patterns of drug use may be possible; however, drugs that are misused or abused can be very dangerous. Chapter 14 focuses on the use and abuse of psychoactive drugs, or those that affect the mind and behavior.

Because alcohol and tobacco are so widely available, chapters 15 and 16 will pay particular attention to their use and abuse. Alcohol and tobacco, though legally obtainable for much of the population, still account for the largest amount of illegal use among all drugs in our society. Additionally, they exact a high toll in terms of disability and years of potential life lost.

Drug Use and Abuse: A Challenge to Well-Being

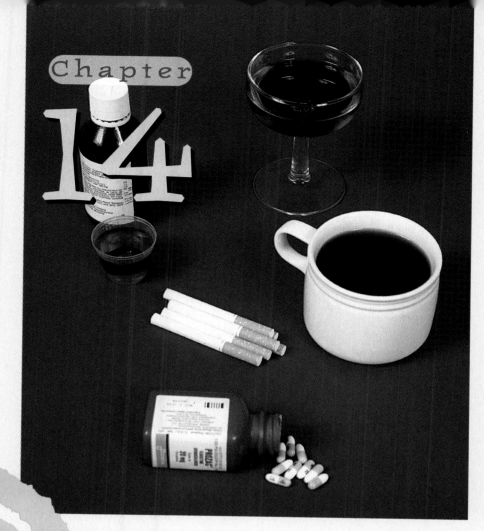

Chapter 14

Student Learning Objectives

Upon completion of this chapter, you should be able to:

1. distinguish between the terms drug and psychoactive drug;
2. distinguish between the five categories of drugs;
3. define the term drug interaction and describe several common forms of interaction;
4. identify five different patterns of drug taking, and describe each;
5. define dependence and list its primary characteristics;
6. distinguish between set and setting;
7. describe the differences between types of OTC analgesics;
8. describe the most common psychotropic prescription drugs;
9. distinguish between recognized and unrecognized drugs;
10. describe the major consequences of caffeine use;
11. describe the primary short- and long-term consequences of cocaine use and abuse;
12. describe the primary short- and long-term consequences of marijuana use and abuse;
13. describe current patterns of heroin abuse;
14. describe the primary short- and long-term consequences of LSD, PCP and inhalants abuse;
15. identify the major issues of drug use and abuse by athletes;
16. describe the problems associated with the use of anabolic steroids;
17. identify major issues related to drug abuse and families;
18. analyze the influence of advertising on drug-taking behaviors;
19. analyze the relationship between drug abuse and crime;
20. define safety issues regarding drug use.

It is hard to imagine a day that passes in which a person does not ingest a drug; yet, many of the substances that are consumed are not typically called drugs. Many substances that we frequently ingest (such as alcohol and tobacco products) contain active ingredients that should properly be called drugs. Many cola beverages that we readily consume contain the drug caffeine, as do some coffees and teas. Cocoa and various chocolates contain an additional drug, theobromine. Both theobromine and caffeine are very potent drugs that stimulate the central nervous system.

Many college students increase their use of drugs, especially during their freshmen year.[1] Some of the more common reasons cited for this increase in drug use and abuse include greater freedom from parental supervision, high levels of stress and anxiety associated with academic and financial pressures, and the availability and peer use of drugs for recreational purposes.

This chapter will focus on the use and abuse of a variety of drugs, especially those that affect a person's mood and behavior. Learning to make responsible choices regarding drug use will help you achieve a higher level of well-being.

What Is a Drug?

Since drugs are readily available to all of us, and since we use them in so many ways, it is important that we look at the dynamics of drug taking in a holistic way. There is no individual who is completely drug free, yet most of us do not have a clear definition of the term *drug*. Defining the term to everyone's satisfaction is difficult. Some people define drugs in terms of their effects, while others think mostly in social terms. For the purpose of this text, however, the term *drug* will be used to describe any substance, other than food and water, that has a direct effect on the structure or function of an individual. A special subcategory of drugs, the **psychoactive drugs,** refers to only those drugs that directly affect a person's mood or behavior. In this regard, penicillin is a drug because it directly affects our ability to function in the presence of an infection;

however, it does not directly affect our mood or cause behavioral changes. Alcohol, on the other hand, is not only a drug, but it is also a psychoactive agent. When we drink alcohol in sufficient quantities, direct effects on both our mood and behavior are observable.

A definition this broad enables us to include virtually everything that we put into our bodies as drugs. At this point, however, do not assume that we are necessarily labeling all of these substances as "good," "bad," or "dangerous." We are merely using the term *drug* in a descriptive sense. As you will see later, the determinant of whether a drug is "good" or "bad" is how the drug is used, and responsible patterns of drug use may be possible for almost all drugs now being used.

Drug Use and Abuse: A Status Report

It appears that the use of alcohol, marijuana and cocaine by children and young adults may be dropping in the U.S. (see figure 14.1). The numbers of people using these drugs, however, still remains quite high. Estimates from the National Center for Health Statistics[2] indicate that, during the past year, 17.4 million people in the U.S. had used marijuana. Lifetime marijuana use estimates are much higher—67.5 million. Additionally, it is estimated that 22.6 million people have used cocaine at some time in their lives. As you can see in figure 14.1, the Substance Abuse and Mental Health Services Administration estimates that, in 1992, 50.3 percent of eighteen to twenty year olds used alcohol, 11 percent of eighteen to twenty-five year olds used marijuana, and 1.8 percent of eighteen to twenty-five year olds used cocaine, all within the past month.

All drugs have the potential to be misused or abused, resulting in significant health problems. The *Healthy People 2000* report recognizes this threat to health and well-being, and outlines specific objectives to decrease alcohol and other drug use and abuse in the U.S. by the year 2000 (see table 14.1). Since there are so many drug objectives, only a sample of them will be presented in this chapter. Where there are specific objectives

Psychoactive drugs: a type of drug that affects primarily a person's moods or behaviors. Alcohol, tranquilizers, and marijuana are examples of psychoactive drugs.

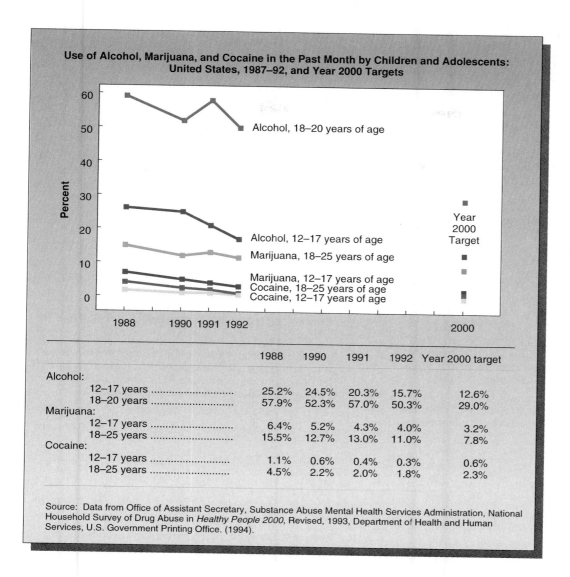

Use of Alcohol, Marijuana, and Cocaine in the Past Month by Children and Adolescents: United States, 1987–92, and Year 2000 Targets

	1988	1990	1991	1992	Year 2000 target
Alcohol:					
12–17 years	25.2%	24.5%	20.3%	15.7%	12.6%
18–20 years	57.9%	52.3%	57.0%	50.3%	29.0%
Marijuana:					
12–17 years	6.4%	5.2%	4.3%	4.0%	3.2%
18–25 years	15.5%	12.7%	13.0%	11.0%	7.8%
Cocaine:					
12–17 years	1.1%	0.6%	0.4%	0.3%	0.6%
18–25 years	4.5%	2.2%	2.0%	1.8%	2.3%

Source: Data from Office of Assistant Secretary, Substance Abuse Mental Health Services Administration, National Household Survey of Drug Abuse in *Healthy People 2000*, Revised, 1993, Department of Health and Human Services, U.S. Government Printing Office. (1994).

Figure 14.1: What Do You Think?

1. What general trend do you see in this graph regarding drug use?
2. Do you think that the U.S. will reach all of its *Healthy People 2000* objectives for alcohol, marijuana, and cocaine use? What evidence do you have to support your position?

related to tobacco or alcohol, those objectives will be presented in the appropriate chapters.

It is worth noting the importance of initiatives targeting members of high-risk groups in the *Healthy People 2000* objectives. Throughout the objectives related to tobacco, alcohol, and other drugs, there is particular attention given to young people.

Categories of Drugs

Drugs are categorized in many ways, but it is helpful to classify drugs according to their availability and sources.[3] These categories include:

1. Herbal drugs, which are not generally regulated by law, such as sassafras, tea, or catnip.

2. Over-the-counter (OTC) drugs, which are legally available without a prescription for self-medication, such as aspirin, some vitamins, and a variety of cough medicines.

3. Prescription drugs, which require a physician's written order, such as tranquilizers, potent cough medications, and sleeping pills.

4. Unrecognized drugs, which are widely available products, some of which have clearly psychoactive effects but are generally not considered to be drugs. Some examples include caffeine-containing soft drinks, nicotine in tobacco, and psychoactive spices such as mace and nutmeg.

1. **Reduce drug-related deaths to no more than 3 per 100,000 people.** (Update: 3.8 per 100,000 in 1991, with no change from the 1987 baseline.)

2. **Reduce drug abuse-related hospital emergency department visits by at least 20 percent to 140.6 per 100,000 people.** (Update: 191.4 per 100,000 in 1992, up from 175.8 in 1991.)

3. **Establish and monitor in 50 states comprehensive plans to ensure access to alcohol and drug treatment programs for traditionally underserved people.** (Baseline: no data as of 1993.)

4. **Extend adoption of alcohol and drug policies for the work environment to at least 60 percent of worksites with 50 or more employees.** (Baseline: 88 percent had alcohol policies and 89 percent had other drug policies in 1992.)

5. **Extend to 50 states administrative driver's license suspension/revocation laws or programs of equal effectiveness for people determined to have been driving under the influence of intoxicants.** (Update: 34 States and D.C. in 1993, up from 38 States and D.C. in 1990.)

6. **Increase by at least 1 year the average age of first use of cigarettes, alcohol, and marijuana by adolescents aged 12 through 17 as follows:**

Substance	1988 Baseline	1992 Update	Target 2000
cigarettes	11.6 years	11.5 years	12.6 years
alcohol	13.1 years	12.6 years	14.1 years
marijuana	13.4 years	13.5 years	14.4 years

7. **Reduce the proportion of young people who have used alcohol, marijuana, and cocaine in the past month, as follows:**

Substance/Age	1988 Baseline	1992 Update	Target 2000
alcohol/12–17	25.2 percent	15.7 percent	12.6 percent
alcohol/18–20	57.9 percent	50.3 percent	29.0 percent
marijuana/12–17	6.4 percent	4.0 percent	3.2 percent
marijuana/18–25	14.5 percent	11.0 percent	7.8 percent
cocaine/12–17	1.1 percent	0.3 percent	0.6 percent
cocaine/18–25	4.5 percent	1.8 percent	2.3 percent

8. **Increase the proportion of high school seniors who perceive social disapproval associated with the heavy use of alcohol, occasional use of marijuana, and experimentation with cocaine, as follows:**

Behavior	1988 Baseline	1992 Update	Target 2000
heavy use of alcohol	56.4 percent	60.8 percent	70.0 percent
occasional use of marijuana	71.1 percent	79.2 percent	85.0 percent
trying cocaine once or twice	88.9 percent	92.2 percent	95.0 percent

9. **Increase the proportion of high school seniors who associate risk of physical or psychological harm with the heavy use of alcohol, regular use of marijuana, and experimentation with cocaine, as follows:**

Behavior	1988 Baseline	1992 Update	Target 2000
heavy use of alcohol	44.0 percent	49.0 percent	70.0 percent
occasional use of marijuana	77.5 percent	76.5 percent	90.0 percent
trying cocaine once or twice	54.9 percent	56.8 percent	80.0 percent

10. **Reduce to no more than 3 percent the proportion of male high school seniors who use anabolic steroids.** (Update: 3.5 percent in 1992, down from 4.6 percent in 1989.)

Source: Data from *Healthy People 2000 National Health Promotion and Disease Prevention Objectives,* 1991; and from *Healthy People 2000 Review, 1993,* 1994. Department of Health and Human Services, Washington, D.C.

---

5. Illicit drugs, which cannot be legally sold, purchased, or in many cases used such as heroin, marijuana, cocaine, crack, and PCP.

These seven categories represent the broad spectrum of drugs with which we come into contact. You should recognize, however, that these five categories include many thousands of drug substances. For instance, there are certainly more than 100,000 OTC drugs readily available in today's marketplace. Add to that perhaps 30,000 to 40,000 medications that can be prescribed legally by physicians and dentists for human consumption. In addition, we can add several thousand herbal preparations containing one or more combinations of the 217 psychoactive ingredients now known, as well as innumerable foods and beverages that have psychoactive properties. We have not yet touched upon illicit drug preparations nor upon two of the most important drugs—alcohol and tobacco products.

Drug Interactions

Virtually everyone is a multidrug user and is affected differently by drug combinations. However, there are some potentially hazardous outcomes when we mix drugs of different kinds. First, drugs may interact in an additive sense; that is, the total effect of the drugs taken is equivalent to the sum of the effects of the individual drugs. Second, one drug may **inhibit** the actions of another; that is, the total effects of two drugs taken together are minimized. Third, drugs may have a **synergistic effect** on one another; that is, the total effects of the two or more drugs are multiplied because of the influence one may have on the actions of the other.

To give you some idea of the magnitude of the potential problem, table 14.2 presents a partial listing of some of the more common drug interactions. This list is not complete, in part because many of the potentially hazardous combinations of drugs are simply not known.

Patterns of Drug Taking

In 1973, the National Commission on Marijuana and Drug Abuse recommended the adoption of another classification system for describing drug-taking behavior.[4] In the Commission's report, five general patterns of drug-taking behavior were described, including the following:

1. **Experimental use,** which implies the short-term use of any one or a combination of drugs. Experimental use seems most often to be a function of individual curiosity or a reaction to peer-group pressure. Experimental use refers specifically to the relatively short-term use of any drugs and is generally associated with low-hazard potential.

2. **Social-recreational use** of drugs refers to the relatively low-risk use of any of a variety of drugs in a social setting to experience euphoria, increase enjoyment of other activities, or serve as a social lubricant (see figure 14.2).

3. **Circumstantial-situational use** refers to a pattern of drug taking that is characterized by short-term use as a coping mechanism to deal with particular situations.

4. **Intensified use** of drugs refers to the regular long-term use of a drug or several drugs in combination as a regular, daily pattern of behavior. Drug dependence is often a characteristic of intensified drug use.

5. **Compulsive use** of a drug or combination of drugs indicates that a person's patterns of use have changed substantially and are no longer tied to pleasure, peer acceptance, or situational issues. This pattern of use reflects loss of control over the use of these drugs.

The American Psychological Association (APA) classifies and describes all mental disorders in its revised third edition reference book entitled *Diagnostic and Statistical Manual of Mental Disorders*. This manual, which is often referred to as the DSM-III-R, does not classify all psychoactive substance use as pathological. Instead, it attempts to distinguish recreational use from substance abuse and substance dependence. The APA considers the latter two patterns of use to be mental disorders. The DSM-III-R is careful to classify only mental disorders, not the individuals who suffer from them. For this reason, the DSM-III-R does not claim that all individuals with a substance use disorder, such as alcohol dependence, will be similar in all psychological characteristics. Such persons may only share the defining features of the disorder.

The essential features of **substance dependence** are (1) impaired control of the use of a psychoactive substance and (2) continued use despite the adverse consequences. The APA identifies nine characteristic symptoms of substance dependence. These symptoms are the same across all classes of drugs, but for some types certain symptoms may be less relevant or not apply at all. For example, one of the nine characteristic symptoms is withdrawal sickness; this is an irrelevant factor in the use of hallucinogens like LSD.

To make the diagnosis of substance dependence, at least three of the nine characteristic symptoms of dependence must be present.[5] If only one or two of the symptoms are present, the diagnosis of substance abuse is probably more appropriate.

1. A person takes a drug and uses it in larger amounts and for longer periods of time than intended. For example, a person may decide to use cocaine until midnight but instead uses it until the sun comes up in the morning.

2. A person admits that his or her substance use is excessive and has attempted to reduce or control it, but has been unable to do so because the drug is available. In some instances a person may want to reduce or control his or her drug use but has not yet attempted to do so.

Synergism: a multiplier effect when certain drugs are used together. A classic example is the multiplied depressant effect when alcohol and barbiturates are taken together.

Substance dependence: impaired control of the use of a psychoactive drug with continued use despite adverse consequences.

TABLE 14.2   A Guide to Common Drug Interactions

This is only a sampling of some of the most common drug interactions.
No action should be taken without checking with your own doctor.

Tranquilizers	Combined with	Interaction
Diazepam derivatives (Librium, Valium, Serax, etc.) and meprobamate (Miltown)	alcohol barbiturate	increases effects of both increases effects of both

Analgesics	Combined with	Interaction
Aspirin	anticoagulant	increases the blood-thinning effect and could cause bleeding

Antihistamines	Combined with	Interaction
Diphenhydramine (Benadryl), chlorpheniramine (Chlortrimeton), dimenhydrinate (Dramamine), promethazine (Phenergan) and others	alcohol barbiturate hydrocortisone	increases sedation nullifies both lessens effect of hydrocortisone

Antibiotics	Combined with	Interaction
Tetracycline	penicillin, antacid, or milk	makes tetracycline less effective
Penicillin G	chloramphenicol (Chloromycetin), antacid, or tetracycline	makes penicillin less effective

Drugs that may interact with alcohol

Antibacterials—inhibits germ-killing action of antibacterials.

Antidiabetic agents (including insulin)—may lower blood sugar to dangerous levels. Insulin also increases the effects of alcohol.

Antihistamines—depresses central nervous system.

Antidepressants—increases the effect of alcohol and depresses the central nervous system.

Tranquilizers—affects coordination and depresses the central nervous system.

Sedatives and hypnotics—causes oversedation and depression of the central nervous system.

Food interactions

Milk and dairy products combined with antibacterials (such as tetracycline) make the antibacterial less effective.

Aged cheese, broad beans, chocolate, bananas, passion fruit, pineapples, tomatoes, and lemon combined with MAO-inhibiting antidepressants cause blood pressure to increase to dangerous levels.

Drugs that may cause skin eruptions when patient is exposed to the sun

Antibacterial sulfas.

Antidiabetic drugs like Orinase and Diabenese.

Tranquilizers, including Librium and Compazine, among others.

Antihistamines, particularly Benadryl.

Antibiotics, including Aureomycin and Terramycin.

Antifungal agents.

Birth-control pills.

Source: Data from the U.S. Government Printing Office

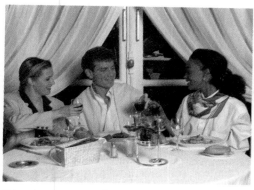

Figure 14.2: What Do You Think?

1. Drugs are often used in a social-recreational context to increase enjoyment and encourage social participation. Do you think that this is an acceptable practice? Explain your rationale.

3. A person spends a great deal of time trying to obtain the substance, using it, and recovering from its adverse effects.

4. A person becomes intoxicated or experiences withdrawal sickness when he or she is expected to fulfill major role obligations, such as those central to being a parent, an employee, or a student. For example, a student goes to class "high" from cocaine or a parent forgets to pick up his or her child from school because he or she is drunk.

5. A person avoids or reduces participation in important social, occupational, or recreational activities because of substance use. That is, a person might withdraw from family activities and hobbies in order to use the substance in private or spend time with substance-using friends.

6. A person ignores the array of social, psychological, and physical problems that occur as a result of high-dose, extended substance use, and continues to use the drug. For example, a person may have a seizure as a result of smoking cocaine but continues smoking the drug the next day.

7. A person develops a tolerance to the effects of the substance. In order for the person to achieve the same desired effect of the drug, larger and larger amounts of the substance need to be ingested.

8. A person develops withdrawal sickness upon cessation of substance use. The severity of this syndrome depends on one's degree of tolerance, length of time of use, general state of health, and use of other substances.

9. A person uses the substance to relieve or avoid unpleasant symptoms when withdrawal sickness occurs. This pattern typically involves using the substance throughout the day, starting in the morning.

These characteristic symptoms highlight features of substance dependence, which the APA attempts to distinguish from substance abuse. This latter term describes the category for classifying pathologic patterns of substance use that do not meet the criteria for substance dependence. **Substance abuse** is indicated by either:

1. continued use despite knowledge of having a persistent or recurrent social, occupational, psychological, or physical problem that is caused or exacerbated by use of the psychoactive substance; or

2. recurrent use in situations in which use is physically hazardous (e.g., driving while intoxicated).

Substance abuse is an appropriate diagnosis only when some of the symptoms have persisted for at least one month or have occurred repeatedly over a longer period of time. It most likely applies to people who have recently started using a substance. It is also frequently used for people who ingest marijuana and hallucinogens. Drugs such as these rarely, if ever, induce physical dependence or the need to use them to prevent withdrawal symptoms.

The Office on Substance Abuse Prevention suggests that the effects of drug abuse are different within special population subgroups in the U.S. These effects may be *biological* (e.g., women become intoxicated more quickly than men do because they generally have more fat and less muscle in their bodies); *genetic* (e.g., Native Americans seem prone to genetic vulnerabilities that make them more sensitive than the general population to the effects of alcohol and that contribute to a greater susceptibility for developing alcoholism); *behavioral* (e.g., people who eat poorly because they may not have access to healthy foods may have more physical problems); or *synergistic* (e.g., people who abuse alcohol and smoke, or who abuse alcohol and are exposed to asbestos or other cancer-causing substances, are more likely to develop alcohol-related cancers).

Substance abuse: using drugs repeatedly in hazardous situations, such as when driving a car. Abuse also occurs when a person continues to use a drug even though they know that it is causing, or making more severe, problems for themselves and others.

Addictive Behaviors

Perhaps most important among other issues at this point is the growing recognition of the similarity in the processes involved in **"addictive behaviors."** Current literature links alcoholism, drug addiction, obesity, smoking, and compulsive gambling under the collected term *addictive behaviors*, and this represents an important step forward in our capacity to deal with the problems produced by these patterns of behavior. Addictive behaviors have been noted to have the following characteristics:[7]

1. The initial behavior, be it taking a drug, eating, or betting, triggers a sensation of pleasure through what is called the reward circuit of the brain;

2. Physical tolerance develops so that an individual must increase the addictive behavior to get the same reward;

3. The individual will go through painful withdrawal if the addictive behavior is stopped;

4. Addictive behaviors lead to a psychological and physical craving for the behavior that is separate from the desire to avoid withdrawal;

5. The resulting addiction results in a variety of changes in the brain including physiological, chemical, anatomical and behavioral;

6. Addictions result in behavioral problems for the individual and society, and eventually lead to an obsession with the addicting behavior;

7. Once addicted, even the process of tolerance, dependence and withdrawal become reinforcing. The cycle of withdrawal followed by a relapse back to the addictive behavior seems to be rewarding in and of itself.

Researchers believe that everyone has the potential to be become addicted to certain behaviors. According to Dr. Steven Childers from the Bowman Gray School of Medicine,[8]

we must all realize that we all share the same circuits of pleasure, rewards, and pain. Anyone who takes cocaine will enjoy it; . . . there is nothing abnormal about getting high on cocaine. Everyone will. There is a natural base of addiction and we need to get away from the concept that only bad or weak or diseased people have problems with addiction. Telling someone to 'just say no' is like telling someone to just say no to eating and drinking and sex. We must begin to see how very human and very hard this is. But it is far from hopeless.

If this view of addictive behaviors becomes more widely accepted, it will have profound effects upon how we treat those addicted to drug taking and other behaviors, as well as how we attempt to prevent such addictions.

Related Concepts

When talking about drugs and their effects, there are several other critical concepts that demand attention. These areas include the effects of user expectations on drug outcomes, the influence of the setting in which drugs are taken, and the dose level consumed.

The term **set** is an extremely important term related to drug use. In the broadest perspective, set refers to the total internal environment of an individual at the time a drug is taken. When describing the complexity of the state of an individual a great deal is involved, including a person's physical health status, nutritional status, mental and emotional state, mood, expectations, and experiences. Of particular importance are the user's expectations regarding a drug's effects.

Setting refers to the external environment of an individual when a drug is taken. Where a person is, what that person is doing, and with whom that person is with are all factors affecting the setting of drug experience (see figure 14.3).

Set and setting play an extremely important role in determining exactly what a person experiences when taking a drug. The likelihood of any individual's set and setting being the same at two different times is very small. Even less likely is the chance that all the variables that affect drug outcomes would be the same in two different individuals at any given time. Because of these differences, individuals may react differently to the same drug and an individual may have somewhat different experiences when taking the same drug at different times. Differences in set and setting explain individual variation in drug experiences. In fact, when we talk about drug

---

Addictive behaviors: behaviors that initially are rewarding but lead to tolerance, craving, obsession with the behavior, and withdrawal if the behavior is stopped.

Set: the total internal environment of an individual at the time a drug is taken. This includes physical, mental, and emotional characteristics.

Setting: the total external environment of an individual at the time a drug is taken. This includes the physical and social environment.

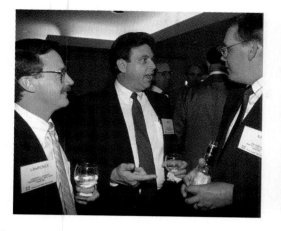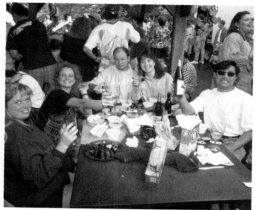

Figure 14.3: What Do You Think?

1. Setting strongly influences the experience of a drug user. What different affects might the two settings portrayed here have on the experiences of the individuals shown using drugs? What evidence are you using to answer this question?

TABLE 14.3 — Some Factors Affecting the Outcome of a Drug Experience

Drug Related	Set		Setting
	Physical	*Mental*	
Which drug	Age	Motivation	Physical environment
Route of administration	Sex	Mood	What a person is doing
Dose level	Body size	Previous experience	Who a person is with
	Basal metabolism	Expectation	
	Heart rate		
	Respiration rate		
	Blood pressure		
	General health		
	Tolerance		
	Genetic endowment		

From R. S. Gold and W. H. Zimmerli, *Drugs: The Fact,* 1973. Reprinted by permission of Kendall/Hunt Publishing Company, Dubuque, Iowa.

effects, we can only refer to likely effects in many cases, and these likely effects are based on averages and probabilities. When we talk about psychoactive drugs, there are few guaranteed effects. You may have experienced some of these differences. Have you seen or heard of times when a person drank a great deal of a particular alcoholic beverage and appeared to tolerate it very well; yet at other times, an equivalent amount resulted in drunkenness? This was probably due to differences in set and setting at the two different times. Table 14.3 illustrates some of the factors that are related to individual variation in drug experiences.

There are several drug-related variables that contribute to the drug's effects—the drug taken, the dose level, and the route of administration. There are two important

terms related to dose level. The **effective dose level** of a drug is the minimal dose required to elicit the desired response. When taken in too large of a quantity, all drugs can be dangerous; therefore, to minimize the potential danger associated with drug taking, it is important that the smallest possible dose be taken to obtain the desired effects. As dose levels increase, the potential for side effects does as well.

The **lethal dose level** of a drug is the required quantity to result in the death of the user. Clearly dose levels approaching these quantities should be avoided.

All drugs have lethal dose levels; overdose is a possibility with any drug. All drugs can be placed in five categories—herbal drugs, over-the-counter (OTC) drugs, prescription drugs, unrecognized drugs, and illicit drugs. Each of these drug categories will be covered in this chapter with an emphasis on psychoactive drugs (those affecting the mind and behavior) and their impact on wellness.

Herbal Drugs

Herbal drugs are plant substances that possess drug effects; legally they can be grown or gathered in the wild by anyone. This is the oldest category of drugs. The first drugs used by humankind were various fruits, seeds, flowers, leaves, and roots with real or imagined drug effects.

In the past two decades, there has been a rebirth of interest in these drugs. Herbal preparations are not only on the shelves of health-food stores but also on supermarket and drug store shelves.

Various herbal drugs that have stimulant effects are available. Caffeine is found in a number of plants, not only the coffee, tea, and cocoa plants but also in American holly, Dahoon holly (or cassina), Brazilian soapberry (or guarana), kola nut, and yerba maté. The Mormon tea plant contains the stimulant ephedrine, and cinnamon has a stimulant effect through an active ingredient that has never been identified. Sassafras contains safrol, which is a stimulant; unfortunately, it is also a carcinogen (a substance that can cause cancer).

Unfortunately, many people believe that herbal drugs are safe because they are "natural." This is nearly the opposite of the truth. Herbal drugs usually contain more than one active drug. Furthermore, the amount of drug present in an herbal preparation may be somewhat unpredictable.

Over-the-Counter Drugs

Over-the-counter (OTC) drugs are big business in the U.S. today. Billions of dollars are spent every year on more than 300,000 different brand-name products.[9] Despite the large number of products, they are actually composed of different combinations of less than 200 basic drugs.

Until 1952, there was almost no regulation of OTC drugs. The 1952 Durham Humphrey Amendment to the 1938 Pure Food and Drug Act required that all drugs being marketed be placed in one of two categories: those that were unsafe for unsupervised use by individuals (prescription drugs) and those that could be used safely without medical supervision (OTC drugs). Ten years later, the 1962 Kefauver-Harris Amendment to the 1938 act mandated a review by the Food and Drug Administration of the safety and effectiveness of OTC drugs.

Since no one ever knew how many OTC products were on the market (estimates ranged from 100,000 to 250,000), the FDA concluded that it could not conduct such a review product by product. Instead the FDA would review the available research on the basic drugs from which the OTC products were compounded. Each of these drugs was to be categorized into one of three groups:[10]

1. Those generally recognized as safe (GRAS) and generally recognized as effective (GRAE),
2. Those known to be either unsafe or ineffective,
3. Those about which not enough was known.

Drugs in the second category would be removed from the OTC market. Those in the third group would be removed from the market unless the drug manufacturers could provide new evidence of their safety before a specific deadline.

Some OTC drugs contain belladonna or other substances capable of producing a state of delirious drunkenness and are occasionally misused for this purpose. The three major types of psychoactive OTC products, however, are the analgesics, sedatives, and stimulants.

Analgesics

Analgesics are drugs that relieve pain. OTC analgesics may be classified into two groups: nonsteroidal anti-inflammatory drugs (NSAIDs), and acetaminophen.

Nonsteroidal Anti-inflammatory Drugs (NSAIDS)

NSAIDS relieve pain by inhibiting the body's production of **prostaglandins.** The most common nonprescription NSAID is **aspirin,** which not only relieves pain but also lowers fever and reduces inflammation and swelling in joints. Aspirin, however, causes unpleasant side effects in some users, including upset stomach, allergic reactions, or irritation of ulcers.

Over-the-counter drugs: commercially produced medications that can be purchased without a physician's approval.

Prostaglandins: a group of compounds produced by the human body that have powerful hormone like effects, and may result in pain.

Aspirin: a common internal analgesic that relieves pain, lowers fever, and reduces inflammation.

In recent years, two new NSAIDs have been put on the market—**ibuprofen** and **naproxen sodium.** Both of these drugs were originally available only by prescription; however, they are now available as over-the-counter medications. Ibuprofen, marketed under names such as Advil, Motrin, and Nuprin, works better than aspirin for pain from menstrual cramps, **inflammation,** or dental work.[11] Ibuprofen is also reported to have fewer side effects than aspirin; however, its use may cause stomach bleeding in some individuals.[12]

Naproxin sodium has been used for years, in its prescription drug form, for treating the pain and inflammation associated with **arthritis.** Recently, it became available in an over-the-counter product called Aleve. Naproxin sodium is marketed as a long-acting drug (eight to twelve hours for one dose), whereas ibuprofen's effects generally last four to six hours. As with ibuprofen, some users of naproxin sodium will experience stomach upset and intestinal bleeding.[13]

Acetaminophen

Acetaminophen, marketed under brand names such as Tylenol and Panadol, is an effective OTC pain reliever and fever reducer but does not have the anti-inflammatory effects of the NSAIDs. Thus, it is not satisfactory for arthritis pain or other pain resulting from inflammation. However, acetaminophen has fewer side effects, especially in terms of stomach upset and bleeding. Long-term effects of consuming large doses of acetaminophen on a regular basis have been documented.[14] Damage to the liver and kidneys is possible. People with known liver or kidney disease, and alcoholics, should not use acetaminophen. Table 14.4 presents detailed information regarding the effects and risks of over-the-counter analgesic use.

Sedatives

Opium was the basic ingredient in many early OTC **sedatives.** Later OTC tranquilizers and sleeping pills were compounded with bromides or belladonna alkaloids as their prime active ingredients. A few of these are still on the market, but their potential for overdose or cumulative poisoning is great enough that today only those containing diphenhydramine are approved.[15]

Most of the current OTC sedatives rely on the depressant side effects of **antihistamines**—antiallergy drugs—such as pyrilamine, doxylamine, and diphenhydramine. Some also contain aspirin or acetaminophen on the assumption that minor aches or pains are a common cause of tension or inability to sleep.

Stimulants

OTC **stimulants** contain a dose of caffeine equivalent to one or two cups of coffee. Some also contain a small amount of vitamin B_{12} for its mythical energizing effects. Large doses of caffeine, whether in the form of OTC products or of beverages such as coffee or tea, can produce the same psychological effects as other major central nervous system stimulants—increased alertness, excitement, nervousness, irritability, and, in very large doses, **paranoia.** The effects of caffeine are more fully discussed in the section on unrecognized drugs. Like many other drugs, OTC preparations should be regarded as potentially dangerous when mixed with other preparations.

Prescription Drugs

Prescription drugs are those that can be administered or sold only by or on the order of a physician—or in some instances a dentist or veterinarian. Drugs are the most commonly used therapeutic modality in the physician's office. An estimated 61 percent of all office visits end with the physician prescribing or providing medications, both prescription and nonprescription pharmacological agents. The three most frequently used categories of drugs are the antibiotics, cardiovascular-renal agents, and analgesics.

Psychotropic drugs (prescription drugs that affect mental and emotional functions, behavior, or experience) include sedative/hypnotics, antidepressants, tranquilizers, and amphetamines. **Sedative/hypnotics,** such as the barbiturates Nembutal, Seconal, and Tuinal, are drugs that have a calming effect in small doses and induce sleep in larger doses. If the user does not yield to the sleep-inducing effects, these drugs will produce a drunken state identical to that induced by alcohol.

Minor tranquilizers, such as Valium and Librium, relax the muscles and relieve anxiety. **Major tranquilizers,** such as Thorazine, Stelazine, and Haldol, relieve the symptoms of schizophrenia—the most severe

Inflammation: a response of the body to infection or injury, often characterized by local redness, swelling, fever, and pain.

Arthritis: a general term referring to an inflammation of the joints. Common symptoms include pain, swelling, and restricted motion. Arthritis has many known causes, such as rheumatic fever and trauma, as well as unknown causes.

Sedatives: depressant drugs that can, at high doses, produce sleep, but ordinarily are used to produce a calming effect on an individual.

Stimulants: substances that excite the central nervous system, the common results of which are increased alertness, rapid reflexes, excitement, nervousness, irritability, and a sense of self-confidence.

TABLE 14.4   OTC Painkillers

Product	Where Effective	Cautions	Comments
Acetaminophen (such as Tylenol or Anacin-3)	Aches, pain, and fever. Useful for children under 16 with chicken pox or flu or those allergic to aspirin. Does not prevent blood clotting.	High doses over long periods may damage liver and kidneys. Should not be used by alcoholics or people with liver or kidney disease (such as hepatitis). Pregnant and breast-feeding women should take only on medical advice. Rare reactions include skin rashes and painful urination.	Will not reduce inflammation, thus not effective for arthritis pain. Does not cause gastrointestinal bleeding.
NSAIDs **Aspirin**	Pain, fever, and inflammation. On medical advice, low dosages daily can prevent heart attack, because aspirin inhibits blood clotting. Possible preventive effect against colon cancer.	Should not be taken by children under 16 with chicken pox or flu symptoms. Not for pregnant women (can cause bleeding); breast-feeding mothers; those with aspirin allergy, ulcers, gout, or stomach bleeding; or people taking anti-coagulants. Frequent use can lead to ulcers. Excessive doses may produce upset stomach or ringing ears.	A highly effective, inexpensive drug. At least 40 percent of people have some stomach bleeding (usually inconsequential) after taking aspirin. Those who experience stomach upset from aspirin may be helped by taking it with food.
Ibuprofen (such as Advil, Motrin, or Nuprin)	Pain, fever, and inflammation. May inhibit blood clotting.	Fewer side effects than aspirin. But those who are allergic to aspirin may experience similar side effects with ibuprofen. In some people, may cause stomach bleeding, like aspirin. May interfere with diuretic and other anti-hypertensive drugs. Children and pregnant or breast-feeding women should take only on medical advice.	Less toxic in large doses than others. Good for menstrual cramps. May be better for fever and muscle aches accompanying a cold, since aspirin or acetaminophen may promote nasal congestion.
Naproxen sodium (Aleve)	Pain, fever, and inflammation. May inhibit blood clotting.	May cause stomach upset and stomach bleeding in some people, but less likely to do so than aspirin or ibuprofen. Not recommended for those with ulcers, asthma, or kidney disease, or for heavy drinkers. Children under 2 should not take. Those under 12 and pregnant or breast-feeding women should take only on medical advice.	Longer-lasting relief; thus good at bedtime. Good for menstrual cramps and postpartum pain. Worth trying if other OTC pain relievers haven't helped. For those over 12, daily maximum is three 200-milligram tablets, with 8 to 12 hours between doses.

Reprinted by permission from the *University of California at Berkeley Wellness Letter,* © Health Letter Associates, 1994.

Opium: a drug extracted from the poppy plant that is classified as a narcotic.

Amphetamines: drugs that stimulate the central nervous system and promote wakefulness and arousal.

of the psychotic mental illnesses. They also are used in smaller doses to control nausea and vomiting.

The term *tranquilizer* was originally coined to describe opium and the tranquil dreamy state it induced in users. **Opium** contains two active ingredients, **morphine** and **codeine,** that are now available, along with several related synthetic substances, as prescription drugs. Known as **opiates** or **narcotic analgesics,** they are used for relief of severe pain. They do not block the sensation

of pain; rather they make the person less aware of and less concerned about the pain.

Amphetamines and other stimulant drugs were once widely prescribed for weight control because of their effect of suppression of appetite. Unfortunately, tolerance to amphetamines develops rapidly and appetite suppression can be sustained only if the dosage is regularly increased. Today, stimulants (because of their ability to increase attention span) are prescribed mainly for the treatment of hyperactive children and narcoleptics (people who suffer from uncontrollable spells of falling asleep). Prolonged and unsupervised use of stimulants can result in a severe paranoid reaction known as "amphetamine psychosis."

As consumers we need to demand more information from health-care professionals regarding the use of these drugs. If they are prescribed for you, you should be certain you know why and how to use these drugs. Your physician or pharmacist should be willing to answer all your questions.

Unrecognized Drugs

Unrecognized drugs are commercial products that have drug effects but are not considered to be drugs by our culture. These substances are produced, sold, and used by people who might be offended if you suggested they were involved with drugs. The unrecognized drugs are one of the major reasons why we may conclude that there are no drug-free individuals in our society—just people who do not realize they are using drugs.

Two of the unrecognized drugs—alcohol and tobacco—are so important in our society that they are covered in chapters of their own (see chapters 15 and 16). The number of other unrecognized drugs is impossible to estimate—it is simply too hard to rise above our cultural definitions and identify how many substances we consider as nondrugs. In this chapter, we will look at one example of unrecognized drugs that illustrates how widely used such substances may be.

Caffeine

Caffeine is probably the most widely used drug in our society. Weidner and Istvan studied the caffeine consumption of a group of 400 men and women over a three-day period.[16] The participants were asked to report on their caffeine consumption from all foods, beverages, and medications. The participants' average daily intake of caffeine was about 400 milligrams. Only eleven of the 400 participants reported no caffeine use during the three-day period. For both men and women, the greatest source of caffeine, by far, was coffee, followed by tea and then soft drinks.

Along with the similar drugs theophylline and theobromine, caffeine is a component found naturally in coffee, tea, and chocolate. Caffeine, on the other hand, is

added to other substances as well. For instance, approximately 95 percent of the caffeine found in soft drinks is added by the manufacturer.[17] Caffeine is an important part of many products. Figure 14.4 contains a summary of the levels of caffeine found in some commonly used beverages, drugs, and foods.

A dose of 100 milligrams of caffeine will stimulate the central nervous system, resulting in feelings of alertness and well-being. The voluntary muscles and heart muscle are stimulated by caffeine, while the involuntary muscles, especially the bronchial muscles are relaxed by it. Heart rate, oxygen consumption, metabolic rate, blood pressure, secretion of acid by the stomach, and urinary output are all elevated by caffeine.

As with other drugs, there are many factors that influence the overall reaction individuals have to caffeine consumption. Among the many factors influencing caffeine effects are age, sex, weight, health status, pregnancy status, diet, smoking, alcohol consumption, and stress. Caffeine intake of as little as 500 milligrams in some people may result in a variety of outcomes, such as insomnia, headache, anxiety, depression, and irritability. Doses twice that large may produce muscle twitching and rambling thoughts and speaking, along with agitation, and **cardiac palpitation.**[18]

Because of its effects on heart rate and blood pressure, caffeine has long been suspected of being a cause of heart disease. Recent reviews of the research literature have concluded that mild to moderate levels of caffeine consumption do not increase the risk for cardiovascular disease.[19]

Caffeine has been found to cause **chromosome** breaks in white blood cells, which has led to suspicions that it might cause birth defects; however, studies have shown that mothers of babies with birth defects are no more likely to be coffee drinkers than are mothers in general.[20] Although human studies have not indicated a relationship between caffeine consumption and birth defects, recent studies have documented potential risks of **infertility** problems,[21] **miscarriage,**[22] and low-birth weight infants.[23] Additionally, caffeine does cross placental barriers. It appears in breast milk, and it has physiological effects on both fetuses and nursing babies. Because of this, it is recommended that pregnant women and

Caffeine: a stimulant drug derived from the dried leaves of tea or the dried seeds of coffee.

Chromosome: a threadlike structure containing genes, found in the nucleus of every cell.

Infertility: the inability to conceive.

Miscarriage: a naturally occurring termination of pregnancy before the fetus is capable of extrauterine life.

Source: Data from "Stimulating Figures" in *American Health*, XIII, (8):29, 1994.

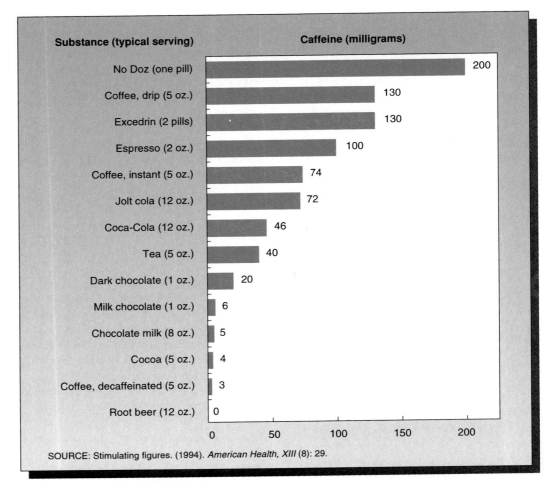

Substance (typical serving)	Caffeine (milligrams)
No Doz (one pill)	200
Coffee, drip (5 oz.)	130
Excedrin (2 pills)	130
Espresso (2 oz.)	100
Coffee, instant (5 oz.)	74
Jolt cola (12 oz.)	72
Coca-Cola (12 oz.)	46
Tea (5 oz.)	40
Dark chocolate (1 oz.)	20
Milk chocolate (1 oz.)	6
Chocolate milk (8 oz.)	5
Cocoa (5 oz.)	4
Coffee, decaffeinated (5 oz.)	3
Root beer (12 oz.)	0

SOURCE: Stimulating figures. (1994). *American Health*, XIII (8): 29.

nursing mothers reduce their caffeine intake to a minimum, or avoid it completely.[24] This includes individuals who are attempting to become pregnant because of the potential infertility effects of caffeine, as well as the effects of caffeine consumption during the first month of pregnancy when most women have not yet discovered that they are pregnant.

There is great concern about the relationship between caffeine consumption and cancer, as well as between caffeine consumption and **fibrocystic breast disease.** Studies have examined the relationship between coffee consumption and cancers of the bladder, pancreas, ovaries, and other organs and fibrocystic breast disease and no significant associations have been found.[25]

Illicit Drugs

The **illicit drugs** are those drugs that are outlawed. It is generally illegal to produce, sell, possess, or use these drugs. This is the youngest and smallest group of drugs. On a nationwide level, there were no illicit drugs in the U.S. until 1914, when Congress in effect outlawed cocaine and heroin (a form of opium used for smoking). Since then, the number of illicit drugs has grown substantially.

Cocaine

Cocaine, also known as "coke," is a crystalline powder extracted from the leaves of the South American Coca plant. Cocaine is both a powerful central nervous system stimulant and a local anesthetic. As an **anesthetic** its effects are essentially the same as those of novocaine or procaine. As a stimulant its effects are basically the same as the amphetamines or caffeine. In fact, mixtures of novocaine or procaine with caffeine or amphetamines have often been sold as cocaine in the illicit street market.

Physically, in addition to acting as a local anesthetic, cocaine increases heart and respiratory rates and blood pressure. It enhances alertness, relieves fatigue, and suppresses appetite. Psychologically, it produces **euphoria,** heightened

Fibrocystic breast disease: a noncancerous breast tumor that consists of fibrous connective tissues and cystic spaces.

Illicit drugs: any drug whose sale, purchase, or use is prohibited by law.

Anesthetic: a substance that reduces or stops sensations, including pain.

self-confidence, and temporary relief from depression. Continued use of large doses leads to weight loss, insomnia, and anxiety. Paranoid delusions and full-blown **psychosis** may result from regular high doses. Another major problem experienced by cocaine users is damage to the lining of the nose and nasal passages resulting from chronic snorting. With long-term use, liver damage is also possible.

Psychological dependence on cocaine can be quite severe, especially where it has been used to cope with chronic depression. Such dependence was once relatively rare, probably because cocaine was too expensive for many people to use it regularly. As cocaine has gotten cheaper, dependence has become more common.

Regular use of cocaine may lead to tolerance of the drug "high" but not to the cardiovascular actions of cocaine. Thus, the user must consume larger doses of cocaine to reach the desired high, which also increases the probability of heart and circulatory damage.[26] Overdoses of cocaine are characterized by respiratory paralysis, heart-rhythm disturbances, and convulsions. Death can occur within minutes from such an overdose.

The effects of cocaine vary according to the way the drug is taken. Cocaine is often inhaled, or **"snorted."** The drug is absorbed into the bloodstream through the mucous membranes in the nasal cavity and reaches the brain within three minutes. The effects of snorting cocaine peak within sixty to ninety minutes.

Some cocaine users inject the drug for quicker absorption. Injected cocaine reaches the brain within fifteen seconds, causing an intense high that peaks in three to five minutes and disappears in approximately thirty to forty minutes.

Smoking cocaine results in an even faster absorption rate and a more intense high. Smoked cocaine reaches the brain within seven seconds. The effects peak within ninety seconds and dissipate within minutes. Frequently, those who smoke cocaine find themselves on cocaine "binges" where they take "hits" of cocaine regularly for hours or even days at a time.

In order to maintain its potency when smoked, cocaine must be purified. A form of cocaine known as **freebase** results from purification with volatile chemicals (usually ether). This is a dangerous process due to the explosive qualities of the volatile chemicals

used. **Crack,** another form of smokable cocaine, results from purification with baking soda and water. Crack is described as "looking like slivers of soap, but having the general texture of porcelain."[27] Crack is a potent and inexpensive form of cocaine. Vials of crack sell for as little as $10 each. Much like the opium dens of the turn of the century, **crack houses** have now become known as a convenient place to buy and use crack. These buildings, apartments, or rooms are often run down, heavily guarded, and now found in most cities in the U.S.

One of the most distressing problems that began to emerge in the mid-1980s and has grown in proportion yearly is **"crack babies."** These are babies whose mothers used crack during pregnancy, and the result is many health problems both at birth and following birth. As yet we are not sure of the full range of consequences of such drug use during pregnancy, but there are certain immediate effects on the baby following birth,[28] and almost certainly long-term consequences on growth and development.

Smoking cocaine (freebase or crack) increases the potential health hazards. In fact, "freebasers" are believed to be at the greatest risk for cocaine overdose. Smoking cocaine often becomes the central focus of living. "Three-quarters of the freebase callers to the 800-COCAINE hot line state that the experience has become more important to them than food, sex, their jobs, and their families. A third say they steal, and a third say they deal to support their use."[29]

It is estimated that there are 3 million occasional users of cocaine in the United States, with an additional 1.3 million "current users" who report using cocaine within the past month.[30] The number of current cocaine users seems to have stabilized in the early 1990s, after peaking at 5.3 million in 1985. However, in 1992, U.S. hospitals saw an 18 percent increase in patients with cocaine-related emergencies.[31] As you can see from this data, cocaine use and its health damaging effects are a major problem in the United States.

Treatment For Cocaine Dependence

There are two distinct phases of treatment for cocaine dependence—initial abstinence and relapse prevention. Initiation of abstinence is the first step of treatment, and during this phase an attempt is made to interrupt the

Euphoria: a general feeling of well-being or satisfaction associated with the use of certain drugs.

Psychosis: a form of mental illness consisting of a loss of contact with reality; hallucinations and delusions are common.

Snorted: the inhalation of a powdered substance through the nose.

Freebase: a smokable form of cocaine that results from purification with volatile chemicals.

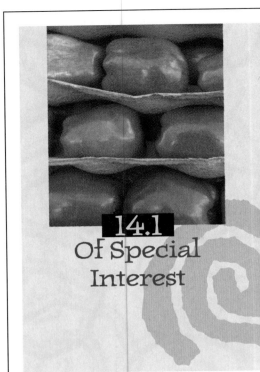

14.1
Of Special Interest

Marijuana and Driving

Cannabis intoxication and chronic marijuana use impairs short-term memory, alters the user's sense of time and space, and impairs overall coordination and motor functioning. The ability to track other vehicles is also impaired and is a major problem in driving a car. Tracking involves judging time, distance, and the speed of other cars. Skills like merging into traffic, making U-turns, and other driving tasks require tracking skills. Adding another drug such as alcohol only makes the situation worse.

Smoking marijuana also makes it very dangerous to operate machinery and other equipment, since perception and timing are off, and the drug may also produce fatigue and drowsiness.

Many persons insist that their driving performance is improved under the influence of marijuana. This is due to their increased sensitivity to enjoying driving, not to a realistic evaluation of driving ability.

A recent study of airplane pilots reported that after smoking marijuana, performance is impaired up to two to three days later, despite the pilots thinking that they did extremely well on simulated tests.

What Do You Think?

1. Do you think that smoking marijuana and driving poses an important public health problem? Explain your rationale.
2. What could be done to prevent the problems that arise from combining alcohol and marijuana consumption with driving?

From Richard Fields, *Drugs in Perspective,* 2nd edition. Copyright © 1995 Brown & Benchmark Publishers. Reprinted by permission of Times Mirror Higher Education Group, Inc., Dubuque, Iowa. All Rights Reserved.

---

cycle of frequent binges for the high that cocaine/crack provides. However, just as with the cigarette smoker or the alcoholic trying to quit, prevention of relapse is critical because it is highly likely that the individual will continue to be exposed to some supplies of the drug.

Marijuana

Long before the city of El Paso, Texas, passed the first law against it in 1914, marijuana had an extensive history as an herbal drug used for medicinal, religious, and recreational purposes. Marijuana comes from the plant Cannabis sativa. The major psychoactive ingredient in marijuana is **delta-9-tetrahydrocannabinol,** or **THC.**

The major psychological effects of marijuana at the most usual dosage levels are much the same as the effects of small doses of alcohol or the sedative-hypnotic prescription drugs. These effects are relaxation, drowsiness, euphoria, lowering of inhibitions, and relief of mild anxiety. More severe anxiety, however, may be worsened by use of marijuana. Unlike alcohol or the sedative-hypnotics, marijuana does not increase aggressiveness; in fact, it suppresses aggressiveness.

One of the most common effects of marijuana is mirthfulness—a tendency to find things funny, often with uncontrolled laughter or giggling. Impairment of short-term memory and loss of train of thought are also common effects of marijuana. Perceptions of space and time may be distorted. Unlike alcohol or any other depressant, marijuana heightens sensitivity to external stimuli. Additionally, complex reaction time is slowed in marijuana users (see Of Special Interest 14.1).

Other physical effects of marijuana are bloodshot eyes, dry throat, cough, and increased appetite and thirst. Heart rate is increased. Blood pressure seems to be lowered when the user is standing, but it remains normal or increases when the user is lying down. (This can result in dizziness or even faintness when a user goes from a lying to a standing position.)

Chronic effects of marijuana on the lungs and heart have been serious concerns in recent years. The best available evidence suggests that respiratory damage from smoking marijuana may be greater than that associated with tobacco. Studies indicate that marijuana cigarettes yield four times more tar than tobacco cigarettes when each are smoked in their usual manner.[32] Tars are the major source of carcinogens in cigarettes, so this high concentration in marijuana is an important health concern. Additionally, marijuana has been shown to decrease the body's ability to exchange oxygen and carbon dioxide in the air sacs of the lungs.[33] The evidence regarding the cardiovascular system indicates that marijuana smoking may increase the risks for cardiovascular problems in those people who already have high blood pressure or hardening of the arteries.[34] Marijuana may increase susceptibility to respiratory infections, and there is some evidence for a general impairment of immune response in marijuana users.[35]

Another concern is the effect of marijuana on reproduction. This concern includes problems with fertility as well as potential damage to the **embryo** or **fetus.** Studies have indicated that male chronic marijuana smokers have reduced **sperm counts** as well as sperm with less motility. Preliminary findings regarding women who regularly use marijuana suggest that **ovulation** is inhibited.[36] Abstinence from marijuana use is recommended for both males and females contemplating pregnancy.

Marijuana (specifically THC) is known to cross the placenta and is suspected to have adverse effects. It is difficult to determine the effects of marijuana on fetal development, however, due to the fact that many women who use marijuana also use other drugs, especially alcohol and tobacco. Several large-scale studies have attempted to control for other drug use in pregnant women. Their findings indicate that marijuana use during pregnancy is associated with lower infant birth weight and length, congenital abnormalities compatible with **fetal alcohol syndrome,** and premature birth.[37] Additionally, it has been shown that THC, the psychoactive ingredient in marijuana, is secreted in the breast milk of lactating women who use marijuana.[38] Further study is needed to determine the effects of THC in breast milk on breast-fed infants.

A final note of caution is important in this discussion of marijuana. According to the National Institute of Drug Abuse, the potency of marijuana increased 275 percent between the mid 1970s and the mid 1980s.[39] Recent street samples of marijuana averaged 6 percent THC. Most research on the effects of marijuana consumption have been done with marijuana that contained 1 to 2 percent THC.[40] This factor should be considered when reading reviews of research studies.

It is estimated that 5.1 million people in the U.S. used marijuana weekly in 1993.[41] This rate has remained stable since 1991 and is significantly lower than the peak rate of 8.9 million weekly users in 1985. However, hospital emergency rooms in the U.S. are reporting an increase in the number of patients they see with marijuana-related health problems.[42] The rate increased 48 percent from 1991 to 1992, and an additional 19 percent in the first half of 1993.[43]

In recent years, we have once again begun to debate whether marijuana and other illicit drugs should be legalized. A Social Perspective 14.1 presents the pros and cons of the current debate.

Heroin

Heroin is a semisynthetic drug produced from morphine. Its effects are the same as those of any other narcotic (such as opium, morphine, codeine, or methadone), but the dose necessary to produce these effects is smaller and the effects may be produced somewhat more rapidly.

Heroin depresses brain activity, producing a dreamy, mentally slow feeling and drowsiness. Experienced heroin users are more likely to experience feelings of depression and unhappiness. A heroin user may, however, experience either reaction to this drug effect the first time or the hundredth time.

Heroin slows the passage of food through the digestive tract, producing chronic constipation in regular users. It slows respiration, reduces urinary output, constricts the pupils of the eyes, and suppresses the cough reflex. Heroin relaxes the muscular walls of the blood vessels in the skin, causing an increased flow of blood to the skin and a slight drop in blood pressure. The rush of blood to the skin may cause itching. The skin will feel warm, but at the same time heat loss through the skin is increased. As a result, body temperature will drop while the user may feel hot and perspire.

Like all narcotics, heroin suppresses aggression, hunger, and sex drive. Contrary to the myth of the sex-crazed dope fiend, heroin addicts are typically passive and uninterested in sex. It is when heroin or a substitute narcotic cannot be obtained that the addict may become violent while trying to get the drug or the money to buy it.

Heroin is rarely seen in its pure form by anyone but the chemist who makes it. The "heroin" that most users buy on the street contains less than 5 percent heroin. The remaining 95+ percent may be milk sugar, quinine, talc, or almost any other powder. Many chronic problems result from these impurities and from unsanitary injection practices.

Embryo: the medical term for the products of conception up to the eighth week of conception.

Fetus: the medical term for an embryo that has developed for at least eight weeks.

Sperm count: the number of sperm found in one ejaculation.

Ovulation: the process by which the ovary releases a mature egg.

Fetal alcohol syndrome: a pattern of abnormalities found in the newborns of women who drank alcohol during pregnancy. This condition consists of a pattern of specific congenital and behavioral abnormalities.

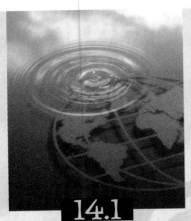

14.1
A Social Perspective

Would Decriminalizing Drugs Reduce Crime and Violence?

KURT SCHMOKE
Mayor of Baltimore

✓ **YES** America's failed national drug strategy is responsible for much of the violence in Baltimore and other urban communities. The enormous profits available from the sale of drugs create crime. Drug traffickers kill to protect or seize drug turf, and addicts commit crimes to get money for drugs. Almost half the murders in Baltimore in 1993 were drug related. . . .

The war on drugs is endangering young people in another way. In Baltimore, AIDS is the No. 1 killer of both young men and young women. Most of these deaths are attributable to intravenous drug use. . . .

That is why I advocate a policy called medicalization. Other advocates for changing national drug policy support setting up a private market like the ones we now have for alcohol and cigarettes. My approach to the problem is health regulatory rather than free market.

Medicalization means giving the public-health system the leading role in preventing and treating substance abuse. Under medicalization, the government would set up a regulatory regime to pull addicts into the public-health system. The government, not criminal traffickers, would control the price, distribution, purity and access to addictive substances—as it already does with prescription drugs. Public-health professionals would have

the authority to maintain addicts, using currently illegal drugs, as part of an overall treatment and detoxification program. Addicts would get counseling, health services and AIDS-prevention information to help break the cycle of addiction, crime and prison. Our communities, in turn, would get relief from the fear and despair that comes from having unremitting violence, addiction and open-air drug markets in their midst. . . .

But changes in Baltimore's drug policy are not enough. We must have a new national drug strategy—a strategy that will reduce crime by taking the profit out of drug trafficking, make our criminal-justice system more effective and increase the availability for treatment.

As a first step toward achieving those same goals, we should set up a new national commission to study how all drugs—legal and illegal—should be regulated. Hundreds of prominent Americans have already signed a resolution calling for the establishment of this kind of commission.

A similar commission was set up in 1929 by President Herbert Hoover to study the prohibition of alcohol. Hoover asked the commission to recommend ways in which Prohibition could be more strictly enforced. But the commissioners came to the conclusion that alcohol prohibition was, in the words of Walter Lippman, a "helpless failure." A similar objective study will likely come to the same conclusion about drug prohibiton.

From *Rolling Stone*, May 5, 1994. Reprinted by permission of Kurt Schmoke, Mayor of Baltimore, and Wenner Media, Inc., New York, NY.

WAYNE J. ROQUES
Demand Reduction Coordinator, U.S. Drug Inforcement Administration

✓ **NO** It is astonishing that Mayor Kurt Schmoke of Baltimore has aligned himself with the drug culture and a small group of elitists and Ivy League intelligentsia (who love social experimentation without regard to the cost in dollars of human tragedy) that promote legalization of an unhealthy, illegal lifestyle.

They simply refuse to learn from the experiences of England and Switzerland. They tried decriminalization/legalization and paid a dear price. Use increased by multiples, as did crime rates and health consequences/costs for the adventure. Switzerland is taking a second run at harm reduction, and the Netherlands, have informally decriminalized hashish. In a few

years, we'll have two more spectacular failures to provide us with the evidence that all drug use outside legitimate medical use is, in fact, abuse. The pseudo public-health, responsible-use, harm-reduction alternative is simply a recipe for a national disaster. . . .

It has been proven that marijuana can cause low birth weights and developmental problems in infants born to users. Some scientists believe that, when all the science is in, it will be proven that there is a Fetal Marijuana Syndrome and Effect, similar to that of alcohol.

Yet, Mr. Schmoke and his band of users, elitists and theorists advocate making this dreadful, toxic substance legally available and, thus, more easily accessible and acceptable. What toll in human tragedy must accrue before they deem their drug of choice unacceptable?

The increase in drug use that would accompany decriminalization/legalization would cause a dramatic rise in health damage and the associated health costs . . . increased random and family violence committed by persons on drugs, accidents caused by drug-impaired drivers/equipment operators, loss of productivity and increased related costs by workers, higher infant mortality and drug-damaged children to care for and to try to educate. The never-to-be-realized mental and physical potential of young and future generations is simply a price too dear to pay for surrender.

The drug culture seeks to confuse, divide and, thus, conquer the so-called straight society. We must act to stop this schizophrenic behavior and work to break the cyle of use, damage and addiction. We need to commit ourselves to expend as much money, time and effort on prevention and treatment as we do on law enforcement. When we mount such a three-pronged attack with the full support of the family, schools, community, churches, employers, health-care providers and all levels and agencies of government, then we will make the inroads and strides necessary to excise the cancer of drug use from our society.

What Do You Think?

Which argument presented above seems to be the most persuasive, in your opinion? What exactly was it that convinced you?

Impairment of lung and liver function is almost universal among heroin addicts for these reasons. Additionally, those heroin users who share needles run a high risk of becoming infected with HIV (the AIDS virus). AIDS is discussed in detail in chapter 11.

Dependence is the most important of the chronic effects of heroin. Heroin produces both physical and psychological dependence. Despite the emphasis placed on physical dependence, the psychological dependence is probably much more important and certainly is far more persistent.

Where an addiction to heroin has been established there is a distinct withdrawal syndrome. A heroin addict begins to crave another dose about four to six hours after the last dose. About eight to twelve hours after the last dose the addict begins to experience nervousness, perspiration, watery eyes, runny nose, yawning, and a craving for sweets. Over the next thirty-six hours, additional symptoms of restlessness, irritability, loss of appetite, muscle aches and pains, tremors, dilated pupils, and "gooseflesh" develop. The withdrawal syndrome hits its peak forty-eight to seventy-two hours after the last dose. At this point, all of the preceding symptoms continue with the addition of nausea, abdominal cramps, vomiting, diarrhea, hot and cold flashes, rapid heartbeat and respiration, elevated blood pressure, sneezing and other cold symptoms, and spontaneous orgasms. Once this peak has passed, the symptoms gradually subside over the next week. Some symptoms may persist for as long as ten weeks.

According to the U.S. State Department the production of heroin has increased by two thirds since 1988. Health experts fear that an increase in the numbers of young heroin users may be seen in the next few years. Evidence of increased health effects has been recently seen in U.S. emergency rooms where heroin-related emergencies increased 44 percent in the first half of 1993.[44] This increase accounted for over half of the total increase in drug-related emergency room visits.

LSD

LSD, a psychedelic drug, is a white, crystalline powder that dissolves readily in water. As a liquid or in large volumes it has a slightly bluish or purplish appearance. It is odorless and tasteless. LSD is the most potent drug known, and the dosage must be measured in micrograms (millionths of a gram) rather than in milligrams (thousandths of a gram). No other psychedelic has an effective dose less than 200 milligrams, but 20 micrograms of LSD will produce effects.

LSD was not the first psychedelic drug—psychedelics played a major role in the development of primitive religions early in human social evolution—but it has been the most important one for the modern U.S. Properly known as lysergic acid diethylamide, LSD was twenty-fifth in a series of lysergic-acid derivatives synthesized by Albert Hofmann in 1938; it came to be known by its laboratory abbreviation, LSD-25. It was not until 1943 that Hofmann accidentally discovered the psychedelic effects of LSD-25. Harvard psychologist Timothy Leary and San Francisco novelist Ken Kesey developed a large following in the 1960s by widely popularizing LSD.

The physical effects of LSD are not extensive for such a notorious drug. It increases heart rate and produces a slight rise in blood pressure and temperature. It increases the activity of the digestive tract and often produces feelings of nausea. Reflexes are speeded up and more easily triggered, muscular twitches or tremors commonly occur, and the pupils of the eyes become dilated. Moderate pain relief is afforded by LSD use. Perspiration, salivation, and tears are all increased.

The psychological effects are considerably more profound. LSD typically produces an exaggerated sense of well-being known as euphoria. Less commonly it may produce the exact opposite effect—an exaggerated sense of wrongness and uneasiness known as **dysphoria.** Although LSD usually reduces anxiety and tension, it may instead increase anxiety.

LSD increases introspection, lowers psychological defense mechanisms, and facilitates focusing on subjective experiences. Aggressiveness is consistently reduced by LSD. Aesthetic appreciation for art or music is usually enhanced by LSD. Users often believe that the drug has enhanced their creativity but objectively this does not seem to be so. Peak or mystical experiences in which the user feels a sense of oneness with nature or the universe are common experiences in LSD use.

Contrary to popular belief, LSD only rarely produces **hallucinations**—perceptions for which there are no actual sensory stimuli. **Illusions** and **closed-eye imagery** do commonly occur. Illusions are distortions of actual stimuli—walls seem to move, faces grow distorted, lights seem to prism into many

Dysphoria: a feeling of discomfort associated with the use of drug substances. Such discomfort may be physical, mental or emotional.

colors or segment into splinters of light. Closed-eye imagery refers to seeing things with your eyes closed. LSD also may produce an effect known as synesthesia in which sensory messages seem to become crossed—sounds are seen, smells are heard, or colors are felt.

LSD's potential for "bad trips" as well as "good trips" is obvious, given its potential for producing dysphoria as well as euphoria and for increasing as well as decreasing anxiety. Borderline psychotics are more likely to have bad experiences with LSD.[45] Flashbacks, in which some elements of an LSD experience recur at a later time without further LSD use,[46] occur in only a relatively small percentage of LSD users.

PCP

Once thought to have medicinal value as an anesthetic, **phencyclidine** (or **PCP**) proved to have side effects that made it unacceptable for medical use. Those side effects were delirium, dysphoria, and hallucinations. PCP did, however, come into widespread use as an animal tranquilizer, especially in fattening hogs for market.

In the 1970s PCP became a street drug when it began to be sold as THC. Actual THC was too expensive to produce and too difficult to store to be a successful street drug, so PCP became a common substitute. Eventually most street-drug users learned of the deception, but many had learned to like PCP and it continued to be sold as "angel dust," "dust," or "tea"—the latter descriptive referring to THC. Angel dust usually refers to a granular crystalline form of PCP that is sprinkled on marijuana or tobacco and then smoked. Tea usually refers to a fine powdered form of PCP that is snorted or sometimes injected.

PCP is a deliriant rather than a psychedelic drug. A typical dose (5 milligrams or less) causes a drunken state similar to that produced by alcohol or a sedative-hypnotic, along with a loss of sensitivity to light pain (such as a pinprick). A dose of 5 to 10 milligrams causes delirium and hallucinations, loss of sensitivity to pain or temperature, and fever accompanied by shivering and possible nausea and vomiting. Larger doses can result in a sudden drop in blood pressure, coma, convulsions, or even death. Soon after taking PCP the user feels an intensification of experience, followed by vivid hallucinations and paranoia. In a later phase the user becomes extremely withdrawn and feels divorced from reality. The user can become so withdrawn as to experience a state of virtual nothingness. Such a state of nothingness seems to be highly appealing to persons who find their ordinary reality extremely unpleasant. Many PCP abusers react with aggression and violence, which has been labeled PCP-rage.

Death due to PCP overdose is distinctly possible. PCP users may also suffer injury due to reduced sensitivity to pain and temperature, lack of coordination, and their own aggressive behaviors.

Inhalants

The use of **inhalants,** or gases that can be breathed into the lungs, appears to be on the rise, especially among young adolescents. One recent survey found that almost 20 percent of eighth-grade students reported that they had used an inhalant at some time in their lives.[47] Among college-age adults the use of inhalants is reported to be less. It is currently estimated that 13.9 percent of young adults have used inhalants at some time in their lives, with 3.1 percent having used them in the last year.[48]

The abuse of glue, solvents, and aerosols from paints, hair spray, nail polish remover and the like are the most common substances inhaled. These substances are not considered by society to contain drugs, and they are not regulated as such. The ease of availability may explain why inhalants are so popular with young adolescents.

When inhalants are breathed into the lungs they are quickly absorbed into the bloodstream and travel to the brain. In low doses these chemicals cause lightheadedness and dizziness, and provide a temporary high. In higher doses, depression of the central nervous system can lead to sleep or coma. The effects of inhalants can be poisonous to the body, resulting in heart rhythm disturbances that can lead to death.

Chronic use of inhalants can lead to permanent damage to the body. Permanent brain damage affecting memory and reasoning abilities, as well as impaired motor ability affecting coordination are special concerns of long-term abuse of inhalants.

Personal and Social Influences on Drug Use Patterns

We have shown that drugs of all kinds are a part of the fabric of our society; most people use drugs of some kind. Current research indicates that by the time a person reaches high school age, he or she will have seen more than 17,000 hours of commercial

Phencyclidine (PCP): an animal tranquilizer, sometimes known as angel dust or tea, that acts as a deliriant in humans.

television programming. Much of that television programming is supported by commercials about psychoactive substances. We would like to turn now to some issues regarding the extent of the influence of drugs in our society today.

Drugs That Enhance Athletic Performance

Ergogenic drugs are substances that can enhance athletic performance. The most commonly used ergogenics are **anabolic steroids** and amphetamines. Other performance-enhancing drugs include caffeine, beta-adrenergic blockers, human growth hormone, levodopa, and dimethyl sulfoxide (DMSO).

Anabolic Steroids

Although there has been a great deal of publicity surrounding the use of ergogenic aids by athletes (steroids to enhance performance), there continues to be evidence that increasing numbers of athletes are using such drugs. A steroid is defined as "any drug or hormonal substance, chemically and pharmacologically related to testosterone (other than estrogens, progestins, and corticosteroids) that promotes muscle growth."[49]

While it is now generally accepted that anabolic steroids can cause increases in body weight and muscle mass that are greater than those achieved through exercise and proper diet, medical authorities conclude that the long-term risks associated with their use exceed any possible short-term benefits. Nonmedical use of steroids is believed to be an addictive habit.[50] Withdrawal symptoms may include decreased **libido** and depression. Steroid users may continue to take the drug to ward off these symptoms or to try to maintain the libido-enhancement and euphoric drug effects offered by initial use of steroids.

Several adverse effects associated with nonmedical steroid use deserve special attention. First, steroids have been shown to stimulate aggression and violent behavior. William Taylor, in a study of health-club athletes who had used steroids for an average of three and one-half years, found that "90 percent confessed to episodes of overaggressiveness and violent behavior that they believed were induced by steroids."[51] Steroid users have labeled these episodes as "roid rage." Secondly, nonmedical use of steroids poses a serious risk for coronary artery disease (CAD).[52] Scientists believe the risk for CAD is related to physiological changes caused by the steroids, including changes in blood-lipoprotein levels, hypertension, and blood-clotting abnormalities. Oral steroids are associated with elevated risk of liver disorders, kidney disease, immune system disturbances, and reproductive system problems. Side effects of steroid use among women include potentially permanent changes in facial hair growth, male pattern baldness, lowering of voice, and enlargement of the clitoris.

It is estimated that two to three million people in the U.S. are nonmedical users of steroids and that most of these users obtain their steroids on the black market, which has become a $300 to $400 million "business" annually.[53]

As a result of the continued problems with steroids and the extensive visibility of the problem, a new federal law, the Anabolic Steroids Control Act (ASCA) of 1990 has been passed. This law makes it a crime to possess, prescribe, or distribute anabolic steroids for any use in humans other than the treatment of specific diseases.[54] According to the new law, steroids will become Schedule III drugs, which carry severe penalties for their violation, including up to five years of prison time and $250,000 fines for first offenses, and up to ten years and $500,000 for subsequent offenses.

Amphetamines

Amphetamines are central nervous system stimulants that have the ability to reduce the effects of fatigue on athletic performance.[55] In one often-cited study of the effects of amphetamines on athletic performance, Smith and Beecher gave the drug to swimmers.[56] They were then timed while performing the event in which they normally competed. It was found that amphetamine produced a 1 percent improvement in their best drug-free times. This small edge may be insignificant to the nonathlete, but for athletes it may mean the difference between finishing first or last in events that are sometimes decided by tenths of a second. The following risks have been associated with amphetamine use:

1. heat exhaustion
2. circulatory collapse
3. paranoid ideation
4. hyperthermia
5. hypertension
6. tachycardia
7. depression following cessation of use.

Anabolic steroids: synthetic derivatives of testosterone, the male sex hormone.

Libido: a term used to describe the level of one's sexual desire.

Drug Use by Athletes

W. A. Anderson suggests five major reasons for carefully examining alcohol and other drug use among athletes.[57]

1. There continues to be extensive coverage by the media regarding drug use by athletes.
2. Since 1985, several well-known college athletes have died in drug-related incidents.
3. In the last five years, alcohol and other drug-use rates among the general population have changed.
4. Many universities have now begun comprehensive drug education programs, targeting their athletes in particular.
5. In 1988, the NCAA instituted a national drug education and drug-testing program. The results of an NCAA study of male and female athletes between 1985 and 1990[58] indicate that alcohol continues to be the most frequently reported drug used by athletes. The study suggests, however, a 12 percent reduction in the use of cocaine/crack, an 8 percent reduction in the use of marijuana, and an 8 percent increase in the use of smokeless tobacco since 1985. They also examined the use of substances designed to improve athletic performance, and found a 5 percent decrease in the use of amphetamines, a 6 percent increase in the use of pain medications, and a slight increase in the use of anabolic steroids. Additionally, they compared patterns of use by athletes with those of other college students and found almost comparable patterns of alcohol use by the two groups, but significantly lower rates of use among athletes for amphetamines, cocaine/crack, and marijuana.

The NCAA has developed guidelines for implementation of drug-testing programs by its member institutions. In 1986, the NCAA began testing for drug use among athletes competing in NCAA championship competitions and postseason football games. The NCAA prohibits athletes from using diuretics, anabolic steroids, marijuana, cocaine, heroin, amphetamines, and caffeine. In addition, the NCAA prohibits blood doping and restricts the use of local anesthetics.[59]

The U.S. Olympic Committee (USOC) sponsors a Drug Control Hot line (1–800–233–0393) to allow athletes opportunities to speak anonymously with a person knowledgeable about drug use in sports. The USOC conducts random drug testing of athletes who are in training and competing for places on the U.S. Olympic team. The USOC follows the International Olympic Committee's extensive list of prohibited substances and attempts to widely distribute this information to U.S. athletes.

In the world of professional sports, several organizations have attempted to introduce mandatory drug testing but such efforts have been met with strong resistance from players' associations. Usually the players' associations maintain that drug testing is an unwarranted invasion of privacy. At this time, mandatory random testing is not conducted by any of the major professional sports organizations in the U.S.; however, each league (football, basketball, and baseball) has implemented drug education/control programs with varying degrees of sophistication and intrusiveness.

Drug Abuse and Families

Drug abuse is not only an individual disorder, but a family disorder as well. There is substantial evidence of the harm done to families resulting from drug abuse by one or more of the family members. There is family instability and higher rates of subsequent alcohol and drug abusing behaviors by other family members. This is particularly true among children of drug abusers.

Parental influences appear to have the greatest effect on children and preteens. Research[60] suggests that positive and warm family relationships, involvement and attachments discourage initiation into drug use. Parental modeling of behavior and attitudes toward alcohol and other drugs also are important determinants of alcohol and drug use. If parents appear to be tolerant of the use of alcohol and other drugs, then the likelihood of their use by children increases.

Peer Influences on Drug Use

Drug use is affected by peer influence in many ways such as pressure to carry out certain behaviors to "belong" to a group, contact with people who have access to such drugs, and having a role model who exhibits drug-taking behavior. Association with drug users during adolescence is one of the strongest predictors of future alcohol and drug use.

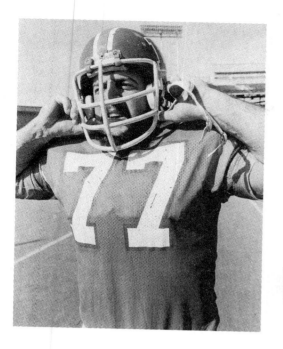

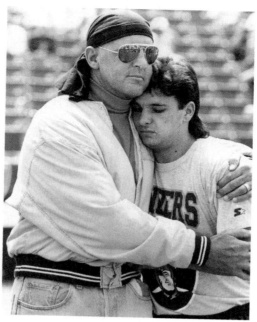

What Do You Think?

1. Drug use and misuse is common in both amateur and professional sports, as illustrated by the case of Lyle Alzado, shown here during his professional career and following the diagnosis of a brain tumor thought to be related to steroid and human growth hormone abuse. What impact do you think celebrities such as Lyle Alzado sharing their steroid-related tragedies with the public will have on steroid abuse in young people? Explain your thinking.

For college students, the freshman year is an especially high-risk time for beginning or increasing drug use and abuse. In a review of the literature on substance use and abuse among college students, Michael Prendergast noted that living arrangements were highly associated with alcohol use and abuse on college campuses.[61] Specifically, students moving away from home to dorms, apartments, or fraternity/sorority houses were much more likely to use and abuse alcohol. It appears that peer influence may be especially important on college campuses.

Community Influences on Drug Use

Influences in the community are often overlooked. Community norms, access to drugs, school policies, and local law enforcement policies are all community influences that affect the potential for drug use among young people.

Global Environmental Influences

When we extend our gaze beyond the person and the immediate environment, we begin to find other factors that have the potential to influence decisions regarding alcohol and other drug use. Such factors include national and state laws regulating access and use, advertising in media, the price of alcohol and other drugs, marketing of alcohol, and television programming and the content of movies. We find that each of these is related to drug-use decisions among young people.

- *State and national laws:* The extent to which minimum age purchase laws are perceived as enforced has been shown to relate to abuse. When weakly enforced, there is greater likelihood of young people unlawfully attempting to buy alcoholic beverages. The same is true for use of other drugs.
- *Price of alcohol and other drugs:* A great deal of research suggests that as the cost of alcoholic beverages increases, overall consumption decreases. Until recently, the federal tax on alcoholic beverages has remained unchanged relative to inflation. It is now felt that if these taxes had increased at the same rate of inflation, there may have been a 32 percent reduction in the number of youth who drink beer frequently.[62] In a related manner, as the cost of street drugs such as "crack" declines, the number of people using such substances increases.
- *Marketing of alcohol:* Wallack[63] estimates that a teenager in the U.S. sees nearly 1,000 advertisements for alcoholic beverages per year. It is clear by viewing any of these advertisements that they are targeted at young people and are aggressive in their attempts to influence individual behavior. These aggressive tactics now extend also to sponsorship of sporting and cultural events to influence even more focused audience segments than general advertisements (see figure 14.5).

1. As the jarring scoreboard
   juxtaposition at Shea Stadium made
   clear, beer was one substance legally
   available at this Mets-Pirates game,
   as it is at games everywhere. Are we
   immersing sport in a sea of
   intoxicating drink?

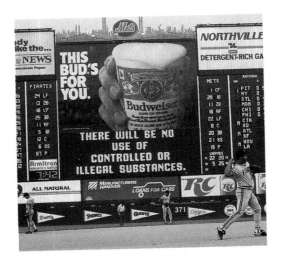

- *Television and movies:* Alcohol-and drug-
  using messages and scenes are portrayed
  frequently and often without regard to
  accuracy. On TV and in movies,
  characters drink alcoholic beverages
  frequently; drinking is often portrayed
  without expression of negative
  consequences; and casual drug use is
  frequently portrayed. Activity for
  Wellness 14.1 will help you assess the
  many ways you come into contact with
  drugs on a typical weekend.

Drug Abuse and Crime

Although many people see the drug abuser as
a criminal, there is evidence of other linkages
between drug abuse and criminal behavior. It
is impossible to say that drug abuse is the sole
cause of criminal behavior because some
would argue that drug abuse is just one of
many aspects of delinquent behavior. It is not
a matter of the drug causing the crime in all
cases, but rather a matter of criminals who
also use drugs. There are, however, two drugs
for which we have evidence of a direct link
between the drug and criminal behavior—
barbiturates and alcohol.[64]

Why Young People Are Legally Prohibited From Using Alcohol and Other Drugs

Infancy through young adulthood are critical
times for healthy human development.
Infants and children depend upon others
both for nurturance and protection, but also
to provide models of appropriate behavioral
patterns. Learning appropriate responses to
situations, and in particular difficult

problems, continues through young
adulthood. The Office of Substance Abuse
Prevention[65] offers the following summary of
these demands:

- Children learn from playing; they learn
  how to share, how to make friends, how
  to cooperate, and so forth.
- Before they enter adolescence, young
  people learn important skills such as how
  to solve problems, how to deal with
  mistakes, how to make decisions, how to
  cope with stress, and how to get along
  with others.
- Teenagers learn how to become
  independent, how to judge whether a
  risk is worth taking, how to deal with a
  new body image, and how to handle
  strong emotions.
- College-age youth prepare for the
  responsibilities of family and jobs. Given
  these challenges, it is important to
  remember that the use of alcohol and
  other drugs makes learning a difficult
  task by affecting concentration, memory,
  attention, thinking, and coordination.
  Moreover, there is some evidence that
  alcohol and other drug abuse can
  interfere with the development of
  autonomy from parents, which is
  necessary for adequate self-identity and
  the capacity to develop other
  meaningful relationships.

Other Drug Use Issues: Responsible Drug Use

Most people in the U.S. are polydrug users.
Their use may include any of the drugs we
have studied in this chapter, including herbal
drugs, over-the-counter drugs, prescription
drugs, unrecognized drugs (including alcohol
and nicotine), and illicit drugs. With any
drug use, be it antihistamines or alcohol, we
must recognize that we have certain
responsibilities. David Duncan and Robert
Gold[66] provide some general guidelines in
three areas: (1) situational responsibilities,
(2) health-related responsibilities, and
(3) safety-related responsibilities.

Situational responsibilities arise out of
circumstances in which drugs are used within
a cultural or traditional context, such as
social gatherings. Because psychoactive drugs,
such as alcohol, are often made available in

How Many Different Ways and Times Do You Come into Contact with Drugs

The purpose of this activity is to examine how often you may be exposed to drugs and drug advertising in an average day. Carry a small notebook everywhere you go for one full weekend—all day Saturday and all day Sunday. In that book make a note each time you see an advertisement for a drug-related product, see drug abuse depicted on TV or in the movies, or see drug taking among those with whom you come in direct contact (e.g., drinking alcoholic beverages, using tobacco products). After the two-day period is over, tally your results on a chart such as this one. Be as thorough and complete as you can.

14.1 Activity for Wellness

		Number of Times	Tobacco/ Alcohol	Illicit Drugs	Other Drugs
Advertisements:	Radio	_____	_____	_____	_____
	TV	_____	_____	_____	_____
	Magazines	_____	_____	_____	_____
	Newspapers	_____	_____	_____	_____
Drug Stories:	TV	_____	_____	_____	_____
	Movies	_____	_____	_____	_____
You See People	Friends	_____	_____	_____	_____
Using Drugs	Family	_____	_____	_____	_____
	Others	_____	_____	_____	_____

As you examine your chart, you should ask yourself some questions. Compare your results with those of your classmates. What are the most frequently advertised drugs? Were you surprised by how many times you saw advertisements for psychoactive drug substances?

Were you surprised by how many different drugs you were exposed to in 48 hours? Were there any patterns that were particularly disturbing to you?

---

these circumstances, there are certain responsibilities that we should be aware of as members of these groups:

1. Be prepared to provide a variety of acceptable models of behavior regarding such use of psychoactive drugs.
2. Respect each individual's decision regarding the use of recreational drugs in a situation if it results in reasonable and responsible behaviors. It should be up to the group to define what is reasonable and responsible in these settings.
3. Recognize that recreational drug use is not the only, nor the most appropriate, social lubricant.
4. Recognize a responsibility for the health, safety, and pleasure of everyone by avoiding severe drug-induced intoxication and by helping others to do the same.
5. Have contingency plans ready to handle cases of severe intoxication if they occur in spite of the group's efforts at prevention. This means, of course, that each member of the group assumes some responsibility for the health and safety of other members of the group.
6. Be aware of the influences of set and setting on psychoactive drug experiences. You should recognize by now that this is quite a complex issue, but since set and setting are so important to the outcomes of drug use, you should:
   a. Not be coerced into using potent psychoactive drugs.

b. Understand your own rationale for using any drug. Make sure that your motivations and rationale are appropriate to the drug, yourself, and your situation.

c. Remember that you cannot take sole responsibility for the outcome of drug use. If you use psychoactive drugs alone, some of the outcomes are left to chance.

7. Encourage your peer group to set reasonable rules and rituals surrounding the use of drugs. We typically find that when groups make a conscious effort to define limits, there tend to be fewer difficulties associated with such drug use.

Health-related responsibilities are those that relate to our own health and the health of others. We can act responsibly for our own health and the health of others by following these guidelines:

1. Choose to abstain from drug use.

2. Heed the advice of a physician either to avoid the use of a particular drug or to use it only as suggested.

3. Recognize that social acceptability does not require drug use.

4. Use prescription and over-the-counter drugs in the manner intended to reduce the potential hazards.

5. Recognize that what some people call recreational drugs are *drugs*, and understand what that means. The outcomes of recreational drug use are substantially determined by the combined influences of set and setting, within the context of the quantity of the drug ingested and the circumstances under which it is taken.

6. Set reasonable limits on the consumption of alcohol that are well within your own capacity; these limits can vary from time to time because of set and setting.

7. Be particularly careful of using combinations of drugs because drug interactions can occur.

8. Remember that the use of some psychoactive drugs may mask signs and symptoms of serious illness or injury. It is thus important to avoid long-term continuous use of any psychoactive drug.

Safety-related responsibilities are an important consideration in any activity.

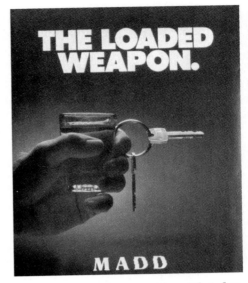

Figure 14.6: What Do You Think?

1. Recreational drug users must always recognize their safety-related responsibility. Have you or a friend or family member ever driven a motor vehicle after drinking too much alcohol?

Because of this, the following safety-related responsibilities are important to consider when using drugs:

1. Avoid situations in which complex tasks must be performed while using drugs such as alcohol. Most specifically, motorized vehicles or large machinery should not be used at these times (see figure 14.6).

2. Avoid situations in which you ride with a driver who is using drugs, and discourage that person from operating motor vehicles.

3. Recognize that your own drug-taking behavior can influence the behavior of others around you, especially children. Always consider carefully whatever actions are taken in the presence of children.

4. Use drugs such as alcohol only in relaxed and responsible social situations.

5. Use drugs such as alcohol in moderation, even if you think that your tolerance for these drugs is high. Remember that set and setting can influence behavioral tolerance to a drug as well as other characteristics of the drug experience.

6. Know basic first-aid techniques, and take responsibility for applying them appropriately in cases of drug emergencies.

Safety-related responsibilities:
responsibilities of drug use that protect individuals using drugs, and innocent bystanders, from injury.

Deciding about Drug Use

List a drug you use now or are thinking about using. Dig out arguments for and against use of this drug. Some of these arguments are personal, others scientific in nature. Write your decision at the bottom of the page.

Drug: _____

For (positive effects)

1. Effect on body _____
2. Effect on mind _____
3. Effect on values _____
4. Legality _____
5. Effect on your human potential _____
6. Effect on family _____
7.
8.
9.
10.

Against (negative effects)

1. Effect on body _____
2. Effect on mind _____
3. Effect on values _____
4. Legality _____
5. Effect on your human potential _____
6. Effect on family _____
7.
8.
9.
10.

Resolution: Write down your decision. Will this decision change as you age? As your social situation changes? As you use other drugs? Or as the amount changes?

_____

_____

_____

_____

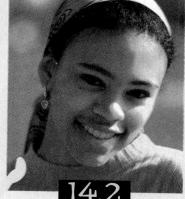

14.2
Activity for Wellness

You may want to come back to this exercise after reading chapters 15 and 16.

From J. M. Corry and P. Cimbolic, *Drugs: Facts, Alternatives, Decisions,* 1985. Copyright © 1985 Wadsworth, Inc., Belmont, CA. Reprinted by permission.

---

7. Avoid the use of unfamiliar drugs, especially when not in the company of others. This is even more important when we consider the consequences of mixing unfamiliar drugs.

Many of these issues are addressed as we make decisions regarding drugs. Activity for Wellness 14.2 is designed to practice such decisions.

Drug Use and Pregnancy

Until now we have focused on some very broadly based issues related to drugs themselves and their use. We have tended to generalize these issues to all drugs. Before we go on, however, it is worthwhile to examine one more general issue in regard to drug use—the relationship between drug use and pregnancy outcomes.

Poor pregnancy outcomes may result from disease, malnutrition, or lack of adequate **prenatal care.** Drug abuse, however, can be added as another potentially causative factor. As you remember from our discussion

of set and setting, the specific effects of any drug taken by an individual cannot be predicted with precision. These factors are multiplied when we consider the difficulties associated with drug interactions, food/drug interactions, and the timing and dosage of drugs taken. In other words, nonmedical use of drugs during pregnancy is questionable and probably never justifiable. The Addiction Research Foundation of Ontario, Canada, lists three main ways in which a drug may influence the outcome of pregnancy.[67]

1. Prior to conception, a drug may alter the mother's bodily processes permanently or it may have a permanent effect on either of the parents' genes. Experiments on the effects of drugs on genes are generally limited to analysis of chromosomes in white blood cells, but it is only if the reproductive cells are damaged that the effect will be transmitted to a child. Most of the current research has been done on such drugs as LSD and cannabis, but proof of their effects on genes is

Prenatal care: actions taken by a future mother and her mate to increase the chances of birthing a healthy baby and reducing the risks of pregnancy and childbirth for the future mother.

inconclusive. More important, a very defective fertilized egg will probably be spontaneously aborted shortly after being fertilized.

2. During early pregnancy (embryonic stage), the use of some recreational drugs may be detrimental. It is especially dangerous during the first two months of pregnancy, since it is during this time that the organs are beginning to form. Drug use at this time may initiate deformities (**teratogenic effects**) in the developing **embryo.**[68] Some critical periods of development include the nervous system (fifteenth to twenty-fifth day); the eyes (twenty-fourth to fiftieth day); the heart (twentieth to fortieth day); and the legs (twenty-fourth to thirty-sixth day).

3. During the later stages of pregnancy (fetal stage), when the fetus is growing and developing, drug use may be related to the potential for physical or mental retardation. We know that most drugs taken by a pregnant woman will reach an embryo or fetus. The placental link between the maternal and fetal blood supplies begins to develop within fourteen days of fertilization of the egg. This placental barrier has some of the same characteristics as other bodily barriers and membranes; that is, it allows the exchange of fat-soluble molecules between the two blood supplies. This, unfortunately, includes most recreational drugs and other drugs used for self-medication.

Many problems are associated with drug use and pregnancy outcomes, regardless of whether drugs are taken prior to actual pregnancy or during the pregnancy itself; however, an embryo or fetus may face other drug-related problems during pregnancy. Perhaps the most important of these other possibilities is the potential for withdrawal from drugs to which the embryo or fetus became accustomed before birth. Such withdrawal, either during pregnancy or at birth, can be serious, especially with drugs such as barbiturates and opiates. We now know that this may also occur with some other common drugs such as alcohol and amphetamines.

Where Do We Go From Here?

One of the most important questions to ask yourself is "is my use or abuse of drugs causing a problem in my life?" Think about the drugs you currently use. Refer back to the beginning of this chapter where we presented the criteria for substance abuse and substance dependence. How many of the criteria mentioned apply to you? Hopefully, none of the criteria fit. However, if you realize that you do have a problem with drugs, there are important steps you can take to improve your level of well-being. Table 14.5 presents suggestions for an effective drug treatment strategy. Additionally, seeking help from health professionals who specialize in drug rehabilitation has been the key to successful drug treatment for many people.

In chapter 1, the stages of behavioral change were discussed in some detail. If you are currently using any drug on a regular basis, especially a psychoactive drug, refer to Activity for Wellness 1.4 to determine which stage of change you are in regarding your use of that drug. Then use the information in table 14.6 to help you improve your well-being through the appropriate use of drugs.

In general, the increasing use of recreational drugs during adolescence and young adulthood results in growing numbers of problems, particularly when these drugs are used as an escape valve from stress or the pressures of life. These drugs produce some negative physical and psychological effects; they also have a dependence-producing potential. A drug user's inability to learn how to cope with reality is an even more substantial problem resulting from such escapism. There are times when the moderate use of socially approved recreational drugs is appropriate, just as there are times when self-administered OTC drugs or supervised use of prescription drugs can be appropriate. But unsupervised, unrestricted, and unrestrained use of any drug diminishes our potential for achieving wellness.

Teratogenic effects: birth defects that result from factors that can affect a growing embryo during its period of rapid growth.

TABLE 14.5   *An Effective Drug Treatment Strategy*

The primary goal of recovery is complete abstinence from drugs/alcohol. The following steps can help those in recovery achieve their goal.

1. *Break the bonds of denial.* Recovery is an ongoing process often facilitated by the support of others—friends, others in recovery from drugs/alcohol, family, or a counselor. All of these people can help addicts/alcoholics work through their denial and maintain sobriety.

2. *Actively work and apply the twelve steps and other Alcoholics Anonymous (AA) principles in recovery.* This provides guidelines, structure, and support for recovery efforts. Developing a relationship with an AA or NA (Narcotics Anonymous) sponsor is a key element in effectively helping the newly recovering person to understand and implement the principles of AA.

3. *Seek nonchemical altered states of consciousness.* The innate human drive to alter one's sense of consciousness can be attained through healthy and balanced activities, not the use of drugs/alcohol. These activities enhance the individual's sense of self and well-being.

4. *Working through negative emotional states and controlling destructive impulses.* Negative life experiences commonly result in emotions that get out of control and end up causing additional problems. The individual in recovery can learn new coping skills and gain support in working through impulses that may lead to destructive decisions and interactions.

5. *Move from passive to active choice making in all aspects of life.* Most addictive behaviors are passive, automatic, ritualistic, and habitual. This includes workaholism, gambling, eating disorders, and many other behaviors that fit our behavioral definition of addiction. Recovering individuals need to be involved and active in their recovery. Most learning comes from doing.

6. *Resist social or peer pressure.* When it endangers welfare or inhibits growth, peer pressure can cause those in recovery to make the wrong choices. Recovery is maintained by being and talking with others in recovery, rather than isolating. Associating with people who don't understand, or more importantly, don't respect the individual's recovery, could require changing relationships. Recovering addicts/alcoholics should develop and maintain relationships that support a healthy drug/alcohol-free lifestyle.

7. *Improve and continue to work on the sense of self.* Those in recovery need to be involved in activities and relationships that promote a positive sense of self. To develop a sense of self, they must believe they are unique, worthwhile individuals with emerging talents and skills; individuals who can accomplish things;

individuals who can trust and be trusted while setting appropriate boundaries in relationships, and avoiding codependency and dysfunctionality.

8. *Deal more effectively with stress.* Recovering addicts/alcoholics must develop awareness in recognizing stressful situations and the need for support (attachments), coping skills, and resources to deal with or adapt to the stress.

9. *Maintain the structure of the recovery program.* Recovering alcoholics and addicts should consistently attend self-help meetings, aftercare, counseling sessions, and other elements of the recovery program.

10. *Have patience and direction.* Those in recovery must have a road map, while maintaining a day-at-a-time perspective in recovery.

11. *Learn how to enjoy life and others.* By developing the capacity to relax, enjoy, and have fun with others, recovering persons can establish leisure activities, hobbies, and explore personal interests.

12. *Maintain a sense of humor.* Those in recovery very much need to keep things in perspective, and remember, "I'm not OK. You're not OK. But that's OK."

13. *Take responsibility for self.* No matter what the event is, those in recovery have the freedom to choose their response to it. Taking responsibility for self leads to awareness, which in turn helps the individual to make effective choices.

14. *Maintain physical, emotional, and spiritual well-being.* Recovering alcoholics/addicts need regular exercise, balanced nutrition, adequate sleep and rest. Recovery also involves effective communication in relationships, especially intimate relationships. One must work on spiritual values in life and strive to experience the joy and creativity of life, while exploring your own sense of spirituality.

15. *Avoid shame.* Mistakes may occur but addicts/alcoholics can return to recovery without a burden of shame. Shame generated by others or themselves inhibits personal recovery and growth from situations that may be painful.

16. *Work on relapse prevention strategies.* Those in recovery need to deal with urges and cravings to use drugs/alcohol, imbalanced lifestyles, negative emotional states, social pressures, high-risk situations, and other factors which may make them vulnerable to relapse.

17. *Adapt to changes in life.* Addicts/alcoholics can remind themselves that they are human and subject to human feelings and emotions. Life is not perfect and always involves change.

Recovery is facilitated by the individual's ability to adapt to change and integrate feelings related to change. Striving for progress rather than perfection is a healthy goal.

 TABLE 14.6   *Tips for Using Drugs Responsibly*

Determining if you have a problem with drug use or abuse and then making changes in your drug-taking habits is not an easy process. You will find that you probably go through a series of steps each time you try to change your drug-taking behaviors. The following tips will help you as you progress through the stages of change for more responsible drug use.

Precontemplation → Contemplation

If you have never thought about whether you have a problem with drug use, and you do not intend to make any changes in your use of drugs during the next six months you might want to consider:

- Assessing your current drug use patterns by keeping a diary of what drugs you commonly use, and in what amounts, for a week. Also keep track of how you feel before, during and after taking the drugs, as well as any problems you notice that relate to your drug use.
- Review the results of your drug use diary and compare those results to the criteria listed in this chapter for substance abuse and substance dependence. Determine if you have a drug taking problem.

Contemplation → Preparation

If you have been seriously considering making some changes in your use of drugs, but have not yet attempted any changes, try to thoughtfully answer the following questions:

- How do I think or feel about taking drugs that interfere with my social, occupational, family, or personal well-being?
- How do I think or feel about making changes in my use of drugs that would result in a higher level of well-being for myself and those I love?

Preparation → Action

If you are ready to make some definite plans for changing your drug use habits during the next month, or if you have already made small changes in the past but were not able to

maintain those changes as a permanent part of your lifestyle, consider the following actions:

- Contact one of the many drug abuse self-help groups or professional drug abuse agencies located in your community; your telephone directory will list the telephone contact numbers for these resources.
- Make a commitment to yourself to attend a self-help support group meeting or visit a local drug rehabilitation center to begin your treatment program. Set a specific date to begin.

Action → Maintenance

If you have recently started to make changes in your drug-taking behaviors, the following tips will help you continue on this healthy path:

- Review and implement the suggestions found in table 14.5, An Effective Treatment Strategy.
- Write a behavioral change contract, such as that found in chapter 1, and find a support person who will help you keep with your plan; have your support person sign your contract.

Maintenance

If you have made important changes in your drug taking behaviors that you have maintained for six months or longer you now need to focus on maintaining your progress every day:

- Rehearse situations in your mind that may tempt you to relapse from your non-drug use lifestyle; for instance, imagine yourself at a party with friends where the drug you are avoiding is being used. How will you deal with this situation so that it does not lead to you using or abusing the drug?
- If you have a day where you lapse back into your old drug-taking pattern, learn to view this as a temporary error rather than a catastrophe. Then go back to following your healthy drug use program. Seek out the help and advice of your support person during this time.

*Based on Prochaska, Norcross and DiClemente's transtheoretical model. See Prochaska, J. O., Norcross, J. C. & DiClemente, C. C. (1994). *Changing for Good.* New York: William Morrow and Company.

Summary

1. We live in a drug-taking culture in which the availability of psychoactive agents is extensive.
2. There is no general agreement on a definition of the term drug, but the soundest approach is to consider the term in its broadest context—as any agent that by its chemical action affects the structure or function of the body.
3. A useful way to categorize drugs is based on their availability and use. This scheme yields five categories including herbal drugs, over-the-counter (OTC) drugs, prescription drugs, unrecognized drugs, and illicit drugs.
4. Individuals use drugs for a variety of reasons. Drug-taking behavior can be classified as experimental, social-recreational, circumstantial-situational, intensified, and compulsive.
5. Many factors affect the outcome of a drug experience, particularly the set (a person's internal environment), setting (the external environment), quantity, and route of administration of a drug.
6. Herbal drugs are plant substances that have drug effects. Herbal drugs can be dangerous because they often contain more than one active drug and the amount of the drugs in an herbal preparation can be unpredictable.
7. Over-the-counter (OTC) drugs are drugs that can be purchased by the consumer without the consent of a physician. The most common psychoactive OTC drugs are analgesics, sedatives and stimulants.
8. Prescription drugs can only be sold by or on the order of a physician, or sometimes by a dentist or veterinarian. The most common psychoactive prescription drugs include the sedative/hypnotics, tranquilizers, and amphetamines.
9. Unrecognized drugs are commercial products that have drug effects but are not recognized by society as drugs. The most commonly used unrecognized drugs are alcohol, nicotine, and caffeine.
10. Illicit drugs are those drugs that are generally against the law to produce, sell, possess, or use. Some of the most commonly used illicit drugs in the U.S. include alcohol (for those under age twenty-one, and in some states by county), cocaine, marijuana, heroin, LSD, PCP, and inhalants.
11. The use of drugs in sports has become an increasing problem, particularly in professional sports leagues. This includes the use of illicit psychoactive drugs as well as ergogenic drugs (substances that enhance athletic performance).
12. Many social factors influence drug taking in our society, including advertising and other media messages, attitudes toward drugs, the availability of drugs, and family and peer influences.
13. Drug use and pregnancy do not mix. Drugs taken prior to or during pregnancy can result in serious health problems for the fetus.
14. Several guidelines for responsible recreational drug use are provided, including situational responsibilities, health-related responsibilities, and safety-related responsibilities.
15. Perhaps more important than looking at the effects of any single drug, it is essential that we recognize the role of drugs in our society. Although drugs are readily available, they can have lifesaving or life-threatening effects. We must learn to make reasonable decisions regarding their use.

Recommended Readings

Carroll, Charles R. *Drugs in Modern Society*, 3d ed. Dubuque, Iowa: Wm. C. Brown Communications, Inc., 1993.

This well-written text covers all of the major psychoactive drugs, with discussions of historical perspectives, pharmacology, and health concerns. Its chapters on drug-abuse prevention and drug education are especially important in light of the current emphasis on the "war on drugs."

Austin, G. Prevention Research Review: Substance Abuse Among Native American Youth. Madison, Wis.: Wisconsin Clearinghouse, University of Wisconsin–Madison, 1990.

Austin, G. A. and M. J. Gilbert. Prevention Research Review: Substance Abuse Among Latino Youth. Madison, Wis.: Wisconsin Clearinghouse, University of Wisconsin–Madison, 1990.

Prendergast, M. L., G. A. Austin, and K. I. Maton. Prevention Research Review: Substance Abuse Among Black Youth. Madison, Wis.: Wisconsin Clearinghouse, University of Wisconsin–Madison, 1990.

These reviews summarize recent information on the problem of adolescent drug abuse among Latino, African-Americans, and Native Americans and the prospects for prevention. It reviews current research, and is designed to provide information to the general population based on that research. Also included is an annotated bibliography of reference materials.

References

1. Fields, R. (1995) *Drugs in Perspective*. Dubuque, Iowa: Brown & Benchmark Publishers.
2. Department of Health and Human Services. (1994). *Healthy People 2000 Review, 1993*. Washington, D.C.: U.S. Government Printing Office.
3. Duncan, D. F. & Gold, R. S. (1982) *Drugs and the Whole Person*. New York: John Wiley & Sons.
4. National Commission on Marijuana and Drug Abuse. (1973) Drug use in America: Problem in perspective. *Second Report of the National Commission on Marijuana and Drug Abuse*, Washington, D.C.: U.S. Government Printing Office.
5. American Psychological Association. (1987). *Diagnostic and Statistical Manual of Mental Disorders*, 3d ed. rev. Washington, D.C.: American Psychological Association, 169.
6. American Psychological Association, *Diagnostic and Statistical Manual of Mental Disorders*, 3d ed. rev., 167.
7. Rodgers, J. E. (1994) Addiction—a whole new view. *Psychology Today* 27 (5):32–38, 72, 74, 76, 79.
8. Rodgers, Addiction—, 79.
9. Schlaadt, R. G. & Shannon, P. T. (1990) *Drugs*, 3d ed. Englewood Cliffs, N.J.:270–271.
10. Schlaadt & Shannon, *Drugs*, 274.
11. "Old drug, new bottle?" (1994) *Consumer Reports on Health* 6:34.
12. "Over-the-counter pain relief." (1994) *UC Berkeley Wellness Letter* 10:3.

13. "Old drug, new bottle?" 34.

14. "Over-the-counter pain relief," 3.

15. Zimmerman, David R. (1983) *The Essential Guide to Nonprescription Drugs* (New York: Harper & Row), 664.

16. Weidner, G. and Istvan, J. (1985) "Dietary sources of caffeine," *New England Journal of Medicine* 313:1421.

17. Lecos, Chris W. (1987–1988). "Caffeine jitters: Some safety questions remain," *FDA Consumer* 21:27.

18. Hanson, Glen & Peter Venturelli. (1995). *Drugs and Society*, 4th ed. (Boston: Jones and Bartlett Publishers), 291.

19. "Caffeine and health: International forum provides research update." (September/October 1993) *Food Insight*, 2.

20. National Institute of Nutrition in Canada. (1987). "Caffeine: A perspective on current concerns," *Nutrition Today* 22:38.

21. Grodstein, F., Goldman, M. B., Ryan, L., & Cramer, D. W. (1993). "Relation of female infertility to consumption of caffeinated beverages." *American Journal of Epidemiology* 137:1353–1360.

22. "Research notes: Caffeine," (1994). *Nutrition Week* XXIV:7.

23. "Research notes: Caffeine," (1993). *Nutrition Week* XXIII:7.

24. "Caffeine: Grounds for concern?" (1994). *UC Berkeley Wellness Letter* 10: 4.

25. "Caffeine: Grounds for concern?" 4; Caffeine and health: International forum provides research update. 2.

26. "Cocaine: The consequences of use," (1988). *Consumer Research*, 18–21.

27. National Institute on Drug Abuse (NIDA). (April, 1986). "Cocaine use in America," *Prevention Networks*, 5.

28. Bateman, D. A., Ng, S. K. C., Hansen, C. A., & Heagarty, M. C. (1993). "The effects of intrauterine cocaine exposure in newborns." *American Journal of Public Health* 83: 190–193.

29. NIDA, "Cocaine use in America," 5.

30. Office of Applied Studies. (1994) "1993 Household Survey: 'Good and bad news'." *SAMHSA News*, 6, 15.

31. "1992 emergency room visits for drug treatment increased by 10 percent." (1994). *Public Health Reports* 109: 145.

32. Ollwenstein, Lori. (1988). "The perils of pot," *Discover* 9: 18.

33. National Institute on Drug Abuse (NIDA). (August, 1986). "Marijuana," *NIDA Capsules*: 1.

34. NIDA, "Marijuana," 1.

35. Allen, W. A., Piccone, N. L., & D'Amanda, C. (1992). *How Drugs Can Affect Your Life*. (Springfield, IL: Charles C. Thomas Publisher), 56.

36. Abel, E. L. (1988). "Effects of marijuana on pregnancy," *Medical Aspects of Human Sexuality* 22: 39–40.

37. DHHS, (1987). "Marijuana and the Cannabinoids." *Drug Abuse and Drug Abuse Research* (Rockville, MD: National Institute on Drug Abuse), 79–80.

38. Abel, "Effects of marijuana on pregnancy," 40.

39. NIDA, "Marijuana," 3.

40. Fields, *Drugs and Alcohol in Perspective*, 114.

41. Office of Applied Studies, "1993 Household Survey: 'Good and bad news'," 6.

42. "1992 emergency room visits for drug treatment increased by 10 percent," 145.

43. "Drug use occupies emergency rooms, public opinion polls." (1994). *Public Health Reports* 109 (4): 586.

44. "Drug use occupies emergency rooms, public opinion polls," 586.

45. Hanson and Venturelli, *Drugs and Society*, 344.

46. Hanson and Venturelli, *Drugs and Society*, 344.

47. Johnston, L., O'Malley, P., & Bachman, J. (1993). *National Survey Results on Drug Use from Monitoring the Future Study*, Vol. 1. Washington, D.C.: National Institute on Drug Abuse.

48. Johnston, et al., National Survey Results on Drug Use from Monitoring the Future Study.

49. Ramotar, J. E. (1991). "Getting tougher on steroid abuse." *The Physician and Sports Medicine* 19: 46.

50. Fultz, O. (1991). Roid rage. *American Health* X: 63.

51. Taylor, W. N. (1987). Synthetic anabolic-androgenic steroids: A plea for controlled substance status. *The Physician and Sports Medicine* 15: 140–150.

52. Fultz, Roid rage, 62.

53. Fultz, Roid rage, 60, 63.

54. Romotar, Getting tough on steroid abuse.

55. McKim, W. A. (1986) *Drugs and Behavior: An Introduction to Behavioral Pharmacology* (Englewood Cliffs, N.J.: Prentice-Hall).

56. Smith, G. M. & Beecher, H. K. (1959). Amphetamine sulfate and athletic performance. *Journal of the American Medical Association* 170: 542–457.

57. Anderson, W. A., et al. (1991). A national survey of alcohol and drug use by college athletes. *The Physician and Sports Medicine* 19: 91–104.

58. Anderson, W. A., et al. A national survey of alcohol and drug use by college athletes.

59. Bell, J. A. & Doege, T. C. (1987). Athlete's use and abuse of drugs. *The Physician and Sports Medicine* 15: 99–108.

60. DHHS. (1993). *Signs of Effectiveness In Preventing Alcohol and Other Drug Problems*. (Washington, D.C.: U.S. Government Printing Office), 7.

61. Prendergast, M. L. (1994). "Substance use and abuse among college students: A review of recent literature." *Journal of American College Health*, 43: 99–113.

62. Office of Substance Abuse Prevention. (1989). *Prevention Plus II: Tools for Creating and Sustaining Drug-Free Communities*. (Rockville, Md.: National Clearinghouse for Alcohol and Drug Information), 29.

63. Wallack, L., Bread, W. & Cruz, J. (1987). Alcohol on prime time television. *Journal of Studies on Alcohol*, 48.

64. White, J. M. (1991). *Drug Dependence* (Englewood Cliffs, N.J.: Prentice-Hall), 200.

65. Office of Substance Abuse Prevention, *Prevention Plus II*, p. 11.

66. Duncan, D. F. & Gold, R. S. *Drugs and the Whole Person*, 216.

67. Addiction Research Foundation. (1979) *Information Review: General Information on Psychoactive Drugs and Pregnancy* (Toronto: Alcoholism and Drug Addiction Research Foundation), 20.

68. Hole, J. W. (1990). *Human Anatomy and Physiology* 5th ed. (Dubuque, Iowa: Wm. C. Brown Publishers).

Tobacco: Smoking and Smokeless Threats to Well-Being

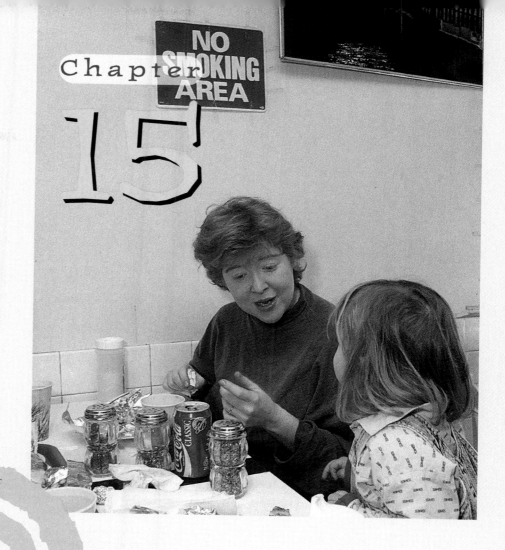

Chapter 15

Student Learning Objectives

Upon completion of this chapter you should be able to:

1. describe the history of tobacco use in the U.S.;

2. describe the variety of smokeless tobacco products;

3. describe the composition of tobacco smoke;

4. identify the risks associated with the ingredients in tobacco smoke;

5. distinguish among the risks associated with different forms of tobacco use;

6. analyze the relationship between level of tobacco consumption and disease risk;

7. identify factors associated with the decision to use tobacco;

8. identify examples of tobacco industry practices which target youth, women, and ethnic minorities in advertising and sales promotions;

9. give illustrations of how the tobacco industry presents its political agenda to promote tobacco use;

10. explain how people can promote regulation of tobacco use through legislative and other political action;

11. identify the benefits of tobacco use cessation as well as the difficulties associated with quitting.

For most people, the decision to begin smoking or to use other forms of tobacco is one that already has been made by the time one enters college. However, the decision to stop being a tobacco user is an important one still well within the grasp of current tobacco users. For nonusers, affirming the decision of being a lifetime nonuser of tobacco may be just as important. This chapter is about tobacco—its history, its use, the health compromising effects associated with its use, its regulation, and tips for cessation. Make no mistake about it; our posture on tobacco use is strongly negative. In taking this stance, we help you to look at some of the social, political, and psychological conditions that contribute to the initiation and maintenance of tobacco use. Since 1964, each Surgeon General of the United States has overseen the careful scientific investigation of tobacco. These reports have accumulated an enormous amount of evidence, and resulted in the production of a large body of literature that links tobacco use to coronary heart disease, lung cancer and other cancers, other forms of lung disease, complications associated with pregnancy, growth disorders, and other negative health consequences.[1] According to a World Health Organization estimate, of all people alive today in the world, 500 million will die from tobacco-related diseases.[2] In *Healthy People 2000,* numerous health-related objectives for the nation that relate to tobacco use have been established (see table 15.1).[3] Studies also have revealed the tobacco industry's deliberate suppression of relevant health data over a period of three decades.[4] Health consequences aside, there is no question but that tobacco has played a significant role historically in the U.S., and has made a remarkable social and economic impact on this nation and others around the globe. How did tobacco in its various forms get to be so much a part of society and culture, and become the basis for debate among public health authorities, smokers' and nonsmokers' rights groups, lobbyists for the tobacco industry, politicians, and others? The answer is found, in part, through a brief examination of U.S. history.

Snuff: a finely ground or powdered form of tobacco that is usually held or clenched in the mouth, or inhaled through the nose; a variety of smokeless or "spit" tobacco.

History of Tobacco Use in the U.S.

Native Americans may have been the first persons to use the various forms of **tobacco.** Consequently, its use in the New World was already established when Christopher Columbus and his sailors set foot on the North American continent. Europeans who settled in territories may have cultivated tobacco plants out of economic necessity. John Rolfe is credited for importing tobacco plants from Trinidad and Caracas in 1611 to save the Jamestown settlement from financial disaster. The imported plants flourished in the mild Virginia climate and, within two years, tobacco became one of the principal exports from the New World. Tobacco was soon in demand in England and elsewhere in Europe. The use of dry, powdered **snuff** became an activity associated with the British aristocracy. Tobacco "snuffing" was not as popular in the American colonies as tobacco chewing, perhaps because the colonials did not wish to be reminded of their British rulers. Tobacco became so valuable as a commodity that during the American revolution, George Washington appealed to his countrymen when supplies were scarce and morale was low, "I say, if you can't send money, send tobacco."[5]

During the nineteenth century and for the first two decades of the twentieth century, the predominant form of tobacco used in the U.S. was **smokeless tobacco** (also called "spit tobacco") and included chewing tobacco and snuff. Popularized by cowboys, farmers, lumberjacks, and other outdoorsmen who worked with their hands, smokeless tobacco was viewed as a convenient and rather harmless, if somewhat aesthetically unpleasant habit.

Even "refined" individuals such as lawyers, politicians, and other professional people dipped snuff or chewed tobacco. It was not uncommon to see women, especially in the South, use dry, powdered snuff. Some people considered the use of smokeless tobacco to be socially displeasing because of the need for the user to spit periodically. In homes and public buildings, spittoons were

TABLE 15.1   *Selected Healthy People 2000 Objectives for the Nation Related to Tobacco Use*

1. **Reduce cigarette smoking to a prevalence of no more than 15 percent among people aged 20 and older.** (Update: 27 percent in 1992, down from 29 percent in 1987.) (Special Target Populations: People with a high school education or less 20 years and over, Blue-collar workers 20 years and over, Military personnel, Blacks 20 years and over, Hispanics 20 years and over, American Indians/Alaska Natives, Southeast Asian males, Females of reproductive age [18–44 years], Pregnant females, Females who use oral contraceptives.)

2. **Reduce the initiation of cigarette smoking by children and youth so that no more than 15 percent have become regular cigarette smokers by age 20.** (Update: 28 percent of youth had become regular cigarette smokers by ages 20 through 24 in 1992, down from 30 percent in 1987.) (Special Target Population: Lower socioeconomic status people 20–24 years.)

3. **Increase to at least 50 percent the proportion of cigarette smokers aged 18 and older who stopped smoking cigarettes for at least one day during the preceding year.** (Update: In 1992, 37 percent of people who smoked in the preceding year stopped for at least one day during that year, up from 34 percent in 1986.)

4. **Increase smoking cessation during pregnancy so that at least 60 percent of women who are cigarette smokers at the time they become pregnant quit smoking early in the pregnancy and maintain abstinence for the remainder of their pregnancy.** (Update: 31 percent quit smoking during pregnancy in 1991, down from 39 percent in 1986.) (Special Target Population: Females with less than a high school education.)

5. **Reduce to no more than 20 percent the proportion of children aged 6 and younger who are regularly exposed to tobacco smoke at home.** (Baseline: more than 39 percent in 1986, as 39 percent of households with one or more children aged 6 or younger had a cigarette smoker in the household.)

6. **Reduce smokeless tobacco use by males aged 12 through 24 to a prevalence of no more than 4 percent.** (Update: 4.8 percent among males aged 12 through 17 in 1992, down from 6.6 percent in 1988; 8.2 percent among males aged 18 through 24 in 1992, down from 8.9 percent in 1988.) (Special Target Population: American Indian/Alaska Native people 18–24 years.)

7. **Establish tobacco-free environments and include tobacco use prevention in the curricula of all elementary, middle, and secondary schools, preferably as part of quality school health education.** (Baseline: 17 percent of school districts totally banned smoking on school premises or at school functions in 1988, antismoking education was provided by 78 percent of school districts at the high school level, 81 percent at the middle school level, and 75 percent at the elementary school level in 1988.)

8. **Increase to at least 75 percent the proportion of worksites with a formal smoking policy that prohibits or severely restricts smoking at the workplace.** (Update: 59 percent of worksites with 50 or more employees in 1992, up from 27 percent in 1985.)

9. **Enact in 50 states comprehensive laws on clean indoor air that prohibit or strictly limit smoking in the workplace and enclosed public places (including health-care facilities, schools, and public transportation).** (Update: 44 states and D.C. had laws restricting smoking in public places; 36 states restricted smoking in public workplaces; but only 16 states had comprehensive laws regulating smoking in private as well as public worksites and at least 4 public places, including restaurants, as of 1992, up from 42 percent, 31 percent, and 13 percent respectively in 1988.)

Source: Data from *Healthy People 2000 National Health Promotion and Disease Prevention Objectives,* 1991; and from *Healthy People 2000 Review 1993,* 1994. Department of Health and Human Services, Washington, D.C.

What Do You Think?

1. Indians of the New World introduced Spanish explorers to tobacco and smoking. From this simple beginning developed an activity that would have profound historic, economic, and medical consequences. If tobacco were just being introduced in the modern world, what do you think its legal status would be?

2. What factors do you think contributed to the popularity of tobacco in Europe and The Americas of the 17th century? Why do you think tobacco is still popular today?

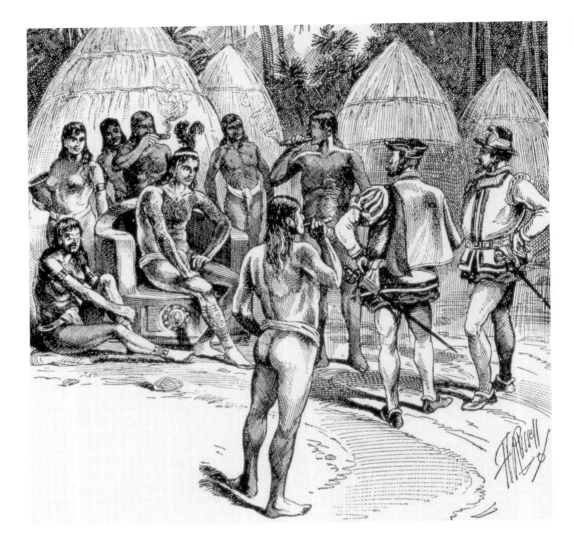

Tuberculosis (TB): an infectious bacterial disease characterized by inflammations, abscesses, calcification of tissue, and other symptoms, affecting the respiratory system and other sites.

common monuments to society's dippers and chewers. Dolly Madison was considered a fine hostess in the White House during the early nineteenth century because she made sure an ample supply of snuff was available. The Capitol in Washington, D.C., along with numerous other government buildings, had communal snuff boxes and cuspidors, many of which remained until nearly 1930. Indeed, a type of smokeless tobacco called "dental snuff" became known as a panacea for a variety of ills. According to some writers, "This form of snuff was said to relieve toothache, to cure neuralgia, scurvy, and bleeding gums, to preserve and whiten teeth, and to prevent decay. It claimed to be the only snuff produced that could be used without injuring the teeth."[6]

It was the need to expectorate, or spit, that eventually led to declining popularity of smokeless tobacco. Spitting was believed to be one of the mechanisms through which

tuberculosis (TB) and other deadly diseases of the day were spread. By the 1920s, cigarettes replaced smokeless tobacco as the predominant form of tobacco in the U.S., largely because it was thought to be a "safe" alternative. It was believed that rolling tobacco in a piece of thin paper and lighting it could not be a hazardous activity. Thus, one health menace declined in popularity but innocently gave rise to one with even greater lethal potential.

Smokeless Forms of Tobacco Consumption

Gregory N. Connolly points out that while cigarette smoking declined 24 percent between 1982 and 1991, the use of oral snuff, a form of "spit" tobacco, increased 60 percent.[7] In the second half of the 1980s, smokeless tobacco use increased 40 percent among college athletes.[8] The National

TABLE 15.2

Percentage of Smokeless Tobacco Users in Selected States and the District of Columbia

High Prevalence		Low Prevalence	
West Virginia	23.1	District of Columbia	0.0
Mississippi	16.5	New Jersey	0.1
Wyoming	15.7	Hawaii	0.2
Arkansas	14.7	Massachusetts	0.2
Montana	13.7	Connecticut	0.3
Kentucky	13.6	Maryland	0.4
Oklahoma	11.0	Rhode Island	0.5
Tennessee	10.3	New York	0.5
New Mexico	10.2	Delaware	0.6

Source: Data from USDHHS, PHS, *Smokeless Tobacco or Health,* NIH Publication No. 93–3461, Government Printing Office, Washington, D.C., 1993.

What Do You Think?

1. Do you notice a pattern in the states represented in the high and low prevalence columns? What factors do you think account for this difference?

2. If your state is not represented in the above list, find out about how many smokeless tobacco users there are. Which set of states is *your* state more similar to?

Collegiate Athletic Association (NCAA) reports that 57 percent of college baseball players use a form of "spit" tobacco.[9] James O. Mason of the U.S. Centers for Disease Control and Prevention reports that overall, smokeless tobacco prevalence in the eighteen to twenty-five age group declined from 12.3 percent in 1987 to 11.6 percent in 1990.[10] The *Healthy People 2000* objective is a prevalence of no more than 10 percent.

Nicotine levels in smokeless tobacco are more than twice those found in cigarettes, making these forms of tobacco cheap sources of nicotine. Smokeless tobacco also contains cancer-causing chemicals, including Polonium-210, benzopyrene, and **nitrosamines** at 20 thousand times the level allowed in food.[11]

Numerous undesirable health effects are now associated with smokeless tobacco use including **nicotine dependence;** pregnancy complications; decreased immunologic response; cancers of the oral cavity, pharynx, and pancreas; acute episodes of elevated blood pressure; recession of the gums; oral infection; and tooth loss—however, most concern is for oral cancer (see figure 15.1). One of the most frequent observations made by dental-health

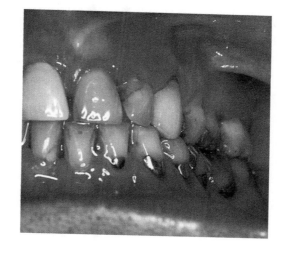

professionals in patients who use smokeless tobacco is the presence of white, patchy lesions, a condition known as **leukoplakia.**[12] These lesions result from irritation of the tissue in the mouth and almost always are associated with the specific area of the mouth where tobacco usually is placed. If the irritant is removed, the oral tissue generally heals itself within a few weeks. While causing pain and discomfort in the affected area, leukoplakia is not usually dangerous; however, these lesions

Figure 15.1: What Do You Think?

1. Consequences of smokeless tobacco use may include leukoplakia (white areas), tooth loss, erosion of the gums, and oral cancer. In light of such serious consequences, what do you think has contributed to the upswing in consumption of "spit" tobacco in the past ten to fifteen years?

2. What factors do you think explain the popularity of "spit" tobacco in some parts of the U.S. and not others, or among groups like athletes and males and not others?

Nicotine dependence: a physical and psychological need to continue using tobacco products containing nicotine.

Leukoplakia: white patchy lesions usually appearing on the mucous membranes of the mouth or on the tongue, considered in some cases to be a precursor to cancer.

Chapter 15: Tobacco: Smoking and Smokeless Threats to Well-Being

15–5

1. Smokeless tobacco products, such as
   (a) snuff and (b) chewing tobacco
   are unfortunately becoming
   increasingly popular among
   adolescents and young adults. How
   do snuff and chewing tobacco differ
   in appearance and use?
2. With what groups do you think snuff
   would be most popular? Which
   groups do you think would prefer
   chewing tobacco? What evidence do
   you base your opinion on?

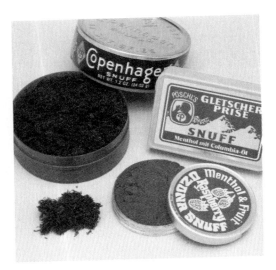

a.

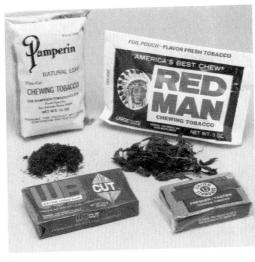

b.

do have the potential to transform into oral cancers. In one study, users of smokeless tobacco experienced eleven times the risk of developing cancers of the mouth and gum as nonusers of any tobacco product.[13]

It is clear that smokeless tobacco use presents threats to wellness, and that it is not a safe alternative to cigarette smoking. Although Public Law 99–252 banned smokeless tobacco advertising on broadcast media in 1986, and required warning labels to be placed on smokeless tobacco products in 1987, some health authorities are concerned that these steps are insufficient to cause users to break the smokeless tobacco habit completely.[14]

Snuff

Snuff comes in "dry" and "moist" varieties (see figure 15.2). The former is inhaled through the nose, where nicotine is absorbed through mucous membranes. It is this form of snuff that was popular among European aristocrats a century or two ago. In this country, its use today is rare outside of the South, where its popularity continues among older women in rural settings. On the other hand, moist snuff is the product primarily responsible for renewed interest in smokeless tobacco, particularly among adolescent and young adult males. One study of university students showed smokeless tobacco was used at least weekly by 14 percent of the males, most of them snuff dippers.[15] There are nearly as many brands of moist snuff as there are brands of cigarettes. Moist snuff packed in cachets, similar to tea bags, is a convenient

way that novice and occasional snuff dippers use this product. Whether in cachet or powdered form, moist snuff is placed in the side of the mouth between the cheek and gum or in the front of the mouth between the teeth and the lower lip. Moisture provided by saliva helps to release nicotine.

Chewing Tobacco

Chewing tobacco has been a tradition among some baseball players for many years, as well as being popular among older adult users of smokeless tobacco. Many youthful individuals have developed an interest in it too—often to emulate athletes, rodeo stars, country and western entertainers, and other people who use chewing tobacco. It typically comes packaged in loose-leaf, plug, or twist varieties. Most people do not actually "chew" these products. Instead, they clamp them between the teeth with just enough pressure to release the juices of the tobacco. As the juices are mixed with saliva in the mouth, nicotine and other constituents of tobacco are absorbed through the mucous membrane linings of the mouth.

Smoking Tobacco

Cigarettes, pipes, and cigars constitute the major methods of smoking tobacco. All of these methods involve the inhalation of hot smoke containing the principal products of combusted tobacco into the smoker's mouth and lungs where these products are absorbed. Most of the issues related to smoking and

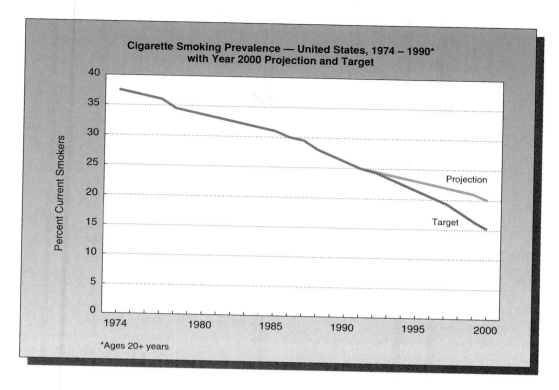

Cigarette Smoking Prevalence — United States, 1974 – 1990*
with Year 2000 Projection and Target

Projection

Target

*Ages 20+ years

Figure 15.3: What Do You Think?

1. What factors have contributed to the downward trend in cigarette smoking during the last 20 years?
2. The projection for year 2000 shows that the level of decline in smoking will not meet the year 2000 objective. What factors might allow the objective to be met early in the 21st century?

Source: Data from James O. Mason, *A Public Health Service Progress Report on Healthy People 2000-Tobacco*, 1992, Centers for Disease Control and Prevention, Atlanta, GA.

health discussed in this chapter are pertinent to all forms of smoking, regardless of mode; however, prospective epidemiologic studies show that persons who smoke only pipes and cigars have mortality rates higher than nonsmokers but lower than cigarette smokers.[16]

An unusual form of cigarette introduced to this country from Indonesia in the 1980s, the clove cigarette, has become popular among some people, particularly youth. Often bearing exotic names and giving off aromatic scents, clove cigarettes, or kreteks, consist of a blend of high **tar** and **nicotine** tobacco, clove oil, cocoa, caramel, and licorice. In addition to having most of the hazardous side effects of regular cigarettes, clove cigarettes can produce acute symptoms in the respiratory system that may even result in death. The combustion properties of some of the components of clove cigarettes have not been studied extensively, so individuals need to be especially cautious about their use, and it is advised to avoid any temptation to try them. Conventional cigarette smoking is the primary mode of tobacco consumption discussed throughout this chapter.

While the percentage of smokers has declined during the past twenty years (see figure 15.3), the percentage of smokers who are heavy smokers (twenty-five-plus cigarettes per day) actually has increased.

Thus, of people who smoke now, more are likely to be heavy smokers, perhaps because it is more difficult for a heavy smoker to quit. Because those who do smoke now are more likely to be heavy smokers, a nonsmoker today who spends a lot of time in the presence of a smoker is probably exposed to more smoke than someone who spent a great deal of time with a smoker thirty or more years ago.[17]

Composition of Tobacco Smoke

Tobacco is an important crop, both economically and agriculturally. Some types of tobacco are grown in almost every country in the world, and tobacco is used everywhere. The plant itself, *Nicotiana tabacum,* was originally found in the Americas. There are more than sixty-five species of tobacco, with variations in the chemical characteristics among species, types, varieties, strains, and grades.

Given these many differences among tobaccos, a lighted cigarette will generate over 4,000 known compounds.[18] The chemical constituents found in the atmosphere, however, are derived from two different sources—**mainstream smoke** and **sidestream smoke.** Mainstream smoke is produced when smoke is drawn through the tobacco during puffing; sidestream smoke

Tar: a thick, brown, sticky substance that forms from the particulate matter resulting from burning tobacco.

Nicotine: the active ingredient in tobacco with addictive potential that acts as a potent central nervous system stimulant.

Mainstream smoke: the smoke drawn into the lungs when a pipe, cigar, or cigarette is inhaled.

Sidestream smoke: smoke that rises from burning tobacco into the environment.

rises from the burning tobacco. We will compare mainstream and sidestream smoke later in this chapter.

Cigarette smoke contains a large number of chemical compounds, including gases, vapors, and small particles. When these particles are condensed, they form tars, which account for approximately 8 percent of the total volume of cigarette smoke. The remaining 92 percent comes from the gases and vapors in the smoke. These tars contain **carcinogens** (cancer-producing chemicals), **cocarcinogens** (substances that can combine with some others to produce cancer), and various other chemicals, such as nicotine, that are suspected to be dangerous in many ways.

According to Allen Vegotsky, at least four substances in cigarette smoke are known to be cancer causing[19] (see table 15.3).

Benzene has been tested carefully on rodents and shown to cause several kinds of leukemias and other cancers (see chapter 11). Similarly, 2-naphthylamine and 4-aminobiphenyl have been shown to produce human bladder cancers. *Polonium-210* is an element that emits alpha radiation. In heavy smokers the accumulation of this element in lung tissue is believed to contribute to the risk of lung cancer. It is speculated that exhaled smoke can contain some of these substances, making them a hazard to nonsmokers as well.

During puffing, temperatures in the burning cone of a cigarette reach 900 degrees centigrade, with some portions of the cone getting as hot as 1,050 degrees centigrade. It is at these temperatures that mainstream smoke (smoke inhaled directly through the cigarette, pipe, or cigar) is produced. Sidestream smoke (smoke from the burning tobacco that enters the environment) is generated when the tobacco smolders at temperatures as high as 800 degrees centigrade. It has been estimated that between 55 and 70 percent of the tobacco of a cigarette is burned between puffs and thus serves as a source for sidestream smoke and ash.[20]

The Coalition on Smoking OR Health reveals that the six major U.S. tobacco companies suppressed information on cigarette additives for more than thirty years.[21] The use of additives in tobacco products has been raised as a potential health concern by authorities over the years. The concern is of particular interest regarding low

tar and nicotine cigarettes whose flavor is chemically enhanced. Although many of the chemicals in question are approved for use in food, their safety when combusted and smoked is unknown. Although the tobacco manufacturers have identified 599 chemical additives used, the actual amounts and specific combinations used remains protected, thus making safety evaluations difficult.

There are many factors that influence the actual content of mainstream or sidestream smoke, including the types of filters used, ventilation, the tobacco variety, the agricultural practices followed in producing the tobacco, the processing methods used in the manufacture of tobacco products, and the nature of the additives combined with the tobacco products (e.g., **burning agents** and **flavoring agents**).[22] Added to this are the complicating factors associated with the type of smoker a person is. Some patterns of behavior alter the amount and content of the smoke puffed. There are several ways to characterize these behaviors including the type of cigarette smoked, the number of cigarettes smoked, the amount of cigarettes smoked, the number of puffs taken from a tobacco product, the depth of inhalation, and the length of inhalation. Each of these factors will ultimately influence the makeup of smoke. Because of this complexity, we will focus here on three major constituents of tobacco smoke and their associated disease risks: nicotine, tar, and carbon monoxide.

Nicotine

Although nicotine can be absorbed from tobacco smoke in the lungs, it can also be absorbed from the mouth cavity from either smoke or the juice of chewing tobacco or snuff. The person who smokes one pack of cigarettes a day takes an estimated 70,000 puffs a year. This frequency of drug ingestion is unmatched by any other type of drug taking.

Nicotine is just one of many substances found in tobacco, but most would agree that it is the most powerful pharmacologic agent in tobacco. Once absorbed, nicotine rapidly enters all major organ systems, tissues, and body fluids. The first effect of nicotine on the nervous system is stimulation, followed by a more lasting depression.[23] Some of the immediate effects of nicotine include increased heart rate and blood pressure, an increased amount of blood pumped by the

Burning agents: chemicals added to tobacco to ensure that the tobacco continues burning once lit. This ensures that a cigarette put down in an ashtray continues to burn.

Flavoring agents: chemicals added to tobacco to make the taste more palatable when a cigarette is smoked.

　　　　　Unit 4: Minimizing Negative Health–Related Behaviors

TABLE 15.3 — Chemicals Identified in Cigarette Smoke*

Constituent	Amount in Mainstream Smoke	Constituent	Amount in Mainstream Smoke
Carbon monoxide	10-23 mg	Anatabine	2-20 µg
Carbon dioxide	20-40 mg	Phenol	60-140 µg
Carbonyl sulfide	12-42 µg	Catechol	100-360 µg
Benezene	12-48 µg	Hydroquinone	110-300 µg
Toluene	100-200 µg	Aniline	360 ng
Formaldehyde	70-100 µg	2-toluidine	160 ng
Acrolein	60-100 µg	2-naphthylamine	1.7 ng
Acetone	100-250 µg	4-aminobiphenyl	4.6 ng
Pyridine	16-40 µg	Benz[a]anthracene	20-70 ng
3-methylpyridine	12-36 µg	Benzo[a]pyrene	20-40 ng
3-vinylpyridine	11-30 µg	Cholesterol	22 µg
Hydrogen cyanide	400-500 µg	γ-butyrolactone	10-22 µg
Hydrazine	32 ng	Quinoline	0.5-2 µg
Ammonia	50-130 µg	Harman	1.7-3.1 µg
Methylamine	11.5-28.7 µg	N-nitrosonornicotine	200-3000 ng
Dimethylamine	7.8-10 µg	NNK	100-1000 ng
Nitrogen oxides	100-600 µg	N-nitrosodiethanolamine	20-70 ng
N-nitrosodimethylamine	10-40 ng	Cadmium	110 ng
N-nitrosodiethylamine	≤25 ng	Nickel	20-80 ng
N-nitrosopyrrolidine	6-30 ng	Zinc	60 ng
Formic acid	210-490 µg	Polonium-210	0.04-0.1 pCi
Acetic acid	330-810 µg	Benzoic acid	14-28 µg
Methyl chloride	150-600 µg	Lactic acid	63-174 µg
1,3-butadiene	69.2 µg	Glycolic acid	37-126 µg
Particulate matter	15-40 mg	Succinic acid	110-140 µg
Nicotine	1.0-2.5 mg	PCDDs and PCDFs	1 pg

*This table is taken from a 1992 EPA report entitled "Respiratory Health Effects of Passive Smoking: Lung Cancer and Other Disorders."

Source: Data from Allen Vergotsky "What the Cigarette Makers Sell" in *World Smoking and Health*, 18.1, 1993, 8–9. U.S. Environmental Protection Agency.

What Do You Think?

1. Which of these substances have you heard of? Do you know what their typical uses are?
2. If food products contained even miniscule levels of some of these substances, there would be a loud protest. Why are people so passive about these substances when they are produced from cigarette smoke?

heart each minute, increased oxygen consumption and coronary blood flow, increased **arrhythmias,** constriction of peripheral blood vessels and bronchial tubes, and increased respiration. In addition nicotine rapidly crosses the placental barrier, causing a number of related effects on the **fetus** during pregnancy, and can be found in the milk of lactating women.[24]

Nicotine is quickly absorbed from the lungs, mouth cavity, or stomach. After absorption, nicotine is metabolized very rapidly in the liver. The half-life of nicotine in the human body is approximately thirty minutes; this might explain why regular smokers seek to replenish the levels of nicotine in their bodies about every half hour when they are awake.[25]

Arrhythmia: any heart beat that is a departure from normal, healthy heart rhythm.

Fetus: the medical term for an embryo that has developed for at least eight weeks.

TABLE 15.4 — Percentage of People in the U.S. Age 18 and Over Who Smoke

	Men	Women
All races	27.5	23.0
African-Americans	32.9	23.2
White Americans	27.0	23.3
Hispanic Americans	25.6	13.4

Source: Data from USDHHS, PHS, *Strategies to Control Tobacco Use in the United States: A Blueprint for Public Health Action in the 1990s*, NIH Publication No. 93–3316, Government Printing Office, Washington, D.C., 1992.

What Do You Think?

1. Although more adult men than adult women smoke, the size of the gap between men and women smokers has narrowed in the past 30 years. What do you think accounts for this narrowing?

2. There seems to be an interactive effect between race and sex. What factors do you think affect this relationship?

It is possible for smokers to experience **nicotine poisoning.** In fact, most people do experience some form of nicotine poisoning when they first begin to smoke or when they smoke too much. Nicotine poisoning causes dizziness, faintness, rapid pulse, cold clammy skin, nausea, and occasionally vomiting and diarrhea. As smokers develop a tolerance to nicotine, these symptoms diminish. In severe cases, however, tremors can occur, followed by convulsions and death. It appears certain that nicotine is the major active agent in tobacco that causes its addiction potential.

A Food and Drug Administration (FDA) panel concluded in 1994 that the amounts of nicotine found in cigarettes on the market then could addict the "typical smoker."[26] The tobacco industry always has denied that cigarette smoking is addictive. Moreover, industry spokespersons have argued that people in the U.S. have the freedom of choice as to whether they smoke or not. If the cigarette is indeed shown to be a "drug delivery system" that in time takes away individual "choice," then the FDA can regulate the amount of nicotine or other drugs in cigarettes.

Tar

Tobacco smoke is composed of gases, vapors, and particles of material; it is these particles that we call tar. Tar is defined as the total of the particulate matter found in smoke, other than moisture and nicotine (see figure 15.4).

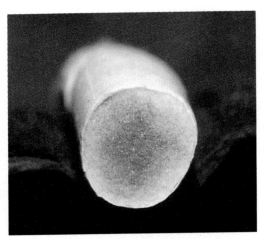

Figure 15.4: What Do You Think?

1. Tar from the smoke of cigarettes, easily seen in this photograph, is believed by scientists to be capable of initiating and promoting tumor growth. What problems occur among people who select low-tar cigarettes to smoke? In what respect is this situation often counterproductive?

2. What evidence exists that relate high tar content to tumor growth?

The tar content of cigarettes varies among brands, and each year the Federal Trade Commission determines and publishes levels for both tars and nicotine in various brands. These two substances, tars and nicotine, exhibit a high degree of association; therefore, the specific effects that each has on the human body is somewhat unclear. As with nicotine, tars are produced by burning tobacco.

The particulate matter found in tobacco smoke has been clearly shown to be related to

- Cancer of the lung
- Chronic obstructive lung diseases (emphysema, chronic bronchitis)
- Cancer of the larynx
- Cancer of the oral cavity
- Cancer of the esophagus
- Ischemic heart disease
- Cancer of the bladder
- Cancer of the pancreas

- Aortic aneurysm
- Ulcers of the stomach and duodenum
- Intrauterine growth retardation
- Low-birth-weight babies
- Unsuccessful pregnancies
- Infant mortality
- Cancer of the kidney
- Cancer of the stomach
- Cerebrovascular disease

What Do You Think?

1. If tobacco were just being introduced to consumers today, do you think it would pass government safety standards? Why or why not?
2. Most people have at least an idea about the risk of lung cancer and heart disease associated with cigarette smoking. What can you do to make people aware of the wider array of health-related issues?

---

increased morbidity. Several mechanisms explain how tars are related to morbidity. Tars have been established as carcinogens or **tumor initiators** in a variety of sites in the human body, particularly the esophagus, the lungs, the pancreas, and the kidney and bladder. At the same time, they are also considered **tumor promoters** in that they help maintain the process of tumor formation when the process has already been established by some other mechanism. Finally, some tars have been shown to be cocarcinogens. That is, the tars cannot by themselves initiate the growth of a tumor, but when combined with other substances that are also cocarcinogens, they can cause tumor growth.

Carbon Monoxide

Other than nicotine, it appears that **carbon monoxide** (CO) from tobacco smoke causes the most noticeable physiological effects. In doses of 10,000 to 50,000 parts per million (approximately 1 to 5 percent of the smoke), CO interferes with the ability of hemoglobin in the blood to carry oxygen. At the same time, CO may also have some ability to impair normal functioning of the nervous system. The CO found in tobacco smoke probably has both acute and chronic effects on the smoker. There is some evidence that the CO levels in smoke are in part responsible for increasing the risk of **heart attack** and **stroke,** and that together with nicotine they increase the risks of all cardiovascular diseases. There are some who believe that CO may contribute to the risk of developing dependence on tobacco; however, there is little evidence to support this view.

Risks Associated with Tobacco

Use of tobacco is associated with risks of both death (mortality) and disease (morbidity).

Mortality Risks

According to former Surgeon General C. E. Koop, "Cigarette smoking is the chief, single, avoidable cause of death in our society, and the most important health issue of our time."[27] Cigarette smoking is a major cause of coronary heart disease in the U.S. for men and women. Overall, cigarette smokers have a 70 percent higher death rate from coronary heart disease than nonsmokers. Cigarette smoking also is associated with stroke, particularly in younger age groups. Smoking acts synergistically with other coronary heart disease risk factors to compound an individual's risk. Compared to nonsmokers, a male smoker between the ages of thirty and forty who smokes forty or more cigarettes per day loses an average of eight years of life. Young men may be at more risk from the

Carbon monoxide: an odorless, colorless gas (CO) with lethal potential that is a byproduct of combustion.

Heart attack: death or impairment of cells of the heart muscle as a result of obstructed blood flow.

Stroke: sudden loss of orientation or consciousness, sensation, or voluntary motion as a result of the rupture or obstruction of an artery in the brain; sometimes called a "cerebrovascular accident" (CVA).

What Do You Think?

1. What does a fetus "inhale" when his or her mother smokes?
2. What are the consequences of maternal smoking on the health of the fetus and the newborn?
3. How are the effects on the fetus of a woman who smokes analogous to the effects on nonsmokers who share space with smokers?

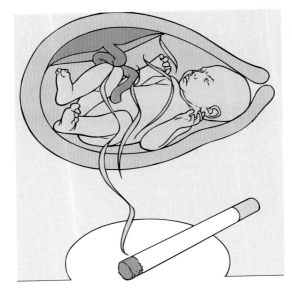

synergistic action of cigarette smoking with another risk behavior, excessive alcohol consumption, than other groups.

Cigarette smoking is causally linked to cancers of the lung, larynx, oral cavity, and esophagus in men and women.[28] Smoking is the major cause of **chronic obstructive lung disease** (COLD) in the U.S. for men and women.

Heavy smokers may face a risk of COLD thirty times that of nonsmokers. Death from COLD generally occurs after an extended episode of illness and disability, with high costs in terms of medical care, lost wages, and premature mortality.

On the average, mortality rates for women who smoke are 1.2 to 1.3 times higher than those for nonsmoking women. Women who smoke forty or more cigarettes per day have a mortality rate 1.63 times that of nonsmoking women. Smoking accounts for about 25 percent of all cancer deaths in women. The risk of heart attack in women who smoke and use oral contraceptives may be increased by a factor of ten. The risk of stroke also may be enhanced.

The overall mortality rate for smokers is actually highest at younger ages and declines slightly with age. This is a relative effect, because death rates from other causes increase significantly as we age. The actual number of excess deaths directly attributable to smoking increases with age for both men and women. Mortality for smokers (for all causes of death) is related to several specific factors for both men and women: (1) the longer a person has smoked, the higher the mortality ratios;

(2) the earlier in life a person started smoking, the higher the mortality ratios; (3) the more someone inhales with each puff, the greater the mortality ratios; and (4) the higher the levels of tar and nicotine in the tobacco smoked, the higher the mortality ratios. Keep in mind, however, that even those who smoke low-tar and low-nicotine cigarettes (less than 1.2 milligrams nicotine and less than 17.6 milligrams tar) have mortality rates more than 50 percent higher than their nonsmoking counterparts.

The *overall* mortality rates of ex-smokers decline with the number of years since smoking.[29] By the time someone has been an ex-smoker for fifteen years, the overall mortality ratio is comparable to someone who has never smoked. Regardless of how long, how much, or what brand a person has smoked, quitting smoking reduces the associated disease risks unless the person is already ill when smoking is stopped.

Morbidity Risks

Regarding morbidity (i.e., development of disease), the risks from smoking tobacco appear to be comparable for both men and women given similar exposure to smoke. Smokers tend to report both more acute and more chronic conditions than those who have never smoked. Specific examples include chronic bronchitis, emphysema, chronic sinusitis, peptic ulcer diseases, influenza, and arteriosclerotic heart disease. There is a strong relationship between the amount smoked and the likelihood of reporting such acute or chronic conditions. The longer an individual has smoked, the higher the tar and nicotine content of the cigarettes smoked, and the more smoke inhaled, the higher the rate of illness.

In a special report by the Surgeon General on the health consequences of smoking for women, some additional problems associated with women's smoking were identified. Babies born to women who smoked during pregnancy are, on the average, 200 grams lighter than babies born to comparable nonsmoking women. The risk of a low-birth-weight (LBW) baby for a light smoker (twenty cigarettes or fewer/day) is increased 53 percent; for a heavier smoker (twenty-one plus cigarettes/day), it is increased 130 percent. Smoking has been found to result in fetal growth retardation manifested as a decrease in body length, chest

Chronic obstructive lung disease (COLD): a category of lung disease characterized by decreased ability of the lungs to perform gas exchanges. Emphysema and chronic bronchitis are common examples.

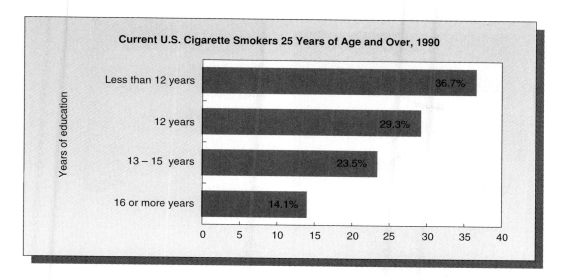

Current U.S. Cigarette Smokers 25 Years of Age and Over, 1990

Years of education:
- Less than 12 years: 36.7%
- 12 years: 29.3%
- 13 – 15 years: 23.5%
- 16 or more years: 14.1%

circumference, and head circumference. The risks of spontaneous abortion, **fetal death,** and **neonatal death** all increase as maternal smoking increases during pregnancy. Up to 14 percent of preterm births are probably due to maternal smoking. Additional studies suggest that smoking by women may impair their fertility.[30] Women who smoke a mean of one pack of cigarettes per day during adulthood will, by menopause, have an average deficit of 5 to 10 percent in bone density, sufficient to predispose them to the brittle bone disorder of osteoporosis[31] (see chapter 18).

An infant's risk of developing **sudden infant death syndrome** is increased with maternal smoking during pregnancy.[32] Additionally, infants and children born to smoking mothers may experience more long-term morbidity than those born to nonsmoking mothers.

Personal and Social Barriers to a Smoke-Free Lifestyle

Approximately 95 percent of adults in the U.S. are aware that smoking increases their chances of getting lung cancer; 88 percent know of the relationship between smoking and cancer of the larynx; 80 percent believe that smoking increases the chance of getting esophageal cancer; and 35 percent are aware that smoking enhances the risk of developing bladder cancer.[33] This does not, however, necessarily translate into nonsmoking behavior. There are many factors to be considered when trying to understand

smoking behavior. Such factors influence the likelihood of starting to smoke, of continuing once started, and of ceasing. Smokers differ in their choices of cigarettes (e.g., low versus high tar and nicotine content), the number of cigarettes smoked (which may range from none to a high of about 100 cigarettes per day), the amount of the cigarette smoked (some people only smoke the first few millimeters of a cigarette while others smoke a cigarette down to the butt end), the number of puffs taken from each cigarette (ranging from one or two to a high of about twenty per cigarette), the depth of inhalation (from the noninhaler to the deep inhaler), and the length of inhalation. Given all of these differences, someone who smokes only ten cigarettes a day could absorb more nicotine, tars, and carbon monoxide than someone who smokes two or three times that amount. Many factors influence a smoker's decisions and habits.

Advertising and the Media

Tobacco retailers spend $4 billion dollars advertising and promoting tobacco use in the U.S. and in other countries.[34] Recently, much of this cigarette advertising has been directed specifically at women, demonstrating such themes as the emancipation of women, romantic love, and the independent single woman. Research indicates that most female smokers have a positive impression of the individuals pictured in these advertisements. Females surveyed who smoke view these images of women in advertisements as attractive (69 percent), enjoying themselves (66 percent), well dressed (66 percent), sexy

Neonatal death: the death of an infant during the first six weeks after birth.

Sudden infant death syndrome (SIDS): the death of a baby from unidentifiable causes. Also known as crib death because the death often occurs at night in a crib.

What Do You Think?

1. Are images always what they seem to be? Does smoking make one "sexier," more "glamorous," or more "at ease?" How much of smoking is initiated or maintained as a consequence of image? Who shapes this image?
2. How does one produce and promote counter images that reflect success, life enjoyment, and glamour associated with nonsmoking?

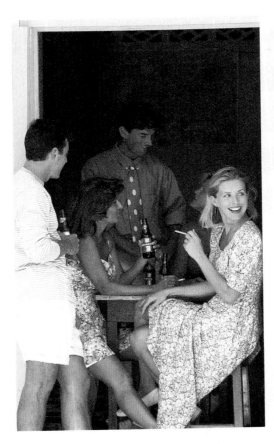

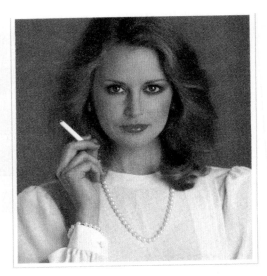

HOW CAN WE REACH YOU?

What Do You Think?

1. Smoking often is depicted as an activity that enhances a woman's glamour, sophistication, and sex appeal. Prevention and cessation efforts are now aimed specifically at women too. Does this antismoking ad have appeal or does it fail to reach out effectively to women who smoke? Explain your reasoning.
2. Since health-promotion campaigns rarely can compete dollar-for-dollar with tobacco advertising, what strategies might enjoy success among college-aged men and women and other adults?

(54 percent), young (50 percent), and healthy (49 percent).[35] The Surgeon General's report stated that:[36] (1) advertisers have been successful in creating a sense of mystery, sophistication, and power around the behavior of smoking; (2) although smoking was once frowned upon for women, people now respond less negatively to a woman smoking; and (3) there is evidence that, for some women, smoking is linked with attitudes and behaviors that comprise a socially valued and successful self-image, and that giving up smoking is a threat to that image.

Although the general argument that advertising influences tobacco use seems compelling, there is still some controversy in a number of areas. There is little empirical research to substantiate the claims that prosmoking advertising increases use or that antismoking advertising decreases use.

On the other hand, Kenneth Warner has suggested that the reduction in media advertising coupled with the antismoking advertising seen in some media may have prevented even greater increases in consumption of tobacco products than we have seen.[37] Others seem to agree that recent reductions in cigarette consumption can be attributed to antismoking ads on television.[38] In any case, the reduction in advertising in the media has been coupled with an increase in advertising at the point of sale, and the specific influence of either change is difficult to determine by itself.

The cigarette industry has stated that the major effect of cigarette advertising appears to be to shift brand preferences rather than to influence decisions whether or not to smoke. It seems clear that advertising does exert some influence on decisions regarding use of tobacco products, as a study of teen smokers found that at least 84 percent who purchase their own cigarettes choose one of the three most heavily advertised brands—Camel, Marlboro, or Newport.[39] Such brand preferences appear to be more tightly concentrated in adolescent smokers than in adult smokers.

Peer Influence

Perhaps the most important determinant of smoking behavior is the number of friends who smoke. This relationship, however, is strongest at younger ages and seems to diminish with age. Peer influence seems only to work when an adolescent belongs to or would like to belong to a group in which smoking is part of the lifestyle. When the peer-group behavior does not include smoking, there may be little pressure on the adolescent to begin to smoke.

These data suggest the importance of peer pressure and conformity in determining whether adolescents will begin smoking. Some studies, however, indicate that adolescents overestimate the number of their peers who smoke. If smoking were considered a behavior to emulate, these overestimates might increase the numbers who actually begin smoking.

Parental Smoking Habits

Parental behavior can have strong influences on the behavior of children—and smoking behavior is one of those areas in which clear empirical evidence of parental influence exists. In families where both parents smoke, 22.2 percent of boys and 20.7 percent of girls also become smokers. In families where neither parent smokes, those rates are reduced to 11.3 percent in boys and 7.6 percent in girls. It appears that parental smoking behavior is the second-best predictor of smoking among junior high and high school students, following the number of friends who smoke.

Government Support

A major barrier to control of tobacco-related disorders is the continuation of government incentives for farmers to produce tobacco. Most tobacco production in the U.S. has been under a federal price support production control program since the early 1930s. Price support is available to eligible tobacco

growers through government loans. To receive support, tobacco growers must certify that their pesticides have been approved by the Environmental Protection Agency and that they have been used in accordance with the label. As long as the government subsidizes cultivation of tobacco, profits for farmers are possible. The economics of several states that grow tobacco as a cash crop are dependent on continued tobacco production, and legislators from these states provide a powerful lobby in Congress. From strictly a health point of view, price supports represent an economic paradox for the government. On the one hand, federal appropriations support numerous health-promotion and disease-prevention efforts. On the other hand, the financial support of tobacco-use prevention programs is meager in comparison to the economic incentives to grow tobacco.

Tobacco and Special Populations

Tobacco use by African-Americans is responsible for nearly 48,000 deaths each year in the United States.[40] The tobacco industry has targeted the African-American community through advertising and promotion, especially in urban, inner-city areas. African-Americans experience more tobacco-related diseases than Whites, and a greater loss of productive years of life.[41]

Tobacco use among Hispanic Americans is less well-documented, but there is reason to believe that it may be increasing from its traditional low levels, especially among Mexican Americans.[42] Studies document a rising lung cancer rate among Hispanic men.[43]

Tobacco advertising has been one of the economic support forces backing publications prepared primarily for distribution to African-Americans. While tobacco advertisements accounted for 6.1 percent of the advertising in 166 consumer magazines in a recent year, it accounted for 10.2, 9.2, and 7.5 percent respectively in three leading African-American-targeted magazines—*Jet, Essence,* and *Ebony*.[44] Similarly, the tobacco industry successfully markets to African-Americans, Hispanics, and Native Americans by sponsoring entertainment, sports, and cultural events. What appears to be a philanthropic activity to promote and celebrate ethnic heritage and cultural diversity has another side to it—one that introduces youthful members of minority communities to health-compromising

1. Cigarette advertising, and the nature of its influence, are controversial issues. Some evidence suggests advertisers are making specific efforts to recruit smokers from ethnic minority groups (note this ad in Spanish). Why do you think the tobacco advertisers segment their audience, targeting their campaigns with specific types of appeals aimed at women, Hispanics, African-Americans, people of generation X, and so on?
2. Do you think that cigarette advertising causes people to begin smoking, or does it only influence people to change brands?

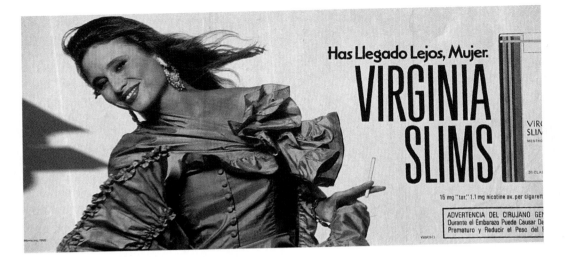

practices.[45] A future challenge for leaders of ethnic minority groups is to achieve their empowerment goals with less risk for the people they try to serve. All Americans can play an important role in this endeavor.

Personal Self-Assessment

Many factors determine who is most likely to become, or continue to be, a tobacco user. Many studies have attempted to determine how many different types of smokers there are.

Although each smoker's habit is unique, the Smokers Self-Test has six categories of smokers, including:[46]

1. *Crutch:* This group uses smoking as a means to reduce tension in their lives. Approximately 30 percent of all smokers fall into this category.
2. *Craving:* These smokers have a psychological dependence upon smoking, and may have some difficulty in quitting if they want to. About 25 percent of smokers are in this group.
3. *Pleasurable relaxation:* Those who fall into this category smoke as a way to relax and enjoy a pleasurable experience. If this smoker is able to identify a satisfactory substitute, there is some indication of a high degree of ability to stop smoking. This group accounts for 15 percent of all smokers.
4. *Habit:* For this group, smoking is done without thought—it becomes an automatic behavior. About 10 percent of regular smokers fall into this category.

5. *Stimulation:* Those who smoke because smoking is stimulating make up approximately 10 percent of smokers.
6. *Handling:* Those for whom the process of smoking is the most important issue account for about 10 percent of smokers.

How the Industry Fights Against Tobacco Regulation

During the 1990s, regulatory efforts at the state and national level have succeeded to some extent in controlling tobacco access and restricting tobacco use to specific areas. The most effective tobacco control strategies probably have arisen at the local level, often as a result of actions by citizen groups.

Previously, the tobacco industry's primary weapon against tobacco control was the grass-roots organization of smokers to fight off regulation. In what has become nothing short of a war between the industry officials and their lobbyists on one side, and health authorities and consumer groups on the other, tobacco companies have moved well beyond "smoker organizing." Michael P. Traynor, Michael E. Begay and Stanton A. Glantz report that the tobacco industry has adopted an aggressive and sophisticated set of strategies to impede further regulation.[47] Among these strategies include:

- Monitoring local government activity by hiring public affairs firms.
- Providing organizational and directional assistance by using "front groups" to defeat local control efforts because of the industry's own low credibility.

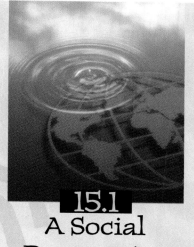

Tobacco Prevention and Control Strategies in the 1990s

Decades of research have documented the health problems associated with tobacco use. Tobacco use, especially cigarette smoking, has been described as the single most important contributing factor to death and disease in the United States. David Satcher and Michael Eriksen write: ". . . we [as a society] are plagued by an entirely preventable problem, and this is the paradox of tobacco control."

Prevention and control efforts may be described in the following categories:

- prevention of the initiation of tobacco use
- treatment of nicotine addiction
- protection of nonsmokers from environmental tobacco smoke
- promotion of nonsmoking messages
- restricting tobacco advertising
- increasing the price of tobacco products
- regulation of tobacco products

Sources: Data from J. Michael McGinnis and William H. Foege, "Actual Causes of Death in the United States" in *Journal of the American Medical Association,* 270 (1993): 2207–2212; David Satcher and Michael Eriksen, "The Paradox of Tobacco Control" in *Journal of the American Medical Association,* 271 (1994): 627–628.

What Do You Think?

1. To what extent can a college student such as yourself become involved in tobacco-control efforts? Which of the above strategies best apply to your own capabilities?
2. Which of the above strategies would be most effective in curtailing tobacco use (a) among college students? and (b) among other population groups by age, sex, and race?

- Supporting referendum petition drives to pass favorable legislation, defeat unfavorable bills, and get issues on the ballot that can be repeated.
- Using election campaigns to endorse and assist candidates who see government regulation of tobacco as the development of unneeded bureaucracy, the waste of taxpayer money, and the creation of unenforceable laws, or ones requiring a special "cigarette police."

The industry plays on people's negative emotions about government control. It calls to mind the era of alcohol prohibition. It points out the expense of government-sponsored programs. It conjures up a sense of laws unnecessarily restricting individual freedoms. Finally, the industry argues that curtailed tobacco consumption hurts farming revenues, diminishes jobs for workers, and depletes funds from government coffers.

Striking Back at the Tobacco Industry

Several tobacco regulatory control measures have been enacted in recent years. Most of these initiatives have one or more of the following features.

Clean indoor air bills prohibit smoking in public places except in specifically designated areas. These laws vary by state. Florida, for instance, requires that restaurants with fifty or more seats designate and post at least 35 percent of the seating area as nonsmoking.[48] Some locales prohibit indoor smoking in *all* public buildings, hospitals, schools, and other establishments.

Child access bills restrict sales to minors. Some laws license tobacco retailers and limit the placement of vending machines to within view of salespersons. Sales to minors laws can be enforced and punished with severe penalty. Some money from fines may be earmarked for prevention education.

Excise taxes raise revenue for local and state treasuries. The per pack federal excise tax on cigarettes in the U.S. is $.46, although during the Clinton Administration a $2.00 excise tax increase was advocated. Most states have enacted their own excise taxes on tobacco in addition to the federal tax (see figure 15.5). Tobacco industry supporters argue that additional excise taxes are regressive and hurt lower socioeconomic groups, especially minorities. Citing Coalition on Smoking OR Health estimates,

TABLE 15.6

Relationship of Proposed Cigarette Price Increases to Smokers' Self-Reported Intentions to Quit

Price per pack	Percentage of smokers reporting they would quit
$7+	91
$6	88
$5	84
$4	78
$3	64

Source: Data from Gallup Poll for SmithKline Beacham, *USA Today,* July 8, 1994, A1.

What Do You Think?

1. To what extent do you think price influences smokers' decisions to purchase cigarettes? On whom would it have the greater effect—new smokers or longtime smokers? What is the rationale for your answer?
2. How much confidence should one have in polls that ask hypothetical questions? Do the above figures represent *overestimates* or *underestimates* of what would happen if such price hikes occurred? What factors besides price determine the decision to quit smoking?

Lynne D. Richardson contradicts the argument, indicating that a $2.00 tax increase would be supported by 66 percent of Whites, 63 percent of African-Americans, and 71 percent of Hispanic Americans.[49] Furthermore, implementing an excise tax of this magnitude could reduce the number of smokers by 7.6 million, save 1.9 million lives, and bring $25 billion in revenue.[50] Former Surgeon General Antonia C. Novello indicates that for every 10 percent increase in the overall cost of cigarettes, there will be a corresponding 4 percent decline in the prevalence of smoking.[51]

In 1994 the Florida Legislature passed a bill authorizing the state to sue cigarette manufacturers for $300 million per year in Medicaid expenses to garner reimbursement for smoking related illnesses.[52] Tobacco companies previously have paid no damages for health claims made against them, so enforcement of this pioneering legislation could make the industry's financial liability virtually automatic. Other states may follow the Florida example, and some U.S. senators contemplate a similar action at the federal level.

The tobacco industry argues that tobacco plays a critical role in a community's economic well-being. The industry attempts to convince legislators, journalists, and the public-at-large that tobacco generates employment and important tax revenues. Economists Kenneth E. Warner and George A. Fulton projected the economic impact on the state of Michigan with and without the sale of tobacco products between the years 1992 and 2005.[53] They concluded that economic and health indicators would make more positive gains in that state in the absence of tobacco sales, thus refuting one of the longstanding tobacco lobby arguments.[54]

Thomas P. Houston, proposes a four-point plan for tobacco control in the United States:[55]

- Increase the federal excise tax on cigarettes by $2.00 per pack.
- Enable regulatory agencies to assume jurisdiction over tobacco products. Thus, the FDA would regulate "drugs" in tobacco; the Federal Trade Commission (FTC), charged with addressing "unfair and deceptive advertising," would investigate advertising claims (see chapter 17); and the U.S. Department of Justice would enforce the ban on televised cigarette advertising currently being broken by tobacco industry sports promotions.
- Protect the public, especially children, from environmental tobacco smoke (ETS) exposure.
- Restrict the tobacco industry's advertising and promotional campaigns that portray smoking as healthy and sexy, and that provide free samples, have gimmicky logo items, use cartoon figures, and target special populations such as children, women, and ethnic minorities.

Medicaid: a federally-sponsored program of health insurance that was established to assist the economically disadvantaged.

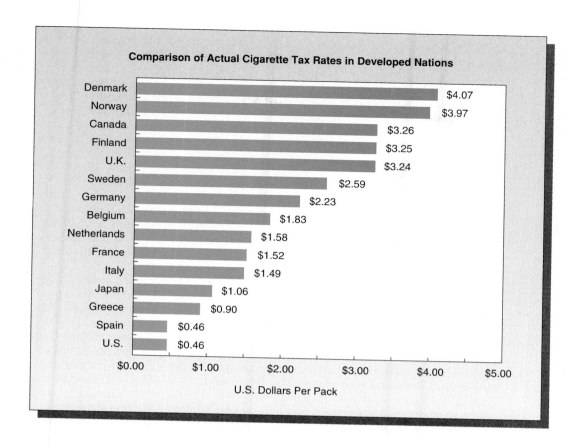

Comparison of Actual Cigarette Tax Rates in Developed Nations

Nation	U.S. Dollars Per Pack
Denmark	$4.07
Norway	$3.97
Canada	$3.26
Finland	$3.25
U.K.	$3.24
Sweden	$2.59
Germany	$2.23
Belgium	$1.83
Netherlands	$1.58
France	$1.52
Italy	$1.49
Japan	$1.06
Greece	$0.90
Spain	$0.46
U.S.	$0.46

Figure 15.5: What Do You Think?

1. What factors are at work that maintain a U.S. cigarette tax rate that is the lowest among industrialized nations of the world?
2. How much money does it cost to be a pack-a-day smoker in the U.S. versus Germany or Denmark? Is life expectancy greater in many of these industrialized nations than in the U.S.? What is the level of cigarette consumption in some of these nations?

From *Tobacco-Free Florida Plan 1994–1995*, Coalition on Smoking OR Health, Washington, D.C.

Former Surgeon General, Antonia Novello, writes that the tobacco industry profited $221 million in a recent year from illegal sales of tobacco to children.[56] Gregory N. Connolly argues that increases in tobacco excise taxes must also apply to smokeless tobacco products, since these tobacco forms are popular in so many places, especially among young adults (see table 15.2).[57]

Quitting Smoking

This section is designed for smokers who want to quit smoking and for nonsmokers who are interested in helping others to quit.

Some Concerns

Smokers vary in terms of the age when they began smoking, the length of time they have been smoking, whether or not they inhale, their choice of cigarette, how much of each cigarette they actually smoke, and how many cigarettes they smoke each day. There are also differences in the motivations of smokers to continue smoking or quit. Because of these differences, there is no single technique for quitting or for long-term maintenance of cessation. Methods that are effective for some smokers may not be useful for others. Some smokers are successful regardless of the technique used, while others are unable to stop smoking with any method. A more realistic approach for the latter group is reduction of smoking, or preparation for cessation.

Arden G. Christen and Kenneth H. Cooper raise several important questions regarding smoking: "(1) In light of the well-known, thoroughly publicized health hazards of smoking, why does this habit continue to have such widespread appeal? (2) Why is it so difficult for many persons to quit smoking once having become habituated? (3) Can a person really do anything to control this tenacious habit?"[58]

In response, Christen and Cooper add two statements: "(1) Smoking provides

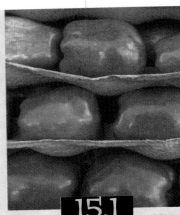

15.1

Of Special Interest

Are Smoking Bans Justified?

AHRON LECHTMAN
Executive Director: Citizens for a Tobacco-Free Society

✓**Yes** If someone came up to you with an aerosol can and sprayed a mist about you containing more than 4,000 chemical compounds, many of which are pharmacologically active, toxic, mutagenic and carcinogenic—what would your reaction be?

Or suppose you were dining in a restaurant and the person at the next table spat upon you, or the waiter slapped you or pinched you? Would you sit idly by while the manager spoke to you about spitters' rights, slappers' rights or pinchers' rights? Would you calmly suggest that these folks be placed in a separate section in the restaurant where they couldn't harm you? No, you'd probably want them arrested and put in jail. That's where people who commit assault and battery are sent.

We haven't done that to smokers. For decades, we've permitted them to smoke virtually anywhere and any time. But tobacco smoke is now widely recognized as the most serious indoor air pollutant—a leading source of toxic chemicals.

The Environmental Protection Agency has declared tobacco smoke a class A carcinogen (the classification reserved for the most lethal environmental hazards, such as asbestos, benzene and radon). The next and most logical step is to protect the public health by banning smoking in all enclosed public places. Smoking should be prohibited from workplaces where most people spend eight hours a day and where it may be impossible to restrict smoking to separate ventilated areas.

Secondhand smoke is a first-class disaster for more than 200 million Americans who have made the decision not to smoke. Despite recent public opinion polls that show overwhelming support for public smoking bans, a rich and powerful tobacco industry has thus far blocked federal bans in places other than the airliner cabin. . . .

The Tobacco Institute—a nonscientific lobby similar to the Flat Earth Society—continues to deny that tobacco smoke is harmful. Only in the bizarre world of the tobacco industry can lobbyists justify the misrepresentation of factual information to make it appear that the controversy over smoking and health remains an open one.

The problem of nonsmokers being forced to breathe secondhand smoke should not be treated as a mere nuisance to be resolved by good manners, but as a severe threat to life and health requiring government action.

People who are addicted to tobacco should be shown compassion and helped to overcome their addiction if they want help, but they should not be permitted to inflict harmful chemicals—the waste products of their addiction—on others who have no choice in the matter.

WALKER MERRYMAN
Vice President: The Tobacco Institute

✓**No** Generally speaking, the American public is a pretty accommodating bunch. They tend to dislike unfair treatment of selected groups in our society. So, it should not be surprising that two public opinion polls in the last year show overwhelming support for treating smokers and nonsmokers fairly.

In December 1991, Gallup Organization researchers indicated, "About two-thirds [of Americans] prefer separate smoking areas . . . rather than a total ban" on smoking. In an interesting twist, the report noted that "support even for these limits has fallen slightly, while backing for no restrictions has grown."

Similarly, when the American Lung Association released another Gallup Poll in June of this year, public preference for no restrictions or separate sections outpaced support for total smoking bans by margins of more than 2 to 1.

Anti-smoking groups will find little support in an article published in the October 1992 issue of the *Journal of the American Medical Association.* The AMA claims that this study is significant because it is the first to use autopsy samples in environmental-tobacco-smoke research.

However, the study's authors state that none of the subjects in the study died of diseases related to cancer. The researchers say they looked at lung tissue samples and observed cell changes they believe "may be lung cancer risk indicators" or were "possibly precancerous lesions." However, the significance of the observed cell changes is unknown. Furthermore, none of the individuals were interviewed for this study before they died to determine if they ever had been exposed to smoking or what other environmental influences they may have encountered in their lives.

This study, like much of the environmental-tobacco-smoke literature, raises many more questions than it answers and adds little to the debate.

In the end, most Americans will continue to reject extreme appeals to banish smokers from society and will instead favor sensibly accommodating smokers and nonsmokers.

Source: From *CQ Researcher*, 2:45, December 4, 1992: 1049–1072. Reprinted by permission of Congressional Quarterly, Inc., Washington, D.C.

What Do You Think?

1. Whose position do you find yourself more in agreement with? Is there a "middle-of-the-road" position on this issue?
2. Is the issue at hand "smoking" or "smokers" or is there a difference? Explain.

TABLE 15.7 — Withdrawal Symptoms and Activities That Might Help

Symptom	Activity
Dry mouth; sore throat, gums, or tongue	Sip ice-cold water or fruit juice, or chew gum.
Headaches	Take a warm bath or shower. Try relaxation or meditation techniques.
Trouble sleeping	Don't drink coffee, tea, or soda with caffeine after 6:00 P.M. Again, try relaxation or meditation techniques.
Irregularity	Add roughage to your diet, such as raw fruit, vegetables, and whole-grain cereals. Drink 6–8 glasses of water a day.
Fatigue	Take a nap. Try not to push yourself during this time; don't expect too much of your body until it's had a chance to begin to heal itself over a couple of weeks.
Hunger	Drink water or low-calorie liquids. Eat low-fat, low calorie snacks.
Tenseness, irritability	Take a walk, soak in a hot bath, try relaxation or meditation techniques.
Coughing	Sip warm herbal tea. Suck on cough drops or sugarless hard candy.

Source: Data from *Quitting Times: A Magazine for Women Who Smoke,* funded by the Pennsylvania Department of Health; prepared by Fox Chase Cancer Center, Philadelphia; in *Clearing the Air: How to Quit Smoking . . . and Quit for Keeps,* National Institutes of Health Publication No. 89–1647, p. 14, February 1989.

powerful, immediate satisfactions for the individual—pharmacological, psychological, emotional, and social. (2) Millions of Americans have successfully quit smoking. It can be done." The following discussion is based on some of these ideas.

Quitting is Not for Everyone

Unlikely as it might seem, there are many individuals who should probably *not* consider quitting smoking at the current time. People who are experiencing some life crisis or emotional difficulties or who are severely depressed should not be considered prime candidates for smoking cessation. Smoking reduction might be a more realistic alternative in some cases than cessation.

All or Nothing

Many people feel that smokers consider quitting an all-or-nothing proposition. Heavy smokers might find a reduction in their intake a more appropriate course of action. About 50 percent of those who successfully quit smoking have done so gradually, with a graded reduction rather than abrupt cessation.

Physiological Withdrawal

Nicotine and some tars actually produce a physical dependence on tobacco products. Two types of withdrawal occur when a person quits smoking. The first is based on the physical dependence on nicotine (**physiological withdrawal**) and the other is based on the psychological dependence that smokers develop for the habit (**psychological withdrawal).** Of the two, physiological withdrawal is the easier with which to deal (see table 15.7). During this time, a person may experience many unpleasant symptoms related to the withdrawal such as headaches, irritability, muscle aches, cramps, increased anxiety, some sleep disturbances, tingling in the fingers, and a craving for tobacco. Although these symptoms may be different for each person, they are generally related to an attempt on the part of the body to eliminate nicotine. This is accomplished by the kidneys flushing the bloodstream and can be helped by drinking lots of fluids—particularly water and fruit juices—during this time.

Physiological withdrawal: the set of physical symptoms experienced when one attempts to stop using a drug to which he or she is addicted.

Psychological withdrawal: the set of psychological or emotional symptoms that is experienced when one attempts to stop using a drug that he or she is addicted to.

- Past failures in trying to quit; expectation to fail again
- Addiction to nicotine
- Fear of gaining weight or past experience with weight gain
- Social pressure to smoke from friends, coworkers, and others
- Smoking in response to stress or anticipated stress
- Grieving over the prospect of being without a psychological comfort
- Lack of social support
- Lack of a plan
- Not knowing how to handle recidivism or "backsliding"

Psychological Withdrawal

Psychological withdrawal is generally the more difficult with which to deal. This type of withdrawal can sometimes last for weeks or years. Some ex-smokers who have not had a cigarette for many years may still experience an occasional yearning for just one. Research seems to indicate that the first several months following cessation are the most critical and this is generally the time when someone will return to smoking. This type of withdrawal is often characterized by changes in behavior and mood and sometimes by a severe craving for tobacco.

Some of the obstacles to quitting smoking are described in figure 15.6.[59] Long-term quitting is a complicated, lengthy process, and coming to grips with the obstacles to quitting involves a great deal of unconscious, constructive, and painful inner conflict. Smoking cessation is a continuous process that requires reinforcement and effort.

Strategies for Smoking Cessation

Many different strategies have been tried in an effort to help people quit smoking. The strategies that have been studied most carefully are drug treatments, hypnosis, and social learning theory and behavior-modification approaches.

One benefit of smoking cessation is the reversal of the accelerated decline in respiratory function experienced by smokers.

Although further decline (other than that due to normal chronological aging) is prevented through cessation, lost function cannot be regained. Nevertheless, among ex-smokers there is a decline in overall death rate as the number of years of cessation increases.

Drug Treatments

A good deal of research has been done in an attempt to find drugs that could minimize the distress of withdrawal and assist people in overcoming their dependence on nicotine and the smoking habit. Nicotine-containing chewing gum has been marketed as an aid to smoking cessation. **Nicotine gum** is a prescription drug that is chewed when a smoker has the urge to smoke. Over time, a smoker gradually cuts down on the amount of gum chewed until it is no longer needed. Nicotine gum has been found to be most effective when used in combination with treatments that address a smokers psychological dependence as well as the physical dependence on nicotine.[60]

Fewer than 10 percent of the 18 million U.S. smokers who try to quit each year are successful.[61] The **nicotine patch** is a device that can provide some help for people preparing to quit or who have taken unsuccessful action before. The patch is an adhesive pad about two inches square that delivers a steady dose of nicotine through the skin. It works eighteen to twenty-four hours per day and is used over a period of eight to twelve weeks. The nicotine dose being delivered is reduced gradually. Use of the patch, accompanied by counseling that stresses early and complete abstinence from smoking, has given success rates of about 26 percent after a period of six months according to Susan L. Kenford and her colleagues.[62] Several key points need to be remembered concerning the nicotine patch:

- The patch is not a "cure" for smoking; it is only an aid to quitting.
- The patch is not for everybody. It should not be used by persons with coronary heart disease or by pregnant women. The best success comes for persons who smoke a pack or more per day, who are highly motivated to quit, and who have counseling in conjunction with use of the patch.

Nicotine gum: a chewing gum product that contains nicotine, used sometimes to assist the tobacco cessation efforts of a person addicted to the nicotine found in tobacco.

Nicotine patch: a pad that adheres to the skin and delivers a measured dose of nicotine to assist the tobacco cessation efforts of a person addicted to the nicotine found in tobacco.

- One must not smoke while using the patch, or else risk a nicotine overdose.
- Some patch users experience adverse effects ranging in scope from minor skin irritations to insomnia and nervousness.
- The patch costs about $4 per day, similar to two packs of cigarettes; some insurance plans reimburse users.

Hypnosis

Although hypnosis was once thought to be a substantial aid to smoking cessation, the research is mixed and leaves some controversy regarding its potential for success. Success rates have ranged from 20 percent to a high of almost 90 percent. It appears, however, that the most effective way that hypnosis can be used is in conjunction with counseling or other therapies. Smokers who want to use hypnosis as a quitting technique should be certain to choose a qualified therapist, such as licensed psychiatrists and psychologists, or an accredited social worker.

Social Learning Theory and Behavior-Modification Approaches

Research in social learning theory and behavior modification has been plentiful and has led to many approaches to smoking cessation. Among the most popular are self-control strategies, such as stimulus control, contingency contracting, and aversion strategies.

Stimulus control provides the smoker with an increased awareness of the expected outcomes and tries to control stimuli and provide skills to deal with those situations in order to accomplish those outcomes. For example, a person who associates a coffee break as a stimulus for a cigarette takes a walk instead. Or, the person for whom a telephone conversation with a friend provides a cue to "light up," stops leaving cigarettes and matches around the phone and limits conversation time. The research in this area has also been mixed, with the most successful programs combining several approaches.

Contingency contracting involves the depositing of sums of money for later disbursement if certain goals are achieved. For instance, the money normally used to purchase cigarettes is placed in a separate bank account and used to finance a special vacation, wardrobe splurge, or other reward. This has produced some encouraging results, but as with stimulus control, the most effective use of contingency contracting appears to be within the context of a much broader program.

Aversion strategies attempt to change behavior by using aversive stimuli. There are three major forms of stimuli used in such approaches, including the use of electric shock, covert sensitization, and cigarette smoke. The first involves the application of electric shocks in order to link smoking with discomfort. Covert sensitization involves the use of methods to produce aversion to smoking by linking smoking with nausea or other discomfort. Cigarette-smoke aversion involves either doubling or tripling consumption prior to withdrawal or forcing someone to puff rapidly on a cigarette to produce unpleasant feelings during smoking. Of the three, it appears that cigarette-smoke aversion holds the most promise when used alone. These approaches are seldom used together, and again research results on their success rates are mixed.

Smoking-cessation programs often utilize many of these social learning theory and behavior-modification techniques together to encourage and support the person trying to give up smoking. This multicomponent approach appears to hold the most potential for success when considering the general population of smokers.

Research indicates that 95 percent of those who have quit smoking have done so without the aid of any organized smoking-cessation program.[63] Moreover, surveys of most current smokers indicate a preference for quitting on their own. They tend to disfavor organized, comprehensive programs.[64]

Nicotine fading involves progressive reduction of nicotine by switching to brands containing less nicotine and tapering off the number of cigarettes smoked. The theory behind this idea is that the body's demand for nicotine will gradually diminish to the point where cessation is possible without major symptoms of withdrawal. R. M. Foxx and R. A. Brown have achieved some success with this particular technique.[65] One of the major drawbacks of this strategy, however, is the tendency for persons to engage in compensatory smoking practices, thereby maintaining the physiological demand for nicotine.

REST (*restricted environmental stimulation techniques*) is based on the theory that removal of external input and cues reduce the need to smoke by creating a "stimulus hunger" and receptivity to new ideas or thoughts. Typical of the REST process would be to place a smoker in a completely dark, soundproof chamber for one to twenty-four hours. Although found to be of some value in selective small studies, the severity of the technique probably reduces its practical utility.

Quitting "Cold Turkey"

Many people who smoke want to quit or have made one or more previous attempts to quit. Altering smoking behavior can require some major lifestyle change because of the physical as well as the psychological addiction associated with smoking. Light smokers and people who have been smoking for only a short period may have an easier time in quitting than heavy smokers who have been smoking for a long period of time—years or even decades. The smoker who attempts to quit **"cold turkey"** may venture back and forth through the stages of behavior change (see table 15.8).

Maintenance of Cessation

Most current studies indicate that maintenance of nonsmoking behavior following quitting is a difficult process. Generally, only 25 percent of the participants of smoking-cessation programs remain abstinent for six months following treatment.[66]

New emphasis on techniques to improve the maintenance phase of cessation promises to improve abstinence rates, with several reports of greater than 50 percent abstinence at follow-ups of six months or longer. To improve maintenance of nonsmoking after intensive treatment programs have ended, reinforcement should be built into the natural environment. Smoking-cessation programs in the workplace may offer an opportunity for this. Social support interventions are also promising. Reliable findings link relapse to social cues and friends and spouses who smoke. The presence of group support, nonsmoking spouses, and professional contact decreases relapse. Providing skills and support to maintain

abstinence following treatment seems to be an important part of the treatment process itself. Activity for Wellness 15.1 offers suggestions to help former smokers stay off cigarettes for good.

Is There a Safe Way to Smoke?

Despite the preponderance of evidence that smoking is hazardous to health, there are still many who smoke and are either not willing or not ready to give it up for their health. For these people, the apparent choices available include all those steps that can be taken to minimize the potential hazards associated with smoking. There appear to be at least four major areas in which this can be accomplished: (1) smoke fewer cigarettes each day, (2) take fewer puffs on each cigarette, (3) reduce the depth of each inhalation, and (4) choose a brand low in tar and nicotine.

Lower-yield tar and nicotine cigarettes have become popular during the past fifteen years. Determining the health hazards of these brands, however, is complicated by the presence of additives and flavoring substances that have been neither identified adequately nor tested for any adverse biological potential. Although low-tar and low-nicotine cigarettes are increasingly popular, the mortality rate among smokers of these cigarettes is still higher than for nonsmokers. Smoking filter cigarettes that are low in tar and nicotine may reduce the risk of cancers of the lung and larynx when compared to unfiltered, high-tar and high-nicotine products, but the risk is still considerably higher than for nonsmokers. While low-tar and low-nicotine cigarettes are designed to decrease the smoker's exposure to the harmful substances produced from burning tobacco, many who switch to these brands engage in a practice called **compensatory smoking** to satisfy nicotine and taste demands. Compensatory smoking behaviors include smoking more cigarettes, inhaling more deeply and for a longer period of time, and puffing more frequently. Ironically, smoking low-tar and low-nicotine brands may, in fact, increase risk if compensatory smoking is practiced.

Some words of caution:

1. There is no safe cigarette and no safe level of consumption.

Cold turkey: a phrase used to describe an approach to smoking cessation where a smoker sets a date to stop smoking and then, on that date, completely gives up smoking cigarettes.

Many smokers have a hard time quitting if they have smoked for a long time, are around others who smoke a lot, and have failed in previous attempts to quit. Some have never thought seriously about quitting. Whatever your status as a smoker, cessation success may be enhanced if you consider some of the points below.

Precontemplation → Contemplation

If you have never thought about how you might become a nonsmoker again, consider:

- Trying to imagine what it would be like for you to be a nonsmoker.
- Keeping a record each time you have a cigarette, recording what you are doing at the time, and how you feel.
- Using the phone book to locate local offices of the American Cancer Society, the American Heart Association, or the American Lung Association, and contacting them concerning publications about smoking cessation.
- Recording how much you spend on cigarettes and other tobacco materials.

Contemplation → Preparation

If you thought about the health and economic costs of smoking but have not prepared yourself for the task of becoming a nonsmoker again, you can try:

- Going more frequently to places that are nonsmoking only.
- Asking your health-care provider about smoking cessation.

Preparation → Action

Having prepared yourself with the know-how to quit smoking, take that all important next step by:

- Identifying a date in the next thirty days when you will carry out your plan to quit smoking, and circling the date on your calendar.

- Viewing quitting as a one day at a time proposition.
- Telling a close friend you are quitting, and letting people know you are not merely "contemplating" action to benefit you—but actually doing it.
- During the week before you quit, deliberately varying your smoking routine, e.g., smoking a different brand, smoking more than usual on one day and less than usual on another.

Action → Maintenance

Having successfully demonstrated success in the early stages of your plan to be a non-smoker again, make smoking avoidance a part of your routine by:

- Avoiding situations and circumstances that "trigger" smoking.
- Diversifying your repertoire of self-care health activities, and letting health consciousness become a way of life.
- Becoming an advocate of nonsmoking among your peers.
- Following the suggestions listed in Activity for Wellness 15.1.

Maintenance

You are on your way to restoring your non-smoking status. Maintain momentum by:

- Rewarding yourself with a gift that represents some fraction of the money you have saved by not purchasing cigarettes or other tobacco products.
- Encouraging a friend who smokes to begin a smoking cessation program.

2. Smoking cigarettes with lower yields of "tar" and nicotine reduces the risk of lung cancer and, to some extent, improves the smoker's chance for longer life, provided there is no compensatory increase in the amount smoked. However, the benefits are minimal in comparison with giving up cigarettes

entirely. The single most effective way to reduce hazards of smoking continues to be that of quitting early.

3. It is not clear what reductions in risk may occur in the case of diseases other than lung cancer. The evidence in the case of cardiovascular disease is too limited to warrant a conclusion, nor is there enough

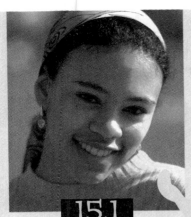

15.1
Activity for Wellness

Staying Off Cigarettes for Good

It might be easy for you to quit smoking for a short period of time, but probably much harder to quit for good. Each year in the United States, nearly 19 million smokers quit for at least one day, but, less than 10 percent of them manage to stay off cigarettes for good. Your quitting program must have a plan to help you stay off cigarettes for life.

Many people believe it only takes willpower to quit smoking. That's not always true. Just like anything you do, it takes practice and experience to be successful at quitting smoking. You have to learn to endure the urges to smoke, and

to bounce back if you slip up. Over time, you will learn how to cope with these stresses, and staying smoke-free will become easier.

A good quit smoking program will include at least a few of the following tips to help you stay off cigarettes for life:

• Be Patient:

Be patient with yourself. Don't panic or give up if you find quitting is difficult. All ex-smokers struggled with quitting at some time, and almost all slipped up at least once. If you can endure the tough times early on, you have a good chance of making it.

• Reward Yourself:

Reward yourself for all your nonsmoking achievements, great or small. Quitting smoking is a big challenge, and you should give yourself encouragement throughout your quit attempt. Celebrate each week and month you stay off cigarettes. Go to a movie. Buy yourself a pair of running shoes. Count the money you've saved by not smoking. Whatever you do, give yourself some kind of reward on a regular basis.

• Be Positive:

While parts of the quitting process can be a little unpleasant, try to focus on the positive aspects of quitting. Besides the immediate and long-term health benefits, you will also be able to exercise more, save money, feel better about yourself, and regain control of your life.

• Get Support From Others:

Social support is very important in helping you stay smoke-free after you've quit. Tell your family, friends, and co-workers that you have stopped smoking—most of them will be supportive. Many of your friends who smoke may want to know how you quit. Talking to them about it will be good for you.

• Avoid "Triggers":

All smokers have certain times, places, and situations that make them want to smoke. For you, it may be on a work break, in your car, or with your morning cup of coffee. Identify these times, and plan to either avoid them or find ways to cope with them.

• Plan Ways to Cope With Stress:

You may slip up and smoke a cigarette when you're feeling stressed or when your guard is down. You can help prevent slips by planning ahead for what you will do in times of stress.

• Don't Be Defeated:

Just because you slip, it doesn't mean you have become a smoker again. Learn from the experience and think about how you will cope the next time you are tempted. Don't feel guilty and don't let your quitting effort go to waste.

Source: Data from *Out of the Ashes: Choosing a Method to Quit Smoking,* Centers for Disease Control Publication No. (CDC) 90–8418, pp. 13–14, July 1990.

information on which to base a judgment in the case of chronic obstructive lung disease. In the case of smoking's effects on the fetus and newborn, there is no evidence that changing to a lower tar and nicotine cigarette has any effect at all on reducing risk.

4. Smokers may increase the number of cigarettes they smoke and inhale more deeply when they switch to lower-yield cigarettes. Compensatory behavior may negate any advantage of the lower-yield product or even increase the health risk.

5. The tar and nicotine yields obtained by present testing methods do not correspond to the dosages that the

individual smokers receive: in some cases they may seriously underestimate these dosages.

6. A final question is unresolved, whether the new cigarettes being produced today introduce new risks through their design, filtering mechanisms, tobacco ingredients, or additives. The chief concern is additives.

You have all heard the advice. If you don't smoke, don't start; if you smoke, quit.

Rights of Nonsmokers

Our discussion so far has focused on the effects of tobacco on those who use it. What about its effects on nonusers?

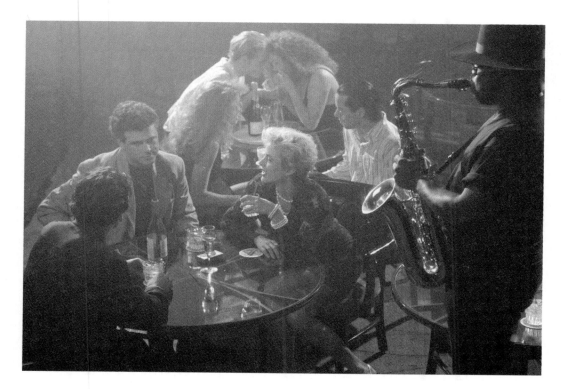

Figure 15.7: A smoke-filled environment's negative effect on nonsmokers is becoming more evident. What Do You Think?

1. Is sidestream smoke a problem of sufficient magnitude to justify its prohibition in restaurants and other public places?
2. In 1995 a prominent chain of restaurants that specializes in the sale of doughnuts announced that its 3000 establishments would thereafter be smoke-free. Will other establishments follow suit? Explain what reasoning such a decision may be based upon.

Mainstream versus Sidestream Smoke

Although the issues related to the health effects of smoking on the smoker have been thoroughly documented and are well known to the general population, this is not the case with the effects of smoke-filled environments on the nonsmoker (see figure 15.7). More information, however, is available.

The acute or immediate health effects of **passive smoking** are irritation of the nose, eyes, and throat. Air cleaning systems that filter out particulate matter cause no apparent reduction in the number of irritating substances that plague many nonsmokers. Allergic reactions, including the onset of **asthma,** are commonly experienced by nonsmokers.

In households where parents smoke, children have more adverse respiratory symptoms, including higher frequencies of **pneumonia** and **bronchitis,** than in nonsmoking households. The magnitude of the effect on children is related, of course, to the number of smokers and the amount smoked. Infants too, experience more respiratory infections if their parents smoke. Moreover, the rate of lung growth and overall development may be retarded in the children of smokers.

An enclosed smoke-filled room may contain up to 4,000 gaseous compounds. The major source of **environmental tobacco smoke** is sidestream smoke emitted from the burning end of a cigarette. The remainder consists of mainstream smoke, which is inhaled by the smoker and subsequently exhaled, and other gases that diffuse through the cigarette paper itself during the smoking process. We now know that many of the constituents of mainstream smoke are also found in sidestream smoke—including the carcinogens, cocarcinogens, and carbon monoxide. What was not known until relatively recently was that these constituents may be in even higher concentrations in sidestream smoke than in mainstream smoke. For example, sidestream smoke contains approximately eight times the levels of carbon dioxide, two and a half times the amount of carbon monoxide, and almost three times the nicotine content as mainstream smoke.

Environmental tobacco smoke (ETS) has been associated with various negative health events including lung cancer, other respiratory diseases, and even brain tumors in children. Passive smoking triggers more frequent and more severe asthma attacks in persons already having the disease (see chapter 11). Peter Boyle estimates that 1500 deaths per year occur in women and 500 in men due to passive smoking.[67] Boyle's figures may be conservative, since the Environmental Protection Agency estimates

Passive smoking: the inhalation of tobacco smoke that comes from the cigarette, pipe, or cigar being smoked by someone else.

Asthma: a chronic condition often of allergic origin marked by labored breathing, wheezing, constriction of the chest, and further manifested by gasping or coughing.

Pneumonia: an inflammation of the lung, usually caused by a bacteria. Symptoms include cough, chest pain, and shadows on a chest x-ray.

Bronchitis: an inflammation of the lining of the bronchi resulting in obscured air flow, arising usually from infection or chronic irritation.

TABLE 15.9   *Intelligent Choice and Smokers' Lines*

"Medical science will find a way someday for people to smoke without contracting cancer."

"Nobody can tell me I'm doing something wrong. Nobody."

"I'm going to die someday, and I think everybody else is, too. It's my own preference."

"I feel like I'm not going to be a smoker all my life." (twenty-year-old woman)

"I think the government should keep their [sic] nose in their own business and out of mine."

"Everything people think of as pleasure, they keep taxing and making more regulations."

"I've been smoking for thirty-five years and have a clean bill of health. My grandmother rolled her own and lived to be 111 years old." (fifty-year-old man)

From Chris Murphy, "Up in Arms Over Their Right to Smoke" in *The Capital Times,* 155.47, 1994. Madison, WI.

What Do You Think?

1. Have you heard these kinds of remarks before? Do they represent rationalizations or hopeful pleas? Are these statements valid?

2. What are smokers' rights and do they have limits? Who decides?

that ETS contributes to 3000 deaths annually due to lung cancer alone.[68] Michael Siegel compared the levels of selected sidestream smoke products in bars and office settings. In bars, carbon monoxide was on average, 3.9 times greater, nicotine 4.8 times greater, and particulate matter 6.1 times greater.[69] Workers in bars are believed to be at significantly elevated risk for lung cancer and other respiratory disease.

Mainstream smoke is inhaled directly into a smoker's body, but sidestream smoke enters the environment; therefore, sidestream smoke is diluted in the ambient air. What is inhaled by the nonsmoker in a smoke-filled environment appears to be less in quantity than what a smoker gets from mainstream smoke; however, the amount of gases and particulate matter from sidestream smoke is greater than mainstream smoke. Inhaling sidestream smoke is called **involuntary smoking** or secondhand smoking. At issue is how dangerous involuntary smoking is.

Indoor **radon,** another environmental pollutant of current public health interest because of its statistical relationship to lung cancer incidence, can make matters even worse. Radon arises primarily from sources other than smoke (e.g., building stone), but can become attached to the particulate components of smoke, thus producing another pathway for its entry into the lungs

and increasing the possibility of cancer developing at that site.

There are many issues and some controversy regarding involuntary smoking. There are some points about which we are sure:

- The potential risk is dependent on many factors, including length and extent of exposure.

- The most dramatic effects appear to be those related to the immediate exposure to the smoke itself and to carbon monoxide.

- Involuntary smoking appears to be distasteful to most people.

Nonsmokers' Bill of Rights

With all of these issues regarding involuntary smoking and its potential effects on health, more people are beginning to demand what is called their dual rights: the right to choose not to smoke, and the right not to have to breathe the smoke of those who choose to smoke. Because of these issues, the following has been proposed:

The Nonsmokers' Bill of Rights.*
Nonsmokers help protect the health, comfort, and safety of everyone by insisting on the following rights:

1. *The right to breathe clean air.* Nonsmokers have the right to breathe clean air, free

Radon: a radioactive gas resulting from the disintegration of radium. Found naturally in certain geographical areas, radon has been implicated in 5 to 10 percent of lung cancers in the U.S.

from harmful and irritating tobacco smoke. This right supersedes the right to smoke when the two conflict.

2. *The right to speak out.* Nonsmokers have the right to express—firmly but politely—their discomfort and adverse reactions to tobacco smoke. They have the right to voice their objections when smokers light up without asking permission.

3. *The right to act.* Nonsmokers have the right to take actions through legislative channels, social pressures, or any other legitimate means—as individuals or in groups—to prevent or discourage smokers from polluting the atmosphere and to seek the restriction of smoking in public places.

The Nonsmokers' Bill of Rights has been proposed by several organizations, including Group Against Smoker's Pollution (GASP) and Your Christmas Seals Association. As a partial result of lobbying efforts by antismoking groups, as of April 23, 1988, the federal government imposed a ban on smoking during all domestic and overseas airline flights of two-hours duration or less. Selected airlines, states, and nations have imposed their own bans covering all flights, regardless of duration.

Smoking is a barrier to wellness that affects both smokers and nonsmokers alike. Advances toward a smoke-free society are also steps toward higher levels of wellness.

A Final Word on Tobacco

Antonia C. Novello, U.S. Surgeon General during the Bush Administration, identifies the relevant tobacco issues for the final years of the 20th century.[70] They are presented here to close out this chapter. She reminds us that:

*Source: Courtesy National Interagency Council on Smoking and Health

- The tobacco industry targets women, children, and members of minority groups in its marketing plan.
- Tobacco use is responsible for the premature deaths of nearly one-half million people in the U.S. every year.
- Smoking is the single most preventable cause of death in the U.S., and it costs in excess of $65 billion per year, more than $1 billion per week.
- Tobacco is the only known product that when used as directed, results in death and disability.

Despite the enormous scientific evidence that identifies the negative health and social consequences of smoking and other forms of tobacco use, a substantial number of people continue to engage in these activities. The 1990s yielded the first year since 1965 in which the percentage of adults in the U.S. who smoke failed to decline. This figure, coupled with the popularity of smokeless tobacco, is disappointing given the strength of the health evidence. Society's commitment to tobacco control as the present century draws to a close will no doubt play a prominent role in determining the health status of the nation as the 21st century unfolds. In February 1995, the State of Florida, citing its 1994 Medicaid Third Party Liability Act, filed a law suit against two tobacco manufacturing conglomerates in an effort to collect reimbursement for monies the state has had to pay out to medically indigent citizens stricken with tobacco-related diseases.[71] Mississippi and other states have similar suits pending. It is indeed ironic that it could be the courts, and not medicine or the scientific community, that ultimately decide the future of tobacco manufacturing and consumption in this country.

Summary

1. Tobacco was used in North America before Europeans ever set foot upon the continent. Early American settlers were introduced to tobacco use, and the habit became fashionable throughout Europe, as well as the Americas.

2. The first common use of tobacco was in its smokeless forms—snuff and chewing tobacco. These forms of tobacco were replaced by cigarettes during the early twentieth century, but began making a comeback in the 1970s and 1980s when the negative health effects of smoking became well known. Smokeless tobacco is not a safe alternative to cigarette smoking, however, and can give rise to a number of adverse oral conditions, the most notable of which is oral cancer.

3. The link between smoking and health has been clearly established. Today, most people realize that smoking cessation is the one activity likely to have the largest impact on the health of our nation.

4. Tobacco smoke in an enclosed room contains more than 4,000 chemical agents with the potential to affect our health negatively. The major constituents include tars, nicotine, and carbon monoxide.

5. Tars are made up of condensed particulate matter and may be both carcinogenic and cocarcinogenic.

6. Nicotine is an addictive drug and perhaps the most powerful agent in tobacco.

7. Carbon monoxide affects our ability to absorb and use oxygen.

8. There are many health risks associated with smoking, including cancer, heart disease, emphysema, respiratory infections, and problems with pregnancy.

9. Among the prominent social barriers to a smoke-free society are advertising and the media, and parental and peer smoking habits.

10. Once begun, the tobacco habit proves difficult to stop. Educational efforts should be focused on preventing use before the habit becomes entrenched.

11. Involuntary smoking from sidestream smoke in the environment can be hazardous to the health of nonsmokers.

12. Health objectives for smoking and other tobacco cessation are established in *Healthy People 2000*.

13. The tobacco industry uses advertising, promotions, and gimmicks to encourage tobacco use. Some of these programs are specially targeted at women, youth, and members of minority groups.

14. Important regulatory efforts are underway at the state and federal level to control tobacco use.

Recommended Readings

American Cancer Society. *Cancer Facts and Figures—1996*. Atlanta, GA: American Cancer Society, 1996.

A publication updated annually with the latest in cancer facts and figures, including advances in prevention, early detection, and treatment. Monitors tobacco use, tobacco-related cancers, and cessation strategies.

U.S. Department of Health and Human Services. *Smokeless Tobacco or Health*. Washington, D.C.: USDHHS, Public Health Service, NIH Publication No. 93–3461, 1993.

Describes the health effects and prevalence of use of smokeless forms of tobacco, along with education programs and strategies for curtailing use.

U.S. Department of Health and Human Services. *Strategies to Control Tobacco Use in the United States: A Blueprint for Public Health Action in the 1990s*. Washington, D.C.: USDHHS, Public Health Service, NIH Publication No. 92–3316, 1992.

Presents a plan for tobacco control strategies in the U.S. through legislation, education, public and professional information campaigns, and behavioral intervention.

References

1. U.S. Department of Health and Human Services, Public Health Service, *Strategies to Control Tobacco Use in the United States: A Blueprint for Public Health Action in the 1990s*, NIH Publication No. 92–3316 (Washington, D.C.: U.S. Government Printing Office, 1992).

2. *University of California at Berkeley Wellness Letter* 9.1 (1992):1.

3. *Healthy People 2000*, National Health Promotion and Disease Prevention Objectives (Washington, D.C.: U.S. Department of Health and Human Services, 1991).

4. Coalition on Smoking OR Health, *Comments on Release of List of Chemical Additives in Cigarettes* (Washington, D.C.: Coalition on Smoking OR Health, April 13, 1994):1.

5. Arden G. Christen et al., "Smokeless Tobacco: The Folklore and Social History of Snuffing, Sneezing, Dipping, and Chewing," *Journal of the American Dental Association* 105 (1982):821, 826.

6. Christen et al., "Smokeless Tobacco," 826, 828.

7. Gregory N. Connolly, "Taxing Other Tobacco Products," *World Smoking and Health* 19.1 (1994):13–14.

8. Connolly, "Taxing Other Tobacco Products," 13–14.

9. Connolly, "Taxing Other Tobacco Products," 13–14.

10. James O. Mason, *A Public Health Service Progress Report on Healthy People 2000—Tobacco* (Atlanta, GA: Centers for Disease Control and Prevention, 1992).

11. Connolly, "Taxing Other Tobacco Products," 13–14.

12. Gregory N. Connolly et al., "The Reemergence of Smokeless Tobacco," *New England Journal of Medicine* 314 (1986):1020–1027.

13. Heather G. Stockwell and Gary H. Lyman. "Impact of Smoking and Smokeless Tobacco on the Risk of Cancer of the Head and Neck," *Head and Neck Surgery* 9 (1986):104.

14. Robert J. McDermott, Barbara J. Clark, and Kelli R. McCormack, "The Reemergence of Smokeless Tobacco: Implications for Dental Hygiene Practice," *Dental Hygiene* 61 (1987):348–353.

15. Robert J. McDermott and Phillip J. Marty, "Dipping and Chewing Behavior among University Students: Prevalence and Patterns of Use," *Journal of School Health* 56 (1986):175–177.

16. U.S. Department of Health, Education, and Welfare, Public Health Service, *Smoking and Health: A Report of the Advisory Committee to the Surgeon General of the Public Health Service*, Publication No. 1103 (Washington, D.C.: U.S. Government Printing Office, 1964).

17. Susan Walton, "Other People's Smoke May Be Risk for You," *National Research Council News Report* 37.1 (1986–87):11.

18. U.S. Department of Health and Human Services, *Smoking Tobacco and Health* (Washington, D.C.: U.S. Government Printing Office, 1989):4.

19. Allen Vegotsky, "What the Cigarette Makers Sell," *World Smoking and Health* 18.1 (1993):8–9.

20. U.S. Department of Health, Education, and Welfare, *Smoking and Health: A Report of the Advisory Committee to the Surgeon General of the Public Health Service*.

21. Coalition on Smoking OR Health, *Comments on Release of List of Chemical Additives in Cigarettes*, 1.

22. U.S. Department of Health and Human Services, Public Health Service, *The Health Consequences of Smoking: The Changing Cigarette: A Report of the Surgeon General*, DHHS Publication No. (PHS) 81–50156 (1981), 5.

23. R. C. Bone, J. R. Phillips, and P. Chodhury, "The Smoking Habit: Physical Dependence on Nicotine," *The Journal of Respiratory Diseases* 2.5 (1981):10–16.

24. U.S. Department of Health and Human Services, Public Health Service, Office of the Assistant Secretary for Health, Office on Smoking and Health, *The Health Consequences of Smoking for Women: A Report of the Surgeon General* (Washington, D.C.: U.S. Government Printing Office, 1980).

25. Bone et al., "The Smoking Habit, 10–16.

26. Marlene Cimons, "Nicotine Is Addictive, FDA Panel Says," *Los Angeles Times* (August 3, 1994):C1.

27. U.S. Department of Health and Human Services, Office on Smoking and Health, *The Health Consequences of Smoking: Chronic Obstructive Lung Disease* (Rockville, Md.: DHHS (PHS) 84–50205, 1984), xii.

28. U.S. Department of Health and Human Services, *Reducing the Health Consequences of Smoking—25 Years of Progress* (Washington, D.C.: U.S. Government Printing Office, 1989):21.

29. U.S. Department of Health and Human Services, *The Health Benefits of Smoking Cessation: A Report to the Surgeon General—Executive Summary* (Washington, D.C.: U.S. Government Printing Office, 1990):9.

30. John R. Sussman and B. Blake Levitt, *Before You Conceive: The Complete Prepregnancy Guide* (New York: Bantam Books, 1989):20.

31. J. L. Hopper and E. Seeman, "The Bone Density of Female Twins Discordant for Tobacco Use," *New England Journal of Medicine* 330.6 (1994):387–391.

32. U.S. Department of Health and Human Services, *Healthy People 2000: National Health Promotion and Disease Prevention Objectives*, 145.

33. U.S. Department of Health and Human Services, Public Health Service, *The 1990 Health Objectives for the Nation: A Midcourse Review* (Washington, D.C.: U.S. Government Printing Office, 1986), 184.

34. Antonia C. Novello, "From the Surgeon General, U.S. Public Health Service," *Journal of the American Medical Association* 270.7 (1993):806.

35. U.S. Department of Health, Education, and Welfare, Public Health Service, National Institutes of Health, National Cancer Institute, *Cigarette Smoking among Teen-age Girls and Young Women: Summary of Findings*, DHEW Publication No. (NIH) 77–1203 (1977), 55.

36. U.S. Department of Health and Human Services, *The Health Consequences of Smoking: Chronic Obstructive Lung Disease*, 326.

37. K. E. Warner, "The Effects of the Anti-Smoking Campaign on Cigarette Consumption," *American Journal of Public Health* 67.7 (1977):645–650.

38. E. Foote, "The Time Has Come: Cigarette Advertising Must Be Banned," in *Research on Smoking Behavior*, eds. M. E. Jarvik et al., National Institutes on Drug Abuse Research Monograph 17, Public Health Service, Alcohol, Drug Abuse and Mental Health Administration, National Institute on Drug Abuse, DHEW Publication No. (ADM) 78–581 (December 1977):339–346.

39. "Tobacco Ads Influence Teens, Says Study," *The Nation's Health* (May-June 1992):18.

40. Harold Freeman, Jane L. Delgado, and Clifford E. Douglas, "Minority Issues" *Tobacco Use: An American Crisis* (Chicago, IL: American Medical Association, 1993), 43–47.

41. Freeman, et al., "Minority Issues," 43–47.

42. Freeman, et al., "Minority Issues," 43–47.

43. Freeman, et al., "Minority Issues," 43–47.

44. Freeman, et al., "Minority Issues," 43–47.

45. Freeman, et al., "Minority Issues," 43–47.

46. D. Horn, "An Approach to Office Management of the Cigarette Smoker," *Diseases of the Chest* 54.3 (1968):203–209.

47. Michael P. Traynor, Michael E. Begay, and Stanton A. Glantz, "New Tobacco Industry Strategy to Prevent Local Tobacco Control," *Journal of the American Medical Association* 270.4 (1993):479–486.

48. Tobacco-Free Florida Coalition, *Tobacco-Free Florida Plan 1994–1995* (Tallahassee, FL: The Tobacco-Free Florida Coalition, 1994).

49. Lynne D. Richardson, "Tobacco Taxes as a Public Health Measure," *World Smoking and Health* 19.1 (1994):4–6.

50. Novello, "From the Surgeon General. U.S. Public Health Service," 806.

51. Novello, "From the Surgeon General, U.S. Public Health Service," 806.

52. Maria Mallory, "Florida May Kick the Tar out of Tobacco," *Business Week* 3379 (July 4, 1994):29.

53. Kenneth E. Warner and George A. Fulton, "The Economic Implications of Tobacco Product Sales in a Nontobacco State," *Journal of the American Medical Association* 271.10 (1994):771–776.

54. Warner and Fulton, "The Economic Implications of Tobacco Sales in a Nontobacco State," 771–776.

55. Thomas P. Houston, *Tobacco Use: An American Crisis* (Chicago, IL: American Medical Association, 1993).

56. Novello, "From the Surgeon General, U.S. Public Health Service," 806.

57. Connolly, "Taxing Other Tobacco Products," 13–14.

58. A. G. Christen and K. H. Cooper, "Strategic Withdrawal from Cigarette Smoking," *CA—A Journal for Clinicians* 29.2 (1979):96–107.

59. Christen and Cooper, "Strategic Withdrawal from Cigarette Smoking."

60. U.S. Department of Health and Human Services, *Out of the Ashes: Choosing a Method to Quit Smoking* (Washington, D.C.: U.S. Government Printing Office, July 1990):9.

61. *University of California at Berkeley Wellness Letter* 9.1 (1992):7.

62. Susan L. Kenford, Michael C. Fiore, Douglas E. Jorenby, et al. "Predicting Smoking Cessation: Who Will Quit with and without the Nicotine Patch," *Journal of the American Medical Association* 271.8 (1994):589–594.

63. U.S. Department of Health, Education, and Welfare, *The Smoking Digest: Progress Report and a Nation Kicking the Habit.* U.S. Department of Health, Education, and Welfare, Public Health Service, National Institutes of Health, National Cancer Institute, Office of Cancer Communications (1977).

64. U.S. Department of Health and Human Services, Public Health Service, Office on Smoking and Health, *The Health Consequences of Smoking: Cancer. A Report of the Surgeon General.* DHHS Publication No. (PHS) 82–50179 (1982).

65. R. M. Foxx and R. A. Brown, "Nicotine Fading and Self-Monitoring for Cigarette Abstinence of Controlled Smoking," *Journal of Applied Behavior Analysis* 12 (1979):111–125.

66. Kenford, et al., "Predicting Smoking Cessation: Who Will Quit with and without the Patch," 589–594.

67. Peter Boyle, "The Hazards of Passive—and Active—Smoking," *New England Journal of Medicine* 328.23 (1993):1708–1709.

68. Environmental Protection Agency, *Respiratory Health Effects of Passive Smoking: Lung Cancer and Other Disorders*, Publication No. EPA/600/6–90/006F (Washington, D.C.: U.S. Government Printing Office, 1992).

69. Michael Siegel, "Involuntary Smoking in the Restaurant Workplace," *Journal of the American Medical Association* 270.4 (1993):490–493.

70. Novello, "From the Surgeon General, U.S. Public Health Service," 806.

71. Lucy Morgan, "Florida Sues Tobacco Industry," *St. Petersburg Times* (February 22, 1995), 1A, 6A; Craig S. Palosky, "State Lawsuit Lights up Tobacco War," *Tampa Tribune* (February 22, 1995), Florida/Metro 1–2.

Alcohol: Risks and Responsibilities

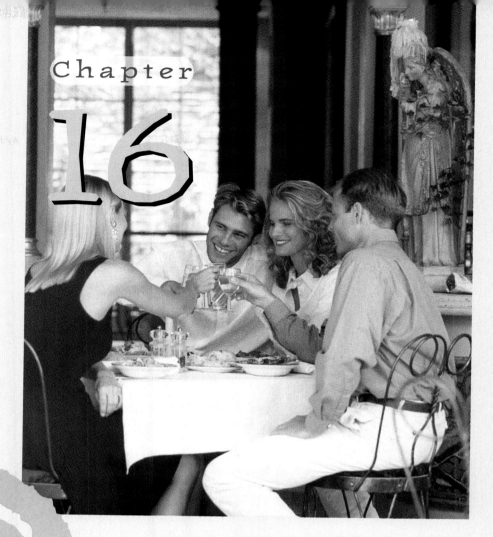

Chapter 16

Student Learning Objectives

Upon completion of this chapter you should be able to:

1. identify the health objectives of the nation for the year 2000 with respect to alcohol consumption and related morbidity and mortality;

2. analyze current and historical patterns of alcohol use in the United States;

3. describe the mechanisms of alcohol ingestion, absorption, and oxidation;

4. interpret the meaning and implications of the term "blood-alcohol concentration";

5. delineate the short-term physiological and psychological effects of alcohol use;

6. evaluate the impact of alcohol use for a woman and fetus during pregnancy;

7. describe alcohol's contribution to death and disability from chronic disease;

8. analyze drinking patterns to determine those that reflect problem behavior;

9. define alcoholism and list its primary characteristics;

10. list some of the secondary consequences of alcohol use;

11. identify the personal and social influences that impact upon responsible versus irresponsible use of alcohol;

12. assess the impact of excessive use of alcohol on health status indicators and mortality among various racial and ethnic groups;

13. provide insights regarding the factors influencing alcohol use and abuse on college and university campuses.

This chapter is about beverage alcohol and its use by different groups in various contexts and circumstances. In presenting our discussion about alcohol, we acknowledge that alcohol is readily available by legal or illegal means to students on the majority of U.S. college and university campuses. In recognizing this fact, though, our position is that illegal, underage consumption of alcohol is an activity to be strongly discouraged. We also are aware that a sizable percentage of people reject the use of alcohol in any and all of its forms, and under any and all circumstances, and even judge occasional drinkers in the harshest of ways. Nevertheless, we are sufficiently attuned to the contemporary pressures and practices at play in many university settings to know that consuming alcohol is often part of the culture of college life, both for older as well as for more youthful students. Thus, while maintaining our position that underage drinking is an inappropriate practice, we wish to foster the development of attitudes and behaviors concerning alcohol that encourage responsible use among those persons who make the decision to drink, regardless of their age. We cannot, however, escape the fact that heavy and abusive consumption of alcohol can initiate or promote the development of severe health and social problems. Because of the variations in drinking behavior, the confounding effect alcohol has on health, and the social significance of alcohol almost since the beginning of recorded history, it is an area of primary emphasis in *Healthy People 2000* (see table 16.1).

Alcohol and its consumption are subjects that are more complex than what they might first appear. Few people argue any longer that alcohol is the most abused drug in U.S. society. Alcohol once was referred to as "the good creature of God" by persons in colonial America, but also as the "demon rum."[1] Before the invention of processes to examine and purify drinking water, the consumption of beer, wine, or distilled spirits may have been a "safer" practice than drinking available well water. The year 1919 brought on the famous period of "prohibition" in the U.S., when the manufacturing, transporting, and sale of alcohol was forbidden by federal law. However, the highly effective and organized distribution of alcohol by "bootleggers," accompanied by loud public outcry to repeal the law, resulted in the relegalization of alcohol. Thus, social and religious indecisiveness about the merits of alcohol use have to a certain extent contributed to some of our present-day ambivalence about alcohol. This ambivalence has been compounded by controversy concerning the health effects of alcohol. While no one denies the negative health consequences of long-term abusive drinking, the problems of alcoholism, and the misuse of alcohol that can lead to serious injury or death, total abstinence from drinking does not necessarily lead to optimal health outcomes.

There is confusion about the amount of drinking that goes on among people in the U.S. Abstainers account for approximately 35 percent of the adult population, and light drinkers account for another 35 percent. By definition, *light drinkers* are persons who consume two drinks a week or less. *Moderate drinkers* average one-half to two drinks per day, and account for 22 percent of people in the U.S. *Heavy drinkers*, 8 percent of the people in the U.S., consume more than two drinks per day.[2] Alcohol is a legal drug that costs the nation far more each year than other drugs regardless of "whatever metric applied; medical, social, economic, or public health."[3] In this chapter we will explore not only the physiological and health effects of alcohol, but also the role of traditions and attitudes on consumption patterns among people young and old alike.

Basic Pharmacology

There are many kinds of alcohols, but only three are commonly used. **Methyl alcohol,** sometimes called wood alcohol, is used in many industrial products such as antifreezes and fuels. It is very toxic to humans even in small quantities. **Isopropyl alcohol** (rubbing alcohol) is used as a disinfectant and solvent. **Ethyl alcohol** (grain alcohol) is consumable. Ethyl alcohol can be produced either synthetically or naturally by a process called **fermentation.** Fermentation is a metabolic form of combustion of grains, with ethyl alcohol as one of the end products.

TABLE 16.1 — Selected Healthy People 2000 Objectives Related to Alcohol and Alcohol Abuse

1. **Reduce deaths caused by alcohol-related motor-vehicle crashes to no more than 8.5 per 100,000 people.** (Update: 6.9 per 100,000 in 1992, down from 9.8 in 1987.) (Special Target Populations: American Indian/Alaska Native males; People 15–24 years.)

2. **Reduce cirrhosis deaths to no more than 6 per 100,000 people.** (Age-adjusted update: 7.9 per 100,000 in 1992, down from 9.2 in 1987.) (Special Target Populations: Black males; American Indians/Alaska Natives.)

3. **Reduce the proportion of high school seniors and college students engaging in recent occasions of heavy drinking of alcoholic beverages to no more than 28 percent of high school seniors and 32 percent of college students.** (Update: 27 percent of high school seniors and 41.4 percent of college students in 1992, down from 33.0 percent and 41.7 percent respectively in 1988.)

4. **Reduce alcohol consumption by people aged 14 and older to an annual average of no more than 2 gallons of ethanol per person.** (Update: 2.46 gallons of ethanol in 1990, down from 2.54 in 1987.)

5. **Establish and monitor in 50 states comprehensive plans to ensure access to alcohol and drug treatment programs for traditionally underserved people.** (No baseline data as of 1994.)

6. **Extend adoption of alcohol and drug policies for the work environment to at least 60 percent of worksites with 50 or more employees.** (Baseline: 88 percent adopted alcohol policies, and 89 percent adopted other drug policies as of 1992.)

7. **Extend to 50 states administrative driver's license suspension/revocation laws or programs of equal effectiveness for people determined to have been driving under the influence of intoxicants.** (Update: 34 states and D.C. in 1993, up from 28 states and D.C. in 1990.)

8. **Increase to 50 states the number of states that have enacted and enforce policies, beyond those in existence in 1989, to reduce access to alcoholic beverages by minors.** (No baseline data as of 1994.)

9. **Increase to at least 20 the number of states that have enacted statutes to restrict promotion of alcoholic beverages that are focused principally on young audiences.** (No baseline data as of 1994.)

10. **Extend to 50 states legal blood alcohol concentration tolerance levels of .04 percent for motor-vehicle drivers aged 21 and older and .00 percent for those younger than age 21.** (Baseline: 0 states in 1990.)

11. **Increase to at least 75 percent the proportion of primary care providers who screen for alcohol and other drug use problems and provide counseling and referral as needed.** (Baseline: 29 percent of pediatricians, 45 percent of nurse practitioners, 34 percent of obstetricians/gynecologists, 63 percent of internists, and 39 percent of family physicians inquire about alcohol consumption in patients 12 years and older as of 1992; 26 percent of pediatricians, 19 percent of nurse practitioners, 24 percent of obstetricians/gynecologists, 33 percent of internists, and 28 percent of family physicians refer patients to alcohol treatment as of 1992.)

Source: Data from *Healthy People 2000 National Health Promotion and Disease Prevention Objectives,* 1991; and *Healthy People 2000 Review 1993,* 1994. Department of Health and Human Services, Washington, D.C.

Fermentation can occur in fruits, vegetables, or grains; therefore, any one of these products can be used to produce drinking alcohol (see table 16.2). The process of fermentation will continue naturally until the concentration of alcohol is sufficiently high to kill the yeast organisms that are responsible for fermentation. Approximately 14 percent alcohol is the natural limit on production by yeast organisms. In order to get an alcohol concentration higher than 14 percent, additional action must be taken, such as distillation or fortification. With either of these two processes, the

TABLE 16.2 — Sources of Alcoholic Beverages

Beverage	Source	Percent Alcohol	Comments
Beer	Malted barley	4–6 percent	—
Ale	Malted barley	6–8 percent	—
Wine			
Dry	Grape juice	12–14 percent	—
Sweet	Grape juice	18–21 percent	Fortified
Whiskey	Malted grains	40–50 percent	Distilled
Brandy	Grape juice	40–50 percent	Distilled
Rum	Molasses	40–50 percent	Distilled
Vodka	Various sources	40–50 percent	Distilled
Gin	Various sources	40–50 percent	Distilled

Figure 16.1: What Do You Think?

1. A can or glass of beer, a glass of wine, and a shot of whiskey all contain the same quantity of absolute alcohol. How many college students do you think know or believe this fact? What is your source of evidence in answering this question?

2. To what extent is preference for a particular type of alcoholic beverage a function of age, gender, or geographical region?

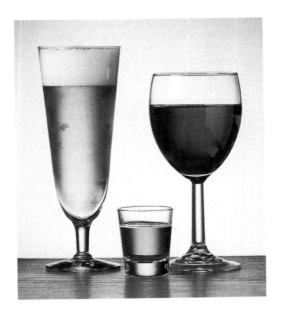

concentration of alcohol produced can be much higher than 14 percent.

In the U.S. today, there are four principal types of alcoholic beverages made from ethyl alcohol: beers (3 to 5 percent alcohol); wines (10 to 14 percent alcohol); fortified wines, such as sherry, port, and vermouth (14 to 20 percent alcohol); and distilled spirits, such as whiskey, rum, and gin (approximately 40 percent alcohol). Based on absolute alcohol, a 12-ounce bottle of beer, a 5-ounce glass of wine, 3 ounces of fortified wine, or 1.5 ounces of distilled spirits all contain the same quantity of alcohol—approximately 0.6 ounces of absolute alcohol (see figure 16.1).

Alcohol Absorption

Ethyl alcohol requires no digestion before it is absorbed into the bloodstream. Approximately 20 percent of the alcohol ingested is absorbed in the stomach while the remaining 80 percent is absorbed in the upper-third of the small intestine (called the **duodenum**). Figure 16.2 illustrates some of the primary absorption sites.

Seven factors influence the rate of absorption at the primary absorption sites. These seven factors are alcohol concentration, rate of consumption, amount of alcohol consumed, chemical present in the alcoholic beverage, condition of the stomach, pylorospasm, and emotional condition.

Alcohol Concentration

The higher the concentration of alcohol, the more rapidly it is absorbed in the digestive tract to an upper limit of approximately 40 percent. After that limit is reached, absorption is slowed.

Rate of Consumption

The more rapidly a person drinks, the greater the quantity of absorption to a point. Overall, however, the rate of absorption is not affected by quantity consumed.

Amount of Alcohol Consumed

The greater the quantity consumed, the longer absorption takes.

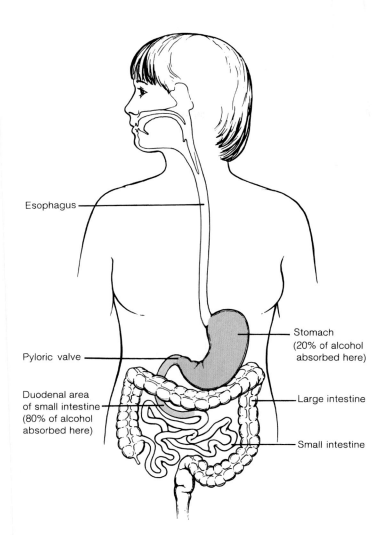

Esophagus

Pyloric valve

Duodenal area
of small intestine
(80% of alcohol
absorbed here)

Stomach
(20% of alcohol
absorbed here)

Large intestine

Small intestine

Figure 16.2: Sites of
alcohol absorption

Source: Data from D. Dennison, et al., *Alcohol
and Behavior*, 1980, C.V. Mosby Company, St.
Louis, MO.

Chemical Present in the Alcoholic Beverage

When nonalcoholic beverages are mixed with alcohol, the absorption process is generally slowed, unless the mixers contain carbonated beverages. Carbonated beverages cause the **pyloric valve** (the ring of muscle separating the stomach and the duodenum) to relax, thereby emptying the contents of the stomach more rapidly into the small intestine. Since the small intestine is the site of the greatest absorption of alcohol, carbonated beverages (such as champagne, other carbonated wines, and drinks mixed with carbonated mixers) increase the rate of absorption by causing a more rapid transition through the stomach (see figure 16.3).

Condition of the Stomach

Many people think that eating will slow absorption of alcohol because the stomach will be coated. It is not uncommon for people

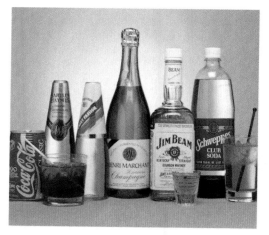

to drink milk or eat before drinking. This will slow absorption of alcohol, but it is not because the stomach is coated, it is because the stomach will not empty its contents into the small intestine until digestion in the stomach is complete. The presence of food in the stomach will slow this emptying into the

Figure 16.3: What Do You Think?

1. Carbonated beverages are absorbed more quickly into the bloodstream. If a person chooses to drink carbonated alcoholic beverages, what precautions should be taken?
2. Are mixed drinks popular among students on your campus? Are they often "mixed" using carbonated beverages? What determines the popularity of beverages?

small intestine and slow down the absorption of alcohol. Not all foods remain in the stomach for the same length of time. Complex chemicals, such as proteins, remain in the stomach much longer than do carbohydrates; therefore, proteins will slow absorption at a greater rate than carbohydrates.

Pylorospasm

Alcohol can be an irritant to the lining of the digestive system. Occasionally, this irritation can cause the pyloric valve to go into a spasm (contraction) called **pylorospasm.** When the pyloric valve is closed, nothing can move from the stomach to the upper small intestine, and absorption is slowed. If the irritation continues, it can cause nausea and vomiting to occur.

Emotional Condition

Set and **setting** are important factors in determining the outcomes of drug experiences. In the case of alcohol absorption, the emotions play an important role in the operation of the pyloric valve and, therefore, affect the rate at which alcohol is absorbed. Stress and tension cause more rapid emptying of the stomach, therefore alcohol is absorbed much more rapidly when people are tense than when they are relaxed.

These factors combined determine the absorption rate of alcoholic beverages by affecting transit time in the digestive system. Those factors that reduce transit time are associated with more rapid absorption of alcohol; those factors that increase transit time slow down the rate of absorption of alcohol.

Alcohol Metabolism

Alcohol is water soluble; therefore, once it is absorbed, distribution to all bodily tissues is complete. Alcohol easily crosses all tissue barriers, including the placental barriers. Once in the bloodstream, **metabolism** of alcohol begins. In humans, the rate of metabolism of alcohol is relatively stable, with approximately 7 to 10 grams (0.31 to 0.44 ounces) of absolute alcohol metabolized per hour. Of all the alcohol consumed, 95 percent must be metabolized by the liver, with the remaining eliminated in the breath, urine, and perspiration.

Blood-Alcohol Levels

Blood-alcohol concentration (BAC) can be defined as the ratio of alcohol to total blood volume. As an example, in an average male (weighing approximately 150 pounds), one drink would produce a BAC of approximately

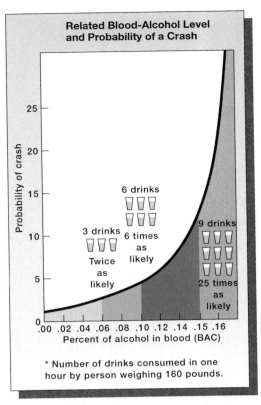

Figure 16.4: One drink can be too many—for safe driving.

Source: Courtesy of AAA Iowa.

0.02 percent (two parts of alcohol to every ten thousand parts of blood). At the 0.07 percent level, people are considered impaired, and at the 0.1 percent level most states consider people to be legally intoxicated. Some states have lowered the legal alcohol limit in the blood to 0.08.[4]

Some people who weigh the same may have different concentrations of muscle and fat, so blood-alcohol concentrations may differ between them. Larger people are generally able to maintain a lower BAC than smaller people who drink the same amount of alcohol at the same rate; however, this is not a hard-and-fast rule. Figures 16.4 and 16.5 provide information regarding blood-alcohol levels and the number of drinks necessary to cause those levels (based on body weight).

Physiological and Psychological Effects

The immediate physiological and psychological effects of alcohol at various levels and their subsequent impact on a person's behavior are of greater importance overall than absolute BAC. Once again, we must recall the importance of individual variation when we consider the overall effects of alcohol. These differences are

Set: the total internal environment of an individual at the time a drug is taken. This includes physical, mental, and emotional characteristics.

Setting: the total external environment of an individual at the time a drug is taken. This includes the physical environment as well as the social environment.

Metabolism: the physical and chemical processes of the body that contribute to the growth, maintenance, repair, and breakdown of body tissues, as well as making energy available.

Unit 4: Minimizing Negative Health-Related Behaviors

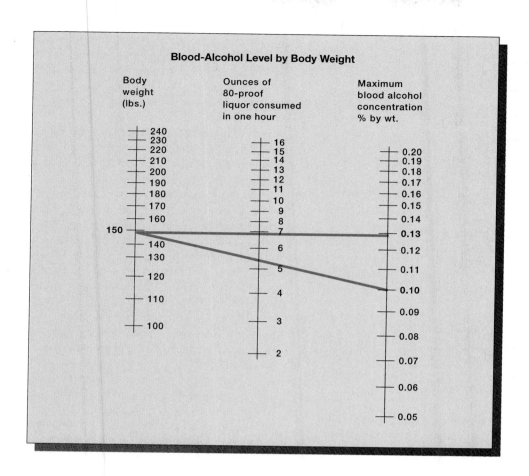

Figure 16.5: The effect of body weight on blood-alcohol concentration
Source: Courtesy of AAA Iowa.

related to set and setting, that is, the biological, psychological, and social differences between individuals; therefore, two different people with a 0.05 percent BAC may exhibit quite different behavior. Table 16.3 contains a summary of the *general* behavior characteristics of most individuals at given blood-alcohol levels.

Alcohol is primarily a depressant. It acts on the **central nervous system** by decreasing its activity over time. The greater the BAC, the greater the effects on the central nervous system. Exactly how alcohol depresses the central nervous system is not yet known; however, the depression is progressive and continuous. At the lowest levels of BAC, the higher centers of the brain are affected first (see figure 16.6). As the number of drinks increases and BAC increases, the depression of the central nervous system continues until the deepest motor areas are affected. Chronic alcohol abuse also can impair memory, possibly by affecting the nerve fibers (white matter) that connect the various regions of the brain.[5]

Impairment of Driving Skills
Alcohol caused or contributed to more than 22,000 motor-vehicle deaths in a recent

year.[6] About half of all pedestrians who are killed have elevated blood-alcohol levels.[7] At some time in their lives nearly 40 percent of people in the U.S. will be involved in an alcohol-related traffic crash.[8] Although the number of alcohol-related motor-vehicle crash deaths among persons aged fifteen to twenty-four years has been on a general decline during the past decade, figure 16.7 illustrates that the level of decline has not yet reached the targeted objective for the year 2000. Studies of the actual blood-alcohol levels in drivers of five different age groups who were involved in fatal motor-vehicle accidents reveal that among sixteen-to nineteen-year-olds, the greatest number of fatalities occurred at much lower BACs than those of persons in older age groups. This may indicate that younger drivers are at greater risk, and pose a greater risk to others, at lower BACs. There are several plausible reasons why this may be so, including the following:

1. The young person who drinks lacks experience in compensating for the effects of alcohol.

Central nervous system: the part of the nervous system consisting of the brain and spinal cord.

Figure 16.6: Alcohol and its effects on the brain

From Betty S. Bergersen and E. E. Krug, *Pharmacology in Nursing*, 12th edition. Copyright © 1973 C. V. Mosby Company, St. Louis, MO.

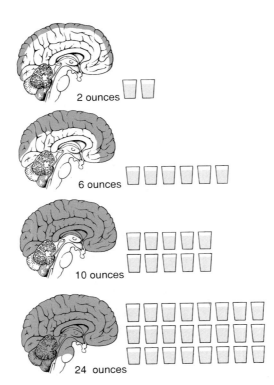

2 ounces

6 ounces

10 ounces

24 ounces

2. The young driver is an inexperienced driver; hence, necessary driving skills are less automatic and more inclined to deteriorate from alcohol's effects.

3. The inclination to take risks, especially strong in young people, may be accentuated by alcohol.

4. On the average, young people weigh less than adults and are therefore more susceptible to the effects of smaller amounts of alcohol.

At a BAC of 0.10 percent, a driver has approximately ten times the likelihood of being involved in a car accident than a driver who has not been drinking alcoholic beverages. At a BAC of 0.15 percent, the probability increases to twenty-five times.

Alcohol and Pregnancy

In 1981, the U.S. Surgeon General issued an advisory that pregnant women should not drink alcohol due to its **teratogenic** (ability to cause birth defects) effects on the developing fetus.

As a pediatric resident, Christy Ulleland found several cases of infants who would not respond to medical care. The infants' failure to thrive prompted Ulleland to search their records in an attempt to identify a cause for their poor development. In each case, she found that the mothers of these infants had been alcoholics during pregnancy. In following up her suspicions, she was able to identify in the medical histories of similar cases, twelve cases with similar circumstances. Of these twelve babies, she found that ten were undersized at birth. Of ten that were tested for normal development, five were retarded, three were borderline, and two were normal.[9]

Problems associated with the consumption of alcohol during pregnancy have been confirmed by many other studies. The specific pattern of deformities associated with **fetal alcohol syndrome (FAS)** was first described in France by Lemoine and others and subsequently confirmed and named fetal alcohol syndrome by Jones and Smith in the U.S.[10]

The three most commonly occurring physical features of FAS are small eye slits, small head circumference, and **prenatal** and **postnatal** growth impairments expressed primarily in deficiency in length at birth and postnatal growth deficiency in length and weight. The most common abnormal developmental characteristic of FAS is mental retardation, which may occur with or without the other associated physical abnormalities.

The effects of FAS are long lasting. When the FAS children, who were originally studied by Jones and Smith, were examined as teenagers, it was confirmed that both the physical and mental handicaps had persisted. All of these children are still below average for weight, height, and head circumference, as well as below-average in intelligence. Additional problems have occurred in these children including hearing, vision, and dental-health problems.

The incidence of fetal alcohol syndrome in the general population is fairly low, with estimates around 2.7 per 1,000 live births;[11] however, smaller amounts of alcohol consumption during pregnancy can also have negative consequences for the developing fetus. Intrauterine growth retardation, causing babies to be small in height and weight as well as in head circumference, and neurobehavioral dysfunction, such as sleep pattern disruptions and lower levels of arousal and attentiveness to the environment may occur. Prenatal exposure to alcohol can produce a wide range of deficits, depending on the amount and timing of the alcohol exposure and individual characteristics and sensitivity of both the mother and

Fetal alcohol syndrome (FAS): a pattern of abnormalities found in the newborns of women who drank alcohol during pregnancy. This condition consists of specific congenital and behavioral abnormalities.

Prenatal: the time from conception to birth.

Postnatal: the time following the birth of a baby.

TABLE 16.3 — Psychological and Physical Effects of Various Blood-Alcohol Concentration Levels*

Number of Drinks†	Blood-Alcohol Concentration	Psychological and Physical Effects
1	0.02 percent–0.03 percent	No overt effects, slight mood elevation
2	0.05 percent–0.06 percent	Feeling of relaxation, warmth; slight decrease in reaction time and in fine-muscle coordination
3	0.08 percent–0.09 percent	Balance, speech, vision, hearing slightly impaired; feelings of euphoria, increased confidence; loss of motor coordination
	0.10 percent	Legal intoxication in most states; some have lower limits
4	0.11 percent–0.12 percent	Coordination and balance becoming difficult; distinct impairment of mental faculties, judgment
5	0.14 percent–0.15 percent	Major impairment of mental and physical control; slurred speech, blurred vision, lack of motor skills
7	0.20 percent	Loss of motor control—must have assistance in moving about; mental confusion
10	0.30 percent	Severe intoxication; minimum conscious control of mind and body
14	0.40 percent	Unconsciousness, threshold of coma
17	0.50 percent	Deep coma
20	0.60 percent	Death from respiratory failure

*For each hour elapsed since the last drink, subtract 0.015 percent blood-alcohol concentration, or approximately one drink.

†One drink = one beer (4 percent alcohol, 12 oz.), one highball (1 oz. whiskey), or one glass table wine (5 oz.).

Source: Modified from data given in Ohio State Police Driver Information Seminars and the National Clearinghouse for Alcohol and Alcoholism Information, Rockville, MD.

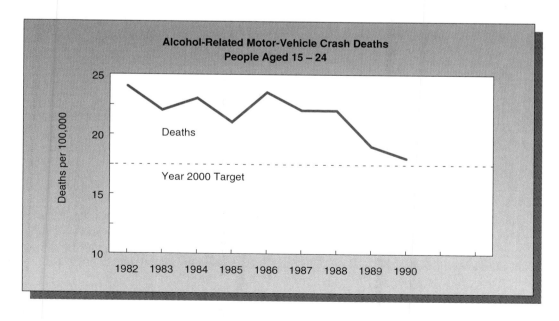

Alcohol-Related Motor-Vehicle Crash Deaths
People Aged 15 – 24

Figure 16.7: What Do You Think?

1. Although progress has been made in reducing the rate of alcohol-related motor-vehicle deaths among youth, current figures suggest that there is still work to be done. What appeals (i.e., types of messages) would be effective to reduce drinking and driving among people in the 15–24-year-old age group?
2. Who would be some effective spokespersons (i.e., same-age peers, sports figures, other celebrities, health authorities) to appeal to this age group?

Source: Data from the U.S. Department of Health and Human Services, 1992.

TABLE 16.4 — Blood-Alcohol Concentration and Driver Impairment

Blood-Alcohol Concentration	Common Effects on Driving Ability	Approximate Amount of Liquor*
0.02 percent	Mild changes occur. Many drivers may have slight change in feelings. Existing mood (anger, elation, etc.) may be heightened. Bad driving habits are slightly pronounced.	1–2 ounces
0.05 percent	Driver takes too long to decide what to do in an emergency. Inhibitions may be influenced. Shows a "so what" attitude, exaggerated behavior and what appears to be loss of finger skills. In most states this blood-alcohol concentration may be considered with other competent evidence in determining whether the person is legally under the influence of alcohol.	2–3 ounces
0.10 percent	Driver exhibits exaggerated emotion and behavior—less concern, mental relaxation. Inhibitions, self-criticism, and judgment† are seriously affected. Shows impairment of skills of coordination. At this blood-alcohol level a driver is presumed "under the influence" in all states—and in many, .10 percent BAC is evidence of being "under the influence."	5–6 ounces
0.15 percent	Shows serious and noticeable impairment of physical and mental functions; clumsy, uncoordinated, should wait 9 to 10 hours before driving.	7–8 ounces
0.40 percent	At this point most drivers have "passed out" (unconsciousness, clammy skin, dilated pupils).	Approximately 15–20 ounces

*Beverages 90 to 100 proof.

†The effect of alcohol on judgment, inhibitions, and self-control, even in the lower blood-alcohol levels, is serious because (1) since self-criticism is affected early, the drinker often is unlikely to recognize any change in his behavior and (2) he often feels more perceptive and skillful and, therefore, is likely to take more chances in passing, speeding, or negotiating curves (self-confidence increases as skill decreases—the worst possible combination).

Reprinted by permission from Table 5, page 41 of *Alcohol: The Crutch That Cripples* by Brent Q. Hafen. Copyright © 1977 by West Publishing Company. All Rights Reserved.

Embryo: the medical term for the products of conception up to the eighth week of conception.

Fetus: the medical term for an embryo that has developed for at least eight weeks.

First trimester: that period of pregnancy beginning with fertilization and continuing to the end of the third month.

Second trimester: that period of pregnancy beginning with the fourth month and continuing to the end of the sixth month.

Third trimester: that period of pregnancy beginning with the seventh month and continuing until childbirth.

Miscarriage: a naturally occurring termination of pregnancy before the fetus is capable of extrauterine life.

embryo/fetus.[12] According to Aronson and Olegard, alcohol abuse will have a greater negative impact on growth and mental development during the **second** and **third trimesters** of pregnancy as compared to exposure during the **first trimester.**[13] Women who drink alcohol during pregnancy have a two times greater likelihood of **miscarriage.**[14]

The specific mechanism by which alcohol exerts its negative effects is unknown, but several theories have been proposed. Alcohol may cause the fetus to receive an insufficient amount of oxygen, and it may have a direct toxic effect on cells through its metabolite **acetaldehyde.**[15]

Current information on FAS can be summarized as follows:

1. Research on the impact of maternal alcohol consumption on human infants has demonstrated that FAS is a clinically observable abnormality.

2. A high blood-alcohol level during a critical time of embryonic development probably is necessary to produce FAS. The average alcohol consumption may not be as important as the maximum concentrations obtained during binge drinking at critical periods during pregnancy.

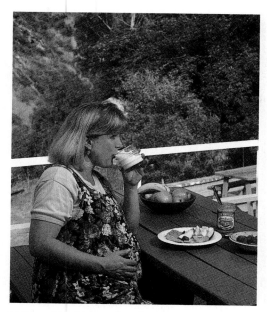

What Do You Think?

1. Pregnancy and drinking alcohol don't mix. What potential side effects is the pregnant woman in this photo protecting her developing child from by choosing to drink nonalcoholic beverages?
2. Do you think that it is primarily alcoholics who drink during pregnancy? Explain the evidence you used to answer this question.

3. The evidence from animal studies is quite compelling and clearly suggests a risk for the human fetus when daily alcohol consumption is three ounces or more. Further animal experimentation and human prospective studies will be required to determine the risk from lower doses of alcohol.
4. Observations of alcohol's effects on physiology and metabolism, particularly as related to the central nervous system, support the view that placental alcohol exposure may impair anatomical and neurological fetal development.
5. The projected incidence of fetal alcohol syndrome makes it the third leading cause of birth defects with associated mental retardation—following only **Down's syndrome** and **spina bifida**—and the only one of the three that is preventable.
6. The physical and mental handicaps associated with FAS appear to persist throughout life.

It is important to recognize that it is difficult to determine the exact consequences of the use of a single substance during pregnancy because it is unusual for humans to use or abuse only one drug. Other drugs, including **nicotine, narcotics,** and **PCP,** have been shown to compromise fetal development to varying degrees.

Clearly, drinking and pregnancy do not mix. The responsible use of alcohol precludes its use during pregnancy.

Alcohol-Related Mortality and Morbidity

The abuse of alcohol carries with it a heavy public health burden, including **alcohol-related mortality (ARM).** The burden, however, is not just in how many deaths occur, but in **years of potential life lost (YPLL)** for people in the U.S. Tables 16.5 and 16.6 contain a summary of ARM and YPLL for the U.S.

For many years it has been thought that alcohol is metabolized mainly in the liver; however, recent evidence indicates that, at times, the stomach also metabolizes alcohol. In fact, a substantial proportion of alcohol is metabolized in the stomach when it is consumed in small amounts. It is hypothesized that this gastric metabolism serves to prevent toxicity associated with occasional moderate to heavy drinking. Chronic alcohol consumption diminishes the effectiveness of gastric metabolism of alcohol.

When alcohol is absorbed, it is distributed throughout the body. If alcohol is used over long periods of time in sufficient quantities, it can adversely affect the performance and health of every organ system in the body. Our focus is on three specific disease risks associated with long-term abuse of alcohol— the risk of developing or aggravating heart disease, the association between alcohol and cancer, and damage to the liver.

Many studies have been done on the relationship between consumption of alcohol and its subsequent impact on health. There is conflict in the results of these studies, and some of the evidence is inconclusive; however, when we look at the total health of a person, data from the Framingham study (a longitudinal study of the risk factors to health) indicate that the relationship between alcohol and health is not linear but

Down's syndrome: a congenital disease caused by the presence of an extra number-21 chromosome, resulting in mental deficiency and a variety of physical defects.

Spina bifida: the most common neural tube defect, in which an infant is born with a spinal column that does not close completely, leaving the spinal cord exposed.

PCP: an animal tranquilizer— phencyclidine—that acts as a deliriant in humans; sometimes known as angel dust or tea.

Alcohol-related mortality (ARM): a cause of death directly attributable to the use of alcoholic beverages.

Years of potential life lost (YPLL): the difference between a person's life expectancy and that person's age at death. This is used as one measure of the consequences of early or premature death.

TABLE 16.5

TABLE 16.5 *Estimated Alcohol-Related Mortality and Male-to-Female Ratio, by Sex and Diagnostic Category—United States*

Diagnostic category	Male No. deaths	(%)	Female No. deaths	(%)	Total No. deaths	(%) deaths	Male: Female ratio
Malignant neoplasms	11,410	(16.3)	4,609	(13.2)	16,019	(15.2)	2.5
Mental disorders	4,192	(6.0)	1,124	(3.2)	5,316	(5.1)	3.7
Cardiovascular diseases	4,604	(6.6)	6,143	(17.6)	10,747	(10.2)	0.8
Respiratory diseases*	1,847	(2.6)	1,842	(5.3)	3,688	(3.5)	1.0
Digestive diseases	13,032	(18.6)	6,524	(18.7)	19,556	(18.7)	2.0
Unintentional injuries	20,637	(29.4)	9,569	(27.4)	30,205	(28.7)	2.2
Intentional injuries	13,644	(19.4)	4,016	(11.5)	17,660	(16.8)	3.4
Other alcohol-related diagnoses	803	(1.1)	1,100	(3.1)	1,903	(1.8)	0.7
Total	**70,168**	**(100.0)**	**34,927**	**(100.0)**	**105,095**	**(100.0)**	

*Includes mortality from respiratory tuberculosis.

Source: Data from *MMWR,* 39(11):175, March 23, 1990.

What Do You Think?

1. What percentage of the total alcohol-related mortality occurs in males as compared to females?

2. What are the top three causes of alcohol-related mortality in females? How does this compare to the top three causes of alcohol-related mortality in males?

Hematologic: a medical term referring to blood and blood-forming tissues.

Electrolytic: a medical term referring to blood concentrations of specific ions, such as sodium, potassium, chloride, and bicarbonate.

Alcoholism: addiction to alcohol, sometimes called alcohol-dependence syndrome, characterized by loss of memory, inability to stop drinking until intoxication, inability to cut down on drinking, binge drinking, and withdrawal symptoms.

Coronary heart disease: a chronic disease condition in which the normal flow of blood through the coronary arteries is reduced or impaired; synonymous with coronary artery disease.

HDL cholesterol: high density lipoprotein cholesterol; a type of lipoprotein that carries cholesterol from the bloodstream to the liver, where it can be excreted from the body. High blood HDL levels may help protect individuals against coronary artery disease.

rather U-shaped. In other words, zero intake of alcohol appears to be less healthful than small to moderate amounts. Intakes higher than the equivalent of two drinks per day, however, are associated with increased rates of nutritional, gastrointestinal, neurological, cardiological, **hematologic,** pulmonary, **electrolytic,** and cancerous problems. The paradox here lies in our inability to determine which individuals are prone to the development of **alcoholism;** therefore, taking these data and making a blanket recommendation for the general public to change its drinking habits would be negligent. Recommending that everyone drink to improve their health would certainly result in an increase in the rate of alcoholism.

Drinking and Coronary Heart Disease

There is evidence that moderate consumption of alcohol reduces the risk of **coronary heart disease** (CHD). Rohan reviewed eleven studies and found that seven of them suggest a reduced risk of CHD following moderate current consumption of alcohol.[16] This

relationship seemed to hold true in one study for up to four to five drinks daily;[17] however, consumption of more than five drinks daily was associated with increased rates of CHD. It should be noted that in the studies that found a relationship between moderate drinking and decreased CHD, none associated alcohol use with decreased mortality.

In addition, Castelli has argued that the apparent protective effect of moderate alcohol consumption against CHD is not due to the pharmacological properties of alcohol but to the lifestyle patterns of those people who drink moderately.[18] Such persons may have less of a tendency to engage in aggression, competition, and other hard-driving behavior associated with CHD; thus, it is probably premature to assume that alcohol decreases the risk of CHD. However, moderate drinking (one-half to one ounce of alcohol per day) does raise the **HDL cholesterol** level that clears fat deposits from the arteries[19] (see chapters 3 and 10).

Drinking and Cancer

Heavy drinkers have a greater risk of developing cancer, and survival rates are

TABLE 16.6 Mean Years of Potential Life Lost (YPLL) for Alcohol-Related Deaths, by Sex and Diagnostic Category—United States

Diagnostic category	Mean YPLL per death		
	Male	Female	Total
YPLL to age 65			
Malignant neoplasms	3.3	2.3	3.0
Mental disorders	12.5	12.6	12.5
Cardiovascular diseases	2.8	1.0	1.8
Respiratory diseases*	1.8	0.8	1.3
Digestive diseases	8.9	7.2	8.3
Unintentional injuries	27.7	21.7	25.8
Intentional injuries	25.7	23.9	25.3
Other alcohol-related diagnoses	3.2	1.7	2.3
Mean YPLL per death	*16.3*	*11.0*	*14.6*
YPLL to life expectancy			
Malignant neoplasms	14.4	15.6	14.8
Mental disorders	24.0	28.9	25.1
Cardiovascular diseases	12.0	10.8	11.3
Respiratory diseases*	10.1	9.8	9.9
Digestive diseases	20.5	22.3	21.1
Unintentional injuries	37.3	35.5	36.7
Intentional injuries	35.7	39.5	36.5
Other alcohol-related diagnoses	13.4	13.7	13.6
Mean YPLL per death	*26.7*	*24.3*	*25.9*

*Includes YPLL from respiratory tuberculosis.

Source: Data from *MMWR*, 39(11):177, March 23, 1990.

What Do You Think?

1. What are the top three mean years of potential life lost to age 65 and to life expectancy for men as compared with women? Which sex loses more years of potential life to alcohol-related deaths?

2. Why is it important to calculate years of potential life lost in addition to knowing the actual numbers of alcohol-related deaths? What additional information does YPLL give us?

substantially lower among heavy drinkers than among the general population. The sites most often affected include the mouth, tongue, pharynx and larynx, esophagus, stomach, liver, lung, pancreas, colon, and rectum.[20] How alcohol may exert a carcinogenic effect is not yet known; however, a number of hypotheses have been proposed to help explain the role of alcohol in cancer causation. The following are several of the more promising theories under study:

1. alcohol-induced immunologic suppression, which reduces the body's ability to defend itself against cancer cells and viruses thought to be cancer-causing,

2. alcohol as a source of cancer-causing contaminants, such as fossil fuel oils and nitrosamines,

3. alcohol as a **cocarcinogen** with tobacco

4. alcohol-induced outcomes (such as malnutrition and **anemia**) as a precursor to cancer,

5. alcohol as a solvent, increasing the entry of cancer-causing substances into cells.

Research has demonstrated a link between moderate levels of alcohol consumption and the development of breast cancer. Studies have shown a 50 percent increase in the risk of breast cancer among

Cocarcinogin: a substance capable of causing cancer only when it is in the presence of another specific substance.

Anemia: a decreased ability of the blood to carry oxygen, due to a decrease in the amount of hemoglobin in the blood.

women who drank more than five grams of alcohol per day, or the equivalent of three drinks per week.[21] Risk of breast cancer increases with increased alcohol consumption.

In one study, when premenopausal women drank about one ounce of pure alcohol daily, they had higher levels of **estrogen** in their blood and urine than when they did not drink. It is possible, therefore, that the link between alcohol consumption and breast cancer is an increased production of estrogen.[22]

The result of the connection between even moderate drinking among women and the increased risk of breast cancer creates a controversy. As indicated above, moderate alcohol intake has an apparent protective role with respect to risk of coronary heart disease. What should a woman do? Unfortunately, irrefutable advice is not available at the present time. Because breast cancer causation is such a complex issue, some authorities advise that there is no health reason for women who are moderate drinkers to alter their habits unless they are planning to become pregnant, are already pregnant, or are nursing.[23]

Drinking and Liver Damage

The greatest health hazard from long-term alcohol abuse is liver disease. The most well-known liver disease associated with long-term alcohol consumption is **cirrhosis of the liver,** one of the top ten causes of death in the U.S. Cirrhosis of the liver is characterized by scarring of tissue in the liver. This scarring interferes with blood flow through the liver and eventually interrupts the liver's major functions of detoxification and metabolism.

Cirrhosis of the liver is the end stage of damage to the liver associated with alcohol abuse. Damage to the liver is a slow process that begins with the accumulation of fatty acids in the liver cells. This process, known as **fatty liver,** is reversible if a person stops drinking. If chronic alcohol abuse persists, **alcoholic hepatitis,** a chronic inflammation of the liver, may develop. Alcoholic hepatitis can be fatal or may progress to cirrhosis.

Other Disease Risks

There is a much greater incidence of several other disorders such as **pneumonia, tuberculosis,** and other respiratory tract infections among heavy drinkers. As with cancer, not only is the incidence rate higher

among heavy drinkers than in the general population, but mortality associated with these conditions is also higher for heavy drinkers.

Alcohol Abuse

The misuse of alcohol is termed **alcohol abuse** and is usually manifested by certain alcohol-related problems. These alcohol-related problems lie in three general areas:

- psychological—involving loss of control over drinking, alcohol dependence and depression, and suicidal states of mind
- medical—involving both acute and chronic illnesses, and injuries
- social—involving antisocial or socially unacceptable behaviors

A great many alcohol-related problems may be the result of excessive use and should not be confused with alcoholism. Although alcoholism directly and indirectly affects many people, there is still considerable controversy over its definition. We will distinguish between alcohol-related disability, alcoholism, and problem drinking in the following paragraphs.

Alcohol-related disability is a broad term that includes alcoholism but doesn't require that alcoholism be present. An alcohol-related disability exists when there is an impairment in the physical, mental, or social functioning of an individual. Impairment includes actual health problems related to a specific drinking bout; injuries, death, and property loss caused by accidents related to drinking; failure of the chronic excessive drinker to fulfill his or her role in the family or on the job; and mental problems, such as depression and anxiety, related to drinking.

Alcoholism is addiction to alcohol. It is also defined as **alcohol-dependence syndrome.** Alcoholism is characterized by symptoms of alcohol dependence that include loss of memory, inability to stop drinking until intoxication, inability to cut down on drinking, binge drinking, and withdrawal symptoms.

A **problem drinker** is a person who drinks alcohol to an extent or in a manner that an alcohol-related disability is manifested. The term *problem drinker* generally is applied to those who demonstrate problems in relation to drinking alcohol.

There are an estimated eighteen million problem drinkers in the adult population (age eighteen and older) in the U.S.[24] This

Estrogen: the primary female sex hormone. This hormone stimulates the development of a female physique and reproductive organs. It also stimulates the female reproductive cycle and maintains the adult female reproductive cycle.

Pneumonia: an inflammation of the lung, usually caused by a bacteria. Symptoms include cough, chest pain, and shadows on a chest x-ray.

Tuberculosis (TB): an infectious bacterial disease characterized by inflammations, abscesses, calcification of tissue, and other symptoms, affecting the respiratory system and other sites.

estimate includes alcoholics. Since as many as 95 percent of those eighteen million problem drinkers are not social isolates, it is quite feasible that the drinking of each one directly affects the lives of as many as four friends, family members, or coworkers. Thus as many as seventy-two million people in the U.S. are either directly or indirectly affected by problem drinking—clearly a public health problem of massive proportions.

What Causes Alcoholism?

Researchers have studied the genetic and environmental factors associated with the development of alcoholism. Alcoholism is

> a primary chronic disease with genetic, psychosocial, and environmental factors influencing its development and manifestations. The disease is often progressive and fatal. It is characterized by impaired control over drinking, preoccupation with the drug alcohol, use of alcohol despite adverse consequences, and distortions in thinking, most notably denial.[25]

In the 1970s, adoption studies suggested that the biological sons of alcoholics were genetically predisposed to becoming alcoholics themselves.[26] In one study conducted in Sweden, Bohman found that male adoptees whose biological fathers were severely alcoholic had a 20 percent incidence of alcohol abuse, compared to only 6 percent of the adopted sons of nonalcoholics.[27] While these studies provide strong evidence of a genetic component in alcoholism, it should be kept in mind that most children of alcoholics do not develop alcoholism themselves. It appears that the susceptibility to alcoholism is genetically transmitted, not the disease itself.[28] Thus, many children of alcoholics may carry this genetic predisposition but may or may not become alcoholics themselves, depending on environmental influences such as family dynamics, peer pressure, and availability of alcohol.

Studies of Swedish adoptees have revealed the existence of at least two different kinds of alcoholism.[29] The most common form is called **Type I** (or milieu-limited) **alcoholism.** This type has been described as occurring in both men and women and is thought to be associated with mild, untreated alcohol abuse in either biological parent.[30] It is also referred to as milieu-limited because its

development depends not only on a genetic predisposition but on environmental factors as well. Type I alcoholics are described as ambitious, sentimental, moody, and dependent on rewards of various types.

The other identified form of alcoholism is referred to as **Type II** (or male-limited) **alcoholism.**[31] Here the genetic predisposition is thought to be much stronger than in Type I alcoholism. Type II seems to appear only in men and accounts for about 25 percent of all male alcoholics. Type II alcoholism is associated with severe alcoholism in the biological father but not in the biological mother. The environment seems to have little impact on the development of this form of the disease. Type II alcoholics are described as impulsive, quick-tempered, excitable, and sensitive to pain.

Only a few years ago, researchers claimed to have located a gene whose examination could predict a person's likelihood of becoming an alcoholic. A controversy ensued as people speculated on the possibility of testing children, job applicants, and even fetuses for possible alcoholism tendencies.[32] If there is legitimacy in the notion of an "alcoholism gene," the prospect of testing is one that is far in the future. Researchers conclude presently that alcoholism has both a genetic and an environmental component. Therefore, alcoholic parents do not always produce children predisposed to alcoholism. Moreover, many alcoholics come from families with no history of alcohol use or alcoholism.[33]

Secondary Consequences of Alcohol Use

There are many other medical, economic, and social consequences that stem from irresponsible use of alcohol. In addition to motor-vehicle accidents, alcohol may play either a direct or indirect role in many other types of events resulting in unintentional or intentional injury, including violent crimes. These problems are tremendously costly to society. Some examples of secondary consequences of alcohol use are listed in table 16.7.

The 1990s have made us aware of the impact that alcohol has on families. We have become attuned to the adult child of the alcoholic, known also as the ACOA. Persons raised in families where alcohol use promotes

TABLE 16.7

Secondary Consequences of Alcohol and Other Drug Abuse

Assault
Child abuse
Disruption of family life and other
  relationships
Homicide
Loss of income
Loss of productivity
Predisposition to high-risk behaviors:
  high-risk sexual behaviors associated
  with unwanted pregnancy and sexually
  transmitted diseases
Rape
Spouse abuse
Suicide
Traffic fatalities
Unintentional injury and deaths
  (e.g., drowning)

anxiety, violence, embarrassment, or other forms of stress learn to adapt to these problems. The adaptation is not always a healthy one, however. The impact of covering up for an alcoholic parent, avoiding conflict, or feeling guilty may be carried into the college years and beyond. Several support groups for children of alcoholics exist, such as Al-Anon and AlaTeen. The Children of Alcoholics Foundation is located at 540 Madison Avenue, New York, NY 10022. If you are an ACOA or know of someone who is, you can write to that address for assistance.

Responsible Drinking Behavior

Irresponsible use of alcohol carries with it an enormous cost in many ways. Since alcohol use is such a traditional part of American society, it is important that people who choose to consume alcohol be responsible users.

1. When you are the host of a gathering in which alcohol will be served, you should:
   a. provide some food as well as drink.
   b. not insist that everyone drink alcohol. Some will prefer other beverages or none at all.
   c. provide alternate nonalcoholic beverages.
   d. make contingency plans for drunkenness.
   e. set reasonable rules regarding levels of consumption for each of your guests.
2. When you are someplace where alcoholic beverages are being served, you should:
   a. drink only when you want to, not when someone else thinks that you should.
   b. be aware of the influences of set and setting and establish reasonable limits for yourself when you choose to drink.
   c. recognize your responsibility for the health, safety, and pleasure of yourself and others.
   d. be aware of the potentially adverse effects of mixing alcohol and other drugs.

You are responsible for your own behavior. Recreational use of alcoholic beverages *can be* perfectly acceptable behavior if you remember to drink responsibly.

Social Influences on the Responsible Use of Alcohol

Six factors have been suggested as important determinants of youthful drinking behavior, including peer influences, familial and parental influences, sociocultural factors, environmental-contextual influences, personality, and behavioral influences. Of these, peer and parental influences may be the most important because of the strong relationship between the drinking practices of young adults and those of their peers and parents.

Parental and Peer Attitudes

We can find direct relationships between parental attitudes toward alcohol and alcohol-related behavior and the attitudes and behavior of their children. Problem drinking among parents is highly related to problem drinking in their children.[34] The pattern of drinking practiced in the home when children are growing up is often the same as the patterns displayed by young adults. Drinking behavior often conforms to what people think their peers find acceptable.

Nonalcoholic Beer: An Alternative for Safer Drinking?

People who like the taste of beer but want to avoid the alcohol and cut down on calories can now turn to any of dozens of brands of nonalcoholic beers made by many of the major domestic and European brewers. Legally these beverages can't be called beer on their labels; instead they're called brews or malt beverages. By law these beers must contain less than 0.5 percent alcohol; some have as little as 0.02 percent (versus beer's usual 4.5 percent alcohol). For most of us, 0.5 percent is an undetectable trace of alcohol that won't interfere with driving, boating, or work. For certain people who are advised to steer clear of alcohol—such as pregnant women, diabetics, and those on certain medications—these brews mean that they don't have to give up beer. Nonalcoholic beer can also be a good way to get the fluid you need before, during, or after exercise (in contrast, the alcohol in regular beer is a diuretic and can thus promote dehydration), provided the carbonation doesn't make you bloated or uncomfortable.

These beers are *not* designed for alcoholics, however, since "nonalcoholic" does not mean alcohol-free. Many researchers believe that such beverages may be the first step back to drinking for many recovering alcoholics. It is unknown whether the danger is psychological or whether it comes from the minute amount of alcohol itself. In addition, these beers are *not* designed for children: some experts in addiction believe that these beverages may serve as "training beers" for kids.

Thanks to modern technology, the taste of these beers has come a long way since the "near beers" of the Prohibition era. In the past, brewers heated the beer to evaporate the alcohol, but this ruined the flavor; now they use more sophisticated methods to remove it. Or they may inhibit fermentation in the first place—for instance, by quickly cooling the hot malt, or else by brewing at a lower temperature. At least one brewer uses a special hybrid strain of yeast that ferments the beverage but produces little alcohol.

Limiting the alcohol eliminates "empty" calories, since each gram of alcohol has seven calories. Nonalcoholic beers have about one-third to one-half the calories of regular beer—anywhere from 50 to 95 calories in 12 ounces, versus the usual 140 to 200 (or about 100 calories in light beers). Like regular beer, nonalcoholic beer is basically carbohydrates (from barley malt and hops), with a small amount of minerals and B vitamins.

Reprinted by permission from the *University of California at Berkeley Wellness Letter,* © Health Letter Associates, 1993.

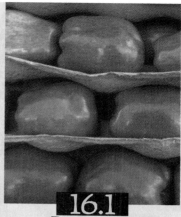

16.1
Of Special Interest

What Do You Think?

1. To what extent do you think nonalcoholic beer is an acceptable alternative for beer drinkers on college and university campuses? for other beer drinkers?
2. Will the absence of the familiar alcohol "buzz" make nonalcoholic beer lack acceptance? Is it a reasonable means to satisfy the issue of being a good host?

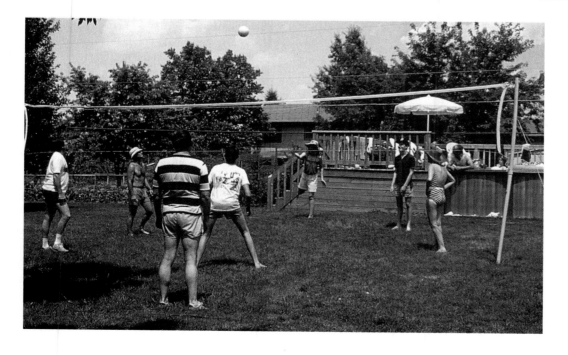

What Do You Think?

1. A party that offers various activities and doesn't focus on drinking encourages the responsible use of alcohol. What does the presence of alcohol at parties say about our culture?
2. How plausible is it in today's culture to host an alcohol-free event at a college or university? at a party with your peers? at a family gathering? Do expectations vary by type of event?

What Do You Think?

1. Children who are introduced early to the responsible use of alcohol tend to experience fewer alcohol-related problems as adults. Yet, many people find it hard to believe that use of alcohol in the home can actually discourage abuse. Why might it discourage irresponsible use?

2. How is alcohol used in different countries and cultures around the world? How does this compare to alcohol use in the U.S.?

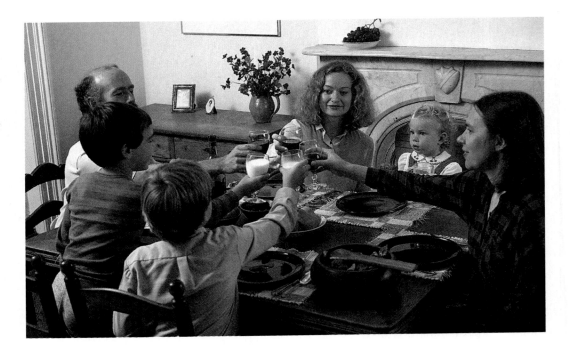

Television Advertising

The presentation of alcohol commercials on television may contribute to acceptance of drinking, even among children and youth, report Joel W. Grube and Lawrence Wallack.[35] They studied awareness of beer advertising on television among ten to fourteen-year-olds. Children who were aware of beer commercials were more knowledgeable about beer brands and slogans, and had more positive beliefs about drinking. They also perceived fewer negative consequences occurring as a result of drinking. Youth who anticipated being frequent drinkers as adults said their peers were more approving of drinking, and also believed their parents drank more frequently.

Patricia A. Madden and Joel W. Grube examined alcohol advertising during televised sporting events over a three-year period.[36] They found that more commercials appear for alcohol products than for any other beverage. Beer commercials are the most predominant alcohol advertisements, and include images that are contrary to recommendations advocated by former Surgeon General C. Everett Koop. In addition to formal commercials, television audiences are exposed to alcohol (and tobacco) advertisements through signs on stadiums, and other brief but recurring written and verbal sponsorship messages. Reminders about moderation in use of alcohol are rare.

The constant audience bombardment seems to affirm the positive aspects of drinking for adults and young people alike.

Alcohol, Health, and Special Populations

Although much diversity in drinking exists within the various racial and ethnic minorities in the U.S., these groups do have collective patterns of alcohol use that differ from the population as a whole.[37] In examining these differences it is important that you remember some important points: (1) few studies have looked at drinking patterns and problems over a long period of time; (2) few studies have examined other relevant variables such as nutritional or health status, socioeconomic status, education, employment status, income, housing conditions, local customs, and shared beliefs about alcohol's symbolic role in a racial or ethnic group's social life.[38]

African-Americans

Although alcohol consumption seems to be lower among Black Americans than among White Americans, Black males may have more drinking-related problems (medical, personal, and social), especially with respect to alcohol dependence.[39] The only problem occurring more frequently among White males is drinking and driving, where White

Decreasing Problems Associated with Alcohol Use: Some Community-Based Responses

What legislative proposals concerning alcohol should you support—through voting, or even by writing to your representatives in Congress and the state legislature? What can communities do to decrease problems caused by alcohol? The following ideas make sense:

1. Alcoholic beverages should be labeled to provide accurate information about ingredients, calories, percentage of alcohol, and number of drinks per container (a drink being defined as 12 ounces of beer, 5 ounces of wine or 1.5 ounces of 80-proof liquor). Every container should carry a toll-free telephone number for information on alcoholism and related problems.
2. Broadcast and print ads should carry warnings that alcohol may be addictive, impairs driving ability, interacts with other drugs, and may harm a fetus—among other health and safety messages.
3. Promotions aimed at minors, such as high school and college students, should be ended, as well as alcohol industry sponsorship of sporting and entertainment events. Malt liquors (beers with high alcohol content) such as Colt 45 and King Cobra have consistently been aimed at the young and others who suffer disproportionately from drug and alcohol problems. The Bureau of Alcohol, Tobacco, and Firearms has been petitioned to exercise its regulatory power to prevent this. For more information, write to the Center for Science in the Public Interest, 1875 Connecticut Avenue NW, Suite 300, Washington, DC 20009–5728.
4. Alcohol advertising in public places—especially billboards—often targets Latino and African-American neighborhoods. For example, one recent survey in Milwaukee showed that billboards advertising alcohol and cigarettes were heavily concentrated where young people, African-Americans, and the poor were most likely to see them. In Chicago, researchers recently noted that of 233 billboards in one Latino neighborhood, 176 advertised alcohol and 40 tobacco. In many cities, neighborhood groups have formed to remove this advertising. The Outdoor Advertising Association of America has proposed "voluntary limits" on the number of billboards advertising products that cannot be sold to minors, and "exclusionary zones" near schools and hospitals.
5. Tax laws should be revised so that alcohol is no longer a deductible business expense.
6. A hike in federal excise taxes could provide revenues for education and research. There's evidence that higher prices would reduce alcohol consumption (and alcohol-impaired driving) among the young, in particular.

Reprinted by permission from the *University of California at Berkeley Wellness Letter,* Health Letter Associates, 1993.

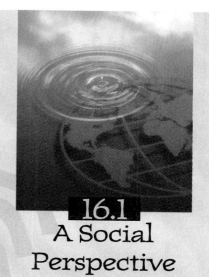

16.1 A Social Perspective

What Do You Think?

1. Does the enactment of such control measures as those described here make good sense, or do they give the government too much authority over its citizenry? By enacting and enforcing such measures does government interfere too much in people's lives? Explain.
2. If people cannot regulate their own behavior and act in ways that threaten the well-being of others, is it government's responsibility to act? Are the negative consequences that still occur despite the current alcohol sales and consumption regulations simply the price we pay to have a free society? Explain.

---

males are 2.5 times more likely to engage in this practice than are Black males. The pattern is reversed among women, where Black females have fewer alcohol-related problems than White females. Furthermore, White females are five times more likely to drive after drinking than are their Black female counterparts. White males aged eighteen to twenty-nine experience more alcohol-related problems than Black males, but problem rates for Black males in their thirties and beyond increase and stay ahead of White males during middle and old age. A possible explanation for the greater level of health problems among Black Americans may be the later onset of heavy drinking. Later-life onset of heavy drinking is associated with a more sustained pattern of drinking. Among White Americans, heavy drinking is more inclined to be a short-term, youth-oriented phenomenon. The apparent high vulnerability of Black Americans to alcohol-related problems may be a reflection of adverse social and economic conditions such as unemployment, poor housing, inadequate heath care, and racial discrimination.[40] The

What Do You Think?

1. Billboards seen at athletic stadiums and viewed on TV provide constant reminders of the social acceptance of alcohol. Should alcohol advertising be banned at sports events? Explain your rationale.
2. Cigarette advertising was banned from TV over 20 years ago. Should alcohol advertising on TV be treated similarly?

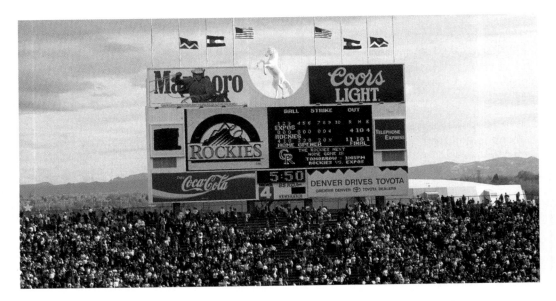

issue of a possible biological predisposition for alcohol-related problems among Black Americans is an interesting question, but one which is far from being answered.

Hispanic Americans

U.S. Hispanics generally have origins in Mexico, Puerto Rico, and Cuba, but come from numerous other countries of Latin America as well. Their diversity in alcohol consumption is reflective of the diversity in their origins. A U.S. Department of Health and Human Services report to the U.S. Congress indicates a striking difference between Hispanic men and women with respect to alcohol consumption.[41] More than 70 percent of Hispanic women either drink less than once per month or not at all. Among men, almost the same percentage are drinkers. As with Black American males, drinking increases dramatically among Hispanic men in their thirties, but declines thereafter. Hispanic women are more likely to engage in heavy drinking during their forties and fifties, but after age sixty the rate of heavy drinking is nearly zero. Mexican-American men and women show the greatest range of drinking patterns among Hispanic Americans. They have higher rates of abstention from drinking as well as heavier use rates of alcohol than men and women of Puerto Rican or Cuban origin.

Health-related problems associated with alcohol use vary by national origin, with the highest rates being among Mexican Americans. The prevalence of alcohol-related problems is higher for Hispanic males than for either Black or White American males. The variations in drinking patterns, as reflected by country of origin, are too diverse to enumerate here. The greater the degree to which Hispanics assimilate with mainstream U.S. culture, the more their drinking patterns seem to reflect those of the U.S. population overall. In general, systematic research on drinking among Hispanics, especially male adolescents, is limited.

Asian Americans

Asian Americans also encompass a broad spectrum of nations and traditions including China, Japan, Korea, Vietnam, the Philippines, India, and other Asian countries. While variations related to country of origin, age, and gender exist, on a whole, Asian Americans have the lowest level of alcohol consumption and alcohol-related problems of all major U.S. racial and ethnic groups.[42] The low rate of alcohol use may be attributed partly to cultural factors and partly to what is known as the *flushing response*. This unusual physiological response is characterized by facial flushing, and may be accompanied by headache, dizziness, increased heart rate, itching, and other discomfort.[43] To the extent that drinking occurs, it is likely to be done with friends and on special occasions. Thus, drinking activity may be performed under more controlled circumstances than what characterizes the U.S. general population. The result is a lower rate of alcohol-related social, personal, and health problems. The effect of acculturation on Asian American drinking patterns is not clear.

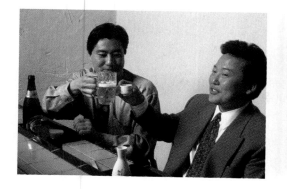
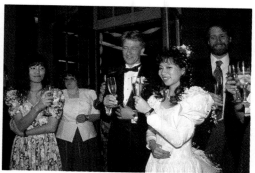

What Do You Think?

1. Cultural traditions may have a strong influence on drinking patterns. Why do you think that alcohol is so important in some traditions and so peripheral to others?
2. What is your family's treatment of alcohol?

American Indians and Alaska Natives

Of all racial and ethnic minorities in the U.S., it is perhaps hardest to generalize the drinking patterns of American Indians and Alaska Natives. Some tribes are mostly abstinent, while others have high levels of alcohol use and abuse.[44]

The extent of alcohol-related problems in this diverse population is reflected in mortality rates among causes that are attributable, in part, to alcohol. Unintentional injuries, chronic liver disease and cirrhosis, homicide, and suicide are among the ten leading causes of death for American Indians and Alaska Natives.[45] This population has a rate of unintentional injury that is 2.2 times higher than for the general U.S. population, and an alcoholism rate that is four times higher. Deaths from alcohol-related causes are three times higher among persons aged twenty-five to forty-four. Binge drinking is problematic, especially among males, and perhaps offers some explanation for the higher rates of unintentional injury and homicide. While women in these populations drink less than men, they may be more susceptible to certain health problems, since they account for nearly half of deaths from cirrhosis of the liver.

Alcohol and College Life

Research shows that alcohol use and abuse is prevalent among college and university students.[46] The precise extent of alcohol use and the patterns of abuse are sometimes difficult to assess accurately because of variations in how drinking behavior is defined, measured, and validated.[47] As indicated in the introduction to this chapter, we all acknowledge that directly or indirectly, alcohol is very much a part of college life and student experience for the majority of persons pursuing higher education. Alcohol use and abuse can contribute to the occurrence of isolated problems for students, or establish a pattern of behavior that relates to quite serious problems (see Activity for Wellness 16.1). As authors of this textbook and as health educators, we have considerable concern for the relationship between alcohol consumption and acts of violence and carelessness that give rise to intentional and unintentional injury, property damage, sexual misconduct, and other problems. We also are concerned about the various promotions that establishments near college and university campuses have that promote heavy and potentially abusive drinking: "Two for one specials 5PM to 7PM nightly," "$1 mixed drinks 6PM 'til closing," "50-cent imported drafts every Wednesday," "$1.95 pitchers during happy hour," "nurses' night every Thursday," "women drink for free 11PM 'til closing," and so on. The combination of reduced prices, extended hours, and specially targeted audiences creates a formula that ultimately can lead to disaster for a lot of people.

People's own insecurities about themselves, combined with society's mixed messages about alcohol, contribute to overindulgence with alcohol. Richard P. Keeling makes an excellent point when he writes:

> The trouble is that the truth of the portent that certain patterns of drinking make assault, or unintended intercourse, or unprotected intercourse more likely shares mental and affective space with other truths that have the validation of cultural approval. Intimacy provokes anxiety, true, and alcohol relieves anxiety (a cover-up rather than a solution, no doubt), true; negotiating takes time and effort, true, and alcohol is faster and easier, true

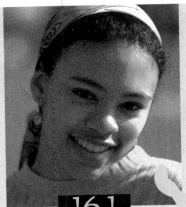

Activity for Wellness

Consequences of Drinking: What Does It Matter Anyway?

What consequences does drinking, especially drinking to excess, have for you? The list which follows contains some unpleasant events that might happen to one who has consumed alcohol. Circle the box corresponding to whether this event happening to you would be **extremely important (EI), somewhat important (SI), neither important nor unimportant (N), somewhat unimportant (SU), or extremely unimportant (EU)** in your life. Compare your results to those of a friend. Which types of circumstances hold the most importance for you: ones that have physical health consequences, ones that have academic consequences, ones that have social consequences, ones that have legal consequences, or ones that have moral or ethical consequences? How many of these events have you or someone you know actually experienced?

1. Have a hangover on one occasion	[EI]	[SI]	[N]	[SU]	[EU]
2. Have a hangover on multiple occasions	[EI]	[SI]	[N]	[SU]	[EU]
3. Have a poor performance on a midterm exam	[EI]	[SI]	[N]	[SU]	[EU]
4. Have a poor performance on a final exam	[EI]	[SI]	[N]	[SU]	[EU]
5. Get into trouble with police or college authorities	[EI]	[SI]	[N]	[SU]	[EU]
6. Engage in property damage after drinking	[EI]	[SI]	[N]	[SU]	[EU]
7. Engage in pranks (e.g., set off fire alarm)	[EI]	[SI]	[N]	[SU]	[EU]
8. Get into an argument	[EI]	[SI]	[N]	[SU]	[EU]
9. Get into a physical fight	[EI]	[SI]	[N]	[SU]	[EU]
10. Vomit	[EI]	[SI]	[N]	[SU]	[EU]
11. Drive a motor vehicle after 1–2 drinks	[EI]	[SI]	[N]	[SU]	[EU]
12. Drive a motor vehicle after 5+ drinks	[EI]	[SI]	[N]	[SU]	[EU]
13. Miss a class	[EI]	[SI]	[N]	[SU]	[EU]
14. Get criticized by a friend	[EI]	[SI]	[N]	[SU]	[EU]
15. Miss an exam	[EI]	[SI]	[N]	[SU]	[EU]
16. Think that I might have a drinking problem	[EI]	[SI]	[N]	[SU]	[EU]
17. Have a memory loss	[EI]	[SI]	[N]	[SU]	[EU]
18. Do or say something I later regret	[EI]	[SI]	[N]	[SU]	[EU]
19. Get arrested for a DUI or DWI	[EI]	[SI]	[N]	[SU]	[EU]
20. Commit sexual assault or be sexually assaulted	[EI]	[SI]	[N]	[SU]	[EU]
21. Have unprotected sexual intercourse	[EI]	[SI]	[N]	[SU]	[EU]
22. Be hurt or injured	[EI]	[SI]	[N]	[SU]	[EU]
23. Receive a failing grade for a course	[EI]	[SI]	[N]	[SU]	[EU]

(remember Ogden Nash? "Candy is dandy but liquor is quicker"). Meeting people is scary, and alcohol might help you lighten up; it is not for no reason that students call beer "liquid courage." All of these truths, like many others about alcohol, are verified not only in the "real-world" context of conscious experience and oral tradition, but also in the normative visualizations and enticements of marketing and entertainment.[48]

Eileen M. Emery and her colleagues confirmed these points when they interviewed students about their reasons for drinking or not drinking, and circumstances surrounding overconsumption.[49] The three most important reasons for drinking were to satisfy their intense need to conform, primarily to peers but also to the society-at-large, to reduce anxiety or stress, and to decrease the fear of inadequacy with respect to social functioning.

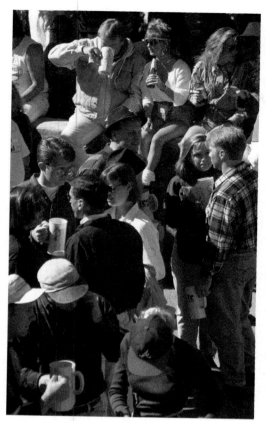

What Do You Think?

1. Some students drink alcoholic beverages to overcome shyness and to gain confidence in social situations. The results can often be harmful. What positive and negative effects of alcohol on personality have you witnessed? Do you think the benefits of using alcohol outweigh the risks?
2. What less-risky alternatives to alcohol exist that can favorably influence confidence, self-esteem, and other personality factors?

For men and women alike, drinking is a way of not having to deal at a conscious level with a possible conflict in values—being sexually "safe" or chaste versus being sexually "free." Keeling surmises that alcohol:

> solidifies men's resolve about finding sexual partners, and beer helps make it happen. Because alcohol advertising (like most other marketing) objectifies women, heterosexual men find in alcohol a sanctioned way to do the same thing. Because beer marketing to gay men objectifies other men (like most other marketing to gay men), gay men similarly find in alcohol a way to avoid dealing with the human elements of a relationship. When, indeed, is one supposed to "say when?" When alcohol is changing your judgment? But that's what you wanted, isn't it? The issue is actually

more complex than the concordance of destructive drinking with the cultural norm; it is that, in the context of that social norm, one can know about alcohol and all of its effects and dangers but not feel too much fear, grief, or pain about those things. And one can feel pretty comfortable without questioning the mix of alcohol and sex too deeply.[50]

It may be easy to envision the following scenario. Eighteen-year-old Heather is a first-year student at college and within the first couple of weeks is invited to a fraternity party, sorority rush, or other social function where there are older students as well as students her own age. Alcohol is being served and regardless of state laws, campus rules, or possible sanctions against Greek organizations, no one is monitoring who is drinking and who is not. Heather feels a bit overwhelmed by the size of the crowd; the freedom of being on her own; the opportunity for friendships; and the potential for meeting new dating partners. While she is a bit anxious and nervous about drinking, refusing to accept a drink that is offered is difficult. What should she do, and is there something that she could have done to prepare for such a moment? How vulnerable is she? Nancy A. Gleason sees such a scenario as having all the ingredients for problem drinking, even against one's will—peer pressure, the desire to relax, the desire to feel sophisticated, and perhaps even the desire to seem seductive.[51] In the scenario above, drinking may help the individual overcome shyness for the moment, and succeed in helping her meet people with a sense of confidence. Alternatively, writes Gleason:

> What may start as drinking to combat shyness, counteract loneliness, join with others and be part of the crowd, be liked and acknowledged, attract and be with either men or women, or reduce inhibitions can provide opportunities for trouble. Alcohol softens the pain of failure in any of these areas—the sense that one cannot meet the expectations of others and of oneself and that one lacks the capacity to enter into satisfying relationships.[52]

Any person, male or female, may drink to bolster courage and self-esteem, or drink to comfort an ailing self-esteem. Either way, it should be clear that an ill-conceived decision to drink might have a powerful influence on one's future social life and experiences with alcohol.

TABLE 16.8   *Tips for Changing the Campus Culture to Alcohol-Free*

As explained earlier, alcohol is sometimes associated with the "culture" of the college or university campus. Therefore, changing that culture is something of a revolutionary idea. It is, after all, easier to conform than to challenge the system. On the other hand, change is possible if people have the courage to take it on.

Precontemplation → Contemplation

If you have never thought about how the campus might be a better place with less emphasis on alcohol consumption, consider the following activities.

- Envision a campus social gathering that is altogether alcohol-free.
- Pay attention to media accounts of socially deviant and violent behavior that may have been triggered, in part, from excessive consumption of alcohol.

Contemplation → Preparation

If you have thought about the problem behaviors associated with excessive alcohol use and are looking for an alternative, try:

- Making a guest list of persons you could invite to an alcohol-free party.
- Developing a list of exotic snacks and beverages that fit an alcohol-free theme.
- If you drink alcohol, keeping a diary of the circumstances under which *you* drink, and the amount that you drink. Tally the calories from these alcoholic beverages.

Preparation → Action

Trying something that is contrary to society's trends can be a scary proposition. Nevertheless, you may increase the likelihood of succeeding in meeting this challenge, if you:

- Tell a close friend that you are planning a health conscious party, and invite him or her to assist you. Make the planning phase a real social experience.
- See if the academic institution or a local radio station will sponsor your event in some way, especially if you are in a residence hall or Greek organization.
- Develop a list of activities and games that fit the alcohol-free theme, (e.g., a campus olympics).
- Set the date of the event in the next thirty days.

Action → Maintenance

First attempts at changing the culture may not be completely successful. You have taken an important first step. The following tips may help you stay involved.

- Avoid circumstances that "trigger" heavy alcohol consumption.
- Plan future social gatherings at locations where there is a wide variety of recreational opportunities, and sites where alcohol use is prohibited.

Maintenance

You have boldly challenged the culture of the campus. Keep the idea alive by:

- Encouraging others to sponsor social events that are alcohol-free.
- Supporting endeavors that make people more aware of the problems associated with alcohol abuse, in conjunction with wellness week, other campus events, or events organized by MADD or SADD.

What seems necessary is to develop an ethic about alcohol and a strategy for changing the "campus culture" without going to the extreme of prohibiting all use of alcohol (see table 16.8). It is no secret that some colleges are identified by the popular press, folklore, and other forms of publicity as so-called "party schools," often to the displeasure of the faculty and administration of those institutions. Some students may in fact have selected their college based more on this criterion than on the school's academic reputation. Redefining the culture of the college setting with respect to alcohol is not easy and not something that is likely to be achieved without mutual cooperation. Gleason concludes:

> The campus is not an island. It must collaborate with other institutions and with the community outside the campus to encourage rational norms. Norms and policies about drinking on one campus will not necessarily prevail at other campuses, and students will seek out the campus that best fits their style. College administrators need to attend to the visitors on their campuses as well as to their own students. Collaborative discussions will also help avoid typecasting, stereotyping, and labeling different campuses.[53]

Alcohol is a drug that, when abused or misused, can cause great problems for individuals and society. But alcohol and wellness can coexist. Acting responsibly when you use alcohol and encouraging similar behavior in your friends will increase your chances of attaining high levels of wellness.

Summary

1. Alcohol is the most abused drug, although its acceptance varies from heavy use to complete rejection.

2. Alcohol use and the health and social problems associated with it are targeted objectives of *Healthy People 2000*.

3. Beverage alcohol is absorbed directly into the bloodstream, and requires no prior digestion.

4. Several factors influence the rate of absorption.

5. Blood-alcohol concentration is a measure of alcohol absorption, and is used to determine whether or not one is legally intoxicated.

6. Alcohol can impair driving and other cognitive and motor skills well below the legal definitions of intoxication.

7. Alcohol use during pregnancy can cause severe abnormalities in the fetus, producing fetal alcohol syndrome and other disorders.

8. Alcohol use is related to the prevention or causation of coronary heart disease, some cancers, liver diseases, especially cirrhosis, and other disorders.

9. Alcoholism may have both genetic and environmental components.

10. Alcoholism is a major disease in the U.S. and worldwide that often goes undiagnosed and untreated.

11. Alcohol use has significant secondary consequences represented by crime and other social problems.

12. Responsible use of alcohol can be motivated in part by being a good host or hostess.

13. Attitudes about alcohol use are influenced by parents, peers, and advertising, and perceptions of cultural norms.

14. Alcohol has various degrees of acceptance and use among different racial and ethnic groups, and contributes to health and social problems that affect these special populations.

15. Alcohol is the drug of choice for many college and university students. Use is often initiated to promote sociability. Abuse can lead to destructive social and health outcomes.

Recommended Readings

Nancy A. Gleason, "College Women and Alcohol: A Relational Perspective," *Journal of American College Health* 42.6 (1994):279–289; Nancy A. Gleason, "Preventing Alcohol Abuse by College Women: A Relational Perspective 2," *Journal of American College Health* 43.1 (1994):15–24.

These two articles bring to the forefront the fact that little research concerning college-aged women and alcohol consumption has been done. The relationship between drinking and physical abuse and other forms of vulnerability is discussed.

Erich Goode, *Drugs in American Society*, 4th edition (New York: McGraw Hill, 1993).

Although about drug use in general, this book gives a good historical account of efforts to control alcohol in the U.S. since the 19th century. Goode identifies the sociocultural factors involved in substance abuse and the comorbidity of alcohol and other drugs.

U.S. Department of Health and Human Services, *Seventh Special Report to the U.S. Congress on Alcohol and Health*, Public Health Service, DHHS Publication No. (ADM) 90–1656, (Washington, D.C.: U.S. Government Printing Office, 1990).

This government document reports on most aspects of alcohol use and abuse, including epidemiologic data, treatment of alcoholism, and alcohol abuse prevention strategies.

References

1. *University of California at Berkeley Wellness Letter* 9.5 (1993):4.

2. *University of California at Berkeley Wellness Letter* 9.5 (1993):4.

3. D. C. Walsh, "The Shifting Boundaries of Alcohol Policy," *Health Affairs* 9.2 (1990):46–62.

4. *University of California at Berkeley Wellness Letter* 9.5 (1993):5.

5. *Consumer Reports on Health* 6.3 (1994):34.

6. *University of California at Berkeley Wellness Letter* 9.5 (1993):4.

7. *University of California at Berkeley Wellness Letter* 9.5 (1993):4.

8. *University of California at Berkeley Wellness Letter* 9.5 (1993):4.

9. Christy Ulleland, "The Offspring of Alcoholic Mothers," *Annals of the New York Academy of Sciences* 197 (May 25, 1972):167–169.

10. P. Lemoine, et al. "Les enfants des parents alcoliques anomalies ovservees. A Popos de 127 cas," *Quest Medical* 21 (1968):276–482; K. L. Jones, et al. "Pattern of Malformation in Offspring of Chronic Alcoholic Mothers," *Lancet* 1 (1973):1267–1271.

11. Elisabeth Rosenthal, "When a Pregnant Woman Drinks," *The New York Times Magazine* (February 4, 1990):30, 49, 61.

12. Rosenthal, "When a Pregnant Woman Drinks," 30, 49, 61.

13. M. Aronson and R. Olegard, "Children of Alcoholic Mothers," *Pediatrician* 14, no. 1–2 (1987):57–61.

14. S. Cooper, "The Fetal Alcohol Syndrome," *Journal of Child Psychology and Psychiatry* 28.2 (1987):223–227.

15. E. A. Abel, "Prenatal Effects of Alcohol," *Drug and Alcohol Dependence* 14 (1984):1–10.

16. T. E. Rohan, "Alcohol and Ischemic Heart Disease: A Review," *Australian and New Zealand Journal of Medicine* 14 (1984):75–80.

17. A. R. Dyer, et al., "Alcohol Consumption and 17-year Mortality in the Chicago Western Electric Company Study," *Preventive Medicine* 9 (1980):78–90.

18. W. P. Castelli, "Epidemiology of Coronary Heart Disease: The Framingham Study," *American Journal of Medicine* 76(Suppl.2A) (1984):4–12.

19. University of California at Berkeley *Wellness Letter* 10.6 (1994):1.

20. American Cancer Society, *Cancer Facts & Figures—1994* (Atlanta: American Cancer Society, 1994), 19.

21. University of California at Berkeley *Wellness Letter* 10.6 (1994):1.

22. University of California at Berkeley *Wellness Letter* 10.6 (1994):1.

23. University of California at Berkeley *Wellness Letter* 10.6 (1994):2.

24. Centers for Disease Control, "Current Trends: Alcohol-Related Traffic Fatalities—United States, 1982–1989," *Morbidity and Mortality Weekly Report* 39.49 (1990):889.

25. University of California at Berkeley *Wellness Letter* 9.5 (1993):6.

26. N. S. Cotton, "The Familial Incidence of Alcoholism," *Journal of Studies on Alcohol* 40 (1979):89–116.

27. M. Bohman, "Some Generic Aspects of Alcoholism and Criminality: A Population of Adoptees," *Archives of General Psychiatry* 35 (1978): 269–276.

28. U.S. Department of Health and Human Services, *Seventh Special Report to the U.S. Congress on Alcohol and Health*, Public Health Service, DHHS Publication No. (ADM) 90–1656, (Washington, D.C.: U.S. Government Printing Office, 1990).

29. C. R. Cloninger, "Genetic and Environmental Factors in the Development of Alcoholism," *Journal of Psychiatric Treatment and Evaluation* 5 (1983):487–496.

30. U.S. Department of Health and Human Services, *Seventh Special Report to the U.S. Congress on Alcohol and Health*.

31. U.S. Department of Health and Human Services, *Seventh Special Report to the U.S. Congress on Alcohol and Health*.

32. University of California at Berkeley *Wellness Letter* 9.5 (1993):6.

33. University of California at Berkeley *Wellness Letter* 9.5 (1993):6.

34. Thomas C. Harford, Mary R. Haack, and Danielle L. Spiegler, "Positive Family History for Alcoholism," *Health and Research World* 12.1 (1987/88):138–143.

35. Joel W. Grube and Lawrence Wallack, "Television Beer Advertising and Drinking Knowledge, Beliefs, and Intentions among Schoolchildren," *American Journal of Public Health* 84.2 (1994):254–258.

36. Patricia A. Madden and Joel W. Grube, "The Frequency and Nature of Alcohol and Tobacco Advertising in Televised Sports, 1990 through 1992," *American Journal of Public Health* 84.2 (1994):297–299.

37. U.S. Department of Health and Human Services, *Seventh Special Report to the U.S. Congress on Alcohol and Health*.

38. B. Lex, "Review of Alcohol Problems in Ethnic Minority Groups," *Journal of Consulting and Clinical Psychology* 55.3 (1987):293–300.

39. D. Herd, "The Epidemiology of Drinking Patterns and Alcohol-Related Problems among U.S. Blacks." In: *The Epidemiology of Alcohol Use and Abuse among U.S. Minorities*. NIAAA Monograph No. 18 DHHS Publication No. (ADM) 89–1435, (Washington, D.C.: U.S. Government Printing Office, 1989).

40. D. Herd, "Rethinking Black Drinking," *British Journal of the Addictions* 82 (1987):219–223.

41. USDHHS, *Seventh Special Report to Congress on Alcohol and Health*, 34.

42. USDHHS, *Seventh Special Report to Congress on Alcohol and Health*, 35.

43. USDHHS, *Seventh Special Report to Congress on Alcohol and Health*, 35.

44. USDHHS, *Seventh Special Report to Congress on Alcohol and Health*, 36.

45. USDHHS, *Seventh Special Report to Congress on Alcohol and Health*, 36.

46. L. D. Johnson, P.M. O'Malley, and J. G. Bachman, *Smoking, Drinking, and Illicit Drug Use Among American Secondary School Students, College Students, and Young Adults, 1975–1991* (Washington, D.C.: National Institute on Drug Abuse, 1992).

47. Stephanie C. Hurlbut and Kenneth J. Sher, "Assessing Alcohol Problems in College Students," *Journal of American College Health* 41.2 (1992):49–58.

48. Richard P. Keeling, "Changing the Context: The Power in Prevention," *Journal of American College Health* 42.6 (1994):243–247.

49. Eileen M. Emery, Gwendolyn P. Ritter-Randolph, Anne L. Strozier, and Robert J. McDermott, "Using Focus Group Interviews to Identify Salient Issues Concerning College Students' Alcohol Abuse," *Journal of American College Health* 41.5 (1993):195–198.

50. Keeling, "Changing the Context: The Power in Prevention," 244.

51. Nancy A. Gleason, "College Women and Alcohol: A Relational Perspective," *Journal of American College Health* 42.6 (1994):279–289.

52. Nancy A. Gleason, "Preventing Alcohol Abuse by College Women: A Relational Perspective 2," *Journal of American College Health* 43.1 (1994):15–24.

53. Gleason, "Preventing Alcohol Abuse by College Women: A Relational Perspective 2," 22.

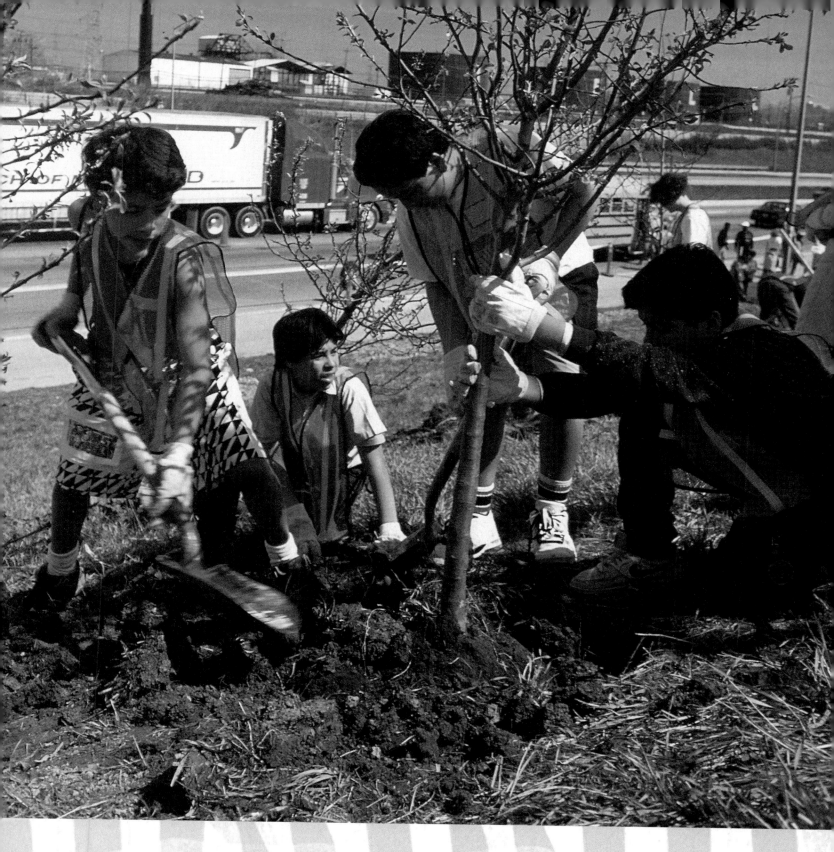

Enhancing Positive Health-Related Behaviors

UNIT

V

In Unit IV, we concentrated on minimizing negative health-related behaviors as one essential part of a wellness lifestyle. You also need to learn to enhance the positive. Unit V will introduce you to some important wellness skills and habits that will be useful to you now and throughout your life.

One prescription for wellness is to become a better health-care consumer. Chapter 17 will help you learn health-related consumer skills such as assertiveness, budgeting, and comparison shopping. In the U.S., there are many different kinds of health-care providers, including physicians, dentists, nurses, physician assistants, and providers of alternative care. There are also various kinds of health-care facilities, ranging from doctor's offices to hospitals, as well as several ways that health-care services are currently financed, including private health insurance and prepaid health insurance plans. Additionally, a great debate has waged over the past several years regarding national health insurance. Chapter 17 will help you understand the current health-care system and proposed changes, giving you a background for making wise health-care consumer decisions.

As we age, a wellness lifestyle becomes even more important. Chapter 18 discusses some of the issues and myths surrounding the aging process. Biological, social, and emotional aspects of aging are highlighted as are recommended health-related behaviors that, if practiced regularly, will help you grow into higher levels of wellness.

Taking responsibility for wellness inevitably leads to concerns about the larger environment. Chapter 19 presents Barry Commoner's Four Laws of Ecology and shows how they relate to current environment health dilemmas such as the proliferation of hazardous waste, and the death and destruction caused by acid rain. Our health-related behaviors, both individually and collectively, have profound implications for our own future and that of generations to come. Chapter 19 discusses the many ways that we can all contribute to making our environment healthier.

Better Consumerism: Rx for Wellness

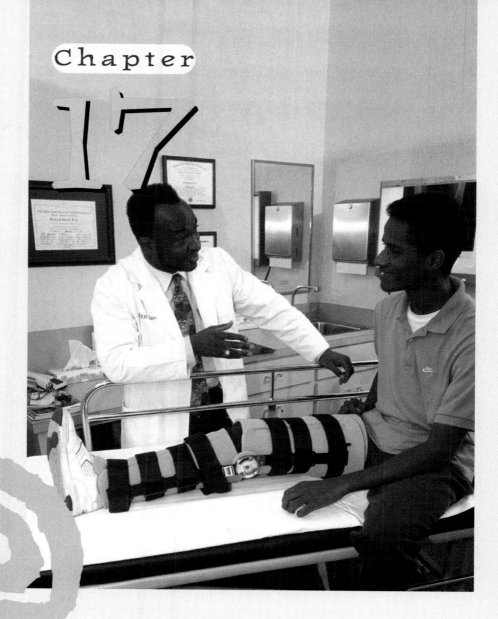

Chapter 17

Student Learning Objectives

Upon completion of this chapter, you should be able to:

1. list the nation's health objectives for the year 2000 with respect to elevating the health-care status of people in the U.S.;
2. list the evaluative criteria for selecting a personal care or family physician;
3. identify several alternative practitioners that provide health-care services;
4. distinguish among primary, secondary, and tertiary levels of health care;
5. explain why some people face numerous barriers to gaining access to health care in the U.S.;
6. describe particular health-care access barriers that are commonly experienced by women in the U.S.;
7. analyze why health-care costs are rising and how these spiraling costs have affected the delivery of care, especially where the health care of racial and ethnic minority groups, the poor, and even the employed middle class are concerned;
8. compare different models for the delivery of health care in the U.S.;
9. assess the components of an ideal health-care system;
10. discuss how fraud affects the poorly informed consumer;
11. list several skills that can assist the consumer in negotiating his or her way through the health-care marketplace;
12. identify several agencies that can provide help for the consumer who has questions or problems that require intervention;
13. write an effective consumer complaint letter.

Attainment of the year 2000 national health promotion and disease prevention objectives requires improved access to clinical services, especially those of a preventive nature[1] (see table 17.1). As a college student you should be acutely tuned in to the decisions about health care that are being made in this country. Significant reform of the health-care system in the U.S. failed to occur during the early years of the Clinton Administration, despite major reform efforts and a myriad of different health-care reform bills. Why should you be concerned about health-care availability, delivery, and spending? Health-care spending surpassed 12 percent of the U.S. gross national product (GNP) in 1991,[2] 14 percent in 1992,[3] and easily could escalate to 20 percent by the year 2004.[4] Not another developed country in the world spends more than 10 percent of its GNP for health-care goods and services.[5] Despite our greater level of spending, we are no healthier as a people than the citizens of comparable developed countries that spend half of what we do, and provide health care for everybody.[6]

Deciding whether or not to purchase health-related goods and services requires us to be informed consumers. Poorly informed consumers may purchase goods and services on faith alone or "gut feelings," a practice that can be detrimental to one's health and one's pocketbook. Wise consumers ask questions, perform background research, and identify people and agencies to whom they can take their questions and complaints.

It might be argued that in no other area of human health and wellness is there greater importance placed on knowledge, assertiveness, and foresight than in our affairs with the health-care delivery system. Astronomical levels of growth and sophistication of medical technology, as well as significant advancements in the preparation of health-care professionals, speak strongly for the capacity of modern science and medicine to diagnose, treat, and rehabilitate most consumers effectively. These advances are not without high price tags. Consequently, to address these rising costs, consumers need to develop some basic skills that will make them more effective in the health-care marketplace.

Most people in the U.S. have personal beliefs about health, health care, health professionals, and health-related institutions and organizations. These beliefs pose no problem unless they are in conflict with reality. Today's reality is not the romantic version of health care that television dramas and soap operas have portrayed over the years. There is fierce competition, and the unaware consumer may make poor decisions. Even well-informed people are subject to error, but being equipped with facts and interactive skills will reduce the probability of the errors being major costly ones.

Health-Care Personnel

The delivery of health care in the U.S. is accomplished through the interaction of a variety of professionals, institutions, and agencies. The most visible element of the system might be those persons who directly provide care. Physicians, dentists, nurses, and other allied health personnel comprise this element of the health-care system.

Physicians

Within the medical profession, there are two approaches to the practice of medicine that we would define as being orthodox. The two are known specifically as allopathy and osteopathy.

Allopathy

Allopathy is the term that is applied to the system of medical care taught at schools of medicine where the doctor of medicine (M.D.) is awarded. The M.D. degree is awarded to an individual following successful completion of four years of schooling at an institution that is accredited by the **American Medical Association (AMA)** and the **Association of American Medical Colleges.** Most states require that graduates of medical schools complete at least one year of hospital internship following graduation. Graduates must also pass either state or national board examinations before they are eligible to be licensed by a state board of medical

Allopathy: a system of medical practice that uses drugs to create effects that specifically oppose the symptoms of a disease.

American Medical Association (AMA): a professional organization whose membership is comprised principally of physicians. The AMA has a variety of functions including continuing education for physicians, lobbying activities, and accreditation of medical schools. The AMA also publishes *JAMA, The Journal of the American Medical Association*.

1. **Increase to at least 95 percent the proportion of people who have a specific source of ongoing primary care for coordination of their preventive and episodic health care.** (Update: 79 percent in 1992, down from 82 percent in 1986.) (Special Target Populations: Hispanics, Blacks, Low-income people.)

2. **Improve financing and delivery of clinical preventive services so that virtually no one in the U.S. has a financial barrier to receiving, at a minimum, the screening, counseling, and immunization services recommended by the U.S. Preventive Services Task Force.** (Update: 17 percent of people under age 65 were without health care coverage in 1990, up from 16 percent in 1989.)

3. **Assure that at least 90 percent of people for whom primary care services are provided directly by publicly funded programs are offered, at a minimum, the screening, counseling, and immunization services recommended by the U.S. Preventive Services Task Force.** (Baseline: For 1991–1992, 10–100 percent of eligible people received immunization services, 40–100 percent of eligible people received counseling, and 10–96 percent of eligible people received screening, from federal programs.)

4. **Increase to at least 50 percent the proportion of primary care providers who provide their patients with the screening, counseling, and immunization services recommended by the U.S. Preventive Services Task Force.** (Baseline: the percent of clinicians routinely providing service to 81–100 percent of patients in 1992 is as follows:

5. **Increase to at least 90 percent the proportion of people who are served by a local health department that assesses and assures access to essential clinical preventive services.** (Baseline proportion of local health departments providing care in 1990: 74 percent health education, 84 percent child health, 92 percent immunizations, 59 percent prenatal care, and 22 percent primary care.)

6. **Increase the proportion of all degrees in the health professions and allied and associated health profession fields awarded to members of underrepresented racial and ethnic minority groups.** (Update of the percent of degrees awarded: 5.7 percent to Blacks, 4.8 percent to Hispanics, and 0.5 percent to American Indians/Alaska Natives in the 1991–92 academic year, up from 5.0 percent, 3.0 percent, and 0.3 percent respectively during 1985–86.)

Service for Children	Pediatricians	Nurse Practitioners	Family Physicians	
Hemoglobin/hematocrit	78 percent	77 percent	52 percent	
Eye exam	64 percent	67 percent	53 percent	
Blood pressure	78 percent	71 percent	42 percent	
Height and weight	96 percent	88 percent	89 percent	
DTP vaccination	86 percent	76 percent	89 percent	
Oral polio vaccination	87 percent	76 percent	89 percent	
Tetanus-diphtheria booster	79 percent	71 percent	70 percent	
Hib vaccination	85 percent	68 percent	74 percent	
Service for Adults	**Ob./Gyn.**	**Nurse Practitioners**	**Family Physicians**	**Internists**
Tetanus-diphtheria booster (18 years and over)	4 percent	38 percent	28 percent	29 percent
Influenza vaccination (65 years and over)	6 percent	42 percent	31 percent	49 percent
Pneumococcal vaccination (65 years and over)	5 percent	33 percent	25 percent	40 percent
Blood pressure	88 percent	82 percent	89 percent	92 percent
Cholesterol level	36 percent	45 percent	61 percent	80 percent
Breast exam (by clinician)	92 percent	78 percent	62 percent	76 percent
Pap smear	95 percent	77 percent	62 percent	67 percent
Mammogram	85 percent	63 percent	53 percent	67 percent

Source: Data from *Healthy People 2000 National Health Promotion and Disease Prevention Objectives,* 1991; and from *Healthy People 2000 Review, 1993,* 1994 Department of Health and Human Services, Washington, D.C.

Allergy: A subspecialty of internal medicine that concerns the diagnosis and treatment of allergic reactions.

Anesthesiology: Administration of drugs to block pain or induce unconsciousness during surgery, diagnostic procedures, or childbirth.

Cardiology: A subspecialty of internal medicine that concerns the diagnosis and treatment of disorders of the heart and blood vessels.

Child psychiatry: A subspecialty of psychiatry that concerns nervous and emotional problems of children.

Colon and rectal surgery (proctology): Diagnosis and treatment of disorders of the lower digestive tract.

Dermatology: Diagnosis and treatment of skin disorders.

Family practice: Provides general medical care to patients and their families.

Gastroenterology: A subspecialty of internal medicine that concerns the diagnosis and treatment of disorders of the gastrointestinal tract.

Internal medicine: Diagnosis and nonsurgical treatment of internal organs and organ systems of the body.

Neurology: Diagnosis and nonsurgical treatment of disorders of the brain, spinal cord, and nerves.

Neurosurgery: Diagnosis and surgical treatment of nervous system disorders.

Nuclear medicine: Use of radioactive substances for the diagnosis and treatment of disease.

Obstetrics and gynecology: Care of women during pregnancy, childbirth and the postnatal period, and/or diagnosis and treatment of disorders of the female reproductive system.

Occupational medicine: Deals with the diagnosis, treatment, and prevention of diseases associated with health risks at the workplace. It is a subspecialty of preventive medicine.

Oncology: Diagnosis and treatment of neoplastic growths or tumors.

Ophthalmology: Medical and surgical care of the eye, including the prescribing of corrective lenses.

Orthopedics: Treatment of diseases, fractures, and deformities of the bones and joints, and diseases of the muscles.

Otolaryngology: Diagnosis and treatment of ear, nose, and throat disorders.

Pathology: Examination of body organs, tissues, body fluids, and excrement to detect disease.

Pediatrics: The medical care of children through adolescence.

Physiatry: The treatment and rehabilitation of physical handicaps.

Plastic surgery: The correction or repair of body or facial structures through surgery.

Preventive medicine: Disease prevention through health habits, immunization, and environmental control.

Psychiatry: Diagnosis and treatment of mental and emotional disorders.

Public health: A subspecialty of internal medicine concerned with the promotion of the general health of the community.

Pulmonary medicine: A subspecialty of internal medicine, concerned with diseases of the lungs.

Radiology: The use of radiation to diagnose and treat disease.

Urology: Diagnosis and treatment of disorders of the urinary tract in both males and females, and the genital organs in the male.

From James H. Price, et al., *Consumer Health: Contemporary Issues and Choices.* Copyright © 1985 Wm. C. Brown Communications, Inc. Reprinted by permission of Times Mirror Higher Education Group, Inc., Dubuque, Iowa. All Rights Reserved.

General practitioner (GP): a physician who provides primary care services to patients. This type of physician is often the first physician seen for an illness or disease. They refer to specialists when necessary, and treat many common health problems that do not require the care of specialists.

examiners. People completing this series of events are referred to as **general practitioners (GP's).**

For individuals wishing to specialize in a particular field of medicine, an additional amount of schooling and internship activity is required. Additionally, students must pass specialty group examinations. Terms such as "board certified," "boarded," and "diplomate" are used to refer to individuals who have

successfully completed this process. Some physician specialists do not complete the entire process of becoming board certified. Consumers can determine if a physician is board certified by checking *The Directory of Medical Specialists*, a national publication containing biographical information on practicing physician specialists. A listing of the various medical specialties can be found in table 17.2.

Osteopathy

Osteopathy is a system of medical practice that emphasizes integrity of the muscular and skeletal systems working in harmony. The training of an osteopathic physician involves four years of medical training following at least three years of preprofessional undergraduate college education. A one-year hospital internship is also required of people graduating from an accredited school of osteopathic medicine. Osteopaths may also choose to specialize in a number of medical fields. Specializing requires additional study and testing following the one-year internship. Osteopathic medicine is recognized as a form of legitimate medical practice in all fifty states.

Choosing and Rating a Physician

An unfortunate aspect of the consumer marketplace is that most consumers are better informed about selecting a refrigerator than about selecting their physician.[7] Some of the most important and useful skills we can possess as health-care consumers come into play when selecting a physician. We not only need to seek out the names of physicians who might be willing to take on new patients but also apply information gathered concerning these individuals as an extension of the selection process. The following information sources may be useful in compiling a list of potential physicians:

Telephone book (Yellow Pages)
Referrals from a former physician
Friends and relatives
American Medical Association (state, county, or other local medical society)
American Board of Medical Specialties

The American Board of Medical Specialties (ABS) can be called to confirm a physician's board certification.[8] The telephone number is 1–800–776–CERT.

Physicians should be board certified, team players (affiliated with hospitals or HMOs), conscientious about following up on advice to increase compliance, recently certified or recertified, nonadvocates of magical solutions to problems (i.e., weight control, cholesterol), highly trained (internship, residency, postdoctoral study), well-groomed and good role models, good communicators, and respected by nurses and other staff members who work with them.[9]

Once a list of potential physicians has been assembled, you can then attempt to rate these persons by acquiring additional information. By gathering information on potential physicians, you increase the probability that the person you select will meet your expectations for high-quality health care. Assuming a passive role in such an important consumer area may result in later dissatisfaction and disappointment.

Other Health-Care Practitioners

Physicians and osteopaths, by virtue of their medical licensing, can perform a full, unlimited range of legitimate medical procedures. Other types of health-care providers are limited in what they can perform. Some of the more common of these practitioners are dentists, podiatrists, nurses, optometrists, clinical psychologists, and physician assistants.

Dentists

The doctor of dental surgery (D.D.S.) and the doctor of medical dentistry (D.M.D.) are concerned with the diagnosis and treatment of diseases and conditions of the teeth, gums, and associated oral structures. Most dentists are general practitioners; however, some specialize in areas such as children's dentistry, treatment of poorly positioned teeth, treatment of tissues supporting the teeth, and treatment of diseases of the inner portion of the tooth. Preventive dentistry, facilitated through the implementation of community **drinking water fluoridation** programs, direct application of fluoride compounds and **sealants** to the teeth, regular toothbrushing and flossing, periodic examinations, and health education, has been an excellent illustration of the cost savings potential brought about through successful health promotion.

Podiatrists

Podiatrists are medical specialists who deal with disorders of the foot. The podiatrist may use surgery, drugs, manipulative therapy, braces, and the like to diagnose and treat foot problems. Podiatrists possess the degree of either **doctor of podiatric medicine (D.P.M.)** or the **doctor of podiatry (D.P.).**

Drinking water fluoridation: a public health practice to help assure that all members of a community receive optimal fluoride exposure to enhance tooth enamel formation and prevent cavities. Community drinking water supplies are modified to attain an optimal level of fluoride, ranging from 0.7 to 1.2 parts per million.

Sealants: a thin coating of plastic material that is put on tooth surfaces. Sealants create a barrier that prevents food and bacteria from accumulating in the pits and grooves of the teeth, thus helping to prevent cavities from forming.

Figure 17.1: What Do
You Think?

1. Nurses are crucial members of the
   health-care team. Do you think the
   specialization of nurses and the
   expanded responsibilities inherent
   with such specialization will improve
   the quality of care received by health
   consumers? Explain your rationale.

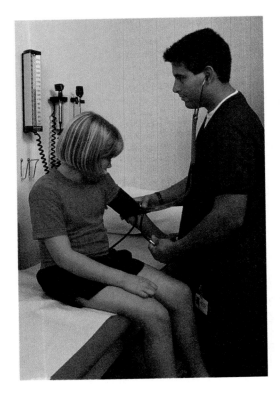

Nursing Occupations

Nurses are licensed health-care workers who perform a variety of duties ranging from administering medication to educating patients and families about self-care techniques (see figure 17.1). Nurses work in a variety of settings, the most common of which include hospitals, clinics, physicians' offices, and skilled nursing homes. Today, nurses, like physicians, have opportunities to specialize. For instance, **nurse practitioners** are professional nurses (R.N.s) who have graduated from specific specialty programs and as a result can engage in a variety of expanded health-care services. Nurse-practitioner programs are increasing rapidly, with the most notable ones being in the area of pediatrics, family health, and obstetrics and gynecology. Nurse practitioners typically work under the direction of an allopathic or osteopathic physician.

In recent years a nursing shortage has occurred in some parts of this country. Inadequate pay for the type of job responsibilities assumed and the wider variety of career options now available to women are two of the major reasons cited for the shortage. Many hospitals are experimenting with innovative nurse recruitment programs. These programs often attempt to give nurses more job autonomy and advancement opportunities as well as giving monetary bonuses to new recruits and to any nurse who recruits a new nurse. The shortage of nurses is not likely to disappear quickly and thus has the potential to impact on the quality of care available to all of us.

Optometrists

An **optometrist** is a professionally prepared person who diagnoses visual problems and improves vision. The work of optometrists primarily involves prescription of glasses and contact lenses.

Clinical Psychologists

Clinical psychologists concern themselves with the nonmedical aspects of human behavior and mental health. Clinical psychologists usually possess an academic doctorate (Ph.D.) in psychology and often specialize in a particular client population or a setting such as schools or worksites.

Physician Assistants

Physician assistants (P.A.s) are usually educated in two-year programs sponsored by medical schools, universities, or technical colleges. They perform routine medical procedures on patients under the supervision and legal obligation of a physician.

Alternative Health Practitioners

In contrast to the orthodox full and limited practitioners discussed, a variety of alternative systems of healing and healers exist. These alternative approaches to medicine are considered somewhat questionable in that the techniques and methodologies have not been subjected to the rigors of scientific testing and evidence. Although these theories and approaches may work for some people with certain ailments, the likelihood that they can cure a wide spectrum of health problems, as professed, is remote. The number of alternative health practices preclude detailed and comprehensive coverage in this chapter. A few of the more common alternative health practices are chiropractic, homeopathy, acupuncture, and naturopathy.

Chiropractic

The **chiropractic** approach to healing is generally characterized as being both drug free and nonsurgical. It is a form of therapy whose theory states that health is contingent upon the structural integrity of the spinal column. Diagnosis is usually made by x ray of the full torso. Then through manipulation of the **vertebrae** by a chiropractor, changes in the health status of the patient are expected to occur. Additionally, many chiropractors administer dietary advice, nutritional supplements, **ultrasound, traction,** hot and cold compress, infrared and ultraviolet light, and professional counsel to their clients. The types of treatment modalities used vary by state and are limited by individual state laws.

Chiropractors are trained in chiropractic colleges, where it takes four years to earn the D.C. degree. Additionally, chiropractors must pass state licensing examinations in order to practice chiropractic. All fifty states have such licensing requirements. Chiropractors and allopathic physicians have traditionally been at odds in their approaches to treating disease, and in regard to each other's professional status. Chiropractors' status has been enhanced as a result of their services being reimbursed by some health insurance plans. Their popularity among consumers has probably never been greater.

Chiropractic is not just a set of techniques for manipulating the spine; it is a belief system that credits the spine with a primary role in health and illness. Allopathic physicians are concerned that this limited view of disease causation and health restoration may cause chiropractors to overlook symptoms or to treat serious conditions through manipulation alone.

What should you do if you have back pain? What course of action should you follow? The following steps are recommended:[10]

- See your physician first to have your symptoms evaluated thoroughly. Some conditions do not respond well to manipulation, and others are, in fact, made worse.

- Get a referral from a reliable source. Call the National Association for Chiropractic Medicine at (713) 280–8262. Since many physical therapists also do manipulation therapy, you may be able to get a referral from a physician.

- Ask questions of the practitioner over the telephone in advance of making an office visit. Some suitable examples of questions include: Do you treat primarily musculoskeletal problems? Can you work with my physician and give him/her updates on my treatment and progress? Can you recommend some at-home exercises for me? About how long (i.e., how many sessions) will treatment require, and at what point will re-evaluation occur?

- Stay alert to warning signs of poor practice such as a chiropractor who takes full-spine or repeated x rays, does not take a comprehensive health history, claims that treatment will improve immune function, cure disease, or prevent disease, solicits other members of your family who are well, or who sells vitamin cures, special nutritional remedies, or other products.

Homeopathy

Homeopaths believe that people who are ill need to be treated with substances and therapies that in a normally healthy person would cause those symptoms. The notion of treating like with like is basic to their profession. Derived in part from herbal medicine, homeopathic remedies are thought to become more powerful when they are diluted to an extreme, even to the point where almost none of the original preparation remains in solution.[11] This theory is in direct opposition to allopathic practitioners who generally treat diseases with opposites. According to the Editors of *Consumer Reports:*[12]

> As it is now practiced, however, homeopathy does pose one clear risk: that of seeing a practitioner who will ignore or misdiagnose early symptoms of a serious disease that needs medical or surgical treatment. Many homeopaths practice out of the medical mainstream or even in direct opposition to it. They may advise patients to avoid appropriate medical care and may prescribe unproven medical treatments in addition to homeopathic remedies. Finally, while these risks are real, there is still no logical scientific case to be made for homeopathy's benefits. The theoretical basis of homeopathy is highly implausible, and what experimental evidence exists is preliminary at best.

Acupuncture

Acupuncture is the ancient Chinese healing art whereby fine needles of varying lengths are inserted at specific points on the body

Vertebrae: the 33 bones that make up the backbone, and through which the spinal cord passes.

Ultrasound: high frequency sound waves, undetectable to the human ear, used to examine the inner structures of the body.

Traction: a medical treatment that applies force to the tissues surrounding a broken bone in order to keep broken bones in a correct position for healing.

1. Acupuncture is an ancient Chinese healing art. Do you know anyone who has experienced acupuncture or acupressure? If so, did they get positive results?
2. Would you consider using alternative forms of medical care such as acupuncture? Explain your rationale.

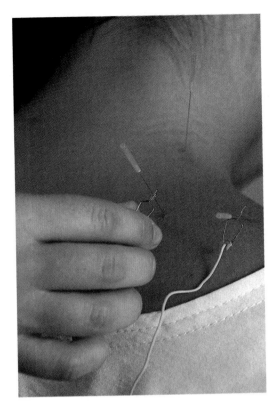

known as loci (see figure 17.2). The insertion of the needles is an attempt to restore a balance to the yin (cold, dark, female, and body interior) and yang (hot, light, male, and body exterior). As the needles are inserted by the acupuncturist and left for a determined period of time, the balance of yin and yang is restored and good health supposedly regained.

While the evidence concerning the efficacy of acupuncture remains controversial, 3,000 U.S. allopathic physicians and osteopaths have studied and used acupuncture, and at least eighty private insurers and Medicaid programs in some states cover acupuncture in the treatment of selected conditions.[13]

Naturopathy

Individuals adhering to **naturopathy** rely on natural elements to restore health to the afflicted. Sunlight, water, electricity, gravity, heat, and herbs are examples of the prescriptions offered for health care. Naturopaths believe that as we get our bodies out of balance with nature we encounter ill health.

Levels of Health Care

A second major component of the health-care delivery system are the various levels of

health care that exist for patients. Usually there is a correlation between the levels of care that are required and the place where that care is received.

Primary Care

Primary care is provided to individuals requiring routine health checkups or those experiencing illness for the first time. Examples of services considered to be primary care include physical examination, immunization, screening, many standard laboratory tests, and basic care for **acute** disorders. Outside of a serious medical emergency, this level of care is typically provided in a practitioner's office or in an outpatient type of care setting.

Secondary Care

Secondary care is usually delivered by physicians who are specialists within a particular area of medicine upon referral from a patient's primary-care physician. Typical services categorized as secondary care include labor and delivery and minor operations such as **appendectomy** or **hernia** repair. This level of care is provided either in the private office or clinic of the health-care provider or in a hospital where more extensive care can be delivered.

Tertiary Care

Tertiary care, the highest level of care, is typically delivered in a hospital. This care is almost always supplied by highly technologically oriented professionals and resources. Tertiary care services include cancer therapy, open heart surgery, and care for other extremely serious, life-threatening illnesses or injuries.

Health-Care Facilities

As we discuss the levels of primary, secondary, and tertiary care, we generally refer to specific places or facilities where such care may be delivered.

Private Practitioners' Offices

Depending on whether the practitioner is considered a primary-care practitioner or a specialist, the types of care will vary in extensiveness. In either case, the care is generally defined as **ambulatory** or outpatient.

Acute: a descriptive term for diseases that have a rapid onset and short duration.

Appendectomy: the surgical removal of the appendix.

Hernia: a condition characterized by part of an organ or tissue protruding outside of the body cavity in which it is normally housed. For example, an hiatus hernia exists when part of the stomach protrudes into the chest cavity through the hole for the esophagus.

Ambulatory: a type of health care synonymous with outpatient care, i.e., no hospital stay required.

Health Clinics

Clinics can be categorized as either private or public. **Public health clinics** may offer the same range of outpatient, ambulatory care services as a private clinic but differ in that public health clinics are supported by either federal, state, or local tax funds. In recent years there has been an expansion of **private health clinics.** These clinics typically provide primary- or secondary-care services and are known by a variety of names such as "medicenters," "urgicenters," "walk-in clinics," and "surgicenters" (see figure 17.3). These centers are often located in or near shopping centers and cater to consumer desires for less costly, more convenient, health-care services.

Hospitals

A variety of institutions are called hospitals. These institutions provide the most extensive level of care, which is usually performed on an inpatient basis. Any institution that attempts to qualify as a hospital is urged to submit to an accreditation process conducted by the **Joint Commission on the Accreditation of Healthcare Organizations (JCAHO).** While such an accreditation process guarantees meeting certain minimum standards for patient care and facilities, it does not guarantee that errors in diagnosing or treating an illness will not occur. The Joint Commission is composed of the American College of Surgeons, the American College of Physicians, the American Hospital Association, and the American Medical Association.

Most hospitals are classified as short-term or acute-care facilities, which means patients are there fewer than thirty days. Hospitals are also classified by the type of treatment rendered (clinical) or by the type of management or ownership.

Nursing Homes

In many instances, nursing homes are referred to as long-term care institutions. Nursing homes are typically classified as either skilled-nursing facilities or intermediate-care institutions. In a **skilled-nursing facility** the patients or residents require daily medical attention by a licensed physician and professional nurses. In an **intermediate-care** institution the residents require assistance but not necessarily professional medical

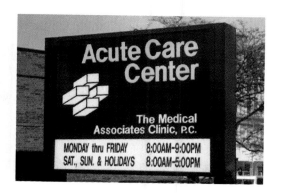

attention. Tender loving care might be one way to describe the care to be rendered to persons in intermediate-care facilities.

Personal and Social Influences on Health Care

Some problems related to the delivery of health care in the U.S. arguably are beyond the influence of the typical consumer, and may act as barriers to effective and efficient delivery of health-care services.

Availability and Accessibility of Services: Time for Reform?

Between 31 and 37 million people in the U.S. are without health insurance or are underinsured.[14] The figure may be as high as 39 million.[15] Consequently, about one in eight persons cannot even access the health-care system.

There is a maldistribution of health-care providers in the U.S., especially with respect to geography. Many physicians and other health professionals are attracted to large cities, places with large, multispecialty clinics and other facilities, and institutions that are affiliated with teaching hospitals and university medical centers. Although people need health care in small, rural towns and cities too, these settings often are viewed as less challenging, and less adequately equipped to permit practitioners to maintain state-of-the-art skills.

The increased specialization among providers further contributes to persons with ordinary kinds of problems not being able to locate a practitioner with necessary skills and interests. Thus, a person's need may be for a family physician or dentist whose practice is general, primary care. However, the only

Figure 17.3: What Do You Think?

1. Walk-in clinics have increased across the United States in recent years. Do you think that consumers receive quality care when using these clinics? What evidence do you have to support your answer?

Figure 17.4: What Do You Think?

1. How might one's cultural traditions and health beliefs affect a person's interactions with the standard U.S. health-care system?

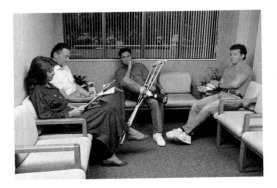

Mammogram: an x ray examination of the breasts used in the early detection of breast cancer.

Pap smear: a microscopic examination of cells of the cervix used as an early detection procedure for cancer of that site.

Exercise stress test: an aerobic exercise test that stresses the cardiorespiratory system. This test can be used, in conjunction with other tests, to diagnose coronary artery disease. It can also be used functionally to determine an individual's maximum heart rate during exercise, which is then used to guide a person in how strenuously they may safely exercise aerobically.

Electrocardiogram (ECG): a medical test that measures and records the electrical activity of the heart, and helps to detect heart disease.

Stroke: sudden loss of orientation or consciousness, sensation, or voluntary motion as a result of the rupture or obstruction of an artery in the brain; sometimes called a "cerebrovascular accident" (CVA).

practitioners available may be specialists in gynecology and obstetrics, allergy, or oral surgery. In locales which have an inadequate supply of general physicians or dentists, other clinicians or allied health professionals may provide services. However, legal restrictions prevent certain types of practitioners (e.g., nurse practitioners, physician assistants, dental hygienists, and other mid-level health-care providers) from carrying out some services.

Language and cultural barriers, restricted hours of service availability, inadequate child-care options, and lack of transportation are additional factors which impede access to health care. These elements affect the poor, the near poor, and racial and ethnic minorities disproportionately.[16] Therefore, they contribute to the burden of excess morbidity and mortality experienced by these groups that has been highlighted throughout this text.

The number of immigrants from Southeast Asia, Latin America, Eastern Europe, and other locations around the globe has again made the U.S. a melting pot of cultures. Not all people subscribe to the same set of beliefs about disease causation, or follow the same tradition of health and sick-role behavior that "Western" medicine dictates. In this country, these groups may feel helpless in the absence of a familiar system of health care. Even racial and ethnic groups that have several generations of familiarity with the U.S. health-care system may feel foreign (see figure 17.4). Major minority groups such as African-Americans, Hispanic Americans, Native Americans, and others are underrepresented in health-care fields such as medicine, dentistry, nursing, pharmacy, allied health professions, and other related occupations.[17]

Even where access to primary care at a reasonable cost is not an issue, the failure of some practitioners to offer certain preventive services can affect one's ability to obtain needed immunizations, baseline measures (e.g., physical examinations), screening tests (e.g., **mammograms, Pap smears, exercise stress tests, electrocardiograms,** and so on), and other services that could have health-enhancing benefits. Although Congress has debated the merits of establishing a financing mechanism for selected prevention activities, many health plans continue to have exclusions concerning preventive care, and therefore, do not reimburse the consumer or the practitioner for such services.[18]

Barriers to preventive care may occur simply as a result of poor management of personnel, facilities, and services within health-care organizations. In some instances, it is the lack of time, or the inadequacy of scheduling that interferes with improving preventive activities. In other public and private clinics, the underemployment or inadequate use of allied health professionals, such as health education specialists, may be blamed for the failure to make care optimal or comprehensive. Inadequate cooperation among providers and agencies may interfere further with well-managed care. The difficulty in interagency sharing of patient records stands in the way of better or more expedient care in some instances. In part, the reluctance to share patient information is based on professional, ethical, and legal constraints involving matters of confidentiality.

Women's Health Issues: Is There Systematic Neglect?

Until recently, women have been excluded from many large-scale studies of health behavior and disease prevention, especially studies of heart disease, cancer, and **stroke,** the leading causes of death in this country.[19] In addition to being excluded as test subjects, their physical complaints often are dismissed as being less serious than men's, or considered to have causes that are more imagined than real.[20]

Women can face special difficulties in navigating their way through the health-care system. Whereas men are likely to be able to meet most of their health-care needs through one provider, the same is not necessarily true for women. Women are more likely to receive either uncoordinated care from several physicians, or receive care from a physician who has little formal professional education about the unique health-care needs of women.[21]

Part of the explanation for this phenomenon is that the medical profession is dominated by male practitioners. Today, male physicians outnumber female physicians four-to-one, a ratio that will still be two-to-one fifteen years from now.[22] There is evidence that male physicians may be less focused on women's health-care needs than their female counterparts. Male physicians are less likely to order Pap smears, mammograms, and other diagnostic procedures than are female physicians. Moreover, they are less apt to perform a thorough evaluation of women who are symptomatic for **coronary heart disease.**[23]

Screening procedures such as mammograms, physical examinations of the breasts, Pap smears, and the like are perceived as invasive, and often arouse anxiety. Fear and discomfort are heightened by the setting and atmosphere of the health-care facility itself, which is likely to be seen as large, impersonal, and lacking in any home-like, soothing ambience. Add to this setting the vulnerability a woman feels when she is wearing a loose-fitting, semi-transparent hospital gown that exposes her body, while positioned on a cold metal table with her feet in stirrups, awaiting someone she scarcely knows and probably cannot see, to probe and penetrate her with strange and foreign instruments. If the practitioner acts aloof in this environment, that further accelerates the rise in the woman's anxiety.

As a result of these experiences, we have seen an increase in the number of facilities that specialize in women's health care (see figure 17.5). These facilities often are designed by women for women, and are staffed by female practitioners. An emphasis is placed on individualized care for women across the life span, where the patient is viewed as a partner in care, thus contributing to the patient's sense of empowerment. Such facilities may take on a less institutionalized appearance, a fact that in itself probably contributes a therapeutic effect on the patient. Health services delivered in such a manner demonstrate that quality care is possible, perhaps even enhanced, when a personal touch is added.

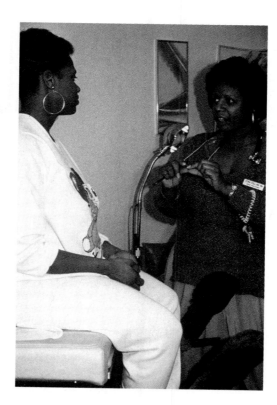

The Cost of Health Care

Why are health-care costs rising? In a recent year, unpaid hospital bills came to more than $8 billion, a figure that may be rising at a rate of 10 percent per year.[24] To recoup the costs of unpaid care, hospitals and physicians simply raise the price tag on services provided by those parties who can pay—individuals, private insurance carriers, and the federal government. In New Jersey, each hospital bill carries a 13 percent surcharge that helps make up the deficit from unpaid services.[25] Such surcharges, in turn, support the need for higher insurance premiums.

Despite the vast sums poured into health care, the U.S. does not perform well in overall health-status measures. Of the twenty-four industrialized nations comprising the Organization for Economic Cooperation and Development (OECD), the U.S. ranks 17th in male **life expectancy,** 16th in female life expectancy, and 21st in **infant mortality.**[26]

An item often cited as accounting for the rise in health-care costs is the proliferation of expensive health technologies. For example, a diagnostic machine known as **magnetic resonance imaging (MRI)** produces images of the body that assist physicians in the diagnosis of conditions without necessitating

Figure 17.5: What Do You Think?

1. New health-care facilities specifically designed to serve women are increasing across the United States. Do you think that these facilities will help to solve the problem of neglect that women have long experienced when trying to access the medical care system? Explain your rationale.

Coronary heart disease: a chronic disease condition in which the normal flow of blood through the coronary arteries is reduced or impaired; synonymous with coronary artery disease.

Life expectancy: the average number of years a group of individuals with common characteristics can expect to live, from birth to death.

Infant mortality: the number of deaths of children under the age of one, per 1,000 live births.

Figure 17.6: What Do
You Think?

1. While expensive, medical
   innovations such as the MRI often
   improve the quality of care available
   to us. Can you give an example of
   how access to MRI technology
   improves quality of care?
2. How important is technology
   development to the health status of
   people in the U.S.? What evidence
   do you have to support your answer?

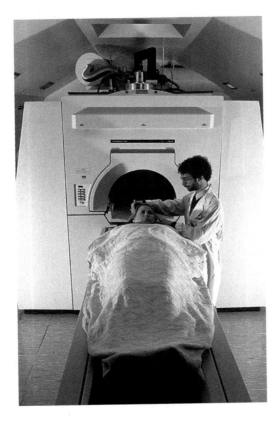

exploratory surgery. Its images are of a higher
quality than its predecessor, the **computer
axial tomograph,** or **CT scan** (see figure
17.6). These high price tag technologies and
others, such as organ transplants, raise ethical
questions about the circumstances of their
use. Should this sophisticated level of
technology, and that which is still to be
developed and tested, be available to
everyone? Should only those who can pay get
access? Should these technologies be
abandoned in order that finite health dollars
can be allocated for delivery of care to
persons less able to pay, thus increasing the
potential for raising the overall health status
of the nation? These are difficult questions to
answer, yet it is someone like you who is
reading this text who will be faced with
making these kinds of judgments.

Disorganization of the Health-Care System

The health-care delivery system is an
extremely large, complex social structure.
Within this structure there appears to be a
significant lack of organization, which
translates into a very fragmented system.
Consumers usually need to travel among a
variety of providers and institutions to

receive necessary care. This situation creates
a very costly and undesirable environment for
the delivery of medical care.

The health insurance industry itself
contributes to the less than desirable situation
through its short-sighted reimbursement
policies. In most instances, insurance
companies refuse payment for outpatient
preventive health services. Providers are
therefore not only encouraged but almost
required to institutionalize patients so that
they can be guaranteed reimbursement and
patients can receive necessary care. This
policy definitely translates into more costly
health care.

Personal Attitudes and Practices

Many of the conditions and situations that
contribute to the high cost of health care are
out of the control of the consuming
population. Many consumer attitudes and
practices, however, may in fact contribute a
great deal to our current dilemma. How
conscientious are you about trying to control
your personal health-care costs?

An increasing number of insurance
companies are identifying occupations and
professions that they are declining to insure.[27]
Why? Because some workers have a higher
risk of filing claims or of changing jobs
frequently (see table 17.3).

Employers are very concerned about the
rising cost of health care, especially as it
relates to the costs of providing adequate
health-care benefits for their workers. Some
employers have found that offering wellness
and disease-prevention programs for their
employees provides a major payoff in the
bottom line of company health-care costs.
Such programs focus on the attitudes and
behaviors of employees and often provide
incentives for staying well. Although wellness
programs will not eliminate the need for
medical insurance, some companies report
that employees with high levels of wellness
require less assistance, on the average, from
the medical-care system. To the extent that
we can assume a greater level of responsibility
for our own well-being, we may be able to
exert some influence over the cost and nature
of health-care services provided.

Financing Health Care

With dramatic increases in all areas of the
system, it is difficult for a rapidly growing

TABLE 17.3

Occupations that Some Insurance Companies May Consider Unacceptable for Health Insurance Coverage

tree trimmers	bartenders
explosives handlers	fry cooks
house painters	janitors
window cleaners	street cleaners
heavy equipment operators	physicians
rodeo performers	lawyers
police officers	professional athletes
doormen	fishermen
models	railroad workers
freelance artists	test drivers
waiters	car wash workers
masseurs	dancers
hospital aides	beauticians
maids	movers
musicians	zoo attendants

Source: Data from "The Crisis in Health Insurance" in *Consumer Reports*, 55.8 (August 1990): 542.

segment of the U.S. population to afford necessary care. With this picture of economic gloom as a backdrop, the third major component of the health-care delivery system becomes more important and visible: specifically, the mechanisms for paying for health care received.

Fee-For-Service or Pay-As-You-Go Health Care

Most people in the U.S. receive health care on a fee-for-service basis. This simply means that we pay either the provider or facility for the actual service rendered. As we witness increases in physicians' fees, hospital costs, drug costs, and auxiliary health services, it becomes readily apparent that most of us desperately need some mechanism to assist us in paying for the care required. Although 25 cents of each dollar spent on health care comes directly from consumers, the vast majority of money (75 cents) is reimbursed by other sources (see figure 17.7).

Private Health Insurers

Private insurance plans are generically referred to as standard indemnity plans. Blue Cross/Blue Shield is an example of such a plan. The insurance usually is written to cover one or more elements of costs incurred. The two costs that are most commonly covered are hospital-cost insurance and medical insurance, which is designed to cover mainly physician-related expenses. Additional forms of private health insurance may be secured, such as major medical insurance (catastrophic), disability, and miscellaneous (which might cover things such as a **prosthesis,** blood, or specialized allied health care).

Prepaid Health Insurance Plans

The concept of prepaid health insurance plans such as **health maintenance organizations (HMOs)** has been around since the 1920s. HMOs provide comprehensive health care to voluntarily enrolled subscribers for a fixed, prepaid fee. The fee may be picked up by an employer, especially if the employer is a large company. In addition to this prepaid fee, there may be an additional **co-payment,** or nominal out-of-pocket fee (no more than $5 to $10 in most instances) which the patient pays upon receiving the services.

The health-care delivery models shown here are all examples of **managed care** systems.[28] The term, managed care, while not a new one at all, is one that has come to the forefront during the debate on health-care reform. In simple terms, it means no more than a plan that finances and delivers health-care services through an organized network of providers.

- **Staff Models**—In a staff HMO, the HMO actually employs a network of physicians and typically pays them on a salaried basis. The HMO often builds and owns the facilities where the care is offered. Most university health centers are staff HMOs. Access to the physician network often is overseen by a primary care provider, usually a general practitioner, who serves as a "gatekeeper" by making referrals for appropriate specialist services.
- **Independent Practice Associations (IPAs)**—In an independent practice association (also known as an individual

Prosthesis: an artificial device that is attached to the body to aid in its function. Examples include artificial limbs, pacemakers, and hearing aids.

Co-payment: a nominal fee provided by a patient to a health-care provider upon delivery of services, usually as part of the patient's contribution to a prepaid health plan.

Managed care: the delivery of health-care services through a coordinated network of providers.

Figure 17.7: The origins and destinations of the nation's health-care dollar.

Source: Data from the Health Care Financing Administration.

Where the nation's health dollar came from

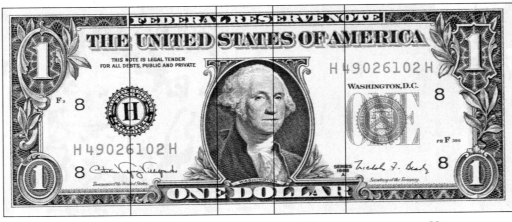

25¢	17¢	11¢	14¢	33¢
Direct patient payments	Medicare	Medicaid	All other state/local government programs	Private health insurance and other private third parties

Where it went

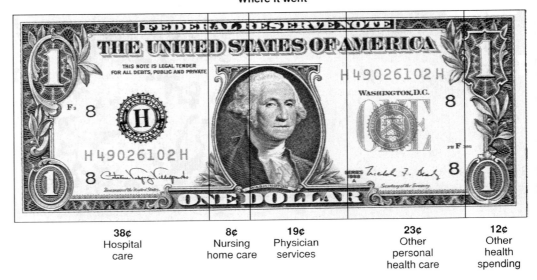

38¢	8¢	19¢	23¢	12¢
Hospital care	Nursing home care	Physician services	Other personal health care	Other health spending

practice association), the HMO contracts with either individual private practicing physicians, or with a legal entity known as an independent practice association to which privately practicing physicians belong, for an agreed-upon fee schedule. In this form of HMO, physicians typically work out of their own offices. Unlike salaried HMO physicians in the staff model, IPA physicians may treat patients from other health-care plans, along with their own fee-for-service patients. A primary care provider

designated by the subscriber may act as a "gatekeeper" in this model of service delivery as well.

• **Point-of-Service (POS) Plans**—In a POS plan, the HMO consists of a network of physicians and facilities that provides an insurance company or an employer with discounts on services. Unlike typical HMO members, subscribers to POS plans have the option of going outside the network of providers to obtain care, in which case the plan reimburses a percentage of the outside fees.

- **Preferred Provider Organization (PPO)**—The PPO is a network of physicians and facilities that provide an insurance company or employer with discounted services. Unlike typical HMO members, patients of a PPO may use any provider within the network, including specialists, whenever they choose.

- **Exclusive Provider Organization (EPO)**—The EPO is a less common health-care plan in which subscribers are eligible to receive benefits only when they use the services of a limited network of care providers. EPOs are similar to HMOs but are regulated under state health insurance laws.

Prepaid health insurance plans have received strong support for development, including passage of the federal HMO Act of 1973. Economic times have reduced the monetary support of the federal government in the development of the programs. The philosophical base of support has remained strong, however, because such plans represent a form of competition in the health-care marketplace.

A unique feature of HMOs is a reimbursement philosophy that stresses more care rendered on an outpatient, ambulatory basis than on an inpatient basis. Most private health insurance companies will not reimburse for a number of procedures unless they are done in a hospital setting. Even casual observers of the system quickly can see that outpatient care should be less costly.

A typical feature of HMOs is that they are operated on a **capitation** basis. That is, a system whereby physicians (or hospitals) are paid a fixed amount for each patient enrolled in the program, regardless of the services actually provided to the patient. Therefore, a well member is an asset to an HMO, as the fewer services required by a member the greater the monetary savings for the HMO. Most HMOs, therefore, are motivated to enhance levels of wellness by providing health maintenance services such as prenatal care, physical fitness, and nutritional counseling. It remains unclear as to whether the traditional HMO model is superior to the IPA or other network models in limiting costs and increasing user satisfaction.[29]

Federal Financing of Health Care

Many people might want to debate what the federal government's role should be

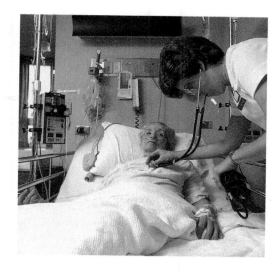

Figure 17.8: What Do You Think?

1. Medicare and Medicaid programs are an important source of health-care financing for the elderly. Why should the government fund health-care services for the elderly?
2. Do Medicare and Medicaid cover the costs of all health-care needs of the elderly? What evidence do you have to support your answer?

concerning matters of health care for the public. Specifically, should government, at any level, sponsor agencies for actually providing health care, or should it pay for care rendered? Presently, outside of special programs for military personnel and their dependents, the government sponsors two programs—Medicare and Medicaid.

For more than thirty years, **Medicare** has been a social program that assists in the payment of health expenses for persons sixty-five years and older who are entitled to social security benefits (see figure 17.8). It is the single largest health insurer in the U.S.,[30] and has been called by some "a lifeline for older Americans" since it pays for about 90 percent of their hospital and physician bills.[31] The Medicare program consists of two parts. Medicare plan Part A provides coverage for inpatient hospital-related expenses, limited nursing home services, and some home health services. It is available to all eligible parties. Medicare plan Part B is a form of optional medical insurance that pays for provider-related expenses (physician and other ambulatory services, durable medical equipment such as wheelchairs, and certain other services). When it was enacted in 1965, Medicare was seen as providing for certain **acute care** needs of older people in the U.S. What has occurred in the past three decades is a shift toward long-term care such as nursing home services, routine eye care, and reimbursement for outpatient prescription drugs. As a result, Medicare has become an enormously expensive venture for the federal government and the taxpayer.

Capitation: a head count of subscribers or enrollees in a prepaid health plan, usually determining the amount of money paid by the plan to the care provider.

Acute care: health care that addresses health issues of short-term or brief duration.

Even with Medicare coverage, a large number of the elderly carry additional private insurance to cover areas that may be exempted by Medicare. Such private insurance is sometimes referred to as a "Medigap" policy. Consumer ignorance surrounding Medicare-supplemental insurance has resulted in insurance companies and some physicians taking advantage of Medicare beneficiaries and the system itself.[32] To discourage fraud, Medicare must rely on the Office of the Inspector General in the Department of Health and Human Services, an office whose budget has been slashed in recent years. Consequently, investigations of fraud have been minimal or abandoned altogether in many parts of the country.[33]

Medicaid is the government-sponsored program of health insurance that was established to assist the socioeconomically disadvantaged, people determined to be in need of such assistance due to a health disability (such as blindness), and the aged poor. This particular program, which covers basic health costs such as hospital expenses, physician expenses, nursing home expenses, and some others, is shared economically with the federal government by the fifty state governments.

Because Medicaid is administered and partly funded by state governments, the scope and quality of Medicaid programs vary by state. Some states contribute more of their monetary resources to Medicaid programs than others; however, even in states with a strong commitment to Medicaid, the health-care needs of the poor are often inadequately met. One estimate is that Medicaid covers medical expenses for only 38 percent of the nation's poor.[34]

Health-Care Reform: Of What Should it Consist?

Even though there is presently no form of nationalized health insurance in the U.S., it is prudent to mention the possibility of its emergence in the future. **National health insurance,** an idea first introduced in the U.S. during the Truman administration, would provide health insurance to all U.S citizens regardless of ability to pay. Prior to the time of the Clinton presidency, Senator Edward M. Kennedy of Massachusetts was the most vocal advocate of a national health insurance program for more than thirty years. A grass-roots effort to reform health care was

responsible, in part, for the election of Bill Clinton to the presidency in 1992. The effort for major reform, including the initiation of universal health insurance coverage, stalled during subsequent Congressional hearings. As the debate continues about health-care reform, consumer input is certainly of critical importance (see table 17.4). National health insurance programs in Germany, Great Britain, and Canada demonstrate that such programs are possible, but have not given conclusive evidence that they have favorably influenced rising health-care costs (see A Social Perspective 17.1).

Self-Care and Self-Diagnosis: Good Ideas?

Consumers today are accepting more personal responsibility for selected health matters (see Of Special Interest 17.1). Among the most popular of the health-care skills are blood-pressure screening and pregnancy testing. Manufacturers have responded by offering accessories to the public to develop these skills. In principle, there is nothing wrong with saving on physician fees, laboratory tests, and avoiding delays in clinic waiting rooms. However, not all of the equipment available may be of sufficient caliber to provide reliable self-assessments.

Blood pressure kits include a **sphygmomanometer** to assess blood pressure and a **stethoscope** for listening to heart sounds. For persons with high blood pressure, home monitoring is an ideal way of saving trips to the clinic, and of staying in touch with their body. One needs to be cautious of low-quality equipment, though. If people must screen their blood pressure, it is worthwhile to invest in professional quality equipment. While it is fun to check blood pressure in coin-operated machines found in shopping malls, results from this type of testing need to be corroborated by a physician.

Home pregnancy tests also are popular self-care items. Their operation is simple. A woman adds a few drops of her urine to a test tube provided in the kit. The test tube contains chemicals that react with the urine if pregnancy has occurred. The reactive substance found in the urine of pregnant women is a hormone known as **human chorionic gonadotropin (HCG).** Kits sell in pharmacies for between $8 and $18.

Sphygmomanometer: a device used, in conjunction with a stethoscope, to measure blood pressure. It consists of an inflatable cuff that is put around the upper arm just above the elbow, and a rubber tube connected to a measuring device (often a tube of mercury). Pressure is applied by the cuff and then gradually released. A stethoscope is used to listen to the pulse just below the cuff; the pressure at which the pulse is first heard and at which it muffles or disappears are recorded as the blood pressure measurement.

Human chorionic gonadotropin (HCG): a hormone produced by the placenta, which keeps the ovaries secreting progesterone. Progesterone secretion will help prepare the uterus for pregnancy and inhibit ovulation during pregnancy.

The subject of health care is a boring topic for many people until they need it and don't have it. A well-rounded college education should prepare one to participate intelligently in the debate about the health-care needs of this country. The following tips may help to inspire your interest.

Precontemplation → Contemplation

If you have not thought about the issues involved or don't know really what they are all about, consider:

- Becoming informed about health-care issues in your state. Read newspaper and magazine articles about health-care issues.

Contemplation → Preparation

If you have read some about health-care issues but can't quite find your way through or around them, you are not alone. It may be time for you to let the politicians hear how you feel. You can:

- Make the decision to take action on a specific health-care issue.
- Identify a date in the next thirty days when you will carry out your plan. Mark the date on your calendar. Tell friends about your idea.

Preparation → Action

You are ready to make some specific plans for action. This is your first step toward what may be a lifetime of political activism about health care as well as other issues. Go ahead and:

- Make a firm appointment (e.g., next Monday at 2:00 P.M.) to assert yourself with respect to an issue.

- Tell others about your intended activity. Let people know that you are not "just thinking about" taking a stance on health care—but actually doing something about it.
- Get the addresses of your Congress person and two U.S. Senators.

Action → Maintenance

If you have started to take action, make advocacy a part of your regular routine by:

- Writing to the President of the United States, The White House, Washington, D.C., 20500.
- Writing to your Congress person and your two U.S. Senators.
- Sending copies of any letters to the Program for Economic Justice, Consumers Union, 101 Truman Avenue, Yonkers, NY, 10703.
- Talking back to the media. Write a letter to the editor of the college newspaper and the local city newspaper indicating your position on health-care reform or other health issues as they arise.

Maintenance

- Keep your momentum by joining an organization that works toward universal access to health care in the U.S. (e.g., Fund for Health Security, Consumer's Union).
- Inviting a roommate, classmate, or other friend to help you with one of your activities that involves a health-care issue.
- Letting your friends and other peers know that health-care issues should not be things of remote interest to them.

There is a certain ill-conceived logic about the use of these kits. Although the tests themselves are sensitive, their results are not always reliable. The tests tend to produce some false-negative results. A woman who gets a negative test result may do one of two things. She might delay seeking prenatal care since she remains unaware of her pregnancy. In the interim, she may use substances such as oral contraceptives, alcohol, or other drugs that can pose a problem for her fetus later. A **false-negative** test also might inspire her to

repeat the test, and therefore, incur added costs without any assurance that the second result is more credible than the first.

A positive pregnancy test produces a similar predicament for the woman. It may lead to a visit to the physician, who will repeat the test and have it interpreted professionally. Thus, the result will be confirmed or refuted, making the original test an unnecessary expense. If you suspect you are pregnant, contact an appropriate medical professional who can schedule a test, if necessary.

False negative: a test result that indicates a person does not have a particular condition, in this case pregnancy, when in fact they do.

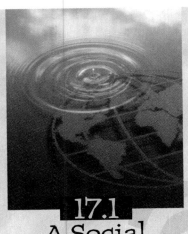

17.1
A Social Perspective

What Is Ideal for Health-Care Reform?

During the early years of the Clinton Administration, several proposals for major reform of health care in the United States were considered. Although none of these bills introduced to the Congress was ultimately acceptable to our elected representatives, it is clear that modification of the current system, however great or small, is a likelihood in the coming years. Lobbyists for the many wealthy and powerful segments of the medical-industrial complex, including the pharmaceutical industry, have been hard at work defending their turf and their profits.* What are the principles or ideals behind health-care reform, whatever its eventual outcome? Some of the major ideals are identified below.**

Universal Coverage
Guaranteed health insurance for everyone, regardless of their employment status, their financial status, their age, or their health status.

Comprehensive Benefits
Inclusive of all medically necessary care, preventive services, and long-term care for the elderly and the disabled.

Consumer Choice
Provides consumers the opportunity to select where and from whom they receive their health care.

Cost Controls
Limit the amount that the country as a whole can spend on medical care. Set fee schedules that limit what physicians and other health-care providers can be paid for service delivery. Establish controls on reimbursement on providers in the private sector similar in principle to what presently exists for Medicare and Medicaid programs in the public sector. Control wasteful paperwork and procedures.

Adequate Financing
Requires a broad-based tax or payroll tax so that employers do not have to shoulder the burden for premiums. Revenue must be sufficiently large to cover all those who presently have some form of insurance as well as those who have little or no insurance.

Public Accountability
Must place patient care above profits. Managed-care organizations must be driven by incentives other than profit if people in true need of care are not to be denied care. System must have consumers well represented on relevant health-care advisory boards and committees.

What Do You Think?

1. Is national health insurance another form of social welfare that is noble in its aim but fails to motivate people to "pull themselves up by the bootstraps?" Has the federal government shown itself to be a good fiscal manager of large-scale programs?
2. Does a society have an obligation to provide for the health-care needs of its most disenfranchised citizens? To what extent is the way in which a society cares for its poor a measure of the greatness of that society?

Sources: Data from Editors of *Consumer Reports*, "Do We Pay Too Much for Prescriptions?" in *Consumer Reports*, 58.10 (1993): 668–674; and Editors in *Consumer Reports*, "What to Watch for in Health Care Reform," in *Consumer Reports*, 59.6 (1994): 396–398.

Buying exercise equipment is another widely practiced consumer activity, and it constitutes the need for sound information and some common sense. People invest in exercise equipment ranging from barbells and exercise bicycles to jogging suits and "designer" sweatbands. There are many high-quality products made and sold by reputable firms, but there are costly items as well, created by phony "experts" that do little, if any, good.

The benefits of exercise depend on the nature of the exercise itself. Weight lifting builds muscle and strength, but has minimal cardiovascular benefit. **Aerobic exercises** like running, swimming, or bicycling can have significant cardiovascular effects and tone muscles as well. It is important to identify your exercise objective before purchasing a host of accessories that may be unnecessary.

Carefully assess ads that promote a product said to be a "total exercise program all by itself." No single product can accomplish that. Have similar skepticism when an ad suggests that you can "see real changes in only moments a day." Products "hawked" in such ads often come with money-back guarantees that appear to enhance the legitimacy of the product prior to its purchase. Many consumers are either too busy to be inconvenienced to return an unsatisfactory product, or too embarrassed to ask for their money back once they have been "taken."

Aerobic exercise: activities that cause a sustained increase in heart rate and use the large muscles of the body continuously for an extended period of time.

In-Home Tests Make Health Care Easier

When it comes to helping people stay healthy, in-home medical tests may be useful. Blood pressure monitors and the new blood cholesterol test, for instance, may play a role in thwarting heart and blood vessel disease. A positive result from a pregnancy test might prompt a woman to go to her doctor sooner, so she gets prenatal care earlier in her pregnancy.

Another device, the home meter for testing blood glucose (sugar) levels can—within seconds—electronically analyze a blood drop from a finger prick, so a person with diabetes knows whether to adjust medicine, exercise, or diet.

"By creating the potential for tight control of diabetes, the blood glucose meter has revolutionized this area of medical practice," says the Food and Drug Administration's Steven Gutman, M.D. "It's a cornerstone of modern diabetic therapy." Gutman is acting director of FDA's division of clinical laboratory devices, Center for Devices and Radiological Health, responsible for reviewing many in-home test devices.

More Benefits

Generally, in-home tests provide easy access to medical knowledge about one's health. In some cases, such as monitoring high blood pressure, home testing reduces the number of times a patient must visit a doctor's office or laboratory, thereby reducing medical costs. People also may feel an increased sense of control over their health.

An over-the-counter (OTC) test performs at least one of three functions:

- doctor-recommended monitoring (*e.g.,* blood pressure, for hypertension; blood glucose, for diabetes control; ovulation, for infertility)
- detecting markers for possible health conditions when there are no physical signs or symptoms (blood cholesterol level, for high cholesterol; hidden [occult] blood in stool, for colon or rectal cancer)
- detecting markers for specific conditions when there are physical signs or symptoms (a specific female hormone in urine after a missed period, for pregnancy).

For any in-home test, the manufacturer must convince the agency not only that the test has value (results will benefit consumers), but also that consumers have the knowledge necessary to decide whether testing themselves is

appropriate, says Jur Strobos, M.D., J.D., director of FDA's Policy Research Staff. "If the firm does not show that consumers can make this judgment," he says, "we assume the test is for screening without preselecting patients. Then, we ask ourselves, is it appropriate for this use?"

Not all tests on the OTC market are equally useful, however, says Philip Phillips, deputy director of FDA's Office of Device Evaluation.

"Some OTC tests that have been marketed for many years," he says, "may not be as useful or acceptable as many consumers believe."

Eye charts, Phillips notes for example, have been sold for decades and are still around in some drugstores, "but you shouldn't rely on them if you think you need eyeglasses or have not had a recent examination." People having eye problems should be examined by a licensed eye-care professional, he says.

Incorrect Results

The more recently approved in-home tests are as reliable as professional tests. Still, all tests can generate false positives (indicating someone has a condition that in fact the person does not) or false negatives (a result that does not identify a condition that is in fact present)—particularly if the user doesn't follow directions.

Instead of signifying colon or rectal cancer, a positive result on a test for hidden blood in stool could reflect such factors as bleeding gums or last night's T-bone steak. Or an untrained person may perform the test incorrectly, causing hidden blood in stool to go undetected.

In other words, it can be risky for consumers to consider test results as a definite diagnosis. Professional follow-up is needed.

A doctor's diagnosis involves evaluation of the patient's medical history and physical examination, often other tests, and sometimes consultation with other medical experts. Further, unlike home testing, professional laboratories must meet quality standards, which provide additional reliability and uniformity to test results.

While no test—OTC or professional—is 100 percent accurate, in a medical setting, Gutman says, "professional, trained people would be expected to interpret test results in a broader context."

The issue of interpreting false results was central to FDA's decision not to grant OTC status to drugs-of-abuse tests, approved for prescription use only. Gutman says scientists are unsure how these tests would affect someone who didn't understand false positives and

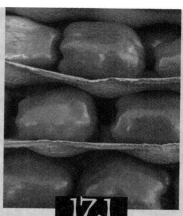

false negatives. Instead of helping people, such a test might hurt them.

"Drugs of abuse," he says, "have a real punch in terms of emotional impact. The harm from a slight error with, say, a cholesterol test is the user might go out and eat a piece of chocolate cake. But a false positive in a test for drugs of abuse might lead to a person being fired or divorced, or a youngster being falsely accused and punished."

Preventing Problems

Interpreting results of the newer OTC tests on pharmacy shelves should not be a problem for consumers. Before FDA will approve OTC sales today, test sponsors must prove that consumers can accurately interpret results.

OTC tests also must be labeled with appropriate warnings. For instance, if a test is not for use by people with diabetes, a large-type warning must state so.

To use in-home tests as safely and effectively as possible, consumers should carefully read the instructions, which FDA makes sure are user-friendly. As Gutman puts it: "Instructions tell how a test works, when it works, when it doesn't, and what to do when it doesn't."

Dixie Farley is a staff writer for FDA Consumer.

What Do You Think?

1. What are the most positive aspects of being able to perform in-home tests that may reflect your health-care status?
2. What are the most negative aspects of performing in-home tests?

Source: From Dixie Farley "In-home Tests Make Health Care Easier" in *FDA Consumer,* 28.10 (1994): 25–28.

Many other health products and devices are sold by mail order, and are advertised on TV or in popular magazines. Consumers may falsely assume that reputable magazines screen out fraudulent advertisements. Products promoted may include sexual pleasure enhancers (vibrators, penis enlargers, erection stimulators) and beauty aids (bustline developers, spot reducers, and hair removers/growers). Any health-related device or gimmick that is available exclusively through mail order ought to be considered dubious.

What kind of medical record keeping should you maintain? You should have a complete and up-to-date set of records. If your primary care provider should retire, die, or relocate to another geographic area, you are prepared to transfer your records to a new care provider. In the past some physicians and other care providers have frowned upon patients obtaining their medical records. About half of all states now guarantee access to medical records.[35] To obtain your records, contact the office or hospital where tests or examinations were performed. Even in states that do not have guaranteed access, most offices will comply with requests, but may require that the request be made in writing and that the person making the request pay a fee for photocopying and mailing. To maintain accuracy and completeness, such a request should be made after each office visit. In the future, technology may permit us to store an entire medical history, including prescription drugs and other pertinent details, on something the size of a credit card. Until that technology is popularized, the wise consumer should be assertive in maintaining records concerning personal health care.

Fraud and the Consumer

In the health marketplace, one will encounter numerous sales pitches, mail-order gimmicks, glamorous and appealing advertisements, and other things to entice a purchase. The unsuspecting consumer can be lured to relinquish hard earned dollars if he or she is unprepared for dubious practices. Below are some of the more common fraudulent schemes of which the consumer should be aware.

A frequently practiced scheme is the **bait-and-switch** tactic. It begins when a retailer advertises a product at an unusually low price to lure customers into the store. Upon arrival, customers learn that the

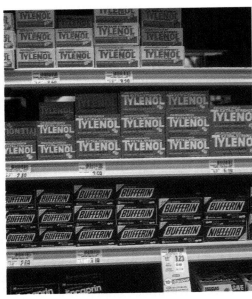

Figure 17.9: What Do You Think?

1. Consumers practicing brand loyalty may pay extra for quality that is no better or only marginally better than less-expensive products. What resources are available to you to help you research when it is worth paying more for a name brand?
2. How often do you research brands before you buy?

advertised merchandise is "sold out" or that it is of inferior quality. A salesman may try to persuade the consumer to purchase a brand that is of "higher quality" but also is higher priced. Retailers concerned about their reputation are not likely to engage in this practice; instead they offer customers "rain checks" to be used when the particular item is restocked. Potential danger exists with this practice too. Once lured to the retail outlet, you may purchase other items simply because you have made a trip. After receiving the rain check, you may return to purchase the original item and again make additional purchases. The retailer gains in either case.

Another technique employed is the **brand loyalty** approach. The retailer or advertiser convinces people that a brand name is the trademark of quality. Well-known products for such items as antacids and pain relievers are usually more expensive but seldom of better quality than more obscure brands or generic products. The key is to read the product label and examine the so-called active ingredients. Be wary of an ad that proclaims: "Buy the name you have come to rely on" or "Accept no substitute." Although the product may be perfectly acceptable, the price tag may be unnecessarily inflated (see figure 17.9).

Another favorite strategy for attracting customers is **product misrepresentation.** Almost everyone has seen a television commercial that begins: "Nine out of ten doctors recommend Brand X for the relief of the headache and congestion of cold and flu." Before rushing out to the corner drugstore, consider such questions as: Which doctors were asked? How were they selected? Were they paid to respond? Obviously, this information is not shared in the commercial. Another common misrepresentation begins: "Studies from a major university reveal Brand Y provides help for hemorrhoidal sufferers." What studies? Which University? Under what conditions and with which research methods? One begins to see how subtle and repetitious media messages can work their way into our repertoire of buying habits.

The wise consumer needs to ask questions and to be on guard for deception, manipulation, misrepresentation, and even complete fraud. Some measure of protection can be attained by identifying reputable retailers who have a long history of service and who provide written guarantees.

Great technological advances are occurring in science and medicine. Consumers, nevertheless, remain vulnerable to quackery because of their lack of adequate knowledge and feelings of hopelessness, helplessness, or despair. Quackery is a lucrative business for its practitioners. Most susceptible to the quack's persuasion are people who are incurably ill, who face surgery, who experience chronic and unending pain, and who have difficulty in adjusting to the prospects of growing older.

For the incurably ill patient, the will to live may be an important determination in the outcome of an illness. Those with the spirit to survive sometimes reach out for any sign of hope that is offered. Often such hope is provided by quacks. The dilemma of the incurably ill patient is a difficult one to comprehend for all but those who have been confronted with a similar situation. The patient must almost hope for a miracle, yet accept the best that medical science has to offer, recognize its limitations, and avoid the temptations of quackery.

Surgery is usually a frightening prospect. Even minor surgical procedures can require anesthesia, hospitalization, and other obtrusive procedures. Some people fear postoperative pain or are dismayed by the reality of the unnecessary surgical procedures that are performed each year. Unless prospective surgical patients receive reassurance both from physicians and family members, they may have severe reservations about proceeding with an operation. If such social support is lacking, the appeal of an alternative practitioner who promises healing without surgery is inviting.

Other people who are confronted with neither terminal illness nor surgery are also susceptible to the hucksters of the health marketplace. These are the chronic pain sufferers whose desperate search for relief opens the door to quackery. Few ailments, for example, cause the physical anguish and mental frustration brought about by **arthritis.** Quacks have exploited this situation by offering such items as "magical" copper bracelets, mineral waters, condensed seawater, and a multitude of other gimmicks and concoctions of no curative value.

The inability to cope with the inexorable process of aging causes still other people to consider quackery. Quacks target both the elderly and the middle aged, offering help for wrinkles, balding, declining interest in sex, or decreasing vigor through cosmetics, diets, drugs, exercises, and other equipment and paraphernalia.

Quackery has survived centuries of exposure and is likely to be around as long as there are vulnerable individuals. Perhaps being aware of times you are most likely to be susceptible to quackery's inviting promises and schemes can direct you towards more beneficial practices.

Consumer Skills and Self-Responsibility

There are some skills that good consumers can develop to defend themselves in the health marketplace or, where appropriate and necessary, to fight back. Corry[36] delineates five important skills, including assertiveness, bargaining and bidding, budgeting, comparison shopping, and data collection.

Assertiveness

Assertiveness sometimes has a negative connotation; it is equated with being exploitative, aggressive, or unnecessarily obnoxious. Being assertive means to stand up for your rights, to be a self-advocate. Unfortunately, many of us are taught not to

Arthritis: a painful inflammation of the joints.

challenge health practitioners. Engaging in constructive confrontation, where appropriate, not only gives the consumer a more positive self-image, but it may benefit the other party as well. Learning to be assertive, like learning to play the French horn, requires practice. Some people fear the prospect of being assertive.

Bargaining and Bidding

These are strategies you can use to pay the lowest reasonable price possible when making a purchase. In some settings, such as at automobile dealerships, bargaining has long been a common and expected practice. A car has a retail price known as the sticker price. A customer makes an offer at something less than the sticker price. The salesperson makes a counteroffer at something between the customer's bid and the sticker price. The familiar process of haggling begins. Perhaps the customer has received an offer from another dealer; that is, has engaged in comparison shopping. At some point, the buyer and the seller agree on a compromise price.

Such a practice has not been common in the health marketplace. It may be that the purchase of practitioner services could become similar to the purchase of a car someday. If that seems improbable, then clearly the prospect of bargaining for a means of paying off practitioners' fees over time, as opposed to a single lump sum due at the time service is performed, is not.

Budgeting

Budgeting is a practice that can save you much anguish and prevent overspending. When you decide to purchase an item or service, establish an upper spending limit. Adhere to it. Such a practice discourages being lured into the bait-and-switch trap.

Comparison Shopping

Comparison shopping saves you money. One of the realities of the health marketplace is that stiff competition exists. The purchase price of both prescription and nonprescription drugs can be moderated by calling different pharmacies. Make phone calls—lots of them. A given prescription drug may be 25 to 40 percent cheaper in the least expensive drug store than in the most expensive one.[37] One particular drugstore may not always be the cheapest for all products though, meaning that if you take more than one product, your greatest savings may come by your shopping at more than one drugstore.[38]

Although it is rarely done, there is no practical reason why the cost of many practitioners' services cannot be given over the telephone. Though cost is not the only criterion to be considered when selecting a service provider, think about the merit of paying $37 for preventive dental services with Dr. Smith compared to $48 for equivalent services from Dr. Jones.

Data Collection

Data collection may be the most tedious and laborious part of being a good consumer. Most of us do not take the time or expend the energy necessary to make the best purchase for our money. It is easier to gamble and keep our fingers crossed. We do not often get burned gambling, so we are tempted to gamble again. When we finally get a bad product and feel stung, we act surprised. The merchandiser knows of this flaw in consumers' characters and exploits it. At the moment we are ready to buy, our only "data" may be what we remember from that television commercial or magazine ad.

What can we do to reduce the chances of being victimized? Any consumer who can read can become a self-advocate. A number of informative and worthwhile publications are widely available. These publications include such periodicals as *Consumer Reports*, *Changing Times*, and *FDA Consumer*. When in a physician's office, a wise consumer should seek information, especially if handed a prescription. Pharmacists are also good sources for information about medications. You can develop the necessary assertiveness to find out what you need and how to find it.

How to Read the Health Literature

How should a good consumer respond to a newspaper or television account of a study that suggests everyone should change their lifestyle habits overnight? Health professionals will tell you that reading the literature must be done with a critical eye. Those who do not critique well may fall into a trap that might be called the *disease-of-the-week syndrome*. This occurrence results when people read about a particular disease or other malady (often a rare disorder) and subsequently believe themselves to be afflicted like the person in the television drama or published case study.

Those persons who are not taken in by this trap might still go on to misinterpret the practical significance of the data that are represented. There are an estimated 40,000 scientific journals which publish more than 1 million articles per year.[39] Beyond these, there are numerous health-related periodicals that are part of the popular press and scores of audience-specific magazines that contribute further to the morass of information that confronts the consumer. There is much confusion, as well as a great deal of skepticism, about the data that are provided to the public. How does one put some order to all of this information?

There are a couple of basic points that can help to put this matter into the proper perspective. First, medical and other scientific journals seldom give advice to the public. Instead, these publications provide a forum for scholars to advance the state of knowledge by attempting to provide evidence that permits themselves and others to arrive at the truth. Second, one isolated study is infrequently the final word on a subject. Rather, the article reports observations that build upon previous studies, either supporting or challenging earlier conclusions. It is, more often than not, the purpose of research to modify current practice and thinking. Science, therefore, is a dynamic process. Moreover, it is one that rarely is able to resolve an issue beyond a shadow of a doubt. There are few clear answers where health matters are concerned. Science has established compelling links between such things as cigarette smoking and hypertension, and subsequent ill health. On the other hand, hypotheses about the merit of using food additives, the long-term effects of air pollution, or the consequences of ozone layer destruction are less adequately resolved.

A responsible and well-informed consumer can be protected from jumping on the bandwagon of a "new" idea by asking a series of important questions. Is this study the first of its kind? Is the research project one of many that have produced similar results? Is the study one of many that have produced conflicting results? Is the study one that assists scientists in reaching a consensus of opinion?

When reading a study or the published account of the study, having a certain degree of skepticism is healthy. Mike Woods[40] offers this advice:

> You don't need absolute certainty to justify minor changes in your behavior—such as cutting down on coffee or alcohol consumption. But you may demand considerably more for major changes, especially those that seriously might decrease your enjoyment of life.

We are so bombarded by health information that it is often difficult to know how to equip ourselves for ordinary health-related events. Thuy and Magda, two college roommates, were discussing what products should be stocked in the medicine cabinet of their apartment. What advice could you offer to them? Activity for Wellness 17.1 is provided to assist you.

Help for the Consumer

As a consumer, you may sometimes feel compelled to complain about the performance of a product or the outcome of a service. Before making a complaint, it is wise to be sure that it is justified. If you failed to follow directions or improperly handled the product, your complaint may not be legitimate. But if you are sure your complaint is justified, be sure you stay coolheaded and diligently follow up on the complaint. There are several private and government agencies to assist consumers.

Private Organizations

Professional associations like the American Medical Association and the **American Dental Association** are instrumental in the war on quackery. State or county affiliates of these groups are usually listed in the telephone book and can address questions about adherence of practitioners to professional and ethical standards. Professional organizations representing other groups such as optometrists and funeral directors exist and also may have local affiliates.

The local **Better Business Bureau** is not an enforcement agency, and does not give legal advice, but it can direct consumers to the most appropriate source of help for their complaint or problem. The Better Business Bureau may be able to provide you with

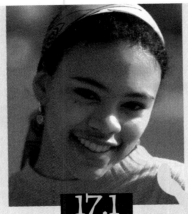

17.1
Activity for Wellness

Can You Take Care of Yourself?

Do you have the necessary supplies on hand to take care of your general daily health and minor emergency medical-care needs? Take this quiz to determine how prepared you are to take care of your personal health needs. Place a check in the box next to each item *you currently keep on hand* in your residence. Then read the answer key to find out if you have the items a wise health-care consumer needs. (Not all of the ingredients listed below are needed by the average consumer.)

❏ 1. sunscreen having an SPF of 8–10

❏ 2. over-the-counter (OTC) decongestant

❏ 3. blood pressure monitor

❏ 4. aspirin, acetaminophen, ibuprofen

❏ 5. gauze bandages & adhesive tape

❏ 6. baking soda (sodium bicarbonate)

❏ 7. OTC cold medications

❏ 8. hydrogen peroxide

❏ 9. rubbing alcohol

Source: From "Can You Take Care of Yourself" in *American Health*, 13.6, 1994:30–31.

❏ 10. syrup of ipecac

❏ 11. laxative tablets

❏ 12. antibiotics

❏ 13. mercurochrome

❏ 14. thermometer

❏ 15. calamine lotion

❏ 16. elastic bandages

❏ 17. cold pack

❏ 18. Imodium (antidiarrheal medication)

Answers:

1. Use a sunscreen with an SPF of 15 if you want reasonable protection. An SPF that is even higher might be warranted for especially fair-skinned persons.
2. OTC decongestants can relieve some cold symptoms, such as stuffy nose, if taken according to the instructions.
3. A blood pressure monitor is probably not worth stocking due to the expense and need for calibration checks. If your blood pressure needs regular checking, have it done professionally.
4. Use these analgesics for relief of mild pain, including headaches. Aspirin and acetaminophen also provide relief from mild fever. Aspirin and ibuprofen are especially useful in treating inflammation.
5. Gauze bandages and adhesive tape are especially useful for large cuts that require control of bleeding or protection.
6. Baking soda is an inexpensive antacid when mixed with water. It should be used cautiously by people with hypertension because of its high sodium content.
7. Some OTC cold medications may contain substances incompatible with other drugs you may take, or they may produce undesirable side effects. Consult a physician before using them.

8. Hydrogen peroxide is a good, inexpensive antiseptic for cleaning minor cuts and scrapes.
9. Rubbing alcohol provides sterilizing capability but should be used according to the instructions on the label.
10. Syrup of ipecac can be used to induce vomiting after poisoning, but *only* after calling the poison control center. Vomiting is *not* the treatment of choice for all ingested poisons. The nearest poison control center telephone number is listed in your telephone directory. To be prepared for an emergency, it is best to post this number next to your telephone.
11. A better choice to treat constipation would be to increase your dietary fiber.
12. Never keep prescription antibiotics "on hand." Use prescription antibiotics according to instructions from the physician or pharmacist. Discard unused medication when the original purpose for it no longer applies. OTC antibiotic ointment or cream can be stored for use on small cuts and scrapes to prevent infection.
13. Mercurochrome is not necessary. Hydrogen peroxide is a less expensive and better product for cleaning minor cuts and scrapes.
14. Keep a rectal thermometer on hand for children under the age of five, and an oral thermometer for others.
15. Calamine lotion is a good product to use to relieve minor, temporary itching from poison ivy, insect bites, sunburn, and minor forms of dermatitis.
16. Elastic bandages (sometimes called Ace Bandages) are useful for treating sprains.
17. A commercial cold pack can be used to control swelling and bruising due to minor injuries. Ice cubes in a plastic bag, wrapped in a towel, can be used as well.
18. Antidiarrheal medication, such as Imodium, successfully controls diarrhea and cramping when used as directed. If symptoms persist a physician should be contacted.

information concerning an establishment's reputation before you spend your money there. It can be a valuable community resource in overseeing consumer satisfaction, arranging for appropriate adjustments when necessary, and acting as an intermediary when a consumer's complaint seems unwarranted.

There are many other private organizations available to aid a troubled consumer. Such organizations are often listed in the telephone book. You can also seek help at the public library, in the local newspaper, or sometimes, by contacting radio and television stations. If all else fails, a comprehensive list of consumer organizations in your state can be obtained from Division of Consumer Organizations, U.S. Office of Consumer Affairs, Washington, D.C. 20201.

Governmental Agencies

Help for the consumer is at hand from three major federal agencies: the **Food and Drug Administration (FDA),** the **Federal Trade Commission (FTC),** and the **United States Postal Service (USPS).**

The FDA is an agency of the Department of Health and Human Services responsible for consumer protection in the areas of falsely represented or worthless drugs, medical devices, and cosmetics. It also protects consumers against food contaminants. The safety and effectiveness of new drugs are regulated by the FDA. Complaints can be addressed to: Director, Consumer Communications, FDA, 5600 Fishers Lane, Rockville, Md 20857.

The FTC provides consumer safeguards against deceptive claims in advertisements. It addresses claims concerning OTC drug products and cosmetics, medical devices, hearing aids, contact lenses, dental appliances, so-called hair restorers and bust developers, and funeral services. Fraud must be evident before the FTC can take legal action. Unfortunately, it may take years before some claims can be completely settled by the FTC. Complaints can be filed by writing: Office of the Secretary, Federal Trade Commission, Washington, D.C. 20580.

The USPS attempts to protect the public from fraud and quackery conducted through the U.S. mail. Conviction of people operating fraudulent businesses or selling worthless products through the mail requires only the proof of product misrepresentation.

If you receive falsely promoted, misrepresented, or unwanted products in the mail, contact your local postmaster or write: Consumer Advocate, U.S. Postal Service, Washington, D.C. 20260.

Writing a Complaint Letter

Resolving a consumer problem to your satisfaction does not always require the help of a consumer advocacy or regulatory agency. Most complaints are settled to everyone's satisfaction through direct communication between parties. Learn to be a self-advocate.

To prepare a letter of complaint, first find out if the company has a local office. If there is no local listing, consult a reference available at most public libraries entitled *Standard & Poor's Register of Corporations, Directors and Executives.* This reference lists the names and addresses of close to 40,000 U.S. businesses.

Type your letter, if possible, and include your name, address, and home and business telephone numbers. Be brief and to the point. Letters that are longer than one page and contain an extensive case history are undesirable. Pertinent facts such as date of transaction, item involved, and the store name should be included. You should state your proposal for a fair and just settlement. Attach documentation to support your claims (sales receipts, canceled checks, etc.). Send photocopies of the documentation rather than originals. It is seldom justified in a first letter to be sarcastic, threatening, or insulting, no matter how tempting it may be. The person reading your letter probably had nothing to do with creating your complaint but may be instrumental in settling it. A sample letter that can be adapted for a variety of situations is shown in figure 17.10.

A Last Word about Consumerism

David Blumenthal[41] writes:

. . . American people will accept major changes in their health-care system when the conditions are right. To achieve those conditions in the modern era, advocates will have to persist in educating the public about options for reform while waiting for Americans to

Figure 17.10: Sample of a complaint letter written by a consumer

Your address
Your city, state, zip

Date

Appropriate person
Company name
Street address
City, state, zip

Dear appropriate person:

Recently I purchased a (name of product with serial or model number or service performed). I made this purchase at (location, date, and other pertinent details of the purchase transaction).

Unfortunately, your product (or service) has not performed in a satisfactory manner (or the service was not adequate) because _____
_____
_____
_____

Therefore, to solve this problem, I am requesting that you (state the specific action you want taken). I have enclosed copies (copies—*not originals*) of my records of this transaction (receipts, guarantees, warranties, cancelled checks, contracts, model or serial numbers, and any other pertinent documents).

I am looking forward to hearing from you and learning how this problem is to be resolved. I shall wait three weeks before seeking third-party assistance. I may be contacted at the above address, or by telephone at (place your home and business numbers here).

Sincerely,

Your name

_____

conclude from personal experience that health-care reform is worth its undeniable risks.

The health marketplace may be perceived by the uninformed consumer as a "jungle." Everyone is likely to have bad experiences from time to time; however, the number of complaints and problems, as well as their eventual outcomes, are often within the consumer's control. By being a self-advocate, you can protect both yourself and others from being victimized (see figure 17.11). A great many problems can be avoided by arming yourself with what it takes to be an informed consumer.

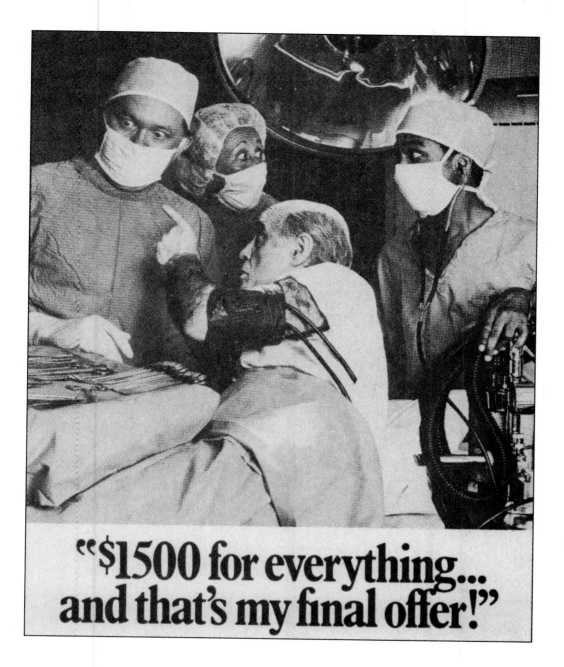

"$1500 for everything... and that's my final offer!"

1. How absurd it sounds—a consumer of medical care who is actually concerned about the price! But while a person such as this may be greeted with amazement by the hospital staff, it is not this person who is amazing—it is the rest of us, who have failed to be better self-advocates. How much did you pay in health-care expenses last year? last month? Do you ask about prices before you purchase health-care services?

Summary

1. Everyone must make decisions about the purchase of health-related goods and services.
2. Consumers need to accept a greater level of responsibility for their well-being and their utilization of the health-care system.
3. Careful selection of health-care professionals is a skill of great importance for enhancing consumer satisfaction with health care. Understanding differences between the various health-care specialties and subspecialties assists consumers in the selection of health professionals.
4. The consumer should be aware of levels of care and their various costs.
5. Health-care spending has continued to skyrocket, accounting for more than 14 percent of the United States gross national product (GNP).
6. The cost of health care remains an important barrier to the average consumer. Other important health-care barriers include the availability of services, the ways health care is currently financed, the organization of the health-care system itself, and certain individual beliefs and practices held by consumers.
7. Consumer knowledge of health-care financing alternatives must be heightened in an effort to aid in cost-control measures.
8. Maintaining a high level of wellness may be one of the most promising methods to control health-care costs.
9. Wise selection and use of health-related products require that a consumer possess both knowledge and common sense.
10. A variety of deceptive or fraudulent sales techniques can mislead unsuspecting and poorly informed consumers. Some common schemes include bait-and-switch, brand loyalty, and product misrepresentation.
11. Vulnerability to quackery and other fraudulent practices can sometimes be predicted and prevented. People most at risk include the incurably ill, those facing surgery, chronic pain sufferers, and those who deal unrealistically with the prospects of advancing age.
12. Certain consumer skills can be learned and practiced to minimize the probability of being defrauded. These skills include assertiveness, bargaining and bidding, budgeting, comparison shopping, and data collection.
13. Consumers have many resources available to assist them. In the private sector, organizations like the American Medical Association (AMA) and the American Dental Association (ADA) can be helpful. The Better Business Bureau can be of great assistance in mediating consumer complaints, though it has no enforcement authority. It can also provide information to consumers prior to both service utilization and product purchase. Federal government agencies such as the Food and Drug Administration (FDA), the Federal Trade Commission (FTC), and the United States Postal Service (USPS) attempt to protect the public from fraud and quackery.
14. Everyone should know how to write a letter of complaint when necessary and to direct it to the appropriate person.
15. Learn to be a self-advocate.

Recommended Readings

Cornacchia, Harold J., and Stephen Barrett. *Consumer Health, A Guide to Intelligent Decisions*. St. Louis: Mosby, 1993.

This well-written text describes the dynamics of the health marketplace, how to separate fact from fiction in advertising, approaches to health care, consumer protection mechanisms, a review of the major health problems affecting the United States, and other issues.

Editors of *Consumer Reports*. "How is Your Doctor Treating You?" *Consumer Reports* 60.2 (February 1995): 81–88.

This article reports the results of a survey completed by more than 70,000 people who assessed their medical care and their physicians. It tells how to be a good patient and how to interact with your health-care provider.

David Himmelstein and Steffie Woolhandler. *The National Health Program Book: A Source Guide for Advocates*. Monroe, Maine: Common Courage Press, 1994.

This book helps the consumer to decode the mystique of the U.S. health-care system. It examines ten of the biggest myths about health care, and explains why a movement in this country toward a Canadian-like system would save enough money to insure the presently uninsured population.

References

1. American Public Health Association, "U.S. Expenditures Pass 12% GNP," *The Nation's Health* 21.7 (1991): 24.
2. The Pepper Commission, *A Call to Action*, (Washington, D.C.: U.S. Government Printing Office, 1990), 5.
3. James F. Fries, "Reducing Need and Demand," *Healthcare Forum Journal* November-December (1993): 18.
4. Editors of *Consumer Reports*, "What to Watch for in Health Reform," 59.6 (1994): 398.
5. Editors of *Consumer Reports*, "Wasted Health Care Dollars," A reprint from the July 1992 issue of *Consumer Reports* magazine, 2.
6. Editors of *Consumer Reports*, "Wasted Health Care Dollars," 1.
7. Nan Silver, "How Good is Your Doctor," *Health* 22.9 (1990): 49.
8. Silver, "How Good is Your Doctor," 50.
9. Janice Hopkins Tanne, "Making Doctor Right," *Health* 22.0 (1990): 52–53.
10. Editors of *Consumer Reports*, "Chiropractors," *Consumer Reports*, 59.6 (1994): 383–390.
11. Editors of *Consumer Reports*, "Alternative Medicine: The Facts," *Consumer Reports* 59.1 (1994): 51–53.

12. Editors of *Consumer Reports*, "Homeopathy—Much Ado about Nothing?" *Consumer Reports* 59.3 (1994): 201–206.

13. Editors of *Consumer Reports*, "Acupuncture," *Consumer Reports* 59.1 (1994): 54–59.

14. Editors of *Consumer Reports*, "The Crisis in Health-Care Insurance," *Consumer Reports* 55.8 (1990): 533.

15. Editors of *Health Policy & Child Health*, "Beyond Insurance . . . Building Primary Care Systems for Children and Youth," *Health Policy & Child Health* (Fall 1994): 1.

16. *Healthy People 2000, National Health Promotion and Disease Prevention Objectives*, (Washington, D.C.: U.S. Department of Health and Human Services, 1991), 530–547.

17. *Healthy People 2000*, 642.

18. *Healthy People 2000*, 530–547.

19. Michele Turk, "The Neglected Sex," *American Health* 12.10 (1993): 54–57.

20. Turk, "The Neglected Sex," 54.

21. Marvin M. Lipman, "What Do Women Need?" *Consumer Reports on Health* 6.5 (1994): 59.

22. Lipman, "What Do Women Need?" 59.

23. Lipman, "What Do Women Need?" 59.

24. Editors of *Consumer Reports*, "The Crisis in Health Care Insurance," 534.

25. Editors of *Consumer Reports*, "The Crisis in Health Care Insurance," 534.

26. Editors of *Consumer Reports*, "Wasted Health Care Dollars," 11.

27. Editors of *Consumer Reports*, "The Crisis in Health Care Insurance," 540–541.

28. Donald Stroetzel and Diana Stroetzel, "HMO's—What You Need to Know," *American Health* 12.5 (1993): 77–80.

29. Robert H. Miller and Howard S. Luft, "Managed Care Plan Performance Since 1980," *Journal of the American Medical Association* 271.19 (1994): 1512–1519.

30. Nancy DeLew, George Greenberg, and Kraig Kinchen, "A Layman's Guide to the U.S. Health Care System," *Health Care Financing Review* 14.1 (1992): 151–169.

31. Editors of *Consumer Reports*, "Filling the Gaps in Medicare," *Consumer Reports* 59.8 (1994): 523–532.

32. Editors of *Consumer Reports*, "Filling the Gaps in Medicare," 423.

33. Editors of *Consumer Reports*, "Medicare Under Siege," *Consumer Reports* 59.9 (1994): 572–576.

34. Editors of *Consumer Reports*, "The Crisis in Health Care Insurance," 533.

35. *University of California at Berkeley Wellness Letter* 10.2 (1993): 1.

36. James M. Corry, *Consumer Health: Facts, Skills and Decisions*, (Belmont, Calif: Wadsworth, 1983).

37. Editors of *Consumer Reports*, "How to Buy Drugs for Less," *Consumer Reports* 58.10 (1993): 675–676.

38. Editors of *Consumer Reports*, "How to Buy Drugs for Less," 675–676.

39. Mike Woods, "Medical Journals Aren't Health Guides," *St. Petersburg Times*, April 20, 1991, A1.

40. Woods, "Medical Journals Aren't Health Guides," A2.

41. David Blumenthal, "Health Care Reform—Past and Future," *New England Journal of Medicine* 332.7 (1995): 465–468.

Aging: Adaptations for Wellness

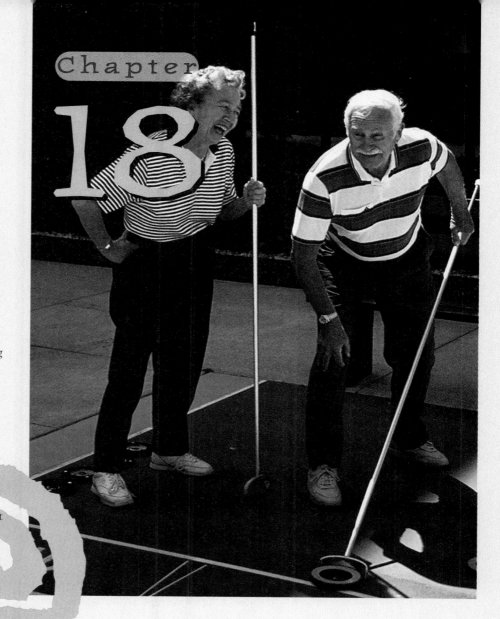

Chapter 18

Student Learning Objectives

Upon completion of this chapter you should be able to:

1. discuss the health status of older people in the U.S. as the year 2000 approaches;

2. identify some commonly believed myths about the elderly;

3. summarize several specific biological changes that occur over time, and correctly attribute them to primary aging versus secondary aging;

4. indicate ways that you are showing signs of the aging process;

5. present the salient features of several theories that try to explain biological processes of aging;

6. compare and contrast different models that describe the social phenomena associated with aging;

7. summarize some specific issues that affect people in the U.S. of different cultural backgrounds disproportionately;

8. identify specific problems that older people in the U.S. face from a safety standpoint;

9. give examples of several lifestyle modifications that can retard aging, enhance adaptations to aging, and increase overall life quality;

10. describe various barriers to wellness in older adulthood and throughout the life span, identifying specific means for overcoming them;

11. evaluate whether it is chronological age, state of mind, social prejudice and stereotypes, or other factors that determine the meaning of "old";

12. assess your readiness to become a supportive caregiver for older people.

As a college student you perhaps have given only passing thought to what it is like to be old. In terms of the future, you may have looked ahead to such events as securing a job, getting married, buying a house, raising a family, and other events that typify existence in the U.S. At this point, even middle age may seem a time far from the present. It is normal to view the future this way. An inevitable part of life, though, is change. Aging can be viewed as a change process that has biological, psychological, sociological, and other dimensions associated with it. How long people live and the quality of life they enjoy has changed dramatically in the U.S. in the twentieth century. Advances in public health, sanitation, nutrition, medical technology, and self-care have contributed to an increase in average life expectancy. Thus, a growing number of persons in the U.S. are living into their eighth and ninth decades and beyond. Although aging is an inevitability for all of us, how we age with respect to the dimensions identified above is unique from person to person.

In 1975 the world had 350 million people over the age of sixty, but by 2050, this number will exceed 1.1 billion. In the U.S. alone, 25 percent of the population will be over the age of fifty-five by the year 2010.[1]

In *Healthy People 2000*, several objectives to improve upon current health status have been identified. Some of these objectives are listed in table 18.1.

Due to technological and other medical advances, one of the implications of an aging society is that one's productive years will also increase.[2] Robert N. Butler[3] identifies five reasons that help to explain the curiosity that social and biological scientists have for studying the elderly. First, there is growing interest in the biology of aging as more becomes known about the genetic and environmental factors that are associated with the aging process. Second, the shift in survival and **life expectancy** has itself driven the inquiry about the social implications. Third, medical science documents the diseases of old age and attempts to moderate their effects. Fourth, an outgrowth of having a "greying society" is the impact that it has on health-care costs.

Finally, psychologists seek to understand the negative attitudes toward the elderly which abound in the 1990s.

Myths about Aging

Many people seem to suffer from a prejudice against old people. Robert Butler describes a societal phenomenon called **ageism** that is, in some ways, similar to racism and sexism.[4] A survey of college students revealed a tendency to view older people as all being alike, with women holding more positive views of the elderly than men.[5] Other studies reveal that when attitudes toward young people and old people are compared, older individuals generally are viewed less favorably.[6]

Philip Slater speaks of a society that tries to "hide" the elderly in institutions.[7] Despite societal prejudice, only a small fraction of the elderly actually are institutionalized.

Other myths about the elderly abound:

- Most old people are senile and incompetent.
- The elderly have no interest in or capacity for sexual relations.
- Old age is a time of depression and waiting around to die.
- The elderly are rigid in their ways and reactionary in their politics.
- Old people experience the aging process in identical ways.
- Most senior citizens are alone or lonely.
- The majority of elderly citizens are poor and without income.

All of these beliefs are false. There is a certain paradox about the way we view the elderly, especially when we take a closer look at how other things which are "old" are seen. An "old" wine is said to be "vintage." An "old" car, piece of literature, or song is said to be "classic." An "old" piece of art or even furniture may be a "collector's item" or a "treasure." But to be an old man or old woman often is seen as having no special status or distinction at all. Thomas R. Cole[8] explains that the origins of ageism may have come about from the decline of social systems where male elders were held in high esteem. In the 19th century for instance, the male hierarchical traditions of the Puritans were replaced by westward migrations, youthful optimism, and material progress that left

Life expectancy: the average number of years a group of individuals with common characteristics can expect to live, from birth to death.

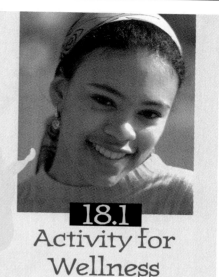

TABLE 18.1   *Selected Healthy People 2000 Objectives Having Implications for Senior Adults*

1. **Reduce to no more than 90 per 1,000 people the proportion of all people aged 65 and older who have difficulty in performing two or more personal care activities, thereby preserving independence.** (Baseline: 111 per 1,000 people 65 years and older in 1984–85.)

2. **Reduce deaths among people aged 65 through 84 from falls and fall-related injuries to no more than 14.1 per 100,000 people.** (Update: 18.0 per 100,000 people 65–84 years in 1991, down from 18.1 per 100,000 in 1987.)

3. **Reduce hip fractures among people aged 65 and older so that hospitalizations for this condition are no more than 607 per 100,000 people.** (Update: 757 per 100,000 people aged 65 and older in 1992, up from 714 per 100,000 in 1988.) (Special Target Population: White females 85 years and older.)

4. **Increase years of healthy life to at least 65 years.** (Update: 63.9 years in 1991, down from 64.0 years in 1990.) (Special Target Populations: Blacks, Hispanics, People 65 years and over [target 14 years of healthy life remaining at age 65].)

5. **Reduce significant hearing impairment among people aged 45 and older to a prevalence of no more than 180 per 1,000 people.** (Update: 215.7 per 1,000 people aged 45 and over in 1990–92, up from 203 per 1,000 in 1986–88.)

6. **Reduce significant visual impairment among people aged 65 and older to a prevalence of no more than 70 per 1,000 people.** (Update: 79.8 per 1,000 people aged 65 and over in 1990–92, down from 87.7 per 1,000 in 1986–88.)

7. **Reduce to no more than 22 percent the proportion of people aged 65 and older who engage in no leisure-time physical activity.** (Update: 29 percent of people aged 65 and older engaged in no leisure-time physical activity in 1991, down from 43 percent in 1985.)

Source: From *Healthy People 2000 National Health Promotion and Disease Prevention Objectives,* 1991; and from *Healthy People 2000 Review 1993,* 1994. Department of Health and Human Services, Washington, D.C.

---

elders out of touch. Respect for old age fell by the wayside. This phenomenon of ageism finds its way in recent years even to the chambers of the U.S. Congress according to gerontologist Slava Lubomudrov,[9] who analyzed 893 statements from the Congressional Record. These men and women who create and enact the policies affecting older people in the U.S. are prone to both positive and negative stereotypes, using such terms as "poor," "socially isolated," "mentally slower," "mostly wise," and "golden agers" to refer to persons sixty-five plus years of age. Television, too, may influence our impressions about the elderly. John Bell[10] analyzed the top ten prime time TV programs having older main characters, and found them portrayed as affluent, influential, and astute. While some

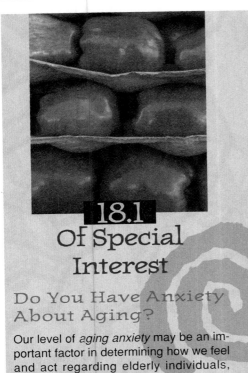

18.1
Of Special Interest

Do You Have Anxiety About Aging?

Our level of *aging anxiety* may be an important factor in determining how we feel and act regarding elderly individuals, as well as being a factor in the eventual adjustment to our own aging process. A recent study by Kathleen P. Lasher and Patricia J. Faulkender suggest that our attitudes and behaviors about aging have several important dimensions. A *physical dimension* includes our perceptions about our physical health status, perceptions about changes in our physical appearance, our ability to perform certain physical tasks, our expression of psychosomatic concerns, and our concerns about sexuality. A *psychological dimension* incorporates perceptions about personal control, dependence versus independence, self-esteem, life satisfaction, and overall psychological well-being. The variables of a *social dimension* are determined by the number and quality of our social contacts, our living arrangement, and feelings of social interaction versus social detachment. Finally, a *transpersonal dimension* challenges our ability in finding meaning with past and present life events, and our ability in coming to terms with death. These four dimensions of anxiety about aging may be expressed by us in specific ways—fear of aging, fear of being old, and fear of old people—among others.

What Do You Think?

1. Do you have a fear of aging or of being old? Do other people you know have such a fear? How do your attitudes differ from other people around you? What accounts for these differences?
2. Do you think that old people are feared by younger members of society? What can be done to bring about better understanding and mutual respect between generations?

Source: Data from Kathleen P. Lasher and Patricia J. Faulkender, "Measurement of Aging Anxiety: Development of the Anxiety about Aging Scale," in *International Journal of Aging and Human Development*, 37.4 (1993): 247–259.

---

of these traits are clearly flattering, one must nevertheless wonder the impact that these portrayals have on us overall.

Although aging can be viewed purely in chronological terms, **gerontologists,** those who study the elderly and the aging process, distinguish three aspects of aging. **Biological aging** refers to the physical changes that occur through time. Clearly, physical change varies among individuals. Genetics plays an important role in the process of biological aging and so do environmental factors. **Sociological aging** refers to changes in a person's familial, occupational, and social roles. Finally, **psychological aging** refers to how one adapts in mind, body, and spirit to the biological and sociological changes and to the passage of time.

Biological Processes of Aging

What are the markers of aging? What distinguishes the periods of life? Are they biological, psychological, or sociological phenomena? Are they a combination of all three? According to Bernice L. Neugarten and Dail A. Neugarten:[11]

The distinctions between life periods are blurring in today's society. The most dramatic evidence, perhaps, is the appearance of the so-called "young-old." It is a recent historical phenomenon that a very large group of retirees and their spouses are healthy and vigorous, relatively well-off financially, well-integrated into the lives of their families and communities, and politically active. The term "young-old" is becoming part of everyday parlance, and it refers not to a particular age but to health and social characteristics. A young-old person may be fifty-five or eighty-five. The term represents the social reality that the line between middle age and old age is no longer clear. What was once considered old age now characterizes only that minority of old persons who have been called the "old-old," that particularly vulnerable group who often are in need of special support and special care. . . . We have conflicting images . . . of age: the seventy-year-old in a wheelchair, but also the seventy-year-old on the tennis court.

There is a distinct difference between chronological age and biological age.[12] Biological age is defined as the ability to adapt

Gerontologist: one who studies any of the multiple aspects of the aged or the aging process.

TABLE 18.2	**Summary of Biological Functional Changes Occurring with Age**
Cardiac output	Declines 30 percent between age thirty and age seventy
Blood pressure	Increases by 20 percent in both systolic and diastolic pressures between age thirty and age seventy
Vital capacity	Decreases 40 to 50 percent between age thirty and age seventy
Residual volume	Increases 30 to 50 percent between age thirty and age seventy
Basal metabolic rate (BMR)	Declines 10 percent on the average between age thirty and age seventy
Muscle mass and strength	Declines by 20 to 25 percent between age thirty and age seventy
Flexibility in joints	Declines by 20 to 30 percent between age thirty and age seventy
Bone mineral	Declines 15 to 30 percent between age thirty and age seventy depending on gender
Sensory ability	Qualitative changes in visual and auditory acuity, taste, and smell
Renal functioning	Decrease in filtration rate by up to 50 percent
Sexual functioning	Qualitative change in lubricating ability of vagina in the female; decreased testosterone production and delayed erection time in the male

to the environment, both the normal situations and the stressors or crises. It is, therefore, virtually independent of chronology. A process called **primary aging** is an unavoidable result of chronology that affects all species sooner or later. Another process, **secondary aging,** occurs as a result of trauma, stress, illness, or neglect. People confuse these two processes and thus reinforce the myth that all old people are sickly. Secondary aging certainly can accelerate primary aging, though it does not cause it.

There comes a time when the elderly experience a marked change in their ability to adapt. What is noted as a sudden loss of ability, however, is really a gradual loss experienced over a period of forty or more years.

Specifically, what biological changes occur over time? Several functional changes are summarized in table 18.2.

Cardiovascular Function

Advancing age brings about significant functional changes in the cardiovascular system. Cardiac output, the ability of the heart to deliver blood to body tissues in a given amount of time, declines by approximately 30 percent between ages thirty and seventy.[13] Cardiac output is a function of two other quantities—

stroke volume (the amount of blood pumped each time the heart beats) and heart rate (the number of heart beats per unit of time). The heart's ability to beat faster, such as during exercise, declines at an annual rate of about .75 percent after age thirty. The contractile force of the heart muscle declines by about the same rate. These changes account for the net loss of function observed over this forty-year span.

In addition, a 20 percent rise in blood pressure is observed in many people. For people whose hereditary pattern predisposes them to hypertension, the increases may be even greater.

Pulmonary Function

Pulmonary function refers to the lungs' ability to move air, exchanging carbon dioxide for oxygen. Two factors affect changes in the lungs during aging—**vital capacity** and **residual volume.** Vital capacity refers to the volume of air that moves when you inhale and exhale at maximum ability. Even when inhaling at the maximum, you do not fill all the available lung space; there is still space not taking part in gas exchange. This quantity is known as the residual volume. In young people, residual volume is small compared to vital capacity. Together, vital

Primary aging: the inevitable changes, especially physical changes, that are associated with the passage of time.

Secondary aging: physical changes beyond those associated with primary aging, that are due to trauma, stress, illness, or neglect.

What Do You Think?

1. The older individual's loss of flexibility often stems as much from lack of exercise as from actual age degeneration. Thinking of people you know over the age of sixty, do you see any correlation between their flexibility and their habits of physical activity?
2. Are you currently increasing the likelihood of well-being in your older age through regular physical activity?

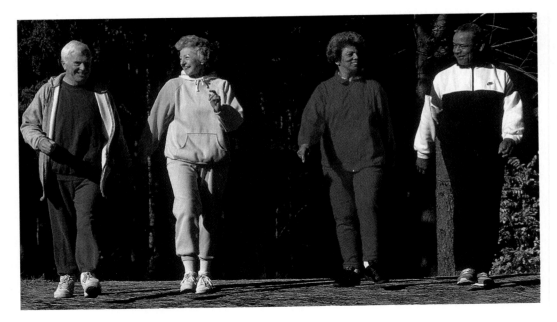

capacity and residual volume comprise the **total lung capacity.** The aging process involves an inversion of these two quantities. Between ages thirty and seventy, vital capacity declines 40 to 50 percent, while residual volume increases 30 to 50 percent.

The elderly person, then, is less able to supply the body with oxygen. This decreased function may go unnoticed when a person is at rest or engaged only in mild activity; however, during vigorous exercise, adequate oxygen supply can only be maintained by breathing more rapidly and by increasing the work load of the heart. The response of the heart during a period of increased work load may not be adequate to maintain the level of activity desired.

Basal Metabolic Rate

The **basal metabolic rate (BMR)** is the rate at which bodily processes are carried out at the cellular level while the body is at rest. The BMR regulates such things as respiration, heart rate, rate of digestion, and body temperature. On the average, BMR declines by a factor of 10 percent between ages thirty and seventy. We have all seen elderly people wearing a sweater or jacket, even on relatively warm days, to maintain comfort. Any discomfort may be a consequence of a lowered BMR. To understand how this 10 percent drop is experienced by the older adult, consider the following situation. Most of us are comfortable in a room where the temperature is controlled at seventy degrees. However, if that temperature is decreased by

10 percent to make it sixty-three degrees, the comfort level changes dramatically.[14] Fingertips, toes, and noses become cold and may even ache slightly. Our ability to concentrate, write, type, or perform other simple activities may be reduced.

Body Composition

Several changes in body composition occur with age. There is a tendency for the overall percentage of body fat to increase over time. The reasons for this change are not completely understood. However, it appears that modification of the body's ability to use dietary protein is a partial explanation of this phenomenon.

Muscle mass decreases with age. The quadriceps, the large muscles of the upper leg, seem to lose mass more rapidly than other muscles in the aging person.[15]

Accompanying the change in muscle mass is a decline in **muscular strength.** Grip strength peaks in males during their mid-twenties and declines thereafter at a gradual pace until age sixty, when the decline becomes steep.[16]

By age seventy, an individual's **flexibility** has declined by 20 to 30 percent due to changes in muscles, ligaments, joints, and tendons. The result is a decreased range of motion for the older individual. It is probable, however, that the lost range of motion or flexibility is a phenomenon stemming as much from disuse of muscles and joints as from actual age degeneration.[17]

Muscular strength: the maximum amount of force that can be exerted by a muscle in a single effort.

Flexibility: the ability of specific joints to move through their entire range of motion.

Changes in Bone

Bone is composed of both organic and inorganic substances. The principal organic component in bone is **collagen,** a protein substance. The inorganic structure of bone is composed of two minerals, *calcium* and *phosphorous.* Approximately 99 percent of the body's calcium and 88 percent of the body's phosphorous are located in the skeleton.[18] It is the change with age in the mineral content of bone that can influence development of a serious health problem.

A significant decline in bone mineral by age seventy is not uncommon. This decline results in a skeletal structure that is weakened and subject to fracture. Particularly affected are the long bones of the leg and the hips with which they articulate, the bones of the forearm and wrist, and the bones that comprise the lumbar and thoracic spine.[19] This condition of decreased bone mass is known as **osteoporosis.**

Osteoporosis produces an enlarged marrow cavity surrounded by porous bone, resulting in loss of bone density and strength. Imagine that you are looking through the end of one of the long bones, as if it were a telescope. In a young person, the marrow cavity appears relatively small and the bone mineral that surrounds it is densely packed. In osteoporotic bone, the marrow cavity is larger and the surrounding bone mineral is less dense (see figure 18.1).

Osteoporosis affects more than twenty million men and women. Bone loss is usually more severe for women and the osteoporotic process occurs earlier in life for women than men. Bone loss in women proceeds at a rate of approximately .75 to 1 percent per year beginning between ages thirty and thirty-five.[20] At the time of menopause, or about age fifty, the loss is accelerated to 2 or 3 percent per year. By age seventy, the loss in bone mass for some women may be as great as 30 percent. This loss threatens the strength of several bones. Osteoporosis contributes to more than 90 percent of the broken hips per year in women over the age of seventy. One occasionally hears of an unfortunate elderly person who falls and breaks a hip. More often than not, the fall was caused by a spontaneous fracture of an advanced-stage osteoporotic bone, rather than the other way around.

Fracture of the wrist and vertebral collapses (dowager's hump) in the spine are additional risks brought about by osteoporosis.

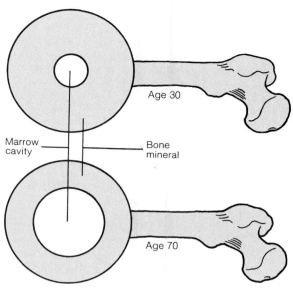

Age 30

Marrow cavity

Bone mineral

Age 70

Figure 18.1:
Osteoporosis causes the densely packed bone mineral surrounding the marrow cavity to become porous, producing an enlarged marrow cavity which results in loss of bone density and strength.

The degree of bone loss can be determined by a technique known as a *dual photon absorptiometry scan.* It is a pain-free and low-cost procedure for persons who may be at risk of osteoporosis. Since women are more at risk for osteoporosis than men, a baseline test in one's mid-thirties and again after menopause can reveal possible fracture spots.

Men experience less of a problem with osteoporosis. Bone loss proceeds at an annual rate about equal to .4 percent but does not begin until around age fifty.[21] Still, a decline in bone mass of 15 percent is possible. The rate appears to remain relatively constant, usually not giving rise to significant problems until men are in their eighties. A mechanism for retarding osteoporosis, or eliminating it as a serious threat to wellness altogether, is suggested later in this chapter.

Sensory Changes

Age also may bring about changes in the nervous system. Reaction time and nerve conduction velocity may decline 10 to 15 percent over the period of time between ages thirty to seventy.[22] Aging brings about significant change in sensory mechanisms, such as hearing, visual acuity, taste, and smell.[23] These alterations sometimes require special early diagnostic, adaptive, or corrective lifestyle steps.

Virtually everyone experiences some degree of hearing impairment by age seventy. Eight percent of the elderly wear a hearing aid, since soft and high-pitched sounds begin to fade from one's hearing repertoire.[24] Increases in the time required to process

Collagen: a type of connective tissue.

Osteoporosis: a disease condition of the bone resulting in a porous appearance and predisposing it to injury and fracture.

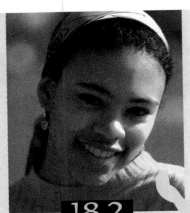

18.2 Activity for Wellness

Are You Placing Yourself at Risk for Developing Osteoporosis?

Twenty million or more people in the U.S. experience the unfortunate effects of osteoporosis. Osteoporosis occurs when minerals, especially calcium, are depleted from the bones, leaving them porous, and vulnerable to collapse and fracture. Certain activities and behaviors place one at risk of developing this debilitating condition. While there are some factors one cannot manipulate, many things that predispose one to developing osteoporosis can be controlled.

If you have several of the following risk factors, you may possess a special susceptibility to this disorder. The greater the number of risk factors possessed, the greater the risk involved.

Uncontrollable Risk Factors

Yes No

____ ____ You are female

____ ____ You have a family history of osteoporosis

____ ____ You have a small skeletal frame

____ ____ You are fair-skinned

____ ____ You are Caucasian or Asiatic in ancestry

____ ____ You are thirty-five years of age or older

____ ____ You have an allergy to milk or milk products

____ ____ You are a woman with early onset of menopause

Partly Controllable Risk Factors

Yes No

____ ____ You are a woman who has never had a baby

____ ____ You are a woman who has had her ovaries removed

____ ____ You are a woman who has breast-fed a baby

____ ____ Your life is stressful

Controllable Risk Factors

Yes No

____ ____ You drink more than a moderate amount of alcohol

____ ____ You have a history of low dietary calcium intake

____ ____ You get little exercise

____ ____ You consume a lot of caffeine-containing drinks

____ ____ Your diet is high in protein

____ ____ Your diet is high in phosphates

____ ____ Your diet is high in sodium

____ ____ You are a smoker

Reprinted with permission from Robert Lindsay, "Managing Osteoporosis: Current Trends, Future Possibilities" in *Geriatrics*, 44 (3): 35–40, 1987. Copyright by Avanstar Communications, Inc. Printed in U.S.A.

---

sounds neurologically necessitates that elderly persons be addressed more slowly, rather than more loudly. Background noise may be particularly distracting to older persons, because it interferes with receiving and processing conversation. Anyone who has been in a room full of people talking and who has tried to focus on hearing a particular conversation can appreciate the dilemma experienced by the elderly person. Hearing loss in the elderly is underreported by hearing impaired persons, their families, and health professionals, possibly because loss is gradual and usually painless. As many as 50 percent of persons over age seventy-five have significant hearing impairment.[25]

Loss of visual acuity is one of several sight-related changes that occur. Problems with

acuity arise from the tendency of the eye lenses to yellow and become harder and less elastic with age, giving rise to a condition called **presbyopia.** The magnitude of this change is heightened further by the presence of glare.

Depth perception is also affected by the aging process. Consequently, elderly people must take extra care in climbing or descending stairs. Even crossing the street necessitates extra caution; the elderly individual must gauge the exact height of the curb to avoid an accidental fall.

Modifications that occur with age alter the ability to see clearly at night. **Night recovery vision** is also affected adversely.[26] Anyone, young or old, knows what it is like to be driving an automobile on a highway at night and suddenly be struck by another

Presbyopia: a visual defect with onset between ages forty and forty-five resulting in loss of ability to focus clearly on near objects. Eye glasses can easily correct for this defect.

vehicle's oncoming headlights. There is a temporary blindness, lasting one to five seconds in most cases. This readjustment period is one's night-glare recovery interval. Older individuals may require eight to ten seconds for complete recovery. This delay makes operating a motor vehicle at night dangerous and frightening. In addition, decreased depth perception further increases the hazard of night driving.

Cataracts can also interfere with visual ability in the older adult. A cataract is a clouding of the lens that interrupts the focusing of light on the retina, resulting in blurred vision. Cataracts tend to develop slowly but become thickened or layered in the process. Unless corrective surgery is performed, vision in the affected eye can become completely occluded.

Another eye disorder that affects many persons in their sixties and seventies (though it can have an earlier life onset) is **glaucoma.** Glaucoma involves an elevation of pressure within the eyeball that produces partial or complete impairment.

Chronic glaucoma is especially dangerous because it has no particular warning signals until the pressure affects the optic nerve directly. It is a painless and progressive cause of unnecessary blindness. Therefore, it is recommended that persons over the age of forty be tested for glaucoma at least every two years. Persons with a family history of glaucoma or a personal history of other eye disorders should be screened more frequently.

The last major areas of sensory change affected by age are those of taste and smell. Modifications in one's sense of taste can have profound effects on food choices and may contribute to obesity.

Taste thresholds for sweeteners and table salt are on the average two to two-and-a-half times higher in the elderly than in young people.[27] Compensation for a reduced capacity to taste sweet things can result in excess sugar. An enhanced sugar intake might aggravate an existing chronic condition such as **diabetes.** Moreover, it can increase caloric intake at a time when one's BMR, and the capacity for and interest in physical activity and exercise, are winding down. In addition, more sugar can increase one's blood triglyceride level, also leading to obesity.

The desire to use more salt to combat food's flat taste (resulting from the sensory losses both of taste and smell) is likely to complicate one's ability to comply with low-sodium diets, which are desirable throughout life but particularly in old age. Dietary salt can, of course, aggravate hypertension and other conditions.

The smell of food is an important component of appetite. The sense of smell is even more vulnerable to the process of aging than is taste. Olfactory thresholds for some food odors, such as cherry, grape and lemon, are eleven times higher for older people.[28] A decreased sensitivity to food odors can result in a lowered appreciation of certain foods. Older people may complain about the bland appeal of food and become less enthusiastic about eating at all. People preparing meals for the elderly need to recognize the possible changes in eating due to modified taste and smell thresholds. Aging also may bring about a decline in one's ability to judge pressure applied by food to the tongue.[29] Thus, food may supply less tactile stimulation in the mouth, which, in turn, may affect interest in eating. Moreover, the absence of feeling on the tongue could have consequences with respect to choking.

Changes in the Kidneys

Several important properties of kidney function may change with age. First, there is a decrease in the overall filtration rate by up to 50 percent.[30] This means that the kidneys filter less blood per unit of time and remove toxic wastes more slowly. Second, there is a decline in blood flow to the kidneys. This decline results in part from the fall in cardiac output and directly affects filtration rate. A third change is reduced reabsorption ability; therefore, some nutrients pass as waste products instead of being used by the body.

Changes in Sexual Functioning

Many people believe that both sexual desire and sexual functioning decline significantly after middle age. Although **menopause** in females and the **climacteric** in males may affect operation of the sexual organs to some extent, these phenomena do not necessarily influence all the psychological desires for physical closeness and participation in sexual intercourse.

The psychological impact of menopause in women, while real and complex, can be exaggerated. Despite stories about menopausal women becoming tearful,

Cataracts: a common occurrence with aging in which the lens of the eye becomes increasingly opaque, resulting in obscured vision.

Glaucoma: a disease of the eye characterized by increased pressure within the eye that is a leading cause of blindness in the United States.

Diabetes: a chronic disease of the pancreas in which the body is unable to utilize sugars and other carbohydrates normally.

Menopause: the age-associated cessation of menstrual activity in women often accompanied by other physiologic changes.

Climacteric: the age-associated decline in sexual functioning, often referred to as the male analogue of menopause.

emotional, unpredictable, and uninterested in sex, the majority of research evidence does not support such stereotypes. Most women feel unchanged after menopause.[31] Many women see the cessation of the menstrual cycle as a welcome relief and report a renewed interest in sexual activity. Some research suggests that a woman's interest in sex following menopause is probably most closely related to her interest in sex earlier in life.[32] Hormonal declines can produce a thinning and drying of the lining of the vagina, sometimes resulting in painful intercourse; however, with the use of an appropriate supplemental lubricant and some patience, there is little reason for age to hinder sexual participation.

There is debate about whether the male climacteric is a biological event or purely a psychological one. It is known that many males undergo a transition period in their lives that may occur anytime between the fourth and seventh decades. This transition, which may affect relationships with a spouse, an employer, or other individuals, is sometimes referred to as the **mid-life crisis.** While a mid-life crisis is often spoken of as a "male event," it is by no means limited just to men. Some researchers believe that although important changes do occur in mid-life, crisis is an avoidable outcome.[33] They conclude that susceptibility to a mid-life crisis hinges on three elements: identity, efficacy, and self-evaluation. Identity is determined by how people view themselves in a variety of contexts—on the job, as a member of a family, as a parent, and so on. Efficacy refers to a person's desire to be effective and competent in these same contexts. Self-evaluation is triggered by such events as birthdays and holidays and causes an individual to reflect on whatever personal successes or failures come immediately to mind. Crisis occurs when a person cannot overcome the loss of efficacy. This can occur when a person is passed over for a promotion, or runs into an old friend who appears as youthful and vigorous as ever, or experiences a loss of sexual potency.

Testosterone production does decrease with age.[34] In conjunction with this event, men may experience a delayed erection time, a reduced ejaculatory volume, and decreased fertility. These changes occur gradually and may go unnoticed. While delayed erection or occasional impotence may be problematic for some men, age also tends to decrease ejaculatory urgency. Thus, while the penis may require a longer time to become erect, intercourse is frequently enjoyed for a longer period.

It is in the areas of sexuality and personal intimacy that ageism again rears its ugly head. Ageists view sexuality among the elderly as an expression of senility or deviance or both. Research by Lionel Corbett showed that the "myth of a sexless old age" prevented married couples residing in some nursing homes from sharing a bedroom or sleeping in anything other than twin beds due to institutional policy.[35] Ageism results in elderly people becoming the butt of tasteless sexual humor. The elderly are portrayed as exhibitionists and "dirty old men" (or women). Evidence shows that in fact society's "dirty old man" is usually in his late twenties. The greatest barrier to successful sexual functioning in old age is probably the extent to which ageism is permitted to be an influence. With the presence of an interesting and interested partner, sexual participation during the seventies, eighties, or nineties can be an important index of good physical and emotional health (see figure 18.2).

Biology, Aging, and the College Student

Can you notice some physical changes that indicate you are aging? Wayne and Derek, two sophomores nineteen and twenty-years-old respectively, see changes in the appearance of their hair. Whereas Derek notices more and more grey among his otherwise brown hair, Wayne sees that while his hair is as fully dark as it has always been, it is receding on both sides of his forehead and thinning in the back.

Three close friends, Kay, Eileen, and Marianne all graduated from the same high school three years ago. Kay notices that her facial skin is much drier and more wrinkled than that of her two friends. Since age thirteen, Kay has always prided herself on her summer tan, and spends much time in the sun and in tanning salons to "perfect" this tan, rarely using a sunscreen. Eileen, who is quite fair-skinned, learned a long time ago how the sun burns her and has taken steps to avoid any unnecessary exposure to it. She looks like she could still pass as a high school student if she dressed the part. Marianne resembles Kay more than she does Eileen, and although she spends time in the sun, she tans slowly and always uses a protective sunscreen. Marianne also looks much like she did as a high school student.

Testosterone: the primary male sex hormone. Testosterone stimulates the development of a male physique and reproductive organs. It also maintains the viability of the adult reproductive organs.

While Kay is not worried about getting old, she is concerned that at age twenty-one she looks more like her mother than her same-age peers. Having read about primary and secondary aging, can you relate these concepts as they may apply to the students just described?

Theories of Biological Aging

Explanations of the processes of biological aging are very much in their infancy. Many a science-fiction story has focused on humankind's search for the potion that would bring immortality. No one is immortal and growing old is as much a fact of life as being born. What are the mechanisms for biological aging? Why does the body change with age (see figure 18.3)?

There are numerous theories of aging, though no single theory is universally accepted. No one theory about aging seems to explain satisfactorily all of the observations made about growing old. Aging is a complex process influenced by heredity, nutrition, disease, and various other factors; however, some interesting and provocative explanations of the aging process keep scientists engaged in debate.

Programmed Endpoint Theory

According to this theory each species is born with a finite amount of genetic material (DNA). When cells "use up" the genetic material, they age and die. Observations reported by Leonard Hayflick showed that certain cells taken from human embryos and maintained in culture underwent a finite number of doublings approximately equal to fifty, after which no more cell reproduction took place.[37] This type of limited survival has been demonstrated for the cells of other species, too. Hayflick concludes that the maximum life expectancy for human beings could be as high as 120 years. Hayflick's programmed endpoint theory has held up to years of intensive scrutiny.[38] Questions concerning how and why some cells cease to duplicate themselves after a point in time, and just what the genetic basis for aging is, remain unanswered.[39]

Not all organs age at the same rate. Thus, a person whose liver is functioning just fine in the eighth decade of life, may have a kidney that is failing. Furthermore, organs age at different rates in different people. One

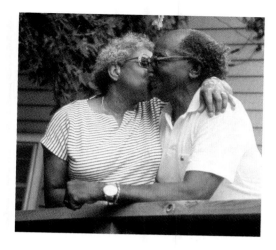

Figure 18.2: What Do You Think?

1. Research tells us that sexual desire and the need for physical closeness do not vanish with age. How could society better support older people and their continued need to express their sexuality?

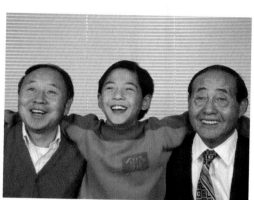

Figure 18.3: What Do You Think?

1. The physical characteristics of aging are often evident when one examines a photograph of three generations of a family. What physical characteristics of aging do you see in this family photograph? What physical characteristics of aging do you notice when you observe several generations of your own family or that of a close friend?

person's hearing mechanism may be healthy and functioning well into the eighth decade of life, while another person's hearing may begin to fail in the fourth decade. While lifestyle plays a vital role in overall functioning, the impact of genetics on subsequent growth and development cannot be denied.

Richard A. Lockshin and Zahra F. Zakeri[40] believe that the programmed death of cells is a response to stress, the breaking of a cell's DNA into tiny fragments, and other developmental changes.

Somatic-Mutation Theory

Howard Curtis and Kimball Miller[41] demonstrated that cells of older mice and guinea pigs contained more chromosomal abnormalities than those of younger animals. They concluded that aging was a result of mutated cells created by chromosomal instructions that got "mixed up." Furthermore, they showed that animals exposed to radiation and certain chemical substances contained more abnormal chromosomes than unexposed animals.

Free-Radical Theory

Free radicals are naturally occurring unstable chemical substances; they react easily with other substances with which they come into contact in order to become stable. Found in some body cells, free radicals react with fats and cause cellular damage. Free radicals are believed to cause cell mutations, and have been linked to cardiovascular disease and cancer.[42]

Wear-and-Tear Theory

The wear-and-tear theory suggests that cells can only deflect a finite number of environmental insults before becoming unable to repair and replace damaged parts. Nerve cells, cardiac cells, and skeletal muscle cells do not divide at all, hence they have no ability to respond indefinitely to accumulated wear and tear.

Autoimmune Theory

The **immune system** contains specialized cells that fight infection and agents identified by the body as foreign. The autoimmune theory suggests that the ability of the body to distinguish its own cellular material from foreign proteins, such as viruses or bacteria, is reduced over time. Consequently, it is possible for the immune system to become confused, to recognize its own proteins as "foreign," and therefore, to attack itself. If this theory is accurate in describing what happens with age, it is not backed by the supportive evidence necessary to explain how. It is, nevertheless, an intriguing theory, and one likely to be the subject of future research.

Sociological Patterns of Aging

Adapting to growing old, and changing social, familial, or vocational roles, are common characteristics of aging. There is no single way to age successfully. In fact, research has delineated at least four predominant patterns of successful aging high in life satisfaction. These patterns are labeled disengagement theory, activity theory, continuity theory, and social-reconstruction theory.

Disengagement Theory

Disengagement theory emphasizes the mutual withdrawal by both society and the individual.[43] Society embraces the disengagement process through such actions as age segregation and mandatory retirement. Disengagement may take on other forms as well, such as moving from a private residence to an institutional setting or parting company with close friends or relatives because of death. Disengagement theory contends that people voluntarily move away from the mainstream to avoid commitments, to let someone else do the work, and to allow more self-investment in their remaining years.

Although disengagement may be satisfying for some people, it is not satisfying for everyone. Forced disengagement may be a source of low life satisfaction, even depression. Critics also contend that disengagement seems to relate more to poor health status, widowhood, decreased income, and retirement than simply to growing older.

Activity Theory

In contrast to disengagement theory, activity theory suggests that older people age successfully by remaining active. Some research supports the notion that a high activity level impacts positively on self-concept, morale, and overall well-being.[44] Activity theory contends that a person's major life satisfaction roles in middle age as worker, parent, spouse, and so on undergo change because of retirement, widowhood, and decreased influence over children. To age successfully and to avoid low life satisfaction, people busy themselves with new types of activities (see figure 18.4).

A clear relationship between level of activity and level of life satisfaction has not been confirmed. Activity theory may be too simplistic an explanation for the complex aging phenomenon. Not all activities adequately replace the lost roles of middle adulthood and help to maintain self-concept. Unless hobbies, pastimes, and other activities of the older adult represent dominant cultural roles, they probably do not lead to role adjustment and high life satisfaction.[45]

Although activity theory has received popular support, research does not consistently support it as a means of extending life. An eight-year study by David J. Lee and Kyriakos S. Markides found no compelling evidence that maintenance of activity in older adulthood correlated with extended longevity.[46]

Continuity Theory

Robert Atchley proposes an alternative theory, the continuity theory, in light of the

Free radicals: unstable, naturally occurring substances which are believed to interfere with healthy cellular functioning, and contribute to aging and disease processes.

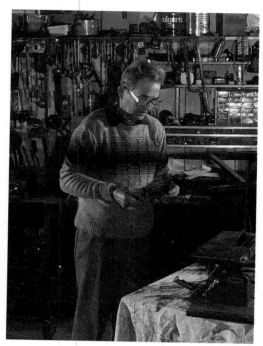

Figure 18.4: What Do You Think?

1. New activities help the elderly stay involved and age successfully. What opportunities exist in your community for older people to become involved in stimulating activities?

limitations of both the disengagement and activity theories.[47] The continuity theory suggests that successful aging is a result of maintaining certain roles of middle adulthood into old age, while withdrawing from other roles. Proponents contend that the commitments and role preferences that contribute most to satisfaction in middle adulthood also provide the basis for satisfaction in later years.

Social-Reconstruction Theory

Social-reconstruction theory holds that low performance expectations on the part of society contribute to the low self-concept and perceived loss of skills experienced by many elderly people.[48] A self-fulfilling prophecy is established when the older adult feels incompetent because of a belief that self-worth is dependent upon a high level of productivity. This theory proposes that successful aging is a function of three things. First, successful adaptation means liberating one's self from the myth of an age-appropriate status. That is, people do not necessarily have to disengage from certain activities because they are seventy, seventy-five, or eighty years old. Second, adaptation depends on one's

ability to access social services. Adequate housing, transportation, and medical services are vital components of successful aging. Third, successful aging requires the ability to control one's own life.

Elderly people can partake in a number of creative activities. Some of these include keeping a personal journal, creating a life history, learning art, performing music, engaging in imagery, or participating in other recreational and leisure tasks. Most of these activities successfully reaffirm competence and stimulate both the physical self and the mind.[49]

Other Sociological Considerations

A criticism of sociological theories of aging is that they focus on trying to define subjective terms such as "life satisfaction," "morale," and "successful aging." In addition, current theories do not account for all of the variation in the social patterns of aging and satisfaction with retirement.[50] Lorraine T. Dorfman, Frank J. Kohort, and D. Alex Heckert found the predictors of retirement satisfaction in order of importance to be: (1) quality of relationships with, and frequency of help from, friends and relatives; (2) involvement in organizations; (3) health status; and (4) financial status.[51] Carol Cutler Riddick's research involving older women found that being employed was associated with greater life satisfaction than simply being a retired homemaker; however, one's level of leisure activity involvement was an important mediator of life satisfaction as well.[52] Karen Seccombe and Gary R. Lee report that women demonstrate less satisfaction with retirement than men, perhaps due to their having lower incomes and their reduced probability of being married.[53]

Thus, an attempt to explain successful aging as a matter of engagement or disengagement, role maintenance, or other factors is difficult at best. Identification of more of the variables affecting the social aspects of aging is anticipated as an increasingly larger proportion of the population reaches older adulthood.

Hirsch S. Ruchlin and John N. Morris found that persons in their sample of adults aged sixty-five to seventy-four who were working expressed higher life satisfaction than their nonworking peers.[54] There does not seem to be a reluctance to work among senior adults, as some "myth holders" about the elderly believe. According to the U.S. Department of Health and Human Services' account of a Louis Harris poll, about 1.9 million Americans fifty to sixty-four years old are ready and able to go back to work, and 67 percent of them would be willing to provide in-home services for older people.[55] In addition, 53 percent would perform clerical tasks, 83 percent would do seasonal work, 60 percent would do work that required standing, 60 percent would be willing to commute more than thirty minutes to get to work, and 54 percent would sacrifice evenings and weekends in order to work. Other researchers have noted that nearly half of nonworking adults aged fifty-five to sixty-four reported that they would prefer to continue working.[56] There is an emerging market for the expertise that comes with being elderly. More than 46 percent of firms hire retirees.[57]

Interpersonal relationships of older adults are likely to be complex, and related to lifelong patterns of relating to other people. Where the elderly are concerned, adult children are more likely to be viewed as confidants than are spouses or friends. On the other hand, spouses and friends may play important companionship roles.[58]

Aging and Diversity

As has been noted throughout this chapter, achieving the status of "senior citizen" sometimes carries with it certain ageist attitudes where the rest of society is concerned. This prejudice may be even further destructive if being old is accompanied by being poor, or being a member of a minority group that is compromised socially, politically, economically, or psychologically.

Elzbieta Gozdziak illustrates this problem using the example of the recently immigrated older adult who came from such distant places as Vietnam, Cambodia, other nations of Southeast Asia, Cuba and other Caribbean countries, as well as from other parts of the world.[59] The nature of the immigration (often as a refugee) may have dissolved the individual's family structure. Even if the family system is left intact, younger generations may become socialized in the U.S. tradition, and thus, "foreign" in a sense to their own family members. Accompanying this situation is the physical and psychological trauma of displacement. Add to this dilemma a language barrier, the absence of formal

education, and the removal of relevant job skills, and one is left with an almost hopeless economic status. The circumstances become even worse if one requires interaction with the U.S. health-care system, since it quite likely will be viewed as strange, fear-arousing, and incomprehensible (as indeed it is even to many people who are raised in this culture). The paradox of being old and being outside the mainstream of social and cultural values can have a major impact on quality of life.

Safety and the Elderly

Persons sixty-five years of age and older in the U.S. comprise a little more than 12 percent of the population but consume over 25 percent of health-care resources related to injuries from falls and other forms of trauma.[60] Falls comprise the leading cause of injury in adults aged sixty-five and older, and the largest single cause of injury-related death.[61] Falls and the resulting injuries can impact negatively on independence and self-confidence, and produce decreased mobility, reduced quality of life, and drain health services that otherwise could go for preventive and other types of care. The study of falls shows that there are modifiable risk factors involved, most of which deal with the home environment. Maxine M. Urton has identified several of these factors which contribute to fall-related injury in older people (see table 18.3). Repeated falls and even the fear of falls can seriously reduce the self-esteem of senior adults.[62]

Marlene A. Young and John H. Stein tell us that there is a curious paradox about crime and the elderly.[63] It seems there may be an inadvertent ageist philosophy applied by law enforcement officials where senior adults are concerned. Justice Department statistics show that persons sixty-five and older are victimized far less often than younger people, which may explain why they often receive less attention and services than other victims. If that explains the relative lack of services for older crime victims, then the statistics have been misused, for crime has very serious consequences for older adults.[64]

Consider these circumstances and the potential impact they might have on the overall well-being of an older individual. First, the fear of crime may be pervasive to the point of being emotionally paralyzing, handicapping, and dangerous. A person may

Table 18.3

Modifiable Factors in the Home Associated with Risk of Falls among the Elderly

Bathroom:	wet, slippery floor and bathtub, absence of grab bars, low toilet seats
Bedroom:	high bed, low-level lighting, sliding throw-rugs, non-locking bed casters, slippery or dusty floor
Stairs:	absence of handrails, inadequate lighting, high steps, worn or absent safety treads on stairs
Dining Room:	slippery floors, inappropriate chair height, absence of armrests, poor lighting
Kitchen:	cabinets out of reach (necessitating chairs to climb on), slippery floors, loose throw rugs, inadequate lighting, distracting glare from floor

Source: Data from Maxine M. Urton, "A Community Home Inspection Approach to Preventing Falls among the Elderly," *Public Health Reports*, 106(2): 192–195, 1991.

be motivated to buy a handgun for "protection" without considering the negative safety implications such a purchase may have. A person who feels at risk may leave a familiar neighborhood, and move to one that is "safer," but does not provide much social support, thus promoting social isolation.

Second, while the elderly are not necessarily victimized directly themselves, they may face the trauma of vicarious crime experience. For instance, they may have to undergo the pain of losing a child or grandchild to homicide, or the grief associated with robbery, injury, rape, or other serious crimes.

Finally, the elderly may bear the burden of injury from crime in a way that is magnified relative to other age groups. For instance, when a crime occurs, an individual can be harmed financially, physically, or emotionally. The financial loss of $50 through robbery may be an unpleasant event for any of us. For an older person on a fixed income, however, this loss can result in a

reduced ability to pay for needed medication, or even food. The theft of a television may all but eliminate some older people's contact with the outside world, and further isolate them from the mainstream of society.

Adaptations for Wellness in Old Age

Although everyone experiences some degree of change as a result of aging, these changes do not necessarily have to impact negatively on mental and physical wellness. Appropriate adaptations reduce the negative effects of aging. We will discuss several of these wellness adaptations.

Adapting to Sensory Change

If corrective sensory devices such as hearing aids and bifocals are affordable to the older adult and can be worn without necessary self-consciousness, many hearing or visual deficiencies can be eliminated. Other supplemental aids are also available. For instance, the hearing-impaired older adult can learn to read lips and visually impaired individuals can develop an ability to respond to auditory and other environmental cues.

A decline in sensory functioning can inhibit other activities such as exercise. Because of visual impairment, a person may not possess the confidence to begin walking or initiate other forms of exercise. In addition, an inability to detect street and traffic noise can undermine one's security about embarking on walks alone. Visual impairment can even interfere with mobility in the home. Climbing stairs, detecting irregularities in carpeting or floor rugs, or locating houseware items can become frustrating chores.

Sensory obstacles can be overcome through common sense and some advance planning.[65] Excess or unnecessary furniture can be removed. Furniture can be arranged to allow optimal mobility. Dishes, silverware, and other household items can be strategically placed for easy access. Practical placement of lamps can help to assure proper room lighting. In general, houses, apartments, or other dwellings serving older adults should be examined for the access and safety of stairs, ramps, thresholds, carpeting, scatter rugs, and other obstacles. Careful placement of safety features and removal of hazardous items can provide critical protective measures for the elderly.[66]

To increase confidence outdoors, the elderly can identify routes of easy and safe access to desired destinations. The ability to see clearly and avoid undue threats in the daylight can be enhanced by simply wearing sunglasses or other corrective lenses that minimize glare.

People whose senses of smell and taste have decreased may show diminished appetites. At meals, large portions of food may intimidate more than stimulate appetite. Substituting small, lightly seasoned portions of food may help elderly people enjoy mealtime. The most important ingredient may be friendly companionship.

Adapting to Biological Change

As indicated previously, some degree of functional change is inevitable as we age. As much as 50 percent of the functional decline seen in the aging population results from lack of use rather than aging.[67] Much of that lost vitality can be maintained into the eighth decade of life through vigorous activity.

Research supports the contention that loss of cardiovascular function need not be an automatic consequence of growing older. In a ten-year study, participants in an experimental exercise program did not show the 1 percent annual decline that was seen in a sedentary control group. The benefits of exercise in promoting oxygen utilization and overall cardiovascular fitness in the elderly have also been shown.[68] Physical activity can moderate both **systolic** and **diastolic blood pressure** in older adults.[69] The most significant outcome of improved cardiovascular fitness may be the performance of routine daily activity with greater ease.

Physical activity may also restore or maintain functions of muscles and joints.[70] Loss of flexibility and range of motion of muscles and joints may be consequences of discontinued use and not functions of aging.

Osteoporosis, the process of bone demineralization, may also be affected by the level of physical activity. A study of male tennis players (mean age 63.8) showed that bone-mineral content of the playing arm was 13 percent more than that of the nonplaying arm.[71] Exercise was also shown to increase total body calcium in postmenopausal women, a group at high risk for osteoporosis.[72] In a nursing-home study, mild exercise significantly increased bone mineral among participants, while sedentary residents

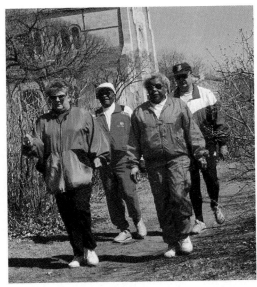

Figure 18.5: What Do You Think?

1. Even modest physical activity can help older adults get fit and stay fit in the seventh and eighth decades of life. What specific physical activities have you observed older adults engaged in? Did they seem to be enjoying themselves?

lost bone mineral at the expected rate.[73] Thus, it appears that physical activity retards the loss of bone mass, helping to maintain both physical and social activity.

In addition to these exercise-derived benefits, Richard Lampman suggests that exercise in older adults can play a role in enhancing glucose tolerance, decreasing fatty substances and increasing **HDL** levels in the blood, increasing lean body mass, and, perhaps, improving the overall quality of life.[74] Other research supports the belief that aerobic exercise can improve self-concept in older people and lead to development of greater self-responsibility for personal health status.[75]

Much of the reluctance of older people to exercise is based on the myth that even moderate activity is destructive. Unless a person has advanced physical disabilities that are multiple in nature, some form of beneficial exercise is available to them. It is not recommended that a person with chronic low back pain take to jogging on hard surfaces; however, the same person can achieve physical improvement by taking up a regular program of walking or stationary cycling (see figure 18.5). Classes for older people offer a wide range of health improvement activities from yoga to swimming. Dancing is recognized as an ideal activity because of its physical as well as social component.

Systolic blood pressure: the highest arterial blood pressure in the cardiac cycle occurring just after the heart contracts (beats).

Diastolic blood pressure: the lowest arterial blood pressure in the cardiac cycle occurring in between heart contractions or beats.

HDL: a type of lipoprotein that carries cholesterol from the bloodstream to the liver, where it can be excreted from the body. High blood HDL levels may help protect individuals against coronary artery disease.

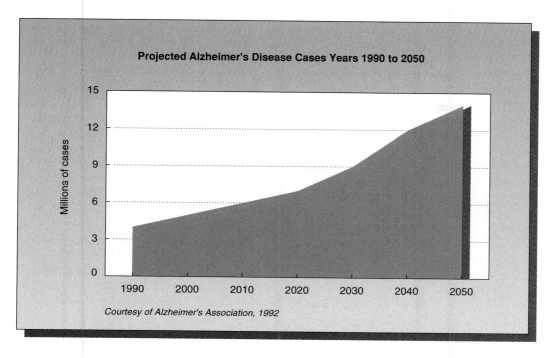

Projected Alzheimer's Disease Cases Years 1990 to 2050

Millions of cases

Courtesy of Alzheimer's Association, 1992

Figure 18.6: What Do You Think?

1. What trend do you see in projected Alzheimer's disease cases?
2. What factors do you think may have contributed to this trend?

Source: Data from Alzheimer's Association, 1992.

Increasing age does not diminish the relationship between health beliefs and health behavior.[76] Marilyn K. Potts and her colleagues studied social support, health beliefs, and health behaviors in 936 elderly men and women. A high level of social support consistently predicted a high level of preventive health practices.[77]

Adapting to Cognitive Change

Most older adults who experience *senility,* also called *dementia* (i.e., loss of memory, attentiveness, and other cognitive functions), do so for one of two reasons. First, they may experience a series of small strokes or **infarcts,** resulting from insufficient oxygen to the brain. When an infarct occurs, the region of the brain having the oxygen deficit ceases to function properly. Multiple small infarcts, or "mini-strokes," can give rise to the array of symptoms identified with senility.

A second cause of senility comes from the presently irreversible degeneration of brain tissue known as **Alzheimer's disease.** It is named for German neurologist Alois Alzheimer, who in 1906 studied the brain tissue of a patient who had shown the characteristic behaviors associated with senility. Examination of the brain revealed a series of twisted nerve cell fibers in numerous small clumps, or **plaques.** It now is suspected that **prions,** viruslike infectious agents containing protein but little nucleic acid, may be implicated in the causation of Alzheimer's disease.[78]

Alzheimer's disease is the fourth leading cause of death among the elderly. In addition, it may account for up to 75 percent of senile dementia in the elderly. Some investigators estimate that 6 percent of people over age sixty-five have Alzheimer's disease.[79] Other authorities estimate the figure to be over 10 percent, with the total number of cases more than doubling by the year 2040[80] (see figure 18.6). About 600,000 of the affected persons reside in nursing homes, and for each Alzheimer's patient in a nursing home, there are four or five living in the community. Onset of the disease is between ages forty-five and sixty-five but has occurred in a person as young as twenty-eight. Its duration may be between one to sixteen years with an average of six to eight years. While more women seem to be affected than men, this difference may be due to women living longer than men on the average. Relatives of people with Alzheimer's disease are four times more likely to develop it than the general population. The occurrence of Alzheimer's disease does not appear to be related to education, occupation, or socioeconomic status.

While individual cases may vary, four phases of the illness are frequently identified.[81] In the first phase, relatives are unsure that anything is wrong. They may notice that the individual has less energy and more difficulty in learning new things. The affected individual may seek familiar people, places, and things. Communication, the

Infarcts: a medical term that means death of tissue. A stroke can be caused by an infarct (or tissue death) in the brain, while a myocardial infarction refers to death of heart tissue (commonly known as a heart attack).

Alzheimer's disease: an age-associated form of dementia and degeneration of brain tissue.

ability to verbalize, and the ability to comprehend instructions may seem impaired.

The second phase of the illness brings more losses. Misunderstandings about what is said or heard in a conversation may become more common. The person may have difficulty planning ahead and making decisions. Forgetfulness and the inability to recognize familiar objects, places, and people occur more frequently. Confusion is seen in the day-night reversal known as the "sundowner syndrome," where the patient is active during the night but sleeps during the day. The person repeats things. Chewing and swallowing food may become difficult tasks to perform, and choking may become a constant danger. Appetite may be excessive or totally absent.

During the early stages of Alzheimer's disease, victims can be assisted greatly if their environment is kept highly structured and predictable. Writes Lenore S. Powell:[82]

> Familiarity is a source of comfort to the patient who becomes more confused in unfamiliar surroundings. An organized room and possessions, plus the labeling of objects that are used regularly, can be very helpful. Placing pictures of stored objects on cabinets is useful. For example, a picture of a pair of socks in the drawer where socks are kept (*sic*). Also useful are lists as reminders of tasks to be done.

Obvious disability is characteristic of the disease's third phase. The victim is not conscious of time, places, or events. People well known to the victim are no longer recognized automatically. The fourth phase of the illness finds the victim apathetic, unable to get around in even a familiar setting, participating in aimless wandering, and requiring help with activities that are part of daily living and self-care. Recent and remote memories fade, perhaps altogether. Syllables and words are repeated as a child just learning language might do. In this final phase, depression, delusions, or delirium all are possible. The loss of memory is accompanied by a loss of personal dignity. Other symptoms, including gait disturbance, feebleness, and incontinence may appear. Victims of Alzheimer's disease are susceptible to progressive paralysis, respiratory illnesses such as pneumonia, other infections, and kidney failure. These disorders comprise the usual causes of death for the Alzheimer's patient.

The financial cost of caring for Alzheimer's disease patients can be substantial and prohibitive for most families. Private insurers, as well as **Medicare,** may not reimburse the cost of care. The available government support specifically for institutionalization of such patients is itself prohibitive, reaching $20 billion a year. By the year 2000, over four million people in the U.S. will have this disease and the cost of care will reach $78 billion.[83] No price tag can be placed on the enormous psychological costs for both the victim and the victim's family.

Duane Lundervold and Lewis M. Lewin note the stress placed on family members who care for a loved one having Alzheimer's disease. They point to the many adverse psychological, physical, and social effects experienced. Caregivers report chronic fatigue and burden, loss of friends and social support, and a lack of time to relax and enjoy social activities.[84] Family members may undergo all of the emotions associated with loss, deprivation, and death (see chapter 13). Anger, fear, and guilt may be overwhelming. It is important, therefore, that medical-care personnel recognize not only the needs of the victim but also the needs of loved ones when addressing this disorder.

There are other causes of senility, as well. About one older adult in five who suffers from memory loss or other indicators of senility does so because of factors that can be modified. The underlying cause of the problem may be related to medications or combinations of drugs that the person takes for another health problem.

Other health-related conditions such as nutritional deficiencies, alcoholism, or changes in endocrine functions may bring about symptoms attributed to senility, simply because they occur in an older person. Persons with failing memories and declining cognitive abilities should be given a thorough physical examination to identify the source of the problem and to learn if corrective procedures are possible.

Lawrence Schonfeld and Larry W. Dupree point out that some older adults experience problems related to the abuse of alcohol.[85] They describe the *early onset* elderly alcohol abuser as a person whose history of abusive drinking started in his or her thirties or forties. This person already may have had extensive contact with the medical profession, social services, and other

Medicare: a federally-funded program that assists in the payment of health expenses for persons aged sixty-five and older who are entitled to Social Security benefits.

community agencies. This person is in contrast with the *late-life onset* person whose problem with alcohol begins in their fifties or sixties. The latter individual is a *reactive drinker*, whose alcohol use is in response to a serious life change or life crisis. For instance, the death of a spouse, retirement, moving, adjusting to a substantially decreased income, or experiencing impaired or declining health may trigger abusive drinking. Such an individual may successfully conceal this behavior by drinking at home, by drinking alone, and by not showing indications of inebriation in public.

Some cognitive changes in older adults may be compensated for simply by restructuring tasks.[86] If short-term memory loss is a problem, a practical solution is the creation of aids such as lists, self-directed notes, special (mnemonic) memory devices, and other techniques. As Susan Whitbourne and David Sperbeck conclude: "Imagination and creative solutions are most likely to come from the individual who must deal with the problem."[87]

Besides dementia, depression is the most frequent psychological disorder in later life.[88] Managing depression that results from ongoing adaptation to chronic illness or from the death of friends and relatives requires considerable skill. Professional help may be required. Managing stress can be a difficult assignment for the elderly as well. Not everyone seems to cope with stress in positive ways. Some adopt a fatalistic attitude that stress and misfortune are parts of growing old. For these people, stress may produce physical illness or chronic depression. Coping with an agonizing condition like **arthritis** can produce changes in mood, personality, and quality of life. Means of managing stress are similar to methods used at other times of life. Transcendental meditation, biofeedback, and relaxation exercises, while foreign to most people at first, can provide stress relief. The elderly may also find relief through prayer and other spiritual measures. The stress that comes from having to get along on limited resources may be reduced through participation in support groups, such as those found in community senior centers.

Personal and Social Issues Related to Wellness

Most people, regardless of age, hope for good health and a comfortable lifestyle; however,

these basic needs are not always easily fulfilled for some older adults. Achieving wellness is thwarted by a host of social, economic, and political forces. A widely accepted means of assessing health status in senior adults is by an examination of the number of days of restricted activity per year.[89] Heart disease, cancer, stroke, diabetes, arthritis, and emphysema account for 81 percent of the days of restricted activity among persons over the age of sixty-five. Note that many of these ailments are ones that involve a significant lifestyle component, and therefore, a degree of choice. Twenty-three percent of noninstitutionalized persons in the U.S. aged sixty-five or over may be functionally limited in performing personal care activities such as bathing, dressing, eating, walking, getting outside, and using the toilet.

Healthy People 2000 indicates that a major health objective of the nation during the next decade is to reduce the amount of restricted activity in senior adults, and to increase their ability to perform essential, routine daily functions.[90]

Health Care

The rising cost of health care is a clear impediment to wellness in the older adult. These health-care costs come at a time when many people are living on diminished or fixed incomes and can least afford added expenses. To further complicate the road to wellness, financial burdens make the older person more vulnerable to quackery, fraudulent insurance schemes, and other gimmicks. Economically disadvantaged elderly people are likely to reap fewer benefits from federal government programs such as Medicare due to inadequate access to, and information regarding, the system.[91]

The experiences of older adults with health-care providers range from highly positive to extremely negative. The nature of the experience clearly can play an important role in whether or not an individual participates regularly in the health-care system. Marie R. Haug and Marcia G. Ory explain that ageist attitudes among health practitioners are prevalent.[92] Moreover, knowledge about traits of elderly patients that affect their taking medication may be lacking among some physicians;[93] however, there has been little systematic research done on the nature of patient traits, provider characteristics, the context of health care,

Arthritis: a general term referring to an inflammation of the joints. Arthritis has many known causes, such as rheumatic fever and trauma, as well as unknown causes.

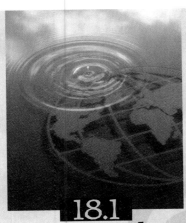
and the complex interactions of these variables. Older patients may be more accepting of disease and therefore less active about seeking health care. Mild symptoms of short or even chronic duration can get attributed to the aging process itself rather than to real but treatable diseases. Consequently, quality of life becomes less than optimal.

Physicians, other health practitioners, and family members of older adults must be mindful of the hesitation to seek health care by some elderly persons. John R. Burton suggests that physicians become more willing to make house calls on behalf of their frail elderly patients.[94] He points out that such a gesture is important to patient care and need not be disruptive of regular office practice or lead to decreased efficiency. Practices that maintain or promote wellness such as health information seeking, self-examination, appointment keeping, and risk avoidance are more likely to be performed by older women than older men and especially so if there is a strongly supportive family environment.[95]

Necessary expenses for prescription and over-the-counter medications can be reduced through the purchase of **generic equivalents.** Most of the time this practice is a good one and favors the elderly consumer. For drugs prescribed for selected conditions, however, generic substances may produce undesirable side effects not seen in their proprietary counterparts.[96] Older persons or their family members should inquire about the use of generic equivalents from both a money-saving and a health perspective.

An "innovation" that has come about as a result of deliberate contamination of drug products on pharmacy and grocery store shelves by sociopathic individuals is the "tamper resistant" package. Though performing its intent quite well, the package unfortunately is often equally resistant to persons with reduced visual acuity or impaired manual dexterity due to arthritis. It may be possible to obtain drugs in packages that are accessible to persons with physical limitations. Inquiries about availability should be made.

Generic equivalent: a drug containing the same active ingredient as one marketed under a trade name, and usually sold at a price less than that of the trade-name variety.

The fact that women live longer than men on the average has health-care financing consequences. Older women are likely to have fewer personal financial resources for health care than their male counterparts, and they must spread these resources out over a longer period of time. Medicare, begun in 1965 to finance health care for elderly persons in the U.S., pays only about 40 percent of average health-care costs. Medicare was designed to reimburse acute, inpatient care rather than the chronic out-patient and long-term care needed by many older people. Among the shortcomings of Medicare are its lack of reimbursement for such things as prescription drugs, eyeglasses, hearing aids, dental services, routine physical examinations, foot care, and long-term home care or nursing-home care.[97] Thus, the illness and disability patterns of a substantial number of older adults are not addressed adequately by the nation's primary health-care reimbursement plan for the elderly. Health-care expenditures not covered by Medicare must come from private insurance or monetary savings of older people themselves. Women especially are affected adversely by this financial dilemma.

Colleen L. Johnson indicates there is growing interest in an emerging group of persons in the U.S. known as the oldest-old, those persons eighty-five or more years of age.[98] She says that the physical and social attributes of this group, as well as the personal competencies and general well-being, are unknown entities since this is the first time that a large group of **octogenarians** has existed. Barbara M. Barer is one gerontologist who has studied the oldest-old.[99] While it is generally true that women outlive men, men who do survive to eighty-five are likely to be in better health and have more years of life remaining than their female counterparts. These men are more likely to have adequate financial resources, and less likely to be widowed than women in this age bracket. These men place a high premium on competency, activity, productivity, independence and self-reliance. Women, in contrast, are more family oriented and content in maintaining the continuity of their domestic role. Future aged cohorts may differ greatly from ones of the 1990s as persons who pioneered new social roles for men and women reach their ninth decade of life.

According to Myrna Lewis, almost 50 percent of older Black women, 25 percent of older Hispanic women, and more than 15 percent of older White women live below the official poverty level.[100] She writes:

> Minority women have a proportionally higher chance of poverty and are the poorest of the poor; but the vast majority of the poor elderly are older White women. A unique feature of old age is that women who were poor all their lives are joined by the "newly poor"—the middle class and even upper class women who may sink to the poverty level, depending on whether they outlive their resources or, more likely, experience catastrophic or chronic illnesses requiring expensive care. Few, for example, can afford the costs of long-term care, in or out of institutions. Nursing home costs alone can amount to $3,000 to $5,000 per month.

While exercise in the elderly typically has shown positive health benefits, significant social and cultural barriers may impede participation, especially for women. According to Sandra J. O'Brien and Patricia A. Vertinsky:[101]

> It is clear that many barriers inhibit older women from increasing their exercise level. Currently, the lack of healthful physical exercise and withdrawal from everyday tasks demanding strength cause too many aging women to be less fit than they need to be. Such stress-inducing situations as fewer valued social roles, lower socioeconomic status, elevated health concerns, lower education levels, social permissiveness for psychological and physical weakness, time constraints, and greater willingness to believe they have health problems, aggravate their unfitness.

Personal Barriers

Inadequate nutrition can constitute a major barrier to wellness for a variety of reasons. The ability to chew, swallow, and digest food can limit what an individual can eat. Half of all people in the U.S. lose their teeth by age sixty-five, and two-thirds lose them by age seventy-five.[102] Diminished senses of taste and smell can cause a loss of interest in

Octogenarians: people between the ages of eighty and ninety.

TABLE 18.4 — Percentage of Persons 65 Years and Older Who Cannot Perform Activities of Daily Living (ADLs)

Care of Body ADLs		Instrumental ADLs	
Bathing	8.9	Using telephone	4.4
Bed/Chair transfer	5.9	Using money	6.3
Dressing	5.1	Shopping	11.1
Toileting	3.5	Getting about community	13.5
Feeding	1.1	Preparing meals	7.5
Walking	7.7	Doing housework	10.1

What Do You Think?

1. To what extent do these percentages reflect your estimate of functional disability among the elderly?

2. Can a person who is unable to perform some of these tasks still experience a high level of wellness? Explain.

Source: Data from Agency for Health Care Policy and Research, *Intramural Research Highlights, Volume 7*, Public Health Service, 1992, Rockville, MD.

eating. The inability to taste salt or sugar can also encourage an excessive use of sweeteners and sodium at a time in life when the body is least able to tolerate it.

Another physical barrier to adequate nutrition is irregular bowel movements. Some people try to regulate themselves by consuming large quantities of mineral oil or other laxatives. This practice can deplete the body's stores of fat-soluble vitamins, upset the electrolyte balance, and lead to dehydration and states of confusion, disorientation, and weakness.[103] A better way to assist regularity is to include high-fiber foods, such as fresh fruit and vegetables, whole grains, and specially fortified cereals, in the diet. These dietary measures add bulk to the stool and promote retention of water in the intestines, thereby softening the stool and speeding up the full digestive cycle. U.S. culture traditionally has not stressed eating these types of foods, making dietary adjustments difficult for some people.

Problems in obtaining and preparing food also create nutritional barriers for the elderly. The cost of food places a limit on what can be purchased. In some cases, this may actually serve a desirable purpose since fattening or expensive foods low in nutritional value may not be affordable; however, a small budget usually means omitting important food items. Immobility or lack of transportation can also affect food purchases (see table 18.4). If transportation to a store is only sporadic, purchased items may consist primarily of nonperishable canned goods. This could lead to a diet low in fresh fruits and vegetables, meat, and dairy products.

There is a common misbelief that milk products are only for children and youth. In fact, we never outgrow our need for milk. The reluctance to use milk products in middle and later adult life may lead to a diminished calcium level and contribute to the osteoporotic process. Low-fat or skim milk provides valuable vitamins and minerals throughout the life span but with fewer calories and less fat than whole milk.

According to W. B. Kannel, the nutritional status of elderly citizens may be influenced by a host of factors, including ignorance of personal nutrition requirements and nutrient properties of foods, poverty, social isolation, physical disability, mental deterioration and depression, alcoholism, and drug taking.[104] Elderly persons least likely to follow optimal eating practices are people living alone, especially men, persons who are disabled, and the most feeble older adults.

Family Barriers

Jean Miller points out that family structures can interfere with wellness in the elderly.[105] One structure is the disengaged family. In this structure family members are so independent that they neither request support from nor respond to the needs of other family members. At the opposite extreme is the enmeshed family, where there is such a strong sense of belonging that persons may lose autonomy or individuality. Although elderly people in the enmeshed group are likely to have their physical needs met, it is often at the expense of their feelings of self-worth. Gail K. Auslander and Howard Litivin found that social support in old age was inversely related to formal help-seeking.[106] That is, persons who sought social services were those least likely to have affective support networks in place.

Two forces that can be destructive to the familial relationship of older people are **parentification** and **infantilization**.[107] In parentification, adult children regress to childlike states when in the presence of their elderly parents and are unable to make decisions without parental consultation and approval. While not particularly destructive to the elder parents, it does usurp the role of the adult child's spouse. Infantilization is the converse of parentification. Infantilization is role reversal where adult children act in the parent role and strip their elders of independence and self-responsibility for maintenance. As Miller indicates: "Such behavior encourages parents to become dependent and to act as children to their children."[108] The identities of adult children and their parents may both be compromised by this practice. As Karen Seccombe points out:[109]

> Data do not support the contention that having children contributes to general happiness in later life for either men or women. In addition, children do not appear to lessen the impact of deteriorating health upon the well-being of the elderly.

Approximately two-thirds of women over age sixty-five are single, but just one-fourth of the men find themselves in this position. When an older woman loses her spouse through death, she loses her lover and companion, an escort for public events, a mate in couple interaction, someone with whom to share household tasks, a familiar lifestyle, and often her married friends.

Environmental Barriers

Affordable housing is a major environmental issue for the elderly. Houses in most locations require winter heating and summer air conditioning. Energy costs are particularly difficult burdens for older persons in the U.S. While there is a tendency, perhaps, to want to move elderly persons into specialized housing projects, many people resist such change. They often achieve more peace of mind in familiar surroundings and in neighborhoods where they feel secure from crime.

Transportation is also a special environmental consideration for the older adult. The elderly depend on adequate transportation for social, recreational, and spiritual activities, as well as for shopping and access to medical care. Community planners must consider three things. First, transportation must be available as well as economical. Inexpensive mass transit is critical for people who do not own or cannot drive automobiles or who cannot afford taxi fares. Second, transportation must be safe. In urban areas, mass transit is often a vehicle for crime. Older people feel too vulnerable to risk using this type of transportation. In rural areas, inexpensive public transportation may be too far away to be of much practical help. Third, transportation must go where older persons are likely to travel. The lack of adequate transportation can be a major reason that people disengage from society, despite their wishes to the contrary.

A Final Word about Aging

As a college student, you can enhance intergenerational understanding by being a supportive caregiver. Some tips for taking on this role are shown for you in table 18.5. The aging process brings changes for you, for your family and friends, and for the social and vocational roles that you hold during your life. The application of wellness strategies throughout the life span can maximize your successful adaptation to aging, and bring about an optimal quality of living in the older adult years. Right now, you can encourage your parents and grandparents to adopt a wellness lifestyle, and support their efforts as you pursue your own wellness endeavors.

TABLE 18.5 — Tips for Becoming A Supportive Caregiver of the Elderly

Sometimes it is difficult for young people and older adults to relate well to each other. You can reduce some of the "generational distance" and be a supportive caregiver at the same time, though, by trying some of the tips provided below.

Precontemplation → Contemplation

If you have never thought about how you might be a supportive caregiver, consider:

- Using the phone book and other resources, develop a list of senior centers, retirement communities, nursing homes, and other facilities where older persons congregate. Contacting places of worship may be of assistance in the identification of key places and people.

Contemplation → Preparation

If you have thought about the value of being a supportive caregiver but have not prepared yourself for the task, try:

- Developing a list of your own personal resources that might be valuable or of use to an elderly person (e.g., "I can drive to the grocery store." "I can mow someone's lawn." "I can apply some safety strips in someone's bathtub or shower." "I can write a letter or send a 'thinking of you' card to my grandparents.").
- Making the decision to take action.

Preparation → Action

Having prepared yourself to be a caregiver by taking inventory of your own abilities and strengths, advance your ambitious plan by:

- Identifying a date in the next thirty days when you will carry out your plan. Circle the date on your calendar.

- Telling others about your activity. Let people know that you are not "just thinking about" helping or becoming friends with an older person—but actually doing it.

Action → Maintenance

Having successfully demonstrated your caregiving ability, you can help to make them part of your regular routine by:

- Celebrating your accomplishment.
- After completing a task involving an elderly person, making a promise to repeat that task or perform another one.
- Making a firm appointment (e.g., next Thursday at 11:00 A.M.) to see the person again.

Maintenance

You are well on your way to being a caregiver. Keep up your momentum by:

- Diversifying your repertoire of activities with the elderly.
- Identifying a new elderly person with whom you can be friends.
- Inviting a roommate, classmate, or other friend to help you with one of your activities or outings that involves an older person. Introduce this peer to the older person.

Summary

1. The health status of older people in the U.S. is better than commonly believed. However, persons over age sixty-five do account for a disproportionate amount of health-care expenditures. Much work still needs to be done to achieve the health objectives of the nation for the year 2000 where the elderly are concerned.

2. Misconceptions about the elderly abound. Part of the wellness challenge is helping to eliminate ageist attitudes and beliefs.

3. Many biological changes occur over time that result in the indicators commonly associated with aging. Little can be done to affect primary aging but conscientious lifestyle decisions can eliminate or minimize the effects of secondary aging.

4. Even by the time you are in college, you can notice physical signs of aging. Some of physical aging results from the negative effects of unwise lifestyle choices.

5. Numerous theories have been advanced to account for the physical indicators associated with aging.

6. Several theories attempt to explain and predict successful adaptation to changing social roles associated with the aging process.

7. Older persons in the U.S. of different cultural backgrounds are affected disproportionately by health and social issues associated with aging.

8. Older persons in the U.S. are often the victims of crime and other events that affect their safety and well-being.

9. Certain lifestyle practices can retard aging and enhance wellness, especially if implemented early in life and maintained through older adulthood.

10. Older persons in the U.S. face many problems that can serve as barriers to achieving high-level wellness. With some creativity and social empowerment, many of these barriers can be overcome.

11. Older persons in the U.S. can adapt to sensory changes of aging by using hearing aids and bifocal eye glasses when necessary, by arranging household items such as furniture, dishes, and lights in easily accessible places, and by having safety features such as hand rails installed.

12. We can adapt more successfully to biological changes of aging by regularly participating in exercise or physical activity such as yoga, walking, swimming, or dancing.

13. Older persons can adapt to cognitive changes of aging by using memory aids such as mnemonic memory devices or self-directed notes. Using stress-management techniques regularly, such as relaxation techniques and support groups, can also help people more successfully adapt to cognitive changes associated with aging.

14. Becoming a supportive caregiver for older persons can reduce some of the self-imposed barriers that limit intergenerational exchange.

15. The term "old" has many meanings and one should avoid making assumptions that may not be valid.

Recommended Readings

Friedan, Betty. *The Fountain of Age*. New York: Simon & Schuster, 1993.

In this highly praised book, Ms. Friedan provides perspective on the paradoxes of old age, the new choices available to people as they age, and fosters the viewpoint that aging is an adventure.

Jackson, James S., Chatters, Linda M., and Taylor, Robert Joseph. *Aging in Black America*. Newbury Park, Calif.: Sage Publishing, 1993.

The authors examine crime, stress, self-esteem, intergenerational support, and life satisfaction from historic and contemporary perspectives among Black Americans in the United States.

Ebersole, Priscilla, and Hess, Patricia, *Toward Healthy Aging*, 4th edition. St. Louis: Mosby, 1994.

Although written primarily for persons in nursing education, this book provides a comprehensive and in-depth review of the health issues facing older persons in the U.S., including chronic conditions, physical and psychological care issues, and other facets of aging.

References

1. Janna B. Herman, "An Overview of Physical Ability with Age: The Potential for Health in Later Life," *Gerontology & Geriatrics Education* 11.1:2 (1990):11–12.

2. Herman, "An Overview of Physical Ability with Age," 11.

3. Robert N. Butler, "Forward to Second Edition," in: C. K. Cassel, D. E. Risenberg, L. B. Sorenson, et al. (eds.), *Geriatric Medicine*, 2nd edition (New York: Springer-Verlag, 1990).

4. Robert N. Butler, "Ageism: Another Form of Bigotry," *The Gerontologist* 9 (1969):243–245.

5. Gregory F. Sanders et al., "Youth's Attitudes toward the Elderly," *Journal of Applied Gerontology* 3.1 (1984):59–70.

6. Mary E. Kite and Blair T. Johnson, "Attitudes toward Older and Younger Adults," *Psychology and Aging* 3.3 (1988):233–244.

7. Philip E. Slater, *The Pursuit of Loneliness* (Boston: Beacon Press, 1970).

8. Thomas R. Cole, *The Journey of Life: A Cultural History of Aging in America* (Cambridge: Cambridge University Press, 1992).

9. Slava Lubomudrov, "Congressional Perceptions of the Elderly: The Use of Stereotypes in the Legislative Process," *The Gerontologist* 27.1 (1987):77–81.

10. John Bell, "The Search of A Discourse in Aging: The Elderly on Television," *The Gerontologist* 32.3 (1992):305–311.

11. Bernice L. Neugarten and Dail A. Neugarten, "The Changing Meanings of Age," *Psychology Today* 21.5 (1987):30.

12. Paula D. Thomas, Philip J. Garry, and James S. Goodwin, "Morbidity and Mortality in an Initially Healthy

Elderly Sample: Findings after Five Years of Follow-up," *Age and Aging* 15 (1986):105–110.

13. Herman, "An Overview of Physical Ability with Age," 17–18.

14. S. P. Tzankoff and A. H. Norris, "Effect of Muscle Mass Decrease on Age-Related BMR Changes," *Journal of Applied Physiology* 43 (1977):1001–1006.

15. Lars Larsson, Gunnar Grimby, and Jan Karlsson, "Muscle Strength and Speed of Movement in Relation to Age and Muscle Morphology," *Journal of Applied Physiology* 46 (1979):451–456.

16. Herman, "An Overview of Physical Ability with Age," 19–20.

17. Kathleen M. Munns, "Effects of Exercise on the Range of Joint Motion," in *Exercise and Aging: The Scientific Basis*, eds. Everett L. Smith, Jr. and R. C. Serfass (Hillside, N.J.: Enslow Publishers, 1981).

18. Everett L. Smith, Jr., "Bone Changes in the Exercising Older Adult," in *Exercise and Aging: The Scientific Basis*, eds. Everett L. Smith, Jr. and R. C. Serfass (Hillside, N.J.: Enslow Publishers, 1981).

19. Everett L. Smith and Catherine Gilligan, "Effects of Inactivity and Exercise on Bone," *The Physician and Sportsmedicine* 15.11 (1987):91–100.

20. Everett L. Smith, "Exercise for Prevention of Osteoporosis: A Review," *Physician and Sportsmedicine* 10.3 (1982):72–80.

21. R. B. Mazess, "Measurement of Skeletal Status by Noninvasive Methods," *Calcified Tissue International* 28 (1979):89–92.

22. Herman, "An Overview of Physical Ability with Age," 20.

23. R. S. Paffenbarger, A. L. Wing, and C. Hsieh, "Physical Activity, All-Cause Mortality and Longevity of College Alumni," *New England Journal of Medicine* 314 (1986):605.

24. Herman, "An Overview of Physical Ability with Age," 17.

25. Enza Ciurlia-Guy, Marlene Cashman, and Brenda Lewsen, "Identifying Hearing Loss and Hearing Handicap among Chronic Care Elderly People," *The Gerontologist* 33.5 (1993):644–649.

26. Herman, "An Overview of Physical Ability with Age," 17.

27. Susan S. Schiffman, "Taste and Smell in Disease II," *New England Journal of Medicine* 308 (1983):1338.

28. Schiffman, "Taste and Smell in Disease II," 1338.

29. James M. Weiffenbach, Carolyn A. Tylenda, and Bruce J. Brown, "Oral Sensory Changes in Aging," *Journal of Gerontology: Medical Sciences* 45.4 (1990):M121–25.

30. Sharon Anderson and Barry M. Brenner, "The Aging Kidney: Structure, Function, Mechanisms, and Therapeutic Implications," *Journal of the American Geriatric Society* 35 (1987):590.

31. Bernice L. Neugarten et al., "Women's Attitude toward the Menopause," *Vita Humana* 6 (1963):140–151.

32. Gloria A. Bachman and Sylvia R. Leiblum, "Sexual Expression in Menopausal Women," *Medical Aspects of Human Sexuality* 15.10 (1981):96B–96H.

33. B. Layton and Ilene Siegler, "Mid-Life: Must It Be a Crisis?" paper presented at the annual meeting of the American Gerontological Society (Dallas, Tex., 1978).

34. Raymond Harris, "Exercise and Sex in the Aging Parent," *Medical Aspects of Human Sexuality* 22.1 (1988):149.

35. Lionel Corbett, "The Last Sexual Taboo: Sex in Old Age," *Medical Aspects of Human Sexuality* 15.4 (1981):117–131.

36. P. Gebhard, W. Pomeroy, C. Christenson, and J. Gagnon, *Sex Offenders: An Analysis of Types* (New York: Harper & Row, 1965).

37. Leonard Hayflick, "Biologic Aging Theories," in: Maddox, G. (ed.), *The Encyclopedia of Aging*, (New York: Springer, 1987).

38. Richard A. Lockshin and Zahra F. Zaker, "Programmed Cell Death: New Thoughts and Relevance to Aging," *Journal of Gerontology: Biological Sciences* 45.5 (1990):B135–140.

39. Robin Holliday, "The Limited Proliferation of Cultured Human Diploid Cells: Regulation or Senescence," *Journal of Gerontology: Biological Sciences* 45.2 (1990):B36–41.

40. Lockshin and Zakrei, "Programmed Cell Death: New Thought and Relevance to Aging," B135.

41. Howard J. Curtis and Kimball Miller, "Chromosome Aberrations in Liver Cells of Guinea Pigs," *Journal of Gerontology* 26 (1971):292–294.

42. C. A. Rice-Evans and R. H. Burdon, *Free Radical Damage and Its Control*, (London: Elsevier, 1994).

43. Elaine Cumming and William E. Henry, *Growing Old* (New York: Basic Books, 1961).

44. R. J. Havighurst, B. L. Neugarten, and S. S. Tobin, "Disengagement and Patterns of Aging," in *Middle Age and Aging*, ed. B. L. Neugarten (Chicago: Univ. of Chicago Press, 1968); G. L. Maddox, "Themes and Issues in Sociological Theories of Human Aging," *Human Development* 13 (1970):17–27.

45. J. F. Gubrium, *The Myth of the Golden Years: A Socio-Environmental Theory of Aging* (Springfield, Ill.: Charles C. Thomas, 1973).

46. David J. Lee and Kyriakos S. Markides, "Activity and Mortality among Aged Persons over an Eight-Year Period," *Journal of Gerontology: Social Sciences* 45.1 (1990):S39–42.

47. Robert C. Atchley, *The Social Forces in Later Life: An Introduction to the Social Gerontology* (Belmont, Calif.: Wadsworth, 1972).

48. J. A. Kuypers and V. L. Bengston, "Social Breakdown and Competence: A Model of Normal Aging," *Human Development* 16 (1973):181.

49. Priscilla Ebersole and Patricia Hess, *Toward Healthy Aging*, 4th edition (St. Louis: Mosby, 1994).

50. Ebersole and Hess, *Toward Healthy Aging*.

51. Lorraine T. Dorfman, Frank J. Kohort, and D. Alex Heckert, "Retirement Satisfaction in the Rural Elderly," *Research on Aging* 7.4 (1985):577–599.

52. Carol Cutler Riddick, "Life Satisfaction for Older Female Homemakers, Retirees, and Workers," *Research on Aging* 7.3 (1985):383–393.

53. Karen Seccombe and Gary R. Lee, "Gender Differences in Retirement Satisfaction and Its Antecedents," *Research on Aging* 8.3 (1986):426–440.

54. Hirsch S. Ruchlin and John N. Morris, "Impact of Work on the Quality of Life of Community-Residing Young Elderly," *American Journal of Public Health* 81 (1991):498–500.

55. U.S. Department of Health and Human Services, "1.9 Million Seniors Ready and Able to Go Back to Work," *Aging* 362(1991):51.

56. T. W. Maloney and B. Paul, *Enabling Older Americans to Work, 1989 Annual Report of the Commonwealth Fund* (New York: The Commonwealth Fund, 1990):37–51.

57. Barbara A. Hirshow & Denise T. Hoyer, "Private Sector Hiring and Use of Retirees: The Firm's Perspective," *The Gerontologist* 34.1 (1994):50–58.

58. Ingrid Arnet Connidis and Lorraine Davies, "Confidants and Companions in Later Life: The Place of Family and Friends," *Journal of Gerontology: Social Sciences* 45.4 (1990):S141–149.

59. Elzbieta Gozdziak, "New Branches . . . Distant Roots: Older Refugees in the United States," *Aging* 359 (1989):2–7.

60. Mark C. Hornbrook, Victor J. Stevens, Darlene J. Wingfield, Jack F. Hollis, Merwyn R. Greenlick, and Marcia G. Ory, "Preventing Falls among Community-Dwelling Older Persons: Results from a Randomized Trial," *The Gerontologist* 34.1 (1994):16–23.

61. Maxine M. Urton, "A Community Home Inspection Approach to Preventing Falls among the Elderly," *Public Health Reports* 106.2 (1991): 192–195.

62. Urton, "A Community Home Inspection Approach to Preventing Falls among the Elderly," 193.

63. Marlene A. Young and John H. Stein, "Elderly Crime Victims," *Aging* 360 (1990):36–37.

64. Young and Stein, "Elderly Crime Victims," 37.

65. Dori Stehlin, "The Silent Epidemic of Hip Fractures," *FDA Consumer* 22.4 (1988):18–23.

66. D. E. Rosenblatt, Edward W. Campion, and Mary Mason, "Rehabilitation Home Visits," *Journal of the American Geriatrics Society* 34 (1986):441–447.

67. G. W. Heath et al., "A Physiological Comparison of Young and Older Endurance Athletes," *Journal of Applied Physiology* 51 (1981):634–640.

68. K. H. Sidney and Roy J. Shephard, "Frequency and Intensity of Exercise Training for Elderly Subjects," *Medicine and Science in Sports and Exercise* 10 (1978):1125–1131.

69. Herbert A. deVries, "Physiological Effects of an Exercise Training Regimen Upon Men Aged 52–58," *Journal of Gerontology* 25 (1970):325–336.

70. David R. Hopkins et al., "Effect of Low-Impact Aerobic Dance on the Functional Fitness of Elderly Women," *The Gerontologist* 30 (1990):189–192.

71. H. J. Montoye et al., "Bone Mineral in Senior Tennis Players," *Scandinavian Journal of Sports Science* 2 (1980):26–32.

72. Smith, "Exercise for Prevention of Osteoporosis," 72–80.

73. Everett L. Smith, Jr., William Reddan, and Patricia E. Smith, "Physical Activity and Calcium Modalities for Bone Mineral Increase in Aged Women," *Medicine and Science in Sports and Exercise* 13 (1981):60–64.

74. Richard M. Lampman, "Evaluating and Prescribing Exercise for Elderly Patients," *Geriatrics* 42.8 (1987):63–76.

75. Samuel Perri II and Donald I. Templer, "The Effect of an Aerobic Exercise Program on Psychological Variables in Older Adults," *International Journal of Aging and Human Development* 20.3 (1984–85): 167–772.

76. Rebecca Ferrini, Sharon Edelstein, and Elizabeth Barrett-Connor, "The Association between Health Beliefs and Health Behavior Change in Older Adults," *Preventive Medicine* 23.1 (1994):1–5.

77. Marilyn K. Potts, Margo-Lea Hurwicz, Michael S. Goldstein, and Emil Berkanovic, "Social Support, Health Promotive Beliefs, and Preventive Health Behaviors among the Elderly," *Journal of Applied Gerontology* 11.4 (1992):425–440.

78. Lenore S. Powell, "Alzheimer's Disease: A Practical, Psychological Approach," in *Health Needs of Women as They Age*, eds. Sharon Golub and Rita Jackaway Freedman (New York: Harrington Park Press, 1985), 57.

79. H. Fenn, V. Luby, and J. A. Yesavage, "Subtypes in Alzheimer's Disease and the Impact of Excess Disability: Recent Findings," *International Journal of Geriatric Psychiatry* 8.1 (1993):67.

80. Pamela Arnsberger Webber, Patricia Fox, and Denise Burnette, "Living Alone with Alzheimer's Disease: Effects on Health and Social Service Utilization Patterns," *The Gerontologist* 34.1 (1994):8–14.

81. Powell, "Alzheimer's Disease," 54–56.

82. Powell, "Alzheimer's Disease," 59.

83. Powell, "Alzheimer's Disease," 58.

84. Duane Lundervold and Lewis M. Lewin, "Effects of In-Home Respite Care on Caregivers of Family Members with Alzheimer's Disease," *Journal of Clinical and Experimental Gerontology* 9.3:201–214.

85. Lawrence Schonfeld and Larry W. Dupree, "Older Problem Drinkers—Long-Term and Late-Life Onset Abusers: What Triggers their Drinking?" *Aging* 361 (1990):5–11.

86. Susan Kraus Whitbourne and David J. Sperbeck, "Health Care Maintenance for the Elderly," *Family and Community Health* 3.4 (1981):11–27.

87. Whitbourne and Sperbeck, "Health Care Maintenance for the Elderly," 11–27.

88. S. Kanowski, "Age-dependent Epidemiology of Depression," *Gerontology* 40(supplement).1 (1994):1–4.

89. Herman, "An Overview of Physical Ability with Age," 14.

90. *Healthy People 2000 National Health Promotion and Disease Prevention Objectives* (Washington D.C.: U.S. Department of Health and Human Services, 1991), 588–591.

91. Douglas C. Kimmel, "Ageism, Psychology, and Public Policy," *American Psychologist* 43.3 (1988): 175–178.

92. Marie R. Haug and Marcia G. Ory, "Issues in Elderly Patient-Provider Interactions," *Research on Aging* 9.1 (1987):3–44.

93. Margaret E. Ferry, Peter P. Lamy, and Lorne A. Becker, "Physicians' Knowledge of Prescribing for the Elderly," *Journal of the American Geriatrics Society* 33 (1985):616–625.

94. John R. Burton, "The House Call: An Important Service for the Frail Elderly," *Journal of the American Geriatrics Society* 33 (1985):291–293.

95. William Rakowski et al., "Correlates of Preventive Health Behavior in Later Life," *Research on Aging* 9.3 (1987):331–355.

96. David T. Lowenthal, "Drug Therapy in the Elderly," *Geriatrics* 42.11 (1987):77–82.

97. Myrna Lewis, "Older Women and Health: An Overview," in *Health Needs of Women as They Age*, eds. Sharon Golub and Rita Jackaway Freedman (New York: Harrington Park Press, 1985), 10–11.

98. Colleen L. Johnson, "Introduction: Social and Cultural Diversity of the Oldest Old," *International Journal of Aging and Human Development*, 38.1 (1994):1–12.

99. Barbara M. Barer, "Men and Women Age Differently," *International Journal of Aging and Human Development* 38.1 (1994):29–30.

100. Lewis, "Older Women and Health," 10–11.

101. Sandra J. O'Brien and Patricia A. Vertinsky, "Unfit Survivors: Exercise as a Resource for Aging Women," *The Gerontologist* 31 (1991):347–357.

102. Nancy Lank and Connie E. Vickery, "Nutrition Education for the Elderly: Concerns, Needs and Approaches," *Journal of Applied Gerontology* 6.3 (1987):259–267.

103. Helen Swift Mitchell et al., *Nutrition in Health and Disease* (Philadelphia: J. B. Lippincott Co., 1976).

104. W. B. Kannel, "Nutritional Contributors to Cardiovascular Disease in the Elderly," *Journal of the American Geriatrics Society* 34 (1986):27–36.

105. Jean R. Miller, "Family Support of the Elderly," *Family and Community Health* 3.4 (1981):51–59.

106. Gail K. Auslander and Howard Litivin, "Social Support Networks and Formal Help Seeking: Differences between Applicants to Social Services and a Nonapplicant Sample," *Journal of Gerontology: Social Sciences* 45.3 (1990):S112–119.

107. S. Minuchin, *Families and Family Therapy* (Cambridge, Mass.: Harvard University Press, 1974), 53.

108. Miller, "Family Support of the Elderly," 42.

109. Karen Seccombe, "Children: Their Impact on the Elderly in Declining Health," *Research on Aging* 9.2 (1987):323.

Ecology: Establishing a Healthy Environment

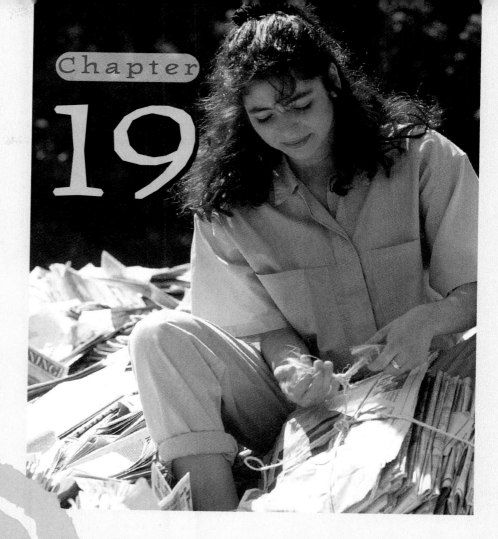

Student Learning Objectives

Upon completion of this chapter you should be able to:

1. define ecology;
2. explain the four "laws of ecology" by providing an example of how each law explains the problem of acid rain;
3. explain the four "laws of ecology" by providing an example of how each law explains the problem of hazardous waste;
4. discuss the special hazardous waste problems affecting communities of color in the U.S. as well as third world countries;
5. evaluate the laws of ecology to a sustainable earth society;
6. describe the adaptation continuum proposed by Robert Russell, and explain what happens as one moves from the ecological to the technological extreme;
7. discuss two U.S. dietary habits that are costly to the environment;
8. list at least five ways in which food energy-consumption patterns can be modified to conserve energy and decrease entropy;
9. give two reasons why synthetic fabrics are costly for the environment, and suggest alternatives that are more environmentally friendly;
10. describe at least four ways to increase environmental sensitivity in the areas of transportation, water use, and solid waste disposal;
11. analyze the relationship between environmental solutions occurring at the policy level (government, industry, or community group) and those solutions that might be undertaken by an individual (personal actions);
12. write an effective environmental advocacy letter.

Environmental issues have received much attention over the past few years, from scientists and consumers alike. The media daily expose us to examples of the environmental crisis. Carbon dioxide levels in the air we breathe are excessively high and may cause dangerous climatic changes in the coming years; the ozone layer is in serious danger of being destroyed, thereby increasing our exposure to harmful radiation from the sun; we are rapidly running out of places to dump our garbage. These seemingly endless crises overwhelm many people, often leading to the attitude that "there is nothing I can do about any of this!" This attitude paves the way for three traps of personal inaction: (1) blind technological optimism—a belief that technology and science will "save" us; (2) gloom-and-doom pessimism—a belief that there is no hope; and (3) apathy—a lack of caring due to a fatalistic outlook.[1]

There is another attitude you can take toward the environment, however. You can accept the challenge of creating a personal lifestyle that is both fulfilling and ecologically sound. Environmental sensitivity of this sort will affect your personal "space," providing valuable support for your wellness lifestyle. Additionally, it will affect the larger environment, fostering higher levels of wellness for your community. As college students, you are in a special position to become the future leaders of your community. Learning to understand and care for the environment will help you to contribute to the well-being of your local community as well as to the global environment.

This chapter will help you to understand the basic concepts of ecology, and provide you with a start on the information and skills necessary for the development of a lifestyle that is ecologically sound. We cannot afford to wait for governments, industry, or technology to solve our environmental dilemmas. As environmentalists Anne and Paul Ehrlich put it, "Human beings already have the power to preserve the Earth that everyone wants—they simply have to be willing to exercise it."[2]

The Laws of Ecology

Ecology, a relatively young science, can be defined as the study of **ecosystems.** Ecosystems consist of interactions between living organisms and the natural environment where they exist. Several generalizations can be made about natural ecosystems. Barry Commoner, director of the Center for the Biology of Natural Systems, has summarized these generalizations in what he terms the *laws of ecology.* Simply stated they are as follows:[3]

1. Everything is connected to everything else.
2. Everything must go somewhere.
3. Nature knows best.
4. There is no such thing as a free lunch.

An understanding of these four laws will be helpful in gaining an overall picture of ecosystems and their functioning.

The First Law: Everything Is Connected to Everything Else

Our planet is composed of ecosystems, or networks, containing numerous interrelated organisms. Every ecosystem consists of two major components: nonliving and living. The nonliving component includes various factors such as the sun (an outside source), wind, heat, rain, and chemicals necessary for life. The living component is usually divided into **food producers** (plants) and **food consumers.** Food consumers can be further divided into **macroconsumers** (animals) and **microconsumers,** or decomposers (bacteria and fungi).

Natural ecosystems are so complex that people often do not see or understand the entire range of connections. As William Allman points out, "The degree of complexity that scientists have so far discovered dwarfs what was imagined even a decade ago. Plankton in the sea exhale chemicals that affect the formation of clouds. Ocean currents such as the Gulf Stream act as a conveyor belt, transporting heat around the world and setting climate patterns that last for centuries at a stretch."[4]

The degree of complexity found in an ecosystem is an important factor in the

Food producers: living components of an ecosystem whose prime responsibility is to make food. Plants are considered to be the main food producers.

Food consumers: living components of an ecosystem that consume food producers. Food consumers consist of animals, bacteria, and fungi, all of which consume plant material.

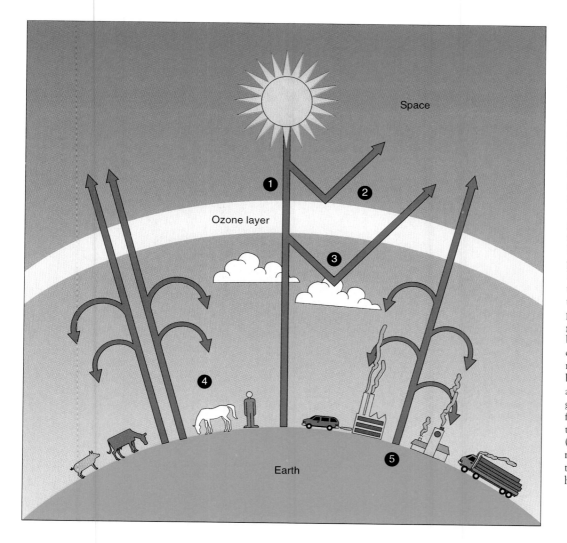

Figure 19.1
The "greenhouse effect" is a natural process that helps to keep the earth's temperature in a range hospitable to human life; it works like this. (1) The sun radiates energy toward the earth. (2) Some of the sun's harmful radiation is deflected by the stratospheric ozone layer 10 to 30 miles above the earth's surface. (3) Of the sun's radiation that passes through the ozone layer, about 30 percent is reflected back into space. (4) Carbon dioxide, and other greenhouse gases that occur in the natural environment, absorb the longer wave length radiation as it passes through to the earth. The long wave length radiation becomes trapped by greenhouse gases near the earth's surface, increasing the planet's temperature. Without the greenhouse effect, the earth would be about 54 degrees colder than our current temperature. (5) This natural process, however, has become overloaded due to the large amounts of "greenhouse gases" generated by the burning of fossil fuels, deforestation, farming, and the use of chlorofluorocarbons (CFCs) in aerosol cans and refrigerants. It is this overloading of the natural greenhouse effect that has environmentalists worried.

ecosystem's ability to cope with natural stressors that may be placed upon it. Consider the case of carbon—sometimes called the backbone of biological chemistry. Carbon, in the form of **carbon dioxide,** is one of the greenhouse gases believed to be contributing to a gradual increase in the earth's temperature. With the burning of fossil fuels, the United States alone adds almost five and one half billion tons of carbon dioxide to the environment each year.[5] Between 1972 and 1992, humans increased the atmospheric concentration of carbon dioxide 9 percent.[6] As illustrated in figure 19.1, atmospheric carbon dioxide, along with other greenhouse gases, form a "blanket" that traps energy near the earth's surface, thus causing global warming. The greenhouse effect is a potentially serious threat to life as we know it. "Even a few degrees' change in the average

temperature of the planet could make Iowa a desert and Alberta a breadbasket, and raise sea levels enough to flood Florida and the Caribbean islands."[7] Some scientists believe, however, that the earth's natural carbon cycle offers a great deal of protection. As described by Allman:

> In a cycle that takes millions of years, carbon is shifted through a series of elaborate feedback loops to counter forces of change that may arise on the planet. For example, an increase in the amount of carbon going into the atmosphere from an outburst of volcanic activity or the burning of fossil fuel will set off a series of compensating changes throughout the cycle, eventually triggering an increase in the rate that carbon is pulled out of the air,

Carbon dioxide: a heavy, colorless, odorless gas that is a byproduct of human respiration. Additionally, carbon dioxide is released into the atmosphere during the burning of fossil fuels, such as oil, gas, and coal.

The Global Balancing Act

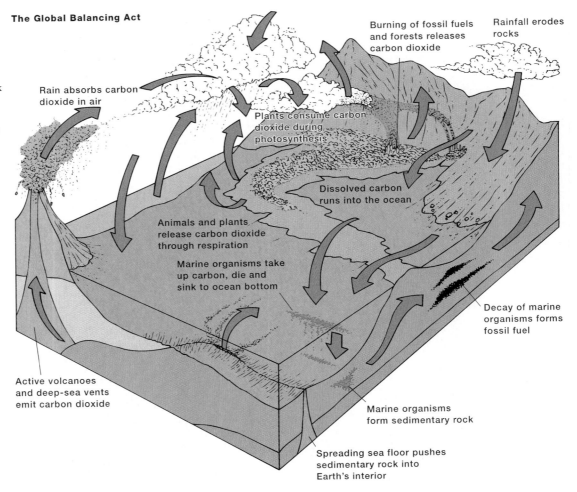

Burning of fossil fuels
and forests releases
carbon dioxide

Rainfall erodes
rocks

Rain absorbs carbon
dioxide in air

Plants consume carbon
dioxide during
photosynthesis

Dissolved carbon
runs into the ocean

Animals and plants
release carbon dioxide
through respiration

Marine organisms take
up carbon, die and
sink to ocean bottom

Decay of marine
organisms forms
fossil fuel

Active volcanoes
and deep-sea vents
emit carbon dioxide

Marine organisms
form sedimentary rock

Spreading sea floor pushes
sedimentary rock into
Earth's interior

dissolved in the ocean and turned to rock on the ocean's floor. Through this cycle, the Earth's carbon-dioxide blanket is regulated so that it keeps the Earth within a temperature range that is hospitable to life.[8] (See figure 19.2.)

Some of these changes work almost instantly, however others take millions of years. At this point in time, no one can say with certainty whether this complex carbon cycle will be able to handle the atmospheric carbon dioxide load we continue to place on it.

In the past, people often have not recognized the importance of ecosystem complexity. It is essential that we begin to view ecosystems as a whole, delineating to the best of our ability the natural interconnectedness found in varying ecosystems and the impact our personal and collective lifestyle will have on each system.

The Second Law: Everything Must Go Somewhere

One of the basic laws of physics, usually referred to as the conservation of matter, states that matter cannot be created or destroyed—it can only be transformed. In terms of ecology, this law clearly informs us that there is no "away" to throw things. Nature's cycles are a true reflection of this ecological law. In nature we find no "waste." Elements excreted by one organism serve as nourishment for another.

Industrialization has created a society based on disposable products, which are designed to be used for a short period of time and then thrown away. As Professor Philip O'Leary and his colleagues have pointed out, "The municipal solid waste produced in this country in just one day fills roughly 63,000 garbage trucks, which lined up end to end would stretch from San Francisco to Los Angeles."[9] The unfortunate illusion created

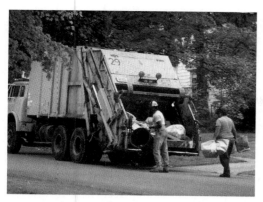

Figure 19.3: What Do You Think?

1. Where does your trash go when the garbage collector takes it "away?"
2. What percentage of your community's solid waste is landfilled? recycled? incinerated?

by this throwaway ethic is a belief that our garbage "goes away" when we set it out for the garbage collector once or twice a week. The second law of ecology, however, tells us that this is not the case (see figure 19.3).

One way to break free of the throwaway illusion is to ask two questions: Where does our waste go? and What is its impact on the ecosphere? In many instances, "away" has meant either dumps and landfills that waste valuable land and contaminate groundwater or municipal incinerators that contribute to air pollution. In any case, the waste products (matter) are not destroyed. They are instead either broken down into varying compounds, many of which are harmful to ecosystems, or in the case of nonbiodegradable waste, they accumulate at various sites on our planet where they do not belong.

The Third Law: Nature Knows Best

It has long been the view of the industrial world that one of technology's greatest merits is its ability to improve on nature. It is now apparent, however, that this may have been an extremely shortsighted view. As Barry Commoner notes in his book *Making Peace with the Planet*, "It is an unbroken rule that for every organic compound produced by a living thing, there is somewhere in the ecosystem an enzyme capable of breaking it down. Organic compounds incapable of enzymatic degradation are not produced by living things. This arrangement is essential to the harmony of the ecosystem."[10] Technology, on the other hand, has repeatedly been responsible for the creation of organic substances that cannot be broken down. Often these **nonbiodegradable** products of technology have created havoc in diverse ecosystems (see Of Special Interest 19.1).

Consider the case of **DDT,** a synthetic chlorinated insecticide that kills insects by attacking biochemical processes in their nervous systems. DDT was hailed as a technological triumph for some years, until Rachel Carson's noteworthy contribution, *Silent Spring.*[11] Carson's book, published in 1962, pointed out the ecological impact of such pesticides on food, wildlife, and humanity.

DDT is a persistent pesticide, sometimes remaining in the environment for as long as fifteen years before degrading. Although DDT is successful for short-term eradication of many pests, it poses several major problems. When sprayed to kill insect pests, DDT also kills the natural predators of that pest. This killing of a broad range of insects tends to simplify ecosystems artificially. Additionally, many insect pests are capable of rapid adaptation, resulting in genetic resistance to DDT. According to the World Health Organization, fifty-one species of malarial mosquitoes have a known resistance to DDT and other similar insecticides.[12] Fish, birds, and other wildlife that consume DDT-infested insects and other contaminated organisms are also affected, often in terms of their ability to reproduce.

An equally disturbing fact is that DDT, which is soluble in fats, has been routinely found in humans.[13] The long-term effects of DDT in humans is inconclusive at this time; however, DDT appears to be a potent cancer promoter.[14] Two recent studies completed in the United States have implicated DDT as a risk factor for breast cancer in women.[15]

In 1972, due in large part to the work of Rachel Carson and other scientists who brought these problems to public attention, the **Environmental Protection Agency (EPA)** banned the use of DDT in the U.S. DDT, however, is still manufactured in the U.S. and is then shipped abroad to underdeveloped nations.[16] When used as pesticides in these underdeveloped nations, DDT continues to poison people, animals, and the environment. Thus, a circle of poison is established as DDT-contaminated products such as coffee, tea,

Nonbiodegradable: substances that do not decay and are not absorbed by the environment.

Environmental Protection Agency (EPA): a federal agency created in 1970 whose major role is to consider and effectively deal with the major environmental problems facing the United States.

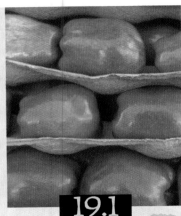

The Degradable Plastics Debate

In theory, one way to make plastics more friendly to the environment would be to produce "degradable" plastics that would gradually decompose into simple molecules such as water and carbon dioxide. If plastics could be broken down either by sunlight (photodegradation) or by microbes (biodegradation), they would pose less of a litter problem and be less harmful in the oceans. When several companies announced in the late 1980s that they had developed biodegradable plastics made with corn starch, consumers were enthusiastic—at first. Garbage bags and diapers labeled "degradable" quickly found a market. Some magazines switched from standard polyethylene mailing bags to bags purported to be degradable.

But the claims of biodegradability were soon challenged. Tests of products made from the new plastic demonstrated that on land, even under ideal conditions, the plastic merely weakened or broke into small pieces, with no appreciable benefit to the environment. And the plastic did not degrade in seawater.

The EPA has said that degradable plastics do not reduce the volume or toxicity of solid waste, partly because the plastics do not degrade completely, and partly because degradable plastics may be weaker than other plastics. That means using more plastic in some products. (Considering the slow degradation rates of organic wastes in today's landfills, even truly degradable plastics may not provide much benefit if landfilled.)

So-called degradable plastics also could derail efforts to prevent littering and to encourage source reduction and recycling by giving people the false impression that plastics disposal is no longer a problem. In addition, the constituents that make plastics more "degradable" make the resins less suitable for recycling. These plastics would have to be treated differently from other plastics in recycling programs, creating added headaches in collection, separation, and processing.

At present, it does not appear that degradable plastics will play a significant role in helping to address the MSW (municiple solid waste) crisis. Only a very few plastics have proven to be completely degradable, and these are expensive and limited to special applications such as soluble surgical threads and protective root coverings for tree seedlings.

The situation could change in the future. The plastics and agriculture industries continue to work on developing truly degradable plastics—partly in response to pressure from state and local governments. For example, 24 states require that six-pack connector rings be degradable. Several companies are researching and developing plastics made from corn, wheat, and rice starches that could begin to fulfill the early promise of degradable plastics. If a new generation of degradable plastics appears, questions regarding the safety of the by-products of the degradation process and the fate of additives such as colorants would need to be answered.

Reprinted from *The Plastic Waste Primer: A Handbook for Citizens,* by The League of Women Voters, by arrangement with the publisher, Lyons & Burford Publishers, 39 West 21st St., New York, NY 10010. Copyright © 1993 The League of Women Voters.

What Do You Think?

1. Do you think we should be using nonrenewable resources to produce plastic products that we use only once for a short period of time? Explain your rationale.
2. What types of "source reduction" strategies could you implement to help you cut down on the use of plastics?

---

bananas, and sugar are shipped back to the U.S. for purchase by the consumer.

The pesticide DDT is only one among many threats to the environment. Any changes people make in the ecosphere are likely to be detrimental to the system. If we are to survive on this planet, we must begin today to cultivate an attitude that regards humanity as a part of nature. We can no longer afford to believe that people can escape from a dependence on the natural environment through technological innovation. We continue on this track only at our own peril.

The Fourth Law: There Is No Such Thing as a Free Lunch

Economic theory provides a sound base for the fourth law of ecology and tells us that for every technological gain there exists an ecological price tag. As is often the case with technological advances, the ecological cost can be delayed for a time. Ultimately, however, it must be paid. This "payment" takes many forms, ranging from actual economic costs to a more qualitative cost in terms of perceived human well-being.

We are now beginning to pay the price for many of the past technological advances that have contributed greatly to the current U.S. standard of living. Automobiles, for instance, have had a tremendous impact on the availability and accessibility of many consumer goods and services. Although more options are available for us in terms of where we choose to work, shop, and play, these options tend to be geographically dispersed. We "need" to drive

1. **Reduce human exposure to criteria air pollutants (ozone, carbon monoxide, nitrogen dioxide, sulfur dioxide, particulates, and lead), as measured by an increase to at least 85 percent in the proportion of people who live in counties that have not exceeded any Environmental Protection Agency standard for air quality in the previous 12 months.** (Update: 78.4 percent in 1992, up from 48.7 in 1988.)

2. **Increase to at least 40 percent the proportion of homes in which homeowners/occupants have tested for radon concentrations and that have either been found to pose minimal risk or have been modified to reduce risk to health.** (Update: 7.4 percent of homes in 1991, up from less than 5 percent in 1989.)

3. **Reduce human exposure to toxic agents by confining total pounds of toxic agents released into the air, water, and soil each year to no more than: 0.24 billion pounds of those toxic agents included on the Department of Health and Human Service's list of carcinogens** (Update: 0.23 billion pounds in 1991, down from 0.48 billion pounds in 1988); **2.6 billion pounds of those toxic agents included on the Agency for Toxic Substances and Disease Registry list of the most toxic chemicals** (Update: 2.16 billion pounds for the 200 most toxic chemicals in 1991, down from 3.5 billion pounds in 1988; 2.70 billion pounds for the 250 most toxic chemicals in 1991, down from 4.48 billion pounds in 1988.)

4. **Reduce human exposure to solid waste-related water, air, and soil contamination, as measured by a reduction in average pounds of municipal solid waste produced per person each day to no more than 3.6 pounds.** (Update: 4.3 pounds per person each day in 1990, up from 4.0 in 1988.)

5. **Increase to at least 85 percent the proportion of people who receive a supply of drinking water that meets the safe drinking water standards established by the Environmental Protection Agency.** (Update: 72 percent of 58,099 community water systems serving approximately 80 percent of the population in 1992, down from 73 percent in 1988.)

6. **Reduce potential risks to human health from surface water, as measured by a decrease to no more than 15 percent in the proportion of assessed rivers, lakes, and estuaries that do not support beneficial uses, such as fishing and swimming.** (Update: 38 percent of rivers, 44 percent of lakes, and 32 percent of estuaries did not support beneficial uses in 1992, up from 30 percent, 27 percent and 29 percent respectively in 1988.)

7. **Eliminate significant health risks from National Priority List hazardous waste sites, as measured by performance of clean-up at these sites sufficient to eliminate immediate and significant health threats as specified in health assessments completed at all sites.** (Update: 1,199 sites were on the list, health assessments have been conducted on 1,452 sites, and 283 sites were listed as public health concerns/hazards in 1992, up from 1,079 sites, 1,379 assessments, and 250 health hazards in 1990.)

8. **Establish programs for recyclable materials and household hazardous waste in at least 75 percent of counties.** (Update: 802 permanent and temporary household hazardous waste recycling programs in 1991, up from 300 programs in 1987; 50 states had at least one program in 1991, up from 28 states in 1987.)

Source: Data from *Healthy People 2000 National Health Promotion and Disease Prevention Objectives,* 1991; and from *Healthy People 2000 Review 1993,* 1994. Department of Health and Human Services, Washington, D.C.

great distances to make use of our options. The ecological price tag attached to our cars is now evident in almost every large city. We find photochemical smog accompanied by nitrogen oxides, hydrocarbons, and **asbestos** particles from brake linings. These and other substances emitted by automobiles have been seriously implicated in disease processes ranging from lung cancer to acute respiratory infections. In addition to the health costs, we have the tremendous economic costs of cleaning our environment and then trying to prevent further deterioration.

As we delay paying ecological costs, the price tag on our environment increases—with interest. If current trends continue, it appears that future generations will be the ones to pay the largest price for our current technological advances. If we are to prevent this mortgaging of future generations we must begin today to ask an important question regarding every human endeavor: Is it worth what it costs?

The number and complexity of environmental problems that we face today, as a planet, preclude us from providing you with a comprehensive coverage of environmental issues here. Instead, we will focus on teaching you to apply the laws of ecology to environmental health concerns. We believe that being able to process, in a meaningful way, the wealth of environmental health information currently available to consumers, is one of the most important skills we could teach. The U.S. Government has delineated several environmental health problems as focus areas in its *Healthy People 2000* report (see table 19.1). We will focus on applying the

Asbestos: a flame-retardant material, used for insulation and other construction, that has been implicated as a factor in the etiology of certain lung diseases.

Source: Data from Jon Naar, *Design for a
Livable Planet*, p. 80, 1990, HarperCollins
Publishing, New York, NY.

Effects of Air Pollution on the Human Body

Dizziness

Headache/migraine

Irritation of eyes

Stuffy nose, sneezing, nasal discharge

Nausea, vomiting

Coughing, sore throat, colds, laryngitis

Constricted airway, asthma,
bronchitis, shortness of breath,
emphysema, chest pains,
pneumonia, lung cancer

Heart disease

Stomach poisoning, stomach cancer

Diseases of blood vessels

Kidney damage

Allergies

laws of ecology to two of these problem
areas—air pollution and toxic waste.

Applying the Laws of Ecology to Air Pollution

Air pollution has been recognized as a
significant health threat for many years. As part
of the Clean Air Act of 1970, the
Environmental Protection Agency (EPA) set
performance standards for and began to monitor
six criteria pollutants (see table 19.2). However,
in spite of the changes required by the Clean Air
Act, air pollution continues to cause health and
environmental problems of great magnitude.

As of 1990, "at least 74 million people
lived in areas that still exceeded at least one
air quality standard. According to the EPA,
as many as 140 million people may have lived
in areas that had ozone levels, or smog, in
excess of national standards during that
year."[17] Air pollutants are associated with a
number of health problems, including lung

cancer, respiratory infections, and heart
disease (see figure 19.4). The American Lung
Association estimates that human exposure
to outdoor air pollution results in health costs
of between $40 and $50 billion a year.
Additionally, they estimate that 50,000 to
120,000 premature deaths are associated with
air pollution each year.[18]

Progress has been made on some fronts.
Lead levels, for instance, have decreased 96
percent since the 1970 Clean Air Act was
enacted. A major factor in this decline was the
switch from leaded to lead-free gasoline to fuel
automobiles. The U.S. has not, however, been
able to meet the 90 percent improvements
mandated by the Clean Air Act for any of the
other criteria air pollutants.[19]

Two of the criteria air pollutants have
received a great deal of attention in recent
years because their release into the
atmosphere results in **acid rain.** The problem
of acid rain can be more easily understood
when analyzed using the laws of ecology.

Acid rain: precipitation with a pH
below 5.6, which is formed when sulfur
dioxide and nitrous oxides are released
into the atmosphere and combine with
water droplets. Acid rain is known to
harm fish, plants, and humans.

TABLE 19.2 — The Common Air Pollutants (Criteria Air Pollutants) of the Clean Air Act

Name	Source	Health Effects	Environmental Effects	Property Damage
Ozone (ground-level ozone is the principal component of smog)	chemical reaction of pollutants; VOCs and NOx	breathing problems, reduced lung function, asthma, irritates eyes, stuffy nose, reduced resistance to colds and other infections, may speed up aging of lung tissue	ozone can damage plants and trees; smog can cause reduced visibility	damages rubber, fabrics, etc.
VOCs* (volatile organic compounds); smog-formers	VOCs are released from burning fuel (gasoline, oil, wood, coal, natural gas, etc.), solvents, paints, glues and other products used at work or at home. Cars are an important source of VOCs. VOCs include chemicals such as benzene, toluene, methylene chloride and methyl chloroform	In addition to ozone (smog) effects, many VOCs can cause serious health problems such as cancer and other effects	In addition to ozone (smog) effects, some VOCs such as formaldehyde and ethylene may harm plants	
Nitrogen Dioxide (one of the NOx); smog-forming chemical	burning of gasoline, natural gas, coal, oil, etc. Cars are an important source of NO_2	lung damage, illnesses of breathing passages and lungs (respiratory system)	nitrogen dioxide is an ingredient of acid rain (acid aerosols), which can damage trees and lakes. Acid aerosols can reduce visibility	acid aerosols can eat away stone used on buildings, statues, monuments, etc.
Carbon Monoxide (CO)	burning of gasoline, wood, natural gas, coal, oil, etc.	reduces ability of blood to bring oxygen to body cells and tissues; cells and tissues need oxygen to work. Carbon monoxide may be particularly hazardous to people who have heart or circulatory (blood vessel) problems and people who have damaged lungs or breathing passages		
Particulate Matter (PM-10); (dust, smoke, soot)	burning of wood, diesel and other fuels; industrial plants; agriculture (plowing, burning off fields); unpaved roads	nose and throat irritation, lung damage, bronchitis, early death	particulates are the main source of haze that reduces visibility	ashes, soots, smokes and dusts can dirty and discolor structures and other property, including clothes and furniture
Sulfur Dioxide	burning of coal and oil, especially high-sulfur coal from the eastern United States; industrial processes (paper, metals)	breathing problems, may cause permanent damage to lungs	SO_2 is an ingredient in acid rain (acid aerosols), which can damage trees and lakes. Acid aerosols can also reduce visibility	acid aerosols can eat away stone used in buildings, statues, monuments, etc.
Lead	leaded gasoline (being phased out), paint (houses, cars), smelters (metal refineries); manufacture of lead storage batteries	brain and other nervous system damage; children are at special risk. Some lead-containing chemicals cause cancer in animals. Lead causes digestive and other health problems	Lead can harm wildlife	

*All VOCs contain carbon (C), the basic chemical element found in living beings. Carbon-containing chemicals are called *organic. Volatile* chemicals escape into the air easily. Many VOCs, such as the chemicals listed in the table, are also *hazardous air pollutants,* which can cause very serious illnesses. EPA does not list VOCs as criteria air pollutants, but they are included in this list of pollutants because efforts to control smog target VOCs for reduction.

From *The Plain English Guide to The Clean Air Act,* April, 1993. United States Environmental Protection Agency.

Figure 19.5: Acid rain.
The simple term "acid rain"
describes a complex mix of both wet
and dry chemical reactions, and
hides the fact that many different
factors combine to produce the
devastating effects that we see
today. Sulphur dioxide (SO_2) and
nitrous oxides (NO_x), released by
our modern industries, begin the
process that ends with the death of
trees and fish. Trees are not killed
directly by the acid, but by toxic
metals that it releases and by lack of
nutrients destroyed or washed away
by the rain. Nor are sensitive fish,
such as trout and salmon, killed by
acid alone, but by an acid-
metal mix.

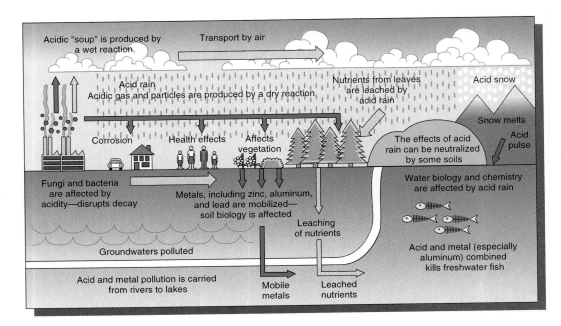

Everything Is Connected to Everything Else

The problem of acid rain begins when **sulfur dioxide** (SO_2) and **nitrous oxides** (NO_x) are released into the atmosphere through the smoke stacks of power plants and industry, and the tail pipes of automobiles (see figure 19.5). Coal-burning electric power plants are responsible for about 70 percent of the sulfur dioxide emissions, while automobiles contribute the largest share of nitrous oxide (about 40 percent).[20] When SO_2 and NO_X come in contact with water they are converted to sulfuric acid and nitric acid respectively. These acids are carried in water droplets or air particles and eventually fall to earth as acid precipitation (rain, snow, and particles).

As you can see in figure 19.5, everything *is* connected to everything else. Acid precipitation follows the natural connections in the ecosystem increasing the acidity of surface and underground water supplies, and damaging both living and nonliving components.

Everything Must Go Somewhere

Industrial processes have long been known for their generation of pollution. Yet, the widespread effects of acid rain have come to our attention over the past twenty years. The second law of ecology helps explain why acid rain is a relatively recent problem.

In the 1960s and 1970s it was painfully clear that many fossil fuel burning industries were causing health problems in their local environments. Thus, in order to solve local air pollution problems industry leaders developed a policy that proclaimed "the solution to pollution is dilution."[21] Power plants and other industry decided that they could get rid of their air pollution problem by building taller smoke stacks that sent the unwanted gases higher into the atmosphere, away from their cities, where they assumed the air pollutants would be safely diluted and dispersed (see figure 19.6). Unfortunately, as the laws of ecology note, there is no *away* to throw things.

Sulfur dioxide and nitrous oxides are carried by the prevailing winds for hundreds or thousands of miles, finally falling to earth as acid rain. This "solution" has created a new set of problems, international in scope (see figure 19.7). Industrial emissions from the U.S., for example, have been carried by the prevailing winds to Canada where they have caused great damage to the environment. One of the most notable effects is the acidification of Canadian lakes, killing fish and other wildlife and damaging the tourist industry—an extremely important economic loss. If only someone had thought about the laws of ecology and asked themselves where these gases would go and what the effects would be!

Nature Knows Best

The third law of ecology reminds us that human-made alterations in natural cycles will result in problems. This is surely the case with acid rain.

Pure water has a pH value of 7, the neutral point on the acid-alkaline scale

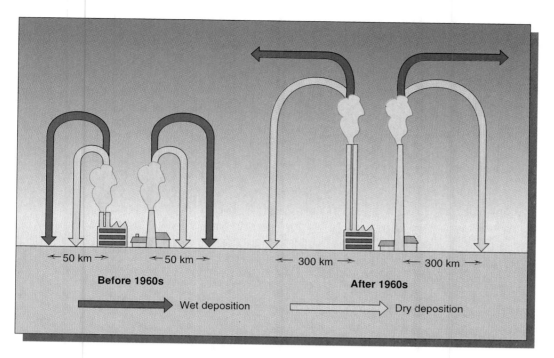

Figure 19.6: Dispersing the problem.
Before the 1960s, smoke from industries polluted their immediate environment. In an attempt to improve the intolerable living conditions created, chimney heights were increased, the view being that the pollutants would thus be dispersed harmlessly in the atmosphere. The result of that miscalculation was international acid rain.

← 50 km → ← 50 km →   ← 300 km →   ← 300 km →

Before 1960s   **After 1960s**

━━━━━━▶ Wet deposition   ───────▷ Dry deposition

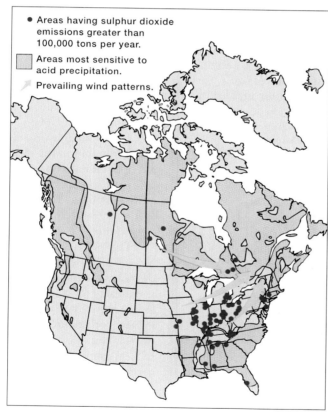

- Areas having sulphur dioxide emissions greater than 100,000 tons per year.

  Areas most sensitive to acid precipitation.

  Prevailing wind patterns.

Figure 19.7: The impact of acid rain in the U.S. and Canada

"Map Depicting the Impact of Acid Rain in U.S. and Canada" from *Design For a Livable Planet*, by Jon Naar. Copyright © 1990 by Jon Naar. Reprinted by permission of HarperCollins Publishers, Inc.

(see figure 19.8). As certain gases, such as sulfur dioxide and nitrous oxides, mix with water vapor in the atmosphere, the pH value becomes more acidic. Normal rain is slightly acidic, measuring 5.6 on the pH scale. Precipitation with a pH below 5.6 is defined as acid precipitation. Some acidic precipitation occurs naturally. It can be triggered by forest fires and volcanic eruptions, for instance.[22] The ecosystem can deal with this level of acid precipitation. Nature has provided natural buffers in some

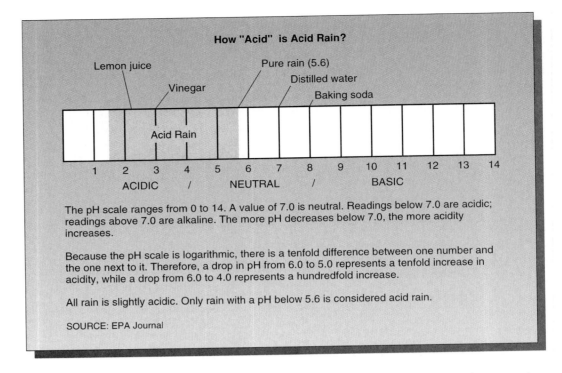

How "Acid" is Acid Rain?

Lemon juice
Vinegar
Acid Rain
Pure rain (5.6)
Distilled water
Baking soda

1 2 3 4 5 6 7 8 9 10 11 12 13 14

ACIDIC / NEUTRAL / BASIC

The pH scale ranges from 0 to 14. A value of 7.0 is neutral. Readings below 7.0 are acidic; readings above 7.0 are alkaline. The more pH decreases below 7.0, the more acidity increases.

Because the pH scale is logarithmic, there is a tenfold difference between one number and the one next to it. Therefore, a drop in pH from 6.0 to 5.0 represents a tenfold increase in acidity, while a drop from 6.0 to 4.0 represents a hundredfold increase.

All rain is slightly acidic. Only rain with a pH below 5.6 is considered acid rain.

SOURCE: EPA Journal

areas that counteract the acidity.[23] Alkaline soil and limestone or sandstone lake beds are examples of natural buffers. These natural buffers, however, cannot handle the magnitude of acid precipitation created by our widespread burning of fossil fuels. Human activity has overwhelmed the natural system.

There Is No Such Thing as a Free Lunch

The fourth law of ecology tells us that for every technological advance there is an ecological price tag. One of the prices of our fossil fuel burning ways is acid rain (see figure 19.5). The price tag for damage in the U.S. is estimated to be at least $10 billion a year.[24]

Possibly the most visible damage from acid rain is the corrosion of architectural structures around the world. In Athens, Greece, the Parthenon and other monuments are threatened.[25] Worldwide, acid rain has the potential to destroy many historical treasures that have existed for thousands of years. Corrosion caused by acid rain can have safety ramifications as well. In Silesia, Poland, trains have had to slow down to 25 mph due to the erosion of railroad tracks.[26]

One of the most widely publicized effects of acid rain is the acidification of lakes making them incapable of sustaining life. Acid precipitation may fall directly into lakes.

Additionally, it may move through the soil leaching metals, such as aluminum, lead and zinc, eventually reaching **groundwater,** rivers, and lakes. It is the combination of metals, such as aluminum, and acidic water that is thought to kill sensitive fish. In acidic water, the "aluminum precipitates in their gills as aluminum hydroxide, reducing the oxygen content in the blood and causing internal salt imbalances."[27] When sensitive fish, such as salmon, trout, and minnows die, it oversimplifies the lake's ecosystem, eventually resulting in lakes that cannot support life.

The health effects of acid rain have become increasingly documented as research continues on the effects of acid rain. Dr. Philip Landrigan, professor of community medicine and pediatrics at Mt. Sinai School of Medicine in New York, estimates that acid rain may be the third leading cause of lung cancer in the U.S., following only active and passive cigarette smoking.[28] Other researchers have found that the increasing level of sulfate and nitrate pollution correlates with increasing hospitalization rates for heart and lung disease.[29] Recent studies have also found that acidic aerosols increase the severity of **asthma.**[30] Additionally, health professionals are concerned that acidic drinking water is corroding water pipes, leading to metal levels in our drinking water higher than EPA safety

Groundwater: water from wells, springs, and large underground reservoirs called aquifers. Groundwater is the major source of drinking water for over half of the U.S. population.

Asthma: a chronic condition often of allergic origin, marked by labored breathing, wheezing, constriction of the chest, gasping, or coughing.

TABLE 19.3 — Common Products that Contribute to Hazardous Waste

The Products We Use	The Potentially Hazardous Waste They Generate. . . .
Plastics	Organic chlorine compounds, organic solvents
Pesticides	Organic chlorine compounds, organic phosphate compounds
Medicines	Organic solvents and residues, heavy metals (mercury and zinc, for example)
Paints	Heavy metals, pigments, solvents, organic residues
Oil, gasoline, and other petroleum products	Oil, phenols and other organic compounds, heavy metals, ammonia, salt acids, caustics
Metals	Heavy metals, fluorides, cyanides, acid and alkaline cleaners, solvents, pigments, abrasives, plating salts, oils, phenols
Leather	Heavy metals, organic solvents
Textiles	Heavy metals, dyes, organic chlorine compounds, solvents

Source: Data from the Office of Solid Waste, U.S. Environmental Protection Agency, 1980.

standards.[31] Long-term ingestion of water polluted with toxic metals has been associated with **Alzheimer's** and **Parkinson's disease,** high blood pressure, kidney damage, and brain damage.[32] Children may be especially vulnerable to these toxic metal concentrations.

Clearly, the medical, economic, social, and emotional costs of acid rain are high. We must, as individual's and as a society, begin to ask ourselves if our current use of fossil fuels is worth what it costs.

Applying the Laws of Ecology to Hazardous Waste

In the late 1970s several communities came to the attention of the nation as they were found to be contaminated with hazardous waste. In Love Canal, New York, toxic chemicals that had been buried for over twenty-five years were found to have contaminated the ground and to have seeped into many basements. Eventually 900 families were evacuated from their homes. In another community—Times Beach, Missouri—oil, unknowingly contaminated with **dioxin,** was spread on dirt roads to keep the dust down. It was later discovered that both the soil and groundwater in Times Beach were contaminated with dioxin, a potent carcinogen. Once again, residents had to be

evacuated from their homes. Today, Times Beach, Missouri is a toxic ghost town.

Incidents such as Love Canal and Times Beach have brought the attention of the nation to focus on the problems of hazardous waste. **Hazardous waste** is defined by the Environmental Protection Agency as "Solid waste (any garbage, refuse, sludge or other discarded material—including liquid, semisolid, solid or contained gaseous material) that because of its quantity, concentration, or physical, chemical or infectious characteristics, may pose a hazard to human health or the environment."[33] The EPA is particularly concerned with four potential hazards—waste that may be ignitable, corrosive, explosive, or toxic.

The public health problems associated with the use and disposal of hazardous substances are numerous and complex. Barry Commoner's Laws of Ecology give us a framework with which to understand the risks associated with hazardous waste.

Everything Is Connected to Everything Else

A great deal of our hazardous waste problem can be traced to the production and consumption of a variety of substances including plastics, pesticides, medicines, paints, leather, textiles, and petroleum products such as oil and gasoline (see table 19.3). The manufacturing process creates the

Alzheimer's disease: a chronic condition physically characterized by structural modifications in the brain's nerve fibers and giving rise to mental infirmity, which is behaviorally manifested by memory loss, hallucinations, and social disorientation.

Parkinson's disease: a chronic, progressive, condition affecting some middle-aged and elderly people, characterized by tremors in the hands, arms, and legs.

Dioxin: the common name for 2, 3, 7, 8-tetrachlorodibenzo (p)dioxin, a potent carcinogen often found in incinerator ash.

Figure 19.9: Hazardous
substances in
your home

From William P. Cunningham and Barbara
Woodward Saigo, *Environmental Science*,
2nd edition. Copyright © 1992 Wm. C.
Brown Communications, Inc. Reprinted by
permission of Times Mirror Higher Education
Group, Inc., Dubuque, Iowa. All Rights
Reserved.

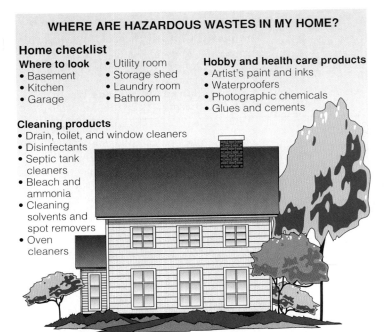

WHERE ARE HAZARDOUS WASTES IN MY HOME?

Home checklist

Where to look
- Basement
- Kitchen
- Garage
- Utility room
- Storage shed
- Laundry room
- Bathroom

Hobby and health care products
- Artist's paint and inks
- Waterproofers
- Photographic chemicals
- Glues and cements

Cleaning products
- Drain, toilet, and window cleaners
- Disinfectants
- Septic tank cleaners
- Bleach and ammonia
- Cleaning solvents and spot removers
- Oven cleaners

Automotive products
- Antifreeze
- Solvents
- Battery acid
- Gasoline
- Rust inhibitor, remover
- Used motor oil
- Brake and transmission fluid

Paint/building products
- Paint thinners, strippers and solvents
- Spray cans
- Lacquers, stains and varnishes
- Wood preservatives
- Acids for etching
- Asphalt and roof tar
- Latex and oil-based paints

Gardening/pest control products
- Sprays and dusts
- Ant and rodent killers
- Flea powder
- Weed killers
- Banned pesticides

bulk of the hazardous waste; however, some products such as pesticides and certain household cleaning substances also create a hazard when used and disposed of by consumers (see figure 19.9).

One of the biggest concerns about hazardous waste disposal is the contamination of groundwater, which is the major source of drinking water for over half of the population in the U.S. and for 95 percent of the U.S. rural population.[34] Groundwater contamination also affects plants, animals, fish and other wildlife. As illustrated in figure 19.10, there are many routes taken by hazardous waste that end in groundwater contamination. **Pesticides** and fertilizers, for instance, are sprayed on farmland to increase crop yield and on our lawns to keep them green and free of pests. Often these pesticides and fertilizers end up in our groundwater as they seep through the soil. In fact, the EPA reports that by 1991, groundwater in most states had been contaminated by 132 different pesticides.[35] Ruth Caplan, in her book *Our Earth,*

Ourselves, challenges us to look for the hazardous waste connections in our everyday life.

For every product in your home, in the supermarket, or in a hardware store, think all the way back to where it came from and all the way forward to where it will end up. Pick up a can of bug spray. Think back: Every pesticide manufacturing plant in the United States is emitting dangerous materials into the air, land, and water. Think forward: Your nearly empty can will end up with millions of others in leaking landfills or polluting incinerators. And don't forget that the actual use of this poison is endangering your health as it settles on your skin and in your lungs. . . . In our intricately connected 'web of life,' all these chemicals sooner or later turn up in the air, soil, groundwater, rivers, lakes, and oceans as well as in our food and ultimately our bodies.[36]

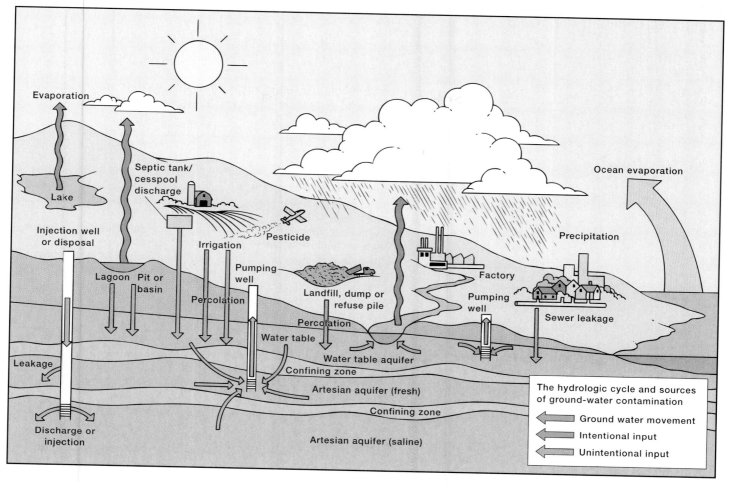

Labels within the figure:

Evaporation

Septic tank/
cesspool
discharge

Ocean evaporation

Lake

Injection well
or disposal

Precipitation

Pesticide

Irrigation

Lagoon | Pit or
basin

Pumping
well

Factory

Percolation

Landfill, dump or
refuse pile

Pumping
well

Leakage

Percolation

Water table

Sewer leakage

Water table aquifer

Confining zone

Discharge or
injection

Artesian aquifer (fresh)

Confining zone

Artesian aquifer (saline)

The hydrologic cycle and sources
of ground-water contamination

Ground water movement

Intentional input

Unintentional input

Everything Must Go Somewhere

Many of the daily conveniences of life are products of the chemical industry. From the styrofoam cup you use to drink a soft drink, to the substances used to dry clean your clothes, to the drugs used to treat you when you are ill, chemicals play a starring role. Yet the manufacturing of such products creates at least 700,000 tons of **toxic** (poisonous) **waste** each day in the U.S.[37] Additional toxic waste is created as the products are used. Where do these toxic wastes go, and what is their effect on the ecosystem when they get there?

Chemical industries dispose of toxic waste in a number of ways; yet, as the second law of ecology tells us, there is really no "away" to throw things. This is especially true of hazardous waste. Most of the disposal methods currently used for hazardous waste threaten our groundwater supply, a natural resource essential for life (see figure 19.10). For a number of years the most common means of disposal was to dump hazardous

waste into pits, ponds, and lagoons. This method is now known to be one of the worst possible ways to deal with hazardous waste in terms of groundwater pollution. Other common disposal methods include **"Secure" landfills** that have a clay and plastic liner, **injection wells** that allow hazardous waste to be pumped into underground wells, and **incineration** which results in toxic air emissions and toxic ash. All of these methods threaten our groundwater with contamination. A 1987 review of what the EPA considers to be the 1,000 worst hazardous waste sites revealed that 80 percent of the sites were leaking toxins into the groundwater.[38]

Not all hazardous wastes end up in hazardous waste sites. Consumers often throw out paint thinner, nail polish remover, and other containers with hazardous waste residues, along with their other "garbage." These hazardous wastes then end up in landfills and incinerators that were never meant to handle hazardous materials. This

Figure 19.10: Sources of ground-water contamination

Source: Data from *Environmental Progress and Challenges: EPA's Update*. U.S. Environmental Protection Agency Publication No. EPA-230-07-88-033, p. 53, August 1988.

Secure landfills: excavated trenches or depressions in the land that are lined with clay and a plastic liner in order to prevent the leakage of hazardous waste from the landfill site.

Injection wells: deep wells, located below groundwater sources, used to store hazardous waste. The effects of such wells on drinking water contamination are debated by both industry and environmentalists.

Incineration: the use of combustion (burning) to dispose of waste.

TABLE 19.4   *Getting Rid of Household Hazardous Wastes*

This is a sampling of the types of products containing chemicals that, when disposed of improperly, can add toxins to our waste stream and water systems.

Product	Hazardous components	Disposal
Plastics	Organic chlorine compounds, organic solvents	Recycle when possible
Pesticides	Organic chlorine compounds, organic phosphate compounds	Use all/share; store for hazardous waste collection
Medicines	Organic solvents and residues, traces of heavy metals	Small amounts down drain
Paints	Heavy metals, pigments, solvents, organic residues	Share, recycle; store for hazardous waste collection
Oil, gasoline; other petroleum products	Oil, phenols and other organic compounds, heavy metals, ammonia, salt acids, caustics	Recycle at approved facility; take to hazardous waste collection site
Metals	Heavy metals, organic solvents, pigments, abrasives, plating salts, oils, phenols	Recycle
Leather	Heavy metals, organic solvents	Reuse; give away
Textiles	Heavy metals, dyes, organic chlorine compounds, solvents	Reuse; give away
Auto batteries	Sulfuric acid, lead	Take to service station or reclamation center
Household batteries	Mercury, zinc, silver, lithium, cadmium	Take to reclamation center or battery store that collects them; keep safely at home until community collection is organized

For more information on the safe disposal of specific products, contact your city or county waste department or the U.S. Environmental Protection Agency, toll free (800) 424–9346. One private firm providing such information is the Environmental Hazards Management Institute, 10 Newmarket Road, P.O. Box 932, Durham, NH 03824; (603) 868–1496, or (800) 446–5256.

poses additional threats to our groundwater and air. Consumers can protect the environment from hazardous waste by cutting down on the number of hazardous substances they use (see table 19.4) and by disposing of hazardous waste in an appropriate manner. Many local governments have established household hazardous waste collection days where citizens can bring such materials to be disposed of in a more controlled and appropriate manner.

The location of hazardous waste disposal sites has recently generated great controversy. Citizens who are threatened with having a hazardous waste landfill or incinerator built in their community have begun to protest in great numbers, taking a NIMBY (Not In My Back Yard) stand. Yet, whose backyards are these facilities currently in? Recent studies indicate that rural, poor communities of color are the most likely sites for hazardous waste disposal.[39] As Alan Durning points out in his paper "Ending Poverty,"[40]

> Three fourths of hazardous waste landfills in the American Southeast are in low-income, black neighborhoods, and more than half of all black and Hispanic Americans live in communities with at least one toxic waste site. In the United States, . . . the rich get richer, and the poor get poisoned.

It is not, however, only the poor in the U.S. who are in danger of contamination from hazardous waste. As U.S. citizens become more vocal against the location of hazardous waste sites in this country, U.S. industries have looked to other countries for hazardous waste disposal. The poor in developing nations are often the new targets for hazardous waste disposal. According to Greenpeace, between 1968 and 1988 more than 3.6 million tons of hazardous waste was shipped from the U.S. to third world countries.[41] Environmentalists note that hazardous waste disposal is much cheaper in developing countries, where there is often an acceptance of such wastes as a means to improve their economies. Some question whether the governments and peoples of these countries understand the environmental and health costs involved in hazardous waste disposal.[42] Clearly, the peoples of the world need to begin to ask themselves where we will put the tons of hazardous waste generated each day, and what the consequences of this action will be.

Nature Knows Best

Many of the hazardous waste materials creating health and environmental problems today are the result of human innovation. Humans set out to create new chemical compounds, and have been extremely successful in reaching that goal. It has been estimated that there are "roughly 12,000 chemical manufacturing plants producing over 70,000 different chemicals, including 37,000 types of pesticides."[43] Most of these chemicals have not been adequately tested for safety, and many are suspected of posing serious threats to human health.

The EPA has stated that, in terms of groundwater contamination, their "major concern is with man-made toxic chemicals such as the synthetic organic chemicals that are pervasive in plastics, solvents, pesticides, paints, dyes, varnishes, and ink."[44] Taking pesticides as an example, it is easy to see that humans have gone outside the natural cycle with our reliance on hazardous chemicals.

Human-made pesticides are now widely used in the U.S. to control insects and weeds. These pesticides contaminate our food sources and our groundwater. Additionally, studies have shown that the targeted insects and weeds develop a resistance to these chemicals, often rendering our chemical-based pest control efforts ineffective, yet leaving a source of poison in our environment. There is, however, a natural method of pest control called **Integrated Pest Management.** With this method, farmers rely on insect predators, crop rotation, mulching, and other planting techniques, as well as natural chemicals such as nicotine and garlic, to control pests. Following the natural cycle allows us to avoid much of the hazardous waste generation and groundwater contamination so prevalent with pesticide use.

There Is No Such Thing as a Free Lunch

One of the greatest costs of our "hazardous chemical" lifestyle is its many threats to health. No one knows for certain what the effects of chronic exposure to a variety of toxins are; however, cancer, neurobehavioral damage, and birth defects are of special concern (see table 19.5).

Another tremendous cost of our reliance on hazardous materials is the money spent to clean up abandoned hazardous waste dumps. In 1980, the federal government enacted the Comprehensive Environmental Response, Compensation, and Liability Act, which created a $1.6 billion, five-year trust fund known as **Superfund.** This money was earmarked for abandoned hazardous waste dump cleanups. What was originally thought to be a short-term problem, however, has turned into an on-going environmental crisis, with new sites continuing to be discovered. Thus, in 1986 Congress passed the Superfund Amendments and Reauthorization Act (SARA), providing an additional $8.5 billion for cleaning up the worst abandoned hazardous waste dumps, and $500 million for the cleanup of leaking underground storage tanks. Just how effective has Superfund been in alleviating hazardous waste dumps? By 1989 it was reported that only thirty-four of the 1,175 hazardous waste dumps on the EPA's National Priorities List (NPL) had been cleaned up, and that the hazardous waste polluters had paid less than one-tenth of the cost.[45] In 1990, the EPA reported that cleanup had been completed at fifty-two of the 1,207 NPL sites.[46] At best, progress has been slow. The EPA reports that over 32,000 potentially hazardous waste sites have been identified in the U.S.—a number that is continually growing. Environmentalists believe that it will take over $750 billion to clean up U.S. hazardous waste sites.[47] Clearly, the cost of cleaning up hazardous waste sites will continue to soar in the years to come.

Integrated Pest Management (IPM): a system of pest control that relies on a variety of techniques that pose the least amount of hazard to both living and nonliving components of the environment. IPM tactics include crop rotation, insect predators, and natural chemicals to control pests.

Superfund: a federal program, first funded in 1980 and refunded in 1986, that authorizes the EPA to respond to hazardous waste spills and clean up abandoned hazardous waste sites in the U.S.

TABLE 19.5

Health Effects of Select Organic Chemicals That May Contaminate Drinking Water

Contaminants	Health Effects	Sources
Organic chemicals		
Endrin	Nervous system/kidney effects	Insecticide used on cotton, small grains and orchards (canceled).
Lindane	Nervous system, kidney and liver effects; possible cancer risk	Insecticide used on seed and soil treatments, foliage applications, wood protection.
Methoxychlor	Nervous system/kidney effects	Insecticide used on fruit trees, vegetables.
2, 4-D	Liver/kidney effects	Herbicide used to control broadleaf weeds in agriculture, used on forests, ranges, pastures, and aquatic environments.
2,4,5-TP Silvex	Liver/kidney effects	Herbicide, canceled in 1984.
Toxaphene	Cancer risk	Insecticide used on cotton, corn, grain.
Benzene	Cancer causing	Fuel (leaking tanks), solvents commonly used in manufacture of industrial chemicals, pharmaceuticals, pesticides, paints, and plastics.
Carbon tetrachloride	Possible cancer risk	Common in cleaning agents and industrial wastes from manufacture of coolants.
p-Dichlorobenzene	Possible cancer risk	Used in insecticides, moth balls, and air deodorizers.
1,2-Dichloroethane	Possible cancer risk	Used in manufacture of insecticides.
1,1-Dichloroethylene	Liver/kidney effects	Used in manufacture of plastics, dyes, perfumes, paints, and SOCs.
1,1,1-Trichloroethane	Nervous system effects	Used in manufacture of food wrappings, synthetic fibers.
Trichloroethane	Possible cancer risk	Waste from disposal of dry cleaning materials. From manufacture of pesticides, paints, waxes and varnishes, paint stripper, and metal degreaser.
Vinyl Chloride	Cancer risk	Polyvinylchloride pipes (PVC) and solvents used to join them. Industrial waste from manufacture of plastics and synthetic rubber.

Source: Data from "You and Your Drinking Water," *EPA Journal,* 12(7) September 1986.

Toxic Release Inventory (TRI): a provision of the 1986 Emergency Planning and Community Right-to-Know Act that requires the EPA to publish an annual inventory of toxic releases and transfers from over 20,000 manufacturing facilities in the U.S.

In addition to SARA, Congress passed the Emergency Planning and Community Right-to-Know Act, known as Title III. The intent of Title III is to inform the public about hazardous chemicals used by industry, and to make certain that local communities are prepared to respond to any potential chemical accidents that might occur. Additionally, it requires **Toxic Release Inventory** reporting to the EPA. Manufacturing industries with ten or more employees, that process over a certain amount of specific chemicals, must report their toxic emissions to air, land, or water.

We depend on synthetic, human-made chemical compounds for many of the essentials and luxuries of the "good life." Yet, it is entirely possible that the costs may be too high. Individually and collectively, we must decide the price we are willing to pay.

Applying the Laws of Ecology to Your Ecosystem

As you go about your daily activities, begin to reflect on these laws of ecology and your place in the ecosphere. Do you step lightly in your ecosystem, becoming part of natural cycles whenever possible? Have you assessed the ecological price tags attached to your lifestyle?

Personal and Social Influences on the Environment

A variety of social factors affect our environment and thus impact on our health and well-being. It is important that we examine these factors, and weigh the consequences of our consumption patterns, in attempting to establish a healthy environment.

Our Consuming Way of Life

Before the industrial revolution, an agricultural lifestyle formed the basis for social and cultural norms. People were capable of producing their own food, clothing, and shelter, so bartering was relatively limited. Industrialization led to a split between the producer and consumer.[48] People began to work at jobs to produce goods for public consumption. After an eight- to twelve-hour day in a factory, workers had little time to produce goods and services for themselves. The market began to dominate society, and the age of the consumer was born.

An important aspect of an industrialized society is its utilization of mass-production processes. Mass production, however, does not function efficiently unless it is accompanied by mass consumption. Therefore, it was essential that industry convince the public to buy and use an endless stream of products.

A quick trip to your local shopping center should be enough to convince you that industry has been quite successful at shaping our needs and desires. The great majority of products for sale are not necessities but rather needs created for us by big business and industry. As Paul Ehrlich and Anne Ehrlich, authors of *The End of Affluence,* state, "People have been persuaded that driving cars everywhere is 'better' than using mass transit, that air conditioning is the way to make things more comfortable in the summer, that disposable everything is better than durable anything, and that embalmed foods are more convenient and just as nutritious as fresh foods."[49]

Alan Durning, a senior researcher at the Worldwatch Institute, believes that people in the U.S. have actually become hooked on consuming. Durning states "Shopping, particularly in the United States, seems to have become a primary cultural activity. Americans spend six hours a week shopping. Some 93 percent of American teenage girls surveyed in 1987 deemed shopping their favorite pastime."[50] In our "need" to consume in ever-greater quantities, we tend to develop sloppy and inefficient consumer habits that contribute little to our personal or community welfare. In addition to impulse buying, we develop a tendency toward wasteful consumption. How many of us, for instance, keep the lights, radio, or air conditioner on in an empty house?

We do not always develop wasteful consumption habits on our own; often they are "sold" to us through advertising. The use of nonreturnable bottles is a prime example. Only thirty years ago 95 percent of the beverages purchased in the U.S. were sold in returnable containers. By the early 1980s this figure had dropped to about 25 percent.[51] To succeed in changing these figures so dramatically, beverage manufacturers in the mid-1960s had to launch massive advertising campaigns to increase public awareness. Advertisers set out to convince consumers that throwaways were better than returnables (see figure 19.11). In the 1990s recycling is once again on the rise, due to the public's recognition of the increasing problems of dealing with solid waste.

Our current consumption patterns have a tremendous impact on the ecosphere. As illustrated in table 19.6, it is estimated that we each throw away 4.2 pounds of trash every day. In terms of the laws of ecology we know there is no "away" to throw these things and that the ecological price tag is quite costly. What are your consuming habits and how do they impact on our environment?

Figure 19.11: What Do You Think?

1. All-aluminum beverage containers first appeared on the market in 1963 as part of the move toward nonreturnable or "throwaway" containers. Today they account for the single largest use of aluminum in the U.S. When you drink out of aluminum beverage cans do you usually throw them away or do you recycle them?

2. Does your campus participate in a formal aluminum container recycling program?

TABLE 19.6

Per Capita Generation* of Municipal Solid Waste, By Material, 1960 to 2000, (in pounds per person per day)

Materials	1960	1970	1980	1990	2000
Paper and Paperboard	0.9	1.2	1.3	1.6	1.7
Glass	0.2	0.3	0.4	0.3	0.3
Metals	0.3	0.4	0.3	0.4	0.3
Plastics	Neg.	0.1	0.2	0.4	0.5
Rubber and Leather	0.1	0.1	0.1	0.1	0.1
Textiles	0.1	0.1	0.1	0.1	0.1
Wood	0.1	0.1	0.2	0.3	0.3
Other	Neg.	Neg.	0.1	0.1	0.1
Total Materials in Products	**1.6**	**2.2**	**2.6**	**3.2**	**3.5**
Food Wastes	0.4	0.3	0.3	0.3	0.3
Yard Trimmings	0.6	0.6	0.7	0.8	0.7
Miscellaneous Inorganic Wastes	Neg.	Neg.	0.1	0.1	0.1
Total MSW Generated	**2.6**	**3.2**	**3.7**	**4.3**	**4.5**

*Generation before materials or energy recovery.

Details may not add to totals due to rounding.

Neg. = Negligible (less than 0.05 pounds per person per day).

Source: Table 1. *Population from Bureau of the Census, Current Population Reports, in EPA, Characterization of MSW,* 1992.

What Do You Think?

1. Table 19.6 gives a detailed presentation of the number of pounds of various types of municipal solid waste (MSW) generated, on average, by each person in the U.S. every day. Looking at the data, what is the greatest source of solid waste generated in 1960? in 1990?

2. How does a rank ordering of the top five sources of solid waste in1960 compare with a rank ordering of the top five solid waste sources from 1990? How do 1960 and 1990 rankings compare with ranking predictions for 2000? What factors do you think account for any changes noted?

3. What trends can be seen in the data presented? Which sources of solid waste have increased over the years and which have decreased? What factors do you think account for any changes noted?

Consumption and Entropy

Where are our excessive consumption patterns leading? It has been suggested that the world has begun a transition toward an age of scarcity. Energy, food, and water shortages have all been predicted. Some of these shortages are already being experienced, at least periodically. The gasoline shortages experienced in the U.S. during the 1970s and the recent famines in Africa are prime examples. Such shortages can be traced back to two prominent laws of physics, commonly known as the laws of thermodynamics.[52]

The first law of thermodynamics, often referred to as the **conservation of energy,** tells us that energy cannot be created or destroyed but only transformed from one form to another. The second law of thermodynamics—the law of **entropy**— specifies the direction in which energy must always be transformed. This law states that energy is always transformed from a usable to an unusable form; from an available to an unavailable form; and from the ordered to the disordered. In other words, energy begins with structure and value and is transformed toward random chaos and waste. We see this daily in the world around us. You know, for instance, that when you leave your house unattended it soon becomes more and more disorderly. This is the law of entropy at work.

Fuels and foods can be used only once to perform useful work. As they are utilized the energy is transformed into an unusable, unavailable, and disordered state. Entropy, then, can be defined as a measure of the amount of energy that is no longer capable of transformation into work. Jeremy Rifkin, author of *Entropy: Into the Greenhouse World*, believes that pollution is another name for entropy, as pollution is the unusable by-product of energy consumption.[53] For instance, gasoline is burned to fuel automobiles, producing hydrocarbons, nitrogen oxide, and other emissions. These emissions are unusable for future work and accumulate in the environment as pollutants. Rifkin challenges his readers to look at entropy in their own lifestyles:[54]

> Take an entire day to observe everything you come in contact with: things you see, hear, touch, smell, feel or consume; things that you change; and things that you exchange. Then try to trace each experience or item in both directions, back to its original source and forward to

its final destination. Chances are better than excellent (in fact guaranteed) that they all started off as some form of raw material (available energy) and that they will all end up somewhere as unusable waste (unavailable energy).

The laws of thermodynamics thus tell us that the energy resources on our planet are finite and that as we use them we unavoidably create pollution. If we continue to consume energy and matter at ever-increasing rates we increase dramatically the ecological price to be paid and head toward drastic shortages and hardship for the peoples of the earth (see table 19.7).

Options do exist to slow down the rate of entropy in our society; however, many ecologists believe that there is little time left to enact such changes. As Rifkin states,

> Now that we are witnessing the transition from an energy environment built upon nonrenewable resources to one built on solar flow and renewable energy sources, great personal and institutional changes will sweep over our society. . . . The transition period will not extend over hundreds of years, as happened during the shift of previous energy environments. . . . Certainly, we can anticipate that the next twenty to thirty years represent the key period in launching the shift in energy environments.[55]

Toward a Sustainable Earth Society

Leading environmentalists have proposed, as one viable future, a move from the throwaway/frontier mentality toward what they term the sustainable earth mentality.[56] A **sustainable earth society** must be founded in the laws of ecology, especially the third law, nature knows best. In the past, people have lived under the illusion that nature could be mastered and controlled, and that people could be relieved of many dependencies on nature. Essential to the sustainable earth society is an adoption of the world view of humanity *and* nature—that is, a cooperation with nature and its laws.

A sustainable earth society is also firmly grounded in the laws of thermodynamics. Slowing entropy through recycling and reusing matter and decreasing our energy consumption are emphasized. This type of society is of necessity decentralized, calling on its people to be more responsible and self-reliant.

Sustainable earth society: a social order based on nature and its laws. In such a society, recycling and reusing matter, decreasing energy consumption, and self-reliant living are stressed.

TABLE 19.7   *Changes in the Earth's Physical Condition*

Indicator	Reading
Forest cover	Tropical forests shrinking by eleven million hectares per year; thirty-one million hectares in industrial countries damaged, apparently by air pollution or acid rain.
Topsoil on cropland	An estimated twenty-six billion tons lost annually in excess of new soil formation.
Desert area	Some six million hectares of new desert formed annually by land mismanagement.
Lakes	Thousands of lakes in the industrial north now biologically dead; thousands more dying.
Fresh water	Underground water tables falling in parts of Africa, China, India, and North America as demand for water rises above aquifer recharge rates.
Species diversity	Extinctions of plant and animal species together now estimated at several thousand per year; one-fifth of all species may disappear over next twenty years.
Groundwater quality	Some fifty pesticides contaminate groundwater in thirty-two U.S. states; some 2,500 U.S. toxic waste sites need cleanup; extent of toxic contamination worldwide unknown.
Climate	Mean temperature projected to rise between 1.5 and 4.5 degrees Celsius between now and 2050.
Sea level	Projected to rise between 1.4 meters (4.7 feet) and 2.2 meters (7.1 feet) by 2100.
Ozone layer in upper atmosphere	Growing "hole" in the earth's ozone layer over Antarctica each spring suggests a gradual global depletion could be starting.

Compiled by Worldwatch Institute from various sources. Reprinted by permission Worldwatch Institute, Washington, D.C.

Figure 19.12: An adaptation continuum

Reprinted by permission of Dr. Robert Russell Southern Illinois University at Carbondale, Carbondale, IL.

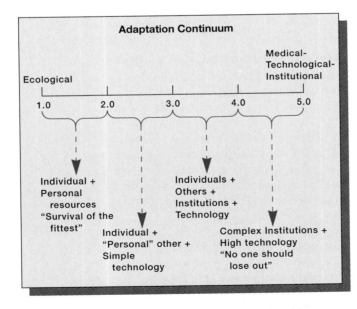

Robert Russell, professor of health education at Southern Illinois University, has developed a theoretical adaptation model that is helpful in understanding humanity in both its frontier and sustainable earth views[57] (see figure 19.12). Russell's Adaptation Continuum is divided into four equal segments, each representing a certain level of human adaptation. The left end of the continuum represents an ecological approach to life; the right end presents a centralized technological approach. At the extreme ecological end (1.0) individuals do all their adapting for themselves, utilizing personal physical, mental, and emotional resources. Moving toward the right, technology and other individuals become involved in the adaptation process, until at the extreme right end (5.0) institutions and technology are providing essentially all adaptation for the individual. Points 1.0 and 5.0 on the continuum are theoretical extremes and would rarely, if at all, exist in the real world. Most people on our planet fall between 2.0 and 4.0; however, our highly affluent and technological society tends more toward the medical, technological, institutional end than many other societies.

While there are many advantages to a highly centralized and technological existence, there are also inherent dangers.

Russell emphasizes two of these dangers in explaining his model. First, when people become dependent on institutions and technology for much of their adapting they may lose (or possibly never learn) the ability to adapt using their own personal resources. Those of us born during or after the baby boom of the late 1940s and early 1950s have probably grown up in an environment where many of our adaptations are made for us. We do not have to grow all of our own food, for example, or make our own clothes, or repair all of our own possessions. Additionally, our education has, in many instances, failed to prepare us for the event of a possible short- or long-term breakdown of the centralized adaptation system. For example, if you needed to, could you feed, clothe, and shelter yourself with your own personal resources and skills?

The second inherent danger revolves around the highly technological adaptations themselves—that is, some of these adaptations may be dangerous in and of themselves. Drugs, for instance, while helping us to adapt to or overcome diseases, all have risks and side effects associated with them.

The further we move to the right on the adaptation continuum the greater is our consumption of energy, which leads to an increase in entropy. A sustainable earth society would tend toward the left on the adaptation continuum, probably locating somewhere between 2.0 and 3.5 indicating a willingness to move back toward more ecological, self-reliant aspects of living.

Changing Our Consumption Patterns

The quality of our environment rests heavily on what you and I, as individuals and in groups, are willing to do. There are many simple changes each of us can make in our consumption of goods and energy that will help in the move toward a sustainable earth society. As you reflect on your personal consumption patterns in several major lifestyle areas and study the suggestions given for reducing consumption, look for several activities you are willing and able to do today. If each of us would take responsibility for our personal environmental actions we would begin to see great advancements in our quest for high-level wellness.

Food

A tremendous amount of energy goes into the production of food for the typical U.S. diet. As with any energy expenditure, food production involves numerous costs to our environment. These costs depend on several major factors. One such factor involves the number of people to be supported by a given area of farmland and the quality of the food they consume. The typical U.S. diet is high in fat and protein. This is due largely to our consumption of meat, which is an energy-expensive way to meet our nutritional needs. Grain products are a more efficient food source as, per acre of land, greater amounts of protein and other essential nutrients can be supplied for human consumption (see figure 19.13). It has been estimated that the 25 percent of the world's population that consumes meat, also consumes 40 percent of the world's grains—"grains that fatten the livestock they eat."[58] As Frances Moore Lappé states, "the production of just one pound of steak requires as much water as a typical household uses in one month. . . . The energy costs are also enormous: to produce a one-pound steak that provides approximately 500 food calories requires the expenditure of 20,000 calories of fossil fuel energy."[59]

Another U.S. dietary pattern raising great environmental concerns is the trend toward the consumption of ever-greater quantities of processed or "fast-food" substances. This trend toward processed food sources utilizes great amounts of our precious energy reserves and contributes to environmental degradation. There are two major environmental concerns related to our consumption of "fast foods": the use of hamburger from tropical rain forests, and the amount of waste generated.

The destruction of tropical rain forests is a global problem causing great concern. One of the reasons for the rain forest destruction is the need to clear the land for cattle ranching. Much of the beef that is raised is sold to U.S. companies where it often ends up in hamburgers at fast-food restaurants. (Several fast-food establishments have stated publicly that they do not use rain forest beef.) The clearing of tropical rain forests plays an important role in the greenhouse effect and leads to widespread destruction of plant and animal species. Species extinction alone will

Figure 19.13: Food efficiency

Source: Data from the U.S. Department of Agriculture, Economic Research Service, Beltsville, MD.

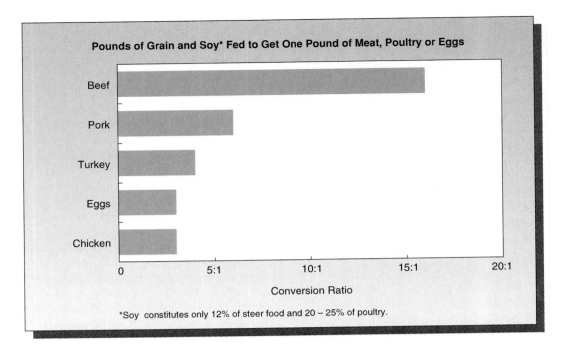

Pounds of Grain and Soy* Fed to Get One Pound of Meat, Poultry or Eggs

Conversion Ratio

*Soy constitutes only 12% of steer food and 20 – 25% of poultry.

have devastating global effects. As pointed out by Jon Naar, author of *Design for a Livable Planet*, "one out of every four pharmaceuticals used by Western chemists comes from tropical plants, (1,400 of which are under review as possible cancer cures). . . . more than 1.2 million species—a quarter of total biological diversity—are expected to vanish within the next 25 years. *No extinction of this magnitude has occurred during the past 65 million years.*"[60]

Fast-food restaurants also contribute a great deal of "trash" to the waste stream in the U.S. Much of this waste is generated by food packaging that is used once for a very brief period of time. Even though many fast-food restaurants are switching to the use of recycled paper for packaging, the sheer volume of packaging materials is still an important solid waste concern.

There are many simple activities easily incorporated into our dietary lifestyle that help to conserve our energy resources and decrease entropy. The following list, adapted from the United States Department of Energy's *Tips for Energy Savers*, should help you begin to assess and modify your food energy-consumption patterns.

- Learn to grow some of your own food by maintaining a small garden, window box, or solar greenhouse.
- Eat fewer meat products; substitute more energy-efficient protein sources such as grains and legumes.

- Eat more unprocessed, fresh foods.
- Consider joining a food co-op, or shop at the local farmers' market (see Of Special Interest 19.2).
- Reduce food waste by serving smaller portions; refrain from throwing food away.
- Thaw frozen foods before cooking.
- Eat cold meals, such as salads, fruits, and vegetables, when feasible.
- Do not preheat ovens.
- Do not buy or use gadget appliances such as hot dog cookers, electric knife sharpeners, and electric can openers.
- Never boil water in an open pan.
- Match the size of the pan to the heating element.
- Use small electric pans or ovens for small meals.
- When using a dishwasher, let dishes air dry by turning off the control knob after the final rinse and propping the door open.

Clothing

Many of us fail to realize the energy expenditures involved in the production and maintenance of our personal wardrobes. The fashion industry is big business. Large sums of money are spent yearly just in advertising efforts to create in the public a need for the latest fad fashion. Fabric and garment production are costly to the environment. Synthetic fibers are one prime example of the costly environmental

From Their Little Plot, a Healthful, Bountiful Harvest

Last year, Jess and Suzanne Unger set aside half an acre of their 160-acre farm in Lovettsville, Va., for organic farming. Using no chemical pesticides, they raised fresh produce for 60 customers. "We grew more than 40 varieties of vegetables," Jess Unger says, "from arugula to zucchini."

The variety of produce that sprouted from the modest plot is not all that distinguishes Brook Farm from many other producers that have adopted organic farming methods. Instead of selling their produce to a store or at a local farmers' market, the Ungers asked their customers to decide what they should raise. "Our customers sign up at the beginning of the year and fill out a questionnaire indicating what types of vegetables they want, and how much," Jess Unger explains. "They pay a lump sum at the beginning for weekly deliveries for 32 weeks from April to November."

The Ungers are among a growing number of farmers who are adopting a marketing strategy called community-supported agriculture. In this reversal of the conventional food-marketing system, consumers contract directly with farmers to grow the commodities they want. The concept, which originated in Europe and quickly became popular in Japan, was introduced in the United States in 1985 with the first group in Massachusetts, Unger says. "From there it has spread throughout the country."

By eliminating the middleman—the grocery store—growers can offer fresher produce, including the more costly organic foods, at prices that often are below grocery-store prices.

"Our Washington customers tell us prices come in under what it costs them to buy at city outlets for organic foods, including the downtown food co-ops," Unger says. "Out here [in suburban Loudoun County], it costs more than Safeway produce, but we feel the cost shows consumers the cost of actually producing the food." Produce sold in grocery stores, Unger says, has hidden costs, such as poor quality and pesticide contamination, that are not readily apparent to consumers.

Although community-supported agriculture today poses little threat to Safeway and the other retail giants, demand for Brook Farm produce is growing. The Ungers are expanding their organic garden to two and a half acres this year. Apart from the lack of chemical residues, Jess Unger says, the main attraction his operation holds out to customers is freshness and the seasonal quality of his produce.

"Why buy something that was grown 2,000 miles away in December," he asks,

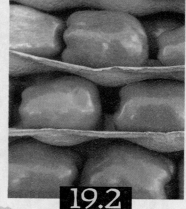

19.2
Of Special Interest

"when you can get the same thing, grown locally, in May or June when it is in season?"

What Do You Think?

1. What do you think are the main attractions of community supported agriculture for consumers?
2. Would you be interested in participating in a program similar to the Unger's? Explain your reasoning.

From "Regulating Pesticides: Do Americans Need More Protection from Toxic Chemicals?" in *CQ Researcher*, 4(4):78, 1994. Reprinted by permission of Congressional Quarterly, Inc., Washington, D.C.

---

impact. Many synthetic fibers, such as nylon, polyester, and vinyls, are made from petroleum and coal. Additionally, the manufacturing processes involved with synthetic fibers require large amounts of energy. Natural fibers such as cotton, wool, and silk, although they are often more expensive to buy, are a better buy in terms of environmental costs.

Each of us must begin today to conserve energy and protect our environment. The following suggestions may increase your environmental sensitivity regarding clothing and assist you in changing your energy-consumption patterns.

- Wear clothes made from natural fibers such as cotton, wool, and silk rather than synthetic fibers.
- Buy few trendy clothes; emphasize fashions that will last and remain attractive for several years.

- Sew or make your own clothes.
- Wash clothes in warm or cold water rather than hot.
- Save energy by drying clothes outdoors on a clothesline.
- Save energy needed for ironing by hanging clothes in the bathroom while you shower, utilizing the shower steam to remove wrinkles.

Transportation

Recent world events, such as the Persian Gulf war, have once again focused national attention on transportation energy-consumption patterns. Although people are more conscious of both the monetary and environmental costs involved, we nonetheless remain extremely dependent on the automobile as a means of maintaining our current lifestyles. In many communities, in fact, it is impossible to work or shop without an automobile.

1. Biking is becoming more popular, both as a means of transportation and as a form of exercise. How often do you or your friends and family use a bicycle as a means of transportation?

2. What barriers prevent you and others in your community from using bicycles more often as a means of transportation and exercise? What solutions can you think of for removing the barriers that exist in your community?

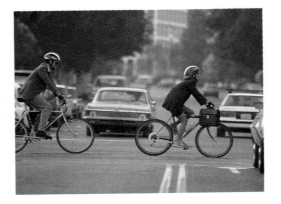

There are many options available to us that would aid in the conservation of transportation energy and decrease the pollution levels inherent in our current systems (see A Social Perspective 19.1). These range from utilizing automobiles and mass transit more efficiently, to making better use of our own muscle power for transportation. Walking and bicycling are becoming more popular, both as forms of exercise and as means of transportation (see figure 19.14).

What changes could you make in your transportation lifestyle that would be conducive to a sustainable earth view?

- Use public transportation, a moped, a motorcycle, a bicycle, or walk to work.
- Join a carpool and share rides.
- Consolidate errands into one trip when possible.
- Eliminate unnecessary trips.
- Rediscover the pleasure of walking, hiking, and bicycling.
- Keep your automobile tuned up.
- Keep your automobile tires inflated at the recommended pressure.
- Drive at a steady pace.

Solid Wastes

Our society is based on a throwaway ethic, with many materials being discarded after just one use. People in the U.S. annually dispose of 56.8 tons of packaging waste alone. "According to the most recent EPA figures, packaging makes up 31.6 percent of U.S. solid waste."[61]

We have many viable options for reducing our production of solid wastes. We can easily accomplish many of them on an individual level. These options range from generating less waste—especially from unnecessary packaging—to making better use of opportunities to reuse and recycle goods. It has been projected that two-thirds of the material resources used in the U.S. yearly could be recycled without important changes in our style of living.

The following list contains suggestions for individual actions aimed at reducing solid-waste generation. As you read these suggestions, pick one or two that would be easily incorporated into your lifestyle. Begin today to experiment with improving the quality of your environment.

- Buy durable goods, such as a leather bag instead of one made from vinyl or plastic. Check consumer guides, such as *Consumer Reports*, for durability information before you purchase.
- Avoid buying and using throwaway products such as paper towels, plates, cups, and disposable razors and diapers.
- When shopping, carry your own cloth or string bags with you to the store (see figure 19.15).
- If you must use paper or plastic bags, reuse them as well.
- Learn to maintain and repair products, rather than replacing them with new items.
- Recycle aluminum cans (see figure 19.16). It takes 90 percent less energy to recycle an aluminum can than to make a new sheet from bauxite ore.[62]
- Compost your food and yard wastes.
- Use a lunch box instead of paper bags.
- Write on both sides of a piece of paper.
- Recycle paper—75 percent of the world's new paper demand could be met by recycling one-half of the paper used today.[63]
- Reuse bottles and cans by purchasing returnable beverage containers: many states have already enacted deposit laws for all beverage containers.

Water

Many people take water for granted, believing it is their right to have an unlimited, clean, and inexpensive source of this natural resource. Environmentalists, however, predict that water shortages are imminent unless we begin to conserve and respect the finite supply of available water.[64] Conservation on an individual level is one obvious component of the solution. Simply turning off the water faucet while brushing your teeth can save an estimated gallon or so of pure drinking water.

Environmental Impact of New Cars Ranked in New Landmark Report

Even though car engines today run much cleaner than 25 years ago, there is little doubt—except perhaps among the automakers themselves—that reasonably priced, "greener" vehicles are possible with existing technologies.

Public Citizen recently released its landmark report, *The Green Buyer's Car Book,* which ranks more than 900 models sold in the United States on their environmental impact. Ratings were based on four criteria: smog and carbon monoxide emissions, global warming caused by fuel consumption, use of ozone-eating CFCs, and recyclability.

The "greenest" vehicle, according to the analysis, was the Geo Metro Xfi. The dirtiest vehicles were an assortment of sport utility trucks, such as the Range Rover Defender 90. The lowest-ranked car was one version of the Pontiac Sunbird, which earned the dishonorable distinction by being among a handful of new vehicles that still use CFCs in air conditioning systems.

"Years ago the auto companies said they couldn't compete if they had to reduce polluting emissions and increase fuel economy," Public Citizen's President Joan Claybrook said at a news conference August 11 at the National Press Club in Washington, D.C. "Although today's cars are cleaner and more efficient than they were in the past, smog still chokes many of our cities, oil spills foul our beaches, solid waste piles up in our landfills, and the global atmosphere itself is being altered. Our pressing ecological problems demand much greener cars, and innovative technologies are available to produce them.

"The auto industry is using the same arguments they used 20 years ago, this time to oppose higher mileage standards and electric cars," Claybrook added. "They were wrong then and they're wrong now."

Author of the study is Christopher Dyson, a researcher with Public Citizen's Critical Mass Energy Project. Dyson relied on the auto manufacturers to provide much of the data for his report because the Department of Transportation maintains only fuel efficiency figures. Most of the companies contacted by Dyson were cooperative, but a handful—including Mazda and Hyundai—refused to provide information about their cars to Public Citizen. That problem, as well as the volume and scope of the work involved, led Claybrook to call on the government to take over the task of providing environmental impact information to prospective new-car buyers.

"What we're hoping is that what this [information] does is lead the Environmental Protection Agency as well as the automakers to look at this issue as one on which cars should compete." said Claybrook. "Just in the way that Lee Iacocca 'got religion' on airbags, and it was a breakthrough in terms of offering them to the public, I think we're going to see that some companies are going to be breakthrough companies. They're going to say 'this is for us' and they're going to adopt

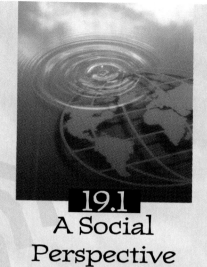

19.1
A Social Perspective

it. As long as there's a rating system and a guide that helps consumers, that encourages manufacturers to behave in this manner."

What Do You Think?

1. Should the auto industry be required to provide consumers with environmental impact data on new cars that they sell in the U.S.? What is the rationale for your answer?
2. Would you consider environmental impact an important consideration if you were in the market to purchase a new car? Explain your reasoning.

From "Environmental Impact of New Cars Ranked in New Landmark Report" in *Public Citizen, 14* (5):21, 1994. Public Citizen Foundation, Washington, D.C.

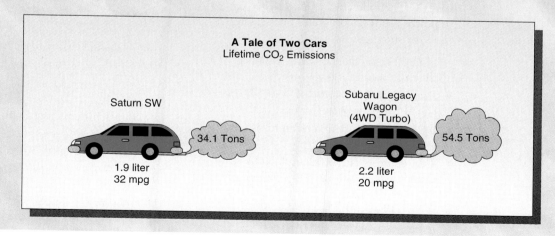

A Tale of Two Cars
Lifetime CO$_2$ Emissions

Saturn SW
34.1 Tons
1.9 liter
32 mpg

Subaru Legacy Wagon (4WD Turbo)
54.5 Tons
2.2 liter
20 mpg

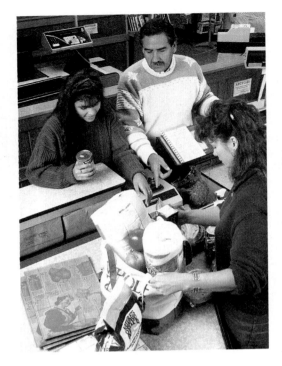

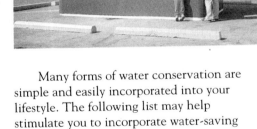

Conservation: using less of a given product.

Energy efficiency: using the least amount of energy to accomplish a given task.

Many forms of water conservation are simple and easily incorporated into your lifestyle. The following list may help stimulate you to incorporate water-saving activities into your style of living.

- Shut off water faucets while washing, shaving, or brushing your teeth.
- Do not boil a full kettle of water for one cup of coffee or tea.
- Do as much household cleaning as possible with cold water.
- Take showers rather than tub baths (this would save an estimated five gallons of water per shower).
- Place a brick in the tank of toilets to reduce the water stored there.

Energy

Energy is the measure of the ability to do work. Humans consume and metabolize carbohydrates, fats, and protein as fuel for bodily energy or movement. We also tap fuel sources such as fossil fuels, wood, solar energy, and nuclear energy to fuel our autos, heat our homes, or generate our electricity. These energy sources, however, are subject to the laws of thermodynamics. That is, once used they are transformed to an unusable, disordered form that we often label pollution. Additionally, most of our fuel sources are in a finite supply on earth. **Conservation** and improved **energy efficiency** are the most desirable approaches to our energy concerns—both in terms of fuel shortages and pollution consequences. In recent years, people in the U.S. have made considerable progress in energy conservation and efficiency. Yet even with these efforts, energy consumption has increased approximately 1.1 percent each year for the past 25 years.[66]

The largest source of residential energy consumption (70 percent) involves the heating and cooling of our homes. Other important sources of energy consumption include heating water, lighting, cooking, and running small appliances. The Department of Energy suggests the following ways to reduce energy consumption:

- For heating, keep your thermostat at sixty-five degrees Fahrenheit during the day and fifty-five degrees Fahrenheit at night.
- Dress in warmer clothing when heat thermostat is turned down.
- Use a window fan for cooling when feasible.
- Set your air conditioner at seventy-eight degrees Fahrenheit.
- Turn off window air-conditioning units when you will be gone for several hours.
- Turn off any lights not being used.
- Keep lamps and light fixtures clean; dirt absorbs light.
- Use compact fluorescent light bulbs whenever possible.
- Use outdoor lights only when necessary.
- Keep your water heater's thermostat at 120 degrees.
- Do not leave appliances, such as a radio or television, running when they are not actually being used.
- When purchasing new appliances pay attention to available energy-conserving features (see table 19.8).

TABLE 19.8   *Increasing Energy Efficiency*

	Energy-Conserving Features Available	*Installation Tips*
Window air conditioner	Check the Energy Efficiency Ratio (EER). An EER below 7 is poor. 7 to 9 is good. 10 or higher is excellent.	Where possible, locate the unit where it will be shaded by trees or awning. If no shade is available, place the unit on the north side of the house when practical.
Dishwasher	An "Energy-Saver" switch lets you bypass the drying cycle. After final rinse, open door and let dishes air dry.	Locate as near as practical to your water heater.
Washing machine	Temperature and water level controls let you select the right amount of water, at the proper temperature, for each load.	Locate as near as practical to your water heater.
Freezer	Chest-type uses less energy than upright models. Manual defrost also saves energy. Magnetic door seal helps prevent leakage. Door-activated interior light helps you find food faster.	Place freezer so that condenser coils have ventilation.
Microwave oven	Uses less energy than conventional oven due to low wattage and shorter cooking times. Oven window and light lets you check food without opening door.	
Electric water heater	Energy efficient models are available in some makes. A special kit for adding insulation is available through most building supply dealers. Ask for low-watt density elements.	Place the water heater in a location central to the major water use centers such as laundry and kitchen. Long pipe runs throughout the house should be avoided, if possible. Insulate hot water pipes running in unheated areas.
Electric clothes dryer	Accessible lint filter for cleaning after each load. Fabric and temperature selection. Automatic timer, responding to air temperature and moisture in clothes, turns dryer off when clothes are dry.	Dryer should be vented to the outside.
Refrigerator	An anti-sweat or "Power-Saver" switch saves on operating costs and energy. Exterior service for ice and water.	Locate refrigerator away from range, dishwasher, and heating ducts.
Electric range	Oven window and interior light cuts down need for opening door to check food. Reflector pans under surface units. Start-stop timers and thermostatically-controlled surface units.	

Note: When buying a major appliance, make sure it is the right size for the job you want it to do. This may be influenced by the size of your family, size and room arrangement of your home, amount of insulation in your walls, floors and ceiling, and by your personal living habits. Your appliance dealer should be able to help you determine the right size equipment.

From Duke Power Company, *A Handbook for the Serious (and Not So Serious) Energy Saver,* Charlotte, NC. Reprinted by permission.

To the Future

Environmentalist and author Garrett Hardin has written extensively on what he calls "The Tragedy of the Commons."[67] The "commons" of this earth are the water, air, and land, which we all need to survive. The environmental concerns we face today are truly global and must be addressed at a policy level by governments and leaders of business and industry; however, policy initiatives must be paralleled by individual initiatives worldwide. It is indeed a tragedy that many people believe their individual impact on the ecosphere to be so small as to be unimportant. In fact, individual actions add up to societal actions.

Individuals can make many contributions on both personal and community levels. Review your own consumption habits and their impact on the environment. There are many alternatives leading to environmental wellness. Begin today to select activities you are willing and able to implement in your lifestyle, and encourage others around you to do the same. This may mean serving as a model of environmental sensitivity or even becoming involved politically. One easy way

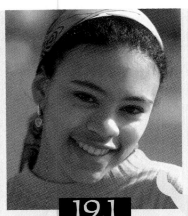

19.1
Activity for Wellness

How to Write an Effective Letter to a Legislator

The right to participate in the political process is one of the most important freedoms we have. One easy way to do this is by communicating your position on issues with your elected officials.

1. **Address it correctly:**
   a. *The President*
      The White House
      1600 Pennsylvania Avenue NW
      Washington, DC 20500
      Dear Mr. President:
   b. *The Honorable. . . .*
      U.S. Senate
      Washington, DC 20515
      Dear Senator. . . .
   c. *The Honorable. . . .*
      U.S. House of Representatives
      Washington, DC 20515
      Dear Representative. . . .

2. **Write first to your own representative** and then to the chair or members of the committee dealing with the legislation you are interested in.

3. **Identify by name and number the bill that deals with the subject you are writing about**—e.g., *Global Warming Prevention Act* (HR 1078) proposed by Representative Claudine Schneider, Republican of Rhode Island.

4. **Keep it brief.** Politicians have short attention spans. Summarize your points and try to confine them to one page.

5. **Be personal.** Identify yourself. Write in your own words. Don't send a form letter. Give your own reasons for supporting or opposing a piece of legislation.

6. **Follow up.** You will almost always get a reply, but it most likely will be a form letter. If you are not satisfied with it, write another letter or, if time is short, send a telegram or make a phone call.

7. **Be courteous.** Don't threaten. When appropriate, thank your legislator for taking positive action.

8. **Phone numbers:** The President: (202) 456–1414; U.S. Senate: (202) 224–3121; House of Representatives: (202) 456–1414.

9. **Get others to write as well;** there is strength in numbers.

"How to Write an Effective Letter to a Legislator" from *Design For a Livable Planet*, by Jon Naar. Copyright © 1990 by Jon Naar. Reprinted by permission of HarperCollins Publishers, Inc.

---

to become politically involved is to monitor pending environmental legislation. Several organizations have telephone hot line numbers that you can call for information on pending legislation. For instance, an environmental publication—*Environmental Action*—has a clean air hot line (call 202–745–4879) that provides a legislative update and information on how to write letters of support. Other groups also provide hot lines: The Sierra Club Hot line (202–547–5550) and The Audubon Society (202–547–9017) are both good sources of information when Congress is in session.

Many environmentalists will tell you that writing letters is one of the most important things you can do to have an influence on environmental issues. "The rule of thumb many congressmen use is: each letter represents the views of at least 100 voters in their district."[68] Activity for Wellness 19.1 provides several important pointers to help you get started in writing effective environmental support letters.

Other activities are also available to help you cast your environmental votes. Keep tabs on how your representatives in Congress vote on environmental issues. The League of Conservation Voters keeps a scorecard of how all U.S. Senators and members of the House of Representatives vote on key environmental issues. (The scorecard is available for $5 from The League of Conservation Voters, 1707 L St. NW, Suite 550, Washington, D.C. 20036 202–785–VOTE.) If your representatives do not support legislation to protect your environment you may want to consider, at election time, voting for a candidate who will.

You also cast environmental votes daily by how you spend your time and money. When you shop, your purchases are votes that influence what manufacturers are willing to provide. Are your choices environmentally sound? Activity for Wellness 19.2 will help you cast your economic votes in a more environmentally friendly manner. Voting with your time is also important. Many worthy environmental projects need volunteers. Table 19.9 will help you increase your involvement in environmental health issues.

Where will we be tomorrow—or next year? Our environmental sensitivity, both individually and collectively, is likely to determine our future.

Shopping Checklist

1. ☐ Do I need this product?
2. ☐ Is the package recyclable or returnable?
3. ☐ Does a similar product come with less packaging?
4. ☐ Can I re-use this disposable product?
5. ☐ Is there a nondisposable alternative?
6. ☐ How many times can I use this product before I throw it away?
7. ☐ How long will this product last?
8. ☐ Can this product be repaired rather than discarded?
9. ☐ If the product is something I seldom use can I borrow or rent it?
10. ☐ Will the disposal of this product be a hazard to the environment? If so, is there a safer alternative?

Reprinted with permission: From H. Patricia Hynes, *Earth Right*, 1990. Prima Publishing, Rocklin, CA.

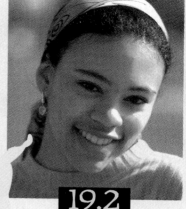

19.2 Activity for Wellness

TABLE 19.9   *Tips for Improving Your Environmental Advocacy Skills*

Increasing your environmental advocacy skills will involve assessing which stage of change you are in (see chapter 1) and then gradually making changes in your involvement with environmental policy decisions. The following tips will help you as you enhance your advocacy skills.

Precontemplation → Contemplation

If you have never thought about taking a political stand on an environmental health issue or you do not intend to take such action within the next six months you might want to consider:

- reading your local newspaper to see what environmental decisions are currently facing your community.
- calling the Sierra Club Hotline or The Audubon Society to learn what environmental issues are currently being considered by the U.S. Congress.

Contemplation → Preparation

If you have been seriously considering becoming involved in environmental advocacy, but have not yet made any actual attempts, try to thoughtfully answer the following questions:

- How much do I value a clean environment that will increase my level of well-being, and that of others in the community, both now and in the future? Am I willing to become involved in finding solutions to our environmental dilemmas?

Preparation → Action

If you are ready to make some definite environmental advocacy plans, or if you have already made small advocacy attempts in the past but were not able to maintain those changes as a permanent part of your lifestyle, consider the following actions:

- Make a resolution to yourself to begin your environmental advocacy with several small steps; for instance, make a commitment to yourself to go to the library and read about an environmental health problem currently facing your community as well as the suggested solutions being considered. Then write a letter to your city council or your local newspaper explaining your perception of the problem and suggested solutions.
- Set a specific date to begin your advocacy activities, for example "On Monday evening I will go to the library to begin my research so that I will be prepared to attend the public hearing in my community being sponsored by the city council."

Action → Maintenance

If you have recently started to take some environmental advocacy actions, the following tips will help you continue on this healthy path:

- Set aside a regular time in your schedule to study environmental problems, write advocacy letters, and attend meetings. A few hours a month may be adequate most of the time. Set objectives for what you hope to accomplish in addressing a particular environmental problem.
- Give yourself rewards *often* for meeting your goals and objectives. Rewards can be material such as a CD you have been wanting, or less tangible such as allowing yourself to sleep in on the weekend. For many people, seeing an environmental problem solved is a great reward in and of itself.

Maintenance

If you have made important changes in your environmental advocacy actions that you have practiced for six months or longer, now you need to focus on maintaining your healthy choices every day:

- Join an environmental group that shares your perspective on environmental problems. Many groups exist in local communities and offer support and resources for your advocacy efforts.

*Based on Prochaska, Norcross and DiClemente's transtheoretical model. See Prochaska, J. O., Norcross, J. C. & DiClemente, C. C. (1994). *Changing for Good*. New York: William Morrow and Company, Inc.

Summary

1. Seeking environmental health involves taking up the challenge to create a personal lifestyle that is both fulfilling and ecologically sound.

2. Environmentalist Barry Commoner has studied natural cycles and summarized them in the four laws of ecology. These laws provide an understanding of ecosystems and their functions.

3. The first law of ecology tells us that everything is connected to everything else. This law points to the necessary complexity of ecosystems. When human beings interfere and oversimplify ecosystems, environmental problems are certain to follow.

4. The second law of ecology states that everything must go somewhere. We must start to ask ourselves where our "waste" is going and what its impact will be on the environment.

5. The third law of ecology tells us that nature knows best. In nature there is no waste; one organism's waste provides nutrients for another. When human beings interfere with natural cycles, environmental problems are invariably the result.

6. The fourth law of ecology states that there is no such thing as a free lunch. For every technological advance there will be an ecological, and often a health-related, price tag. We must begin to ask ourselves if the price of various technologies is worth what they cost.

7. Air pollution is a serious threat to human health. U.S. policy changes, such as the Clean Air Act, have improved air quality for some pollutants; however, other pollutants continue unchecked. Respiratory diseases and heart disease are some of the important health problems resulting, in part, from air pollution.

8. Acid rain is a form of air pollution caused by the release of sulfur dioxide and nitrous oxides into the atmosphere from industry and automobiles. These gases are vented high in the atmosphere where they travel to distant places and fall to earth as acid rain. Acid rain kills fish and other wildlife, destroys forests, and is associated with human lung cancer, asthma, and heart disease.

9. Hazardous waste is another important environmental health threat. Disposal of such wastes results in groundwater contamination, polluting a major source of drinking water in the U.S. Incineration of hazardous waste results in toxic air emissions.

10. Hazardous waste disposal is a particularly important problem for minority communities of color and impoverished third world countries. These people are more likely to have hazardous waste disposal systems, such as landfills and incinerators, in their neighborhoods than are wealthy communities and countries.

11. The EPA is responsible for identifying, assessing the health risks of, and overseeing the cleanup of abandoned toxic waste sites in the U.S. A monetary fund from the U.S. Government, known as Superfund, is used to pay for the assessments and to attempt to track down the businesses responsible for the abandoned sites.

12. The U.S. is a society of consumers. Since industrial consumption patterns are often wasteful and do not follow nature's patterns, they have a great negative impact on the environment. Thus, consumption patterns of people in the U.S. need to change.

13. One viable future proposed by environmentalists is the sustainable earth society. This society would be based on a philosophy of people cooperating with nature. Recycling and reusing matter, energy conservation, and reducing consumption of material goods would be emphasized.

14. You can cast your environmental vote through political involvement, wise consumer choices, and support of worthy environmental projects and groups.

15. We cannot afford to wait for governments and business and industry, or the "other guy" to act on environmental issues. We must each take the challenge—the opportunity—to move toward environmental wellness.

Recommended Readings

Naar, John. (1990) *Design for a Livable Planet: How You Can Help Clean Up the Environment* (New York: Harper and Row).

A practically oriented book, *Design for a Livable Planet* addresses what individuals and groups can do to improve the environment. Naar covers the problems of solid and toxic waste, water and air pollution, acid rain, deforestation, global warming, and radiation. He also addresses a variety of actions that can be taken to solve these concerns including environmental law, organizational strategies, and consumer choices.

Starke, Linda, ed. (1994) *State of the World 1994*. (New York: W. W. Norton and Company).

This report, sponsored by the Worldwatch Institute, presents annually the worldwide progress made toward achieving a sustainable earth society. The environmental concerns addressed vary each year and are based on the latest research findings. The 1994 report addresses the earth's carrying capacity, redesigning the forest economy, safeguarding oceans, reshaping the power industry, reinventing transportation, using computers for the environment, assessing environmental health risk, cleaning up after the arms race, rebuilding the World Bank, and facing food insecurity.

The League of Women Voters Education Fund. (1993) *The Plastic Waste Primer: A Handbook for Citizens.* (New York: Lyons & Burford, Publishers).

This well written handbook for consumers provides an excellent overview of our use of plastics, including both the benefits and hazards associated with their production and use. Many practical tips are included, such as how to shop environmentally and how to become active in policy formation at the local level.

References

1. Miller, G. Tyler. (1992) *Living in the Environment,* 2nd ed. (Belmont, Calif.: Wadsworth Publishing Co.), 481.

2. Ehrlich, Anne H., and Paul R. Ehrlich. (1987) *Earth.* (New York: Franklin Watts), 252.

3. Commoner, Barry. (1990) *Making Peace with the Planet.* (New York: Pantheon Books).

4. Allman, William F. (October, 1988) "Planet Earth: How it works—how to fix it." *U.S. News & World Report.*

5. Silver, Cheryl Simon. (1993) "Greenhouse warming." In World Resources Institute, Ed. *The 1993 Information Please Environmental Almanac.* (Boston: Houghton Mifflin Company), 319.

6. Brown, Lester R. (1993) "A new era unfolds." In Starke, Linda, ed. *State of the World 1993: A Worldwatch Institute Report on Progress Toward a Sustainable Society.* (New York: W. W. Norton & Company), 4.

7. Allman, "Planet Earth."

8. Allman, "Planet Earth."

9. O'Leary, Philip R., Patrick W. Walsh, and Robert K. Ham. (1988) "Managing solid waste." *Scientific American* 259 (6): 36–42.

10. Commoner, *Making Peace with the Planet,* 11–12.

11. Carson, Rachel. (1962) *Silent Spring.* (Boston: Houghton Mifflin).

12. Goldsmith, Edward, and Nicholas Hildyard. (1988) *The Earth Report.* (Los Angeles: Price Stern Sloan), 175.

13. Caplan, Ruth, and the staff of Environmental Action. (1990) *Our Earth, Ourselves.* (New York: Bantam Books), 122–123.

14. Commoner, *Making Peace with the Planet,* 74.

15. Misch, Ann. (1994) "Assessing environmental health risks." In Starke, Linda, ed. *State of the World 1993: A Worldwatch Institute Report on Progress Toward a Sustainable Society.* (New York: W. W. Norton & Company), 119.

16. "Regulating pesticides: Do Americans need more protection from toxic chemicals?" (1994) *The CQ Researcher* 4 (4): 79.

17. Silver, Cheryl Simon. (1993) "Air pollution." In *The 1993 Information Please Environmental Almanac* ed. World Resources Institute. (Boston: Houghton Mifflin Company). 89.

18. Department of Health and Human Services, (1991) *Healthy People 2000: National Health Promotion and Disease Prevention Objectives* (Washington, D.C.: U.S. Government Printing Office), 321.

19. Commoner, *Making Peace with the Planet,* 39.

20. Hinrichsen, Don. (1988) "Acid rain and forest decline." In *The Earth Reports,* eds. Edward Goldsmith and Nicholas Hildyard (Los Angeles: Price Stern Sloan).

21. Hinrichsen, "Acid rain and forest decline."

22. Hinrichsen, "Acid rain and forest decline."

23. Hinrichsen, "Acid rain and forest decline."

24. Naar, *Design for a Livable Planet,* 98.

25. Naar, *Design for a Livable Planet,* 101.

26. Naar, *Design for a Livable Planet,* 101.

27. Naar, *Design for a Livable Planet,* 101.

28. Caplan et al., *Our Earth, Ourselves,* 92.

29. Naar, *Design for a Livable Planet,* 98.

30. Misch, "Assessing environmental health risks," 131.

31. Naar, *Design for a Livable Planet,* 98.

32. Caplan et al., *Our Earth, Ourselves,* 92.

33. EPA, (August, 1988) *Environmental Progress and Challenges: EPA's Update* (Washington, D.C.: Office of Policy Planning and Evaluation [PM-219] EPA-230-07-88-033): 82.

34. "Progress and Challenges: Looking at EPA today," (1990) *EPA Journal* 16 (5): 21.

35. "Regulating pesticides," 88.

36. Caplan et al., *Our Earth, Ourselves,* 120, 144.

37. Naar, *Design for a Livable Planet,* 38.

38. Carpenter, Betsy, et al. (1991) "Is your water safe?" *U.S. News & World Report* 111 (5): 53.

39. Cotton, Paul. (1994) "Pollution and poverty overlap becomes issue, administration promises action." *JAMA* 271 (13), 967–970.

40. Durning, Alan B. (1990) "Ending poverty." In *State of the World 1990,* ed. Lester R. Brown (New York: W. W. Norton & Company), 148.

41. Chepesiuk, Ron. (1991) "From ash to cash: The international trade in toxic waste," *E: The Environmental Magazine* 11 (4): 32.

42. Chepesiuk, "From ash to cash," 36.

43. Caplan et al., *Our Earth, Ourselves,* 117.

44. EPA, *Environmental Progress and Challenges,* 52.

45. Naar, *Design for a Livable Planet,* 46.

46. "Progress and Challenges," 24.

47. Brown, "A new era unfolds," 10.

48. Pollock, Cynthia. (1987) "Realizing recycling's potential." In *State of the World 1987,* ed. Lester R. Brown, et al. (New York: W. W. Norton & Company, 1987), 102–103.

49. Ehrlich, Paul R., and Anne H. Ehrlich. (1974) *The End of Affluence.* (New York: Random House).

50. Durning, Alan. (June, 1991) "Enough is enough: Assessing global consumption." *Dollars & Sense:* 15–18.

51. Lobell, John. (1981) *The Little Green Book.* (Boulder, Colo.: Shambhala Publications), 374.

52. Ehrlich and Ehrlich, *Earth,* 39.

53. Rifkin, Jeremy. (1989) *Entropy.* (New York: Bantam Books), 49.

54. Rifkin, *Entropy,* 73.

55. Rifkin, *Entropy,* 284–285.

56. Durning, "Enough is enough:," 15–18.

57. Russell, Robert. (1969) "Toward a functional understanding of ecology for health education." *Journal of School Health* 39 (10): 702–708; Russell, Robert. (1972) "Effects of ecological thinking on health education." *School Health Review* 3 (4): 3–5.

58. Durning, "Enough is enough:," 15–18.

59. Lappé, Frances Moore. (1990) "Choose to eat low on the food chain." In *Green Lifestyle Handbook: 1001 Ways You Can Heal the Earth*, ed. Jeremy Rifkin (New York: Henry Holt & Company), 60.

60. Naar, *Design for a Livable Planet*, 115.

61. Mast, Terry Stutzman. (1993) "Wastes." In *The 1993 Information Please Environmental Almanac* ed. World Resources Institute. (Boston: Houghton Mifflin Company), 57.

62. Golden Aluminum Company, a subsidiary of the ACX Technologies.

63. Pollock, "Realizing recycling's potential," 111.

64. "Water quality: Should safety standards for drinking water be tougher in the U.S.?" (1994) *CQ Researcher* 4 (6): 123.

65. Prugh, Thomas. (1993) "Energy." In *The 1993 Information Please Environmental Almanac* ed. World Resources Institute. (Boston: Houghton Mifflin Company), 67.

66. Prugh, "Energy," 72.

67. Hardin, Garrett. (1968) "The tragedy of the commons." *Science* 162 (3859): 1243–1248.

68. The Earth Works Group. (1991) *The Next Step: 50 More Things You Can Do to Save the Earth*. (Berkeley, Calif.: Earthworks Press), 36.

Appendix

Food and Nutrition Board, National Academy of Sciences—National Research Council Recommended Dietary Allowances,[a] Revised 1989

Designed for the maintenance of good nutrition of practically all healthy people in the United States

Category	Age (years) or Condition	Weight[b] (kg) (lb)		Height[b] (cm) (in)		Protein (g)	Fat-Soluble Vitamins				Water-Soluble Vitamins		
							Vitamin A (µg RE)[c]	Vitamin D (µg)[d]	Vitamin E (mg α-TE)[e]	Vitamin K (µg)	Vitamin C (mg)	Thiamine (mg)	
Infants	0.0–0.5	6	13	60	24	13	375	7.5	3	5	30	0.3	
	0.5–1.0	9	20	71	28	14	375	10	4	10	35	0.4	
Children	1–3	13	29	90	35	16	400	10	6	15	40	0.7	
	4–6	20	44	112	44	24	500	10	7	20	45	0.9	
	7–10	28	62	132	52	28	700	10	7	30	45	1.0	
Males	11–14	45	99	157	62	45	1000	10	10	45	50	1.3	
	15–18	66	145	176	69	59	1000	10	10	65	60	1.5	
	19–24	72	160	177	70	58	1000	10	10	70	60	1.5	
	25–50	79	174	176	70	63	1000	5	10	80	60	1.5	
	51 +	77	170	173	68	63	1000	5	10	80	60	1.2	
Females	11–14	46	101	157	62	46	800	10	8	45	50	1.1	
	15–18	55	120	163	64	44	800	10	8	55	60	1.1	
	19–24	58	128	164	65	46	800	10	8	60	60	1.1	
	25–50	63	138	163	64	50	800	5	8	65	60	1.1	
	51 +	65	143	160	63	50	800	5	8	65	60	1.0	
Pregnant						60	800	10	10	65	70	1.5	
Lactating	1st 6 months					65	1300	10	12	65	95	1.6	
	2nd 6 months					62	1200	10	11	65	90	1.6	

Reprinted with permission from *Recommended Dietary Allowances,* 10th edition. © 1989 by the National Academy of Sciences. Published by National Academy Press, Washington, D.C.

[a] The allowances, expressed as average daily intakes over time, are intended to provide for individual variations among most normal persons as they live in the United States under usual environmental stresses. Diets should be based on a variety of common foods in order to provide other nutrients for which human requirements have been less well defined.

[b] Weights and heights are actual medians for the U.S. population of the designated age. The use of these figures does not imply that the height-to-weight ratios are ideal.

Category	Water-Soluble Vitamins					Minerals						
	Riboflavin (mg)	Niacin (mg NE)[f]	Vitamin B_6 (mg)	Folate (μg)	Vitamin B_{12} (μg)	Calcium (mg)	Phosphorus (mg)	Magnesium (mg)	Iron (mg)	Zinc (mg)	Iodine (μg)	Selenium (μg)
Infants	0.4	5	0.3	25	0.3	400	300	40	6	5	40	10
	0.5	6	0.6	35	0.5	600	500	60	10	5	50	15
Children	0.8	9	1.0	50	0.7	800	800	80	10	10	70	20
	1.1	12	1.1	75	1.0	800	800	120	10	10	90	20
	1.2	13	1.4	100	1.4	800	800	170	10	10	120	30
Males	1.5	17	1.7	150	2.0	1200	1200	270	12	15	150	40
	1.8	20	2.0	200	2.0	1200	1200	400	12	15	150	50
	1.7	19	2.0	200	2.0	1200	1200	350	10	15	150	70
	1.7	19	2.0	200	2.0	800	800	350	10	15	150	70
	1.4	15	2.0	200	2.0	800	800	350	10	15	150	70
Females	1.3	15	1.4	150	2.0	1200	1200	280	15	12	150	45
	1.3	15	1.5	180	2.0	1200	1200	300	15	12	150	50
	1.3	15	1.6	180	2.0	1200	1200	280	15	12	150	55
	1.3	15	1.6	180	2.0	800	800	280	15	12	150	55
	1.2	13	1.6	180	2.0	800	800	280	10	12	150	55
Pregnant	1.6	17	2.2	400	2.2	1200	1200	320	30	15	175	65
Lactating	1.8	20	2.1	280	2.6	1200	1200	355	15	19	200	75
	1.7	20	2.1	260	2.6	1200	1200	340	15	16	200	75

[c]Retinol equivalents. 1 retinol equivalent = 1 μg retinol or 6 μg β-carotene.

[d]As cholecalciferol. 10 μg cholecalciferol = 400 IU of vitamin D.

[e]α-Tocopherol equivalents. 1 mg d-α-tocopherol = 1 α-TE.

[f]NE (niacin equivalent) is equal to 1 mg of niacin or 60 mg of dietary tryptophan.

Glossary

A

accident A sequence of events that results in unintended injury, death, or property damage.

acetaldehyde A by-product of the metabolism of alcohol.

acetaminophen An analgesic which relieves pain and lowers fever, but does not have the anti-inflammatory effect of aspirin.

acid rain Precipitation with a pH below 5.6. Acid rain is formed when sulfur dioxide and nitrous oxides are released into the atmosphere and combine with water droplets.

acrosome A structure covering the head of a sperm cell that contains an enzyme capable of breaking down the coating of cells that surround the egg, thus enabling the sperm to penetrate it.

acupuncture An ancient Chinese healing art whereby fine needles are inserted at specific points on the body in order to restore health.

acyclovir An antiviral drug that has demonstrated some favorable results in treating the acute symptoms of herpes infection.

addictive behaviors Behaviors that initially are rewarding, but lead to tolerance, craving, obsession with the behavior, and withdrawal if the behavior is stopped.

additive A form of drug interaction where the total effect of the drugs taken is equivalent to the sum of the effects of the individual drugs.

adipose cells Fat-storing cells.

adrenal glands Endocrine glands located on the tops of the kidneys.

adrenalin A hormone secreted by the adrenal glands during the stress response. (Also known as epinephrine.)

adrenocorticotrophic hormone (ACTH) A hormone released by the pituitary glands that activates the adrenal glands.

aerobic exercise Activities that cause a sustained increase in heart rate and use the large muscles of the body continuously for an extended period of time.

affirmation A verbal description of a desired condition stated as if it were present reality; a technique for promoting mental wellness by "psyching" oneself into thinking in positive terms about the present and the future.

afterbirth Comprises the placenta and fetal membranes that are expelled from the uterus following the birth of the child.

ageism A systematic way of regarding the elderly with contempt, ignoring contributions they can make, or engaging in practices that exclude them from access to certain rights and privileges.

AIDS Acquired immune deficiency syndrome; a condition in which the immune system becomes severely compromised and the body comes under attack by disorders usually proving lethal.

AIDS dementia complex Neurologic complications from AIDS involving memory loss, erratic behavior, and other symptoms.

alarm stage The first stage of the General Adaptation Syndrome, during which the body awakens to a stressor and gears up to deal with it. Typical signs and symptoms include muscle tension, a pounding heart, butterflies in the stomach, and the like.

alcohol Beverage produced by fermentation of natural sugars that have intoxication properties.

alcohol abuse The misuse of alcohol resulting in alcohol-related psychological, medical, and social problems.

alcohol-dependence syndrome Addiction to alcohol, often known as alcoholism, characterized by loss of memory, inability to stop drinking until intoxication, inability to cut down on drinking, binge drinking, and withdrawal symptoms.

alcoholic hepatitis A chronic inflammation of the liver due to chronic alcohol abuse.

alcoholism Addiction to alcohol, sometimes called alcohol-dependence syndrome, characterized by loss of memory, inability to stop drinking until intoxication, inability to cut down on drinking, binge drinking, and withdrawal symptoms.

alcohol-related disability Refers to an impairment in the physical, mental, or social functioning of an individual when that impairment can be shown to be related to alcohol consumption.

alcohol-related mortality (ARM) A cause of death directly attributable to the use of alcoholic beverages.

alpha fetoprotein blood test A maternal blood test that can detect birth defects of the brain and spinal cord.

alveoli Compartmentalized air sacs in the lungs that exchange oxygen and carbon dioxide during normal breathing.

Alzheimer's disease A chronic condition physically characterized by structural modifications in the brain's nerve fibers and giving rise to mental infirmity, which is behaviorally manifested by memory loss, hallucinations, and social disorientation.

AMA *See* American Medical Association.

ambulatory A type of health care synonymous with outpatient care, i.e., no hospital stay required.

amenorrhea A lack of menstrual periods.

American Dental Association A professional organization whose membership is comprised principally of dentists.

American Medical Association   A professional organization whose membership is comprised principally of physicians.

amino acids   Nitrogen containing chemicals that are the building blocks of protein.

amino acid supplements   A product sold in many health-food stores that contains amino acids. Often in tablet or powder form, these supplements are touted as having the ability to increase muscle mass, and thus athletic performance. Scientific evidence does not support these claims, and there are dangers in taking these supplements in high doses.

amniocentesis   The testing of amniotic fluid to discover genetic disorders in the developing fetus.

amniotic fluid   Fluid found in the amniotic sac that acts as a barrier to physical shock and helps maintain proper temperature.

amniotic sac   A clear, fluid-filled membrane that develops during the embryonic period and surrounds the embryo, and later the fetus, providing a protective and nurturing environment until birth.

amphetamine   A class of drugs that stimulates the central nervous system and promotes wakefulness and arousal. Tolerance develops rapidly, requiring ever increasing doses to maintain its effects. Prolonged use may lead to dependence.

anabolic steroids   Synthetic derivatives of testosterone, the male sex hormone.

anaerobic exercise   Activities requiring an intense, maximum burst of energy and which are done for short time intervals (ten to ninety seconds).

analgesic   A drug that relieves pain. Such pain relief may be accomplished by both external or internal administration of analgesics.

androgens   Male sex hormones, such as testosterone.

androgyny   The adoption of behaviors that exhibit high levels of both male and female characteristics.

anemia   A decreased ability of the blood to carry oxygen, due to a decrease in the amount of hemoglobin in the blood.

anesthetic   A substance that reduces or stops sensations, including pain.

aneurysm   A "ballooning" or outpocketing of an artery resulting from a diseased and weakened arterial wall.

angina   Severe chest pain resulting from restricted blood flow through the coronary arteries; synonymous with angina pectoris.

angina pectoris   Severe chest pain resulting from restricted blood flow through the coronary arteries.

angioplasty   A procedure in which a balloon catheter is inserted into a blocked coronary artery. The balloon is then inflated in order to stretch the plaque and allow more blood to flow through the artery.

anomie   A state of confusion, disorientation, and anxiety.

anonymous test   A test performed whose outcome is revealed through assignment of a number rather than an identity.

anorexia nervosa   An eating disorder characterized by a loss of at least 25% of original body weight, preoccupation with food, preoccupation with diet and body image, fear of fat, reduced sexual activity, loss of menstrual periods, and hyperactivity.

anorgasmia   The inability to reach orgasm.

antibiotics   A substance produced to inhibit or kill microorganisms, directed primarily at pathogenic ones.

antibodies   Immunoglobulin proteins that have been changed into plasma cells (cells that make up the fluid portion of the blood). The transformation from immunoglobulin to antibody occurs in order to counteract a specific antigen of an invading pathogen.

antibody-mediated immunity   Immunity produced through the action of the B-cells.

anticoagulant   A substance that impedes blood clot formation.

antigen   Any substance whose introduction to the body is capable of producing the immune response.

antihistamines   Drugs used to treat symptoms of allergy.

antioxidants   Substances that prevent the formation of free radicals, or atoms in which there is an unpaired electron. Free radicals are natural by-products of the body burning oxygen (oxidation). By inhibiting the formation of free radicals, antioxidants are thought to decrease the risk of developing a variety of chronic diseases including heart disease and some cancers.

anus   A small opening at the lower end of the intestines, below the rectum, through which feces is discharged.

aorta   The large arterial trunk that carries blood from the heart to the arterial and capillary network of the body; the largest artery in the body.

appendectomy   The surgical removal of the appendix.

arrhythmia   Any heart beat that is a departure from normal, healthy heart rhythm.

arteries   The vessels that carry blood from the heart to the body.

arterioles   Small arteries that branch from larger ones and lead to capillaries.

arteriosclerosis   A chronic and progressive disorder whereby the walls of the arteries thicken, harden, and lose their elasticity.

arthritis   A general term referring to an inflammation of the joints. Common symptoms include pain, swelling, and restricted motion. Arthritis has many known causes, such as rheumatic fever and trauma, as well as unknown causes.

artificial insemination   Using means other than a penis to introduce semen into the female vaginal tract.

artificially acquired active immunity Immunity resulting from the development within the body of substances stimulated by inoculation with a vaccine.

artificially acquired passive immunity Temporary immunity acquired through the delivery of the gamma globulin fraction of blood.

asbestos A flame-retardant material used for insulation and other construction that has been implicated as a factor in the etiology of certain lung diseases.

aspartame An artificial sweetener used in some diet soft drinks and other food and beverage products that is marketed as Equal® or Nutrasweet®.

aspirin The most common internal analgesic, this drug relieves pain, lowers fever, and reduces inflammation and swelling of the joints.

Association of American Medical Colleges One of the accrediting bodies for U.S. medical schools.

asthma A chronic condition often of allergic origin marked by labored breathing, wheezing, constriction of the chest, and further manifested by gasping or coughing.

atherosclerosis A particular type of arteriosclerosis whereby the walls of the arteries become clogged with deposits of fats and other substances, forming plaques.

atrium The upper chamber of each half of the heart.

autoimmune reaction An abnormal body response where T-cells attack the body's own healthy cells and tissues.

autonomic nervous system A part of the nervous system that regulates body functions usually not under voluntary control, such as heart rate, breathing rate, etc.

avoidance A defense mechanism whereby a person stays away from situations that are perceived to be distressful.

AZT *See* zidovudine.

B

bacterial pneumonia Also known as pneumococcal pneumonia, this infectious disease is caused by the bacteria *Streptococcus pneumoniae*, and is transmitted through respiratory secretions.

bait and switch A sales tactic whereby the retailer lures a customer into a store with a specially advertised offer and then substitutes a different, and usually more costly, product.

Bartholin's glands Glands found in the external female reproductive system, one on each horizontal side of the opening of the vagina, that secrete a mucus prior to female orgasm.

basal body temperature The lowest body temperature naturally reached by a healthy person.

basal body temperature (BBT) method An ovulation prediction method of birth control that uses measurement of body temperature to predict ovulation.

basal metabolic rate (BMR) The energy required to maintain basic life functions, such as heart rate, digestion, and breathing for a person at rest.

B-cell Lymphocytes that develop in the bone marrow and protect against disease and infection.

behavior modification A set of techniques used by psychologists to help facilitate behavior changes through a process of describing the behavior to be changed, replacing and controlling established behaviors, and reinforcing or rewarding successful changes.

benign Usually in reference to a tumor, meaning noncancerous or nonmalignant.

beta-endorphin A compound occurring in the brain that appears to have a pain-suppressing action, and which may be responsible for the "high" associated with long-distance running.

bile salts A major component of bile, these molecules aid in the digestion and absorption of fats.

bioelectrical impedance analysis (BIA) A method of estimating body composition using a painless electrical current introduced into the body that measures the conductivity of lean body mass. The validity of this body fat measurement technique is uncertain.

blood alcohol concentration A measure of the amount of alcohol found in the blood of an alcohol user.

blood-cholesterol The amount of cholesterol circulating in one's circulatory system. It is a high blood cholesterol level that constitutes a major risk for coronary artery disease.

body composition The amount of an individual's body that is fat versus fat-free tissue.

body mass index (BMI) A measure of body composition that is highly correlated with percent body fat measures. To calculate BMI, you divide weight (in kilograms) by body height (in meters) squared.

brain death The cessation of electrical activity in the brain; in the absence of oxygen to brain tissue it takes the brain about fifteen minutes to die completely.

brand loyalty A sales tactic whereby the retailer attempts to convince a potential customer to buy a familiar brand name that may be more costly, but no more effective, than a less expensive or less known brand.

breasts As part of the external female reproductive system, fatty tissue structures containing fifteen to twenty milk ducts each, all of which open to the external nipple.

breast self-examination (BSE) The systematic exploration and palpation of the breasts with the hand to identify normal and abnormal or irregular features, a self-care early detection procedure for breast cancer.

breech births Babies not born in the head-first position. These births include buttocks first, legs first, or shoulder first presentations.

bronchi The two tube-like passageways branching from the trachea (windpipe) and leading to the lungs.

bronchitis An inflammation of the lining of the bronchi resulting in obscured air flow, arising usually from infection or chronic irritation.

bulbourethral glands   Two glands found in the male reproductive system connected to the urethra as it enters the penis. These glands release an alkaline secretion that may neutralize any urine in the urethra prior to ejaculation.

bulimia nervosa   An eating disorder characterized by binge eating, often followed by self-induced vomiting or purging.

burning agents   Chemicals added to tobacco to ensure that the tobacco will continue burning once lit. These agents are added to make sure that when a cigarette is put down in an ashtray, it will continue burning.

C

caffeine   A stimulant drug derived from the dried leaves of tea or the dried seeds of coffee.

calcium   Mineral which in its ionic form is critical for bone growth, muscle contraction, and other metabolic functions; in its solid state it comprises about 85% of the mineral matter in bones.

calendar method   An ovulation prediction method of birth control that keeps track of menstrual cycles in order to predict ovulation.

calorie   A unit of measure of the amount of energy derived from food.

Campylobacter   A common type of food-borne infection caused by eating food contaminated with the *campylobacter bacterium*; symptoms include muscle pain, nausea, vomiting, fever, cramps, and occasionally bloody diarrhea.

cancer   A collection of diseases characterized by the presence of malignant tumors of potentially unlimited growth that expand locally by invasion and systemically by metastasis.

Candida albicans   A yeast infection usually of the oral or genital area; becoming increasingly more common as a confounding disease in persons with AIDS.

candidiasis   An infection caused by C. albicans; not necessarily of sexual contact origin, but can be transmitted sexually; increasingly, an opportunistic infection associated with AIDS.

capillaries   The smallest blood vessels connecting arterioles and venules forming networks throughout the body.

carbohydrate loading   A diet regimen practiced by some athletes that consists of depleting body stores of carbohydrates through exercise, followed by several days of dietary carbohydrate restriction, and finally by several days of high dietary carbohydrate intake. The goal is to increase glycogen stores in the body.

carbohydrates   A nutrient composed of carbon, hydrogen, and oxygen, which is the body's preferred form of energy, supplying four calories per gram.

carbon dioxide   A heavy, colorless, odorless gas that is a by-product of human respiration. Additionally, carbon dioxide is released into the atmosphere during the burning of fossil fuels, such as oil and coal. It is believed to be one of the "greenhouse gases" responsible for global warming.

carbon monoxide   An odorless, colorless gas (CO) with lethal potential that is a by-product of combustion. CO is a component of smoke formed when tobacco is burned.

carcinogen   Any substance or factor that has cancer-causing potential.

carcinoma   A cancer arising from epithelial tissues that line organs.

cardiac arrest   Complete cessation of the heart beat.

cardiac catheterization   A procedure in which a small flexible tube (catheter) is inserted into an artery or vein in the arm or leg and fed through the vascular system to the heart.

cardiac palpitation   An awareness of one's heartbeat.

cardiopulmonary resuscitation (CPR)   Mouth-to-mouth resuscitation combined with closed (external) heart massage to maintain breathing and circulation.

cardiorespiratory endurance   The ability of the circulatory and respiratory systems to supply the necessary oxygen for sustained strenuous activity.

carotid arteries   Arteries, located along the side of the neck that ascend and supply blood to various structures in the neck, face, jaw, scalp, and to the brain.

cataract   Common occurrence with aging in which the lens of the eye and/or its capsule becomes increasingly opaque, resulting in obscured vision.

cell-mediated immunity   Immunity occurring primarily from response of the T-cells.

Centers for Disease Control (CDC)   A series of offices and divisions at the national level in the U.S. whose personnel study the cause, distribution, and treatment of disease.

central nervous system   The part of the nervous system consisting of the brain and spinal cord.

cerebral arteries   Arteries that carry blood, oxygen, and nutrients to the brain. Blockage in one of these arteries gives rise to a stroke.

cerebral thrombosis   The blockage of a cerebral artery in the brain by a blood clot, resulting in a stroke.

cervical cap   A thimble-sized and -shaped device, placed over the cervix, that prevents fertilization by not allowing sperm to enter the uterus and fallopian tubes.

cervical mucus method   An ovulation prediction method of birth control that uses changes in the consistency of the female's cervical mucus to predict ovulation.

cervix The opening of the uterus which connects with the vagina.

cesarean section The surgical opening of the abdomen and uterus for childbirth.

chancre The self-limiting sore or lesion that characterizes the primary stage of syphilis.

chancroid An STD limited primarily to tropical or subtropical areas of the world, producing early symptoms similar to those of syphilis.

chemical abortions A type of induced abortion that relies on the use of toxic substances introduced into the amniotic sac resulting in premature delivery of a dead fetus.

chemical birth-control methods Methods that use chemicals that prevent fertilization (spermicides) or prevent ovulation or end implantation (birth-control pills).

chemotherapy The treatment of disease by use of drugs; usually mentioned in reference to the treatment of cancer.

chewing tobacco A preparation of tobacco leaves in looseleaf, plug, or twist forms mixed with flavoring agents that is held in the mouth clenched between the teeth; a variety of smokeless tobacco.

chickenpox A highly communicable infectious disease caused by a herpes virus; the most notable symptom is itchy, dark red bumps that cover the entire body; a new vaccine has been introduced to prevent this common childhood disease.

child abuse The maltreatment of children, which includes sexual maltreatment, as well as physical and emotional injury caused by improper care and discipline or neglect.

childbirth supervisor The person in charge of childbirth; this person may be a physician, nurse midwife, lay midwife, or layperson.

child neglect A type of child abuse that consists of failing to provide for the essential physical needs of a child, such as not providing adequate food or clothing.

chiropractic An alternative approach to healing that is founded on the theory that health is contingent upon the structural integrity of the spinal column.

chlamydia trachomatis A microorganism responsible for several STD infections sharing certain properties and traits.

cholera A communicable infectious disease caused by the bacteria *Vibrio cholerae* transmitted through food or water contaminated with infected feces. Common symptoms include severe diarrhea and vomiting, often resulting in dehydration and circulatory collapse. If treated promptly and properly, the fatality rate is low. Without such care the fatality rate may exceed 50 percent.

cholesterol A fatty substance found in animal products and manufactured by the body. Its presence in high amounts is associated with an elevated risk of cardiovascular disease.

chorionic biopsy A procedure where a sample of the chorionic tissue is taken through the vagina of a pregnant woman. This procedure can provide information on possible fetal genetic defects as early as the seventh week of pregnancy.

chorionic tissue A membrane that completely surrounds an embryo once implantation occurs.

chromosome A threadlike structure containing genes, found in the nucleus of every cell.

chronic obstructive lung disease (COLD) A category of lung disease characterized by decreased ability of the lungs to perform gas exchanges. Emphysema and chronic bronchitis are common examples.

cilia Tiny hairlike projections that line certain parts of the body, such as the respiratory tract, whose constant motion helps to sweep away foreign particles and prevent the introduction of pathogens.

circumcision An operation to remove the prepuce or foreskin from the penis.

circumstantial-situational drug use The short-term use of a drug as a coping mechanism to deal with particular situations.

cirrhosis of the liver Scarring of tissue in the liver that interferes with blood flow through the liver, eventually interrupting the liver's major functions of detoxification and metabolism.

climacteric The cessation of the female's reproductive cycle or the corresponding period of lessening sexual activity in the male.

clinical death Cessation of heartbeat and respiration that will be permanent if not reversed within approximately four minutes by CPR or other emergency procedures.

clinical psychologist A health-care professional who possesses a Ph.D in psychology and focuses his or her practice on mental health and human behavior.

clitoris A small erectile organ located in the female at the top of the labia minora and labia majora; corresponds to the penis of the male.

closed-eye imagery Seeing things with your eyes closed.

cocaine A crystalline powder extracted from the leaves of the South American coca plant, this drug is a powerful central nervous system stimulant and a local anesthetic.

cocarcinogen A substance capable of causing cancer only when it is in the presence of another specific substance.

codeine An analgesic derived from morphine.

cohabitation Describes a living arrangement in which two people who are not married to each other share both bed and board.

cohabiting *See* cohabitation.

coitus interruptus A technique used by some individuals to prevent pregnancy, sometimes referred to as 'withdrawal'; during vaginal intercourse the penis is withdrawn from the vagina prior to ejaculation; failure rates are high.

coitus *See* vaginal intercourse.

cold turkey A phrase used to describe an approach to smoking cessation where a smoker sets a date to stop smoking and then, on that date, completely gives up smoking cigarettes.

collagen A fibrous insoluble protein found in connective tissue, including skin, bones, ligaments, and cartilage; it comprises 30% of the total body protein.

collateral circulation Tiny blood vessels that connect with major arteries and provide a limited backup system for obtaining blood flow to tissue when an artery is blocked; collateral blood vessels will dilate and attempt to carry greater blood flow in the event of blockage of an artery.

colostrum A substance secreted by the breasts prior to milk production. Colostrum contains several antibodies that protect newborns from illness, allergies, respiratory diseases, and diarrhea.

commitment As used to define love, commitment is described as a short-term decision to love someone and a long-term decision to maintain that loving relationship.

compensatory smoking A side-effect of a smoking cessation effort whereby the person smokes more than usual to satisfy the body's demand for nicotine.

complete protein Any food containing all eight of the essential amino acids.

complex carbohydrate A form of carbohydrate consisting of three or more simple-sugar molecules bonded together in varying patterns. Common complex carbohydrates include starch, fiber, and glycogen.

compulsive drug use A pattern of drug use that reflects loss of control over the use of these drugs.

computed-axial tomograph (CT scanner) A diagnostic machine that produces images of the body in a noninvasive manner.

condoms Cylindrical sheaths made of rubber, animal skin, or polyurethane that are placed either over the male's penis (male condom) or in a woman's vagina (female condom) to prevent fertilization by trapping semen.

condyloma acuminata Synonymous with venereal warts; benign tumors in the genital area from viral infection acquired sexually.

confidential test A test performed whose outcome and the identity of the person tested is known only to the person and the health-care provider.

congenital heart malformations Defects in the heart that are present at birth.

congenital syphilis Syphilis that results from transmission of disease across the placenta to a fetus.

congestive heart failure Heart failure in which the heart is unable to maintain adequate circulation of blood through the body, or to pump out venous return blood.

conjunctivitis Inflammation of the conjunctiva of the eye due to any irritation or infection, frequently mentioned in reference to a complication of gonorrhea.

conservation Using less of a given product.

conservation of energy The first law of thermodynamics; energy cannot be created or destroyed, but only transformed from one form to another.

constructive self-talk A personality engineering strategy that involves talking pleasantly to oneself, repeating statements that focus on positive aspects of one's life.

contact investigation A mechanism for reducing the likelihood of an epidemic by asking persons treated for STDs to identify sexual partners who can be traced, examined, and successfully treated, if necessary.

contraindications Health conditions in which a particular birth-control method represents a serious health risk to the user.

cooldown Gradually slowing down at the end of an exercise session in order to keep blood from pooling in the lower extremities and to aid in the removal of waste products that may have built up in muscles during exercise.

coronary arteries The two arteries, one right and one left, that arise from the aorta and supply the heart with oxygen.

coronary artery bypass surgery A surgical procedure that reroutes the blood supply in a coronary artery around a severe blockage.

coronary artery disease A chronic disease condition in which the normal flow of blood through the coronary arteries is reduced or impaired; synonymous with coronary heart disease.

coronary heart disease *See* coronary artery disease.

coronary thrombosis The blockage of a coronary artery by a blood clot, resulting in a heart attack.

corpus luteum The temporary endocrine gland in the ovary that secretes hormones. Its purpose is to prevent menstruation during pregnancy.

corticosteroids Steroid hormones secreted by the adrenal cortex, including hydrocortisone and aldosterone. These hormones are sometimes used as a prescription medication to treat a variety of conditions.

corticotropin releasing factor (CRF) A hormone released by the hypothalamus that activates the pituitary glands.

crack A smokable form of cocaine that results from purification with baking soda and water.

crack babies Babies whose mothers used crack during pregnancy. These babies often experience substantial health problems during birth, early in life, and perhaps throughout life.

crack house A location where crack cocaine or other drugs are available for purchase or use.

creativity   The production of new and effective thoughts, actions, or things.

cremation   The burning of a dead body to a state of ashes.

cues to eating   A behavior modification term describing activities or events associated with initiation of food consumption.

cunnilingus   The oral stimulation of the female's genitals.

cyclamates   Artificial sweeteners implicated by some research in the cause of bladder cancer.

cytomegalovirus   A salivary gland inhibiting virus that can affect numerous sites in the body.

D

daily reference values (DRVs)   The amount of fat, saturated fatty acids, cholesterol, total carbohydrates, fiber, sodium, potassium, and protein adults and children over four should consume daily for maintenance of good nutrition. These values are based on a 2,000 calorie diet, and are listed on the "Nutrition Facts" food label.

DDT   A synthetic insecticide that kills insects by attacking biochemical processes in their nervous systems.

defense mechanisms   A natural, often unconscious, psychological response used to defend oneself against distress.

defensive driving skills   Specific skills necessary to reduce the likelihood of motor vehicle crashes. These skills include specific acts taken with the assumption that other drivers or road and environmental conditions are likely to increase the risk (e.g., waiting to see if a car stops at a red light before proceeding through an intersection).

delta-9-tetrahydrocannabinol (THC)   The active ingredient in marijuana that is responsible for the common effect of the drug.

denial   A defense mechanism whereby a person refuses to accept reality.

dental caries   The process through which teeth decay. Commonly known as cavities.

dental plaque   A gummy mass of microorganisms on the crowns of teeth, spreading to the roots, that makes teeth susceptible to decay.

deoxygenated blood   Blood returned to the heart from the body to be replenished with oxygen in the lungs.

Depo-Provera   An injectable, synthetic progesterone birth-control method; one injection will prevent ovulation for twelve weeks.

depression   A state of altered mood ranging in severity and duration; in its mild form, it consists of sadness and discouragement, usually of brief duration. In more severe forms, it consists of prolonged or recurrent mental incapacitation, possibly with thoughts of self-destruction or death.

DES   Stands for diethylstilbestrol, a drug formerly prescribed during pregnancy, that gave rise to reproductive system cancers primarily in the daughters of those who took it; still used as a morning-after birth-control pill in cases of rape or incest.

diabetes   A metabolic disorder caused by lack of insulin or resistance to insulin, resulting in the body not being able to metabolize sugar for energy. Diabetes can be controlled through diet, exercise, and medication. Uncontrolled diabetes can result in life-threatening complications.

diabetes mellitus   *See* diabetes.

diaphragm   A shallow rubber dome inserted into the vagina, covering the cervix, that prevents fertilization by not allowing sperm to enter the uterus and fallopian tubes.

diastolic   The lowest arterial blood pressure in the cardiac cycle occurring just before contraction of the left ventricle.

dietary cholesterol   Cholesterol that is consumed in food products. Some foods such as liver, egg yolks, cheesecake, and soft-serve ice cream are high in cholesterol. The American Heart Association and the U.S. Daily Reference Value recommend that people consume less than 300 mg of cholesterol daily.

dietary fiber   The part of food that is not digested by enzymes in the small intestine. The major forms of dietary fiber include soluble and insoluble fiber.

dilated   Enlarged or expanded.

dilation and evacuation   A type of induced abortion that requires dilation of the cervix before using suction and scraping to remove the uterine contents.

dimorphic   A species (like humans) that has two distinct reproductive forms, a male and a female.

dioxin   The common name for 2, 3, 7, 8-tetrachlorodibenzo(p)dioxin, a potent carcinogen often found in incinerator ash.

diphtheria   A highly communicable infectious disease caused by the bacteria *Corynebacterium diphtheriae*. Common symptoms include a sore throat, weakness and mild fever, followed by a constriction of the air passage causing difficulty in breathing. Toxin produced by the bacteria can cause death from heart failure if not treated promptly.

direct contact   The spread of a disease-causing organism from one person to another through intimate association.

disability days   The number of days during a year when a person is not able to engage in his or her usual activities because of an injury or illness.

disaccharide   A sugar formed by the union of two simple sugars or monosaccharides.

disease prevention   Activities undertaken to decrease the likelihood of the occurrence of a disease, to detect disease as early as possible, or to rehabilitate people when disease occurs.

distress   Intense, prolonged, or unrelenting stressors that can upset one's physical and psychological balance.

diuretics   Drugs that increase the amount of urine produced and excreted. Diuretics are often used to treat edema.

diverticular disease   A disease characterized by the formation and inflammation of sacs opening off of the colon.

Doctor of Podiatric Medicine (D.P.M.)   A degree possessed by medical specialists who deal with disorders of the feet.

Doctor of Podiatry (D.P.)   A degree possessed by medical specialists who deal with disorders of the feet.

domestic violence   Violence that is committed by and directed toward members of one's family or other individuals with whom there is an intimate relationship. Domestic violence includes partner abuse, rape, child abuse, elder abuse, and the like.

Down's syndrome   A congenital disease caused by the presence of an extra number-21 chromosome, resulting in mental deficiency and a variety of physical defects.

drinking water fluoridation   A public health practice to help assure that all members of a community receive optimal fluoride exposure to enhance tooth enamel formation and prevent cavities. Community drinking water supplies are modified to attain an optimal level of fluoride, ranging from 0.7 to 1.2 parts per million.

drug abuse   Using a drug in such a way as to greatly increase the hazard or impair the ability of the individual to function normally.

drug use   Using a drug in such a way as to ensure that the sought-for effects are attained.

duodenum   The upper third of the small intestine.

durable power of attorney (DPA)   The legal authority to represent another person whose own ability, by reason of mental or physical disorder, has become impaired.

dysmenorrhea   Painful menstruation.

dyspareunia   A medical term for painful sexual intercourse.

dysphoria   A feeling of discomfort associated with the use of drug substances. Such discomfort may be physical, mental, or emotional.

E

eclampsia   A condition affecting some pregnant women consisting of preeclampsia, convulsions, and coma.

E coli O157:H7   A common type of food-borne infection caused by eating food contaminated with the E coli O157:H7 bacterium; symptoms include bloody diarrhea, cramps, and low-grade fevers; complications may occur and include kidney failure, strokes, seizures, brain damage, and death.

ecological perspective   A philosophical view of life and death that sees all life forms as equivalent and that professes the nonexistence of an afterlife.

ecology   The study of ecosystems.

ecosystems   The interactions between a community of living organisms and their natural environment.

ectopic pregnancy   Occurs when an embryo develops outside the uterus. Ectopic pregnancy occurs most frequently in the fallopian tubes.

edema   The swelling of body tissue due to fluid retention.

effective dose level   The minimal dose of a drug that is required to produce a specific effect.

effectiveness rate   The chance of procreating if you use a particular method of birth control.

ejaculate   The fluid component discharged from the male reproductive tract at ejaculation that contains sperm cells; commonly known as semen.

ejaculation   The expulsion of semen from the urethra, usually accompanied by orgasm.

elder abuse   Any maltreatment of elderly individuals, including sexual maltreatment, as well as physical and emotional injury caused by improper or violent care and neglect.

electrocardiogram (ECG)   A medical test that measures and records the electrical activity of the heart and helps to detect heart disease.

electrocoagulation   A form of tubal ligation that uses electricity to seal a portion of each fallopian tube.

electroencephalograph (EEG)   An instrument for recording the electrical activity of the brain, also used to determine brain death.

electrolytic   A medical term referring to blood concentrations of specific ions, such as sodium, potassium, chloride, and bicarbonate.

electronic fetal monitoring (EFM)   A device inserted into the vagina of a pregnant woman during labor, used to monitor fetal vital signs.

embalmers   People who preserve dead bodies with chemicals.

embryo   The medical term for the products of conception up to the eighth week of conception.

emphysema   A progressive loss of function or rupture of the alveoli of the lung, resulting in increased respiratory distress.

enabling factors   Skills and resources that help one implement a health promotion plan.

endemic   Diseases that occur frequently or commonly in a particular location or population.

endocardium   Inner surface of the lining of the heart.

endocrine pathway hormones   Substances released directly into blood or body fluids from the endocrine system. An important function of these hormones is to increase body metabolism during the stress response.

endocrine system   All glands that secrete hormones directly into the blood or body fluids. This system consists of the pituitary, thyroid, parathyroid, and adrenal glands, as well as the pancreas, ovaries, testes, pineal gland, and thymus gland.

endometriosis   A condition in which a piece of the endometrium is attached to reproductive organs adjacent to the uterus. It is a common cause of infertility.

endometrium   The innermost layer of the uterus that secretes fluids and nutrients for the developing embryo.

energy   A measure of the ability to do work.

energy-balance equation   A theory of obesity causation that suggests that obesity results, over a period of time, from consuming more calories than one expends.

energy efficiency   Using the least amount of energy to accomplish a given task.

entropy   The second law of thermodynamics that specifies the direction in which energy must always be transformed from usable to unusable, from ordered to disordered, and from available to unavailable.

Environmental Protection Agency (EPA)   A federal agency created in 1970 whose major role is to consider and effectively deal with the major environmental problems facing the U.S.

environmental tobacco smoke   Smoke emitted from the burning end of a cigarette; also known as sidestream smoke.

enzyme   A protein substance that speeds up biochemical reactions.

enzyme immunoassay (EIA or ELISA)   A quantitative in vitro test for an antigen or antibody; with AIDS, EIA seeks the presence of AIDS antibodies.

epidemic   A disease or condition affecting many individuals in a population, community, or region at the same time.

epidemiology   The study of the distribution and causes of disease.

epididymis   A structure in the male reproductive system located over the testes whose major function is the temporary storage of sperm.

epidural   An anesthetic administered to some women during labor and delivery to reduce pain associated with the birthing process.

episiotomy   The surgical cutting of some tissue between the anal and vaginal openings in order to prevent this tissue from tearing during childbirth.

epithelial structures   Components of the body with epithelial tissue. Epithelial tissue is a type of tissue that lines all body surfaces, such as the outer layer of skin, and the inside lining of the digestive tract.

erectile dysfunction   Inability of a male to have an erection; sometimes referred to as impotence.

ergogenic drugs   Drug substances used for the purpose of giving athletes an edge in competition; such use is often illegal or ill-advised because of the potential for harm to the athlete.

erogenous zones   Areas of the body that are especially receptive to sexual stimulation, such as the mouth, ears, inner surfaces of the thighs, the breasts, and the genitals.

essential amino acids   Eight of the basic nitrogen-containing building blocks of protein that must be consumed preformed from food each day to maintain optimal growth and maintenance of body tissues.

essential fat   Fat stored in major body organs and tissues and necessary for normal, healthy functioning of the human body.

estrogens   The primary female sex hormones. They stimulate the development of a female physique and reproductive organs. Estrogens also stimulate the female reproductive cycle and maintain the adult female reproductive organs.

ethyl alcohol   The type of alcohol that is consumable. Also called grain alcohol.

euphoria   A general feeling of wellness or satisfaction associated with the use of certain drugs.

eustress   A term coined by Hans Selye to designate desirable stress.

euthanasia   The withholding of treatment or the removal of equipment that would prolong life through employment of heroic measures.

excitement phase   The first phase of sexual response; characterized in the female by vaginal lubrication and vasocongestion in the vagina, cervix, and vulva; characterized in the male by erection of the penis and movement of the testicles closer to the body.

exercise stress test   An aerobic exercise test that stresses the cardiorespiratory system. This test can be used, in conjunction with other tests, to diagnose coronary artery disease. It can also be used functionally to determine an individual's maximum heart rate during exercise, which is then used to guide a person in how strenuously they may safely exercise aerobically.

experimental drug use   The short-term use of any one or a combination of drugs.

experimental freedom   A characteristic of Rogers' fully functioning person involving the ability to make choices freely between different courses of action.

F

fallopian tube   A tube found in the internal female reproductive tract that lies between the ovaries and the uterus. With rare exceptions, these tubes are the site of fertilization.

false negative result   An erroneous test outcome that implies a person does not have a disorder when in fact he or she may.

false positive result   An erroneous test outcome that implies a person has a disorder when in fact he or she may not.

fat   A body tissue, sometimes called adipose tissue, composed of fat cells. Fat cells contain stored fat in the form of triglycerides.

fat-cell theory   A theory of obesity causation that suggests that people gain fat cells only during three specified periods of time. As adults, weight gain or loss is usually a result of expanding or contracting the content of fat cells, rather than adding or subtracting numbers of fat cells.

fats   A major nutrient that is the body's second major source of energy (calories) and is a preferred means of storing energy. Fat can supply or store approximately nine calories per gram.

fat-soluble vitamins   Vitamins that are transported and stored in lipids. Because the body stores these vitamins (A, D, E, and K), they can build up to toxic levels if great quantities are consumed.

fat substitute   A variety of compounds used in the production of processed foods that imitate the taste and texture of fat. Whey, oat flour, egg whites and milk proteins are some of the more common components of currently available fat substitutes.

fatty acids   An organic substance that serves as a building block for fat molecules.

fatty liver   The accumulation of fatty acids in liver cells.

FDA   Food and Drug Administration; an office of the U.S. Department of Health and Human Services having numerous responsibilities including approval and regulation of cosmetics and drugs.

fellatio   The oral stimulation of the male's genitals.

female condom   A disposable, lubricated polyurethane cylindrical tube with flexible rings at each end. The female condom is inserted into the vagina and prevents the passage of sperm into the uterus.

fermentation   Metabolism of grains, with one of its end products being ethyl alcohol.

fertilization   The creation of a zygote.

fetal alcohol effect (FAE)   Any congenital defect (birth defect) caused by the mother's consumption of alcohol during pregnancy.

fetal alcohol syndrome (FAS)   A pattern of abnormalities found in the newborns of some women who drank alcohol during pregnancy. This condition consists of a pattern of specific congenital and behavioral abnormalities. Current research suggests even low to moderate alcohol consumption may be problematic.

fetal death   Death of a fetus in utero.

fetus   The medical term for an embryo that has developed for at least eight weeks.

fibrillation   Very rapid irregular contractions of the muscle fibers of the heart resulting in a lack of synchronism between heart beat and pulse.

fibrocystic breast disease   A noncancerous breast tumor that consists of fibrous connective tissues and cystic spaces.

fimbriae   Fingerlike projections on the end of fallopian tubes nearest the ovaries, responsible for "picking up" an egg as it leaves the ovary.

first stage of labor   The period of childbirth beginning with the onset of uterine contractions and extending until the cervix is completely dilated.

first trimester   That period of pregnancy beginning with fertilization and continuing to the end of the third month.

flavoring agents   The hot smoke from burning tobacco has a distinctive taste and flavor. This taste may be chemically modified by a cigarette, pipe or cigar manufacturer to make the taste more palatable.

flexibility   The ability of a specific joint to move through its entire range of motion without pain.

fluoride   An anticaries agent contained in some toothpastes, mouthwashes, and community drinking water supplies.

folacin   *See* folic acid.

folic acid   A B vitamin, also known as folacin, that aids in the formation of hemoglobin in the red blood cells and is necessary for the production of genetic material. Recently, daily consumption of 0.4 mg. of folic acid by pregnant women has been associated with a reduction in neural tube defects in newborns.

follicle-stimulating hormone (FSH)   A hormone secreted by the pituitary that in females stimulates the ovaries to produce eggs, and in males stimulates the testes to produce sperm.

food consumers   Living components of an ecosystem that consume food producers.

food producers   Living components of an ecosystem (plants) whose prime responsibility is to make food.

foreskin   Loosely fitting skin that covers the glans of the penis, technically referred to as the prepuce.

freebase   A smokable form of cocaine that results from purification with volatile chemicals.

free radical   Naturally occurring, unstable chemical substance believed to be involved in cell mutations, contributing to the biologic aging process.

frequency   Referring to the number of times per week an individual exercises.

FTC   Federal Trade Commission; a federal agency that regulates certain products and services for consumer protection.

full-term pregnancy   Pregnancy that lasts until the ninth month.

fully functioning person   A concept offered by Carl Rogers, indicating that an individual is able to be open to new experiences, live life to its fullest, accept intuition as a legitimate source of information, make rational choices from alternatives, and engage in creative thought and activity.

funeral director   An individual professionally prepared in providing funeral services such as aspects of mortuary science, grief counseling, and preparation of the deceased for burial, cremation, or other final disposition.

G

gallstones   Cholesterol crystals hardened by inorganic salts that may form in the gallbladder, producing pain.

gamma globulin   A protein fraction of blood rich in antibodies.

gender   The sociocultural expression of one's masculinity or femininity; consists of both gender identity and gender role.

gender identity   An individual's interpretation of what is masculine and feminine.

gender role   A group or societal view of what is masculine and feminine.

gender-role stereotype   An oversimplified and often greatly distorted idea of how each gender should think, feel and behave. Gender-role stereotypes are often sanctioned and rewarded by the dominant culture.

general adaptation syndrome (GAS)   A predictable response of the body to stress, consisting of the alarm stage, the stage of resistance, and the stage of exhaustion.

general practitioner   A physician who provides primary care services to patients. This type of physician is often the first physician seen for an illness or disease. They treat many common health problems and refer to specialists when necessary.

generic equivalent   A nonproprietary drug, i.e., not protected by a trademark; a drug containing the same active ingredient as one marketed under a trade name, and usually sold at a price less than that of the trade-name variety; in the U.S., generic drugs are required to meet the same bioequivalency test as the original trade-name products.

genital warts   A sexually transmitted disease caused by the human papilloma virus; common symptoms include warts, varying in size and shape, frequently clustered in the genital and anal areas.

gerontologist   An individual who studies one or more of the facets of aging, including physiological, psychological, economic, and sociological dimensions.

gestation   The time from the formation of a zygote until childbirth. In humans, the average gestation is 266 days.

glans   The head of the penis.

glaucoma   Disease of the eye characterized by increased intraocular pressure, resulting in atrophy of the optic nerve and blindness.

glucose   A form of carbohydrate (simple sugar) that is the major energy-supplying molecule for the brain.

glycogen   Stored sugar, found mainly in the liver and voluntary skeletal muscles, which can be used as a ready source of energy in emergency situations.

gonadotropin-releasing hormone (GnRH)   GnRH is secreted by the hypothalamus and causes the release of two other hormones, luteinizing hormone (LH) and follicle-stimulating hormone (FSH). FSH stimulates the testes to produce sperm and the ovaries to produce eggs. LH stimulates the testes to produce testosterone and the ovaries to produce estrogens.

gonorrhea   A sexually transmitted disease caused by a type of bacteria called *Neisseria gonorrhoeae*. Common symptoms include painful urination and a discharge of pus from the penis or vagina. If untreated, severe chronic diseases such as arthritis, inflammation of the heart valves, or sterility may result.

graafian follicle   A small, estrogen-secreting gland in the ovary, containing a maturing egg. When the egg is fully matured, the graafian follicle ruptures, releasing the egg, a process known as ovulation.

GRAE   Those drugs categorized by the Food and Drug Administration (FDA) as being generally recognized as effective.

GRAS   Those drugs categorized by the Food and Drug Administration (FDA) as being generally recognized as safe.

groundwater   Water from wells, springs, and large underground reservoirs called aquifers. Groundwater is the major source of drinking water for over half the U.S. population.

H

hallucinations   Perceptions that have no basis in reality or external stimuli.

hazardous waste   Solid waste (including liquid, semisolid, solid, or contained gaseous material) that because of its quantity, concentration, or physical, chemical, or infectious characteristics may pose a hazard to human health or the environment.

HCG   Human chorionic gonadotropin; a hormone whose presence in a woman's urine is a positive indicator of pregnancy.

HDL   *See* high-density lipoprotein.

HDL cholesterol *See* high-density lipoprotein cholesterol.

health maintenance organization (HMO) A prepaid group health-care plan that offers comprehensive medical services, often in one location.

health promotion Activities geared toward enhancing the quality of life and preventing disease and disability.

health-related responsibilities Responsibilities of drug use that relate to the health of oneself and others.

heart attack Death or impairment of cells of the heart muscle as a result of obstructed blood flow.

heart murmur The abnormal sound made by the heart, particularly a heart valve, when blood passes through a damaged or constricted area as may occur following an episode of rheumatic fever.

hematologic A medical term referring to blood and blood-forming tissues.

hepatitis Inflammation of the liver caused by reactions to drugs, toxic agents, excess alcohol intake, bacteria, or viruses.

herbal drugs Plants that have drug effects and whose use is not generally regulated by law.

hernia A condition characterized by part of an organ or tissue protruding outside of the body cavity in which it is normally housed. For example, an hiatus hernia exists when part of the stomach protrudes into the chest cavity through the hole for the esophagus.

heroin A semisynthetic, psychoactive drug produced from morphine.

herpes simplex virus Type I (HSV-I) The herpes virus usually associated with cold sores on or around the mouth and lips.

herpes simplex virus Type II (HSV-II) The virus usually implicated in genital herpes.

high-density lipoprotein (HDL) A type of lipoprotein that carries cholesterol from the bloodstream to the liver, where it can be excreted from the body. High blood HDL levels may help protect individuals against coronary artery disease.

HIV *See* human immunodeficiency virus.

homeopaths Persons who practice homeopathy, or the disease treatment systems that employ drugs that produce symptoms similar to the treated disease if given to a healthy person. This system is based on the notion of treating like with like.

homeostasis A normal or balanced state of the body that aids in optimal functioning.

homicide The killing of a human being by the illegal actions of another human being.

hormones A substance secreted by an endocrine gland and transported in the blood or other body fluids.

hospice A concept of care for the terminally ill that allows the dying person to be as free from physical and psychological discomfort as possible.

human chorionic gonadotropin (HCG) This hormone is released by the implanted embryo. The detection of this hormone is used for several pregnancy tests.

human immunodeficiency virus The virus that causes the symptoms associated with AIDS.

humanistic perspective A philosophical view of life and death that sees human life as the highest life form, and one to be preserved until such point that continuation of life is no longer dignified; it also professes no existence of an afterlife.

human papilloma virus (HPV) A virus that is responsible for causing one or more sexually transmitted diseases.

hydrogenation A manufacturing technique whereby hydrogen is added to unsaturated fats, thus making them more saturated (with hydrogen) than they would be naturally.

hymen A membrane which partially covers the vaginal opening.

hypertension Abnormally high arterial blood pressure of a chronic nature, generally identified in persons with a diastolic pressure above 90 mm Hg, or a systolic pressure above 140 mm Hg.

hypoglycemia An abnormally low blood glucose level (sometimes referred to as low blood sugar).

hypothalamus A small part of the forebrain, located below the cerebrum, that is linked to both the thalamus and the pituitary gland; involved in a number of body functions including water metabolism, temperature regulation, appetite, thirst, blood sugar level, growth, sleep, certain emotions such as anger, and cycles of the reproductive system. It is also the center of the autonomic nervous system.

hysterotomy A type of induced abortion that is identical to a small cesarean section. A small incision is made in the female's lower abdomen and uterus and the fetus is removed.

I

ibuprofen A nonsteroidal antiinflammatory drug marketed under names such as Advil, Motrin, and Nuprin; works especially well for treating pain from menstrual cramps, inflammation, or dental work; may cause stomach bleeding in some individuals.

illicit drugs Any drug whose sale, purchase, or use is prohibited by law.

illusion A distortion of ordinary perception that results in a misinterpretation of reality.

immune system The system of body responses to substances that are foreign or that are interpreted as being foreign; the system that fights disease and infection and is compromised in acquired immunodeficiency syndrome (AIDS).

immunity The state of being able to resist a particular disease by counteracting the potential effects of a foreign substance or pathogen.

immunoglobulin Protein substances in the blood serum that produce antibodies.

immunotherapy The treatment of disease by bolstering the body's natural immune system response; usually mentioned in reference to the treatment of cancer.

implantation The attachment of the zygote to the uterus.

improvement-conditioning stage The second stage of progress for individuals who want to improve their cardiovascular endurance. Duration of exercise sessions and target heart rate are both systematically increased during this phase, creating a state of overload that leads to a cardiovascular training effect.

incest Sexual relationships between close blood relatives, such as a father and daughter, or a brother and sister.

incineration The use of combustion (burning) to dispose of hazardous waste. Ash containing dioxin, a powerful carcinogen, is one hazardous by-product of incineration.

incubation period The time span between the exposure to a disease-producing vector and the onset of symptoms.

individual differences A principle of fitness that points out that individuals attain the many benefits of physical fitness at varying rates.

induced abortion Medical termination of a pregnancy before the fetus is capable of extrauterine life.

infant mortality The number of deaths of children under the age of one, per 1,000 live births.

infection The state produced by the establishment of a pathogen in a susceptible host.

infertile A label given to a person or couple who cannot naturally conceive or maintain a pregnancy after attempting for a year or more.

infertility The inability to conceive.

inflammation A response of the body to infection or injury, often characterized by local redness, swelling, fever, and pain.

influenza A highly contagious viral disease producing fever, aches and pains, and upper respiratory distress.

inhalant Gases that can be inhaled into the lungs, such as from glues, solvents, aerosols from paints, hair spray, and nail polish remover; when inhaled in light doses these chemicals cause lightheadedness and dizziness and provide a temporary high; in higher doses depression of the central nervous system can lead to sleep or coma, and heart rhythm disturbances may lead to death.

inhibit A form of drug interaction where one drug decreases the effects of another drug when taken together.

initial-conditioning stage The beginning stage of progress for individuals starting a vigorous aerobic exercise program. This stage usually lasts from four to six weeks and gradually prepares an individual to safely participate in more strenuous physical activity.

injection wells Deep wells, located below groundwater sources, used to store hazardous waste. The effects of such wells on drinking water contamination are debated by both industry and environmentalists.

insoluble fibers Materials from the cell walls of plants that cannot be digested by the human body.

insulin A hormone secretion of the pancreas necessary to convert carbohydrates into energy and sometimes used therapeutically to control diabetes.

insulin-dependent diabetes mellitus *See* Type I diabetes.

insulin theory A theory of obesity causation that suggests that high blood insulin levels can increase fat tissue as well as keep people hungry, thus affecting their ability to lose fat weight.

intellectualism A defense mechanism whereby a person transforms their feelings into thoughts, in order to avoid feelings of distress.

intensified drug use Regular long-term (daily) use of a drug or several drugs in combination.

intensity How strenuously an individual exercises for a given period. Usually measured by taking an exercise heart rate and comparing it to a prescribed target heart rate.

intentional injury Physical, emotional, or social damage or suffering that is the result of homicide, suicide, or other violent acts.

interferon An antiviral protein naturally produced by the body that assists in the immune response, thought to play a future role in the treatment of various diseases.

intermediate-care institution A nursing home where patients require assistance but not necessarily professional medical attention.

intestate To die without having created a valid will, resulting in the laws of the state governing how and to whom property of the deceased person is distributed to heirs.

intimacy As used to define love, intimacy is described as the emotional aspect including closeness, sharing, communication, and support.

intrauterine device (IUD) A plastic device that is inserted into the uterus through the vaginal tract by a physician and ends implantation of any zygote that may enter the uterus.

introitus The opening of the vagina.

invasive birth-control methods Methods that involve entering the body in order to surgically alter any internal reproductive organs or to end a pregnancy (sterilization, abortion).

in vitro fertilization (IVF)   A procedure in which a mature egg is removed from an ovary, fertilized in a laboratory dish, incubated, and then placed inside the uterus to allow implantation to occur.

involuntary smoking   Inhalation of sidestream smoke; synonymous with secondhand smoking.

ischemia   A lack of sufficient blood flow to an organ resulting in an inadequate oxygen supply to that organ.

isopropyl alcohol   A form of alcohol that is used as a disinfectant. Also called rubbing alcohol, this form is not consumable.

J

jaundice   A yellowing of the skin due to the presence of too much bile pigment in the blood.

JCAH   Joint Commission of the Accreditation of Hospitals, a group that insures that hospitals meet set standards for providing care and conducting business.

K

Kaposi's sarcoma   A rare type of cancer associated primarily with persons infected by the AIDS virus.

killer T-cell   A T-cell that destroys a cell (such as a tumor cell) identified as foreign or unnatural to the body.

L

labia   Two paired folds of skin that surround the female's vaginal and urethral openings and extend to the clitoris.

labia majora   Paired folds of tissue found in the female reproductive system that surround the clitoris, urethral opening, and vaginal opening.

labia minora   Paired folds of tissue found in the female reproductive system that extend along the vestibule.

labor   A series of contractions of the uterus and abdominal muscles that help to expel the fetus, placenta, and membranes during childbirth. The average length of labor ranges from eight to twelve hours.

lacto-ovo vegetarian   A type of vegetarian who consumes dairy foods and eggs, but no animal flesh.

lacto-vegetarian   A type of vegetarian who consumes dairy foods, but not eggs or animal flesh.

laparoscopy   An outpatient technique for performing tubal ligation that involves making a tiny incision just below the naval, inserting a lighted instrument into the abdominal cavity so that the physician can see the fallopian tubes while he cuts and ties them, clips them, or cauterizes them.

latent stage   A stage of syphilis lasting up to twenty years where obvious disease symptoms may not be present.

late-stage syphilis   Synonymous with tertiary stage syphilis; systemic involvement with severely compromised health, leading to death.

LDL cholesterol   *See* low-density lipoprotein cholesterol.

lean   All body tissues other than fat, sometimes called fat-free tissue.

lethal dose level   The minimum dose of a drug that will cause death in the user.

leukemia   A cancer arising in the blood-forming tissue, principally the bone marrow and spleen.

leukoplakia   White, patchy lesions usually appearing on the mucous membranes of the mouth or on the tongue, considered in some instances to be a precursor to cancer.

leydig cells   Special cells in the testes which produce testosterone.

libido   A term used to describe the level of one's sexual desire.

life-after-life perspective   A philosophical view independent of religion that sees death as a joining of the deceased person with previously deceased ancestors for continued spiritual existence.

life expectancy   The average number of years a group of individuals with common characteristics can expect to live, from birth to death.

life management   Everything a person does to adapt and attain optimal functioning. Life management involves channeling stress so that it leads to higher levels of wellness.

lifestyle factors   Individual practices that are part of an established pattern of long-term behavior. Lifestyle factors may be habits or cultural practices, and often affect health status and wellness levels. Examples include food consumption patterns, exercise habits, drug use and abuse, stress management techniques, and the like.

lipids   A fat compound that usually has fatty acids as a part of its structure.

lipoproteins   Special molecules, consisting of protein and lipids, that carry cholesterol in the bloodstream.

Listeria   A rare, but potentially fatal, type of food-borne infection caused by the bacterium *listeria monocytogenes;* symptoms include flu-like fever and chills; can cause spontaneous abortions and stillbirths, as well as severe illness in newborns and immune-suppressed people.

living will   A quasi-legal document prepared by an individual usually to inform relatives, physicians, and other concerned parties about the extent to which measures are to be taken to prolong life in the event of accident or serious illness.

low-density lipoprotein (LDL)   A type of lipoprotein that carries cholesterol from the digestive tract to other body cells. High levels of blood LDL are associated with an increased risk of coronary artery disease.

lower-body obesity   A type of obesity characterized by greater fat stores in areas of the body such as the thighs, hips, and buttocks. These fat cells are believed to be greater in number, and to store fat in a captive manner.

LSD   A white, crystalline powder that is a potent psychedelic drug, producing heightened and distorted sensory experiences.

luteinizing hormones (LH)   A hormone secreted by the pituitary gland that in males stimulates the testes to produce testosterone and in females stimulates the ovaries to produce estrogen.

Lyme disease   An inflammatory disorder of the skin and other body systems whose causative organism is carried by certain varieties of ticks.

lymph nodes   Small, encapsulated oval bodies occurring in clusters in various parts of the body. Their primary functions are to filter lymph fluid and produce lymphocytes, playing an important role in the body's immune system.

lymphocyte   White blood cells circulating in lymph fluid that perform basic surveillance functions against disease.

lymphogranuloma venereum (LGV)   A sexually transmitted disease caused by a type of bacteria called *Chlamydia trachomatis*. Symptoms include a small, painless sore on the penis or vulva, inflammation of surrounding lymph nodes and tissue, fever, chills, headache and joint pain.

lymphoma   A cancer that arises from lymph cells.

M

macroconsumers   Animals; a type of food consumer.

macrophage   A phagocytic tissue cell derived from a monocyte that protects against infection.

magnetic-resonance imager (MRI)   A diagnostic machine that produces images of the body in a noninvasive manner.

mainstream smoke   The smoke drawn into the lungs when a pipe, cigar, or cigarette is inhaled.

maintenance stage   Referring to an exercise program, the final stage of progress for individuals participating in a vigorous aerobic exercise program. During this stage the individual continues at a frequency, intensity, and duration of aerobic exercise that they have become accustomed to in the improvement-conditioning stage. They do not continue to overload for improvement, but rather maintain the level of physical fitness attained.

major minerals   Those minerals that each account for 0.05% or more of body weight. These include calcium, phosphorus, magnesium, potassium, sulfur, sodium, and chloride.

major stressor   Stressor that tends to evoke an intense stress response. Examples of major stressors include the death of a loved one, moving to a new residence, becoming pregnant or fathering a child, etc.

major tranquilizers   Drugs used to control schizophrenia and, in smaller doses, to control nausea and vomiting.

malignant   Usually in reference to a tumor, meaning cancerous and of life-threatening potential.

mammogram   *See* mammography.

mammography   X ray examination of the breasts used in the early detection of breast cancer.

marijuana   A drug from the plant Cannabis sativa, the psychoactive ingredient is delta-9-tetrahydrocannabinol, or THC.

marker events   Changes or events specific to developmental stages of growth, as well as the social and cultural factors influencing them that are intense stressors when experienced.

masturbation   Self-stimulation of one's own body for the purpose of sexual pleasure.

mausoleum   A large vault or tomb for the dead.

maximal heart rate   The highest heart rate reached during an all-out aerobic effort.

measles   A highly communicable infectious disease caused by a virus; the most notable symptom is pink, slightly elevated rash; a vaccine is available.

mechanical birth-control methods   Methods which prevent fertilization (condom, diaphragm, cervical cap, sponge) or end implantation (IUD).

Medicaid   A federally sponsored program of health insurance that was established to assist the socioeconomically disadvantaged, and certain others.

medical treatment   As related to a category of stress-management strategies, this group of strategies involves consultation with health-care providers because of stress-induced pain or body dysfunction.

Medicare   A federally funded program that assists in the payment of health expenses for persons sixty-five years and older who are entitled to Social Security benefits.

medicated childbirth   Childbirth in which one or more drugs are used by the mother during delivery.

megadose   Referring to vitamins and minerals, doses in excess of ten times the RDA.

melanin   Pigment-producing cells of the skin.

melanoma   A serious type of skin cancer of the pigment-forming cells.

memory cell   A T-cell sensitized to a specific antigen by having been exposed to it previously.

menarche   The first female reproductive cycle, and is marked by the female's first menstruation.

menopause   The cessation of the female's reproductive cycles.

menstruation   The cyclical bleeding that signifies the beginning of the next reproductive cycle.

mercy killing   A deliberate act performed either voluntarily or involuntarily to hasten death.

metabolism   The physical and chemical processes of the body that contribute to the growth, maintenance, repair, and breakdown of body tissues, as well as making energy available.

metastasis   The spread of a previously localized cancer to new sites in the body, thereby increasing the lethal potential of the disease.

methyl alcohol   Also called wood alcohol, this form of alcohol is used in such industrial products as antifreezes and various fuels.

microconsumers   Bacteria and fungi; a type of food consumer.

mild tranquilizers   Drugs which relax the muscles and reduce anxiety; sometimes called minor tranquilizers.

minerals   Inorganic substances, found naturally in the earth, that play a vital role in human metabolism. Some minerals, such as iron and zinc, are needed in only small amounts and are known as trace elements. Other minerals, such as calcium and sodium, are required by the body in larger amounts and are called major minerals.

minilaparotomy   An outpatient technique for performing tubal ligation that involves making a tiny incision just above the pubic hairline, inserting an instrument to lift the fallopian tubes and bring them out of the abdominal cavity so they can be cut and tied, clipped, or cauterized.

minipill   A type of birth-control pill containing progestin only. This pill is believed to both prevent fertilization and end implantation.

minor stressor   Stressors one encounters and adapts to on a regular or daily basis.

minor tranquilizers   Drugs which relax the muscles and reduce anxiety.

miscarriage   A naturally occurring termination of pregnancy before the fetus is capable of extrauterine life.

mittelschmerz   Pain, discomfort, or pressure experienced by females around the time of ovulation.

mode of transmission   A mechanism that facilitates the transfer of disease from an infected host to a previously uninfected new host.

moderate obesity   A level of obesity (fat excess) commonly associated with risk factors, such as hypertension, elevated blood cholesterol, and diabetes.

monoclonal antibodies   Special factors which bolster the body's response to disease, especially by carrying targeted drugs and radiation to specific disease sites.

monocyte   A large phagocytic white blood cell in the body.

monophasic birth-control hormones   Birth-control pills that release the identical dose of estrogen and progestin each day.

monosaccharides   A simple sugar, such as glucose, fructose, and galactose, that is the basic structural unit of carbohydrates.

monounsaturated fat   A type of fatty acid with one double bond between its carbon atoms.

morbidity rate   The proportion of a disease in a given geographical area.

morbid obesity   An extreme level of obesity (fat excess) at which death and debilitating diseases, such as coronary artery disease and diabetes, occur at very high rates.

morning sickness   Nausea and vomiting a pregnant female may experience throughout the day or night.

morphine   A major derivative of opium; an effective analgesic for most types of pain.

mortality rate   The proportion of deaths in a given geographical area.

multiphasic birth-control hormones   Birth-control pills that release varying doses of estrogen and progestin each day.

multiple sclerosis   A chronic disease of the nervous system characterized by a variety of nervous system abnormalities such as shaky limbs, being unsteady or stumbling when walking, or having problems pronouncing words.

mumps   A viral infection typically occurring in young children. The most distinct symptom of mumps is the presence of swollen salivary glands on the sides of the face. If the infection spreads to the testicles it can cause sterility.

muscular endurance   The ability to lift light to moderate amounts of weight repeatedly over a period of time. In weight training this would be many repetitions with less weight.

muscular fitness   The strength and endurance capability of an individual's muscles.

muscular strength   The amount of weight that an individual can safely lift in one all-out effort. For weight training this would be high weight with few repetitions.

myasthenia gravis   A chronic disease characterized by excessive fatigue and weakness in certain muscles, often so severe the muscles are temporarily paralyzed.

myocardial infarction (MI)   A heart attack; death or impairment of cells of the myocardium as a result of obstructed blood flow.

myocardium   The middle muscular layer of the heart wall.

myometrium   The muscular layer of the uterus, essential for menstruation and childbirth.

myotonia   The tightening of the reproductive organs during sexual stimulation.

N

naproxen sodium   A nonsteroidal antiinflammatory drug marketed under the name Aleve; this long-acting drug (8–12 hours for one dose) is often used for treating the pain associated with arthritis; may cause stomach upset and intestinal bleeding in some people.

narcotic analgesics   Another term for opiates, or drugs that relieve pain by reducing a person's awareness of pain.

narcotics *See* narcotic analgesics.

national health insurance A federally sponsored insurance plan that would, if enacted, provide health insurance to all U.S. citizens regardless of their ability to pay. Such an insurance does not currently exist in the U.S.

natural birth-control methods Techniques that estimate when a female is ovulating so that abstinence can be practiced in order to prevent fertilization of an egg.

natural childbirth Childbirth in which the mother uses no drugs during delivery.

naturally acquired active immunity Immunity acquired as a result of exposure to a pathogen and subsequent development of the disease; or temporary immunity acquired by a fetus by flow of maternal antibodies across the placenta.

naturally acquired passive immunity A temporary form of immunity found in newborns; acquired from antibodies that passed from the maternal bloodstream to the fetal bloodstream in utero, and from breast milk to the infant during breast-feeding.

naturopathy A disease treatment system that relies on only natural elements to restore health.

near-infrared interactance (NIA) A method of estimating body composition using a painless infrared light beam introduced into the body that measures the degree of infrared energy absorption as it passes through the body. The validity of this body fat measurement technique is uncertain.

neonatal death Death of an infant during the first six weeks after birth.

neoplasm A new growth of tissue serving no physiological function; synonymous with tumor.

neurotransmitters Chemicals that transmit nerve impulses from one nerve cell to another. The neurotransmitters thought to be related to depression include serotonin, norepinephrine, and dopamine.

neutrophil The chief type of phagocytic white blood cell in the body.

nicotine The active ingredient in tobacco with addictive potential. Nicotine acts as a potent central nervous system stimulant, and is considered to be a drug.

nicotine dependence A physical and psychological need to continue using tobacco products containing nicotine. Nicotine is the active ingredient in tobacco products responsible for the compulsion to continue using these products.

nicotine gum A chewing gum product that contains nicotine. Such gum products are sometimes used during withdrawal to assist a person who is addicted to tobacco products.

nicotine patch A pad that adheres to the skin and delivers a measured dose of nicotine to assist the tobacco cessation efforts of a person addicted to the nicotine found in tobacco.

nicotine poisoning The toxic effects of nicotine inhalation or ingestion characterized by dizziness, faintness, rapid pulse, nausea, and other symptoms; potentially fatal in small children.

nitrosamine A chemical compound found in tobacco, certain foods, and other substances; some nitrosamines have been shown to be cancer-causing.

nitrous oxides One of the waste gases released into the atmosphere during the burning of fossil fuels, especially by automobiles. Nitrous oxide is one of the gases linked to acid rain.

nonbiodegradable Substances that do not decay and are not absorbed by the environment.

nongonococcal urethritis (NGU) A sexually transmitted disease with symptoms like those produced in gonorrhea, but of different microorganism origin.

non-insulin dependent diabetes Sometimes referred to as Type II or adult-onset diabetes, this form of diabetes is usually diagnosed in persons over age forty; in this type of diabetes the body does not make enough insulin, the cells are not as sensitive to the insulin, or both.

nonoxynol-9 A spermicidal agent that may also protect against some sexually transmitted diseases such as HIV infection; used to lubricate certain brands of condoms.

nonspecific urethritis (NSU) An infection of the urethra whose cause cannot be tied to a single microorganism but is linked to many; may be sexually transmitted.

nonspecific vaginitis (NSV) An infection of the vagina whose cause cannot be tied to a single microorganism but is linked to many; may be sexually transmitted.

noradrenalin A substance released from the ends of some nerve fibers. One of the action preparation hormones that gears the body for fight or flight during the stress response.

normal In a mental health context, the state of mind and behavior shared by most people at a particular point in time.

Norplant A series of surgically implanted rods, placed just under the skin, that are designed to leak a progestin into the surrounding tissue, to accomplish birth control.

nurse midwife A registered nurse who has received advanced training in assisting women through pregnancy and childbirth.

nurse practitioners Registered nurses who have additional specialized training equivalent to a master's degree and are able to engage in a variety of expanded health-care services.

nurses Licensed health-care workers who perform a variety of duties ranging from administering medication to patient education.

O

obesity A condition whereby too great a proportion of the body tissue is fat. A variety of standards for obesity exist including body weight, body mass index, and percent body fat. Values considered as obese vary by sex, and sometimes by age.

obstetrician A physician who specializes in pregnancy and childbirth.

omega-3 fatty acids A type of fatty acid found mostly in the oils of cold-water fish such as salmon, halibut, mackerel, herring, and lake trout.

oncogene A bit of genetic material or "gene" that plays a role in promoting the development of certain types of cancers.

opiates A drug and its derivatives, extracted from the poppy plant, that relieve pain by reducing a person's awareness of pain.

opium A drug, extracted from the poppy plant, classified as a narcotic.

opportunistic disease Any otherwise rare disease that attacks a person whose immune system has been severely compromised, as during AIDS.

optometrist A health professional trained to diagnose visual problems and improve vision through prescription glasses and contact lenses.

organismic trusting A characteristic of Rogers' fully functioning person involving the ability to trust one's own judgments and intuitions.

orgasm The climax of sexual excitement, consisting of sudden muscle contractions followed by a distinct release of sexual tension.

orgasmic phase The third phase of sexual response; characterized in both sexes by orgasm.

osteopathy The treatment of disease by manipulation of the skeleton and muscles, as well as by drugs and surgery.

osteoporosis A condition affecting mostly the elderly, especially women, resulting from a decline in bone mineral content, making bones susceptible to fracture.

otitis media An inflammation of the middle ear that can be caused by either bacteria or virus. Common symptoms include severe pain and a high fever.

ovarian follicles A cavity in the ovary where the ova or egg develops.

ovaries The primary female reproductive organs that produce mature eggs and estrogen, the female hormone.

overload Exercising the body at a level of activity greater than that to which it is accustomed, as a way to increase physical fitness.

over-the-counter drugs Commercially produced medications that can be purchased without a physician's approval.

overweight Being over the normal weight for your height; usually determined by weighing oneself on a scale and comparing the result to a standardized height/weight table.

ovo-vegetarian A type of vegetarian who consumes eggs but no other dairy foods or animals.

ovulation Occurs when the ovary releases a mature egg.

oxidation The process of burning oxygen for fuel.

P

pacemaker An electrical device for stimulating or steadying the heart beat or reestablishing the rhythm of a heart in cardiac arrest.

Pap smear A microscopic examination of cells of the cervix used as an early detection procedure for cancer of that site.

Pap test *See* pap smear.

paranoia A rare, chronic mental disorder characterized by systematic irrational beliefs labeled delusions.

particulate matter Small particles found in the smoke of burning tobacco.

passion As used to define love, passion is described as the motivational aspect of love that leads to physiological arousal.

passive anal sex During an act of anal sex, having a penis inserted into one's anus.

passive smoking The inhalation of tobacco smoke that comes from cigarettes, pipes, or cigars smoked by other people.

pathogen An organism that can produce disease in a host.

PCP *See* phencyclidine.

pediculosis pubis Infestation of the pubic hair and pubic region by crab lice.

pelvic inflammatory disease (PID) A general infection of the female reproductive tract, usually as a complication of an undiagnosed or untreated STD, and having the potential to cause permanent sterility.

penis The external male reproductive organ that contains the urethra through which both sperm and urine are discharged.

percentage of body fat The proportion of one's body tissue that is fat or adipose tissue, usually measured by underwater weighing or skinfold techniques.

percutaneous umbilical blood sampling (PUBS) A prenatal test for birth defects that requires a physician to insert a needle into one of the blood vessels in the umbilical cord to draw a blood sample.

perimetrium The outermost layer of the uterus.

perineum   An area of the female external genitals that extends from the introitus to the anus.

periodic abstinence   A method of birth control designed to estimate when ovulation is occurring in a woman, and abstain from vaginal intercourse during this 'unsafe' time.

period of communicability   The stage of an infectious disease during which it is most easily transmitted from one host to another.

pernicious anemia   A type of anemia (a decreased ability of the blood to carry oxygen) that results from a genetic defect that interferes with the body's ability to absorb vitamin B12.

personality engineering strategies   Techniques that help to reduce the stress response by deliberately modifying some aspect of one's personality.

pertussis   A communicable infectious disease caused by the bacterium *Bordetella pertussis;* usually affects children; common symptoms include an excessive secretion of mucous from the respiratory tract, mild fever, and a cough with a characteristic whooping sound; also known as whooping cough.

pesco-vegetarian   A type of vegetarian who consumes dairy food, eggs, and fish, but no other animal flesh.

pesticides   Chemicals used to kill insect "pests."

phagocytosis   The process whereby white blood cells "eat" bacteria or other pathogens, by engulfing them and digesting them.

phencyclidine   An animal tranquilizer that acts as a deliriant in humans; also known as PCP, angel dust or tea.

phosphorous   Along with calcium, this element comprises the hardened structure of bones and teeth in the body.

physical fitness   The ability to function efficiently defined in terms of cardiorespiratory endurance, muscular strength and endurance, flexibility, and body composition.

physician assistant   A health professional who has completed a two-year program sponsored by a medical school, university, or technical college, and is trained to perform routine medical procedures under the supervision of a physician.

physiological withdrawal   The set of physical symptoms experienced when one attempts to stop using a drug to which he or she is addicted.

PID   *See* pelvic inflammatory disease.

pituitary gland   An endocrine gland the size of a pea, located beneath and attached to the hypothalamus in the brain. The pituitary gland secretes various hormones when it receives hormone-releasing factors from the hypothalamus.

placenta   A temporary organ that transfers nutrients and oxygen from mother to developing embryo/fetus. This organ also secretes hormones that maintain the pregnancy.

place of exit   A pathway open to a pathogen for leaving one host and entering another.

plaque   In an artery, a yellowish, swollen area in the arterial lining formed by deposition of lipids in the area; in the brain, a series of twisted nerve cell fibers occurring in clumps, characteristic of Alzheimer's disease; on teeth, a gummy mass of microorganisms on the crowns, spreading to the roots that makes teeth susceptible to decay.

plateau phase   The second phase of sexual response; characterized in the female by swelling and narrowing of the vagina and changes in skin color when orgasm is imminent; characterized in the male by increasing size of the penis and testes and the release of a small amount of seminal fluid from the penis.

***Pneumocystis carinii* pneumonia**   An inflammation in the lungs caused by a protozoan; occurs in individuals with suppressed immune systems, such as persons with AIDS.

pneumonia   An inflammation of the lung, usually caused by a bacteria. Symptoms include cough, chest pain, and shadows on a chest X ray.

podiatrist   Medical specialists who deal with disorders of the foot.

polio   The short name for poliomyelitis, an infectious disease caused by a virus; symptoms include muscle stiffness, weakness, and sometimes paralysis; a vaccine is available.

polyunsaturated fat   A type of fatty acid with two or more double bonds between carbon atoms.

portal of entry   A pathway open to a pathogen that allows its introduction from a reservoir or host to a new host.

post natal   The time following the birth of a child.

postpartum   The first few days following the birth of a child.

PPNG   Acronym for penicillinase-producing Neisseria gonorrhea, a strain of gonorrhea-causing bacteria that does not respond to treatment with penicillin.

predisposing factors   Knowledge, attitudes, beliefs, values, and confidence levels that serve as either motivators or barriers to practicing health-related behaviors.

pre-eclampsia   Pregnancy-induced hypertension (high blood pressure), with associated swelling of the face, neck, and upper extremities due to fluid retention.

premature ejaculation   Dissatisfaction with the duration of sexual intercourse due to the male's loss of erection following orgasm.

premenstrual syndrome (PMS) A condition ranging in severity that some women experience several days before the onset of menstruation that is characterized by some of the following symptoms: tension, anxiety, mood change, depression, headache, breast tenderness, water retention, and other symptoms. Severity usually diminishes close to onset of the menstrual period. Exact causes of PMS are unknown but may relate to changes in estrogen and progesterone during the menstrual cycle.

prenatal The time from conception to birth.

prenatal care The actions a future mother and her mate take to increase the chances of birthing a healthy baby and reducing the health risks of pregnancy and childbirth for the future mother.

preparatory depression For a terminally ill person, the obsessive thoughts of a future that he or she will not be a part of and the final separation from all things that are familiar.

prepuce Loosely fitting skin that covers the glans of the penis, sometimes referred to as foreskin.

presbyopia A visual defect with onset between ages forty and forty-five resulting in loss of accommodation of near point; occurs from lost elasticity of the lens of the eye.

prescription drugs Commercially produced medications that cannot be purchased without a physician's approval.

primary aging The inevitable physical and physiological consequences of growing older, resulting usually in measurable functional changes in performance.

primary amenorrhea The absence of menstruation by age sixteen.

primary birth control Methods that prevent fertilization.

primary care A level of health care consisting of routine health checkups and care for individuals experiencing an illness for the first time.

primary prevention Activities undertaken to decrease the probability of the occurrence of disease.

primary stage The first stage of syphilis, characterized by the appearance of a chancre at the site of infection.

private health clinics Outpatient, ambulatory health-care settings not funded by tax revenues.

problem drinker A person who drinks alcohol to an extent or in a manner that an alcohol-related disability occurs.

product misrepresentation A sales tactic whereby the retailer advertises selective information about a product that leads a consumer to make faulty assumptions about the product's worth or effectiveness.

progesterone A steroid hormone responsible for the preparation of the inner lining of the uterus for possible pregnancy. If pregnancy occurs, it maintains the uterus and prevents ovulation.

prostaglandins A group of compounds that have powerful hormone-like effects.

prostate gland A small gland found in the male reproductive system at the base of the bladder. This gland secretes a fluid with a neutralizing action that protects sperm as they travel through the male and female reproductive tracts.

protein A major nutrient composed of carbon, hydrogen, oxygen, and nitrogen and whose major function is the growth, maintenance, and repair of body tissues.

psychoactive drug Type of drug that primarily affects a person's moods or behaviors. Alcohol, tranquilizers, and marijuana are examples.

psychological withdrawal The set of emotional symptoms experienced when one attempts to stop using a drug to which he or she is addicted.

psychosis A form of mental illness consisting of a loss of contact with reality; hallucinations and delusions are common.

psychotropic drugs Drugs which affect psychic functions, behavior, or experience.

public health clinics A health-care setting for outpatient, ambulatory care that is supported by either federal, state, or local tax revenues.

pus A yellowish white fluid comprised of white blood cells, tissue debris, and microorganisms following the body's response to localized infection or injury.

pyloric valve The ring of muscle separating the stomach and the duodenum.

pylorospasm Contractions of the pyloric valve.

Q

quickening The first movement of a fetus felt by the mother.

R

radial artery Arteries that travel along the thumb side of the arm from the forearm to the wrist.

radiation Energy emitted or radiated in the form of waves or particles implicated in the cause of certain cancers, but also used in the treatment of some cancers.

radiotherapy The X ray treatment of tumors, especially of a cancerous nature, to reduce their size and potential lethality.

radon A radioactive gas resulting from the disintegration of radium. Found naturally in certain geographical areas, radon has been implicated in 5 to 10 percent of lung cancers in the U.S.

rape The act of forcing someone to have sexual intercourse when he or she does not want to.

RDA Recommended dietary allowance, or the amount of various nutrients, recommended by the Food and Nutrition Board of the National Research Council considered to be adequate for the maintenance of good nutrition in most healthy persons in the U.S.

reactive depression For a terminally ill person, the depression felt from such radical life changes as loss of job, inability to care for one's family, and other changes.

rectum The end segment of the large intestine that connects to the anal canal and stores feces prior to defecation.

reference daily intakes (RDIs) Formerly known as the USRDA, the amount of certain vitamins and minerals that should be consumed daily by adults in the U.S. The current RDIs are identical to the USRDA established in 1968.

refractory period Following an orgasm, the period of recovery time needed by males before a second orgasm can be experienced.

registered nurses (R.N.) A nurse who has passed state licensing requirements.

reincarnation perspective A philosophical view that sees existence as a continuous stream of experience spanning many lifetimes, and death as merely a pathway to a new life and continued existence.

reinforcing factors Feedback that either rewards or punishes certain behaviors, thus enhancing or diminishing the likelihood that the behavior will be continued.

relaxation training Techniques taught to people so they can systematically induce a physiological condition that is almost the complete opposite of the stress response.

religious perspective A philosophical view of life and death that sees these phenomena as being determined by a supreme being; persons who live a good earthly life are rewarded in death by being granted happiness for all eternity.

reservoir An environment conducive to the maintenance of pathogenic organisms.

residual volume The volume of lung capacity that does not take part in exchange of gases during breathing.

resistance stage The second stage of the General Adaptation Syndrome, during which the body adapts to the stressor and attempts to return to a state of homeostasis.

resolution phase The fourth phase of human sexual response, following the orgasmic stage, characterized by the loss of sexual tension and a return to a preexcitement stage.

resolution stage *See* resolution phase.

respite care Temporary professional care provided for disabled individuals, with the intention of giving family caretakers a brief rest from caregiving responsibilities.

reversibility A principle of fitness that stresses that once benefits of regular exercise have been attained, a person must continue to exercise on a regular schedule or he or she will begin to lose the benefits.

rheumatic heart disease Damage done to the heart, particularly the heart valves, following one or more attacks of a strep bacterial-induced disease, rheumatic fever.

rheumatoid arthritis A form of arthritis (inflammation of the joints) most commonly affecting the joints of the fingers, wrists, feet, ankles, hips, or shoulders.

reversibility rates Estimate a person's ability to become a biological parent after discontinuing the use of a particular birth-control method.

rigor mortis A temporary condition following death in which the muscle tissue of the body undergoes chemical change resulting in stiffness.

risk factors Variables that, when present, increase the probability that disease or injury will occur in the future.

risks The perception of the likelihood of injury, damage, or other negative consequences following an action.

RU-486 A drug also known as mifepristone or the French abortion pill; this antiprogesterone drug interrupts the normal development of the endometrium and placenta resulting in a chemically-induced abortion.

rubella A virus-induced infection that, if acquired by a woman during pregnancy, may result in fetal malformations.

S

safety The application of knowledge, skills, and attitudes in any situation to minimize risks.

safety-related responsibilities Responsibilities of drug use that protect individuals using drugs, and innocent bystanders, from injury.

saline A solution used in chemical abortions that contains sodium chloride.

salmonella A common type of food-borne infection caused by eating food contaminated with the salmonella bacterium; symptoms include nausea, vomiting, diarrhea, cramps, fever, and headache beginning six to forty-eight hours after eating contaminated food.

sarcoma A cancer that arises from connective tissues, such as bone and cartilage.

saturated fat A type of fatty acid with all carbon atoms joined by single bonds, allowing the maximum number of hydrogen atoms to bond to the molecule. Usually found in animal sources, saturated fats are usually solid at room temperature. Consumption of foods containing saturated fats increases one's total and LDL blood cholesterol, increasing the risk of cardiovascular disease.

scabies An infestation of the body, particularly of the pubic hair, by mites.

scrotal skin Skin that forms a sac that is suspended in the groin of males and houses the two testes.

scrotum A skin sac suspended in the groin area of the male that houses the two testes.

sealants A thin coating of plastic material that is put on tooth surfaces. Sealants create a barrier that prevents food and bacteria from accumulating in the pits and grooves of the teeth, thus helping to prevent cavities from forming.

secondary aging Loss of functional capacity due to disuse, neglect, illness, or trauma that exceeds what would be expected due to primary aging alone.

secondary amenorrhea The absence of menstruation for six months or longer, in a female who has previously established a normal pattern of menstrual cycles.

secondary care A level of health care consisting of care delivered by specialists, often in a private clinic or hospital.

secondary prevention Screening for the early detection of disease, with the aim of decreasing death and disability.

secondary sex characteristics Physical changes that lead to sexual maturity, such as the growth of breasts in females.

secondary stage The stage of syphilis following disappearance of primary symptoms characterized by rash, mild flulike symptoms, and other vague symptoms.

second stage of labor The period of childbirth beginning with the complete dilation of the cervix and ending with the birth of the infant.

second trimester That period of pregnancy beginning with the fourth month and continuing to the end of the sixth month.

secure landfills Excavated trenches or depressions in the land that are lined with clay and a plastic liner in order to prevent the leakage of hazardous waste from the landfill site.

sedative A class of depressant drugs that at low doses produce a calming effect, and at higher doses produce sleep; an overdose may cause death through depression of the central nervous system resulting in cessation of breathing.

sedative hypnotics *See* sedative.

self-actualization A concept popularized by Abraham Maslow, the self-actualized person is one who is able to achieve his or her full potential. Self-actualization sits atop the pinnacle of a series of needs that begin with basic human physiologic needs, the need for security, the need for love and acceptance, and the need for self-esteem.

self-efficacy A person's sense of personal adequacy or competency; one's confidence in being able to attain goals through individual effort.

semen The fluid component discharged from the male reproductive tract at ejaculation. The fluid contains sperm, fructose to supply the sperm with an energy source, and prostaglandins that are thought to help move sperm to the fallopian tubes for possible fertilization of an egg.

seminal fluid The fluid component discharged from the male reproductive tract during ejaculation. This fluid contains sperm, fructose to supply the sperm with an energy source, and prostaglandins that are thought to help move sperm through the fallopian tubes.

seminal vesicles Two small glands found in the male reproductive tract at the end of each vas deferen. These glands produce fluid that contains a simple sugar which provides nutrients for the sperm. Additionally, they produce prostaglandins that help in stimulating sperm locomotion as well as stimulating contractions of the female's reproductive tract, both of which aid in the transport of sperm through the female reproductive tract.

seminiferous tubules Highly coiled tubes, found in the testes, which are the site of sperm production.

semi-vegetarian A type of vegetarian who consumes dairy foods, eggs, chicken, and fish, but no other animal flesh.

senility Mental or physical weakness that may be associated with old age.

serotonin A naturally occurring and potent neurotransmitter chemical and vasoconstrictor found in the body; thought to be important in neural mechanisms, sleep, and sensory perception. Persons with altered serotonin levels are believed to be more susceptible to depression and self-destructive behavior.

set The total internal environment of an individual at the time a drug is taken. This includes physical, mental, and emotional characteristics.

set-point theory A theory of obesity causation that suggests that fat storage is determined by a thermostatic mechanism in the body that acts to maintain a specific amount of body fat.

setting The total external environment of an individual at the time a drug is taken. This includes the physical environment as well as the social environment.

sexual abstinence A premeditated decision not to have sexual intercourse for a specific period of time.

sexual abuse Any maltreatment of an individual that involves sexual coercion. This includes rape, incest, and any sexual activity between a child and an adult.

sexual dysfunction A medical term used to refer to a variety of sexual performance problems.

sexuality Includes our awareness of and reaction to our own maleness or femaleness and that of everyone with whom we interact.

sexually transmitted disease (STD) Any of a host of diseases that has the potential to be transmitted interpersonally through sexual or other intimate body contact.

sexual orientation A term that describes one's sexual attraction to members of the same- and opposite-sex; often conceptualized as a continuum ranging from purely homosexual orientation to purely heterosexual orientation.

shock A situation in which blood flow is inadequate to return sufficient blood to the heart for normal function; associated with injury, trauma, heart attack, and other conditions; produces rapid but weak pulse, and shallow breathing; can be life-threatening if not addressed by proper first aid and advanced care.

sickle-cell anemia   A hereditary disease that primarily affects people of African descent. Defective hemoglobin causes the red blood cells to become sickle shaped, resulting in anemia and often severe complications such as kidney or heart failure.

sickle cell disease   *See* sickle-cell anemia.

sidestream smoke   Smoke that rises from burning tobacco into the environment.

simple sugars   The basic building blocks of carbohydrate, technically termed monosaccharides, consisting of glucose, fructose, and galactose.

sinusitis   An inflammation of the sinus cavities located in the facial bones; common symptoms include headache, tenderness around the sinuses, and a mucous discharge from the nasal passage.

situational responsibilities   Responsibilities of drug use that arise from circumstances in which drugs are used recreationally within a cultural or traditional context, such as social gatherings.

skilled-nursing facility   A nursing home where the patients need daily medical attention from licensed physicians and nurses.

smallpox   A now extinct contagious infection that was caused by a virus and was transmitted through respiratory secretions or direct contact with skin sores. Its symptoms included high fever and a rash that left patients with scars.

smokeless tobacco   Chewing tobacco, snuff, or other forms of tobacco that are not burned and smoked.

snorted   The inhalation of a powdered substance through the nose.

snuff   A finely ground or powdered form of tobacco that is usually held or clenched in the mouth, or inhaled through the nose; a variety of smokeless tobacco.

social engineering strategies   Stress management strategies based on the assumption that certain stressors cannot be changed and that managing the stress response calls for modifying one's position or response to such a stressor. Brainstorming and evaluating alternate responses is one well-known example.

social norms   Behavior expected, exhibited, and rewarded by a given culture.

social-recreational drug use   The use of any of a variety of drugs in a social setting to experience euphoria, increase enjoyment of other activities, or as a social lubricant.

sodium   A macromineral that helps regulate blood and other body fluids, aids in nerve-impulse transmission and heart action, and helps in the metabolism of carbohydrates and protein. Excess consumption of sodium is associated with hypertension.

sodium chloride   Table salt, the primary form of sodium consumption in American diets.

sodomy   The term often used legally to define unnatural sex acts that may be determined by a state to be illegal. Anal intercourse, as well as oral-genital stimulation and sex with animals, are usually listed as sexual behaviors prohibited as sodomy.

soluble fibers   Materials from plant sources that remain undigested in the small intestine but are digested and absorbed in the large intestine.

species-specific resistance   A term that describes the fact that some species never are affected by certain organisms that are pathogenic or even lethal if encountered by other species.

specificity   A principle of fitness that indicates that physiological adaptations to activity are specific to the type of activity and overload.

sperm banks   Organizations that solicit and store sperm donations for use in artificial insemination.

sperm count   The number of sperm found in one ejaculation.

spermicidal condoms   A condom that is laced with a spermicide.

spermicides   Chemicals that prevent fertilization by destroying sperm.

sphygmomanometer   A device used to measure blood pressure.

Spina bifida   The most common neural tube defect, in which an infant is born with a spinal column that does not close completely, leaving the spinal cord exposed.

spirochetes   A type of bacteria that has a spiral shape.

spleen   An organ of the lymph system located on the left side of the abdominal cavity. The primary functions of the spleen are to assist in the production of lymphocytes, filtering of blood, and destroying old red blood cells. In infants, it is also an important producer of red blood cells.

stage of exhaustion   The third stage of the General Adaptation Syndrome that occurs after extended exposure to a stressor. In this stage, symptoms of stress are experienced, organ systems become less effective and break down, and death can occur.

starch   A plant source of complex carbohydrate, such as whole-grain foods, potatoes, rice, beans, and vegetables.

stenosis   The constriction of a blood vessel or a heart valve.

sterility   The inability to have children.

sterilization   A permanent method of birth control, usually accomplished by cutting and closing off the vas deferens in males and the fallopian tubes in females.

stethoscope   A device used to monitor heart beat and arterial sounds.

stillbirth   The birth of a fetus at or later than twenty-eight weeks gestation, that has no heart beat or respiration.

stimulants   Substances that excite the central nervous system, the common results of which are increased alertness, rapid reflexes, excitement, nervousness, irritability, and a sense of self-confidence.

storage fat   Fat that accumulates in adipose or fat cells. Some storage fat is necessary to serve as padding for internal organs and insulation during extreme cold.

stress   The body's response to a stimulus or stressor, either pleasant or unpleasant, consisting of a mobilization of bodily resources for adaptation.

stressor   The stimulus that elicits the stress response.

stress test   *See* exercise stress test.

stroke   Sudden loss of orientation or consciousness, sensation, or voluntary motion as a result of the rupture or obstruction of an artery in the brain; sometimes called a "cerebrovascular accident" (CVA).

stroke volume   The amount of blood discharged with each ventricular contraction (i.e., heart beat).

subcutaneous fat   The storage fat found just beneath the skin.

substance abuse   Continued use of a drug or drugs, despite knowledge of having a persistent or recurrent social, occupational, psychological, or physical problem that is caused or exacerbated by use of the substance; or recurrent use in situations in which use is physically hazardous.

substance dependence   Impaired control of the use of a psychoactive substance with continued use despite adverse consequences.

sudden infant death syndrome (SIDS)   The death of a baby from unidentifiable causes. Also known as crib death because the deaths often occur at night in a crib.

suicide   The intentional act of taking one's own life.

suicide clusters   A group of suicides that are related in some way (i.e., occurring among a group of friends or acquaintances, or in one geographic location in a short period of time).

sulfur dioxide   One of the waste gases released into the atmosphere during the burning of fossil fuels, especially by coal-burning power plants. Sulfur dioxide is one of the gases linked to acid rain.

sun protection factor (SPF)   A rating assigned to tanning and sunscreen products, indicating the relative level of protection from solar radiation. Any of the compounds that block the ultraviolet radiation of the sun to prevent or minimize burning, risk of skin cancer, and premature wrinkles.

superfund   A federal program, first funded in 1980 and refunded in 1986, that authorizes the Environmental Protection Agency (EPA) to respond to hazardous waste spills and clean up abandoned hazardous waste sites.

suppositories   A type of drug in solid form that is intended to be inserted into the vagina or rectum.

suppressor gene   A bit of genetic material or "gene" that plays a role in preventing abnormal cell growth of the type associated with cancer, and whose malfunction may contribute to the formation of some cancers.

surrogate mothers   Paid or unpaid female volunteers who make their reproductive organs available for procreation and pregnancy through artificial insemination. Surrogate mothers agree to give the child to the prospective parents following childbirth.

susceptible host   An individual whose ability to fight off disease is compromised for some reason.

Sustainable Earth Society   A social order based on nature and its laws. In such a society, recycling and reusing matter, decreasing energy consumption, and self-reliant living are stressed.

symptothermal methods   An ovulation prediction method of birth control which combines the calendar, basal body temperature, and cervical mucus methods to predict ovulation.

synergism   A multiplier effect when certain drugs are used together.

syphilis   One of the classic STDs with congenital potential caused by the spirochete *Treponema pallidum*, which if untreated, runs a three-stage clinical course over a period of many years.

systemic lupus erythematosus   A chronic inflammatory disease of connective tissue, of unknown cause, that affects the skin, joints, kidneys, nervous system, and mucous membranes.

systolic   The highest arterial blood pressure in the cardiac cycle occurring just after contraction of the left ventricle.

T

tar   Thick, brown, sticky substance that forms from the particulate matter resulting from burning tobacco.

target heart rate   A measure of the recommended intensity of an aerobic exercise. The American College of Sports Medicine recommends that an individual's target heart rate be between 60 percent and 90 percent of their estimated maximum heart rate.

T-cell   Lymphocytes that mature in the thymus and protect against disease and infection.

teratogenic effects   Factors that can cause congenital malformations by affecting an embryo during its period of rapid growth.

tertiary care   A level of health care consisting of care delivered in a hospital by health-care specialists, often using the latest medical technology.

tertiary prevention   Activities or treatments undertaken once a disease has occurred that aim to return a person to the highest level of functioning (wellness) possible.

tertiary stage   Synonymous with late-stage syphilis; systemic involvement with severely compromised health, leading to death.

testator   Anyone who makes a will that expresses how and to whom property should be distributed in the event of his or her death.

testes   The primary male reproductive organs, also known as testicles, that produce sperm and testosterone.

testicular self-examination (TSE)   The systematic exploration and palpation of the testicles with the hand to identify normal and abnormal or irregular features; a self-care early detection procedure for testicular cancer.

testosterone   The primary male sex hormone. This hormone stimulates the development of male reproductive organs and secondary sex characteristics such as muscle development and beard growth. It also stimulates the female reproductive cycle and maintains the adult female reproductive cycle.

tetanus   An acute infectious disease caused by the bacterium *Clostridium tetani*; infection occurs when the bacterium enters a wound, multiplies, and produces a nervous system toxin; symptoms include muscle stiffness, spasm, and muscle rigidity beginning in the neck and jaw; death rates are high in untreated cases, however a vaccine is available; also known as lock jaw.

thanatology   The scientific study of death and dying.

THC   Delta-9-tetrahydrocannabinol, the psychoactive ingredient in marijuana.

T-helper cell   A T-cell that assists another T-cell or a B-cell in responding to a specific antigen or that activates some other kind of cell.

theoretical effectiveness rate   The estimated maximum effectiveness of a birth-control method if there is no human error.

thermocoagulation   A form of tubal ligation that uses heat to melt away a portion of each fallopian tube.

third stage of labor   The period of childbirth following the birth of the infant; the uterus continues to contract and expels the placenta and remains of the fetal membranes, sometimes referred to as the afterbirth.

third trimester   That period of pregnancy beginning with the seventh month and continuing until childbirth.

thyroxine   A hormone secretion of the thyroid gland that regulates the basal metabolic rate and increases the synthesis of protein in some organs of the body.

time   In terms of exercise, the third FIT guideline; refers to the amount of time an individual needs to devote to vigorous aerobic activity in order to achieve cardiovascular endurance benefits.

tobacco   A plant used to make smoking (cigarettes, cigars) and smokeless (chewing tobacco, snuff) products.

tonsillitis   Inflammation of the tonsils, usually caused by a viral or bacterial infection; symptoms include a sore throat, difficulty swallowing, and fever.

total lung capacity   The sum of vital capacity and residual volume; the maximum volume available in the lungs.

toxemia   Pregnancy-induced hypertension (high blood pressure), with associated swelling of the face, neck, and upper extremities due to fluid retention.

Toxic Release Inventory   A provision of the 1986 Emergency Planning and Community Right-to-Know Act that requires the Environmental Protection Agency (EPA) to publish an annual inventory of toxic releases and transfers from over 20,000 manufacturing facilities in the U.S. Currently, over 300 toxic chemicals are tracked by the EPA and reported to the Toxic Release Inventory.

toxic shock syndrome (TSS)   A bacterial infection usually established in the vagina and associated with products and devices that block the vaginal tract. However, the causes of TSS are not entirely clear, and premenarchial girls and men have contracted the infection.

toxic waste   Solid waste that is poisonous to humans or the environment.

Toxoplasma gondii   The causative agent in toxoplasmosis, a disease with mild to severe symptoms that can include fatigue, muscle pain, and swollen lymph glands.

trace elements   Those minerals that each account for 0.005% or less of body weight. These include iron, zinc, manganese, copper, iodine, and cobalt.

traction   A medical treatment that applies force to the tissues surrounding a broken bone in order to keep broken bones in a correct position for healing.

training effect   Cardiovascular conditioning from an aerobic exercise program designed to build a thicker and stronger heart muscle that can pump more blood per beat than an untrained heart. A cardiovascular training effect results from regular, vigorous aerobic activity.

tranquilizers   Substances that produce a mild depression of the central nervous system, relax the muscles, and cause general calming effects.

trans-fatty acids   A form of fatty acids derived from the process of hydrogenation. These fatty acids, when consumed in foods, are believed to increase total and LDL cholesterol, and decrease HDL cholesterol, thus increasing a person's risk for coronary artery disease.

transient ischemic attack (TIA)   A small stroke-like event that lasts only for a short time and is caused by a partially blocked blood vessel in the brain. A person having a TIA acts confused, dizzy, or loses short-term memory temporarily.

trichomoniasis   A protozoan-induced infection with the potential for being transmitted by sexual means and passed back and forth between sexual partners until both partners are treated with effective medication.

triglycerides A lipid that consists of three fatty acid molecules attached to a glycerol molecule. Triglycerides are stored in fat cells; elevated blood triglyceride levels are associated with an increased risk of cardiovascular disease.

tropical oils Certain tropical plant oils (coconut oil, palm oil, and palm kernel oil) that are highly saturated fats.

T-suppressor cell A T-cell that suppresses the response of B-cells or other T-cells to an antigen resulting in tolerance for the antigen.

tubal ligation A form of sterilization for females that involves the cutting or tying of the fallopian tubes.

tuberculin skin test A test that determines whether a person has been in contact with the bacteria that causes tuberculosis.

tuberculosis (TB) An infectious bacterial disease characterized by inflammations, abscesses, calcification of tissue, and other symptoms, affecting the respiratory system and other sites.

tumor An abnormal mass of cells arising from preexisting tissue, and serving no useful purpose; synonymous with neoplasm.

tumor initiator A substance or factor that can give rise to cancer; a synonym for carcinogen.

tumor promoter A substance or factor that contributes to the process of tumor formation.

Type A personality A personality type exhibited by a person who feels an urgency about time, is competitive, impatient, and is driven to complete tasks as quickly as possible.

Type B personality A personality type exhibited by a person who is more easy going and less concerned with time pressures.

Type I alcoholism Milieu-limited alcoholism, or alcoholism occurring in both men and women, thought to be associated with mild, untreated alcohol abuse in either biological parent.

Type II alcoholism Male-limited alcoholism, or alcoholism occurring only in men, thought to be associated with severe alcoholism in the biological father but not in the biological mother.

Type I diabetes Diabetes arising from destruction of the pancreative beta cells that produce insulin.

Type II diabetes Diabetes arising from changes in insulin secretion or sensitivity of the body to insulin.

typhoid fever A communicable infectious disease caused by the bacteria *Salmonella typhi*, transmitted through food or water contaminated with infected feces or urine. Common symptoms include fever, headache, weakness, red rash on the chest and abdomen, and a nonproductive cough.

U

ultrasound High frequency sound waves, undetectable to the human ear, used to examine the inner structures of the body.

umbilical cord A cordlike structure that connects the embryo/fetus to the placenta.

unintentional injury Physical, emotional, or social damage or suffering that is the result of motor vehicle crashes, falls, poisoning, drowning, and residential fires.

unrecognized drugs Commercially available products that function as drugs, but are not generally regulated as drugs.

upper-body obesity A type of obesity characterized by greater fat stores in the abdominal area. These fat cells are believed to be larger and to store the fat in a manner that is easily mobilized. It is this form of obesity that is associated with a greater risk of diabetes, stroke and coronary artery disease.

urea The chemical form of nitrogen that is excreted in urine.

urethra A tube that conducts urine from the bladder to the exterior of the body. In men, the urethra also conducts semen from the male reproductive system to the exterior of the body during sexual arousal.

urinary tract infections (UTIs) Sometimes called bladder infections, UTIs occur when pathogenic organisms, such as bacteria, enter the urethra and migrate to the bladder.

use-effectiveness rate The estimated effectiveness of a birth-control method that considers human error. Use-effectiveness rates are derived from an actual population of people who have used a particular birth-control method.

USPS United States Postal Service; a federal agency whose consumer protection duties include preventing fraud perpetrated through the mail.

uterus A hollow, muscular, pear-shaped organ found in the internal female reproductive system. This organ is the preferred site for implantation of a zygote.

UV-A rays Long wavelength ultraviolet rays, more intense than their UV-B counterparts, that can penetrate and damage soft tissues of the body.

UV-B rays Short wavelength ultraviolet rays associated with sunburn, skin cancer, and premature wrinkling of the skin.

V

vaccine A preparation that is delivered to stimulate an immunity to a particular disease.

vacuum aspiration An abortion technique that requires the dilation of the cervix followed by insertion of a suction tube to remove the uterine lining.

vagina A tubular organ that leads from the uterus to the vestibule of the female reproductive system.

vaginal intercourse Sexual activity in which there is insertion of the penis into the vagina.

vaginal sponge A soft, polyurethane pad containing a spermicide that is inserted into the vagina, covering the cervix. It prevents fertilization by killing sperm, blocking the cervix, and absorbing sperm.

vas deferens A structure of the male reproductive system that originates in the scrotum, circles the bladder, and eventually joins with the urethra. Its function is to transport sperm from the epididymis to the urethra.

vasectomy A form of sterilization for males that involves the cutting and tying of the vas deferens.

vasocongestion When organs become filled with blood, such as the penis or vulva during sexual stimulation.

vegans A type of vegetarian who avoids both animal food sources and dairy products.

vegetarians Individuals who consume the majority of their calories from plant foods. Some vegetarians eat only plant foods, while others may consume a combination of plant foods and dairy products, fish, or poultry.

veins Blood vessels that receive blood from venules and return it to the heart.

venereal warts *See* genital warts.

ventricle The lower chamber of each half of the heart; the left ventricle pumps blood to the body for general circulation; the right ventricle pumps blood to the lungs to exchange carbon dioxide for oxygen.

venules Small veins that branch from larger systemic veins connecting them with the capillaries.

vertebrae The thirty-three bones that make up the backbone, and through which the spinal cord passes.

vestibule The area of the female external genitals enclosed by the labia minora.

vital capacity The breathing capacity of the lungs upon full inspiration of air.

vitamins Organic substances that play a vital role in human metabolism; their absence from the diet results in deficiency diseases. (Thirteen vitamins have been identified thus far.)

vulva The anatomical name for the female external genitalia. The vulva consists of two paired folds of skin that surround the female's vagina and urethral openings and extend to the clitoris.

W

warm up Slowly beginning an exercise session with brisk walking and some limited stretching to gradually increase the blood flow to active muscles, as well as slowly increasing internal body temperature.

wasting syndrome Sometimes called "Slim Disease," this syndrome consists of severe weight loss, chronic diarrhea and weakness, and a persistent cough.

water-soluble vitamins Vitamins that are dissolved in water within the body. These vitamins (B complex and C) are not stored by the body in any significant quantity.

wellness A process of optimal functioning and creative adapting that involves the total person (physical, mental, emotional, social, and spiritual dimensions) and strives for an ever-increasing quality of life.

Western Blot test A confirmatory test for AIDS antibodies having a low incidence of false negatives.

white blood cells A component of blood, also called leukocytes, capable of leaving the capillaries of the circulatory system in order to reach an infection site where they play a variety of roles in attacking the pathogen.

World Health Organization (WHO) An international agency responsible for studying and controlling disease on a global basis.

Y

years of potential life lost (YPLL) The difference between a person's life expectancy and that person's age at death. This is used as one measure of the consequences of early death.

Z

zidovudine A drug that has demonstrated an ability to retard progress of disease in some persons having AIDS.

zygote The term for a human egg (ovum) that has been fertilized by a sperm cell (spermatozoon) before the process of cell division begins.

Credits

Photos

Part Openers

Unit I: © Index Stock Photos; Unit II: © Walter Bibikow/The Image Bank; Unit III: © Martha McBride/Unicorn Stock Photos; Unit IV: © Mark Antman/The Image Works; Unit V: © Cathlyn Melloan/Tony Stone Images.

Activity for Wellness Boxes

© David R. Frazier Photolibrary.

Of Special Interest Boxes

© Digital Stock Professional.

A Social Perspective Boxes

© Corel Professional Photos.

Chapter 1

Opener: © Index Stock Photos; Figure 1.7: © Hank Morgan/Science Source, Photo Researchers, Inc.; Figure 1.10: © Sullivan/Index Stock Photos; Figure 1.11: © Tony Freeman/PhotoEdit.

Chapter 2

Opener: © Index Stock Photos; Figure 2.1: © Michael Newman/PhotoEdit; Figure 2.2: © Ron P. Jaffe/Unicorn Stock Photos; Figure 2.3: AP/Wide World Photos; p. 37: © Bob Daemmrich/Tony Stone Images; Figure 2.5: © Dave Schaefer/The Picture Cube; Figure 2.6: © Bob Daemmrich/The Image Works; Figure 2.9: © Tom McCarthy/Unicorn Stock Photos; Figure 2.10: © T. Michaels/The Image Works; Figure 2.11: © Dennis MacDonald/Unicorn Stock Photos.

Chapter 3

Opener: © John P. Kelly/The Image Bank; Figure 3.2: Courtesy of FDA Consumer; Figure 3.3: © Bob Coyle; Figure 3.7A&B: © James L. Shaffer; Activity for Wellness 3.2A: © Andy Sacks/Tony Stone Images; Activity for Wellness 3.2B: © Andrew McClenaghan/SPL, Photo Researchers, Inc.; Figure 3.8: © Felicia Martinez/PhotoEdit; Figure 3.9: Courtesy of FDA Consumer; Figure 3.11: © Tony Freeman/PhotoEdit.

Chapter 4

Opener: © David Young-Wolff/Tony Stone Images; Figure 4.3A: © James L. Shaffer; Figure 4.3B: © A. Kaye Photo/Index Stock Photos; Figure 4.4: © S. Gazin/The Image Works; Figure 4.5: © John Anderson/Southern Stock Photos; Figure 4.8: © Skjold Photographs; Figure 4.11: © Bob Coyle; p. 147: "Losing Weight: What Works, What Doesn't" © 1993 by Consumers Union of U.S., Inc., Younkers, NY 10703–1057. Reprinted by permission from CONSUMER REPORTS, June 1993.

Chapter 5

Opener: © Jeff Smith/The Image Bank; p. 167: © Karen Holsinger Mullen/Unicorn Stock Photos; Figure 5.3A: © Lori Adamski Peek/Tony Stone Images; Figure 5.3B: © Martha McBride/Unicorn Stock Photos; Figure 5.3C: © Edward Lettau/Photo Researchers, Inc.; Figure 5.4: © David Young-Wolff/PhotoEdit; Figure 5.5: © Dennis MacDonald/Unicorn Stock Photos; p. 179: © A. Reininger/Unicorn Stock Photos; Figure 5.6A&B: © Bob Coyle.

Chapter 6

Opener: © Index Stock Photography; Figure 6.1 (top): © Steve Skjold/PhotoEdit; Figure 6.1 (bottom): © Bill Bachman/PhotoEdit; Figure 6.6A: © Myrleen Ferguson Cate/PhotoEdit; Figure 6.6B: © Cleo Photography/PhotoEdit; Figure 6.6C: © David Young-Wolff/PhotoEdit; Figure 6.10A: © Robert Brenner/PhotoEdit; Figure 6.10B: © David Young-Wolff/PhotoEdit; Figure 6.11: © Larry Mangino/The Image Works.

Chapter 7

Opener: © Dann Coffey/The Image Bank; Figure 7.9: © Sandy King/The Image Bank; Figure 7.10: © Alexander Tsiaras/Science Source/Photo Researchers, Inc.; Figure 7.11: © Garuis Keriman/Peter Arnold, Inc.; Figure 7.13: © Myrleen Ferguson Cate/PhotoEdit; Figure 7.14: © Blair Seitz/Photo Researchers, Inc.; Figure 7.15: © Diana Rashe/Tony Stone Images.

Chapter 8

Opener: © Michael Newman/PhotoEdit; Figure 8.5: © Chris Grajczyk/Viewfinders; Figure 8.6& 8.7: © Bob Coyle; Figure 8.9: © James L. Shaffer; Figure 8.10A: © TMHEG/Bob Coyle, Photographer; Figure 8.10B: © SIU School of Medicine/Bruce Coleman, Inc.; Figure 8.11: © Benn Mitchell/The Image Bank; Figure 8.12: © John Griffin/The Image Works.

Chapter 9

Opener: © Greg Greer/Unicorn Stock Photos; Figure 9.1: © A. Ramey/ Unicorn Stock Photos; Figure 9.2: AP/Wide World Photos; Figure 9.4: © TRW, Inc.; Figure 9.5: © Eric R. Brendt/Unicorn Stock Photos; p. 335 (both): Rueters/Bettmann; p. 329: © Karen Holsinger-Mullen/Unicorn Stock Photos.

Chapter 10

Opener: © Michael Newman/PhotoEdit; Figure 10.3: © Bob Daemmerich/The Image Works; Figure 10.4: © Blair Seitz/Photo Researchers, Inc.; p. 355 (left): © Ken Huang/The Image Bank; p. 355 (right): © McLaughlin/The Image Works; p. 359: © Philippe Gontier/The Image Works.

Chapter 11

Opener: © Bob Garas/Unicorn Stock Photos; Figure 11.1: © Bob Coyle; Figure 11.2: © Don Smetzer/Tony Stone Images; Figure 11.3A: © David Vance/The Image Bank; Figure 11.3B: © Alan Becker/The Image Bank; p. 383: © Mahaux/The Image Bank.

Chapter 12

Opener: © Ellen Going Jacobs/The Image Bank; Figure 12.5: Reuters/Bettmann; Figure 12.7A: © Biophoto Associates/Photo Researchers, Inc.; Figure 12.7B: © Center for Disease Control, Atlanta, GA; Figure 12.10A: © Dr. John Wilson/Photo Researchers, Inc.; Figure 12.10B: © Health, Education and Welfare; Figure 12.11: © Bob Daemmrich/The Image Works; p. 402 (both): Reuters/Bettmann.

Chapter 13

Opener: UPI/Bettmann; p. 434: Historical Picture Service; p. 436 (both): © Richard Anderson, M.D.; p. 440: © James L. Shaffer; p. 441: © Wayne Floyd/Unicorn Stock Photos; Figure 13.3: AP/Wide World Photos.

Chapter 14

Opener: © James L. Shaffer; Figure 14.2: © Campolungo/The Image Bank; Figure 14.3A: © Bob Daemmrich/The Image Works; Figure 14.3B: © Jim Shippee/Unicorn Stock Photos; Figure 14.5: © Jerry Wachter/Photo Researchers, Inc.; Figure 14.6: © Michael Siluk; p. 479 (both): AP/Wide World Photos.

Chapter 15

Opener: © Robert Brenner/PhotoEdit; p. 492: North Wind Picture Archives; Figure 15.1: © Lester V. Bergman, Cold Spring, NY; Figure 15.2A&B: © TMHEG/Bob Coyle Photographer; Figure 15.4: © Michael Gadomski/Bruce Coleman, Inc.; p. 502 (left): © Fernando Diez/Image Bank Chicago; p. 502 (right): © Courtesy of the American Cancer Society; p. 504: © Bob Daemmrich/The Image Works; Figure 15.7: © Stewart Cohen/Index Stock Photography.

Chapter 16

Opener: © Christopher Bissell/Tony Stone Images; Figure 16.1: © David Young-Wolff/PhotoEdit; Figure 16.3: © TMHEG/Bob Coyle Photographer; p. 531: © Amy C. Etra/PhotoEdit; p. 537: © Doris Brooks/Unicorn Stock Photos; p. 538: © James Marshall; p. 540: © Jim Steinberg/Photo Researchers, Inc.; p. 541 (left): © Michael Newman/PhotoEdit; p. 541 (right): © Leslye Borden/PhotoEdit; p. 543: © Chuck Schmeiser/Unicorn Stock Photos.

Chapter 17

Opener: © Bob Daemmrich/Tony Stone Images; Figure 17.1: © Jonathan Nourok/PhotoEdit; Figure 17.2: © Willie Hill, Jr./The Image Works; Figure 17.3: © James L. Shaffer; Figure 17.4: © Tom McCarthy/Unicorn Stock Photos; Figure 17.5: © Suzanne Arms/The Image Works; Figure 17.6: © Hank Morgan/Science Source/Photo Researchers, Inc.; Figure 17.8: © Ken Sherman/Bruce Coleman, Inc.; Figure 17.9: © Bob Daemmrich/The Image Works; Figure 17.11: © AETNA Life Insurance Company.

Chapter 18

Opener: © Myrleen Ferguson/PhotoEdit; **p. 584:** © Will and Deni McIntyre/Photo Researchers, Inc.; **p. 589 (top):** © CLEO/PhotoEdit; **Figure 18.2:** © Myrleen Ferguson/Photo Edit; **Figure 18.3:** © CLEO/PhotoEdit; **p. 591:** © James L. Shaffer.

Chapter 19

Opener: © Maria Taglienti/The Image Bank; **Figure 19.3:** © D. Wells/The Image Works; **Figure 19.11:** © Chen/Index Stock Photography; **Figure 19.14:** © Nathon Bilow/Allsport USA; **Figure 19.15:** © Bob Daemmrich/The Image Works; **Figure 19.16:** Courtesy of Golden Aluminum.

Illustrations

Chapter 1

Figure 1.4: From H. L. Blum, *Planning for Health-Developmental Application of Social Change Theory,* 1974. Reprinted by permission of Human Science Press, New York, NY.

Chapter 2

Figure 2.8: Figure 3, page 39 from *Stress Without Distress* by Hans Selye, M.D. Copyright © 1974 by Hans Selye, M.D. Reprinted by permission of HarperCollins Publishers, Inc.

Chapter 3

Figure 3.10: Copyright © 1994, Center for Science in the Public Interest. Reprinted by permission.

Chapter 4

Figure 4.2: Reproduced with permission, from T.V. Van Italie, *Annals of Internal Medicine,* 1985; 103:983–988. American College of Physicians, Philadelphia, PA. **Figure 4.9:** From "Facts About Fat, Take a Look at the Inside . . ." from *Medical Times* Patient Education Chart. Reprinted by permission of Romaine Pierson Publishers, Inc., Port Washington, NY. **Figure 4.10:** From "Facts About Fat, Take a Look at the Inside . . ." from *Medical Times* Patient Education Chart. Reprinted by permission of Romaine Pierson Publishers, Inc., Port Washington, NY.

Chapter 6

Figure 6.1: From Jerrold S. Greenberg, et al., *Human Sexuality: Insights and Issues,* 2nd edition. Copyright © 1989 Wm. C. Brown Communications, Inc. Reprinted by permission of Times Mirror Higher Education Group, Inc., Dubuque, Iowa. All Rights Reserved. **Figure 6.4:** From Jerrold S. Greenberg, et al., *Human Sexuality: Insights and Issues,* 2nd edition. Copyright © 1989 Wm. C. Brown Communications, Inc. Reprinted by permission of Times Mirror Higher Education Group, Inc., Dubuque, Iowa. All Rights Reserved. **Figure 6.5:** From Jerrold S. Greenberg, et al., *Human Sexuality: Insights and Issues,* 2nd edition. Copyright © 1989 Wm. C. Brown Communications, Inc. Reprinted by permission of Times Mirror Higher Education Group, Inc., Dubuque, Iowa. All Rights Reserved. **Figure 6.6:** From *Human Sexual Response,* © 1966 Masters &

Johnson Institute, St. Louis, MO. Reprinted by permission. **Figure 6.7:** From *Human Sexual Response,* © 1966 Masters & Johnson Institute, St. Louis, MO. Reprinted by permission. **Figure 6.11:** From Curtis O. Byer, et al., *Dimensions of Human Sexuality,* 2nd edition. Copyright © 1988 Wm. C. Brown Communications, Inc. Reprinted by permission of Times Mirror Higher Education Group, Inc., Dubuque, Iowa. All Rights Reserved.

Chapter 7

Figure 7.2: From John W. Hole, Jr., *Human Anatomy and Physiology,* 4th edition. Copyright © 1987 Wm. C. Brown Communications, Inc. Reprinted by permission of Times Mirror Higher Education Group, Inc., Dubuque, Iowa. All Rights Reserved. **Figure 7.3:** From Kent M. Van De Graaff, *Human Anatomy,* 3rd edition. Copyright © 1992 Wm. C. Brown Communications, Inc. Reprinted by permission of Times Mirror Higher Education Group, Dubuque, Iowa. All Rights Reserved. **Figure 7.4:** From John W. Hole, Jr., *Human Anatomy and Physiology,* 4th edition. Copyright © 1987 Wm. C. Brown Communications, Inc. Reprinted by permission of Times Mirror Higher Education Group, Inc., Dubuque, Iowa. All Rights Reserved. **Figure 7.5:** From Kent M. Van De Graaff, *Human Anatomy,* 3rd edition. Copyright © 1992 Wm. C. Brown Communications, Inc. Reprinted by permission of Times Mirror Higher Education Group, Dubuque, Iowa. All Rights Reserved. **Figure 7.6:** From John W. Hole, Jr., *Human Anatomy and Physiology,* 4th edition. Copyright © 1987 Wm. C. Brown Communications, Inc. Reprinted by permission of Times Mirror Higher Education Group, Inc., Dubuque, Iowa. All Rights Reserved. **Figure 7.7:** From John W. Hole, Jr., *Human Anatomy and Physiology,* 4th edition. Copyright © 1987 Wm. C. Brown Communications, Inc. Reprinted by permission of Times Mirror Higher Education Group, Inc., Dubuque, Iowa. All Rights Reserved. **Figure 7.8:** From Kent M. Van De Graaff and Stuart Ira Fox, *Concepts of Human Anatomy and Physiology,* 3rd edition. Copyright © 1992 Wm. C. Brown Communications, Inc. Reprinted by permission of Times Mirror Higher Education Group, Dubuque, Iowa. All Rights Reserved. **Figure 7.12:** From Kent M. Van De Graaff, *Human Anatomy,* 3rd edition. Copyright © 1992 Wm. C. Brown Communications, Inc. Reprinted by permission of Times Mirror Higher Education Group, Dubuque, Iowa. All Rights Reserved. **Figure 7.16:** Data from Earl Ubell, "Encouraging News for Childless Couples" in *Parade Magazine,* May 6, 1984, as appeared in John W. Hole, Jr., *Human Anatomy and Physiology,* 5th edition. Copyright © 1990 Wm. C. Brown Communications, Inc. Reprinted by permission of Times Mirror Higher Education Group, Inc., Dubuque, Iowa. All Rights Reserved.

Chapter 8

Figure 8.3: From Kenneth L. Jones, *Dimensions of Human Sexuality,* Copyright © 1985 Wm. C. Brown Communications, Inc. Reprinted by permission of Times Mirror Higher Education Group, Inc., Dubuque, Iowa. All Rights Reserved. **Figure 8.13:** From John W. Hole, Jr., *Human Anatomy and Physiology,* 4th edition. Copyright © 1987 Wm. C. Brown Communications, Inc. Reprinted by permission of Times Mirror Higher Education

Group, Inc., Dubuque, Iowa. All Rights Reserved. **Figure 8.14:** From Curtis O. Byer and Louis W. Shainberg, *Dimensions of Human Sexuality,* 4th edition. Copyright © 1995 Wm. C. Brown Communications, Inc. Reprinted by permission of Times Mirror Higher Education Group, Inc., Dubuque, Iowa. All Rights Reserved.

Chapter 10

Figure 10.1: From John W. Hole, Jr., *Human Anatomy and Physiology,* 6th edition. Copyright © 1993 Wm. C. Brown Communications, Inc. Reprinted by permission of Times Mirror Higher Education Group, Inc., Dubuque, Iowa. All Rights Reserved.

Chapter 11

Figure 11.4: From Kent M. Van De Graaff, *Human Anatomy,* 2nd edition. Copyright © 1988 Wm. C. Brown Communications, Inc. Reprinted by permission of Times Mirror Higher Education Group, Dubuque, Iowa. All Rights Reserved.

Chapter 12

Figure 12.2: From John W. Hole, Jr., *Human Anatomy and Physiology,* 7th edition. Copyright © 1996 Times Mirror Higher Education Group, Inc., Dubuque, Iowa. All Rights Reserved. Reprinted by permission. **Figure 12.3:** From *The Sexually Active and VD,* 1979 by the American Social Health Association, Research Triangle Park, NC. Reprinted by permission.

Chapter 13

Figure 13.2: Reprinted by permission of Choice In Dying, 200 Varick Street, New York, NY 10014. 212/366–5540.

Chapter 15

Figure 15.5: From *Tobacco-Free Florida Plan 1994–1995,* Coalition on Smoking and Health, Washington, D.C.

Chapter 16

Figure 16.6: From Betty S. Bergersen and E.E. Krug, *Pharmacology in Nursing,* 12th edition. Copyright © 1973 C.V. Mosby Company, St. Louis, MO.

Chapter 19

Figure 19.2: Copyright, October 31, 1988, *U.S. News & World Report.* **Figure 19.7:** "Map Depicting the Impact of Acid Rain in U.S. and Canada" from *Design For a Livable Planet,* by Jon Naar. Copyright © 1990 by Jon Naar. Reprinted by permission of HarperCollins Publishers, Inc. **Figure 19.9:** From William P. Cunningham and Barbara Woodworth Saigo, *Environmental Science,* 2nd edition. Copyright © 1992 Wm. C. Brown Communications, Inc. Reprinted by permission of Times Mirror Higher Education Group, Inc., Dubuque, Iowa. All Rights Reserved. **Figure 19.12:** Reprinted by permission of Dr. Robert Russell, Southern Illinois University at Carbondale, Carbondale, IL.

Index

Arrhythmia, 497
    characteristics of, 352
    management of, 352
Arteries, functions of, 346
Arterioles, functions of, 346
Arteriosclerosis, characteristics of, 349
Arthritis, 569, 597
    over-the-counter medication for, 467
Artificial insemination, 231, 267
Artificially acquired active immunity, 399
Artificially acquired passive immunity, 399
Artificial sweeteners, cancer risk from, 371–72
Aruffo, J. F., 413
Asbestos, health risks from, 369, 613
Ascherio, A., 84
Ashley, J. M., 125
Aspartame, 372
Aspirin, prevention of cardiovascular disease, 359
Assisted suicide, 449
Association of American Medical Colleges, 550
Asthma, 515, 618
    characteristics of, 389
    management of, 389
    triggers of, 389
Atchley, R. C., 591
Atherosclerosis, 349
    and hypertension, 349–50
Athletes, 110–11
    carbohydrate loading, 111
    dietary guidelines for, 111
    drugs used by, 477–78
Atkins, S. A., 263
Atrium, 346
Auslander, G. K., 601
Autoimmune disease, 399–400
    mechanism in, 400
    types of, 400
Autoimmune reaction, 400
Autoimmune theory, of aging, 590
Automobile accidents, 320–24
    and air bags, 320–21
    defensive driving skills, 321, 322–23
    preventive measures, 320–21
Automobiles, ranking of energy efficient vehicles, 633
Autonomic nervous system, and stress, 47
Aversion strategies, for smoking cessation, 511
Avoidance, defense mechanism, 61
Azar, V., 302
AZT, 405

B

Bachman, G. A., 588
Bachman, J., 476
Bachman, J. G., 541
Back pain, steps to take, 555
Bacterial pneumonia, 403
Bait-and-switch tactics, health products, 568
Ballor, D. L., 145
Barer, B. M., 599
Barrett, T. C., 327
Barrett-Connor, E., 595
Barrs, J., 444
Bartholin's glands, 241–42
Basal body temperature, definition of, 282
Basal body temperature method, birth control, 282–83
Basal metabolic rate (BMR), and aging, 584
Bateman, D. A., 471
Bateman, P., 332
B cells, and immune response, 398–99
Becerra, J., 253
Bechhofer, L., 331, 332
Becker, L. A., 597
Beckman, I. M., 250

Beecher, H. K., 477
Begay, M. E., 504
Behavior modification
    of eating behaviors, 146–48
    of exercise behavior, 148
    smoking cessation, 511–12
Behavior therapy, for depression, 43
Bell, J., 581
Bell, J. A., 478
Bem Sex-Role Inventory, 203
Benenson, A. S., 402, 403, 417, 421
Bengston, V. L., 591
Benign tumors, 368
Bennett, W., 141
Bennion, L. J., 124, 130, 132, 133, 138, 152, 153, 191
Benson, R. C., 245, 292, 304
Berkam, L. F., 12
Berkanovic, E., 595
Berland, T., 152
Beta-endorphins, and physical activity, 167
Better Business Bureau (BBB), 571, 573
Bierman, E. L., 124, 130, 132, 133, 138, 152, 153, 191
Bile salts, 85
Bioelectrical impedance analysis, body fat measurement, 129
Biofeedback training, 59
Biological aging, 582
Birth control
    abortion, 278, 299, 301–4
    basal body temperature method, 282–83
    birth control pills, 292–93
    calendar method, 282
    cervical cap, 285–86
    cervical mucus method, 283
    chemical methods, 277
    coitus interruptus, 277
    cost factors, 280–81
    Depo-Provera, 295, 297
    diaphragm, 284–85
    effectiveness of, 279–80
    female condoms, 288–89
    future view, 296
    intrauterine device (IUD), 290–92
    invasive methods, 278
    male condoms, 287–88
    mechanical methods, 277
    natural methods, 276–77
    Norplant, 294–95
    reversibility, 281
    safety factors, 280
    sexual abstinence, 281–82, 284
    and sexually transmitted diseases (STDs), 280
    social/personal influences, 304
    spermicides, 277, 290
    sterilization, 278, 297–99
    symptothermal method, 284
    vaginal sponge, 286–87
Birth control pills, 292–93
    medications affecting effectiveness, 294
    risks/benefits, 293
    types of, 292
Bisexual orientation, 208
Blackburn, G., 125
Bladder cancer, 377
Blair, S. N., 175
Blood-alcohol concentration (BAC), 321, 324, 526–28
    by body weight, 527
    and driving, 530
    psychological/physical effects, 529
Blood pressure, systolic and diastolic pressure, 349
Blood transfusion, and HIV/AIDS prevention, 410–11
Blum, S., 240
Blumberg, J. B., 112

Blumenthal, D., 87, 573
Bobak, M. D., 250, 258, 259
Boccher-Lattimore, D., 424
Body composition
    and aging, 584
    meaning of, 171
Body fat measurement, 127–29
    bioelectrical impedance analysis, 129
    near-infrared interactance, 129
    percentage of body fat, 127
    skin-fold measurement, 127–28
    underwater weighing, 127
Body Mass Index (BMI), 130
Body weight measurement, 129–30
    Body Mass Index (BMI), 130
    ideal weight charts, 129–31
Bohman, M., 535
Bolden, S., 368
Bone, R. C., 496, 497
Bone mass, and aging, 585
Botulism, 107
Bouchard, C., 175
Bourgoin, B. P., 102
Bowel health, and elderly, 600
Bowers, F. R., 51, 441
Boyle, P., 515
Brain death, 435–36
Brand loyalty approach, health products, 568
Braud, R. J., 355
Bread, W., 479
Breast cancer, 375–76
    early detection of, 376
Breast-feeding, 263–64
    advantages of, 263
    and drug use, 250
Breasts, anatomy of, 242
Breast self-examination, 376, 382, 384
Breathing rhythm skills, 59
Breech birth, 258
Brendt, D. A., 250
Brendt, R. L., 250
Brenner, B. M., 587
Brent, R. L., 250
Breslow, L., 12
Brody, J., 89
Bronchi, 388
Bronchitis, 515
Brooks, J. A., 354
Brothers, J., 331
Brown, B. J., 587
Brown, L. R., 622, 623, 625
Brown, L. T., 609
Brown, R. A., 511
Brownell, K. D., 149, 153
Bruess, C. E., 252
Bryan, M. H., 263
Buchner, D., 175
Bulbourethral glands, 239
Bulimia nervosa, 154–57
    behavior in, 155–56
    health risks of, 156–57
Bullock, L., 335
Bupropion, 43
Burdon, R. H., 374, 590
Burkman, R., 292
Burnette, D., 595
Burning agents, in tobacco, 496
Burton, J. R., 598
Buss, D. M., 211, 212
Butler, R. N., 580
Butterworth, S. W., 358
Byer, C. O., 200
Byers, T., 95

C

Cabral, R. J., 304
Cadenhead, C., 336
Caffeine, 469–70
    adverse effects of, 469–70
    and pregnancy, 250
    sources of, 469
Calcium, 99–102
    absorption factors, 102
    facts about, 97
    food sources, 101, 102
    functions of, 99
    optimal intake, 99–100
    and osteoporosis, 100–101
    supplements, 101–2
Calendar method, birth control, 282
Calories, meaning of, 69
Calvo, M. S., 102
Campbell, S. M., 124, 125
Campion, E. W., 593
Campylobacter, food contamination, 103, 106
Cancer
    and alcohol use, 532–34
    biological factors, 372–74
    bladder cancer, 377
    breast cancer, 375–76
    categories of, 369
    causes of, 368
    cellular mechanisms in, 368
    cervical cancer, 376
    colorectal cancer, 375
    and diet, 371–72
    early detection, 382–85
    leukemias, 376
    lung cancer, 374–75
    lymphomas, 378
    medical factors, 370
    metastasis, 368, 369
    and minorities, 378, 379
    occupational factors, 369
    oral cancer, 377
    ovarian cancer, 376–77
    pancreatic cancer, 377–78
    prevention of, 380–81
    prostate cancer, 377
    skin cancer, 376
    social factors, 370–71
    and sun exposure, 372
    testicular cancer, 376
    uterine cancer, 376
    warning signs, 387
Cancer treatment
    chemotherapy, 379–80
    immunotherapy, 380
    quack treatments, 380
    radiotherapy, 378–79
    surgery, 378
Candida albicans, 406
Candidiasis, 421–22
    complications from, 421
    treatment of, 422
Cantwell, J. D., 174
Capillaries, functions of, 346
Capitation, 563
Caplan, R., 611, 618–20, 623
Carbohydrate loading, 111
Carbohydrates, 76–82
    complex carbohydrates, 78, 80–82
    functions of, 76
    simple carbohydrates, 76–78
Carbon dioxide, 609
Carbon monoxide, 499
Carcinogens, 496, 533
    and fiber consumption, 80
Carcinomas, nature of, 369
Cardiac arrest, 351
Cardiac catheterization, 363
Cardiopulmonary resuscitation (CPR), 437
    nature of, 351

Cardiovascular disorders
    and alcohol use, 532
    angina, 351–52
    arrhythmia, 352
    arteriosclerosis, 349
    aspirin in prevention of, 359
    and cigarette smoking, 353–54
    congenital heart disease, 353
    congestive heart failure, 352
    cost of medical procedures for, 363
    and fat intake, 354–55
    high blood pressure, 349–51
    and hypertension, 354
    and physical inactivity, 357–58
    rheumatic heart disease, 353
    risk prediction charts, 360–63
    stroke, 352–53
    and Type A personality, 355–57
Cardiovascular endurance
    and aerobic exercise, 173–83
    meaning of, 171
Cardiovascular system
    and aging, 583
    physical activity benefits, 167–69
Carmelli, D., 137
Carnett, J. R., 102
Carotid arteries, 180–81
Carpenter, B., 621
Carr, C. A., 440
Carson, R., 611
Cashman, M., 586
Cassel, C. K., 580
Castelli, W. P., 532
Cataracts, 250, 403, 587
    and antioxidants, 91
Cates, W., 288
Cell-mediated immunity, 399
Centers for Disease Control and Prevention
    (CDC), 394
Central nervous system
    and alcohol use, 527
    and stress, 47–48
Cerebral arteries, 352
Cerebral thrombosis, 349
Cervical cancer, 376
Cervical cap, 285–86
    risks/benefits, 286
Cervical mucus method, birth control, 283
Cervix, 204, 243, 283
Cesarean section, 265–66
    and maternal herpes, 421
Chakraborty, R., 137
Chancres, 417
Cheadle, A., 164
Chemical abortion, 303
Chemotherapy
    cancer treatment, 379–80
    meaning of, 363
Chepesiuk, R., 623
Chewing tobacco, 494
Chi, I., 298
Chicken pox, 400
Chideya, F., 302
Child abuse, 333–34
    prevention of, 334
Childbirth, 262–63
    breech birth, 258
    cesarean section, 265–66
    childbirth supervisor, 264–65
    electronic fetal monitoring (EFM), 265
    facilities for, 265
    labor, stages of, 262–63
    Lamaze method, 265
    multiple births, 258
    nurse midwife, 264
    pain relief in, 266
    witnesses to, 266
Childbirth supervisor, 264–65
Childhood disease, 400

Child neglect, 333–34
Chiodo, G. T., 335
Chiropractors, 554–55
Chitkarn, U., 259
Chlamydia-related infections, 419–20
    types of disorders, 419–20
Chlorine, facts about, 97
Chodhury, P., 496, 497
Cholera, 399
Cholesterol, 85–86
    and coronary artery disease, 85–86
    dietary cholesterol, 85
    and fiber consumption, 80
    food sources of, 85, 86
    functions of, 85
    HDL cholesterol, 83, 85
    LDL cholesterol, 83, 85
Chorionic biopsy, 259
Chrebet, J., 124
Christen, A. G., 490, 507, 510
Christenson, C., 588
Chromosomes, 236
    and caffeine, 469
    and gender determination, 200
    and sexual orientation, 207
Chronic bronchitis, characteristics of, 389
Chronic disease
    asthma, 389
    chronic bronchitis, 389
    diabetes, 385, 387–88
    emphysema, 388
Chronic obstructive lung disease, 369
    and cigarette smoking, 500
Cigarette smoking. *See* Smoking cessation;
    Tobacco; Tobacco use
Cilia, 239
Cimons, M., 354, 498
Circumcision, 240
Cirrhosis, 534
Ciurlia-Guy, E., 586
Clark, B. J., 377, 494
Clean Air Act, 614
Clean indoor air bills, 505
Clearwater, H. E., 317, 319
Clifton, T., 302
Climacteric, 587
Clinical death, 437
Clinical psychologists, 554
Clitoris, 204
Cloninger, C. R., 535
Clostridium perfringens, food contamination, 106
Clothing production, and environment, 630–31
Clove cigarettes, 495
Cobalt, facts about, 97
Cocaine, 470–72
    crack, 471
    physiological effects, 470–71
    routes of administration of, 471
    treatment for dependence, 471–72
Cocarcinogens, 496
Codeine, 468
Coffman, S. L., 440
Coffman, V. T., 440
Cognitive therapy, for depression, 42
Cohabitation, 226
    meaning of, 218
    reasons for, 226
Cohan, A., 334
Coitus interruptus, 277
Cold turkey, smoking cessation, 512, 513
Cole, T. R., 580
Collagen, 585
Collateral circulation, 351
College students, and alcohol use, 541–44
Colon cancer, and fat intake, 372
Colorectal cancer, 375
Colostrum, 263

Linder, C. W., 336
Linderman, J., 136
Lingard, S. M., 102
Lino, M., 246
Lipids
    and exercise, 143
    nature of, 82
    See also Fats
Lipman, M. M., 559
Listeria, food contamination, 107, 108
Litivin, H., 601
Liver disease, and alcohol use, 534
Living will, 448
Lobell, J., 625
Lockshin, R. A., 589
Long, P., 111
Lonnqvist, J., 327
Loss, emotions related to, 433
Loucks, A., 421
Love, parental, 249
Loveless, P. A., 335
Love relationships
    commitment in, 208
    companionate love, 209
    consummate love, 209
    factors for success, 211
    intimacy, 208
    measurement scale, 212–13
    partner selection, 211–14
    passion, 208–9
    romantic love, 209
    ten rules for, 210
Low-calorie diets, 138–40, 145
    effects of, 138, 140
Lowenstein, A., 441
Lowenthal, D. T., 598
Lower-body obesity, 133–34
Low-fat/high-carbohydrate diet, for weight control, 146
LSD, 475–76
    physiological effects, 475
Lubomudrov, S., 581
Luby, V., 595
Lucas, A. R., 153
Luft, H. S., 563
Lundberg, G. D., 335
Lundervold, D., 596
Lung cancer, 374–75
    and women, 375
Luteinizing hormone (LH), functions of, 237–38
Lyman, G. H., 377, 494
Lyme disease, 403–4
Lymph nodes, and immune response, 398
Lymphocytes, 398
Lymphogranuloma venereum, 419, 420
Lymphomas, 378
    nature of, 369
Lynn, T. D., 358

M

Macera, C. A., 175
Macroconsumers, 608
Macrophages, 398
Madden, P. A., 538
Maddox, G. L., 590
Magnesium, facts about, 97
Magnetic resonance imaging (MRI), 559–60
Magnus, M. H., 164
Mainstream smoke, 495, 515–16
Maintenance stage, physical activity program, 187–88
Major minerals, 96, 97
Major stressors, 45
Male reproductive system, 238–41
    bulbourethral glands, 239
    ejaculation, 240–41
    epididymis, 239

penis, 240
prostate gland, 239
scrotum, 238–39
semen, 239
seminal vesicles, 239
sperm, 240
urethra, 239
vas deferens, 239
Malignant tumors, 368–69
Mallory, M., 506
Maloney, T. W., 592
Mammography, 376, 382, 558
Managed care, 561–63
    See also Health maintenance organizations (HMOs)
Mandel, L. D., 78
Manganese, facts about, 97
Manson, J. E., 354
MAO inhibitors, 43
Marcus, B. H., 175
Margarine, 83
Marijuana, 472–73
    adverse effects from, 472–73
    fetal effects, 473
    legalization issue, 474
    physiological effects, 472
Mark, M. B., 51, 441
Markides, K. S., 590
Marriage, 227
    benefits of, 227
    and divorce, 227–29
    marital status of population, 228
Marty, P. H., 494
Marty, P. J., 382
Maslow, A., 17, 34
Mason, J. E., 84
Mason, James O., 493
Mason, M., 302, 593
Massage, 59
Massey, L. K., 102
Masters, W. H., 203
Mastdt, S., 632
Masturbation, 216
Maximal heart rate, meaning of, 180
May, 293
Mazess, R. B., 585
McArdle, W. D., 138
McBride, G., 94
McCauley, A. P., 295
McCormack, K. R., 377, 494
McDermott, R. J., 377, 382, 494, 542
McDonald, R., 116
McFarlane, J., 335
McHenry, P. C., 327
McKim, W. A., 477
McLean, D. A., 412, 413
McLearn, G. E., 137
McWilliams, M., 116
Measles, 399
Meat, low fat choices, 87
Medicaid, 506, 564
Medicare, 563–64, 599
Medigap policies, 564
Meditation, 59
Megadose, vitamins, 90
Meisind, R. P. M., 83
Melanin, 372
Melanoma, 372, 376
    warning signs, 377
Menarche, 245
Menopause, 587–88
    meaning of, 242
    psychological factors, 587–88
Menstrual cycle, 244–45
    disorders of, 245
    menarche, 245
    premenstrual syndrome, 245

Menstruation, 244
Mental diversion skills, 59
Mental health problems
    depression, 38–44
    stress, 44–51
Mental wellness
    and acceptance of stereotypes, 62
    and career advancement, 64
    characteristics of, 30–31
    and defense mechanisms, 61–62
    definitional problems, 31–32
    expanding through awareness, 60–61
    expanding through experience, 61
    and family life, 62
    and fully functioning person, 33–34
    and pace of society, 62–64
    and poverty, 62
    and self-actualized person, 34–36
    sound mind, sound body concept, 36–37
    stress management, 51–60
Menzies, D., 427
Mercy killing, 451
Mesind, R. P. M., 83
Metabolism
    of alcohol, 526
    and exercise, 141
    nature of, 89
Metastasis, 368, 369
Methyl alcohol, 522
Meyer, M., 420
Michael, R. T., 206, 208, 213, 215–18, 220, 222, 224
Microconsumers, 608
Mid-life crisis, 588
Miller, D. R., 112
Miller, G. T., 608
Miller, J. R., 600, 601
Miller, K., 589
Miller, R. H., 563
Miller, S., 302
Miller, W. C., 136
Minerals, 96–102
    calcium, 99–102
    listing of, 97
    major minerals, 96, 97
    sodium, 96, 98–99
    trace elements, 96, 97
Minilaparotomy, 298
Minipills, 292
Minorities
    and aging, 592
    and alcohol use, 538–41
    and cancer, 378, 379
    and HIV/AIDS, 412–13
    and infant mortality, 4, 5
    and life expectancy, 13
    and obesity, 124–25
    and physical activity, 164–65
    and suicide, 325–26
    and tobacco use, 503–4
Minor stressors, 45
Minuchin, S., 601
Miscarriage, 288, 469
Misch, A., 611, 618
Mishell, D. R., 297
Mishell, D. R., Jr., 423
Mitchell, H. W., 600
Mittelschmerz, 293
Moderate obesity, 137–38
Monoclonal antibodies, 380
Monophasic birth control pills, 292
Monosaccharides, 76
Monounsaturated fat, 82
Montoye, H. J., 594
Moody, R. A., Jr., 437
Morbidity rates, meaning of, 4
Morbid obesity, 137–38
Morgan, K. C., 327

Pate, R. R., 175
Pathogens, 220, 287
    in communicable disease, 394–96
    and enzymes, 397
Patrick, K., 175
Patrono, C., 359
Paul, B., 592
PCP, 476, 531
    death from, 476
    physiological effects, 476
Peak experiences, and self-actualized person, 35
Pearson, D., 164
Pedersen, N. L., 137
Pediculosis, 422
Peers
    and alcohol use, 536
    and drug abuse, 478–79
    and tobacco use, 503
Pelletier, K. R., 36, 37
Pelvic inflammatory disease (PID)
    and cervical cap, 286
    and infertility, 416
    signs of, 287
Pendergrast, R. A., 336
Penis, 200
    anatomy of, 240
Percentage of body fat, body fat measurement, 127
Percutaneous umbilical blood sampling, 259
Perimetrium, 243
Perineum, 241
Pernicious anemia, Vitamin B12 deficiency, 95
Pernoll, M. L., 245, 292, 304
Perri, S., II, 594
Personality engineering approach
    affirmations, 56
    constructive self-talk, 56
    stress management, 55–57
    and Type A behavior, 56
Personal wellness contract, 25
Pertussis, 399
Pesticide use, 611–12
    DDT, 611–12
    versus integrated pest management, 623
Peto, R., 369
Pfost, K. S., 441
Phagocytosis, meaning of, 398
Phillips, J. R., 496, 497
Phosphorus, facts about, 97
Physical activity
    cardiovascular benefits, 167–69
    and disease prevention, 169–70
    injuries, types of, 189
    making time for, 191–92
    and minorities, 164–65
    psychological benefits, 166–67
    and weigh control, 169
Physical activity program
    improvement-conditioning stage, 187
    initial conditioning stage, 187
    maintenance stage, 187–88
    play-oriented approach to, 165
    starting program, 183, 187
Physical fitness
    aerobic exercise, 173–83
    anaerobic exercise, 174
    components of, 171
    definition of, 171
    and individual differences, 173
    overload principle, 171–72
    reversibility principle, 173
    specificity principle, 172
Physicians, 550–53
    allopathy, 550, 552
    choosing/rating of, 553
    medical specialties/subspecialties, 552
Physicians assistants, 554

Physicians offices, 556
Physiological withdrawal, smoking cessation, 509
Piccone, N. L., 473
Pierce, E. F., 358
Pi-Sunyer, F. X., 124
Pituitary gland, functions of, 237
Placenta, 257, 302
Planned Parenthood v. Casey, 301
Plaque
    in Alzheimer's disease, 595
    in arteries, 349
    dental, 77
Plateau phase, human sexual response, 204
Pleasure, and health behavior, 17
Pneumocystis carinii pneumonia, 406
Pneumonia, 515, 534
Pober, B., 250
Podiatrists, 553
Poehlman, E. T., 145
Point-of-service (POS) plans, 562
Polio, 399
Polland, R. L., 240
Pollard, P. M., 443
Pollock, C., 625, 632
Pollock, M. L., 175
Polyunsaturated fat, 82
Pomeroy, W., 588
Poppy, J., 320
Population growth, 305
Posner, B. M., 112
Postpartum period, 276
Potassium, facts about, 97
Potts, M. K., 595
Poverty
    and health status, 15
    and mental wellness, 62
    and nutrition, 113
    and obesity, 124
Powell, K. E., 336
Powell, L. S., 595, 596
Powers, S. K., 128, 132, 134, 143, 167
Pratt, M., 175
Pratt, W., 276
Predisposing factors, 15–16
    created need as, 17
    fulfillment of needs as, 17
    knowledge as, 16–17
    meaning of, 16
    pleasure/pain as, 17
Pre-eclampsia, 259
Preferred provider organizations (PPO), 563
Pregnancy, 249–62
    and alcohol use, 528, 530–31
    and caffeine use, 469–70
    childbirth, 262–63
    and cigarette smoking, 500–501
    complications of, 258–59
    dietary guidelines, 111–12
    HIV/AIDS transmission to fetus, 411
    indicators of, 258
    and marijuana use, 473
    physiological maternal changes, 258–59
    prenatal care, 249–53
    prenatal development, 253, 256–58
    prenatal testing, 259, 262
    sexual activity during, 252
    trimesters of, 256
Prejudice, negative aspects of, 62
Premature ejaculation, 223
Premenstrual syndrome (PMS), 245
    treatments for, 245
Prenatal care, 249–53, 483
    benefits of, 252–53
    drug use, avoiding, 250, 252
    genetic counseling, 249

    nutrition, 251–52, 254–55
    physical health status of mother, 249
    ultrasound monitoring of fetus, 253
    vitamins, 250, 253
Prenatal development, 253, 256–58
    embryonic period, 256–57
    fetus, 257–58
    implantation, 256
    trimesters, 256
Prenatal testing, 259, 262
    alpha fetoprotein blood test, 259
    amniocentesis, 259
    for Down's syndrome, 259
    percutaneous umbilical blood sampling, 259
Prendergast, M. L., 479
Prentice, A. M., 129, 130
Presbyopia, 586
Prescription drugs, 459, 467–69
    amphetamines, 468–69
    psychotropic drugs, 467
    sedative/hypnotics, 467
    tranquilizers, 467–68
Primary aging, 583
Primary care, health care, 556
Primary prevention, meaning of, 4
Private health insurance, 561
Prochaska, J. O., 21, 24, 26
Pro-choice argument, 301
Product misrepresentation, health products, 568
Progesterone, functions of, 133, 242
Programmed endpoint theory, of aging, 589
Progressive muscle relaxation, 59
Pro-life argument, 301
Prostaglandins, 466
    and abortion, 303
Prostate cancer, 377
Prostate gland, 239, 419
Protein, 88–90
    and amino acids, 88
    complete protein, 89
    functions of, 88–89
    protein-rich food combinations, 91
    sources of, 89–90
Prothrow-Stith, D., 329
Prozac, 42
Prugh, T., 634
Psaty, B. M., 164
Psychoactive drugs
    nature of, 458
    See also Illicit drugs
Psychological aging, 582
Psychological withdrawal, smoking cessation, 510
Psychotherapy, for depression, 42
Psychotropic drugs, 467
Pulmonary function, and aging, 583–84
Purtilo, D. T., 353
Purtilo, R. B., 353
Pyloric valve, 525
Pylorospasm, 526

Q

Quattrone, A. J., 102
Quickening, 257

R

Raczynski, J. M., 164
Radial artery, 181
Radiotherapy, cancer treatment, 378–79
Radon, 516
Ragland, D. R., 355
Rahe, R., 51
Rakowski, W., 598
Ramesy, S. A., 30
Ramorar, J. E., 477